G. Wallach

Epidural Analgesia

Philip R. Bromage, *M. B., B. S. (Lond.)*
F. F. A. R. C. S., F. R. C. P. (C)

Professor of Anesthesiology and
Professor of Obstetrics and Gynecology,
Duke University Medical Center,
Durham, North Carolina;
Formerly, Professor and Chairman,
Department of Anesthesia, McGill University,
Montreal, Canada

W. B. SAUNDERS COMPANY Philadelphia • London • Toronto

W. B. Saunders Company: West Washington Square
Philadelphia, PA 19105

1 St. Anne's Road
Eastbourne, East Sussex BN21 3UN, England

1 Goldthorne Avenue
Toronto, Ontario M8Z 5T9, Canada

Library of Congress Cataloging in Publication Data

Bromage, Philip Raikes.

Epidural analgesia.

Includes index.

1. Peridural anesthesia. I. Title. [DNLM: 1. Anesthesia, Epidural. WO305 B868e]

RD85.P4B76 617'.964 77-79389

ISBN 0-7216-2005-1

Epidural Analgesia ISBN 0-7216-2005-1

Last digit is the print number: 9 8 7 6 5 4 3 2

Dedication

To the memory of David Langhorne, F.R.C.S., of Chichester, England, good friend and surgeon, who loved life yet met death with a smile.

Preface

Twenty-three years have elapsed since the preliminary version of this work was published under the title *Spinal Epidural Analgesia*. During the intervening period a great deal of new information has become available on the pharmacology of local anesthetics, the basic mechanism of epidural analgesia and the clinical applications of the technique. Epidural analgesia is used more widely now than ever before, in spite of the immense popularity of the muscle relaxant techniques combined with light general anesthesia. Epidural blockade is recognized as a necessary skill for every consultant anesthesiologist, especially if he is engaged in obstetrical practice or in the management of chronic pain.

Valuable work from both clinical and laboratory sources is widely reported in the literature, and this book attempts to bring together what I consider to be the more important aspects of both fields, in the hope that clinicians and laboratory workers may see things slightly differently when one group looks through the eyes of the other.

Unfortunately, in the natural progress of growth the book has suffered the fate of so many second editions, having lost its youthful silhouette to chunky middle age. It has been completely rewritten. The chapter on anatomy has been expanded to include new work on neuroanatomy and the structure and relationships of the meninges and perineural membrane, as well as the vasculature of the spinal canal as it affects epidural blockade. A new chapter on pharmacology has been added, not as a complete treatise on local anesthetic agents, but as a basis for the logical use of these drugs in practice. The section on physiology has had to be enlarged to deal with the wealth of information that has accumulated on the respiratory, cardiovascular and metabolic effects of epidural blockade. Chapters have also been included on caudal analgesia, on epidural analgesia for obstetrics and on diagnostic and therapeutic applications. The chapter on complications and contraindications has been greatly enlarged. The reason for this expansion is twofold. First, since every medical act, including masterly inactivity, carries the seeds of possible disaster, the risks must be known and faced if they cannot be avoided. Second, there has been much confusion between natural and iatrogenic causes in accidents associated with epidural analgesia, and in our present unsatisfactory medicolegal climate it is necessary to keep the issues as clear as possible. Finally, a critique on extant audiovisual teaching aids has been added in the hope that my own subjective bias will encourage the viewer to use these aids as critically as possible, for nothing is perfect.

PHILIP R. BROMAGE

Acknowledgments

The earlier version of this book would never have seen the light of day without the support of my colleagues in Chichester and Portsmouth, England, especially the warm encouragement of the late Mr. David Langhorne, F.R.C.S., to whose memory this edition is dedicated.

I have been most fortunate in enjoying exceptionally pleasant professional relationships favorable to developing this work on both sides of the Atlantic. Under the National Health Service in Britain, the South West Metropolitan Regional Hospital Board granted generous study leave. Research facilities were made available at McGill University and the Royal Victoria Hospital, Montreal, and grants from many agencies have supported the work over the years, especially those from the Medical Research Council of Canada and Astra Pharmaceuticals, Inc. At McGill University, Dean Patrick Cronin generously supported my application for sabbatical leave to write this book at a time when my absence was inconvenient.

I would like to express my gratitude to Professor J. Gordon Robson, Professor Leon Wolff, Professor Samuel Solomon and Professor Kris Krnjevic for their patient guidance in laboratory techniques, to the late Dr. Aldo Truant for help and advice, and to my colleagues who cheerfully shared the work and were co-authors in many of the papers that form the backbone of this book, especially Dr. Robert T. Pettigrew, Dr. Douglas Crowell, Dr. André Joyal, Dr. John Binney, Dr. Michael F. Burfoot, Dr. Michael J. Cousins and Dr. R. Stuart B. Bramwell.

I am particularly grateful for the help of two colleagues who assumed my professional responsibilities while I was absent on sabbatical leave to write this book. Dr. Paul E. Otton relieved me as Anaesthetist-in-Chief at the Royal Victoria Hospital, Montreal, and Dr. T. McCaughey as Chairman of the Department of Anaesthesia at McGill University. Their staunch support was indispensable.

The illustrations owe their existence to Mrs. Margaret Wherry and her staff in the Department of Medical Art at the Royal Victoria Hospital, who skillfully interpreted my rough sketches and added artistry to them, and to Miss Pat McKenna and Mr. Charlie Hodge, who gave expert photographic assistance, both in the studio and under demanding clinical conditions.

Thanks are due to the many authors and publishers who have kindly allowed their work to be quoted and reproduced in the text.

Mr. Jack Hanley of W. B. Saunders Company has been a wise and patient adviser in overseeing all phases of the publication, and it has been a constant pleasure to work with him.

Lastly, I thank my wife Meg for her inspiration and guidance, for it was she who typed, criticized and nursed the manuscript while keeping me fed, happy and encouraged throughout this work.

Contents

Chapter 9

Chapter 10

Chapter 11

Chapter 12

chapter 1
Introduction

The terms "extradural," "peridural" and "epidural" are synonymous. Although the first of these is the most correct etymologically, keeping as it does a purity of Latin in its parts, "epidural" is the shortest and falls most readily from the tongue. It would be pedantic to insist on excluding the other two synonyms on the grounds of mixed Greek and Latin parentage, for the Romans themselves were not averse to such mixtures. Throughout this book all three terms will be used freely and interchangeably, and preference for one or another in any situation will only be given for reasons of custom and euphony.

The epidural space, region of fat and blood vessels lying between the dural envelope of the spinal cord and the bony walls of the spinal canal, began to attract attention at the turn of the last century. Within this narrow space, injected solutions track up and down, as well as outwards through the intervertebral foramina, offering clinical opportunities to the radiologist and the anesthesiologist. The space may be entered either between the laminae of the vertebral arches, usually termed the "spinal" epidural route, or from below through the sacral hiatus—the "caudal" route.

HISTORY

Corning has been credited with being the first to use epidural analgesia in 1885. Corning had the idea that medications injected within the spinal canal might be taken up by the rich plexuses of blood vessels in the neighborhood and be carried into the substance of the spinal cord, thus allowing direct medication of the cord, either for treatment of neurological disease or for providing surgical analgesia. However, from his own description of the two experiments he carried out, it is evident that he neither intended nor achieved a genuine epidural injection. Nevertheless, it is ironic that Corning's hypothesis of spinal cord uptake was discredited and dismissed as unscientific. After the passage of nearly 100 years, the original idea now seems remarkably close to the truth, and all the available evidence points to the cord as an important site of action of epidural blockade.

Epidural analgesia has been practiced, by one technique or another, since 1901 when Sicard and Cathelin of France independently popularized the caudal approach. After the favorable reports of Sicard and Cathelin, Tuffier attempted epidural analgesia by the lumbar approach later in the same year, but his lack of success, and the natural difficulties of locating a narrow space 2 to 4 mm wide at a depth twenty times that amount, discouraged all further attempts for many years. In 1913, Heile tried to revive the idea of high epidural blocks by entering the spinal canal laterally through the intervertebral foramina instead of by midline puncture. Heile used this approach for surgical and therapeutic purposes, but his method does not seem to have had much following outside Germany. In the meantime, the caudal route became established as the only safe approach to the epidural space, and there was a tendency to limit the field of analgesia to the area supplied by the cauda equina (Läwen, 1911), since efforts to carry the block higher met with quite variable results, owing to the individual differences in the anatomy of the sacrum and its foramina.

This state of affairs continued until 1921 when Fidel Pagés renewed interest in the midline lumbar approach, pointing out the increased ease of access and wider applicability of this route as compared with the caudal route. Pagés' method of identifying the epidural space was primarily tactile, demanding great dexterity from the operator in order to detect the "feel" of the needle passing from the ligamentum flavum into the epidural space. The degree of skill required for Pagés' method was clearly a limiting factor to the technique, and other workers set about establishing mechanical substitutes for manual dexterity. These refinements gradually developed, and it is now possible to obtain a very high success rate in lumbar epidural analgesia without possessing an unusual sensitivity of touch.

Although the mode of action of epidural blockade remained conjectural, there was no lack of theories for its possible site of action, and for many years the technical aspects of epidural analgesia were dictated by clinical impressions and qualitative observations rather than by systematic measurements. There were a few notable exceptions to this, particularly in the works of Dogliotti (1939) and Gutierrez (1939), but the bulk of the literature on the subject was based on clinical results, without too much attention being paid to careful analysis of the many variables encountered between different drugs and different patients; therefore, it was not surprising that confusion and disagreement arose over details of technical management when the fundamental principles underlying these matters were so poorly understood.

Thus, because the majority of practicing anesthesiologists came to regard the method as unreliable and even frankly dangerous in unskilled hands, it was relegated to the status of a museum piece, to be dusted and shown the light of day from time to time at examinations and scientific meetings, but for the most part not to be regarded too seriously except perhaps in the hands of a few enthusiasts who, somewhat inexplicably, made it their hobby.

With the advent of neuromuscular blocking agents in 1946, local injection techniques of every sort suffered a sharp decline, and any form of regional analgesia had to be able to withstand severe scrutiny in order to justify itself in competition with intravenous relaxant drugs, which were safe, convenient and efficient. It seemed that the very lightest of general anesthesia was sufficient for even the boldest and most protracted surgery, provided neuromuscular blockade was maintained and somatic responses were prevented. The patients appeared to withstand their operations well, and the results spoke as loudly as was needed to bury forever the lingering ideas of "anoci-association" that had been common parlance since Crile proposed them in 1915 (Crile and

Lower, 1915). Before the days of curare it had seemed obvious, as Crile had suggested, that patients were in better condition after operation under regional analgesia, or combinations of regional analgesia and light general anesthesia, than after operation under the deep levels of anesthesia that had been necessary to obtain satisfactory muscle relaxation using general anesthesia alone. Now that curarization could be induced independently, it seemed clear that deep general anesthesia was the deleterious factor and not the bombardment of afferent input that Crile had thought. It was argued that patients did equally well under regional analgesia or neuromuscular blockade, provided the need for *deep* general anesthesia was removed.

Nothing withstood the power of curare and its congeners. From open heart surgery to vaginal delivery and correction of ingrown toenails, the story and the technique were much the same: a rapid induction, a paralyzed patient with a watertight endotracheal airway, artificial ventilation and rapid emergence at the end. The logic and the results seemed unassailable. Nevertheless, for obscure reasons of tradition, stubborness or perhaps just an indefinable "hunch," the proponents of regional analgesia clung to their eccentric ways and their untenable position, stripped of all rational defenses in the face of the overwhelming success of relaxant techniques. The regionalists argued that some unidentified but precious qualitative difference existed between patients under regional analgesia and those under muscle relaxants, and one could only appreciate the difference by working with both techniques. After regional anesthesia patients were alert, cooperative and functional in a way that had to be seen to be believed.

Once again anesthetic thought became polarized between the de-efferenting majority and the de-afferenting minority. In the meantime, however, the teaching of regional anesthesia suffered an eclipse that produced a generation of anesthesiologists who were trained largely in ignorance of regional anesthesia. In some centers this ignorance was almost militant in its rejection of deafferenting thought.

Epidural analgesia managed to escape the general decline in regional techniques when it was given a fresh impetus by the introduction of the Tuohy needle and the indwelling epidural catheter. With these technical refinements it became possible to maintain analgesia continuously, or intermittently, for very long periods extending to days or even weeks, if necessary. For the first time, prolonged surgical, obstetrical and therapeutic interventions came within the range of practical deafferentation. This gave this technique an important advantage over the relaxant, de-efferenting techniques, for now it was theoretically possible to relieve pain and yet maintain voluntary function in a way that was impossible after even the lightest general anesthesia. The relaxant techniques could provide good operating conditions only so long as complete muscle paralysis existed, but afterward they did nothing to relieve the burden of pain, nor could they restore voluntary function in the postoperative period.

Polarization between de-efferentation and deafferentation was now complete. With the muscle relaxant techniques the patient was committed to endotracheal intubation, artificial ventilation and awakening to a period of postoperative pain that would interfere with rest and at the same time arouse protective reflex responses that inhibited normal movement and respiratory function. In contrast, with prolonged deafferentation normal respiratory function could be preserved during operation, if desired, and after major abdominal surgery the patient could be maintained both comfortably rested and almost fully functional to such an extraordinary extent that it was possible to permit immediate pain-free ambulation within an hour or so of leaving the operating room (Cleland, 1949).

In childbirth, this sort of analgesic capability opened the door to revolutionary changes in obstetrical methods. No longer were centrally depressant analgesics and anesthetics required. Labor could be pain free from start to finish without the need for any pharmacological depression of the fetus, and with the judicious use of elective induction, "daylight obstetrics" became a practical possibility.

RECENT DEVELOPMENTS

For many years epidural analgesia had been practiced empirically, and apart from the obvious fact that it produced a segmental type of analgesia, the anatomical and pharmacological bases for its mechanism of action were virtually unknown. Moreover, the physiological results were seen only in their broadest outlines. Consequently, clinical results were often unpredictable and imprecise. During the past two decades new analytical tools have brought precise measurements to many fundamental aspects of the technique that were not clear before. The synthesis of ideas from systematic clinical observations and from research in related disciplines has lifted epidural analgesia out of its former state of empiricism to a new level of versatility and clinical safety.

In the field of neuroanatomy, electron microscopy has brought about a renaissance of thought comparable to the impact of the telescope on medieval astronomy. The membranes guarding the nervous system and the ways through them can now clearly be seen. Key junctional points between the peripheral and central nervous systems have been scrutinized by transmission and scanning electron microscopy, and the strategic zones for penetration of epidural anesthetics have been identified. Within the nervous system itself, enumeration of nerve fibers has yielded some surprising results that undoubtedly will have a profound effect on future developments in practical neural blockade. The shadowy minority of unmyelinated fibers that lurked beyond the fringe of light microscopy are now seen to be a vast host of slender filaments peculiarly resistant to the blocking effects of cold and dilute solutions of local anesthetics. Traveling in unfamiliar pathways, these tiny C-fibers dictate the destiny of sensation and autonomic function, and possibly some aspects of muscular function as well. Among these unmyelinated fibers are the prime messengers of pain; therefore, effective analgesic blockade must reckon with them, above all other types of fiber, and new drugs must be sought to deal preferentially with their ubiquity and resistance.

While neuroanatomy has identified prime target structures and their location in the peripheral and central nervous system, parallel advances in pharmacology have enabled the uptake, disposition and site of action of epidural drugs to be plotted with great accuracy by means of gas chromatography and radioisotopic tracers. It is now possible to follow the principal pathways of uptake and distribution of local anesthetic drugs from the epidural space into the nervous system and the body as a whole, as well as to determine the proportion of drug that reaches the fetus in obstetrical cases. In addition, many of the factors that influence potency and toxicity have become known and subject to pharmacological manipulation. New local anesthetic agents with widely differing properties have been introduced, and the extent and intensity of chemical blockade can now be chosen with a degree of versatility and predictability that was impossible 20 years ago.

The physiological responses to epidural blockade fall into two main categories. First are the obvious results of autonomic blockade that follow interruption of the sympathetic outflow, with consequent effects on vascular beds and cardiac performance, as well as effects on other visceral structures. Second are the less obvious but clinically more important effects that follow interruption of somatic pain pathways, with consequent restoration of functions that would otherwise be inhibited by reflex response to pain. Both of these physiological outcomes of epidural blockade have been studied extensively during the past 20 years, and the relevant details are discussed in subsequent chapters dealing with the basic and applied aspects of epidural analgesia.

CHOICE

What of the difficulties and dangers of the method and the incidence of failure? That there is a definite failure rate cannot be denied, but it is, or should be, a very small one. Accidental puncture of the dura, or "wet-tap," is the commonest difficulty, but this can be reduced to vanishing point by correct technique. My own incidence of dural puncture, using a Tuohy or a Hustead needle and a rigorously standardized technique, has been six "wet-taps" in the last 3,000 cases—an incidence of 0.2 per cent. In an earlier series of 1,500 cases in which an ordinary straight needle with an obtuse bevel was used, the incidence was between 1 and 1.5 per cent. This technical improvement appears to be related to the use of the Tuohy needle and is probably explicable in terms of the peculiar hydrodynamics of its Huber tip, which will be discussed more fully in Chapter 9.

Later in this book, emphasis will be placed on the need for the anesthesiologist to make things easy for himself; that and the ability to be scrupulously careful constitute the only formula for successful epidural puncture. A technical failure rate of less than 1 per cent is acceptable from a practical viewpoint. However, if successful epidural puncture cannot be assured in more than 95 per cent of cases, the method is probably not worth retaining for everyday clinical use, and physicians who are unable to maintain this level of success are best advised to avoid the method in the interests of their patients and surgical colleagues. A failed epidural is a disappointment to the patient and a source of wasted time and irritation to the surgeon and the operating team who are kept waiting unnecessarily for the case to begin.

The complications of the technique are dealt with very fully in Chapter 14. The list is formidable and daunting unless read with a sense of proportion and some realization that *all* complications, whether real or apparent, must be seen against a control background of the risks and dangers that lie in the alternative options, including the option of doing nothing. This viewpoint is best illustrated in the field of obstetrics in which the alternative choices are quite well documented. There, the risks of general anesthesia for vaginal delivery are known and considered by most specialist anesthesiologists to be unwarranted, if satisfactory alternative methods of regional analgesia exist. Also, the danger of doing nothing, that is to say "natural" childbirth, is becoming more clearly recognized, and there is mounting evidence that labor and delivery are less traumatic to the newborn, both physically and biochemically, under well-managed epidural analgesia. In addition, there is increasing documentation of inherent neurological risks of labor to the mother that occur spontaneously, with an incidence of about 1 in every 2,000 to 3,000 deliveries, even in the absence of regional anesthesia (see Chapter 12).

Without these "control" vital statistics of inherent complication rates it is impossible to arrive at an accurate assessment of the risks of any technique. For then the true balance of therapeutic gain versus technical complications remains hidden behind a rickety scaffolding of impressions, anecdotes and unrecognized disasters from a "control" population whose neglected natural history and detailed outcome escape the scrutiny of rigorous documentation. These shortcomings of current methods of control data collection and the errors arising from them will be considered more fully in Chapter 14.

In certain fields, as in obstetrics, it is possible to put numbers, or at least approximate numbers, against some parameters for the immediate and remote benefits of epidural analgesia. In some areas it is less easy to do this, and there, as in so many branches of medicine, therapeutic evaluation has not yet evolved from a qualitative state to the more sophisticated level of quantitative measurement. In these poorly lit areas, art and irrationality linger, and science is not yet fully in command. In the succeeding chapters an attempt is made to identify those points where controversy stems from the failure of imperfect methodology to unravel a complex tangle of variables and where uncertainty still reigns. When the profit and loss balance in this incomplete state of knowledge is being weighed, clinical impressions must be the guide as they have been in the past, although one should keep in mind that impressions are highly subjective and in need of continuous critical review.

CLINICAL SCOPE AND PRACTICALITY

Epidural analgesia has practical applications in three main areas—surgery, obstetrics and chronic pain relief—and each of these is dealt with separately in Chapters 11, 12 and 13. Any major anesthesiology department should be active in all three of these aspects of the specialty, although with modern policies of regionalization, obstetrics may become increasingly concentrated in special units. While it would be possible to run an effective surgical anesthesia unit without employing regional anesthesia of any description, the overall quality of service would inevitably suffer by such a restricted policy.

It is in obstetrical and pain clinic activities that epidural analgesia is absolutely indispensable. At the time of writing, continuous epidural blockade is the most efficient and satisfactory method available for pain relief in labor and delivery, and no modern obstetrical unit would be complete without epidural facilities on a 24-hour basis. Similarly, the technical capabilities of any pain clinic should include epidural analgesia among its therapeutic options, with staff able to induce blockade reliably and safely at any spinal level.

Epidural analgesia should not be used indiscriminately, but it is a good method of pain relief for many purposes, and in certain circumstances it is the best. It is a technique that demands the serious attention of all anesthesiologists who are prepared to give the care necessary for its satisfactory employment.

REFERENCES

Cathelin, M. F.: Une nouvelle voie d'injection rachidienne. Méthode des injections épidurales par le procédé du canal sacré. Applications à l'homme. C. R. Soc. Biol. Paris *53*:452, 1901.

Cleland, J. G. P.: Continuous peridural and caudal analgesia in surgery and early ambulation. Northwest Med. J. *48*:26, 1949.

Corning, J. L.: Spinal anaesthesia and local medication of the cord. N.Y. Med. J. *42*:483, 1885.

Crile, G. W., and Lower, W. E.: Anoci-Association. Philadelphia, W. B. Saunders Company, 1915, p. 108.

Dogliotti, A. M.: Anesthesia, S. B. Dubour, Chicago, 1939.

Gutierrez, A.; Anestesie Extradural. Rev. Cirug. Buenos Aires, 1939.

Heile, B.: Der epidurale Raum. Arch. Klin. Chir. *101*:845, 1913.

Läwen, A.: Uber Extraduralanästhesie fur chirurgische Operationen. Dtsch. Z. Chir. *108*:1, 1911.

Pagés, F.: Anestesia metamerica. Rev. Sanid. Mil. Madr. *11*:351, 385, 1921.

Sicard, A.: Les injections médicamenteuses extra-durales par voie sacro-coccygienne. C. R. Soc. Biol. Paris *53*:396, 1901.

Tuffier, T.: Analgésie cocaïnique par voie extradurale. C.R. Soc. Biol. Paris *53*:490, 1901.

chapter 2
Anatomy

For now we see through a glass darkly; but then face to face: now I know in part. . . .

I Corinthians 13:12
(King James Version 1611)

Within the cranium the endosteal and meningeal layers of dura mater are closely united, but below the foramen magnum the two layers separate, the outer becoming the periosteal lining of the spinal canal and the inner forming the spinal dura mater. Between these two layers lies the epi-, extra- or peridural sac. The spinal canal is triangular in cross section, and the epidural space is widest in the midline posteriorly, in the lumbar region averaging about 5 mm between the ligamentum flavum and the posterior surface of the spinal dura. Owing to the obliquity of the vertebral laminae, the depth is increased slightly in close proximity to the inferior border of the lamina.

The boundaries of the epidural space are:

Above:	The foramen magnum where the periosteal and spinal layers of dura fuse together
Below:	The sacrococcygeal membrane
In front:	The posterior longitudinal ligament covering the posterior aspect of the vertebral bodies and the intervertebral discs
Behind:	The anterior surface of the vertebral laminae and the ligamenta flava
Laterally:	The pedicles of the vertebrae and the intervertebral foramina

The ligamentum flavum is an important landmark for technical identification of the extradural space during induction of epidural analgesia. It is composed of tough elastic fibers disposed in a vertical direction connecting the upper and lower borders of adjacent laminae. It is thinnest in the cervical region, becoming progressively thicker lower down the spine, and is thickest in the lumbar region. The interspinous ligament, lying immediately superficial to the ligamentum flavum in the median plane, is another landmark which is thickest and best defined in the lumbar region (Fig. 2–1).

Techniques for penetrating the epidural space are determined by the anatomical peculiarities of the spinal column at its various levels. The epidural space is entered most easily and safely in the mid-lumbar region. In newborn infants the spinal cord terminates at the lower border of the third lumbar vertebra, but the tip of the cord ascends during growth as the spinal column lengthens, and by adolescence the end of the cord comes to lie opposite the lower border of the first lumbar vertebra or upper border of the second. Thus, in adults the conus medullaris is usually safe from accidental trauma if puncture is made below the second lumbar vertebra. Also, the lumbar spines and interspinous ligament are widest in the mid-lumbar region, making an easy landmark for insertion of the epidural needle. Below the fourth lumbar verte-

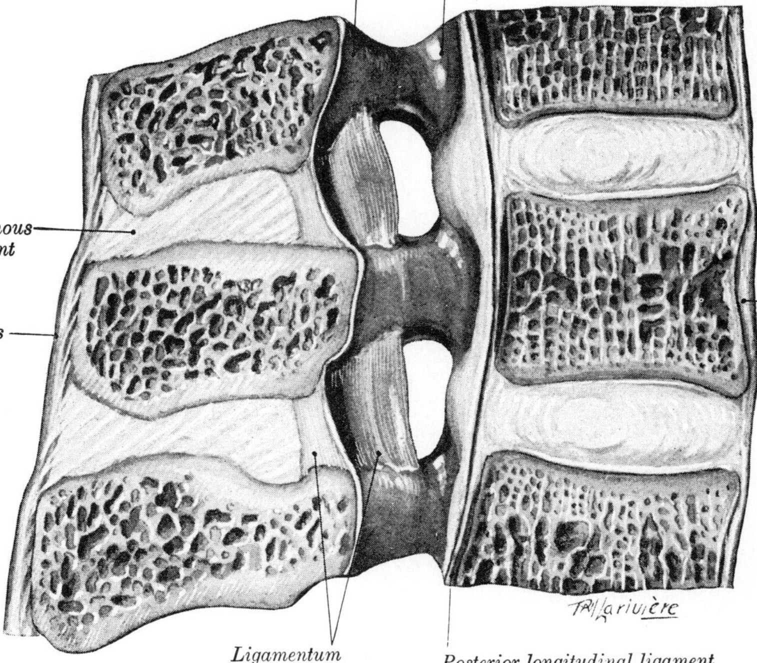

Figure 2–1. Median sagittal section through a portion of the lumbar region of the vertebral column. (Gray's Anatomy.)

bra the interspinous ligament becomes narrower and more tenuous, and technical difficulties in placing the epidural needle increase somewhat.

In the mid-thoracic region, overlap of the lamina and spines makes midline puncture technically more difficult, and epidural needles must usually be insinuated between the laminae by an oblique paramedian approach (see Chapter 6). Above the fourth thoracic vertebra, the spines slope progressively less and the interspinous ligament becomes wider. Midline puncture becomes feasible again in this section and technically very easy at the interspace between the seventh cervical (vertebra prominens) and the first thoracic spines.

Useful surface markings are found at the following sites (Fig. 2–2):

1. *Seventh cervical spine* (vertebra prominens), at the lower end of the nuchal furrow: easily seen and felt, especially on flexion of the neck.

2. *Tip of third thoracic spine,* opposite the roots of the scapular spines, when the arm is by the side.

3. *Tip of the seventh thoracic spine,* opposite the inferior angle of the scapula, when the arm is by the side.

4. *Third lumbar interspace,* on a level with the intercristal line (i.e., line drawn between the highest points of the iliac crests).

5. *Posterior superior iliac spines,* on a level with the spine of S_2 and the termination of the dural sac.

The segmental dermatomes or cutaneous receptive fields of each spinal root are shown in Figure 2–3. The anesthesiologist must have a good working knowledge of the spinal dermatomes, so that he can assess the progress

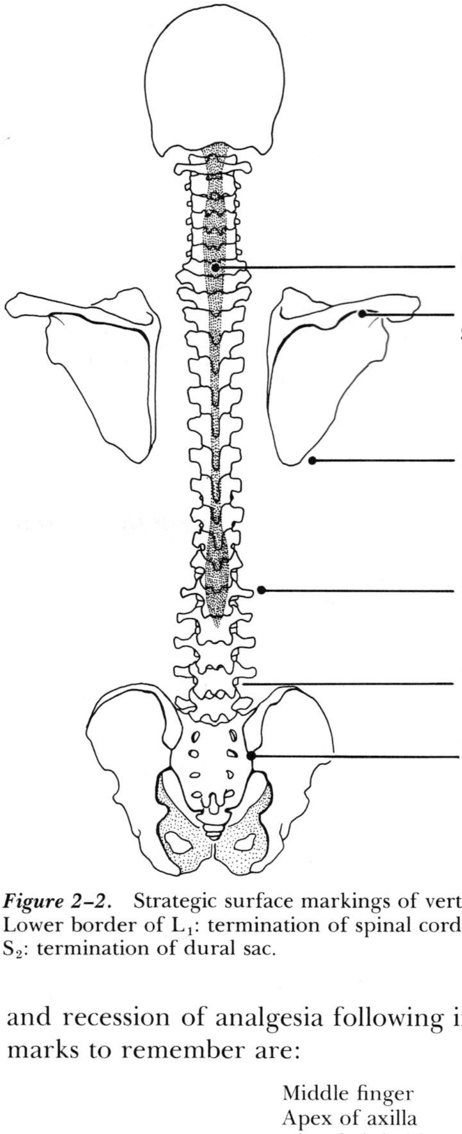

Figure 2–2. Strategic surface markings of vertebral spines. Lower border of L_1: termination of spinal cord. Lower border of S_2: termination of dural sac.

and recession of analgesia following induction of epidural blockade. Key landmarks to remember are:

Middle finger	C_7
Apex of axilla	T_3
Tip of xiphoid cartilage	T_7
Umbilicus	T_{10} (approximately)
Inguinal ligament	T_{12}
Front of knee	L_3
Medial side of calf	L_4
Outer side of calf	L_5
Outer border of foot	S_1
Back of knee	S_2

CONTENTS OF THE EPIDURAL SPACE

The epidural space between the dural tube and the walls of the spinal canal is a potential space filled with fat, blood vessels and lymphatics. Each of these occupants can take up more or less room within the spinal canal, depending on circumstances and especially on the cardiovascular dynamics prevailing from moment to moment.

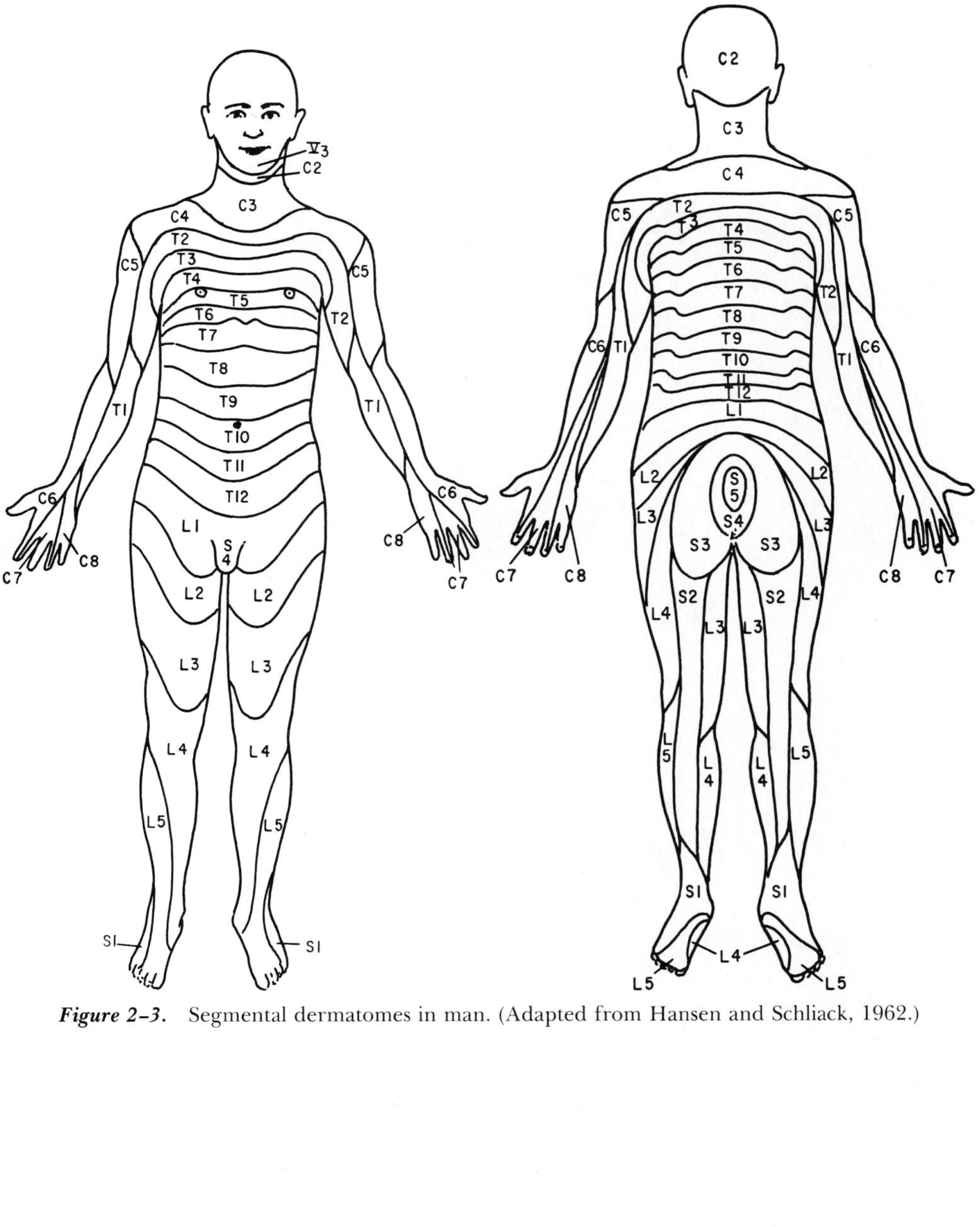

Figure 2–3. Segmental dermatomes in man. (Adapted from Hansen and Schliack, 1962.)

Spinal Dural Sac

The dural tube, with its lateral prolongations covering each pair of spinal nerve roots, extends from the foramen magnum to the lower border of the second sacral vertebra. Beyond this point the tubular sheath of the filum terminale continues as a strand of tissue and is attached to the back of the first segment of the coccyx. Occasionally the dural tube descends lower in the sacrum to within 2 to 3 cm of the sacrococcygeal membrane; this anomaly increases the rare hazard of accidental dural puncture during caudal analgesia.

The dural tube tends to hug the anterior wall of the spinal canal, so that the anterior portion of the epidural space is narrow, while posteriorly the space is much wider. The dura is thickest posteriorly (Fig. 2–4). Fibrous strands pass from the posterior longitudinal ligament to the anterior aspect of the

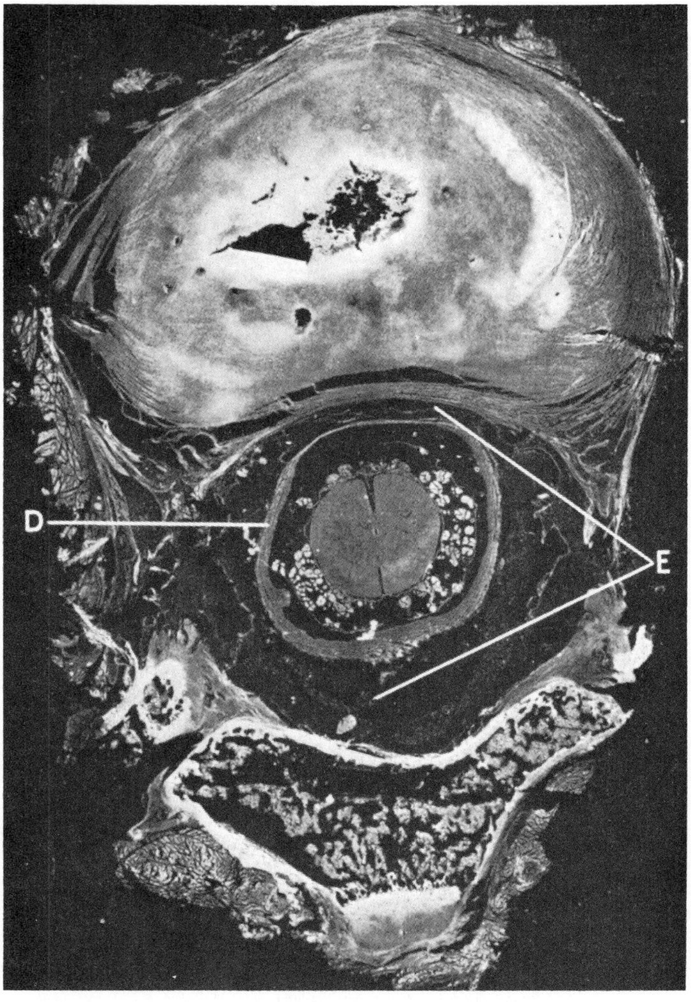

Figure 2–4. Transverse section of spine between first and second lumbar vertebrae of three-year-old child (× 3.5). (D) Dura mater, thickest posteriorly; (E) epidural space, wider posteriorly than in front. Note that the sacral cord is still present at this level in a young child. (Courtesy of Professor R. Walmsley.)

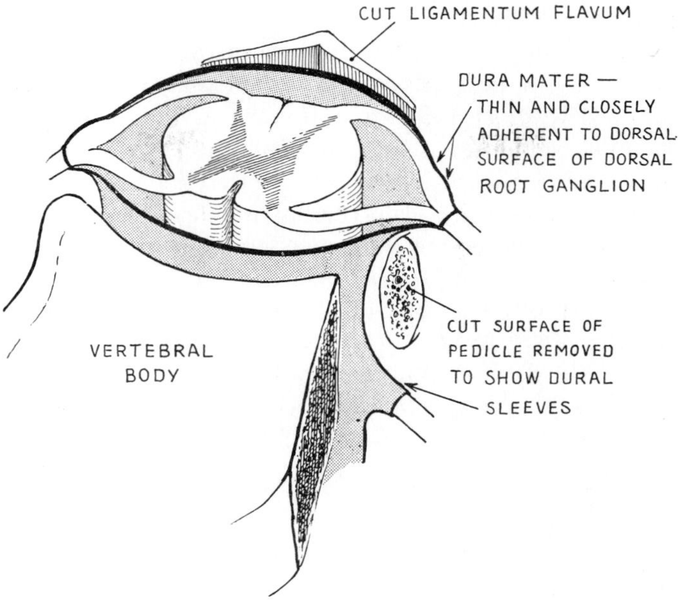

Figure 2–5. Diagram of the dural cul-de-sac surrounding a pair of spinal nerve roots.

dura, anchoring it in place and tending to divide the anterior epidural space into two longitudinal compartments. In the upper cervical region the spinal nerve roots and their dural coverings pass horizontally to their respective intervertebral foramina, but lower down they become more inclined, owing to the discrepancy between the length of the spinal cord and the spinal canal, until the lower lumbar and sacral roots are almost vertical. Dural prolongations sheathe each pair of spinal roots, enclosing a small subarachnoid cul-de-sac, and end by adhering closely to the distal portion of the spinal ganglion at the point where the anterior and posterior roots fuse to form the "nerf de conjugaison" or first part of the mixed nerve; here the dura is slightly thinner posteriorly. Beyond this point the dura is contiguous with the epineurium (Fig. 2–5). The termination of the dural cuffs occupies different positions in relation to the intervertebral foramen at different levels. In the cervical region this termination is within the gutter of the foramen; in the thoracic region it is related to the internal aspect of the foramen; and in the lumbar and sacral regions it lies entirely within the spinal canal.

Distance Between Ligamentum Flavum and Dura

The width of the posterior epidural space varies, depending on the capacity of the spinal canal, in relation to the size of the cord and its coverings at each level. Two major enlargements of the cord, the cervical and lumbar, corresponding to the neuromeres serving the limbs, make for slightly more crowded conditions at their respective levels. The cervical enlargement extends from the third cervical to the second thoracic vertebra, its widest diameter being at the sixth cervical where the cord is largest, with dimensions of 13 to 14 mm (transverse) × 8 to 9 mm. Flexion of the neck moves the cord and this cervical enlargement upward slightly within the spinal canal. The lumbar enlargement begins at the ninth thoracic vertebra, reaches its greatest width at the twelfth thoracic vertebra (12 mm × 7 mm) and then tapers rapidly into the conus medullaris. Between these two enlargements with their correspondingly thick nerve roots, the cord is slender (9 to 10 mm × 6.5 to 7.0 mm), and the mid-thoracic rootlets are proportionately fine.

The greatest distance between the ligamentum flavum and the dura is found in the midline at the second lumbar interspace, where the distance is about 5.0 to 6.0 mm in adult males. In the mid-thoracic region the distance is somewhat less, in the range of 3.0 to 5.0 mm at the midline. In the lower cervical region the distance narrows to 1.5 to 2.0 mm, but below the seventh cervical vertebra it widens again, especially during flexion, and at the first thoracic interspace the distance is about 3.0 to 4.0 mm when the neck is acutely flexed.

Fat

The contents of the spinal canal lie cushioned in a packing of semi-fluid lobulated fat. Solutions injected into the epidural space track up and down between the lobules of this fatty areolar tissue. The amount of fat in the epidural space tends to vary with that elsewhere in the body, obese patients having a well-stuffed and capacious epidural space. Epidural fat is highly vascular, with many capillary walls appearing in serial microscopic sections (Tretjakoff, 1926; Ramsey, 1959). The greater part of the epidural fat lies free and unattached in the spinal canal, but collagen bundles become increasingly numerous in the region of the nerve roots, and a considerable amount of connective tissue is intermingled with the fat within the intervertebral foramina.

The epidural fat constitutes an important pharmacological "space" and depot for injected local anesthetic agents, and it is one of the three main competitors for its share of drug, the other two competitors being nervous tissue of the spinal roots and cord, and blood vessels within the spinal canal. Drugs with high lipid solubility and lipoprotein binding characteristics will tend to enter the fat phase and remain there for periods of time, depending on their pharmacodynamics and on the briskness of local blood flow competing for uptake (Morikawa et al., 1974).

Spinal Arteries

Arteries derived embryologically from the intersegmental arteries enter the intervertebral foramina to supply the osseoligamentous spinal canal and the spinal cord. In the adult these arteries arise from the vertebral, the ascending cervical, deep cervical, intercostal, lumbar and iliolumbar arteries. They anastomose with their neighbors above and below, as well as across the midline, and lie chiefly in the lateral parts of the epidural space. The vascular supply to the cord will be dealt with in greater detail later in this chapter.

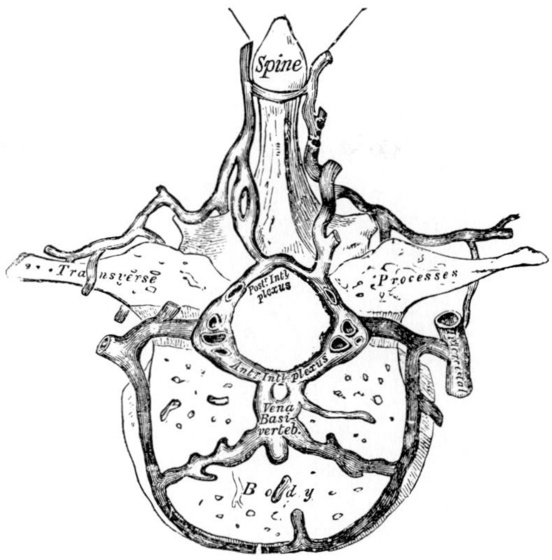

Figure 2–6. Transverse section through a thoracic vertebra, showing the vertebral venous plexuses. (Gray's Anatomy.)

Epidural Veins

The internal vertebral venous plexus, draining both cord and canal, lies mainly in the anterolateral parts of the epidural space (Fig. 2–6). It has rich segmental connections at all levels and opens into the intervertebral veins, which pass out through the intervertebral foramina and end in the vertebral, posterior intercostal, lumbar and lateral sacral veins. Through this venous network increased intra-abdominal and intrathoracic pressures (as in coughing and straining) are transmitted to the epidural space. Under the stress of these pressures the valveless epidural veins distend and diminish the effective volume of the epidural space, so that epidural solutions tend to spread more widely than usual if coughing or straining occurs during or immediately after injection.

Above, the vertebral plexuses communicate with the occipital, sigmoid and basilar sinuses within the skull, as shown by the early diagram of Willis (1664) (Fig. 2–7). This primitive venous network forms a vascular highway between the pelvic and cranial cavities, and it provides an important alternative to the caval drainage system from the pelvis whenever obstruction of the inferior vena cava occurs for any reason. The veins of the cord and the internal vertebral venous plexus will also be dealt with in greater detail later in this chapter.

Lymphatics

Lymphatic networks surrounding and draining the dural cul-de-sacs of the dural root sleeves run anteriorly from each intervertebral foramen and empty into longitudinal channels in front of the vertebral column (Field and Brierley, 1948a). These share a vital sanitation role with the arachnoid villi (vide infra) in eliminating debris from the subarachnoid space. The lymphatic drainage system responds rapidly to the challenge of foreign material in the subarachnoid space. Particulate matter, such as fine India ink suspensions with

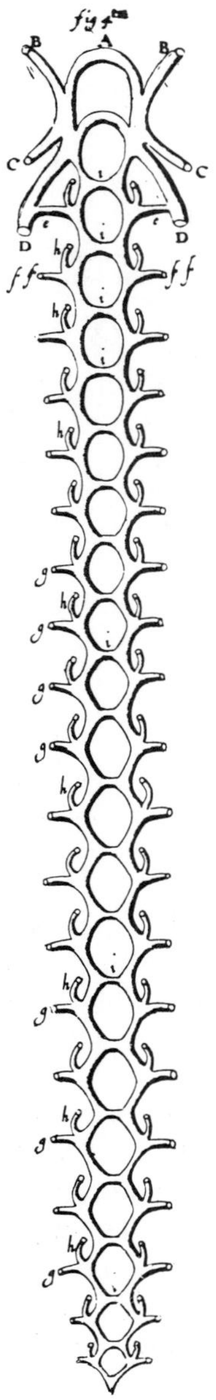

Figure 2–7. Diagram from Thomas Willis' book "Cerebri Anatome" (1664), showing the connections of the internal vertebral (epidural) venous plexuses.

A.	Venous loop at the level of the foramen magnum
BB.	Connections between the vertebral plexuses and the cranial sinuses (occipital, sigmoid and basilar)
CC.	Channels connecting the junction of the vertebral plexus and vertebral veins to the internal jugular vein
DD.	Vertebral veins
ee.	Tributaries from the vertebral plexus to the vertebral veins
ffff. gggg.	Intervertebral veins
hhhh.	Veins of the spinal cord connecting with the internal vertebral plexus
iiii.	Segmental commissural vessels opposite each vertebra

particle sizes between 0.4 and 1.5 μ, is rapidly scavenged into the leash of lymphatic vessels surrounding the dural sleeves and from thence to the regional lymph glands (Brierley and Field, 1948a). With colloidal carbon this passage takes less than 30 minutes (Woollam and Millen, 1953).

MENINGES

Much of the confusion that has existed in the past about the unpredictable mode of spread and variable effects of epidural blockade can be traced to the rather incomplete knowledge of spinal anatomy prior to the application of electron microscopy.

The behavior of solutions in the epidural space was envisaged in simple geometrical and hydrodynamic terms, based on the volume of solution injected in relation to the volume of the epidural space. The extradural space is sealed at the base of the skull by the fusion of dura mater with periosteum, and so the space was likened to a leaky cylinder within which anesthetic solutions could travel up and down to an extent mainly determined by the quantity injected. If the holes in the cylinder—that is, the intervertebral foramina—were large, then appreciable amounts of solution would leak out and little would be left to spread up and down inside the cylinder. On the other hand, if the intervertebral foramina were caulked up by fibrous tissue and leakages were negligible, spread would be extensive inside the canal, and many more spinal segments would become anesthetized. By good fortune the dural seal at the base of the skull would prevent an epidural overdose from ever reaching the intracranial contents, and this natural anatomical barrier was thought to confer a high degree of safety upon the technique of epidural analgesia (Pagés, 1921; Dogliotti, 1933; Odom, 1940; Dawkins, 1945; Foldes et al., 1956). In this simple schema, with its built-in safety barrier, increased concentrations of local anesthetic would obviously produce more intense neural blockade, while spatial dermatome spread would have to be achieved by injecting larger volumes of solution.

We now know that the facts do not fit this simple view of things, as we shall see in later chapters. Unfortunately, the barrier at the base of the skull is anatomical rather than functional, and it provides no insurance against the intracranial effects of gross overdosage. Experiments with radioactive local anesthetics in dogs have shown that the material passes freely from the extradural space into the cerebrospinal fluid and spinal cord and may reach as high as the medulla, the cerebellum and even the occipital cortex (Bromage et al., 1963). The number of spinal segments blocked is determined not only by the volume, but also by the concentration of local anesthetic. As a corollary, increased concentrations of local anesthetics do not necessarily increase the intensity of neural blockade. Moreover, certain physiological and pathological states exaggerate the segmental spread of epidural anesthetics to an extent that would be difficult to explain fully in simple hydraulic terms.

Some working hypothesis must be found to reconcile these awkward observations, and in seeking one we are forced to look more closely at the anatomical features of the extradural space, especially at the integuments of the nerves and spinal cord which normally insulate these aristocratic ectodermal structures from the surrounding mesenchymal masses. This and succeeding chapters will try to put together a reasonably convincing picture to explain the facts, sometimes rather bizarre, as we find them.

The fragile delicacy of the central nervous system and the limpid purity of its waters are so striking to the eye, and so dramatically different from the rest of the body, that the dullest observer cannot fail to ask what manner of barrier it is that preserves this extraordinary dreamlike realm, so effectively cloistered from contact with the workaday surrounding flesh. The connective tissue coverings of the spinal cord and nerves have been a matter of conjecture and controversy for more than two centuries, and only now under the tremendous power of the transmission and scanning electron microscopes are the speculations of many decades taking coherent shape in a schema that includes answers to questions first asked 200 years ago. Some of these answers have also helped to provide an anatomical basis for explaining the mode of action of epidural analgesia.

Dura Mater

The dura mater gives compliant mechanical support and protection to the delicate structures inside its boundaries, and there its function seems to end. It is a mesenchymal membrane consisting mainly of collagen fibers with some elastic fibers as well, sandwiched between layers of flattened fibroblasts on its inner and outer surfaces (Waggener and Beggs, 1967). On electron microscopy the inner surface of the dura is characterized by electron dense cells alongside the contrasting more lucent arachnoid components. Normally, no obvious space exists between the two membranes, but the arachnoid and the dura are quite easily separated to form an artifactual subdural space.

The dural root sleeves covering the dorsal and ventral roots are pierced by blood vessels and lymphatics passing to and from the underlying subarachnoid space and neuraxis, and this "cuff" region is extremely important in the drainage of spinal cerebrospinal fluid and in the elimination of particulate matter from the subarachnoid space. Beyond the root sleeve area the dura extends outward as the epineurium, the connective tissue sheath that binds the peripheral nerve fascicles into their common bundles.

Arachnoid Mater

The arachnoid membrane lining the dura mater is a looser and metabolically more active structure with overlapping cellular tiers sparsely intermingled with connective tissue trabeculae. Subcellular organelles with active metabolic concerns are numerous in the clear cytoplasm (Waggener and Beggs, 1967). Embryologically, the arachnoid mater arises from a primary mesenchyme of epiblastic origin. It is stratified with complex cellular interdigitations and "closed-contact" intercellular junctions in its most superficial layer, suggesting a barrier function, perhaps to the escape of cerebrospinal fluid (McLone and Bondareff, 1975). This appearance led to the view that the arachnoid membrane was impermeable to the passage of red cells or particulate matter (Alksne and Lovings, 1972). However, large empty vacuoles are a common feature in many cells lining the arachnoid mater, some of which communicate directly with the subdural space (Tripathi, 1973). Tripathi and Tripathi (1974) have suggested that these giant vacuoles represent a dynamic system of transcellular channels or pores for bulk drainage of cerebrospinal fluid, in a manner similar to the outflow of aqueous humour from the eye (Tripathi, 1971). These arachnoid cells go through a cycle of vacuolation, leading to the formation of discrete but temporary channels passing right through the cells and allowing macromolecular and particulate matter to escape from the subarachnoid space (Fig. 2–8).

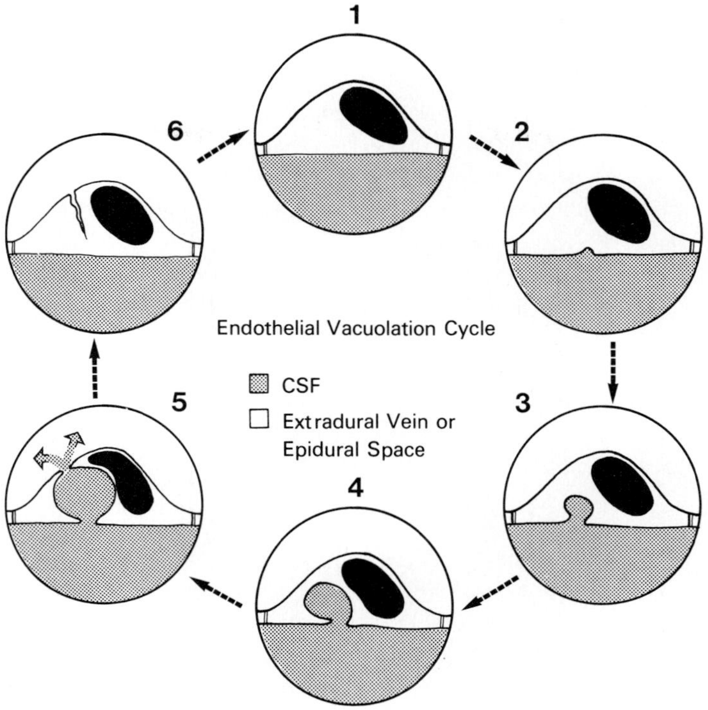

Figure 2–8. The endothelial vacuolation cycle of the arachnoid mater. (After Tripathi and Tripathi, 1974.)

Pia Mater

The pia mater is a smooth layer of epithelium composed of extremely flat overlapping cells covering a layer of connective tissue fibers running randomly in all directions over the surface of the cord (Morse and Low, 1972). The pia can be stripped off the underlying cord with relative ease, except where it dips into crevices and follows blood vessels for short distances into the cord. The scanning electron microscope reveals a smooth surface with scattered white microvilli and a few blebs probably covering underlying macrophages. There are occasional bare spots or fenestrations where the surface cells are missing, exposing the underlying layer of connective tissue fibers (Cloyd and Low, 1974). In these bare areas the neural basement membrane is all that separates the subarachnoid space from the cells of the glial and nervous tissue lying beneath (Morse and Low, 1972).

Subdural Space

A potential space exists between the dura mater and the pia-arachnoid membrane. Contrast media frequently enter this space during diagnostic myelography, with a varying incidence of 1 to 13 per cent, depending on technique used and length of needle employed (Schultz and Brogdon, 1962;

Jones and Newton, 1963; Taveras and Wood, 1972). Partial subdural injection may be a cause of failure in subarachnoid anesthesia (Sechzer, 1963; Cohen and Kallos, 1972). Accidental subdural injection can also occur as a rare complication of attempted epidural puncture, especially if the anesthesiologist inserts the needle unskillfully and rotates the bevel repeatedly, risking unnecessary trauma to the dura. Boys and Norman (1975) have obtained radiographic evidence of a case of accidental placement of an epidural catheter in the subdural space. Injected solutions spread slowly but quite extensively in the subdural space, and this particular anatomical error may be a cause of occasional cases of unexplained massive extradural analgesia (Dawkins, 1969).

COVERINGS OF PERIPHERAL NERVES

Epineurium

The epineurium is a peripheral extension of the dura mater mainly composed of collagen fibers, most of which are orientated in the long axis of the nerve sheath. Interspersed among the collagen fibers are a few elastic fibers and scattered fibroblasts.

The epineurium is quite freely permeable, and it does not constitute a diffusion barrier to local anesthetics. At one time there was considerable confusion over this point. Lorente de Nó (1950) held firmly to the belief that the connective tissue sheaths of peripheral nerves were ineffective as diffusion barriers, while others held contrary views. The argument was settled by a clear definition of what was meant by "nerve sheath." Lorente de Nó was correct insofar as the epineural component was concerned, and it is clear that this outer connective tissue layer does not constitute an appreciable barrier to local anesthetics. However, the next layer, the perineurium, is an effective barrier; in isolated nerve preparations it was shown that local anesthetics act 2 to 50 times faster when the perineurium has been stripped off together with the overlying epineurium than when the nerve is intact (Feng and Liu, 1949; Crescitelli, 1951; Causey and Palmer, 1953; Krnjevic, 1954a, 1954b).

Perineurium

The perineurium is composed of 3 to 15 concentric layers of flattened cells disposed in a lamellar fashion around the nerve trunk, deep to the epineurium (Thomas, 1963; Sunderland, 1965). These cells have a characteristically well-defined basement lamina that distinguishes them from other tissues. The cells are of pavement epithelial type with "closed contact" margins, thus forming a series of continuous and apparently impermeable sheets investing the underlying nerves. The perineural cells have two additional features of interest, one possibly contractile and the other possibly excretory by nature, somewhat analogous to the cyclic vacuolations described by Tripathi in arachnoid cells.

When a nerve is cut the severed ends retract. Electron microscopy at a magnification of 60,000 diameters shows short areas of fine filaments within the perineural cells, similar in appearance and organization to the myofibrils of smooth muscle, and Ross and Reith (1969) have suggested that these are contractile elements responsible for retraction and for adaptation of nerve length during body movements.

Small vesicular invaginations of cell membrane and intracellular vesicles are also common features of the perineural cell (Novikoff, 1967; Ross and Reith, 1969), as shown diagrammatically in Figure 2–9. Although speculative at present, it seems likely that these micropinocytotic vesicles are performing some sort of selective transport function similar to the cyclic vacuolation seen in arachnoid cells. Tracer substances of quite large molecular weight, such as ruthenium red and horseradish peroxidase (MW 40,000), applied to the outer surface of a nerve travel inward through the perineurium by this micropinocytotic mechanism, with a rapid time course of 30 minutes to 6 hours (Singer et al., 1972; Krishnan and Singer, 1973).

Shanthaveerappa and Bourne (1962, 1963, 1966) have described the perineural membrane as a direct peripheral extension of the pia-arachnoid, reaching out to the extreme limits of the peripheral nervous system, covering all motor and sensory nerve endings and effectively separating the entire aristocratic nervous system from the baser masses of the flesh. This concept is outlined in Figure 2–10 taken from Shanthaveerappa and Bourne's work. In this schema a continuous potential space is considered to exist under the perineural membrane of the peripheral nerves extending centrally as the subpial space next to the cord. Thus, solutions injected under the subperineural membrane of a peripheral nerve would be able to travel centripetally and

CONTRACTILE AND EXCRETORY ELEMENTS IN PERINEURAL CELLS

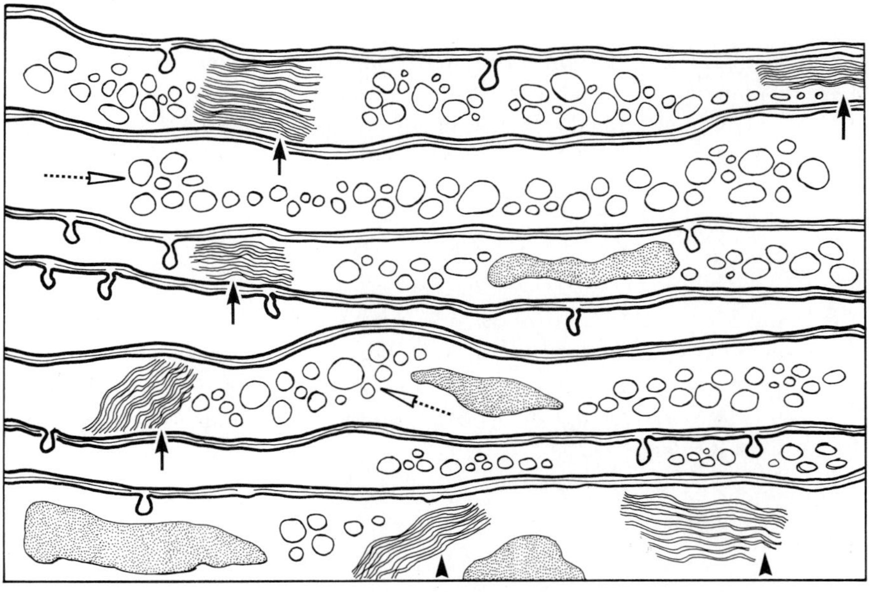

Figure 2–9. Diagram of electron microscopic appearance of perineural cell layers. These cells have a well-defined basement lamina. Short lengths of myofibril-like filaments are present in the cells, together with numerous micropinocytotic vesicles. Symbols. ➞ contractile elements in perineural cell; ······▷ micropinocytotic vesicles. (After Ross and Reith, 1969.)

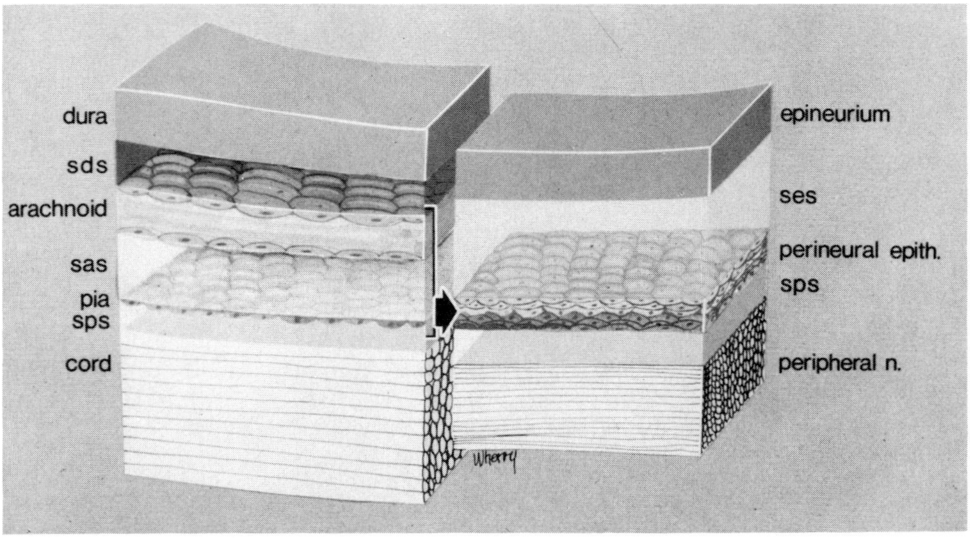

Figure 2–10. The meninges and their peripheral extensions. (After schema of Shanthaveerappa and Bourne, 1966.)

s.d.s. = subdural space
s.a.s. = subarachnoid space
s.p.s. = subpial space and subperineural space
s.e.s. = subepineural space

reach the surface of the spinal cord rapidly and with great ease. Recent studies by Andres (1967) and by Low and his associates (McCabe and Low, 1969; Haller and Low, 1971) have suggested some modification of this schema. Low's work suggests that the arachnoid and the perineurium are two distinct structures, joined in the region of the root sleeves and interleaved somewhat like the taper joints in a system of farm drainage pipes. However, these detailed histological differences remain consistent with Shanthaveerappa and Bourne's general proposition of a functionally continuous diffusion barrier clothing the whole nervous system, like a close-fitting inner skin separating its own delicate milieu internale from the coarser external mesodermal world all around it.

Endoneurium

The endoneurium is the innermost portion of the nerve sheath composed of a delicate layer of fine collagen fibers and clear fibrocytes devoid of basement laminae, investing the underlying neural tissue (Sunderland, 1965).

The endoneurium does not appear to behave as a barrier to the diffusion of local anesthetics.

THE ROOT SLEEVES

Anatomical connections between the subarachnoid space and the epidural space are richest in the region of the dural root sleeves covering the dorsal and ventral roots, as they make their exit through the intervertebral foramen. Here vessels enter or leave the subarachnoid space, and the root sleeve is covered by a pampiniform plexus of small veins. In this area the dura is pierced by many vascular channels, both arterial and venous; in addition, numerous outpouchings of the arachnoid mater poke their heads through the dural sleeves like mushrooms growing on a hillside, some of them as large as 3 mm in diameter, and may invaginate the walls of adjacent extradural vessels (Woollam and Millen, 1958a). These arachnoid outpouchings are most numerous in the lumbosacral areas both in man (Rexed and Wennström, 1959) and in marsupials (Attwood and Wooley, 1974), and they become more numerous with advancing age.

This is a region of fundamental importance to drainage of cerebrospinal fluid and to sanitation of the subarachnoid space, as well as one of the most strategic points for penetration of local anesthetics and for mechanism of action of epidural blockade. Communication between the root sleeve area and the vascular system has been studied extensively for many years. Weed's experiments with Prussian (Berlin) Blue in 1914 led to a number of other experiments that have developed our present concept of an effective and rapid transport system between the spinal subarachnoid recesses and the vascular and lymphatic systems (Weed, 1914a, 1914b). Only a few of these works will be described here, and the interested reader is referred to the quoted sources for a wider review of the relevant literature.

The possibility of communications between the subarachnoid space and the lymphatic system was suggested by the work of Mortensen and Sullivan (1933), who showed that contrast material appeared in the cervical lymph nodes of dogs within 90 minutes of injection into the cisterna magna. Between 1948 and 1951 Brierley and Field published several papers in which they examined the possibility of connections between the subarachnoid space and surrounding tissue spaces by injection of particulate matter of various sizes into the subarachnoid space of rabbits, as well as by intraneural injection of radioactive tracers (Brierley and Field, 1948, 1949; Field and Brierley, 1948b; Brierley, 1950; Field, 1951). India ink suspension with a particle size of 0.4 to 1.5 μ readily passed out of the subarachnoid space through the root sleeves, suggesting the term "ink-cuff area." Ink particles stained the surrounding epidural fat and passed to the regional lymph nodes, as shown in Figure 2–11 (Brierley and Field, 1948). In animals that survived for 48 hours a speckling of carbon particles could be seen among the cells of the dorsal root ganglion (Brierley, 1950). Using particles of even smaller size in colloidal carbon, Woollam and Millen (1953) found that passage from the subarachnoid space to the regional lymph glands was very rapid, and staining could be seen within 30 minutes of subarachnoid injection.

Arachnoid Granulations and Arachnoid Villi

Rapid transport of particulate matter from the spinal subarachnoid space to the epidural fat and regional lymph nodes is effected by the outpouchings of arachnoid mater that protrude through the dura into the epidural space. Some of these are microscopic nubs of arachnoid tissue, while others are large

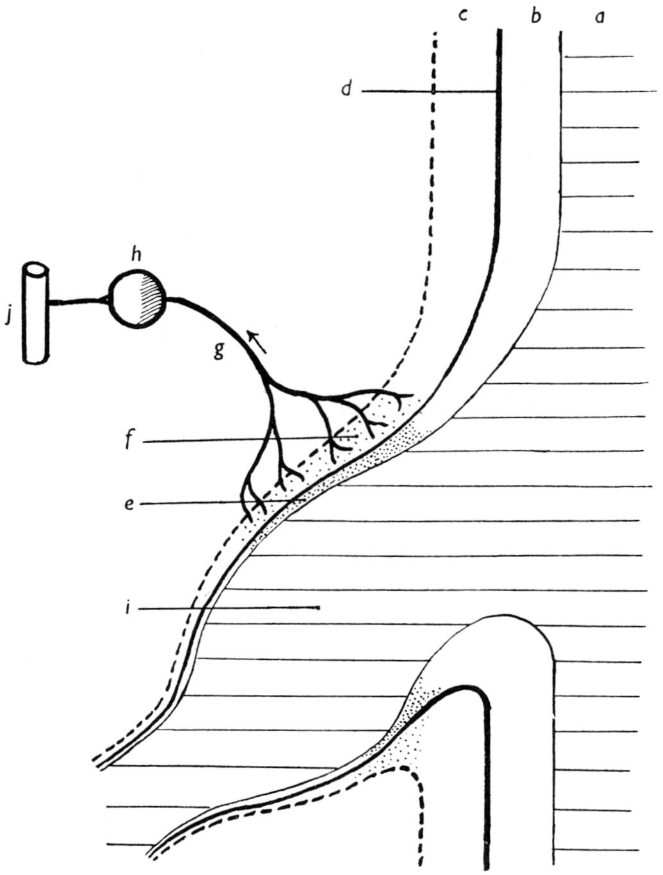

Figure 2–11. Diagram of spinal root (rabbit) and its surrounding "ink-cuff," following injection of India ink into the subarachnoid space.
(a) spinal cord
(b) subarachnoid space
(c) epidural connective tissue
(d) dura mater
(e) ink particles in subarachnoid cul-de-sac
(f) ink particles in epidural connective tissue
(g) fine lymph channels draining epidural tissue
(h) lymph nodes of body wall
(i) spinal nerve
(j) longitudinal lymph channel
(From Brierley and Field: The connexions of the spinal sub-arachnoid space with the lymphatic system. J. Anat. *82*:153, 1948.)

enough to be seen by the naked eye. The larger granulations appear as stalked tufts or villi up to 3 mm in diameter, and many of them invaginate the walls of adjacent veins. Le Gros Clark (1920) noted that the cranial arachnoid villi increase in number with advancing age and that they become enlarged and distended in states of raised intracranial pressure—features that also apply to the spinal arachnoid protrusions.

Cranial arachnoid protrusions or pacchionian bodies were originally noted by Thomas Willis in 1664, but they were named eponymously after Pacchioni, who described them in greater detail in 1712. Their role in the absorption of cerebrospinal fluid was studied by Weed (1914) using the Prussian Blue reaction to precipitate particles of ferric ferrocyanide in the subarachnoid space. Later, Elman (1923) used a similar technique to investigate the possible outflow of cerebrospinal fluid in the region of the root sleeves. During the course of these experiments he noticed cell tuftings and outpouchings of arachnoid mater at the subarachnoid angle that were quite analogous to the arachnoid granulations of the cranial sinuses. Moreover, Elman was able to trace the passage of Weed's Prussian Blue from the subarachnoid space through the arachnoid granulations into the lumen of surrounding epidural veins, showing that a pathway for outflow of cerebrospinal fluid probably existed in this region.

These myxomatous-looking arachnoid granulations of the spinal root sleeves have exactly the same structure as the arachnoid villi of the cranial sinuses (Hassin, 1930), but as late as 1959 some authorities considered them to be of pathological origin (Rexed and Wennström, 1959). In the spinal canal the arachnoid granulations show three principal variations (Welch and Pollay, 1963), outlined in Figure 2–12.

1. They may remain within the dura, usually in close apposition to one of the thin-walled leash of veins draining the spinal cord.

2. They may penetrate the dura mater and lie with their heads free in the epidural fat.

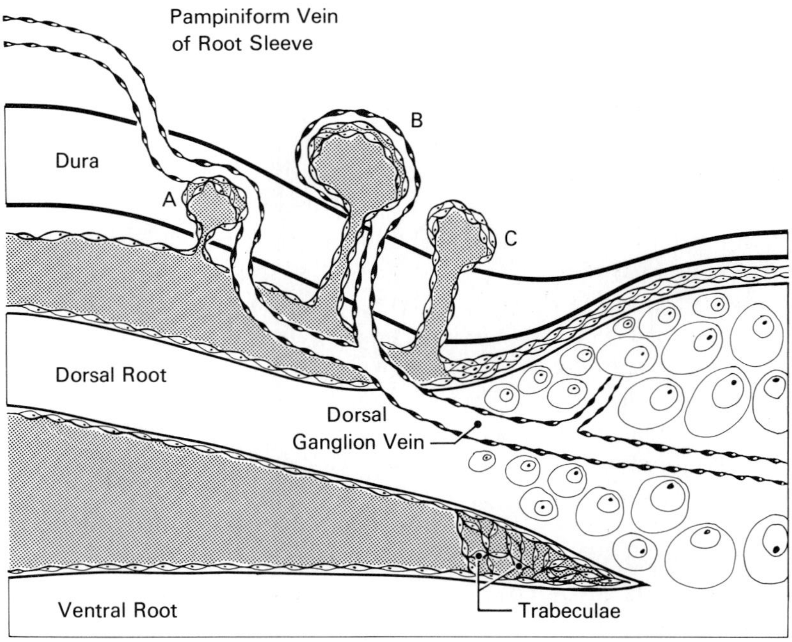

Figure 2–12. Diagrammatic representation of the three principal types of arachnoid protrusions in the spinal root sleeves.

(A) Growth of arachnoid cells in close apposition to thin-walled vein draining the spinal cord running in the wall of the dura mater.

(B) Protrusion of arachnoid villus into one of the pampiniform veins covering the root sleeve.

(C) Arachnoid protrusion penetrating dura mater and lying free in the epidural fat.

(After Welch and Pollay, 1963.)

3. They may extend further as a stalked villus and invaginate into one of the numerous extradural veins of the delicate pampiniform plexus covering the dural root sleeves.

Their business is to drain cerebrospinal fluid (Davson et al., 1973) and to remove debris from the subarachnoid space, unloading it either into the blood stream (Howarth, 1952) or into the regional lymphatic system (Brierley and Field, 1948; Woollam and Millen, 1958; Millen and Woollam, 1962).

The precise mode of transfer was in doubt for many years, and the available evidence was conflicting. Under electron microscopy the epithelial cells of arachnoid villi had the appearance of being completely impermeable, with tightly joined cells and "closed-contact" junctions (Alksne and Lovings, 1972), yet earlier work by Simmonds (1953) and Bradford and Johnson (1962) had shown that intact labeled red cells could pass from the cerebrospinal fluid into the blood stream quite rapidly. Similar experiments by Adams and Prawirohardjo (1959) showed that 25 per cent of tagged red cells injected into the subarachnoid space were absorbed directly into the blood stream, while the remainder became enmeshed in the arachnoid (Shabo and Maxwell, 1968). Welch and Pollay (1961) examined the behavior of a variety of particulate matter in the cerebrospinal fluid and found that rigid polystyrene particles of up to 1.8 μ in diameter could pass freely through perfused arachnoid villi, with perfusion pressures well within the normal physiological range.

All these experiments showed that the arachnoid villi must possess some peculiar faculty that belies their convincing outward appearance of rigid impermeability. The villi appear as if they ought to be completely impermeable, and yet in fact they allow small rigid microspheres and larger but conformable red cells to pass with relative ease. The paradox of villous function was finally resolved by the classic work of Tripathi, who showed that a system of transcellular transport is responsible, and that the same basic mechanism exists to drain both the subarachnoid space and the anterior chamber of the eye (Tripathi, 1971, 1973; Tripathi and Tripathi, 1974). Serial section analysis of arachnoid villi showed that a process of cyclic vacuolation takes place, starting on the basal (subarachnoid) surface of the epithelial cells and then spreading through the cell body to form temporary transcellular channels 2.3 to 3.5 μ in diameter and large enough for particulate debris, red cells or macrophages to pass out of the subarachnoid space (see Fig. 2–8 and Arachnoid Mater, page 18). Arachnoid villi invaginating epidural veins discharge their effluent directly into the blood stream (see Fig. 2–12). Those without vascular contact empty their contents into the interlobular areolar tissue of the epidural fat, and from there particulate matter is taken up by the network of local lymphatic channels and carried to the regional lymph glands, as shown in Figure 2–11. At present, it is not known whether the choice of ejection site is a random phenomenon or if some biological signal determines whether specific sorts of subarachnoid rubbish are selectively directed to either the venous or the lymphatic drainage system. It can readily be appreciated that the delicate arachnoid protrusions make an ideal site for epidural local anesthetics to penetrate the meningeal defenses and reach the subarachnoid space, or possibly even to travel retrogradely along the spinal veins toward the spinal cord if local venous dynamics are favorable.

Fine Structure of the Root Sleeves and Nerve Coverings

In 1950 Brierley speculated that the subdural space (i.e., the potential space between the dura and the arachnoid) was in direct continuity with the subperineural space of the peripheral nerve. However, Shanthaveerappa and Bourne's extensive studies of the perineural membrane modified this view and suggested instead that the pia-arachnoid fuses to form the perineural epithelium, and that a continuous space exists under this epithelial barrier, extending centrally as a potential space under the pia mater, completely covering the spinal roots and the spinal cord (Shanthaveerappa and Bourne, 1962, 1963; Shantha and Bourne, 1968; Shantha and Evans, 1972), as shown diagrammatically in Figure 2–10.

More recently, electron microscopy analyses by Andres (1967) and by Low and his colleagues have revealed details of the root sleeves and their contents that indicate some slight modifications should be made in Shantha and Bourne's original schema (McCabe and Low, 1969; Haller and Low, 1971; Haller et al., 1972). These studies seem to show that the perineural epithelium extends centrally only as far as the subarachnoid angle, where the layers split to form an outer and an inner component. The outer component ends between the dura and the arachnoid layers of the root sleeve, while the inner layer continues as an irregular fenestrated sheet covering the spinal roots, with only its basal membrane in complete continuity, as shown diagrammatically in Figure 2–13.

The loose, fenestrated structure of the root sheath does not suggest an arrangement that constitutes the efficient sort of diffusion barrier described by Shantha and Bourne. Rather, there appears to be an opportunity for seepage from the endoneurial space to the subarachnoid space over a considerable portion of the root sheath.

Scanning electron microscopy of the subarachnoid angle shows that the arachnoid membrane is heavily involved in a series of entanglements across the lateral recess between the dorsal and ventral roots (Malloy and Low, 1974). These pictures reveal a scene of eerie beauty (Fig. 2–14), in which fenestrated

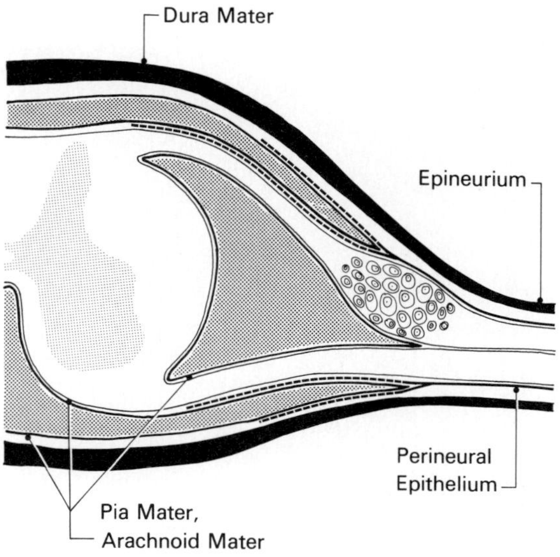

Figure 2–13. Diagram of central extension of the perineural epithelium. The perineural epithelium splits at the level of the subarachnoid angle, and the outer layer gradually disappears between the dura and the arachnoid. The inner layer continues as a fenestrated sheet over the spinal roots with only the basement membrane in complete continuity. (After Haller and Low, 1971.)

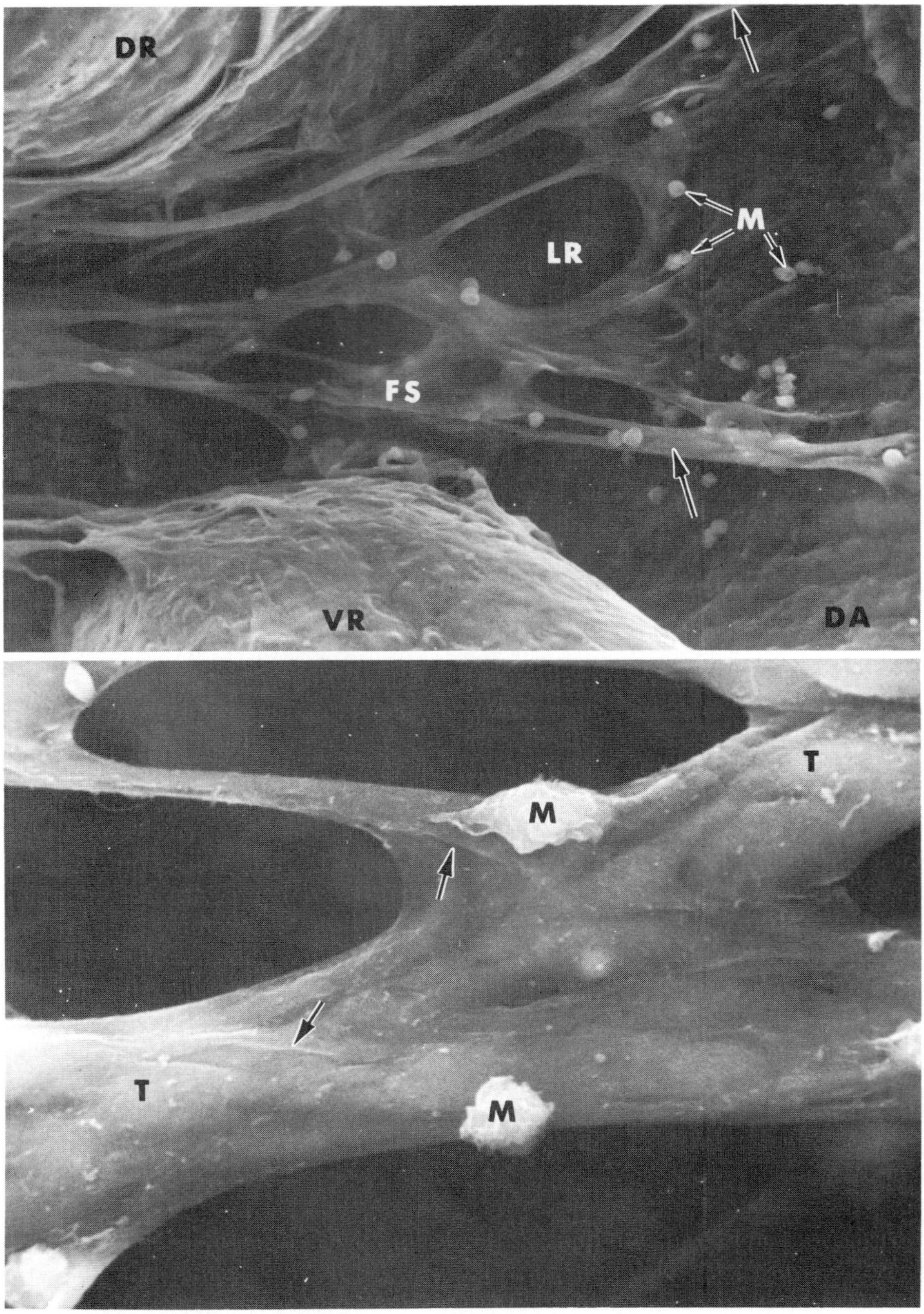

Figure 2–14. *A*, Subarachnoid angle. Scanning electron microscopy × 390. Lateral recess between dorsal and ventral roots looking outward. A dorsal root (DR) and a ventral root (VR) approach their common exit. Arachnoid trabeculae (arrows) arise from the dura-arachnoid (DA) adjacent to the exit. Some trabeculae join to form a fenestrated sheet (FS); the lateral recess (LR) is beyond. Numerous macrophages (M) roam the area. *B*, Scanning electron microscopy × 1800. Arachnoid trabeculae (T) have smooth surfaces with cell boundaries (arrows) appearing as low ridges. Macrophages (M) patrol the trabeculae. (From Malloy, J. J., and Low, F. N.: Scanning electron microscopy of the subarachnoid space in the dog. J. Comp. Neurol. *157*:87, 1974.)

curtains and weblike trabeculae of gleaming white arachnoid hang like tattered shrouds in the narrowing passes where the rootlets and the dural cuffs converge toward the outermost limits of the lateral subarachnoid recess. Subarachnoid debris litters the recess (Himango and Low, 1971), and squads of free-moving macrophages roam the entanglements, patrolling this vulnerable border area like soldiers around the portcullis of a medieval castle.

The whole complex structure enclosed by the dural root sleeve is clearly a vital but pharmacologically weak point in the meningeal fortifications. It is an area preoccupied with the dual roles of busy interchange and defense-in-depth against microbial invasion, and it is here that the fenestrations and loose overlapping of tissue barriers allow local anesthetics preferential access to the underlying neural tissue (see Chapter 4, Mechanism of Action of Epidural Blockade).

TISSUE SPACE CONNECTIONS

It is important to appreciate the relationships of the tissue spaces around the spinal cord and peripheral nerves in order to understand the paths of least resistance that an epidural anesthetic solution is likely to take, with consequent blockade of neural sites along the route.

Connections Between Peripheral and Central Integumental Spaces

The existence of connections between the tissue spaces of peripheral nerves and the subarachnoid space has been argued for more than two centuries. In 1764 Domenico Cotugno published a commentary on the sciatic nerve in which he examined the question of whether the subarachnoid root sleeves were in direct continuity with the sheaths of the peripheral nerve. He concluded that there was a direct connection, on the basis of mercury injections into the subarachnoid space that spread out beyond the dorsal root ganglia under the coverings of the spinal nerves. These crude beginnings, using overwhelming physical pressures, started a controversy that has only recently been clearly resolved (Cotunnius, 1775).

At the dorsal root ganglion the neural integuments are tightly bound around the underlying nerve (Sicard and Cestan, 1904). Sicard and Cestan pointed out that the barrier is usually intact during life but that it can be broken down artificially by high pressures, such as were applied by Cotugno in his original experiments with metallic mercury 200 years ago. Similarly, injections made into the subperineural space of the peripheral nerve can also break through the barrier at the "nerf de conjugaison" to reach the subarachnoid space. The capacity and physical compliance of the subarachnoid space are relatively large, so volumes of many milliliters can be injected before the cerebrospinal fluid pressure rises high enough to rupture the barrier. On the other hand, the capacity of the subperineural space is extremely small, and very small volumes injected under the perineural epithelium will therefore cause disproportionately high pressures to develop within the restricted space; thus rupture into the subarachnoid space can occur after quite minute volumes of tracer material have been injected into the subperineural space (Sullivan and Mortensen, 1934; Mulder, 1938; Chen, 1945).

The critical pressure at which rupture occurs between the subarachnoid and subperineural space is far above the normal range of cerebrospinal fluid (5 to 37 mmHg) and beyond the limits encountered in disease. Key and Retzius (1876) observed passage of Prussian Blue from the subarachnoid space to the peripheral nerve with pressures of about 60 mmHg. Cerebrospinal fluid pressures of this order are higher than would be obtained in any reversible disease situation and are high enough to jeopardize blood flow in the cord. Somberg (1947) examined the effect of injection pressure by giving subarachnoid injections of methylene blue to 12 moribund patients, followed by extensive post mortem dissection of the spine in six of the patients who died. When injection pressure was kept below 15 mmHg, this highly neurotoxic dye was found to be arrested at the arachnoid reflection in the root sleeve, on a level with the proximal part of the dorsal root ganglion. However, when pressures of 44 mmHg were sustained for about 30 minutes, the dye broke past the root sleeve and spread outward along the peripheral nerves under the nerve sheaths. In dogs, French and his colleagues (1948) found that high pressures of the order of 130 to 200 mmHg were required to break through the subarachnoid angle, either from the subarachnoid space into the subperineural space or in the reverse direction from the subperineural space into the subarachnoid space. In chronic preparations, subarachnoid particulate matter may find its way through the lateral recess of the root sleeves into the subperineural space after several days (Quincke, 1872; Brierley, 1950; Steer and Horney, 1968), but the slow passage is probably brought about by macrophage ingestion and migration.

The conditions required for centripetal spread of injected solutions from the subperineural space to the subarachnoid space depend on accurate intraneural injection through the perineural epithelium with fine-gauge obtuse beveled needles. Under these circumstances it is relatively easy to attain sufficient subperineural pressure to cause retrograde spread, with rupture of the arachnoid barrier and passage into the cerebrospinal fluid, resulting in massive subarachnoid block (Chen, 1945). The danger of accidental transverse myelitis from neurolytic agents inadvertently forced along this pathway has been clearly pointed out by Moore and his colleagues (1954).

These longitudinal connections of integumental spaces around the spinal roots and nerves are of great interest in elucidating the possible pathways and mechanism of action of epidural analgesia. However, the demonstration of a normal tissue barrier at the arachnoid reflexion in the root sleeves suggests that subperineural spread is probably not a major factor in allowing local anesthetics to reach the spinal roots and the cord. The prime portal of entry to the subarachnoid space and its contents is almost certainly the highly vascular, sievelike root sleeves, where so many small vessels and arachnoid granulations penetrate the meningeal defenses. From there, access to the cerebrospinal fluid, the spinal roots and the surface of the cord is relatively unhindered. Any local anesthetic that does reach the subperineural space of the peripheral nerve is likely to do so after penetration of the thin sheaths around the spinal roots, then by seepage under the pia and outward beneath the perineural epithelium.

Connections Between Extradural and Paraspinal Tissue Spaces

The epidural space is not a closed system. Many of the tissue planes around the spinal canal connect to form an extended system of tracks through which injected solutions and tracer dyes can spread in a variety of directions (Kumar et al., 1971). Macintosh and Mushin (1947) showed that if paravertebral needles are placed on both sides of the spine, fluid injected into the needles on one side will often drip out of the needles on the opposite side. The route of connection between the two is through the intervertebral foramina and the epidural space lying between. Evans, Dobben and Gay (1967) used radiopaque dyes to show even more diverse connections through the retroperitoneal space, as well as through the epidural space.

At the turn of the century Sicard (1901) was the first to investigate the physical spread of solutions in the epidural space. He continued his work over the next 25 years with other collaborators (Sicard and Cestan, 1904), most notably Forestier (Sicard and Forestier, 1921, 1926), who made a special study of the intervertebral foramina as they provided physical escape routes from the epidural space (Forestier, 1922). There are 58 foramina in all, and the areolar tissue around the exits of these intervertebral foramina varies in density according to age. In the young it is soft and tenuous, but with age it undergoes increasing condensation, forming a definitely recognizable structure. In his thesis of 1922, Forestier described it thus: "As the nerve trunk leaves the intervertebral foramen it encounters an easily dissectable fibrous sheet which forms a sort of fibrous operculum to the external orifice of the intervertebral foramen." With advancing age these opercula thicken and block off the intervertebral foramina more effectively than in young subjects. Then, solutions injected into the epidural space are confined within the spinal canal, and they escape less readily along the neurovascular bundles into the paravertebral spaces. Peridurograms with Lipiodol show a characteristic outward spread in young subjects, with radiopaque oil extending laterally through the intervertebral foramina into the paravertebral spaces and along the neurovascular bundles. In old subjects there is very little lateral spread, and the radiopaque oil climbs much higher within the spinal canal, as shown in Figure 2–15.

Until quite recently it was thought that anatomical spread of solutions within the epidural space and beyond into the paravertebral spaces played a major role in the mechanism of action of epidural blockade. In 1939 Gutierrez considered that the dura was impermeable and that the site of blockade lay entirely beyond the boundaries of the spinal canal after the local anesthetic had escaped through the intervertebral foramina to act on the mixed nerves in the paravertebral spaces. At the time this was not an unreasonable assumption on the basis of the evidence available, for there was a fairly close correspondence between the anatomical volume of the epidural space and the large amounts of anesthetic solution that were used to produce a satisfactory level of segmental blockade. Using sodium iodide solution as a contrast medium

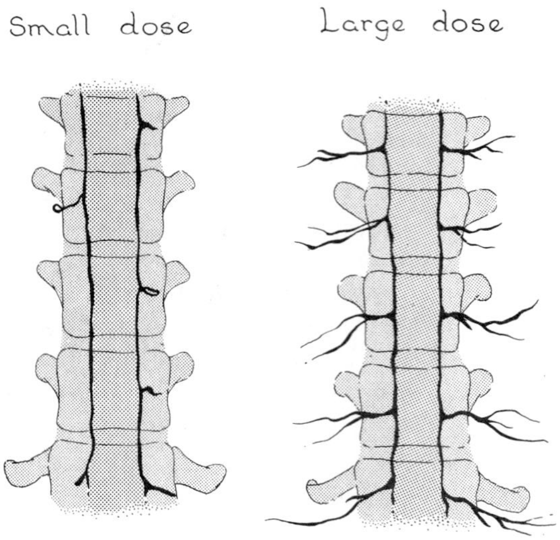

Figure 2–15. Pattern of epidurograms in old and young subjects.

for peridurograms in fresh cadavers, Farr (1926) found that a volume of about 118 ml was required to fill the entire epidural space from the sacral canal to the base of the skull, while a volume of 89 ml extended up to the fourth thoracic segment. These anatomical volumes were not very different from the large quantities of rather feeble concentrations of procaine and tetracaine (Pontocaine), in the range of 40 to 80 ml, that were used for epidural analgesia at that period of anesthetic history (Schlimpert, 1911; Farr, 1926), and it seemed an acceptable assumption that these large volumes might be acting in the paravertebral spaces to produce a multiple paravertebral block of the mixed nerves. However, as more powerful local anesthetics became available, smaller volumes of solution were needed, and it became increasingly evident that these new doses were far too small in volume to provide effective blockade at multiple paravertebral sites. It seemed more likely that the prime site of action must be some point within the spinal canal, not beyond in the contiguous paravertebral spaces (Bromage, 1967a). As laboratory and clinical data accumulated, the evidence pointed more and more strongly to a primary site of action within the spinal meninges at the spinal roots and the surface of the spinal cord (Bromage, 1975). This evidence is also discussed in Chapter 4 on Mechanism of Action. Here we will consider some of the relevant properties and anatomical dispositions of nerve fibers and tracts within the spinal roots and cord as they influence the neurological outcome of epidural blockade.

SPINAL ROOTS

Dorsal Roots

The spinal roots vary greatly in size and thickness. The thoracic roots are thin and delicate structures, compared to the heavy cables of the cervical and lumbosacral enlargements subserving the limbs, where the largest roots are found. The great differences in size and neural populations within the roots have interested anatomists for more than 100 years (Kölliker, 1850; Stilling, 1859). In 1903 Ingbert performed a very exhaustive enumeration of the size and population of the dorsal roots taken from the body of a healthy middle-aged man who had died in an accident. Ingbert's findings are summarized in Figure 2–16, in which the cross-sectional area and the medullated population of the dorsal roots are shown on the same axes. It can be seen that the root size and neuronal population are very closely associated. At that time, long before electron microscopy became a reality, enumeration of nerve fibers lacked the exquisite precision of today, and large Remak bundles of unmyelinated fibers were probably interpreted as single myelinated fibers under the light microscope. Nevertheless, Ingbert's measurements confirmed and refined the general trend of earlier work by Kölliker and by Stilling, and they showed very clearly the twin peaks of maximum fiber population at C_8 and S_1.

Recently, Galindo and his colleagues (1975) repeated some of these earlier measurements of root size in the lumbosacral region, with somewhat similar but more limited results:

Nerve Root	*Diameter (mm)*
T_{12}	2.2
L_2	3.0
S_1	3.8 (range 3.1 to 5.0 mm)
S_2	3.4
S_3	2.3
S_4	1.5
S_5	1.0

Although the size of the dorsal roots remains fairly constant during adult life, the population of neurons declines steadily with age (Hodge, 1894; Corbin and Gardner, 1937; Semenowa, 1941; Rexed, 1944; Shock, 1962); by

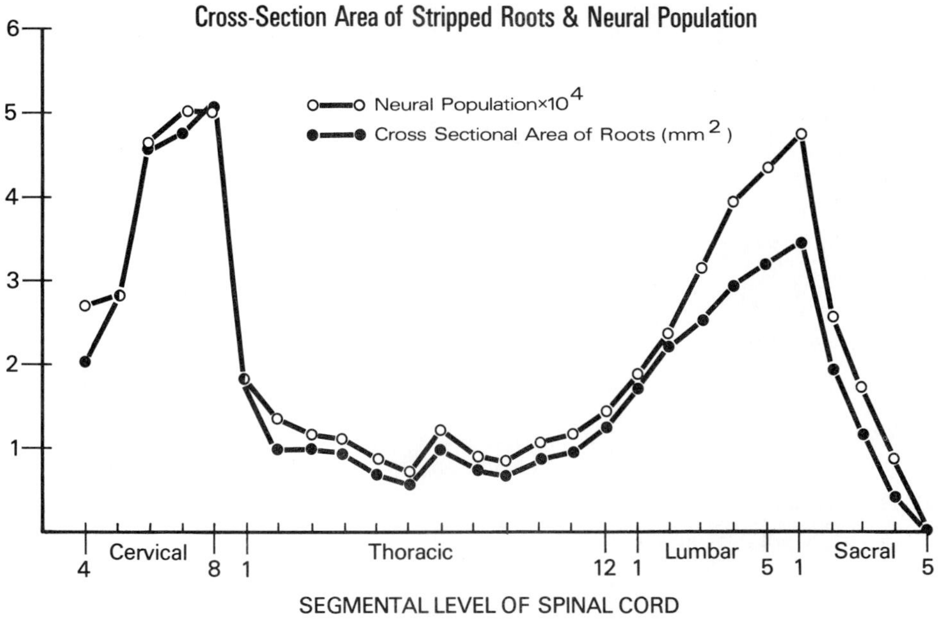

Figure 2–16. Cross-sectional area of spinal dorsal roots in sq mm. Medullated neural population shown in 10,000's. (After Ingbert, 1903.)

the ninth decade about one third of the neuronal population has died. The lost neurons become replaced by connective tissue, so that the ratio of connective tissue to neurons gradually increases. The quality of the connective tissue also deteriorates; intercellular amorphous substance becomes replaced by fibrous elements, and injected dyes spread through the tissues more rapidly than in the young (Ham and Leeson, 1961).

Ventral Roots

Coggeshall and his associates (1974) have carried out a most interesting and detailed analysis of the number and type of nerve fibers in the ventral roots throughout the length of the human spinal cord, using both light microscopy (LM) to count myelinated fibers and electron microscopy (EM) to count unmyelinated fibers. This analysis also confirms that the largest number of fibers is present opposite the cervical and lumbosacral enlargements, but a much more intriguing finding has been the very high proportion of unmyelinated fibers in the ventral roots at all levels of the cord, a proportion that is very much higher than hinted at by Sherrington in 1894 (Fig. 2–17).

In cats, many of these unmyelinated fibers in the ventral roots have sensory functions, some with cutaneous receptive fields (Clifton et al., 1974). Aguayo's EM studies have suggested that many of the unmyelinated fibers in the ventral roots of man are what were formerly thought to be "B-fibers," that is, preganglionic sympathetic efferent fibers, while others are destined to end in muscle spindles, with functions that are at present undetermined (Aguayo, 1975, personal communication).

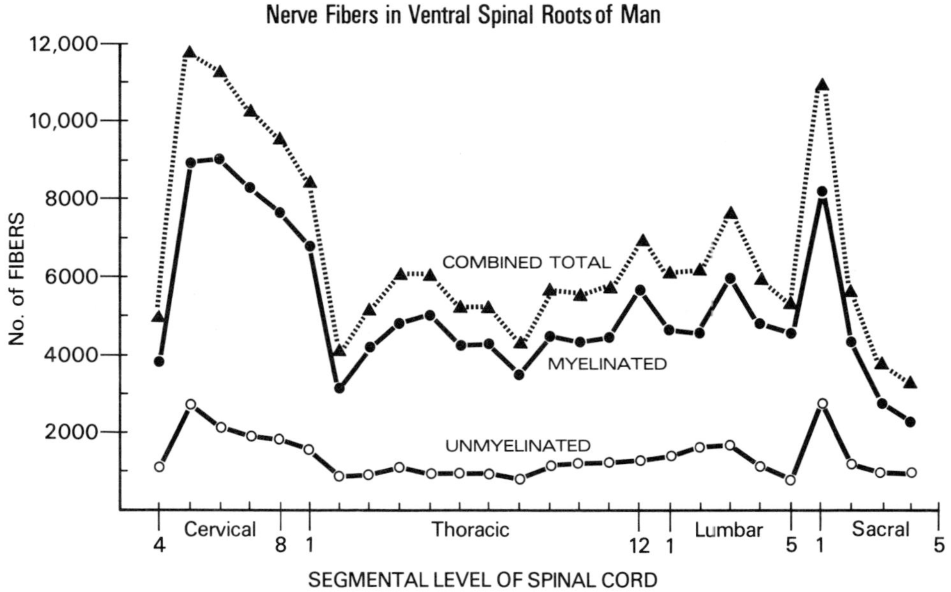

Figure 2–17. Total nerve fiber counts in ventral spinal roots of man, showing proportion of unmyelinated fibers (EM count) and myelinated fibers (LM count). Enumerations are the average from three fresh cadavers. (After Coggeshall et al., 1975.)

Thus, Magendie's law no longer survives to provide intellectual comfort by dividing the dorsal and ventral roots into tidy sensory and motor compartments, dictating as it did an entire epoch of neurological thought and neurosurgical execution.

The very large diameter and the high neural population of the dorsal and ventral roots of the first sacral segment are associated with great resistance to epidural blockade. Prolonged latency and poor analgesia of the first sacral segment are common with most orthodox local anesthetic agents except the carbonated solutions (Bromage et al., 1967; Bromage, 1967b). This association of large root diameter and numerous fiber population with imperfect analgesia suggests that poor penetration of local anesthetic is the cause and that an adequate blocking concentration fails to reach fibers that are deeply placed at the core of the root. Only the most highly penetrating agents, such as carbonated solutions, are able to reach the central fibers in sufficient amounts to produce consistent and reliable blockade of these very large, heavily populated and resistant roots.

Each dorsal root divides into approximately six separate rootlets as it approaches the spinal cord. Each of the rootlets carries a complete spectrum of fiber size and sensory modality, arranged in an apparently random fashion. However, within a few millimeters of the cord, the fibers reorganize themselves into two distinct groups. The large fibers move medially toward the dorsal columns, while the smaller fibers turn laterally to occupy the ventrolateral part of the rootlet, before entering the tract of Lissauer at the lateral margin of the dorsal horn (Sindou, Quoex and Baleydier, 1974).

Intersegmental Connections

The classic boundaries of segmental innervation are less pure than commonly imagined. Frequent intersegmental nerve filaments can be seen running between neighboring nerves, roots or dorsal ganglia (Pallie, 1959; Jacob and Jacob, 1971). Usually these connections are fine filaments running between adjacent dorsal roots, but they may occur between a dorsal ganglion and a ventral root of an adjacent segment, and they may carry up to 28 per cent of the population of a dorsal root. The filaments linking dorsal root ganglia and ventral roots carry an abnormally high proportion of unmyelinated nerve fibers (Jacob and Weddell, 1975). Clearly, these cross-segmental arrangements allow for a considerable amount of overlap in adjacent cutaneous receptive fields, and they are likely to blur the precision with which a clinical level of cutaneous analgesia can be related to neural blockade occurring at a root level during epidural blockade.

NERVE FIBER SIZE IN ROOTS AND CORD: INFLUENCE ON EPIDURAL BLOCKADE

Knowledge of neuroanatomy and neurophysiology is developing at an accelerating pace. Articles devoted to these subjects are appearing in a number of specialized journals, some of which publish over 2,000 pages of new material each year. Old wiring diagrams for the central nervous system are undergoing frenetic reorganization as each day brings fresh and often unexpected data from the powerful experimental tools available. Much of this new work touches on the mechanisms and the logical application of epidural blockade, and in the sections that follow I have attempted to select what seems to me the more relevant information from the masses of material available. In doing so I have also tried to avoid straying too far into the many attractive side issues that could expand this volume into unmanageable proportions. Current theories on pain mechanisms are dealt with very briefly in the text, and then only insofar as they concern the immediate anatomical problems of epidural analgesia at the level of the first order afferent nerves and their ascending connections in the cord.

Theories of epidural and subarachnoid analgesia have been founded on three simple premises. First, that sensory blockade occurs at first-order afferent nerve fibers before they enter the spinal cord, while motor blockade occurs in lower motor neurons in the ventral spinal roots, or beyond, after they leave the spinal cord. Second, that afferent and efferent fibers are neatly segregated into their respective dorsal and ventral spinal roots. And third, that large nerve fibers are more resistant to blockade than small ones. Unfortunately, all three of these anatomical premises are only half-truths, and so technique and practices founded upon them reveal a number of inconsistencies and shortcomings that can only be corrected when all the facts are recognized and properly applied.

Epidural analgesia is almost never complete. Unlike subarachnoid block, some motor function nearly always remains. Indeed, retention of motor activity is one of the main attractions of the technique, for in many clinical situations it is desirable to retain functional capabilities in the presence of pain relief, as we shall see in Chapter 11 on Surgical Applications. The problem of neural blockade and of the manipulation of sensory and motor activity as separate entities is therefore of prime interest to the practicing anesthesiologist in his efforts to exploit some degree of differential blockade for clinical purposes.

Nerve fibers differ in size, function and anesthetic susceptibility. In any given fiber, anesthetic blockade is a function of many different variables, including concentration, pH, pCO_2, length of nerve exposed to the anesthetic and duration of exposure. The literature on the subject of differential blockade is often confusing if the reader does not appreciate the interplay of the many factors involved, for these are complicated enough when the action of a single nerve is being studied under controlled laboratory conditions, but many times more complicated in the living subject. Moreover, much of the underlying microanatomy is still unknown.

ANATOMY OF NERVE FIBERS AND MORPHOLOGICAL DETERMINANTS OF LOCAL ANESTHETIC ACTION

Nerve fibers can be divided into two main morphological groups—*myelinated* and *unmyelinated.* Unmyelinated or C-fibers are small and very numerous and account for about 75 to 80 per cent of all fibers in peripheral sensory nerves and about 95 per cent of preganglionic autonomic fibers (Aguayo and Bray, 1975). The two types of fiber have marked morphological, histochemical

TABLE 2–1 Classification of Peripheral Nerves in Relation to Size and Function (Pre-1973)

Type	*Diameter (microns)*	*Conduction Velocity (m/sec)*	*Internodal Distance* (mm)*	*Function*
A alpha	13–22	70–120	1.2–1.6	Motor, muscle, proprioception
A beta	8–13	40–70	0.8–1.3	Joint afferents, pressure
A gamma	4–8	15–40	0.5–0.9	Touch, muscle spindle efferent
A delta	1–4	5–15	0.2–0.4	Pain, heat, cold, pressure
B	1–3	3–14	0.1–0.4	Preganglionic autonomic efferent
C	0.1–2.5	0.2–1.5	Inter–Schwann cell distance 0.1–0.5	Pain, ?heat, ?cold, ?pressure

*After Coppin and Jack (1972).

and functional differences that are of importance in local anesthetic blockade. Table 2–1 lists the various types of nerve fibers according to their relative size, conduction velocity, internodal distance and function.

The total spectrum of fiber size for axons of all diameters extends from 0.1 μ for the smallest unmyelinated C-fibers to 22 μ for the largest myelinated motor fibers. A typical distribution spectrum for a sensory nerve is shown in Figure 2–18. Larger fibers in the range of 13 to 22 μ are confined to muscle proprioceptors and to motor nerves. The relative proportion of myelinated to unmyelinated axons in a peripheral sensory nerve is roughly 1:4, as shown in Figure 2–19. The proportion of smaller fibers increases with advancing age in both peripheral somatic nerves and in autonomic nerves (Ochoa and Mair, 1969b; Appenzeller and Ogin, 1973).

Myelinated Nerve Fibers

Myelinated fibers range from about 2 μ to 22 μ in diameter, and the distance between the nodes of Ranvier is proportional to the diameter of

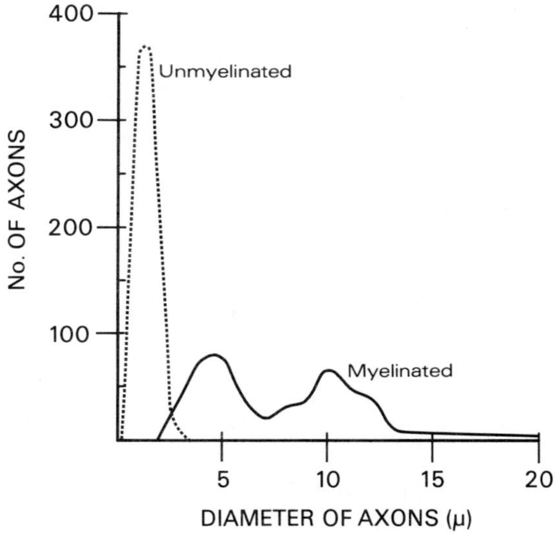

Figure 2–18. Size-frequency spectrum of unmyelinated and myelinated nerve fibers in a peripheral sensory nerve (sural). (Data from Ochoa and Mair, 1969a.)

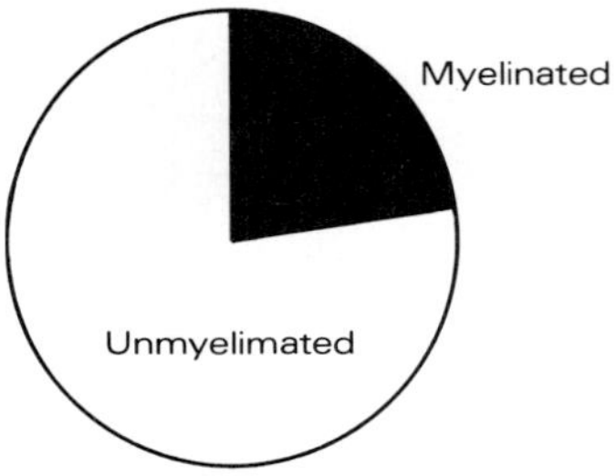

Figure 2–19. Proportion of myelinated and unmyelinated fibers in sural nerve. (After Aguayo et al., 1971.)

the fiber. Internodal distances range from 0.2 mm to 1.6 mm. The ratio of diameter to internodal distance varies with age and is about 1:100 at 18 years and 1:80 at 65 years (Lascelles and Thomas, 1966; Appenzeller and Ogin, 1973). This shortening of internodal distance reflects a gradual loss of large-diameter fibers with advancing age.

The myelin sheath acts as an efficient insulator. Saltatory or "jumping" conduction in myelinated fibers depends on ionic flow and exchange at the nodes of Ranvier. Examination of the nodal and paranodal region by electron microscopy has revealed a remarkably complex and metabolically active apparatus well suited for ionic exchange (Elfvin, 1961). It has also been shown that this region is a highly specialized acceptor site for cations (Landon and Langley, 1971) and hence for charged cationic local anesthetics.

The region of the node of Ranvier is referred to as the nodal-paranodal apparatus (Williams and Landon, 1963; Landon and Williams, 1963), and it has the following features, as shown diagrammatically in Figure 2–20.

1. Crenation of the paranodal myelin sheath with longitudinal fluting of the subjacent axon into five or six segments (Elfvin, 1961; Williams and Landon, 1963; Landon and Williams, 1963).

2. Accumulation of Schwann cell cytoplasm between the fluted seg-

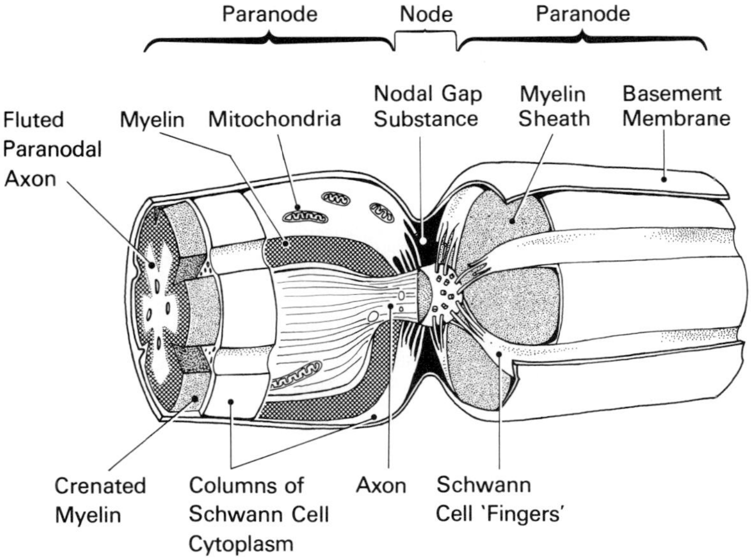

Figure 2–20. The nodal-paranodal apparatus of a node of Ranvier in a large unmyelinated nerve. (After Williams and Landon, 1963, and Landon and Langley, 1971.)

ments of the axon membrane. This region of folded grooves is rich in mitochondria, reflecting a potential for vigorous metabolic activity (Williams and Landon, 1963; Berthold, 1968).

3. Cytoplasmic columns of the Schwann cell end in microvillous fingers, attached somewhat like guy-ropes of a tent to the axon membrane and embedded in nodal gap substance to the Schwann cell basement membrane (Landon and Williams, 1963).

4. Nodal gap substance contains a high content of protein-linked carboxylated mucopolysaccharides (Abood and Abul-Haj, 1956; Landon and Langley, 1971). Landon and Langley (1969, 1971) have shown that mucopolysaccharides of the nodal region are rich in electrostatic binding sites, bearing anionic charges. These anionic sites attract cations of all sorts, and they are presumably an important region for attachment of cationic local anesthetics. Special staining techniques show that certain cations, such as barium, are also bound in a thin layer along the external surface of the adjacent myelin sheath, and this layer may extend inward to involve the whole terminal bulb after prolonged exposure to concentrated solutions.

Unmyelinated Fibers (C-fibers)

Unmyelinated fibers form the most numerous neural element in peripheral nerves, and they account for about 80 per cent of the axonal population. In preganglionic sympathetic nerves they may account for as much as 95 per cent of the fibers (Aguayo, Martin and Bray, 1972).

Unmyelinated axons range from 0.1 μ to 2.5 μ in diameter. Whereas small A delta myelinated axons are insulated in their individual myelin sheaths, the tiny C-fibers are encased in bundles of 1 to 24 fibers wrapped around by a continuous invaginated envelope formed by chains of Schwann cells. These fascicular bundles are known as Remak bundles* and have a diameter of 2 to 4 μ, with a space approximately 100 to 150 Å wide lying between the invaginated Schwann cell membrane and the enclosed C-fibers (Fig. 2–21).

---

*After R. Remak, the Polish neurologist who first described the light microscopy appearance of C-fiber bundles in his doctoral thesis of 1838 while working in Johannes Muller's laboratory in Berlin.

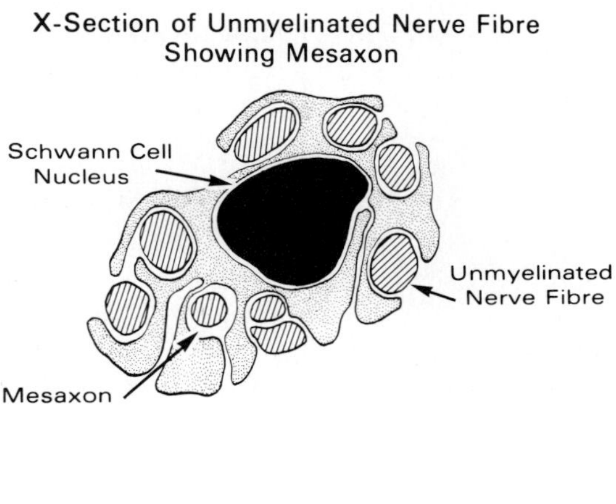

Figure 2–21. Diagram of cross section of Remak bundle showing eight C-fibers encased by invaginations of a single Schwann cell.

The mesaxon forms a channel of connection with the extracellular space outside the nerve bundle.

The ratio of axon diameter to Schwann cell internuclear distance is quite variable but roughly comparable to that of myelinated fibers, lying between 1:50 and 1:200 (Peyronnard et al., 1973; Carlsen et al., 1974). As with myelinated fibers, advancing age is accompanied by a loss of larger caliber fibers and a resultant shift of spectral distribution of fiber size toward a population of smaller diameter (Ochoa and Mair, 1969b). Also, unmyelinated C-fibers survive ischemic compression better than the larger myelinated fibers. If both types of fiber are injured by compression, the unmyelinated axons regenerate by sprouting very fine fibers 0.1 to 0.2 μ in diameter, and the spectrum of fiber size is shifted toward a relatively greater population of very small axons (Fowler and Ochoa, 1975). This phenomenon of altered fiber spectrum may perhaps play a part in the origin of causalgic states following nerve injury.

Effects of Aging on Neural and Perineural Tissue

Advancing age is accompanied by deterioration within the spinal cord, spinal roots and peripheral nerves. The neural population declines steadily after the age of 18 to 20 years, and a parallel deterioration occurs in the connective tissue surrounding the nerves. These changes have profound effects on epidural dose requirements, and they may be summarized as follows:

Decrease in neural population

With advancing age the myelinated fibers in the dorsal and ventral roots lose their youthful contours on cross section and decline in number, so that by the ninth decade one third of the myelinated population has disappeared, leaving a smaller number of survivors to compete for any local anesthetic drugs that may be presented to them (Hodge, 1894; Semenowa, 1941; Rexed, 1944). Indeed, the population curve for myelinated fibers in dorsal roots is very similar in shape to the curves relating epidural dose requirements to age shown in Chapter 3. Both reach a peak at about 20 years and then decline steadily thereafter (Corbin and Gardner, 1937; Bromage, 1969a).

Decrease in conduction velocity

After the third decade there is a steady slowing of conduction velocity in peripheral nerves, amounting to about 0.4 m per second per year (Downie and Newell, 1961; La Fratta and Canestrari, 1966).

Decrease in inter-Schwann cell distance

In myelinated fibers this is expressed by a decrease in internodal distance. Thus, more nodes are present per unit length of nerve, with proportionally more cationic acceptor sites available for electrostatic attachment of ionized local anesthetic drugs. In unmyelinated fibers there is also a decrease in

Schwann cell internuclear distance with increasing age, but the relationship of charged sites to morphology is less well understood for C-fibers than for myelinated axons.

CHANGES IN PERINEURAL CONNECTIVE TISSUE

With increasing age the mucopolysaccharides of connective tissue ground substance undergo qualitative changes that render the extraneural connective tissue barriers increasingly permeable to the passage of dyes and other diffusible agents (Meyer and Rapport, 1951; Kirk and Laursen, 1955; Ham and Leeson, 1961). Myelin sheaths also show increasing deterioration with age, and there is increased thickening and PAS staining of the walls of the vasa nervorum (Fagerberg, 1957, 1959).

All these factors are accelerated by arteriosclerosis. Angiopathy from diabetes or arteriosclerosis has the effect of caricaturing and exaggerating the morphological changes that accompany the normal aging process in the neuraxis and its integuments (Bromage, 1962).

Generally speaking, large fibers are more resistant to blockade than small ones. Gasser and Erlanger's classic work on fiber size and nerve blockade gave rise to the idea that susceptibility to anesthetic blockade was simply a matter of surface-to-volume ratio, and that small fibers with large surface areas in relation to their volume would absorb relatively more local anesthetic than larger fibers with greater bulk in relation to their surface area (Gasser and Erlanger, 1929; Heinbecker, Bishop and O'Leary, 1934). While this rule does apply to the *myelinated* fibers (Matthews and Rushworth, 1957), it does not apply to the *unmyelinated* fibers. The very small C-fibers with diameters of 0.1 to 2.5 μ (Gasser, 1955; Sykes and Coggeshall, 1973) are more resistant to block by cold or by weak concentrations of local anesthetics than preganglionic B-fibers or the smallest A delta fibers with diameters 2 to 30 times larger than those of the C-fibers (Douglas and Malcolm, 1955; Nathan and Sears, 1961; Paintal, 1967; De Jong, 1970; Heavner and De Jong, 1974; Franz and Perry, 1974).

At very weak dilutions of local anesthetic, the unmyelinated C-fibers seem remarkably tough and resistant. After prolonged soaking for more than 30 minutes in a weak solution of 0.02 per cent procaine (1 mM procaine), C-fibers may continue firing even when A-fibers of all diameters have been blocked (Franz and Perry, 1974). Thus, at extremes of anesthetic dilution, such as may exist in some neuronal sites during epidural analgesia, C-fiber activity may be expected to escape blockade from time to time and allow some impulses to reach the central nervous system when all other sensory activity has been interrupted. This may explain the bizarre type of tourniquet pain that often breaks through an apparently effective epidural or subarachnoid block even when dermatome analgesia extends well above the segmental representation of the limb (Leatherdale. 1956; De Jong and Cullen, 1963).

The peculiar resistance of the C-fiber is probably related to its anatomy. The loose system of insulation of the Remak bundle seems to provide better protection against cold blockade and local anesthetic penetration than the close-fitting myelin sheaths of the A delta fibers with their vulnerable nodes of Ranvier (Douglas and Malcolm, 1955; Heavner and De Jong, 1974). Clearly, this resistant arrangement is a great practical handicap tending to thwart clinical attempts at differential blockade, and the clinician's hopes of retaining movement and kinesthesia through unblocked large myelinated fibers while blocking small pain fibers is almost doomed at the outset by the existence of these dogged tiny messengers.

One further peculiarity of the C-fiber is perhaps worth mentioning, if only to share ignorance of its significance. In 1955 Gasser noted the curious fact that unmyelinated C-fibers in dorsal roots are about half the size and twice as numerous as C-fibers distal to the dorsal root ganglion. Also, the packaging arrangements in the Remak bundles are different. In the peripheral nerve, unmyelinated fibers are tightly stuffed into the sheath of the Schwann cells, while in dorsal roots they are packed more loosely, with much more unoccupied space around them in the Schwann cell cytoplasm (Gasser, 1955). Gasser interpreted these findings to represent branching of the proximal axons of the dorsal root ganglion cells. However, another interpretation with relevance to differential blockade in spinal roots is possible. For many years physiologists have suspected that some sensory fibers may travel in the ventral roots, ever since Sherrington proposed the idea in 1894 (Sherrington, 1894; Kato and Tanji, 1971). White and Sweet discuss this possibility very thoroughly in their book *Pain Mechanisms* (White and Sweet, 1955). Recent electron microscopy counts by Coggeshall and his associates show that the population of unmyelinated fibers in ventral roots is much higher than suspected and that up to one third of all axons in the anterior lumbar roots are unmyelinated C-fibers, performing duties of an unspecified nature (Coggeshall, Coulter and Willis, 1973, 1974; Sykes and Coggeshall, 1973). It is possible that an appreciable number of these fibers may be sensory rather than motor in function. This interpretation is speculative, but if it is shown to be correct and if a large proportion of the ventral root is indeed devoted to afferent duties, then clearly a revision of established neurosurgical and neuropharmacological techniques for pain relief will be required. Analgesic procedures directed specifically to deafferenting the dorsal roots alone will be only partially effective. With a sizable proportion of small fiber afferents in the ventral roots, a more logical approach would lie in blockade of *both* dorsal and ventral roots whenever conditions permitted, or as Coggeshall and his colleagues have suggested, in a direct attack on the unmyelinated cell stations in the dorsal root ganglion (Coggeshall et al., 1975).

Anatomical Determinants of "Minimum Effective Concentration" (C_m)

In epidural analgesia the final assault on target axons is done by scattered remnants of the original analgesic force, after heavy losses from vascular absorption or from quantities of local anesthetic being held prisoner in binding sites along the way. Thus, we are concerned with the blocking capabilities of these scattered remnants in very dilute solution at some points, and because of the thin dispersion of anesthetic molecules in the tissues, we must think of their aggregate mass and their effect both in space and time as well as in concentration.

Lord Adrian was the first to show that the rate of onset of conduction blockade is dependent on the length of nerve affected, and he found that alcohol vapor took twice as long to block 4.5 mm of frog nerve as it did a length of 9.0 mm (Adrian, 1912). There has been a general appreciation of the importance of nerve length since that time (Kato, 1936), but a critical analysis of the reasons for this importance was long in coming. During the second world war Huruyama, in Japan, drew attention to the importance of the nodes of Ranvier as the primary site of blockade (Huruyama, 1941), and it is mainly from this source and the subsequent work of Tasaki that our present understanding stems (Tasaki, 1953).

Anesthetic blockade of myelinated fibers takes place only at the nodes of Ranvier, where the axon membrane is bare of myelin sheath. The nodes occupy only about 0.02 per cent of the total length of the nerve, and the distance between nodes is proportional to the diameter and conduction velocity of the nerve. A conducted impulse will be slowed by blockade of one or two adjacent nodes, but it can jump a gap of that size and carry on as a normally propagated impulse beyond such a minor hurdle. *For complete blockade at least three adjacent nodes must be blocked* (Tasaki, 1953). In large A alpha fibers conducting at 120 m/sec the internodal distance may be as great as 1.6 mm (Coppin and Jack, 1972), so for blockade of these fibers at least 3.2 to 3.5 mm of axon length must be exposed to local anesthetic or they will never become effectively blocked (De Jong, 1970; Franz and Perry, 1974). In large nerve bundles in which interfascicular penetration is patchy or irregular, even greater lengths of nerve must be bathed with local anesthetic (Brown, Stumpf and Roth, 1969). Rud showed that for uniform comparison of drug activity a length of 32 mm was required before one could be sure of eliminating variables arising from inadequate longitudinal exposure (Rud, 1961).

Therefore, for blockade to occur, three things are necessary. The concentration of the drug must be sufficient; there must be enough time for the anesthetic molecules to arrive at their target sites on the axon membranes; the anesthetic solution must bathe a sufficient length of nerve. These factors can be put together in a three-dimensional diagram, as shown in Figure 2–22. This general relationship will hold for all local anesthetics.

To summarize, with concentrated solutions of very penetrating agents, little time and only short lengths of nerve sufficient to expose three ad-

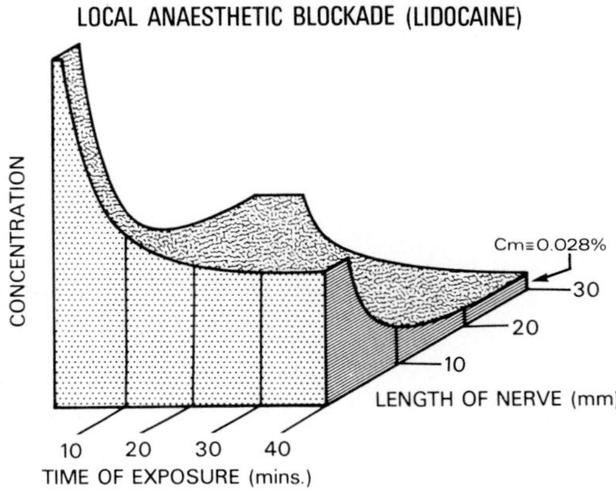

Figure 2–22. Local anesthetic blockade (lidocaine). Relationship of concentration, time of exposure and length of nerve required for complete blockade. Cm: minimum effective concentration.

jacent nodes are needed, but with increasing dilution more time is required for blockade, and the anesthetic solution must be able to reach greater lengths of axon. Under laboratory conditions lidocaine has a minimum effective concentration (C_m) of about 0.02 per cent (i.e., 1 mM/L or 0.28 μg/ml), provided plenty of time is available (up to 40 minutes) and an adequate length of axon is bathed (De Jong, 1970; Franz and Perry, 1974). At these extreme dilutions the length of nerve needs to be about ten times greater than at higher concentrations, and the critical length increases to over 30 mm (Rud, 1961).

Differential Blockade

In light of the available data of fiber size and resistance to blockade, it is difficult to be optimistic about producing an effective and predictable differential block in peripheral nerves and spinal roots. If the block is tenuous enough to let large A alpha activity through, it will probably also let some of the resistant C-fiber activity past as well. At low levels of painful stimulation, analgesia may be satisfactory if the traffic of afferent impulses over C-fiber pathways is light enough. However, with increasing stimulation more C-fibers will be recruited, and some of them may elude blockade; then characteristic diffuse aching pain will be felt in and around the stimulated area (Collins et al., 1960). Consequently, adequate analgesia can only be achieved by abandoning attempts at differential blockade and administering a greater mass of local anesthetic to ensure interruption of both large and small axons, with subsequent loss of motor activity.

In epidural analgesia not all local anesthetics confer the same sort of differential blockade. Some, like bupivacaine, produce quite an effective differential block with the clinically desirable pattern of good analgesia and very little loss of motor activity (Bromage, 1969b), although motor blockade does become more intense when the concentration of bupivacaine is increased from the usual strength of 0.5 per cent to 0.75 per cent (Nolte et al., 1974). This performance could be satisfactorily explained on the basis of blockade at spinal roots. The drug is doing what it should do, blocking small fibers and sparing the large ones, and by some fortunate biochemical chance it is also performing the laudable task of blocking troublesome C-fibers. However, other agents such as tetracaine and etidocaine produce the reverse pattern of differential blockade, particularly in weak concentrations, with marked motor block but relatively poor analgesia (Bromage et al., 1974). In terms of spinal roots or peripheral nerves, this is an unlikely situation and difficult to interpret unless one invokes some special affinity for large fibers. However, there are no solid biochemical grounds for such an idea, and some explanation must be sought, not only for the adverse behavior of tetracaine but also for the more favorable performance of bupivacaine.

There is no satisfactory explanation for these variations in sensory dissociation in terms of first-order afferent fibers. To resolve this paradox we must direct our search centrally beyond the first-order afferent fibers and trace their connections into the cord, to see if an acceptable explanation may lie there. Available laboratory and clinical evidence suggests that the answer may indeed lie in the anesthetic action on pathways within the spinal cord, and later sections will develop this argument more fully. For the moment we must consider the nature of these pathways.

ORGANIZATION OF AFFERENT AND EFFERENT PATHWAYS IN THE CORD

Figure 2–23 shows stylized representations of the main ascending (afferent) and descending (motor) pathways in the cord. In real life, tract territories overlap to a considerable extent. On entering the cord afferent fibers send branches up and down Lissauer's tract surrounding the base of the dorsal root. This tract often shows signs of demyelination after subarachnoid injections of neurolytic agents for relief of intractable pain. The dorsal columns constitute a fast conducting pathway for large fibers, rapidly alerting central nervous connections via the cuneate and gracile nuclei and the medial lemniscus. Large fast conducting fibers also travel in the dorsolateral tract on the same side. Some large fibers also pass deep into the dorsal horn to form synapses with neurons crossing to the lateral funiculi on the opposite side.

Smaller slowly conducting fibers enter the tip of the dorsal horn and almost immediately form relays of synapses with small cells in the substantia gelatinosa (lamina II) and then in turn act upon large neurons placed more deeply in the gray matter of the dorsal horn (Pearson, 1952). The latter project into superficial ascending pathways on the ipsilateral side (ventral spinothalamic tract), and many of these seem to be C-fibers specifically concerned with noxious stimuli (Manfredi and Castelucci, 1969; Pomeranz, 1973). The majority cross over in the anterior commissure to the lateral spinothalamic tract on the opposite side, as well as to the ventral spinothalamic tract lying superficially next to the anterior median fissure (Kerr, 1975). Note that both the anterior and lateral spinothalamic pathways are very superficially placed at the periphery of

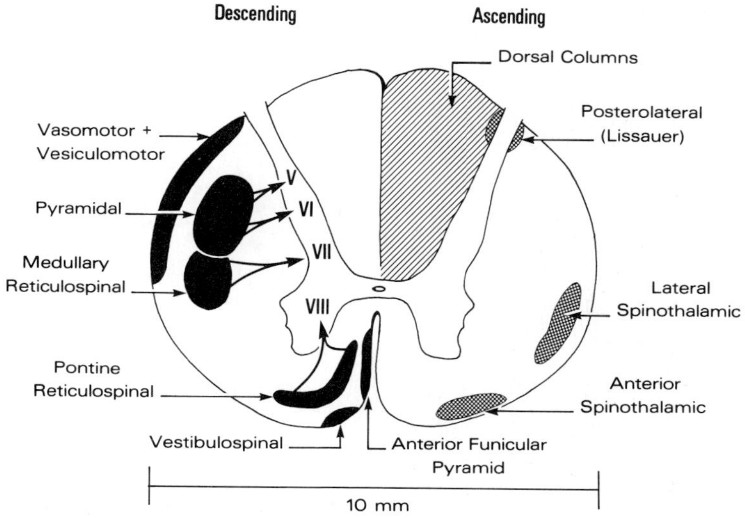

Figure 2–23. Ascending and descending spinal pathways.

the cord. A few slowly conducting fibers also find their way into the dorsal and dorsolateral columns.

Integration of sensory input and motor output takes place in the spinal gray matter, which is arranged in layers that are structurally distinct and also functionally distinct. Rexed's classic paper of the cytoarchitectonic organization of the spinal cord in the cat has been generally adopted as the descriptive basis for the cellular architecture of the spinal gray matter (Rexed, 1952). This nomenclature described ten layers or laminae, as shown in Figure 2–24.

Lamina I consists of a thin layer of large, sparsely scattered neurons, at some points represented only by the thickness of a single cell covering the margin of the dorsal horn. Some of these cells appear to project directly to the spinothalamic tract (Kumazawa et al., 1975). Below the posteromarginal cells of lamina I lie the two layers of smaller cells of laminae II and III. Lamina II was formerly known as the substantia gelatinosa of the dorsal horn. Laminae II and III cells appear to be concerned with modulation and integration of efferent input (Melzack and Wall, 1965). Lamina IV is concerned with relays to lamina V, together with a large number of cells projecting rostrally. Lamina V, and to a lesser extent lamina VI, are the principal layers containing large cells concerned with rostral projection of sensory stimuli (Trevino, Coulter and Willis, 1973). Laminae VII and VIII receive a considerable number of projection fibers from the reticulospinal tract (Kuypers, 1964; Nyberg-Hansen, 1966).

Descending pathways travel at varying depths from the surface. Among the most superficial are the reticulospinal and anterior longitudinal fascicular pathways and the uncrossed pyramidal fibers in the anterior funiculus, projecting to laminae VII and VIII.

Descending autonomic pathways subserving visceromotor function, such as bladder control and vasoconstriction, travel in the most peripheral part of the dorsolateral funiculus just below the pia, between the dorsal root and the dentate ligament, as shown in Figure 2–25 (Kerr and Alexander, 1964; Illert and Gabriel, 1972; Foreman and Wurster, 1973, 1975). Inhibitory vasomotor fibers lie somewhat deeper in the cord at a greater depth from the surface (Illert and Gabriel, 1972; Coote and MacLeod, 1974). Some of these descending autonomic pathways bypass the medulla and become integrated at a relatively low spinal

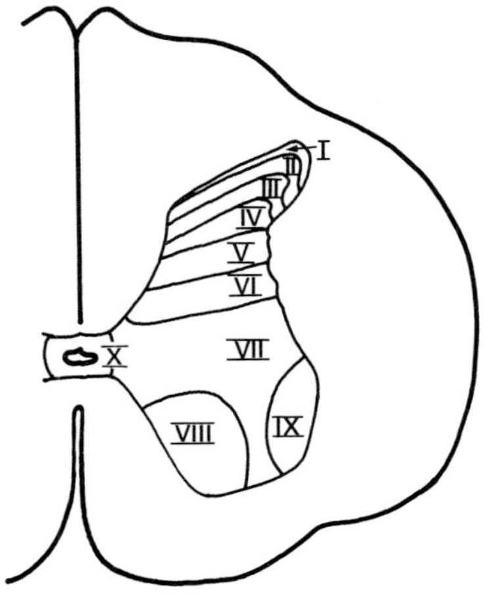

Figure 2–24. Rexed's laminae in the gray matter of the spinal cord. (After Rexed, 1964.)

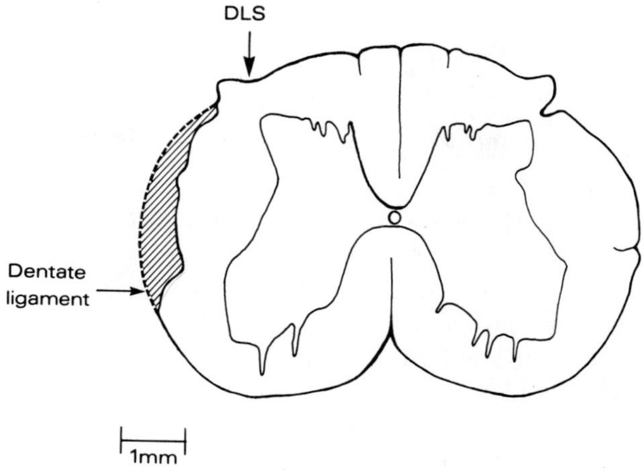

Figure 2–25. Cross section of spinal cord at C_8–T_1 to show extent of lesion necessary to interrupt descending sympathetic *excitatory* pathways in dorsolateral funiculus. DLS: dorsolateral sulcus. (After Foreman and Wurster, 1975.)

level, in contrast to the generally accepted classical concept of an integrated medullary center controlling vasomotor function (Coote and MacLeod, 1974). The crossed pyramidal and rubrospinal tracts are more deeply placed in the lateral funiculus, and these project to laminae V and VI (Fig. 2–26).

At the level of the cervical and lumbar enlargements the cord is almost 14 mm wide, and the crossed pyramidal tracts are several millimeters below the surface, but in the mid-thoracic region where the cord thins down to a transverse diameter of 9 to 10 mm, these fibers are only 1 to 2.5 mm below

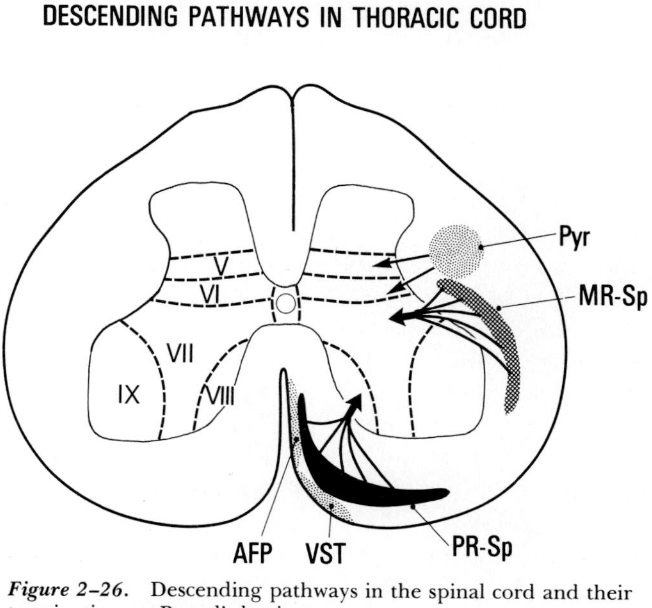

Figure 2–26. Descending pathways in the spinal cord and their termination on Rexed's laminae.

Pyr = pyramidal tract
MR-Sp = medullary reticulospinal fibers
PR-Sp = pontine reticulospinal fibers
VST = vestibulospinal tract
AFP = anterior funicular pyramid

(After Nyberg-Hansen, 1965, 1969, and Kuypers, 1964.)

the surface and within easier range of local anesthetics penetrating inward from the circumference of the cord.

The interaction of these pathways will be discussed further in Chapter 4 on Mechanism of Action.

Sensory Modulation in the Spinal Cord

Almost immediately after entering the spinal cord, the first-order afferent neurons fall under the influence of an extremely elaborate propaganda system devoted to a policy of expediency and physical action (Bromage and Melzack, 1974). At each synapse the messages they carry are subject to censorship, with the possibilities of amplification, suppression or distortion upon instructions from above. Wildly distorted interpretations of external events are possible by internal manipulation of incoming data, and final patterns of sensation may bear little relation to the quality of spatial distribution of the initial stimulus (Melzack and Wall, 1965; Melzack, 1973). The greater part of this internal censorship system seems to lie in the reticular formation of the brain stem and its distal extension as the substantia gelatinosa (laminae II and III) of the dorsal horn. The most potent office of this censorship system lies in the periaqueductal gray matter and median raphe, and here localized stimulation can completely suppress intense levels of noxious stimulation and abolish pain (Reynolds, 1969; Akil et al., 1972; Liebeskind et al., 1973; Oliveras et al., 1974). In the dorsal horn laminae V and VI seem to be particularly important instruments for local distribution of propaganda information decreed from above, and most of the cells projecting to the lateral spinothalamic tract arise from these laminae (Dilly, Wall and Webster, 1968; Trevino et al., 1973).

Detailed mapping of these sensory control systems has only been feasible since the development of micropipette techniques in the 1950's when it became possible to record the activity of single cells within the neuraxis. With this powerful experimental tool the relationships of living nerve cells can be traced with a beauty and precision unattainable before. In 1954, Hagbarth and Kerr showed that stimulation of bulbar and brain reticular formation could suppress ascending spinothalamic volleys resulting from stimulation of the dorsal roots, and Lindblom and Ottoson (1957) demonstrated electrical changes in the dorsal parts of the cord and the dorsal horn on stimulation of descending pyramidal pathways. Since that time a number of descending pathways have been shown to modify afferent input in a tonically active, ongoing fashion (Taub, 1964; Wall, 1967).

Anatomical studies by Kuypers (1964) and Nyberg-Hansen (1966) had shown that two principal descending tracts, the crossed pyramidal in the lateral funiculus and the reticulospinal tract in the anterior funiculus, terminate on different layers in the spinal gray matter, the pyramidal tract ending on laminae IV, V and VI, and the reticulospinal projecting to laminae V, VI and VII. Electrical recording confirms these distributions, and laminae V and VI respond to pyramidal stimulation in the medulla (Wall, 1967), while laminae VI and VII will respond to stimuli from higher cortical centers (Besson and Rivot, 1973). Not only does pyramidal stimulation affect the quantity of information that is allowed to pass, by determining the size of peripheral receptive fields, but also it can switch the quality or modality of sensation from touch to proprioception (Wall, 1967; Hillman and Wall, 1969). Figure 2–27, adapted from Wall's paper of 1967, summarizes the basic neural connections involved in these pyramidal sensory transactions. Blockade of the descending pathways by externally applied cold (Wall, 1967), or by depletion of their neurotransmitter content (Nobin et al., 1973; Vogt, 1974), abolishes tonic control from above. With normal censorship removed, segmental receptive fields expand, allowing an unbridled torrent of afferent traffic to pour upward along ascending pathways to the brain stem and beyond. The net result of this sensory bombardment is an antianalgesic state, as shown by diminished responses to the analgesic effects of morphine (Vogt, 1974).

At the present time there is insufficient evidence to say which descending tracts are most important for restraining incoming sensory traffic. Clearly, however, it is possible to imagine that with partial or patchy blockade of these pathways and their ascending neighbors, a whole spectrum of results could follow, from complete restraint of sensory input to complete license.

Although there is good evidence that epidural blockade involves the peripheral parts of the cord (Bromage et al., 1963; Bromage, 1975), existing data do not extend to quantitative differences of penetration by various local anesthetic agents. However, there are strong presumptive grounds for believing that different agents do penetrate to different depths, with characteristically distinct clinical effects. The hypothesis of circumferential cord blockade is put forward as a possible explanation for some of the clinical inconsistencies that have been observed with various local anesthetic agents used in epidural blockade. This hypothesis will be developed more fully in Chapter 4 on Mechanism of Action.

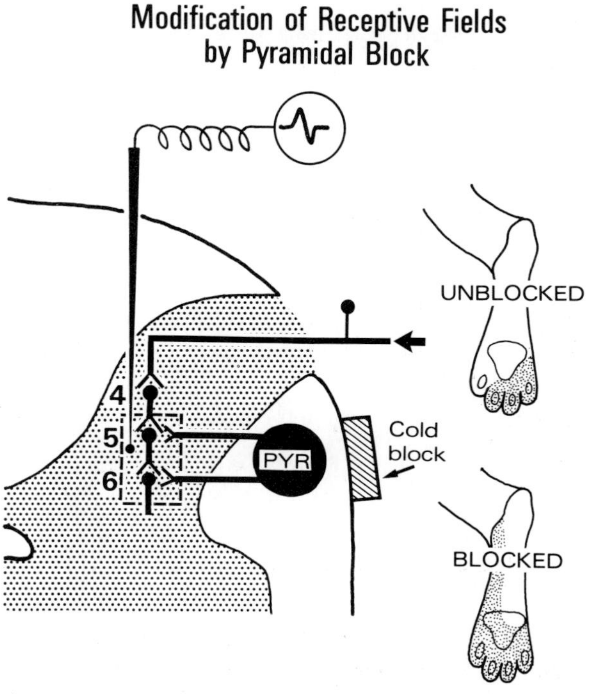

Figure 2–27. Cutaneous receptive fields from hind limb of cat, and effect of pyramidal pathways (PYR). Numbers 4, 5 and 6 designate Rexed's laminae in dorsal horn. Intracellular recordings.

Unblocked pyramidal tracts: Cells in laminae 5 and 6 respond to a relatively small area of stimulated skin.

Blocked pyramidal tracts: Cutaneous receptive field is greatly expanded when pyramidal tract is reversibly blocked by cold, and cells in laminae 5 and 6 now respond to a much wider area of skin stimulation.

(Adapted from Wall, 1967: "The laminar organization of dorsal horn and effects of descending impulses.")

ARTERIAL SUPPLY OF THE SPINAL CORD

The blood supply of the cord is richest and most plentiful where the neuronal population is greatest, that is, opposite the cervical and lumbosacral enlargements, and it is most tenuous in the thin mid-thoracic region where the cord is least populated with neurons (Woollam and Millen, 1958b). The profile of arterial density in the central parts of the cord closely reflect the profile of neural population in the spinal roots along the length of the cord, as can be seen by comparing Figure 2–17 with Figure 2–28, which shows the number of central spinal arteries per centimeter of cord (Lazorthes et al., 1962).

Developmentally, the cord has advanced through three stages: (1) from a primitive state, in which all its nutrient supply came from investing pial vessels entering at the circumference (Hibbard, 1963), (2) through a stage in which anterior and posterior segmental arteries penetrated more deeply into the substance of the cord, (3) to the present stage in which large areas have lost their segmental arrangement and the anterior and the deeper parts of the cord are supplied by a single anastomotic channel running longitudinally in the anterior median fissure (Lhermitte and Corbin, 1962). The three primary areas of distribution are evident on cross section, as shown in Figure 2–29. The peripheral parts of the cord are supplied by a pial network of small surface vessels, while the posterior columns and dorsal horns receive a segmental supply through the paired posterior spinal arteries. The anterior horns and funiculi and deeper parts of the lateral funiculi, including the corticospinal tract, are supplied entirely by arborizations arising from the anterior spinal artery.

Anterior Spinal Artery

The anterior spinal artery extending along the length of the anterior median fissure is really a composite vessel made up of anastomosing segments

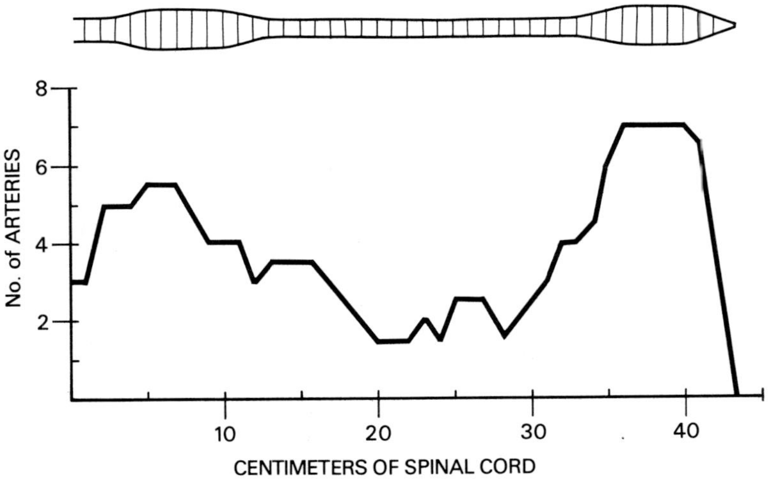

Figure 2–28. The number of central arteries to the cord per centimeter of length: longitudinal profile. (After Lazorthes et al., 1962.)

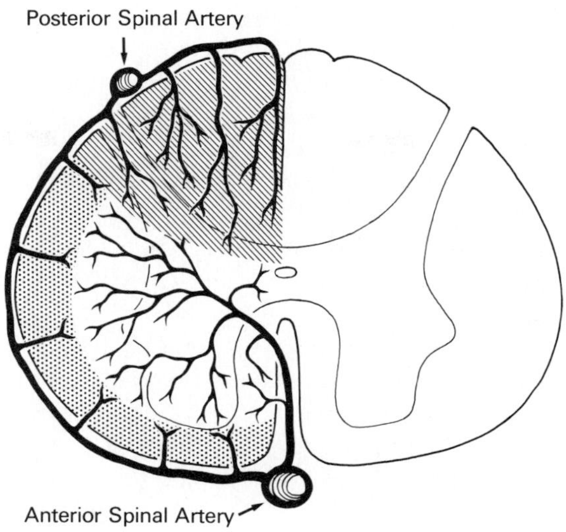

Figure 2–29. Arterial territories of the spinal cord on cross section. (After Lhermitte and Corbin, 1962.)

of ascending and descending midline branches arising from vertebral, intercostal and iliac arteries (Woollam and Millen, 1955; Gillilan, 1958). Small segmental arteries supply the cord through each of the intervertebral foramina, but at certain points along the vertebral column larger vessels enter to feed the anastomotic system of the anterior spinal artery (Fig. 2–30). Considerable individual variation exists in this arrangement, and the wide range of variability makes it impossible to predict where points of ischemia will arise when arterial flow is jeopardized by disease or surgical trauma to intercostal vessels or by profound and prolonged hypotension. For this reason, "accidents and operations which are harmless in one patient are perilous in another" (Henson and Parsons, 1967).

Spinal cord damage after epidural analgesia is extremely rare, but

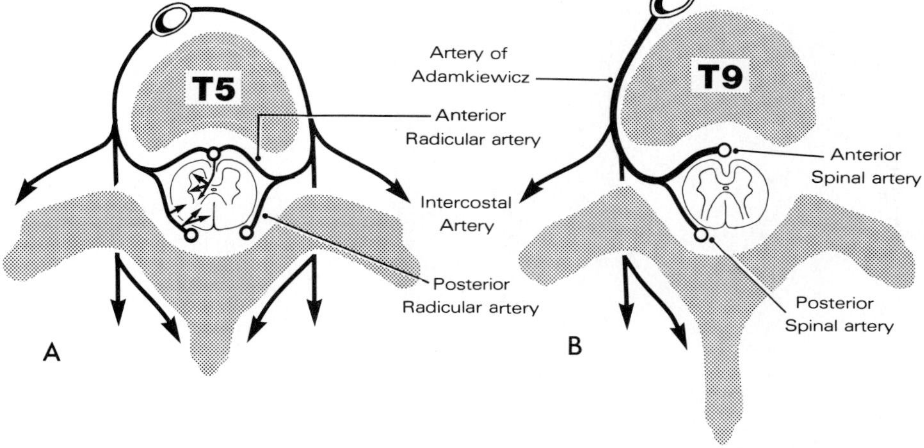

Figure 2–30. Diagram of arterial supply to the spinal cord. *A*, General segmental arrangement with anterior and posterior radicular arteries feeding the anterior and posterior spinal arteries. *B*, Major nonsegmental feeder to anterior spinal artery, i.e., artery of Adamkiewicz at T_9.

when it does occur it usually takes the form characteristic of the "anterior spinal artery syndrome"—that is, symptoms and signs arising from vascular insufficiency of the anterior horns and anterior funiculi. The clinical picture, therefore, is essentially one of motor loss due to damage of the deeper parts of the cord, with sparing of the peripheral and sensory elements. Because of the very variable nature of the anterior arterial supply to the cord, there is also a wide variation in the clinical picture that may result from thrombosis or embolism of a section of the anterior spinal artery and its tributaries. Some knowledge of the relevant vascular distribution is therefore necessary when one is faced with the problem of a neurological deficit after surgery. Although the majority of neurological mischances are due to factors unrelated to an epidural anesthetic, nevertheless post hoc ergo propter hoc arguments tend to point a finger of suspicion at the anesthetic, and such preconceived suspicions can only be dispelled by solid evidence obtained from a thorough neurological history and examination (see Chapter 14 on Complications and Contraindications).

The territory supplied by the anterior spinal artery is divided into

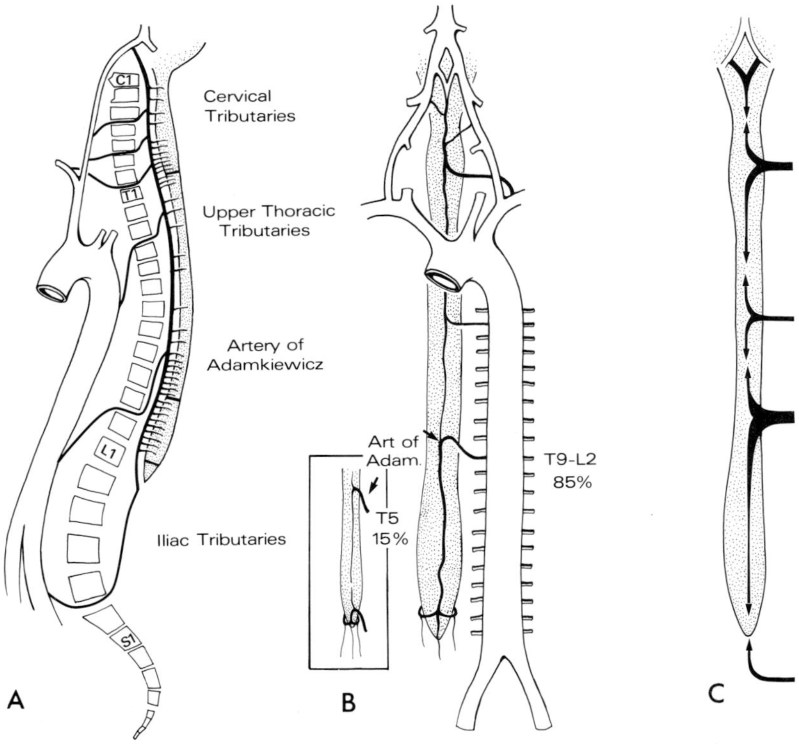

Figure 2–31. Diagram to show components of the anterior spinal artery.
A, Lateral view.
B, Anterior-posterior view, showing origins of artery of Adamkiewicz.
85% cases: origin between T_9 and L_2.
15% cases: high take-off at T_5, associated with important contribution from the iliac arteries to tip of conus medullaris.
C. Schematic representation of direction and volume of flow from nutrient vessels supplying the anterior spinal artery: size of arrows proportional to flow contribution.
(After Lazorthes et al., 1962, 1966.)

three functionally distinct levels, each fed by one or more nonsegmental nutrient arteries (Fig. 2–31) in the following pattern:

Cervicodorsal

Small anastomotic arteries derived from the intracranial portions of the vertebral arteries descend in front of the cord to meet ascending branches from the subclavian artery, carried by the vertebral, thyrocervical and costocervical arteries. These supply the cervical enlargement of the cord as far down as the level of the fourth thoracic vertebra.

Intermediate or Mid-thoracic

The small caliber of the midthoracic segments of the cord is matched by a meager arterial supply usually arising from one of the intercostal arteries between the fourth and the ninth thoracic vertebrae.

Lumbosacral

The main blood supply to the lower section of the anterior spinal artery comes from a single large vessel arising from one of the intercostal arteries between T_8 and L_3, known eponymously as the artery of Adamkiewicz, who called it the "arteria radicularis anterior magna" (Adamkiewicz, 1882); its simplest and most apt name is "the artery of the lumbosacral enlargement" (Lazorthes et al., 1957, 1962). This is one of the most important spinal arteries, and it has the largest territorial commitment within the spinal cord. The segmental origin of this major vessel is quite variable, but it is most commonly left sided (in 80 per cent of cases) and at the segmental level of T_8 to T_{10} in 50 per cent of cases.

Arteriograms of the artery of Adamkiewicz show a hairpin-shaped contour (Fig. 2–32), with a small ascending branch supplying the lower part of the thoracic cord and a larger descending branch running all the way down to the tip of the conus, where it anastomoses with loops from the posterior spinal arteries. A supplementary blood supply to the conus ascends from the internal iliac arteries, via the lateral sacral arteries, to join the descending loop of the artery to the lumbosacral enlargement. The size of this contribution varies according to the level of Adamkiewicz's artery: it is large when the take-off is high with a long slender descending branch, and it is smaller when Adamkiewicz's artery is placed unusually low (Lazorthes et al., 1966). Selective arterial angiography of the cord may be helpful in determining the level of these nutrient vessels, especially in cases of arteriovenous malformation of the cord, or of atheroma, when accurate anatomical data is crucial to planning appropriate surgical treatment (Doppman et al., 1969; Djindjian et al., 1970, 1972).

The end results of spinal cord ischemia are heavily dependent on the causes of ischemia and the individual arterial anatomy of the cord in question (Lazorthes et al., 1966). In general, the brunt of the damage falls upon the territory of the anterior spinal artery: "within the spinal cord susceptibility to hypoperfusion increases caudally, is more marked in anterior horns than in

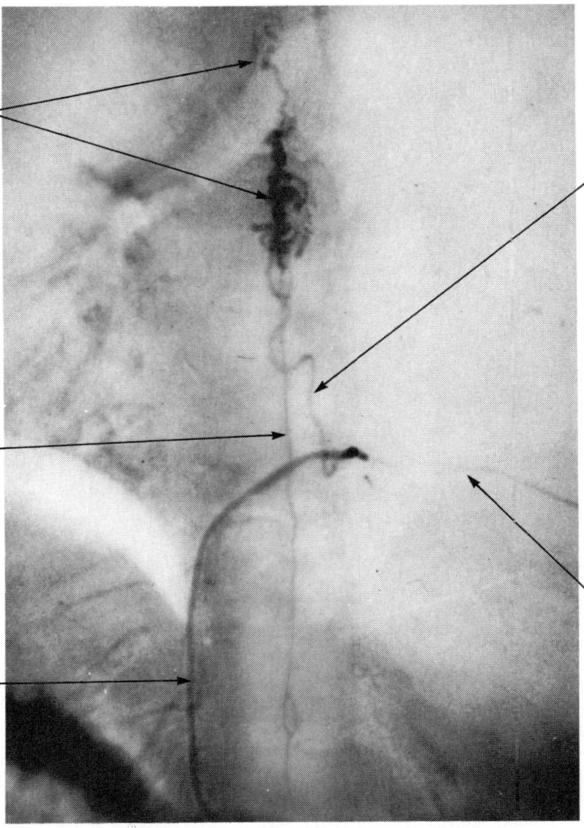

Figure 2–32. Subtraction arteriogram of thoracic spine, with transfemoral catheter placed in left ninth intercostal artery, showing arteriovenous abnormality extending from T_1 to T_9. Note ascending branch of artery of Adamkiewicz feeding the arteriovenous abnormality. Descending branch to lumbosacral enlargement (retouched) is faint and tenuous owing to arterial "steal" by arteriovenous abnormality. (Case history described in Chapter 14, page 680.) (Courtesy of Dr. Andrew A. Eisen.)

posterior horns, and is more prominent deep within the individual nuclei" (Gilles and Nag, 1971). Interneurons and anterior horn cells are particularly susceptible to ischemic anoxia (Krogh, 1945; Van Harreveld and Khattab, 1967; Silver and Buxton, 1974). The lumbosacral enlargement seems peculiarly vulnerable to acute or chronic hypotension (Turnbull, 1973). Gilles and Nag (1971) describe the spinal cords of six children under two years of age in whom transient cardiac arrest and hypotension had preceded death by some hours and in whom ischemic damage was confined to the territory of the descending branch of Adamkiewicz's artery, that is, the anterior horns and neighboring gray matter in the lumbosacral enlargement.

Thus, when one is confronted with a postoperative neurological deficit originating in the cord, careful enquiry must be made into the most likely causes, whether surgical from trauma to nutrient intercostal vessels (Usubiaga et al., 1970; Pasternak et al., 1972), or medical from factors creating low flow states within the circulation. Severe arterial hypotension is probably the commonest precipitating factor (Garland et al., 1966; Henson and Parsons, 1967; Silver and Buxton, 1974). The effects of arterial hypotension are exaggerated if there is a coincidental rise of venous pressure, for then the net perfusion pressure across capillary beds in the spinal cord is reduced still further (Bromage, 1974).

Space-occupying masses, such as hematomas in the epidural space, probably exert a complex vascular effect. Radiopaque perfusion studies with inflatable balloons in the spinal canal of dogs show variable results, depending on the positions of the mass in relation to the spinal cord (Ramsey and Doppman, 1973). Laterally placed epidural masses produce relatively little obstruction to longitudinal flow in the anterior spinal artery or to flow in the substance of the cord. However, anteriorly or posteriorly placed masses cause much greater interference with cord blood flow. Surprisingly enough, they appear to have little or no effect on longitudinal flow in the anterior spinal artery itself, but they do obstruct central perforating vessels arising from it at the level of the artificial tumor. Using a similar compression technique, Griffiths (1975) found edema and capillary leakage in the intermediate gray matter and the dorsolateral columns.

Intermittent Vascular Spasm: Cervical Spondylosis

Many theoretical explanations have been proposed to account for the myelopathy that is frequently associated with cervical spondylosis, including narrowing of the spinal canal and direct pressure effects on the cervical enlargement (Crandall and Batzdorf, 1966). The neurological lesion has a peripheral distribution in the lateral and anterior columns, suggesting ischemia of the superficial pial vessels (Bedford et al., 1952), but without obvious arteriosclerotic changes in the segmental vessels concerned (Breig et al., 1966). Gooding (1974) has proposed the interesting and rather plausible hypothesis that mechanical irritation of the segmental lateral spinal arteries may cause reflex spasm and intermittent disturbances of autoregulation and blood flow in the cervical cord. This vascular hypothesis remains unproven, but clinical evidence does tend to support the idea. We have seen marked clinical improvement resulting from repeated cervical epidural injections of hydrocortisone acetate suspensions in dilute solutions of local anesthetic. A possible explanation of the beneficial effect might lie in the alleviation of the type of reflex vascular spasm proposed by Gooding.

EPIDURAL VEINS

The internal vertebral venous plexus has a powerful influence on the dispersion, uptake and distribution of epidural drugs, as well as on blood flow through the cord and on venous return to the heart. An understanding of the functions and behavior of the extradural venous plexus is of fundamental importance in the clinical management of patients receiving epidural blockade.

During the past 35 years interest has been awakened in the extradural venous system as a vascular highway possessing important functions in health and disease and in the normal vascular readjustment of pregnancy. Although the unity of this system was shown by Willis in 1664 (see Fig. 2–7) and by other anatomists over the years (Breschet, 1829), its full significance was not widely appreciated until Oscar Batson of Philadelphia published his classic paper on "The Function of the Vertebral Veins and Their Role in the Spread of Metastases" in 1940. Because of anatomical and dynamic relationships with other compartments of the venous circulation, it is impossible to picture the behavior of the epidural veins in isolation from these connections, and in the description which follows it will be necessary to consider them as a functional part of the venous system as a whole.

Developmentally the epidural venous system is an archaic arrangement of meandering plexuses rich in segmental connections. Apart from some rudimentary cusps at the junction of the posterior intercostal and vertebral veins (Bowsher, 1954), there are no valves in this complex of venous channels which connects all segments of the body from the pelvis to the cranium by anastomotic linkages involving the caval and azygos systems, and to a lesser degree the portal and pulmonary systems as well. Through this vast network, venous pressures can be equalized in all the major body cavities, and embolic material can travel freely on its tides up and down the spine from one compartment to another, depending on the pressure differences that may exist between them from moment to moment. Venous blood is able to circulate in this system, not only in the strictly Harveian sense of continuous circular motion but also in the ancient Galenical conception of ebb and flow (Herlihy, 1947; Batson, 1957; Dommisse, 1975).

In deep diving mammals, such as the seal and the whale, the extradural venous system is very large and highly specialized. In these mammals a large midline vein runs in the dorsal part of the extradural space, with tributaries from capacious venous sinuses in the thorax and abdomen. These storage spaces appear to be concerned with accommodating the venous return during the periods of remarkable bradycardia and reduction of cardiac output that accompany diving (Franklin, 1937; Irving et al., 1942; Harrison and Tomlinson, 1956).

In man and non-diving mammals, the internal vertebral plexus lies mainly in the anterolateral parts of the epidural space, conveniently placed away from the normal path of a needle entering the epidural space in the midline (Bowsher, 1954; Worthman, 1956). The epidural venous plexus drains both the cord and the vertebral canal, as well as the cerebrospinal fluid from the subarachnoid space. Above, it communicates with the occipital, sigmoid and basilar sinuses of the brain, while below, anastomotic channels via the sacral canal form a connecting system between the vertebral plexus and the inferior vena cava. At each spinal segment a pampiniform plexus of veins invests the dural root sleeve as it travels toward the intervertebral foramen (Woollam and Millen, 1958b; Bowsher, 1960; Millen and Woollam, 1962), and it is this plexus that receives the filtered effluent from the cerebrospinal fluid via the arachnoid granulations, as described earlier in the chapter. From there, veins emerge from the intervertebral foramina to end in the vertebral, posterior intercostal, lumbar and lateral sacral veins, and these in turn empty into the azygos system. The azygos vein ascends in the right chest, arches over the root of the right lung and ends in the superior vena cava just before it enters the pericardium (Fig. 2–33).

Thus the epidural plexus forms a venous network between the pelvis and the brain that can act as an alternative pathway to the caval system. In his

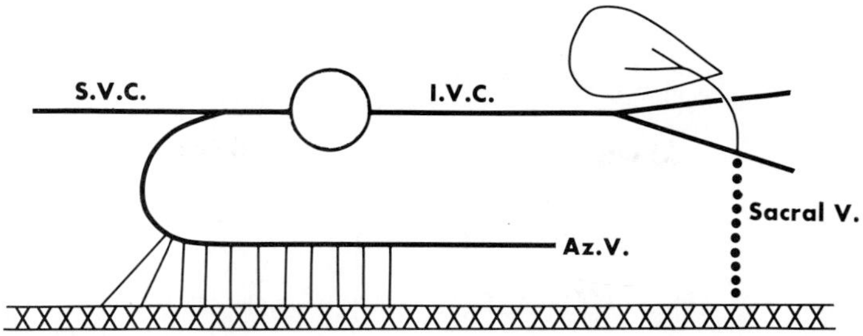

Figure 2–33. Diagram of vertebral venous drainage into the azygos system and the superior vena cava. Caval-vertebral venous connections: intercostovertebral veins and azygos system in thorax; sacral venous plexus links uterine and iliac veins to vertebral venous plexus in pelvis. S.V.C. = superior vena cava; I.V.C. = inferior vena cava; Az. V. = azygos vein.

original paper of 1940, Batson showed that radiopaque material injected into the dorsal vein of the penis can be made to travel directly up into the cranial sinuses without passing through the venae cavae. This alternative route to the caval drainage of the pelvis may explain the frequency of malignant or infective cerebral emboli and vertebral metastases from primary lesions in the pelvis.

Figure 2–34 summarizes in diagrammatic form the main communications that can exist between the various compartments of the venous system and which may be called upon in disease. Fresh thoroughfares are opened up if the pressure in one compartment is raised for a sufficiently long time, and then the localized high pressure system is led off into neighboring low pressure areas, which in turn share the burden of venous distension (Marchand et al., 1950; Pump, 1963). For example in Figure 2–34 the dotted line joining the pulmonary and portal systems represents a network of anastomotic channels that may develop in either severe pulmonary hypertension (e.g., mitral stenosis) or severe portal hypertension (Laennec's cirrhosis). In the former case arterialized blood may flow into the portal circulation, while in cirrhosis there is a venous admixture of portal blood in the left auricle, causing a fall of arterial oxygen saturation (Calabresi and Abelmann, 1957; Williams, 1960).

Acute changes of intra-abdominal or intrathoracic pressure, as in coughing or straining or a voluntary Valsalva maneuver, are also transmitted to the epidural space through the venous networks outlined in Figure 2–34. Thus, in any condition that causes acute or chronically raised venous pressure, the anesthesiologist should visualize in his mind's eye a distension and ballooning of the epidural veins. Venous distension diminishes the effective volume of the epidural space and probably increases the absorptive area of venules and capillaries coursing through it.

Obstruction of the inferior vena cava from any cause has profound effects on the hemodynamics of the epidural veins, especially in pregnancy when anastomotic channels have had time and opportunity to open up through the network of connecting sacral veins. In the face of caval obstruction, venous return from the legs and pelvis is forced to seek the alternative pathway through the vertebral-azygos system. Then, not only are the epidural veins distended, but also flow through them is markedly increased. Under these circumstances a small dose of local anesthetic injected accidentally into an epidural vein will

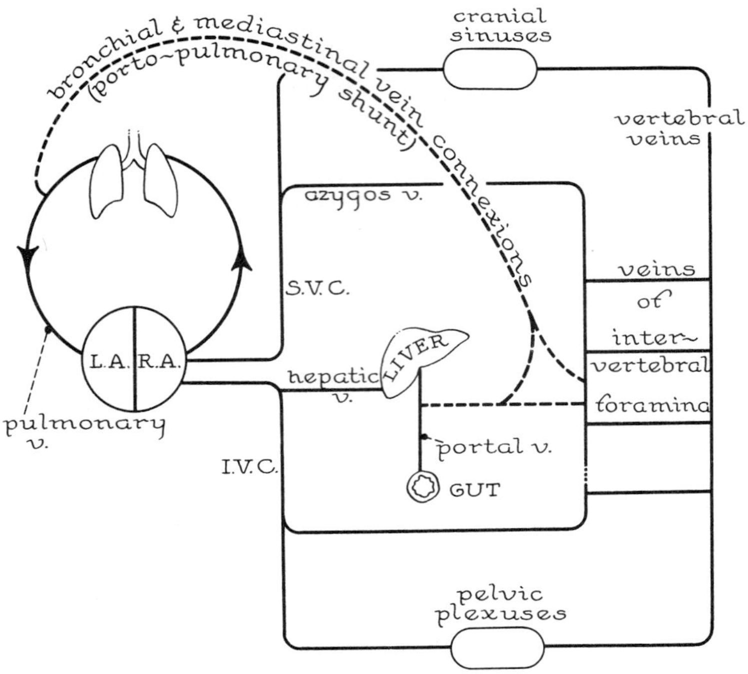

Figure 2–34. The venous compartments and their potential interconnections.

have its relative toxicity increased. Normally, at rest, flow through the epidural veins is sluggish, and accidentally injected solutions are distributed into a large volume of blood moving slowly through an extensive network of anastomotic channels. When the inferior vena cava is obstructed, however, epidural and azygos flow are sharply increased and probably channeled, and any accidentally injected agent will travel as a bolus directly to the right atrium and arrive at the heart in a concentration many times greater than under conditions of free unobstructed caval flow. This is probably the anatomical basis for the increased toxicity of local anesthetic solutions that are accidentally injected into an epidural vein during the course of active labor, when the gravid uterus presses on the inferior vena cava, particularly when the mother is lying in the supine position (see Chapter 12 on Epidural Analgesia for Obstetrics).

Epidural Phlebography

The epidural veins can be displayed radiographically by a variety of techniques. Perey et al. (1956) used a balloon catheter inserted into the inferior vena cava via the saphenous vein before injecting a large bolus of 20 to 40 ml of contrast material distal to the occluding balloon. This method was replaced by the interosseous route, in which radiopaque solution was injected into one of the lower lumbar vertebral spines while the vena cava was occluded by abdominal compression or by a forceful Valsalva maneuver (Schobinger et al., 1961).

Under these conditions 25 ml of contrast medium spreads into the epidural veins and outlines the epidural plexus for a few vertebral spaces adjoining the injection site. More recently, transfemoral catheterization of an ascending lumbar vein by the Seldinger technique has made the process simpler and less painful for the patient (Bücheler et al., 1968; Doppman et al., 1969; Gargano et al., 1974). Normally, the epidural veins appear as a continuous ladder of venous structures in the frontal plane and as a wavelike pattern in the lateral projection, as shown in Figure 2–35.

Epidural masses, such as protruded intervertebral discs, appear as filling defects in the normal ladder pattern of epidural veins. The method of visualization seems to be reliable in skilled hands, and Schobinger et al. (1961)

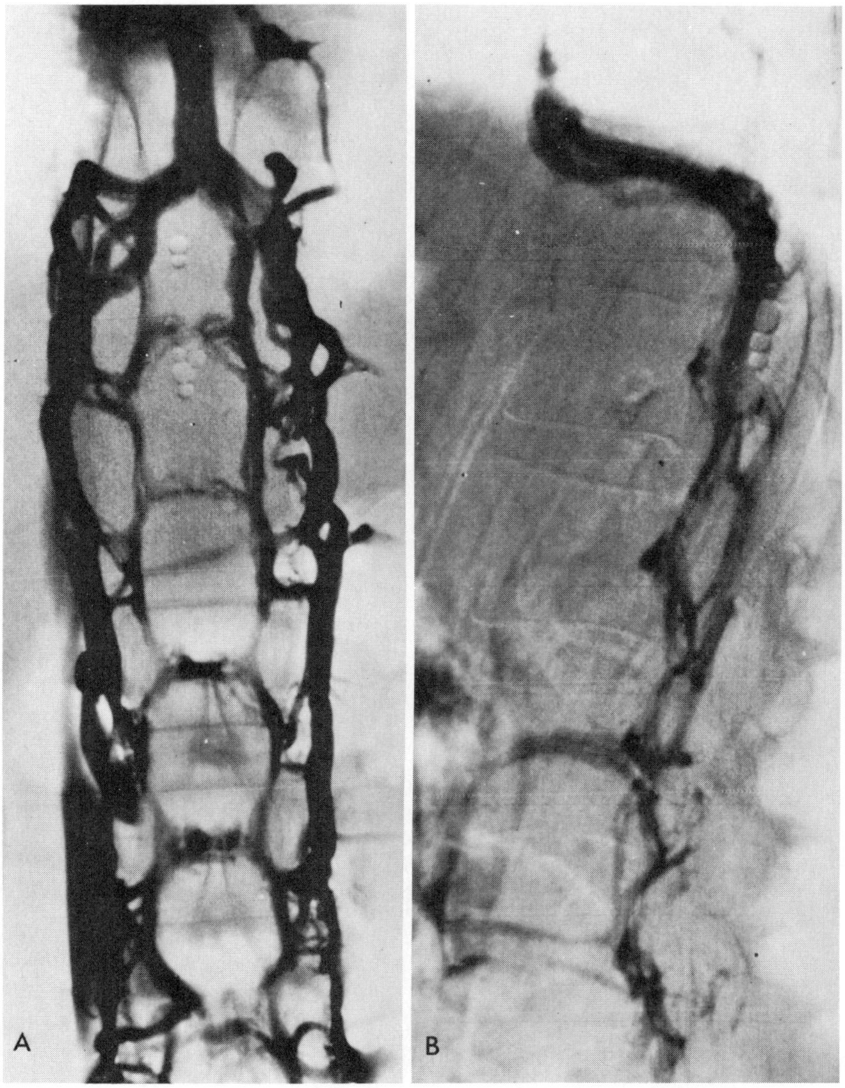

Figure 2–35. Frontal and lateral projections of normal epidural venogram. (From Doppman, J. L., DiChiro, G., and Ommaya, A. K.: Selective Arteriography of the Spinal Chord. St. Louis, Mo., Warren H. Green, Inc., 1969.)

and Gargano et al., (1974) have reported a higher incidence of correct diagnoses with Hypaque epidural venography than with Pantopaque myelography.

From the anesthesiologist's point of view, these radiographic studies confirm the anatomy and general disposition of the epidural veins very beautifully, and they emphasize two facts that have an important bearing on the technical outcome of epidural blockade:

1. Obstruction of flow in the inferior vena cava by compression or by a Valsalva maneuver forces blood into the vertebral plexus and distends the epidural veins.

2. During epidural puncture, care should be taken that the needle point pierces the ligamentum flavum as close to the midline as possible, in order to avoid the large longitudinal epidural veins that hug the lateral walls of the spinal canal.

REFERENCES

Abood, L. G., and Abul-Haj, S. K.: Histochemistry and characterization of hyaluronic acid in axons of peripheral nerve. J. Neurochem. *1*:119, 1956.

Adamkiewicz, A.: Die Blutgefässe des menschlichen Rückenmarkes. II. Die Gefässe der Rückenmarksoberfläche. S. B. Heidelberg. Akad. Wiss. *85*:101, 1882.

Adams, J. E., and Prawirohardjo, S.: Fate of red blood cells injected into cerebrospinal fluid pathways. Neurology *9*:561, 1959.

Adrian, E. D.: On the conduction of subnormal disturbances in normal nerve. J. Physiol. *45*:389, 1912.

Aguayo, A. J.: Personal communication, 1975.

Aguayo, A. J., and Bray, G. M.: Experimental pathology of unmyelinated nerve fibres. *In* Dyck, P. J., Thomas, P. K., and Lambert, E. H. (eds.): Peripheral Neuropathy. Philadelphia, W. B. Saunders Company, 1975, p. 363.

Aguayo, A. J., Nair, C. P. V., and Bray, G. M.: Peripheral nerve abnormalities in the Riley-Day syndrome. Findings in a sural nerve biopsy. Arch. Neurol. *24*:106, 1971.

Aguayo, A. J., Martin, J. B., and Bray, G. M.: Effects of nerve growth factor antiserum on peripheral unmyelinated nerve fibers. Acta Neuropath. (Berl). *20*:288, 1972.

Akil, H., Mayers, D. J., and Liebeskind, J. C.: Comparaison chez le rat entre l'analgésie induite par stimulation de la substance grise périaqueducale et l'analgesia morphinique. C. R. Acad. Sci. (Paris) *274*:3603, 1972.

Alksne, J. F., and Lovings E. T.: The role of the arachnoid villus in the removal of red blood cells from the subarachnoid space. An electron microscope study in the dog. J. Neurosurg. *36*:192, 1972.

Andres, K. H.: Über die Feinstruktur der Arachnoidea und Dura mater von Mammalia. Z. Zellforsch. *79*:272, 1967.

Appenzeller, O., and Ogin, G.: Myelinated fibres in the human paravertebral sympathetic chain; quantitative studies on white rami communicantes. J. Neurol. Neurosurg. Psychiat. *36*:777, 1973.

Attwood, H. D., and Wooley, P. A.: Arachnoid villi in the spinal cord of Dasyurid Marsupials. J. Comp. Neurol. *155*:343, 1974.

Batson, O. V.: The function of the vertebral veins and their role in the spread of metastases. Ann. Surg. *112*:138, 1940.

Batson, O. V.: The vertebral vein system. Amer. J. Roentgen. *128*:195, 1957.

Bedford, P. D., Bosanquet, F. D., and Russell, W. R.: Degeneration of the spinal cord associated with cervical spondylosis. Lancet *2*:55, 1952.

Berthold, C–H.: Ultrastructure of the node-paranode region of mature feline ventral lumbar spinal-root fibres. Acta Soc. Med. Uppsala *73*:37, 1968.

Besson, J. M., and Rivot, J. P.: Spinal interneurones involved in presynaptic controls of supraspinal origin. J. Physiol. *230*:235, 1973.

Bowsher, D.: A comparative study of the azygos venous system in man, monkey, dog, cat, rat and rabbit. J. Anat. *88*:400, 1954.

Bowsher, D.: Cerebro-Spinal Fluid Dynamics in Health and Disease. Springfield, Ill., Charles C Thomas, Publisher, 1960, p. 38.

Boys, J. E., and Norman, P. F.: Accidental subdural analgesia. Brit. J. Anaesth. *47*:1111, 1975.

Bradford, F. K., and Johnson, P. C.: Passage of intact iron-labeled erythrocytes from subarachnoid space to systemic circulation in dogs. J. Neurosurg. *19*:332, 1962.

Breig, A., Turnbull, I., and Hassler, O.: Effects of mechanical stresses on the spinal cord in cervical spondylosis: A study on fresh cadaver material. J. Neurosurg. *25*:45, 1966.

Breschet, G.: Recherches anatomiques, physiologiques et pathologiques sur le système veineux, et spécialement sur les canaux veineux des os. Thèse. Paris. 1829.

Brierley, J. B.: The penetration of particulate matter from the cerebrospinal fluid into the spinal ganglia, peripheral nerves, and perivascular spaces of the central nervous system. J. Neurol. Neurosurg. Psychiat. *13*:203, 1950.

Brierley, J. B., and Field, E. J.: The connexions of the spinal sub-arachnoid space with the lymphatic system. J. Anat. *82*:153, 1948.

Brierley, J. B., and Field, E. J.: The fate of an intraneural injection as demonstrated by the use of radio-active phosphorus. J. Neurol. Neurosurg. Psychiat. *12*:86, 1949.

Bromage, P. R.: Exaggerated spread of epidural analgesia in arteriosclerotic patients. Dosage in relation to biological and chronological ageing. Brit. Med. J. *ii*:1634, 1962.

Bromage, P. R.: Physiology and pharmacology of epidural analgesia. Anesthesiology *28*:592, 1967a.

Bromage, P. R.: Improved conduction blockade in surgery and obstetrics: Carbonated local anesthetics. Canad. Med. Assoc. J. *97*:1377, 1967b.

Bromage, P. R.: Ageing and epidural dose requirements. Segmental spread and predictability of epidural analgesia in youth and extreme age. Brit. J. Anaesth. *41*:1016, 1969a.

Bromage, P. R.: An evaluation of bupivacaine in epidural analgesia for obstetrics. Canad. Anaesth. Soc. J. *16*:46, 1969b.

Bromage, P. R.: Spinal thrombophlebitis after hypotensive anaesthesia. New Zealand Med. J. *80*:519, 1974.

Bromage, P. R.: Mechanism of action of extradural analgesia. Brit. J. Anaesth. *47*:199, 1975.

Bromage, P. R., and Melzack, R.: Phantom limbs and body schema. Canad. Anaesth. Soc. J. *21*:267, 1974.

Bromage, P. R., Joval, A. C., and Binney, J. C.: Local anesthetic drugs: Penetration from the spinal extradural space into the neuraxis. Science *140*:392, 1963.

Bromage, P. R., Burfoot, M. F., Crowell, D. E., and Truant, A. P.: Quality of epidural blockade. III. Carbonated local anaesthetic solutions. Brit. J. Anaesth. *39*:197, 1967.

Bromage, P. R., Datta, S., and Dunford, L. A.: Etidocaine: An evaluation in epidural analgesia for obstetrics. Canad. Anaesth. Soc. J. *21*:535, 1974.

Brown, D. A., Stumpf, W. E., and Roth, L. J.: Location of radioactively labelled extracellular fluid indicators in nervous tissue by autoradiography. J. Cell. Sci. *4*:265, 1969.

Bücheler, von E., Düx, A., and Venbrocks, H. P.: Die direkte vertebrale Venographie bei lumbalen Bandscheibenhernien. Fortschr. Geb. Röntgen. *109*:593, 1968.

Calabresi, P., and Abelmann, W. H.: Porto-caval and porto-pulmonary anastomoses in Laennec's cirrhosis and in heart failure. J. Clin. Invest. *36*:1257, 1957.

Carlsen, F., Knappeis, G. G., and Behse, F.: Schwann cell length in unmyelinated fibres of human sural nerve. J. Anat. *117*:463, 1974.

Causey, G., and Palmer, E.: The epidural sheath of a nerve as a barrier to the diffusion of phosphate ions. J. Anat. (Lond). *87*:30, 1953.

Chen, C. J.: The perineural space of the peripheral nerve. M. S. Thesis, McGill University, Montreal, 1945.

Clark, W. E. Le Gros: On the Pacchionian bodies. J. Anat. (Lond). *55*:40, 1920.

Clifton, G. L., Vance, W. H., Applebaum, M. L., Coggeshall, R. E., and Willis, W. D.: Responses of unmyelinated afferents in the mammalian ventral root. Brain Res. *82*:163, 1974.

Cloyd, M. W., and Low, F. N.: Scanning electron microscopy of the subarachnoid space in the dog. J. Comp. Neurol. *153*:325, 1974.

Coggeshall, R. E., Coulter, J. E., and Willis, W. D.: Unmyelinated fibers in the ventral root. Brain Res. *57*:229, 1973.

Coggeshall, R. E., Coulter, J. D., and Willis, W. D.: Unmyelinated axons in the ventral roots of the cat lumbosacral enlargement. J. Comp. Neurol. *153*:39, 1974.

Coggeshall, R. E., Applebaum, M. L., Fazen, M., Stubbs, T. B., and Sykes, M. T.: Unmyelinated axons in human ventral roots, a possible explanation for the failure of dorsal rhizotomy to relieve pain. Brain *98*:157, 1975.

Cohen, C. A., and Kallos, T.: Failure of spinal anesthesia due to subdural catheter placement. Anesthesiology *37*:352, 1972.

Collins, W. F., Nulsen, F. E., and Randt, C. T.: Pain and nerve fibre size. Arch. Neurol. *3*:381, 1960.

Coote, J. H., and Macleod, V. H.: The influence of bulbospinal monoaminergic pathways on sympathetic nerve activity. J. Physiol. *241*:453, 1974.

Coppin, C. M. L., and Jack, J. J. B.: Internodal length and conduction velocity of cat muscle afferent nerve fibres. J. Physiol. *222*:91P, 1972.

Corbin, K. B., and Gardner, E. D.: Decrease in number of myelinated fibers in human spinal roots with age. Anat. Rec. *68*:63, 1937.
Cotunnius, D.: A treatise on the nervous sciatica, or, nervous hip gout. J. Wilkie, St. Paul's Churchyard, 1775, p. 53.
Crandall, P. H., and Batzdorf, U.: Cervical spondylosis and vascular changes. J. Neurosurg. *25*:57, 1966.
Crescitelli, F.: Nerve sheath as a barrier to the action of certain substances. Amer. J. Physiol. *166*:229, 1951.
Davson, H., Domer, F. R., and Hollingsworth, J. R.: The mechanism of drainage of the cerebrospinal fluid. Brain *96*:329, 1973.
Dawkins, C. J. M.: Discussion on extradural spinal block. Proc. Roy. Soc. Med. *38*:299, 1945.
Dawkins, C. J. M.: An analysis of the complications of extradural and caudal block. Anaesthesia *24*:554, 1969.
de Jong, R. H.: Physiology and Pharmacology of Local Anesthesia. Springfield, Ill., Charles C Thomas, Publisher, 1970, p. 103.
de Jong, R. H., and Cullen, S. C.: Theoretical aspects of pain: Bizarre pain phenomena during low spinal anesthesia. Anesthesiology *24*:628, 1963.
Dilly, P. N., Wall, P. D., and Webster, K. E.: Cells of origin of the spinothalamic tract in the cat and rat. Expl. Neurol. *21*:550, 1968.
Djindjian, R., et al.: Angiography of the Spinal Cord. Baltimore, University Park Press, 1970, pp. 14, 16, 24.
Djindjian, R., Rey, A., Guilmet, D., Godlewski, S., and Houdart, R.: Etude des deux premiers cas opérés d'ischémie médullaire par sténose athéromateuse de l'artère d'Adamkiewicz. Rev. Neurol. (Paris) *127*:471, 1972.
Dogliotti, A. M.: Segmental peridural spinal anesthesia. Amer. J. Surg. *20*:107, 1933.
Dommisse, G. F.: The Arteries and Veins of the Human Spinal Cord From Birth. Edinburgh, Churchill Livingstone, 1975, p. 94.
Doppman, J. L., DiChiro, G., and Ommaya, A. K.: Selective Arteriography of the Spinal Cord. St. Louis, Miss., Warren H. Green, Inc., 1969, p. 3.
Douglas W. W., and Malcolm, J. L.: The effect of localized cooling on conduction in cat nerves. J. Physiol. *130*:53, 1955.
Downie, A. W., and Newell, D. J.: Sensory nerve conduction in patients with diabetes mellitus and controls. Neurology *11*:876, 1961.
Elfvin, L. G.: The ultrastructure of the nodes of Ranvier in cat sympathetic nerve fibers. J. Ultrastruct. Res. *5*:374, 1961.
Elman, R.: Spinal arachnoid granulations with especial reference to the cerebrospinal fluid. Johns Hopkins Hosp. Bull. *34*:99, 1923.
Evans, J. A., Dobben, G. D., and Gay, G. R.: Peridural effusion of drugs following sympathetic blockade. J.A.M.A. *200*:573, 1967.
Fagerberg, S-E.: Studies on the pathogenesis of diabetic neuropathy. III. Diabetic neuropathy in relation to diabetic vessel complications. Acta Med. Scand. *159*:59, 1957.
Fagerberg, S-E.: Diabetic neuropathy. Acta Med. Scand. Suppl. *345*:1, 1959.
Farr, R. E.: Sacral anesthesia: Some practical and experimental points. Arch. Surg. *12*:715, 1926.
Feng, T. P., and Liu, Y. M.: The connective tissue sheath of the nerve as effective diffusion barrier. J. Cell. Comp. Physiol. *34*:1, 1949.
Field, E. J.: Observations on the passage of Weed's prussion blue mixture along the axis cylinders and inter-fibre fluid of nerves. J. Neurol. Neurosurg. Psychiat. *14*:11, 1951.
Field, E. J., and Brierley, J. B.: The lymphatic connexions of the subarachnoid space. Brit. Med. J. *1*:1167, 1948a.
Field, E. J., and Brierley, J. B.: The lymphatic drainage of the spinal nerve roots in the rabbit. J. Anat. *82*:198, 1948b.
Foldes, F. F., Colavincenzo, J. W., and Birch, J. H.: Epidural anesthesia: A reappraisal. Curr. Res. Anesth. Analg. *35*:33, 1956.
Foreman, R. D., and Wurster, R. D.: Localization and functional characteristics of descending sympathetic spinal pathways. Amer. J. Physiol. *225*:212, 1973.
Foreman, R. D., and Wurster, R. D.: Conduction in descending spinal pathways initiated by somatosympathetic reflexes. Amer. J. Physiol. *228*:905, 1975.
Forestier, J.: Le Trou de Conjugaison Vertebral et l'Espace Epidural. Paris, Jouve et Cie, 1922, p. 105.
Fowler, T. J., and Ochoa, J.: Unmyelinated fibres in normal and compressed peripheral nerves of the baboon: A quantitative electron microscopic study. Neuropath. Appl. Neurobiol. *1*:247, 1975.
Franklin, K. J.: A Monograph on Veins. Springfield, Ill., Charles C Thomas, Publisher, 1937.
Franz, D. N., and Perry, R. S.: Mechanisms for differential block among single myelinated and non-myelinated axons by procaine. J. Physiol. *236*:193, 1974.

French, J. D., Strain, W. H., and Jones, G. E.: Mode of extension of contrast substances injected into peripheral nerves. J. Neuropath. Exp. Neurol. 7:47, 1948.
Galindo, A., Hernandez, J., Benavides, O., Ortegon deMuñoz, S., and Bonica, J. J.: Quality of spinal extradural anaesthesia: The influence of spinal nerve root diameter. Brit. J. Anaesth. *47*:41, 1975.
Gargano, F. P., Meyer, J. D., and Sheldon, J. J.: Transfemoral ascending lumbar catheterization of the epidural veins in lumbar disk disease. Radiology *111*:329, 1974.
Garland, H., Greenberg, J., and Harriman, D. G. F.: Infarction of the spinal cord. Brain *89*:645, 1966.
Gasser, H. S.: Properties of dorsal root unmedulated fibers on the two sides of the ganglion. J. Gen. Physiol. *38*:709, 1955.
Gasser, H. S., and Erlanger, J.: The role of fiber size in the establishment of a nerve block by pressure or cocaine. Amer. J. Physiol. *88*:581, 1929.
Gilles, F. H., and Nag, D.: Vulnerability of human spinal cord in transient cardiac arrest. Neurology *21*:833, 1971.
Gillilan, L. A.: The arterial blood supply of the human spinal cord. J. Comp. Neurol. *110*:75, 1958.
Gooding, M. R.: Pathogenesis of myelopathy in cervical spondylosis. Lancet *2*:1180, 1974.
Griffiths, I. R.: Vasogenic edema following acute and chronic spinal cord compression in the dog. J. Neurosurg. *42*:155, 1975.
Gutierrez; A.: Anestesia Extradural. Rev. Cirug. Buenos Aires, 1939, p. 34.
Hagbarth, K-E., and Kerr, D. I. B.: Central influences on spinal afferent conduction. J. Neurophysiol. *17*:295, 1954.
Haller, F. R., and Low, F. N.: The fine structure of the peripheral nerve root sheath in the subarachnoid space in the rat and other laboratory animals. Amer. J. Anat. *131*:1, 1971.
Haller, F. R., Haller, A. C., and Low, F. N.: The fine structure of cellular layers and connective tissue space at spinal nerve root attachment in the rat. Amer. J. Anat. *133*:109, 1972.
Ham, A. W., and Leeson, T. S.: Histology. Philadelphia, J. B. Lippincott Company, 1961, pp. 136, 146.
Hansen, K., and Schliack, H.: Segmentale Innervation. Stuttgart, Thieme Verlag, 1962, p. 97.
Harrison, R. J., and Tomlinson, J. D. W.: Observations on the venous system in certain pinnipedia and cetacea. Proc. Zool. Soc. Lond. *126*:205, 1956.
Hassin, G. B.: Villi (pacchionian bodies) of the spinal arachnoid. Arch. Neurol. Psychiat. *23*:65, 1930.
Heavner, J. E., and De Jong, R. H.: Lidocaine blocking concentrations for B− and C− nerve fibers. Anesthesiology *40*:228, 1974.
Heinbecker, P., Bishop, G. H., and O'Leary, J.: Analysis of sensation in terms of nerve impulse. Arch. Neurol. Psychiat. *31*:34, 1934.
Henson, R. A., and Parsons, M.: Ischaemic lesions of the spinal cord: An illustrated review. Quart. J. Med. *36*:205, 1967.
Herlihy, W. F.: Revision of the venous system: The role of the vertebral veins. Med. J. Aust. *1*:661, 1947.
Hibbard, E.: The vascular supply to the central nervous system of the larval lamprey. Amer. J. Anat. *113*:93, 1963.
Hillman, P., and Wall, P. D.: Inhibitory and excitatory factors influencing the receptive fields of Lamina 5 spinal cord cells. Exp. Brain Res. *9*:284, 1969.
Himango, W. A., and Low, F. N.: The fine structure of a lateral recess of the subarachnoid space in the rat. Anat. Rec. *171*:1, 1971.
Hodge, C. F.: Changes in ganglion cells from birth to senile death. Observations on man and honey-bee. J. Physiol. (Lond.) *17*:129, 1894.
Howarth, F.: Observations on the passage of a colloid form from cerebrospinal fluid to blood and tissues. Brit. J. Pharmacol. *7*:573, 1952.
Huruyama, M.: The relation between the time to failure of the nervous conduction and the number of nodes of Ranvier affected by the narcotic. Keio Igaku *21*:201, 1941.
Illert, M., and Gabriel, M.: Descending pathways in the cervical cord of cats affecting blood pressure and sympathetic activity. Pflügers Arch. *333*:109, 1972.
Ingbert, C.: An enumeration of the medullated nerve fibers in the dorsal roots of the spinal nerves of man. J. Comp. Neurol. *13*:53, 1903.
Irving, L., Scholander, P. F., and Grinnell, S. W.: The regulation of arterial blood pressure in the seal during diving. Amer. J. Physiol. *135*:557, 1942.
Jacob, M., and Weddell, G.: Neural intersegmental connection in the spinal root and ganglion region of the rat. J. Comp. Neurol. *161*:115, 1975.
Jacob, S., and Jacob, M.: Intersegmental anastomoses between adjacent dorsal roots of spinal cord in the human. Neurology (India) *19*:51, 1971.
Jones, M. D., and Newton, T. H.: Inadvertent extra-arachnoid injections in myelography. Radiology *80*:818, 1963.

Kato, G.: On the excitation, conduction and narcotisation of single nerve fibres. Cold Spring Harbor Symp. Quant. Biol. *4*:202, 1936.
Kato, M., and Tanji, J.: Physiological properties of sensory fibers in the spinal ventral roots in the cat. Japan. J. Physiol. *21*:71, 1971.
Kerr, F. W. L.: The ventral spinothalamic tract and other ascending systems of the ventral funiculus of the spinal cord. J. Comp. Neurol. *159*:335, 1975.
Kerr, F. W. L., and Alexander, S.: Descending autonomic pathways of the spinal cord. Arch. Neurol. *10*:249, 1964.
Key, E. A. H., and Retzius, G.: Studien in der Anatomie des Nervensystems und des Bindgewebes. Stockholm, Samson & Wallin, 1876.
Kirk, J. R., and Laursen, T. J. S.: Diffusion coefficients of various solutes for human aortic tissue. With special reference to variation in tissue permeability with age. J. Gerontol. *10*:288, 1955.
Kölliker, A.: Microscopische Anatomie. Leipzig, 1850, p. 433.
Krishnan, N., and Singer, M.: Penetration of peridoxase into peripheral nerve fibers. Amer. J. Anat. *136*:1, 1973.
Krnjevic, K.: The connective tissue of the frog sciatic nerve. Quart. J. Exp. Physiol. *39*:55, 1954a.
Krnjevic, K.: Some observations of perfused frog sciatic nerves. J. Physiol *123*:338, 1954b.
Krogh, E.: Studies on the blood supply to certain regions in the lumbar part of the spinal cord. Acta Physiol. Scand. *10*:271, 1945.
Kumar, A., Battit, G. E., Froese, A. B., and Long, M. C.: Bilateral cervical and thoracic epidural blockade complicating interscalene brachial plexus block: Report of two cases. Anesthesiology *35*:650, 1971.
Kumazawa, T., Perl, E. R., Burgess, P. R., and Whitehorn, D.: Ascending projections from marginal zone (lamina 1) neurons of the spinal dorsal horn. J. Comp. Neurol. *162*:1, 1975.
Kuypers, H. G. J. M.: The descending pathways to the spinal cord, their anatomy and function. Prog. Brain Res. *11*:178, 1964.
La Fratta, C. W., and Canestrari, R. E.: A comparison of sensory and motor nerve conduction velocities as related to age. Arch. Phys. Med. *47*:286, 1966.
Landon, D. N., and Langley, O. K.: The local chemical environment of nodes of Ranvier. A study of cation binding. J. Anat. *108*:419, 1971.
Landon, D. N., and Williams, P. L.: Ultrastructure of the node Ranvier. Nature *199*:575, 1963.
Lascelles, R. G., and Thomas, P. K.: Changes due to age in internodal length in the sural nerve in man. J. Neurol. Neurosurg. Psychiat. *29*:40, 1966.
Lazorthes, G., Poulhes, J., Bastide, G., Roulleau, J., and Chancolle, A. R.: Recherches sur la vascularisation artérielle de la moelle. Applications à la pathologie médullaire. Bull. Acad. Nat. Méd. *41*:2123, 1957.
Lazorthes, G., Poulhes, J., Bastide, G., Chancolle, A. R., and Zadeh, O.: Le vascularisation de la moelle épinière (etude anatomique et physiologique). Rev. Neurol. *106*:535, 1962.
Lazorthes, G., Gouazé, A., Bastide, G., Soutoul, J.-H., Zadeh, O., and Santini, J.-J.: La vascularisation artérielle du renflement lombaire. Etude des variations et des suppléances. Rev. Neurol. (Paris), *114*:109, 1966.
Leatherdale, R. A. L.: Phantom limb pain associated with spinal anaesthesia. Anaesthesia *11*:249, 1956.
Lhermitte, F., and Corbin, J. L.: Discussions des rapports (de Lazorthes, G.). Rev. Neurol. *106*:648, 1962.
Liebeskind, J. C., Guilbaud, G., Besson, J.-M., and Oliveras, J.-L.: Analgesia from electrical stimulation of the periaqueductal gray matter in the cat: Behavioural observations and inhibitory effects on spinal cord interneurones. Brain Res. *50*:441, 1973.
Lindblom, U. F., and Ottoson, J. D.: Influence of pyramidal stimulation upon the relay of coarse cutaneous afferents in the dorsal horn. Acta Physiol. Scand. *38*:309, 1957.
Lorente De Nó, R.: The ineffectiveness of the connective tissue sheath of nerve as a diffusion barrier. J. Cell Comp. Physiol. *35*:195, 1950.
Macintosh, R. R., and Mushin, W. W.: Observations on the epidural space. Anaesthesia *2*:100, 1947.
Malloy, J. J., and Low, F. N.: Scanning electron microscopy of the subarachnoid space in the dog. II. Spinal nerve exits. J. Comp. Neurol. *157*:87, 1974.
Manfredi, M., and Castellucci, V.: C-fiber responses in the ventrolateral column of the cat spinal cord. Science *165*:1020, 1969.
Marchand, P., Gilroy, J. C., and Wilson, V. H.: An anatomical study of the bronchial vascular system and its variations in disease. Thorax *5*:207, 1950.
Matthews, P. B. C., and Rushworth, G.: The relative sensitivity of muscle nerve fibres to procaine. J. Physiol. *135*:263, 1957.
McCabe, J. S., and Low, F. N.: The subarachnoid angle: An area of transition in peripheral nerve, Anat. Rec. *164*:15, 1969.

McLone, D. G., and Bondareff, W.: Developmental morphology of the subarachnoid space and contiguous structures in the mouse. Amer. J. Anat. *142*:273, 1975.

Melzack, R.: The Puzzle of Pain. Harmondsworth, Middlesex, England, Penguin Education, 1973.

Melzack, R., and Wall, P. D.: Pain mechanisms: A new theory. Science *150*:971, 1965.

Meyer, K., and Rapport, M. M.: The mucopolysaccharides of the ground substance of connective tissue. Science *113*:596, 1951.

Millen, J. W., and Woollam, D. H. M.: The Anatomy of the Cerebrospinal Fluid. London, Oxford University Press, 1962, pp. 23, 104, and 115.

Moore, D. C., Hain, R. F., Ward, A., and Bridenbaugh, L. D.: Importance of the perineural spaces in nerve blocking. J.A.M.A. *156*:1050, 1954.

Morikawa, K. I., Bonica, J. J., Tucker, G. T., and Murphy, T. M.: Effect of acute hypovolaemia on lignocaine absorption and cardiovascular response following epidural block in dogs. Brit. J. Anaesth. *46*:631, 1974.

Morse, D. E., and Low, F. N.: The fine structure of the pia mater of the rat. Amer. J. Anat. *133*:349, 1972.

Mortensen, O. A., and Sullivan, W. E.: The cerebrospinal fluid and the cervical lymph nodes. Anat. Rec. *56*:359, 1933.

Mulder, J. D.: An experimental and critical study on the spreading of foreign substances in the nerve. Acta Neerl. Morph. *1*:289, 1938.

Nathan, P. W., and Sears, T. A.: Some factors concerned with differential nerve block by local anaesthetics. J. Physiol. *157*:565, 1961.

Nobin, A., Baumgarten, H. G., Björklund, A., Lachenmayer, L., and Stenevi, U.: Axonal degeneration and regeneration of the bulbospinal indolamine neurons after 5,6-dihydroxytryptamine treatment. Brain Res. *56*:1, 1973.

Nolte, H., Meyer, J., Kopf, B., and Zenz, M.: Klinische und elektrophysiologische Parameter zur Differenzierung der Wirkung von Lokalanaesthetica. Der Anaesthesist *23*:165, 1974.

Novikoff, A. B.: Enzyme localization and ultrastructure of neurone. *In* Hyden, H. (ed.): The Neuron. New York, Elsevier, 1967, p. 272.

Nyberg-Hansen, R.: Functional organization of descending supraspinal fibre systems to the spinal cord. Anatomical observations and physiological correlations. Ergbn. Anat. EntwGesch. *39*:1, 1966.

Nyberg-Hansen, R.: Sites and modes of termination of reticulo-spinal fibers in the cat. An experimental sutdy with silver impregnation methods. J. Comp. Neurol. *124*:71, 1965.

Ochoa, J., and Mair, W. G. P.: The normal sural nerve in man. I. Ultrastructure and numbers of fibres and cells. Acta Neuropath. *13*:197, 1969a.

Ochoa, J., and Mair, W. G. P.: The normal sural nerve in man. II. Changes in the axons and Schwann cells due to ageing. Acta Neuropath. *13*:217, 1969b.

Odom, C. B.: Epidural anesthesia in resumé and prospect. Curr. Res. Anesth. Analg. *19*:106, 1940.

Oliveras, J. L., Beeson, J.-M., Guilbaud, G., and Liebeskind, J. C.: Behavioral and electrophysiological evidence of pain inhibition from midbrain stimulation in the cat. Exp. Brain Res. *20*:32, 1974.

Pacchioni, A.: Dissertatio Epistolaris de Glandulis Conglobatis Durae Meningis Humanae. Frankfurt, C. Riefel, 1712, p. 139.

Pagés, F.: Anestesia Metamerica. Rev. Sanid. Milit. (Madrid) *11*:351, 385, 1921.

Paintal, A. S.: A comparison of the nerve impulses of mammalian nonmedullated nerve fibres with those of the smallest diameter medullated fibres. J. Physiol. *193*:523, 1967.

Pallie, W.: The intersegmental anastomoses of posterior spinal rootlets and their significance. J. Neurosurg. *16*:188, 1959.

Pasternak, B. M., Boyd, D. P., and Ellis, F. H.: Spinal cord injury after procedures on the aorta. Surg. Gynecol. Obstet. *135*:29, 1972.

Pearson, A. A.: Role of gelatinous substance of spinal cord in conduction of pain. Arch. Neurol. Psychiat. *68*:515, 1952.

Perey, O., Lind, J., and Wegelius, C.: Phlebography of the intervertebral plexus. Acta Ortho. Scand. *25*:228, 1956.

Peyronnard, J.-M., Aguayo, A. J., and Bray, G. M.: Schwann cell internuclear distances in normal and regenerating unmyelinated nerve fibers. Arch. Neurol. *29*:56, 1973.

Pomeranz, B.: Specific nonciceptive fibers projecting from spinal cord neurons to the brain: A possible pathway for pain. Brain Res. *50*:447, 1973.

Pump, K. K.: The bronchial arteries and their anastomoses in the human lung. Dis. Chest *43*:245, 1963.

Quincke, H.: Zur Physiologie der Cerebrospinalflüssigkeit. Arch. f. Anat. Physiol. u. Wissen Med. 153, 1872.

Ramsey, H. J.: Fat in the epidural space in young and adult cats. Amer. J. Anat. *104*:345, 1959.

Ramsey, R., and Doppman, J. L.: The effects of epidural masses on spinal cord blood flow. An experimental study in monkeys. Radiology *107*:99, 1973.

Remak, R.: Observationes anatomicae et microscopicae de systematis nervosi structura. Thesis, Berlin, 1938.
Rexed, B.: Contributions to the knowledge of the postnatal development of the peripheral nervous system in man. Acta Psychiat. Neurol. Suppl. 33, 1944.
Rexed, B.: The cytoarchitectonic organization of the spinal cord of the cat. J. Cell. Comp. Neurol. *96*:415, 1952.
Rexed, B. A., and Wennström, K. G.: Arachnoidal proliferation and cystic formation in the spinal nerve-root pouches of man. J. Neurol. *16*:73, 1959.
Reynolds, D. V.: Surgery in the rat during electrical analgesia induced by focal brain stimulation. Science *164*:444, 1969.
Ross, M. H., and Reith, E. J.: Perineurium: Evidence for contractile elements. Science *165*:604, 1969.
Rud, J.: Local anesthetics: An electrophysiological investigation of local anesthesia of peripheral nerves, with special reference to Xylocaine. Acta Physiol. Scand. *51*(Suppl.):178, 1961.
Schlimpert, H.: Hohe und tiefe extradural Anästhesien. Z. Gynäk. *35*:477, 1911.
Schobinger, R. A., Krueger, E. G., and Sobel, G. L.: Comparison of intraosseous vertebral venography and Pantopaque myelography in the diagnosis of surgical conditions of the lumbar spine and nerve roots. Radiology *77*:376, 1961.
Schultz, E. H., and Brogdon, B. G.: The problem of subdural placement in myelography. Radiology *79*:91, 1962.
Sechzer, P. H.: Subdural space in spinal anesthesia. Anesthesiology *24*:869, 1963.
Semenowa-Tjan-Schanskaja, W.: Die Morphologischen Veränderungen der peripheren Nerven beim Menschen im Geisenalter. Z. Neurol. Psychiat. *172*:587, 1941.
Shabo, A. L., and Maxwell, D. S.: Electron microscopic observations on the fate of particulate matter in the cerebrospinal fluid. J. Neurosurg. *29*:464, 1968.
Shantha, T. R., and Bourne, G. H.: The perineural epithelium—A new concept. *In* Bourne, G. H. (ed.): The Structure and Function of Nervous Tissue. New York, Academic Press, 1968, p. 379.
Shantha, T. R., and Evans, J. A.: The relationship of epidural anesthesia to neural membranes and arachnoid villi. Anesthesiology *37*:543, 1972.
Shanthaveerappa, T. R., and Bourne, G. H.: The "perineural epithelium," a metabolically active, continuous, protoplasmic cell barrier surrounding peripheral nerve fasciculi. J. Anat. Lond. *96*:527, 1962.
Shanthaveerappa, T. R. and Bourne, G. H.: The perineural epithelium: Nature and significance. Nature *199*:577, 1963.
Shanthaveerappa, T. R., and Bourne, G. H.: Perineural epithelium: A new concept of its role in the integrity of the peripheral nervous system. Science *154*:1464, 1966.
Sherrington, C. S.: On the anatomical constitution of nerves of skeletal muscles; with remarks on recurrent fibres in the ventral spinal nerve-root. J. Physiol. *17*:211, 1894.
Shock, N. W.: The physiology of aging. Sci. Amer. *206*:100, 1962.
Sicard, A.: Les injections médicamenteuses extra-durales par voie sacrococcygienne. C. R. Soc. Biol. Paris *53*:396, 1901.
Sicard, J. A., and Cestan, R.: Etude de la traversée méningo-radiculaire au niveau du trou de conjugaison, Le nerf de conjugaison (nerf radiculaire spinal). Quelques déductions cliniques. Bull, Mem. Soc. Méd. Hop. Paris *21*:715, 1904.
Sicard, A., and Forestier, J.: Radiographic method for exploration of the epidural space using Lipiodol. Rev. Neurol. *28*:1264, 1921.
Sicard, J. A., and Forestier, J.: Roentgenologic exploration of the central nervous system with iodised oil (Lipiodol). Arch. Neurol. Psychiat. *16*:421, 1926.
Silver, J. R., and Buxton, P. H.: Spinal stroke. Brain *97*:539, 1974.
Simmonds, W. J.: The absorption of labelled erythrocytes from the subarachnoid space in rabbits. Aust. J. Exp. Biol. *31*:77, 1953.
Sindou, M., Quoex, C., and Baleydier, C.: Fiber organization of the posterior spinal cord-rootlet junction in man. J. Comp. Neurol. *155*:15, 1974.
Singer, M., et al.: Penetration of ruthenium red into peripheral nerve fibers. Anat. Rec. *173*:375, 1972.
Somberg, H. M.: The relation of the spinal subarachnoid and perineurial spaces. J. Neuropath. Exp. Neurol. *6*:166, 1947.
Steer, J. C., and Horney, F. D.: Evidence for passage of cerebrospinal fluid along spinal nerves. Canad. Med. Assoc. J. *98*:71, 1968.
Stilling, B.: Neue Untersuchungen über den Bau des Rückenmarks. Germany. Cassel, H. Hotop, 1859, p. 346.
Sullivan, W. E., and Mortensen, O. A.: Visualization of the movement of a brominized oil along peripheral nerves. Anat. Rec. *59*:493, 1934.
Sunderland, S.: The connective tissues of peripheral nerves. Brain *88*:841, 1965.
Sykes, M. T., and Coggeshall, R. E.: Unmyelinated fibers in the human L_4 and L_5 ventral roots. Brain Res. *63*:490, 1973.

Tasaki, I.: Nervous Transmission. Springfield, Ill. Charles C Thomas, Publisher, 1953.
Taub, A.: Local, segmental and supraspinal interaction with a dorsolateral spinal cutaneous afferent system. Exp. Neurol. *10*:357, 1964.
Taveras, J. M., and Wood, E. H.: Myelography: Technical errors. *In* Robbins, L. L. (ed.): Golden's Diagnostic Roentgenology. Baltimore, The Williams & Wilkins Company, 1972, p. 836.
Thomas, P. K.: The connective tissue of peripheral nerve: An electron microscope study. J. Anat. (Lond.) *97*:35, 1963.
Tretjakoff, D.: Das epidurale Fettgewebe. Zeit. f. Anat. *79*:100, 1926.
Trevino, D. L., Coulter, J. D., and Willis, W. D.: Location of cells of origin of spinothalamic tract in lumbar enlargement of the monkey. J. Neurophysiol. *36*:750, 1973.
Tripathi, R. C.: Mechanism of aqueous outflow across the trabecular wall of Schlemm's canal. Exp. Eye Res. *11*:116, 1971.
Tripathi, R. C.: Ultrastructure of the arachnoid mater in relation to outflow of cerebrospinal fluid. Lancet *ii*:8, 1973.
Tripathi, B. J., and Tripathi, R. C.: Vacuolar transcellular channels as a drainage pathway for cerebrospinal fluid. J. Physiol. *239*:195, 1974.
Turnbull, I. M.: Blood supply of the spinal cord: Normal and pathological considerations. Clin. Neurosurg. *20*:56, 1973.
Usubiaga, J. E., Kolodny, J., and Usubiaga, L. E.: Neurological complications of prevertebral surgery under regional anesthesia. Surgery *68*:304, 1970.
Van Harreveld, A., and Khattab, F. I.: Electron microscopy of asphyxiated spinal cords of cats. J. Neuropath. Exp. Neurol. *26*:521, 1967.
Vogt, M.: The effect of lowering the 5-hydroxytryptamine content of the rat spinal cord on analgesia produced by morphine. J. Physiol. *236*:483, 1974.
Waggener, J. D., and Beggs, J. The membranous coverings of neural tissues: An electron microscopy study. J. Neuropath. Exp. Neurol. *26*:412, 1967.
Wall, P. D.: The laminar organization of the dorsal horn and effects of descending impulses. J. Physiol. *188*:403, 1967.
Weed, L. H.: Studies on cerebro-spinal fluid. II. The theories of drainage of cerebro-spinal fluid with an analysis of the methods of investigation. J. Med. Res. *31*:21, 1914a.
Weed, L. H.: Studies of cerebro-spinal fluid. III. The pathways of escape from the subarachnoid spaces with particular reference to the arachnoid villi. J. Med. Res. *31*:51, 1914b.
Welch, K., and Pollay, M.: The spinal arachnoid villi of the monkeys *Cercopitheus aethiops sabaeus* and *Macaca irus*. Anat. Rec., *145*:43, 1963.
Welch, K., and Pollay, M.: Perfusion of particles through arachnoid villi of the monkey. Amer. J. Physiol. *201*:651, 1961.
White, J. C., and Sweet, W. H.: Pain, Its Mechanisms and Neurological Control. Springfield, Ill. Charles C Thomas, Publisher, 1955, p. 36.
Williams, M. H.: Hypoxemia due to venous admixture in cirrhosis of the liver. J. Appl. Physiol. *15*:253, 1960.
Williams, P. L., and Landon, D. N.: Paranodal apparatus of peripheral myelinated nerve fibres of mammals. Nature *198*:670, 1963.
Willis, T.: "Cerebri anatome." Tab. XIII. Fig. IV. London, 1664.
Woollam, D. H. M., and Millen, J. W.: An anatomical approach to poliomyelitis. Lancet *i*:364, 1953.
Woollam, D. H. M., and Millen, J. W.: Observations on the production and circulation of the cerebrospinal fluid. *In* Wolstenholme, G. E. W., and O'Connor, C. M. (eds.): Ciba Foundation Symposium on the Cerebrospinal Fluid. London, J. & A. Churchill, Ltd., 1958a, p. 124.
Woollam, D. H. M., and Millen, J. W.: The anatomical background to vascular disease of the spinal cord. Proc. Roy. Soc. Med. *51*:540, 1958b.
Worthman, R. P.: The longitudinal vertebral nervous sinuses of the dog. II. Functional aspects. Amer. J. Vet. Res. *17*:349, 1956.

chapter 3
Pharmacology

Biological function appears to be more a correlate of macromolecular geometry than chemical detail.

Anfinsen, 1973

Hypothesis is the opiate of the scientist.

Danielli, 1972

We should not think of pharmacology, physiology and anatomy as three separate aspects of a trinity but rather as a convenient way of looking at a unitarian whole. At a distance they seem separate, but the closer we look the more the margins blur, and at the molecular level at which pharmacology operates, we are concerned with questions of ultramicroscopic anatomy involving the shape, texture and mechanics of cell membranes. At this level chemistry has become anatomy, and anatomy has become chemistry.

THE CELL MEMBRANE

During the past 50 years an enormous amount of investigation has been carried out on the properties of natural cell membranes and on artificial lipid and lipoprotein membranes, but the precise architecture of living biomembranes is still speculative. An excellent and detailed review of the subject up to 1972 by experts in the field is to be found in a symposium published by the New York Academy of Sciences on Membrane Structure and Function (Green, 1972).

The fluid mosaic model of Singer and Nicholson (1972) appears to be the one that is most consistent with theoretical and experimental requirements. In this model a fluid phospholipid bilayer is organized with hydrophilic polar groups pointing outward and hydrophobic fatty acid residues directed inward along the lines proposed in the earlier model of Gorter and Grendel (1925). Floating in this lipid matrix are cholesterol molecules and globular protein molecules of varying size. The globular proteins are postulated to be amphipathic, as are the phospholipids—that is, with an ionic and polar exterior facing outward in contact with water and a hydrophobic interior region embedded in the lipid membrane (Singer and Nicholson, 1972). Calcium is associated with the proteins (Kwant and Seeman, 1969).

It is further suggested that transmembrane channels are associated with the larger helical protein molecules that span the full width of the membrane. Water fills the space within these large protein molecules, forming channels of varying size that allow ion fluxes to pass across the membrane. The size of these water-filled channels will vary with conformational stresses within the membrane. Artificial membrane models confirm this postulate (Urry, 1972).

Figure 3–1 illustrates a model biomembrane of an excitable cell in diagrammatic form. Charged polar (phosphate) groups of phosphatidyl choline (or serine) face outward, while the nonpolar fatty acid residues face inward, with cholesterol molecules floating between the fatty acid chains. Protein molecules intrinsic to the membrane also float in the lipid bilayer. Some are unipolar with a single charged surface facing outward, while others are bipolar, spanning the lipid bilayer. Some of these larger protein molecules contain a helical water-filled channel that can function as an ion pore. These pores bear surface charges and are distributed sparsely over the membrane. There also appears to be a single negatively charged group within the channel, lying about one third of the way in from the surface (Hille, 1975). This anionic group is probably a carboxylic acid, and it binds with protons which then block the

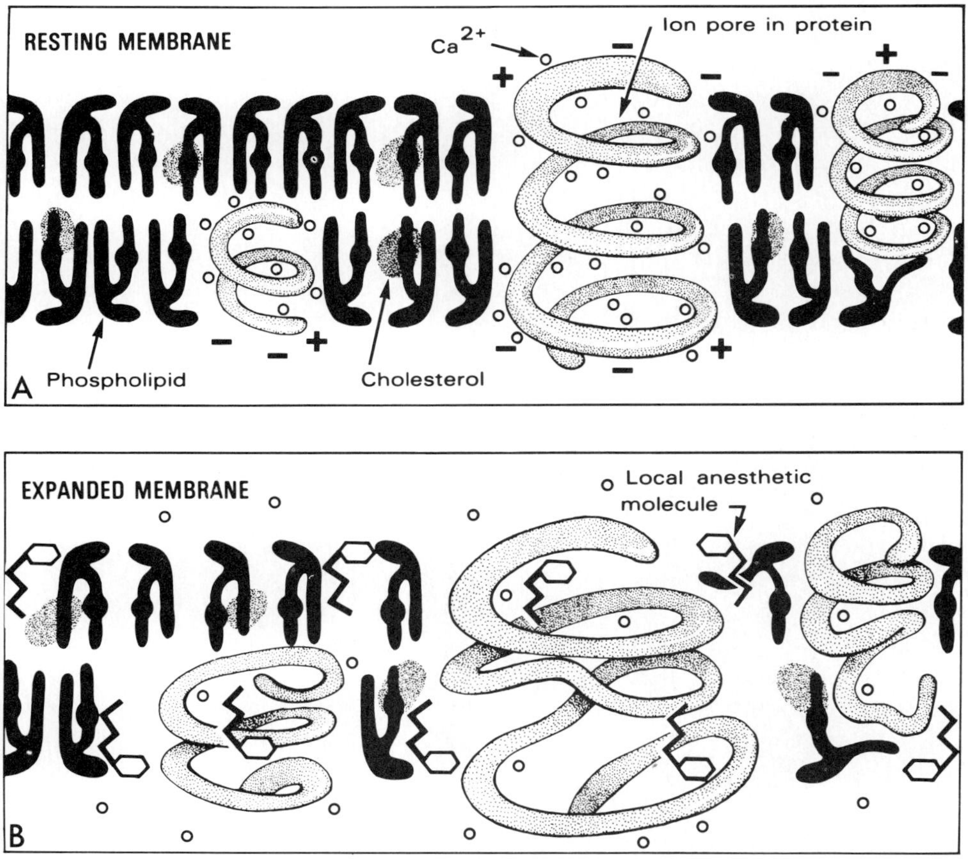

Figure 3–1. Diagrammatic and theoretical representation of an axon membrane based on the fluid mosaic model of Singer and Nicholson (1972). A phospholipid bilayer contains calcium, as well as cholesterol and protein molecules. Some protein molecules span the width of the membrane and enclose helical ion pores. *A*, Resting state. *B*, Expanded membrane after application of local anesthetic (see text for explanation).

channel, preventing the passage of Na^+ ions through the membrane (Woodhull, 1973). Studies with tetrodotoxin suggest that there are less than 75 channels large enough to carry sodium and rather fewer potassium channels per square micron of membrane surface (Moore et al., 1967; Keynes et al., 1971). Sodium channels behave as if they were about 3Å × 5Å (Hille, 1971) in cross section, while potassium channels are narrower (Keynes, 1972). Thus, a very tiny portion of the membrane is occupied by ion pores, and the ratio of pores to total surface is about 1:500,000.

During the resting state the ion pores of an excitable membrane are relatively closed, maintaining the internal and external ionic imbalance that determines the electrical potential or polarization of the membrane. This potential is normally about −70 mV relative to the exterior. During excitation the ion pores open for about 3 msec, and sodium moves into the cell while potassium moves out. A current passes and the cell is briefly depolarized, becoming repolarized as sodium is pumped out and potassium leaks back to restore the original ionic differential.

In spite of vigorous research efforts and intense speculation, the precise method of "gating" the ion pores remains unproven, although conformational changes within the membrane and the protein molecules of the ion pores seems the most likely explanation. Calcium ions are involved, but probably indirectly rather than directly. An earlier theory that the divalent calcium cations sat astride and blocked negatively charged ion channels is too simplistic. Instead, calcium probably contributes to electrical fields both at the surface and inside the membrane which in turn bend or deform the protein ion channels. Other alkaline earth elements can substitute for calcium in this mechanism, and magnesium and lanthanum also "stabilize" the membrane pores; however, lanthanum, being trivalent, exerts a more forceful and tenacious effect (Lettvin et al., 1964). Hydrogen ions also inhibit the passage of sodium through the nerve membrane by occupying anionic sites within the sodium channels (Woodhull, 1973). This action is very fast, and it may possibly be involved to some extent in the rapid activity of the carbonated local anesthetic solutions that will be discussed later.

The phospholipids of biological membranes provide numerous negatively charged sites for cation exchange, and there is a high concentration of calcium in excitable membranes (Nash and Tobias, 1964). Local anesthetics compete with cations such as Na^+ or Ca^{2+} for negatively charged (anionic) binding sites in the membrane. Thus, among their other effects local anesthetics displace Ca^{2+} from the membrane (Blaustein and Goldman, 1966), while their blocking action is partially antagonized by increased concentrations of calcium (Aceves and Machne, 1963; Feinstein, 1966) or sodium (Condouris, 1961, 1963) outside the membrane. Local anesthetics with long hydrophobic side chains, such as the butylene chain of tetracaine, penetrate more deeply into the hydrophobic parts of the membrane and displace more Ca^{2+} than anesthetic agents without long side chains (Cerbón, 1972; Fernandez and Cerbón, 1973).

Depot sites for anions involved in the excitation process are placed at strategic points over the surface of the excitable membranes. Electron probe microanalysis has shown that calcium is stored, probably as a bound form, in packages between the Schwann cell and the axon membrane (Hillman and Llinas, 1974; Oschman et al., 1974). In addition, the nodal matrix at the nodes of Ranvier of medullated nerves is rich in polyanionic charged sites for ion exchange and electrostatic storage of cations (Langley, 1969; Landon and Langley, 1971). Na^+ and Ca^{2+} are held in large amounts at these exchange sites, presumably in readiness for entry and escape from the membrane during passage of an impulse. Both sodium and calcium are competitively displaced from these sites by cationic local anesthetics (Langley, 1973), and the resultant depletion of readily available Na^+ may be an important factor in lowering the amplitude of the action potential (Condouris, 1961, 1963).

The axon membrane can be rendered partially or completely depolarized and inactive by manipulating the external ionic environment. For example, low sodium (hyponatremia) or high potassium (hyperkalemia) outside the nerve both reduce ionic gradients across the membrane and lower the membrane potential (Huxley and Stämpfli, 1951; Nathan and Sears, 1962). This mechanism has been put to use in the clinical field by adding potassium salts to local anesthetic solutions with the idea of intensifying the quality of blockade (Hoffmann and Kochmann, 1912; Meecker, 1925; Lechat et al., 1964). The desired effect is indeed achieved, and anesthetic blockade is intensified, but unfortunately depolarizing phenomena in the form of twitches and muscle cramps render it a dubious practice (Bromage and Burfoot, 1966).

Action of Local Anesthetics on Excitable Membranes

Local anesthetics stabilize excitable membranes and block the flux of sodium and potassium through the ion pores of axon membranes.

Historically, man is late to stumble on the trick of inactivating excitable membranes by prolonged stabilization; a number of species of plankton and reptilia have been in the business of sodium channel blockade for millions of years, probably since Mesozoic times. A large family of reptile and fish toxins has defensive uses, some for survival of the individual and some for survival of the species, as in the case of the newt *Taricha torosa* which covers its eggs with a layer of tetrodotoxin to deter predators (Mosher et al., 1964). Both tetrodotoxin from the puffer fish and saxitoxin from the "red tide" Dinoflagellata *Gonyaulax catanella* block sodium channels at the outer surface of the membrane by hydrogen bonding (Dettbarn, 1971). The molecules of these toxins are comparable in size to those of cocaine, but they attach firmly to the surface charges of the nerve membrane, and the resultant blockade is extremely prolonged. Only about 30 to 100 molecules of tetrodotoxin are needed to produce complete blockade of one square micron of cell membrane. By contrast, about 250,000 molecules of local anesthetic are required to do the same job (Seeman, 1972).

Surface versus deep interactions

While the feral blocking agents of fish and reptile toxins act mainly at the surface of the axon membrane, pharmacological local anesthetics appear to have a more complex mode of action both at the surface of the axon membrane and deep within the lipid matrix. The precise details of local anesthetic action have been debated for many years, with particular attention to the question of whether the charged ionized form or the uncharged nonionized

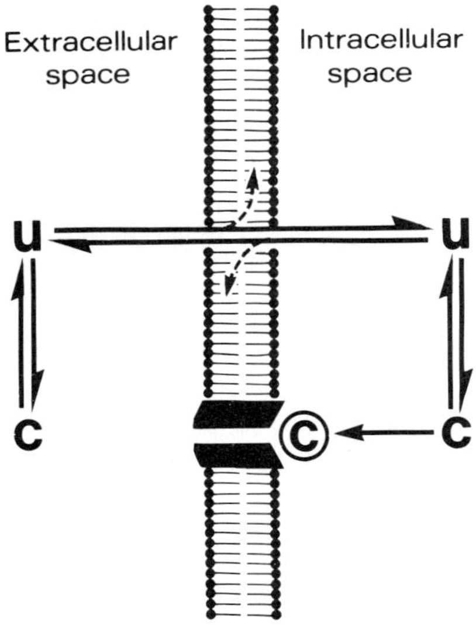

Figure 3–2. Action of charged (C) and uncharged (U) moieties of local anesthetic on excitable membrane.

form is responsible for blockade (Ritchie and Greengard, 1961). More will be said about the question of ionization later in the section dealing with penetration of local anesthetics. For the moment we need only consider the fact that at physiological pH the local anesthetics in common use exist partly as an ionized or positively charged cationic form and partly as a nonionized electrically neutral molecule. The charged cationic form is capable of forming electrostatic bonds at the surface of the charged membranes, while the nonionized form is not. However, the uncharged form can penetrate readily into the hydrophobic depths of the lipid bilayer and occupy space between the hydrophobic parts of the lipid molecules. Skou (1961) observed that this penetrating action caused a physical expansion of the membrane, and Shanes (1963) suggested that the resulting conformational changes would effectively hold the ion pores closed.

Later, it appeared that the two actions of surface electrostatic effect and lipid penetration had quite independent significance. Penetration of the membrane by the uncharged form was considered to be merely a stage on the journey of the local anesthetic to its target, while the charged cationic form was responsible for actual blockade of the membrane through occupation of charged receptor sites on the surface (Ritchie, Ritchie and Greengard, 1965a, 1965b). Work done by Narahashi et al. (1970), Armstrong et al. (1973) and Strichartz (1973) suggested that most of the surface blocking effect of local anesthetics takes place at the *inner* surface of the axon membrane after passage of the uncharged form through the lipid phase, as shown in Figure 3–2. It now seems clear that *both* the charged and uncharged forms of local anesthetic molecules play their own but different roles in the process of conduction blockade (Ritchie and Ritchie, 1968; Strobel and Bianchi, 1970; Ritchie, 1975), and two long-standing and sometimes opposed theories have been reconciled.

Surface (Cationic) Blockade and Membrane Expansion

Interactions of local anesthetic cations with surface charges on the membrane can be illustrated by Feinstein's proposed model of complex formation between tetracaine and acidic phospholipids, as shown in Figure 3–3 (Feinstein, 1964). In this model, polar aromatic nitrogen and the positively charged tertiary alkyl nitrogen of tetracaine are shown orientated toward the negatively charged phosphate groups of two phosphatidyl serine molecules. Artificial membrane models suggest that the positively charged portion of the local anesthetic molecule remains anchored at the surface, as proposed by Feinstein, while any lipophilic tail on the end of the anesthetic molecule becomes orientated parallel to the fatty acid residues of the phospholipids and buried in the membrane. With this sort of orientation, agents such as tetracaine, dibucaine and bupivacaine will have their butylene chain buried deep in the hydrophobic parts of the membrane with their methyl terminal level with the seventh or eighth methylene group of the fatty acid residues (Singer, 1974).

As early as 1957, Spyropoulos showed that large increases of hydrostatic pressure (7,000 psi) could reverse the blocking action of 3 to 7 per cent ethanol on squid axons, suggesting that physical expansion of the membrane might underly the process of blockade. Shortly after this, Skou (1961) and Shanes (1963) speculated that local anesthetic action could be explained by expansion of the cell membrane following solution of the nonionized drug in the lipid phase. This idea was shelved after the work of Ritchie and his colleagues demonstrated the overriding importance of the cationic form of tertiary amine drugs, such as lidocaine and procaine, in the blocking process (Ritchie and Greengard, 1961; Ritchie, Ritchie and Greengard, 1965a, 1965b). However, further work by the Ritchies pointed out that cationic behavior only intensified the activity of local anesthetics and that true anesthetic activity resided in the lipophilic part of the molecule (Ritchie and Ritchie, 1968). Since then, interest

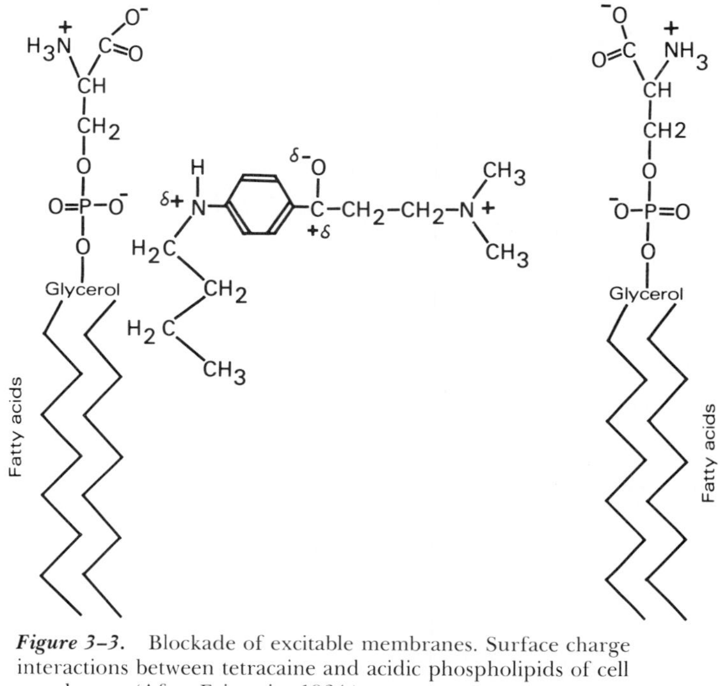

Figure 3–3. Blockade of excitable membranes. Surface charge interactions between tetracaine and acidic phospholipids of cell membrane. (After Feinstein, 1964.)

has swung back to the earlier theories of membrane expansion as a physical basis for conduction blockade.

In a large series of experiments with red cell "ghosts" as a membrane model, Seeman has demonstrated a number of interesting physical changes accompanying treatment by local and general anesthetics, and the subject is very thoroughly reviewed in Pharmacological Reviews *24*:583–655, 1972. All anesthetics expand cell membranes. At concentrations that cause general anesthesia, the membrane is expanded 0.4 to 0.6 per cent. At concentrations sufficient for conduction blockade, the membrane expands 2 to 3 per cent. At higher concentrations sufficient to cause a 5 to 7 per cent expansion, the membrane buckles inward and disrupts (Seeman, 1974a, 1974b).

The expansion of biomembranes is about ten times greater than the actual volume occupied by the anesthetic molecules. Moreover, the specific volume expansion of biological membranes is many times greater than for artificial lipid membranes, and this strongly suggests that the cause of the phenomenon may lie in changes of shape and spatial distribution of the membrane proteins (Seeman, 1974a). The maximum uptake of local anesthetic by the membranes and the maximum uptake of Ca^{2+} are very similar, and it is possible that competitive displacement of Ca^{2+} may be one of the important factors leading to conformational changes of membrane proteins (Kwant and Seeman, 1969), as shown in Figure 3–1 *B*.

Recently, Lee (1976) has sought to reconcile the lipid-soluble and cationic effects of local anesthetics in a unitary model for action that involves both aspects but emphasizes the effects of solubility in the membrane lipids rather than changes of shape in the membrane proteins. This model postulates that the sodium channels are surrounded by a ring of lipid (not protein), which is in a crystalline or gel state that is rigid enough to keep the channel open. Solution of local anesthetic base in the lipid triggers a change from the rigid gel state to a fluid liquid state that relaxes the ion channel and allows it to close. In addition, there is the evidence already presented to suggest that anions, both monovalent (Na^+) and divalent (Ca^{2+} and Mg^{2+}), are most plentiful on the outside of the membrane, with depots between the Schwann cell and the axon membrane. Lee points out that this concentration of anions at the outer surface leaves a relatively greater abundance of available negatively charged lipid sites on the inside of the membrane to which cationic local anesthetics can attach themselves, thus explaining Narahashi's finding that cationic local anesthetic action appears to be at the inner surface of the axon membrane, after the lipid-soluble local anesthetic base has penetrated through the lipid phase (Narahashi et al., 1970).

Secondary events accompany the process of membrane expansion and "stabilization." The membrane becomes less permeable, not only to cations but also to larger particles, such as glucose molecules (Clausen et al., 1973). In addition, a slight reduction of oxygen consumption has been observed in nerve tissues exposed to local anesthetics (Geddes and Quastel, 1956; Pietra, 1963). However, this change probably reflects depressed oxidative metabolism in the underlying axoplasm rather than in the axon membrane, as will be discussed later in this chapter.

In summary, local anesthetics act by solution of the nonionized base in the lipid phase of the membrane and by cationic attraction to anionic sites on the inner surface of the membrane. There they compete with divalent ions associated with the membrane proteins and either deform the proteins or possibly cause a phase change in the lipids, as proposed by Lee. This in turn leads to expansion of the membrane, closure of ion pores and reduced permeability to anions and to glucose. Local anesthetic molecules with long hydrophobic (lipophilic) side chains, such as bupivacaine, dibucaine, tetracaine and etidocaine, will penetrate into the hydrophobic depths of the membrane and exert more powerful calcium-displacing effects than molecules with short side chains.

Local anesthetics in excessive concentration cause overdistension of the membrane and disruption of its architecture, with buckling and finally lysis of the membrane.

From a practical point of view, a local anesthetic must produce its blocking effect quickly to be of use in the clinical field. Therefore, the qualities of rapid penetration and intense cationic activity at the membrane surface are likely to be of equal or greater importance than solution in the lipid phase and subsequent expansion of the membrane.

Molecular shape

At this point we need to look at the structure and shape of local anesthetics to see how their geometry and ionic characteristics enable them to stick onto charged membranes.

The naturally occurring anesthetic toxins cocaine and tetrodotoxin have relatively large molecules that contain certain atomic groupings common to all local anesthetics in clinical use. Each has a positively charged polar nitrogen atom, enabling it to engage in a strong electrostatic interaction between the positive nitrogen and negative oxygen atoms at phosphate groups on the surface of excitable membranes. Also, each of these toxins has one or more carbonyl groups in the molecule. The carbonyl group C=O is a trademark of all the local anesthetics in use today, and it confers great ionic reactivity to the molecule by enabling electron transfer to occur along the chain of atoms oscillating between the ketonic and enolic forms, thus:

Ketonic Enolic

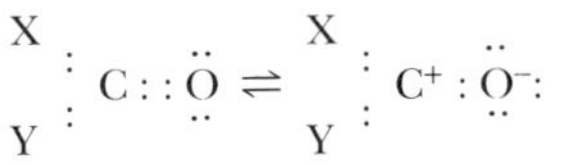

Within a molecule such as procaine the chain movement will be:

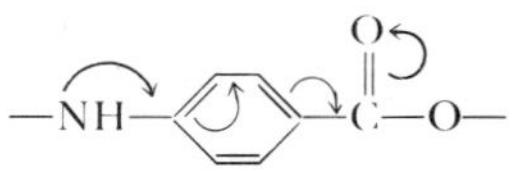

Electron transfer along the molecule is a key function determining the binding characteristics and clinical qualities of a local anesthetic agent. A few instances of molecular geometry will be given below to illustrate the principles involved. For more detailed study the reader is referred to articles by Perlia (1967) and Büchi (1967) and to Chapter 4 on "Drugs that depolarize nerve membranes" in *Fundamentals of Cell Pharmacology* (Narahashi, 1975), as well as *Local Anesthetics* (de Jong, 1977).

Efficient local anesthetics must behave like guerrilla fighters in some respects. They must penetrate defensive positions very rapidly, make contact with their target, occupy it for an appropriate time and then disengage. However, unlike guerrillas they must inactivate their target but leave it totally unharmed and fully operational when they retire. This is a demanding task, for many of the steps that fulfill these requirements are mutually exclusive. Therefore, it is understandable that the right balance of gentleness and aggression is so seldom found among the host of local anesthetics that have been tried but found wanting in some respects.

Local anesthetics have their target in membranes that are polar by nature, part hydrophobic and part hydrophilic, so it is not surprising that their molecules also should be polar. At the target, the task is to bend or bridge terminal charged chains in such a way that sodium channels are blocked. Thus, the distance between charged or bonding sites on the molecule is likely to be critical and related to the distances between polar groups at the membrane surface. In fact, 5Å to 9Å seems to be the critical distance between the polar parts of an effective local anesthetic molecule, and this critical section is referred to as the "intermediate chain," a name that lacks the forcefulness of its functional importance. The so-called intermediate chain is in fact crucial for many fundamental characteristics. For example, the potent carbonyl grouping is located here, and additions or branches to the chain may alter dramatically the physicochemical and clinical properties of the molecule. The difference between lidocaine and etidocaine is a classic example of this type of change brought about by adding an ethyl branch to the intermediate chain (see Chapter 9).

The polar parts of the molecule must be considered next:

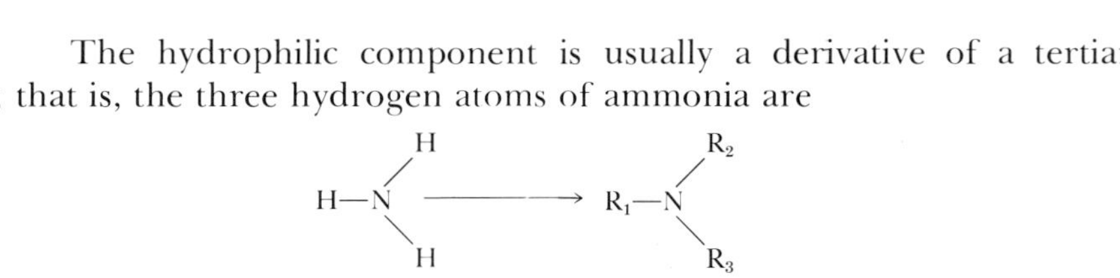

The hydrophilic component is usually a derivative of a tertiary amine; that is, the three hydrogen atoms of ammonia are

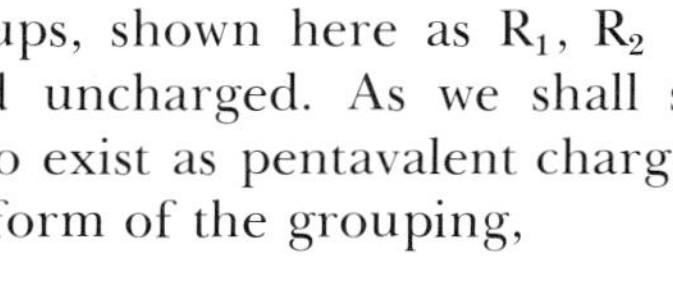

replaced by organic groups, shown here as R_1, R_2 and R_3. In this form the nitrogen is trivalent and uncharged. As we shall see later, the uncharged trivalent nitrogen can also exist as pentavalent charged nitrogen in the "dissociated" electrically active form of the grouping,

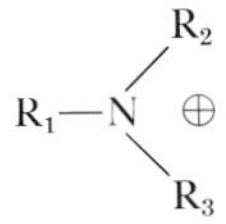

depending on the pH of its environment. This change of valency and electrical activity is fundamental to the clinical properties of local anesthetics and will be considered more fully in the next section. Quaternary compounds with

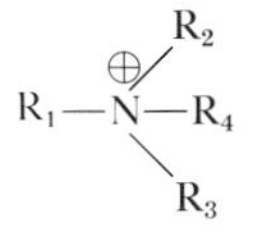

an additional organic group and a constant charge on the amino nitrogen also have local anesthetic properties, but they are only able to block sodium channels when applied *directly* to the inner surface of the axon membrane, for their electrical charge prevents penetration of the axon membrane, and they are relatively ineffective for clinical purposes.

Lengthened hydrocarbon chains on the lipophilic component, as in tetracaine, bupivacaine and etidocaine, confer heightened attractive forces with stronger protein binding and longer duration of action. Unfortunately, these alluring binding sites are not selective for the favors of axons alone, and many competitors, free-roving in plasma or lurking in other membranes on the way, may entrap the local anesthetic molecules as they pass by, leaving only a handful of starters to reach the journey's end.

The lipophilic component, usually a derivative of benzoic acid or aniline, is combined with an amino alcohol, or an amino acid in the case of aniline, to form either an ester or an amide linkage. The two typical agents illustrating ester and amide linkage are procaine and lidocaine.

Procaine

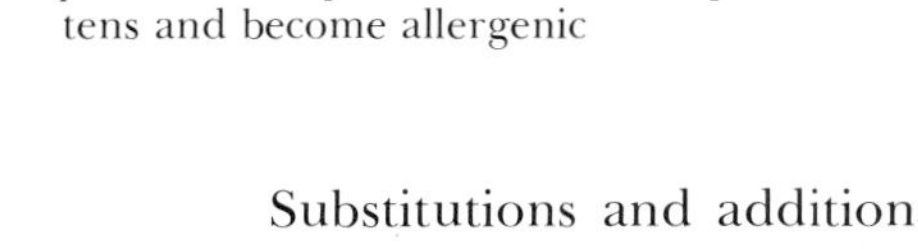

1. Ester linkage rapidly broken down by hydrolysis or by cholinesterase in the plasma
2. *p*-Amino compounds can form haptens and become allergenic

Lidocaine

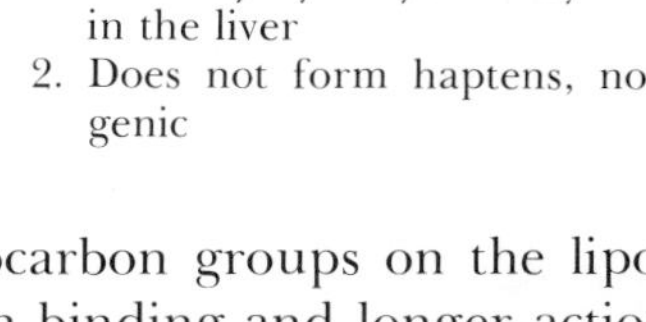

1. Amide linkage very slowly broken down by hydrolysis or by amidases in the liver
2. Does not form haptens, nonallergenic

Substitutions and additional hydrocarbon groups on the lipophilic component may also confer increased protein binding and longer action. For example, short-acting procaine becomes the longer acting and more potent tetracaine by substituting a butyl group on the para-amino nitrogen and shortening the hydrophilic ethyl groups to methyl groups.

This brief introduction will serve as a basis for appreciating some of the ionic and structural principles that underly the wide divergence in clinical performance that may exist between two closely related local anesthetic agents of quite similar structure.

Penetration of local anesthetics

A difficult journey stretches between the site of injection and the axon membrane, with its polar groups guarding the target ion channels. Two alternating and incompatible phases of lipoprotein and water recur successively in the membrane barriers and the spaces between them, and the local anesthetic agent must pass easily across them all, equally at home and soluble in both media.

Swift changes of valency in the hydrophilic amino nitrogen are the key to this journey. Only in its trivalent uncharged form can the molecule become electrically incognito, slip through the hedge of negative charges guarding each membrane surface and pass freely through the lipid matrix to reach the next layer of water. At the water's edge, however, it must change back to pentavalent nitrogen and to its positively charged water-soluble form for the next stage of the journey. This transition is expressed as:

$R{\equiv}N + H^+$	$\rightleftharpoons$	$R{\equiv}NH^+$
(uncharged base)		(charged cation)
Lipid-soluble		Water-soluble
Insoluble in water		Insoluble in lipid (Fig. 3–4)

The efficiency of this flip-flop behavior from a charged (ionized) to an uncharged (nonionized) form and back again depends on the dissociation constant (Ka) of the drug and the concentration of hydrogen ions in the surrounding water phase. Local anesthetics are weakly basic, and the dissociation constant expresses the following relationship:

$$Ka = \frac{[H+]\ [\text{Uncharged Base}]}{[\text{Charged Cation}]}$$

or, converted to logarithms,

$$pKa = pH - \log \frac{[\text{Base}]}{[\text{Cation}]}$$

hence,

$$\log \frac{[\text{Cation}]}{[\text{Base}]} = pKa - pH$$

This logarithmic relationship is shown graphically in Figure 3–5. It can be appreciated that when the pH equals the pKa, the relationship of cation to base is poised and balanced, with equal proportions of both moieties (Fig. 3–5). Small alterations of hydrogen ion concentration on either side of the balance point will produce large differences in the two ionic species. In alkaline solution, when $pKa - pH < 0$ there is more base available and precipitation will probably occur, whereas in acid solution, when $pKa - pH > 0$ more of the soluble charged cation is available. Clinically effective local anesthetics have their pKa above the physiological range of pH; all local anesthetic solutions are manufactured on the acid side of the pKa to maintain water solubility, and the expression $pKa - pH$ is always greater than zero.

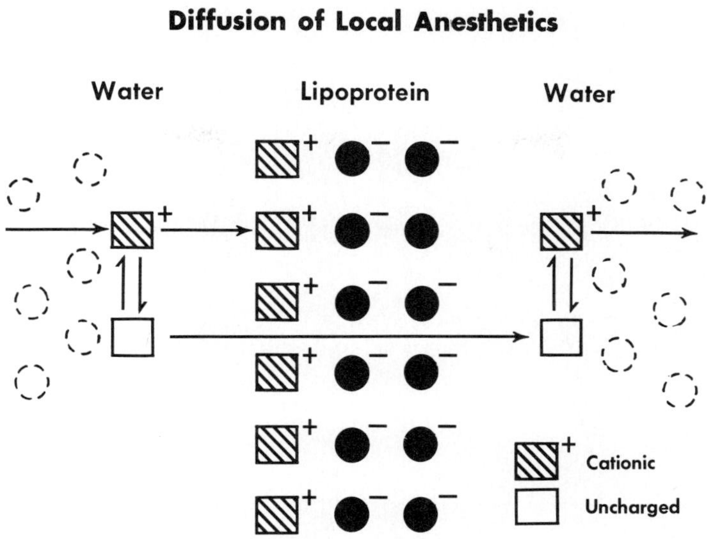

Figure 3–4. Passage of local anesthetic through lipoprotein membrane. Charged cationic form is held by net negative charge on surface of membrane and is unable to penetrate. Uncharged lipid-soluble form can enter and cross to water phase on other side, where dissociation again takes place.

For example, the pKa of several local anesthetic agents is given below:

Mepivacaine	7.65
Lidocaine	7.87
Tetracaine	8.50
Bupivacaine	8.05
Etidocaine	7.74
Procaine	8.92

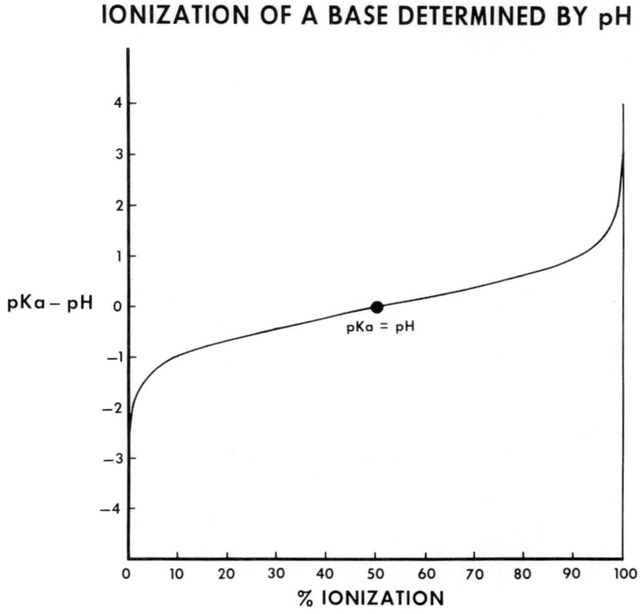

Figure 3–5. Relationship of pH, pKa and degree of ionization of a local anesthetic.

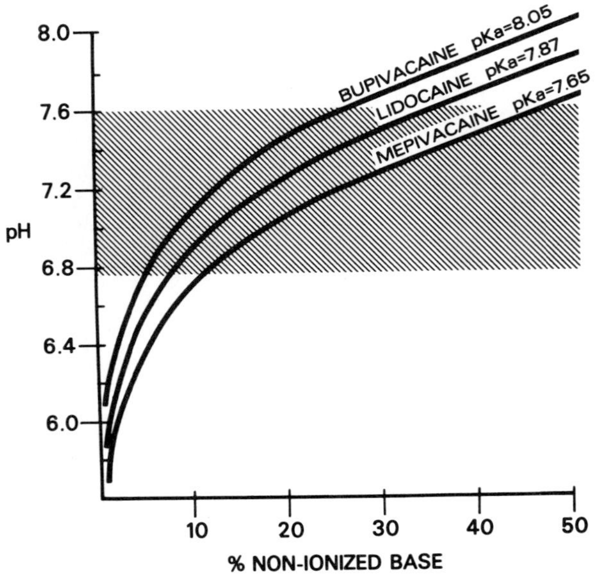

Figure 3–6. The pH, pKa and ionization of local anesthetics; relationship of pH to percentage concentration of diffusible, nonionized base for bupivacaine, lidocaine and mepivacaine. Hatched area represents approximate physiologically viable limits of pH. Note that bupivacaine has the least and mepivacaine the most diffusible base present at any given pH.

Therefore, at physiological pH (pH = 7.4) water solubility is assured and relatively little nonionized base is present and available for diffusion across lipid membranes. The relationship of nonionized base to pH for bupivacaine, lidocaine and mepivacaine is shown in Figure 3–6. It can be seen that at any given pH within the hatched area, bupivacaine will have the least nonionized base, while mepivacaine will have the largest proportion of diffusible base. In the case of lidocaine, the proportions of nonionized base and cation at various levels of pH will be those shown in Table 3–1. In the alkalotic situation at pH 7.62, twice as much nonionized lidocaine base is present as at pH 7.22, and this extra amount of base is sequestered in the lipid phase. In the physiologically acidotic situation of pH 7.22, 27 per cent more ionized cation is available to occupy surface binding sites on the membrane.

These principles can be put to practical use by manipulating the acid-base environment to mobilize local anesthetics into or out of body compartments. For example, anesthetic uptake can be hastened by creating a cationic trap, as shown by the hypothetical situation in Figure 3–7. Here, imaginary values for pH and pKa are given in round numbers for ease of demonstrating

TABLE 3–1. Effect of pH on Proportions of Charged and Uncharged Lidocaine (pKa = 7.87)

		Percentage as:	
Tissue pH	*pKa − pH*	*CATION*	*NONIONIZED BASE*
7.42 (normal)	+ 0.45	73.8	26.2
7.62 (alkalosis)	+ 0.25	64.01	35.99
7.22 (acidosis)	+ 0.65	81.7	18.3

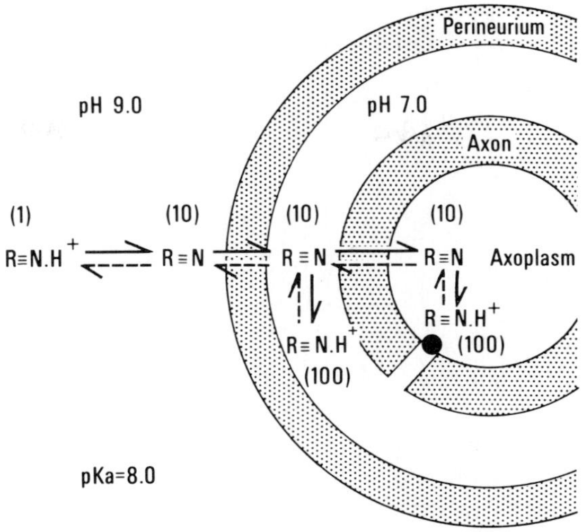

Figure 3–7. Ionization of local anesthetics: penetration and blockade. Hypothetical situation to illustrate "cationic trap" effect of diminishing pH across tissue membranes, supposing an extraneural pH of 9.0 and a local anesthetic with pKa of 8.0. A tenfold change of nondiffusible cation accompanies each unit difference of pH.

the resulting logarithmic changes. The relative amounts of uncharged base and cation are given in brackets. Two units of difference in pH on the two sides of the membrane will make a hundredfold difference in the amount of cation concentrated inside the membrane (Ritchie et al., 1965b). A reverse situation can be exploited to eliminate absorbed local anesthetic from the blood stream into the urine (Eriksson and Granberg, 1965), as shown in Figure 3–8. Here, acidification of the urine will trap water-soluble cation in the renal tubules and prevent reabsorption into the blood again.

In vivo, some degree of cationic trap probably exists around every nerve, with a slightly lower pH inside the axoplasm than outside, owing to metabolic activity of the nerve cell. Thus, there will be a general tendency for

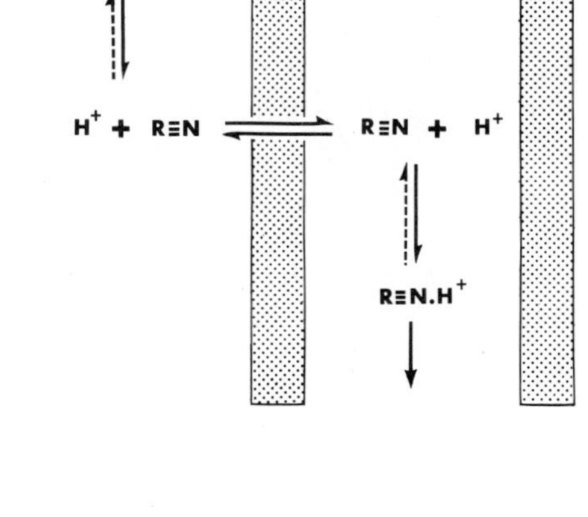

Figure 3–8. Renal elimination of local anesthetic in an acid urine. (After Eriksson and Granberg, 1965.)

local anesthetics to migrate toward the axon. This normal tendency can be exaggerated by the use of carbonated local anesthetics, that is, local anesthetic solutions in which the anesthetic base has been made water-soluble as a salt of carbonic acid instead of the orthodox salt of hydrochloric acid. The introduction of carbonated local anesthetics is an interesting example of serendipity—the happy exploitation of a chance observation by an informed mind—and it is worth relating how it happened.

CARBONATED LOCAL ANESTHETICS

In 1963, Mr. George Nordstrom, production engineer for Astra Pharmaceuticals, Inc., Worcester, Massachusetts, was examining a selection of gaseous vehicles for topical local anesthetic sprays. Carbon dioxide was among the gases under consideration, and he sought firsthand experience by spraying mixtures of lidocaine on his own lips. To his surprise he found that a spray propelled by carbon dioxide had a more intense effect than other sprays with inert propellants. It was a short distance down the corridor to the office of the Research Director, the late Dr. Aldo P. Truant, and there possible explanations were chalked out on the blackboard. Laboratory evidence already existed from at least three separate sources that carbon dioxide penetrates membranes extremely rapidly and has profound effects on bioelectric events in living tissue. Arvanitaki and Chalazonitis at Monaco (1954) and Caldwell in London (1958) had shown that raising the external pCO_2 of squid or lobster nerves produced a rapid decline of internal pH and partial membrane depolarization within a matter of seconds. Halpern and Binaghi (1959) in Paris also found similar falls of pH across other biological membranes in the presence of a high external pCO_2. There was enough respectable evidence to suggest that Nordstrom's observation might be not just a chance event but a real and predictable augmentation of local anesthetic effect in the presence of carbon dioxide. Nordstrom had shown that it was possible to dissolve lidocaine base as a salt of carbonic acid by bubbling carbon dioxide through a watery emulsion of the base in the cold. In this way a solution of carbonated lidocaine could be prepared and bottled in ampules, without the addition of hydrochloric acid and with a pH of about the same as the plain hydrochloride solution at 6.5. The solution had a pCO_2 of about 700 mmHg and was slightly "pétillant" when an ampule was opened. I was fortunate enough to be invited to try the new mixture, and I performed a number of digital and lateral femoral cutaneous nerve blocks on myself and several colleagues, with encouraging results. Onset of blockade was fast, the quality of analgesia was intense and there were no ill effects. Clinical trials seemed in order, and these were started in December, 1963, with a series of epidural blocks, the carbonated and hydrochloride salts of lidocaine and prilocaine being compared. The results were unequivocal and showed that the carbonated salts were indeed a major advance in local anesthesia. There was a 30 per cent increase in effectiveness, in terms of both shorter latency and more intense quality of sensory and motor blockade (Bromage, 1965; Bromage et al., 1967).

The train of reactions accompanying the formation and action of the carbonated solutions may be represented as:

$$H_2O + CO_2 \rightleftharpoons H_2CO_3 \rightleftharpoons H^+ + HCO_3^- \tag{1}$$

$$\begin{array}{c} H^+ + HCO_3^- \rightleftharpoons H_2CO_3 + R{\equiv}N \rightleftharpoons R{\equiv}NH^+ + HCO_3^- \\ \upharpoonleft\downharpoonright \\ H_2O + CO_2 \end{array} \tag{2}$$

The right hand parts of equations (1) and (2) occur during the preparation of the agents, while equation (2) proceeds to the left after release and injection. Carbon dioxide diffuses extremely rapidly across tissue membranes, releasing base at the site of injection and probably exaggerating a series of cation traps, as shown in Figure 3–9, increasing the *speed* of uptake of local anesthetic by neural tissue. Release of H^+ ions near the outside of the axon membrane may also contribute to enhanced blockade through attachment of H^+ ions to anionic sites within the sodium channels (Woodhull, 1973) and on the surface of the membrane (Seimiya and Ohki, 1973). We have no evidence that the *quantity* of drug taken up by neural tissue is any greater than usual. Epidural injection with ^{14}C-labeled agents was done in dogs to see if there was a measurably greater uptake in spinal nerves and their coverings with carbonated solution than with the hydrochloride salts, but our studies did not show any significant difference in this animal preparation (Bromage and Burfoot, 1964).

The mechanism of action of the carbonated solutions is probably quite complex, involving not only pH changes and shifts of local anesthetic cation but also secondary alterations of ionization of Ca^{2+} in the membranes, and further work needs to be done to elucidate their precise action. In vitro data by Catchlove (1973) at McGill support the belief that carbon dioxide does more than just create a cationic trap for ionizable local anesthetics, since the blocking potency of *n*-butanol, a nonionized anesthetic, is also augmented in the presence of carbon dioxide. This suggests that carbon dioxide has a direct effect on the axon membrane over and above its tendency to trap cations, possibly through release of H^+ at the axon surface, as suggested by Woodhull (1973).

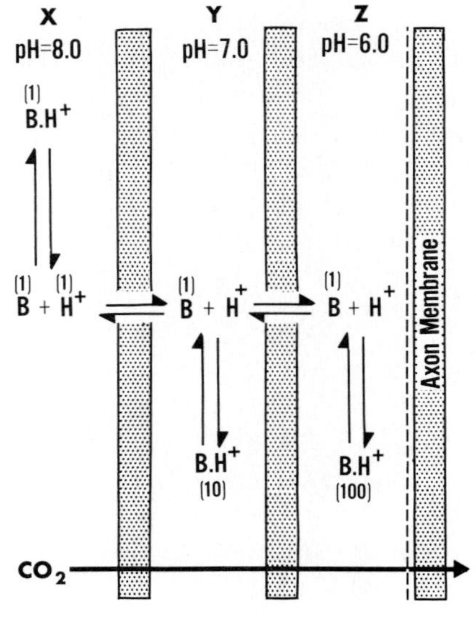

Figure 3–9. Carbonated local anesthetic solutions: diffusion of carbon dioxide facilitates "cationic trap" effect. Assuming the hypothetical values of a pKa of 8 and pH values of 8, 7 and 6 in compartments X, Y and Z, respectively, a hundredfold concentration of cation will occur at Z. Inward diffusion of CO_2 increases the *speed* of cationic concentration.

Effect of CO_2 on Potency of Lidocaine (1 mM)

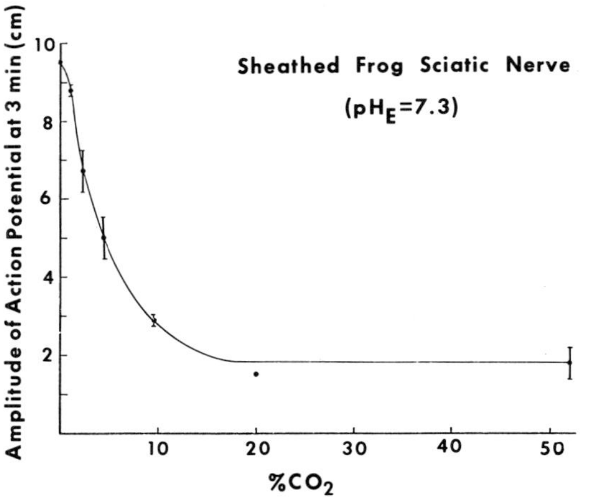

Figure 3–10. In vitro effect of carbon dioxide on potency of lidocaine at dilution of 1 mM (i.e., 0.028%). Blockade of sheathed and buffered frog sciatic nerve becomes more effective as concentration of CO_2 increases: maximum effect of CO_2 at about 15% (From Catchlove, McGill MSc. Thesis, 1971.)

The preparation of carbonated local anesthetics is a tedious, expensive process, and clearly it would be simpler to use the orthodox hydrochloride salt equilibrated with carbon dioxide at the required partial pressure. In 1964, Condouris and Shakalis showed markedly augmented blockade in rat sciatic nerves when exposed to hydrochloride local anesthetic solutions gassed with varying concentrations of carbon dioxide between 2.5 per cent and 20 per cent. Later, Catchlove (1971, 1972) showed the same mechanism in buffered frog sciatic nerves (Fig. 3–10). However, simple gassing of hydrochloride solutions with carbon dioxide does not seem to be so successful in clinical situations. We studied a series of epidural blocks using lidocaine hydrochloride equilibrated with carbon dioxide at 700 mmHg, and although there was a slight improvement over the ungassed hydrochloride solutions, the results were not as effective as with the carbonated base (Bromage et al., 1967). The superiority of the carbonated base over the gassed hydrochloride solution is probably due to a difference in the initial pH values of the injected solutions and different availability of diffusible base. For example, the carbonated solution of lidocaine base at a pCO_2 of 700 mmHg and the ungassed hydrochloride solution are both relatively alkaline in the range of pH of 6.2 to 6.5, respectively. However, gassing the hydrochloride solution with carbon dioxide reduces its pH by about 1.6 units from 6.5 to 4.9, with proportionally less base available for diffusion from the site of injection.

pH OF PLAIN SOLUTIONS AND EPINEPHRINE-CONTAINING SOLUTIONS

Plain solutions of most amide drugs, such as lidocaine, mepivacaine and bupivacaine, are stable and resistant to hydrolysis at hydrogen ion concentrations close to physiological levels. For example, plain lidocaine (Astra Pharmaceuticals) is manufactured at a pH of 6.5, and at this pH as much as 4.25 per cent of the drug is in the nonionized diffusible form. However, epinephrine-containing solutions are manufactured with an antioxidant (0.1 per cent sodium bisulphite) to prevent oxidation of the epinephrine, and these solutions are more acid, with a pH of about 4.5; then practically all the drug is present in the ionized cationic form and only 0.1 per cent as diffusible base. Thus, solutions manufactured with epinephrine in them are likely to have slower latencies because of the time required for buffering of the acid injectant to a point at which adequate amounts of diffusible base are released for penetration.

SYSTEMIC UPTAKE AND DISTRIBUTION OF LOCAL ANESTHETICS FROM THE EPIDURAL SPACE

The neuronal uptake of epidural anesthetics is considered in Chapter 2, and at this point we will deal only with the systemic uptake.

Competition for local anesthetic between nerve, blood and fat occurs at any injection site. In the epidural space the competition is fierce, and the nerves hidden behind layers of membranes receive only a relatively small share of the available drug. Direct measurement of vascular uptake from the epidural space is technically difficult among the network of vessels entering and leaving the space, and sampling of venous drainage gives only a rough estimate of relative changes. Diving mammals with large longitudinal veins in the dorsal part of the extradural space might make a useful laboratory preparation for measurements of vascular uptake, but these have not been tested. However, a major portion of the extradural vascular effluent drains into the azygos collection system, and sampling from the azygos vein gives a useful approximation of events. In dogs, a collecting catheter can be inserted into the azygos vein quite easily via an intercostal vein. Using this technique we were able to obtain comparative estimates of the proportion of labeled drug taken up by the azygos vein after extradural injection under various conditions (Burfoot and Bromage, 1971).

We found that only a small proportion of the injected drug (about 9 per cent in 30 minutes) could be accounted for by azygos sampling, but the proportion was markedly affected by the presence or absence of epinephrine 1/200,000 in the epidural solution. Figure 3–11 shows the average concentrations of ^{14}C-labeled mepivacaine in azygos blood after injection of 100 mg at the thoracolumbar level of the epidural space. The peak concentration is about 2½ times greater with the plain solution than with the epinephrine-containing solution.

This mirrors what is seen clinically in terms of analgesic effect and peripheral blood concentrations of local anesthetic (see Chapter 9). Early measurements of lidocaine uptake in 1961 using colorimetric methods (Bromage and Robson, 1961) have since been confirmed by more sophisticated gas chromatographic methods for a number of agents (Braid and Scott, 1965), and there is general agreement that peak blood concentrations are reduced 20 to 50 per cent by adding 1/200,000 epinephrine, even when powerful binding agents, such as bupivacaine, are used (Reynolds and Taylor, 1971; Scott et al., 1972; Mather et al., 1976).

When these studies are taken in conjunction with data of clinical effectiveness, there seems to be overwhelming evidence that epinephrine re-

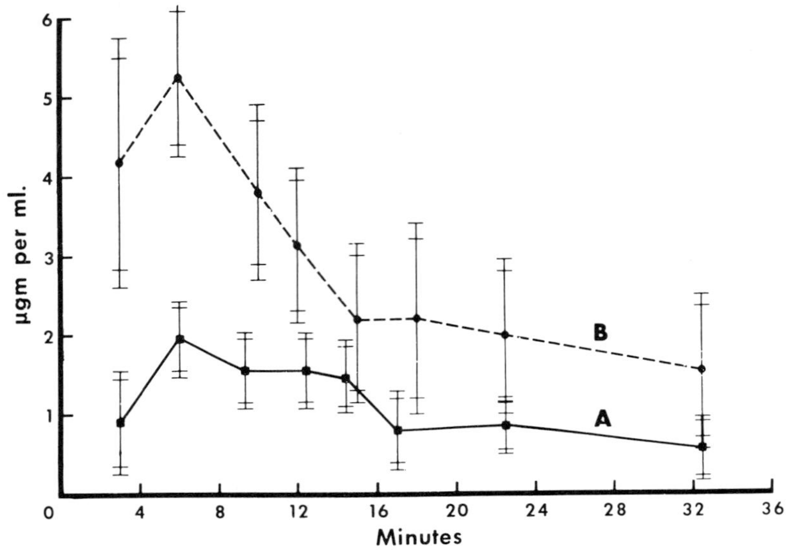

Figure 3–11. Effects of epinephrine on vascular absorption of local anesthetic from the epidural space of dogs. Net concentrations of mepivacaine in the azygos vein after epidural injection of 100 mg of 2 per cent ^{14}C-labeled mepivacaine.
Curve A: mepivacaine + 1/200,000 epinephrine
Curve B: mepivacaine plain
(Means ± 90 and 95 per cent confidence limits)
(From Burfoot and Bromage, Anesthesiology, 1971.)

duces vascular absorption and sways the competition for uptake in favor of more intense neural blockade. Other vasoconstrictors, such as octapressin, have similar effects, but to date, epinephrine still appears to be the superior agent for clinical use.

The time course of vascular uptake from the epidural space varies from agent to agent, depending on the diffusion characteristics and dosage of the drug and the presence or absence of epinephrine. In man, peak concentrations in the blood occur 15 to 25 minutes after injection, and the systemic effects of the injected material will be most apparent during this period. Obviously, very high and very rapid peak levels will be attained if injection is made accidentally into an extradural vein instead of into the epidural space.

Hyaluronidase

The gel of intercellular ground substance is a minor component of the barrier to diffusion and spread of local anesthetics across tissue planes. Hyaluronic acid, an important constituent of the mucopolysaccharides in this gel, is structurally altered by the depolarizing action of hyaluronidase, thus reducing the effectiveness of the intercellular cement as a tissue barrier. Hyaluronidase has been used to increase vascular uptake from injection sites (Mushin, 1956), and Scott (1956) reported on it favorably as a means to shorten the onset of epidural blockade. However, Bromage and Burfoot (1966) found hyaluronidase to be quite unsuitable as an additive for epidural blockade, as it caused no appreciable shortening of latency, and the quality of sensory and motor blockade was markedly impaired.

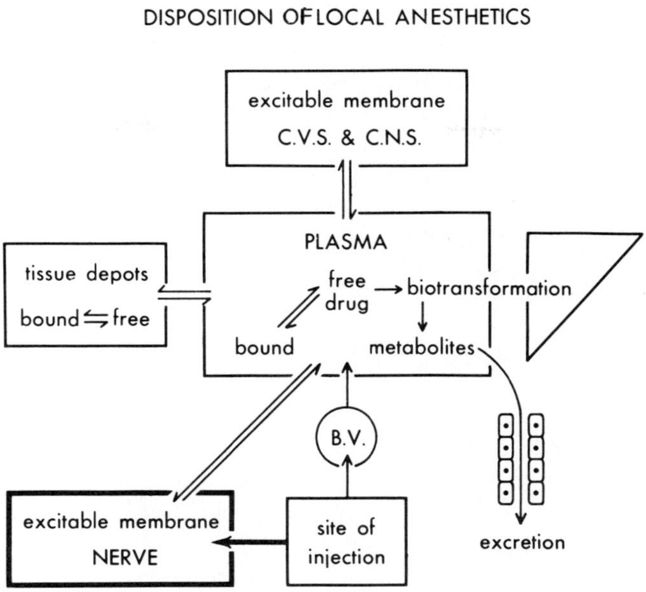

Figure 3–12. Outline of disposition and elimination of local anesthetics. Uptake into nerves and blood vessels (B.V.) leads to distribution into plasma, tissue depots and potentially toxic sites in CNS and CVS. Biotransformation occurs in plasma and/or liver. Elimination of metabolized and some unchanged drug occurs in urine.

Disposal

Figure 3–12 outlines the general scheme of uptake and elimination of local anesthetic drugs from the epidural space. In continuous epidural anesthesia, we are concerned with the rate at which local anesthetic will accumulate in the body, and it is important to have some idea of the variables that will determine safe blood concentrations during prolonged administration.

Depots

Uptake by fat and protein binding sites is greater with agents that exhibit high lipid solubility and strong protein binding. For example, lidocaine is removed from the circulation and bound to depot sites at about twice the speed of procaine (although procaine is broken down faster in the blood) (Sung and Truant, 1954). Among the amide-type agents, bupivacaine and etidocaine have greater binding capabilities than lidocaine or mepivacaine, as shown in Table 3–2.

TABLE 3–2 Binding of Amide-Type Local Anesthetics in Adult Human Plasma (Drug Concentration in Plasma = 2.0 μg/ml)

Drug	*Percentage Binding at pH 7.4*
Etidocaine	92
Bupivacaine	95.6*
Lidocaine	64.3*
Mepivacaine	77.5*

*Data from Tucker et al. (1970a and b).

Thus, bupivacaine and etidocaine are removed from the free unbound state onto plasma proteins and other binding sites very rapidly, and free plasma levels are kept low. Other substances in the plasma with strong protein binding affinities may compete for binding sites and displace local anesthetic molecules. Competitive binding of this sort may lead to unexpectedly high levels of free local anesthetic in the blood and greater toxicity (Ghoneim and Pandya, 1974). An example of this is the presence of bilirubin in the fetal blood, which in a concentration of 3 mg/100 ml reduces the binding affinity of plasma proteins by about 50 per cent (Chignell et al., 1971).

BIOTRANSFORMATION (METABOLIC BREAKDOWN)

Ester-type anesthetics, such as procaine and tetracaine, are hydrolyzed and rapidly inactivated by plasma cholinesterase in the blood stream. The rate of hydrolysis depends on molecular configuration. Chloroprocaine appears to be a very safe agent in this regard, while tetracaine persists unchanged for much longer (Table 3–3).

Amide-type anesthetics are broken down predominantly in the liver. The process is relatively slow, so these agents tend to persist unchanged (although bound) for longer than the ester-type agents.

Hydrolysis

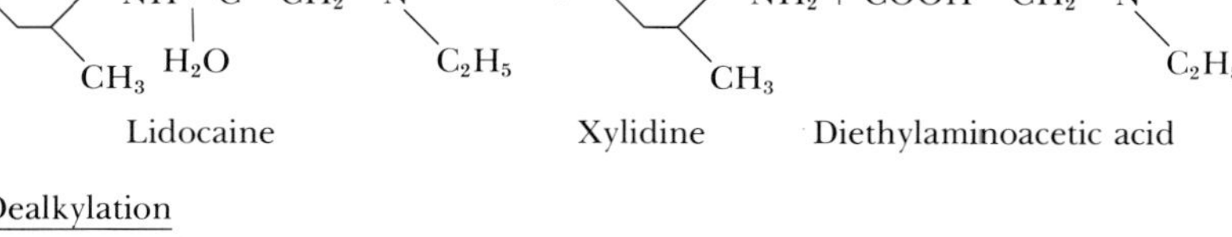

Lidocaine — Xylidine — Diethylaminoacetic acid

Dealkylation

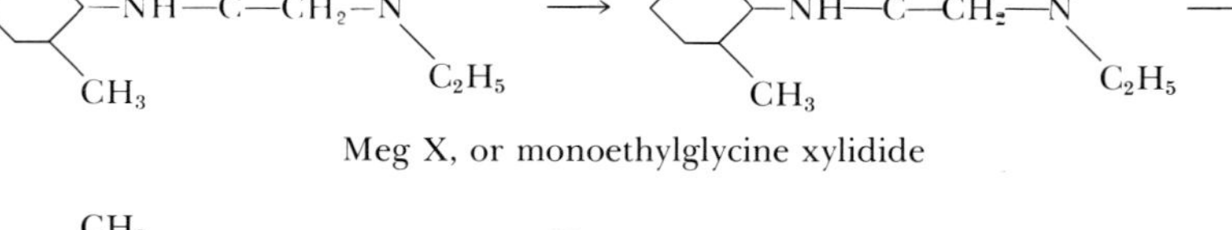

Meg X, or monoethylglycine xylidide

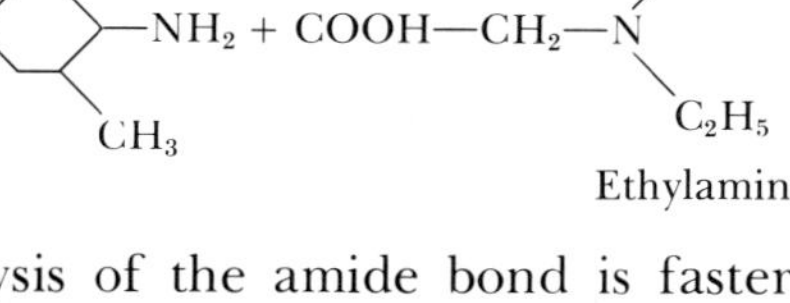

Ethylaminoacetic acid

Hydrolysis of the amide bond is faster after dealkylation or when only one methyl group protects the amide link, as in prilocaine (Citanest).

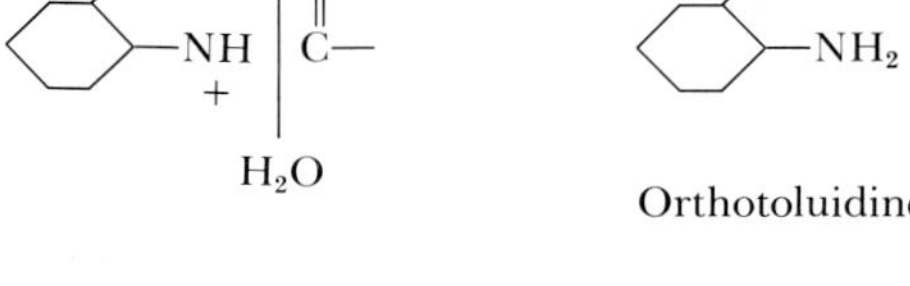

Orthotoluidine

TABLE 3–3 Rate of Hydrolysis (Ester-type Agents)*

Agent	*Hydrolysis Rate (μM/ml/hour)*
Tetracaine	0.3
Procaine	1.1
Chloroprocaine	4.7

*Foldes et al., Clin. Pharmacol. Ther. *6*:328, 1965.

The orthotoluidine residue from prilocaine enters red cells and allows hemoglobin to become oxidized to methemoglobin (Geddes, 1967). With small doses of prilocaine, methemoglobinemia is not clinically apparent, but doses of over 600 mg in 70-kg adults should be avoided. Fetal hemoglobin is unusually susceptible to oxidation, and as little as 200 mg of prilocaine administered as a paracervical block to the mother at delivery has been associated with clinical methemoglobinemia in the newborn (Harley and Celermajer, 1970).

Excretion

Breakdown products and unchanged drugs are excreted wherever secretions are formed. Significant amounts of cation are excreted unchanged from the stomach, bile and urine. In man only about 5 to 10 per cent of unchanged lidocaine is excreted in the urine (Sung and Truant, 1954; Beckett, Boyes and Appleton, 1966). The amount of renal clearance is markedly affected by changes in urinary pH, greater quantities being excreted by the "cationic-trap" mechanism of an acid urine (Eriksson and Granberg, 1965), as shown in Figure 3–8.

While the ester-type local anesthetics are rapidly cloven by hydrolysis to *p*-aminobenzoic acid and then excreted in the urine, the amide local anesthetics are much more slowly eliminated from the body. Therefore, although the amide local anesthetics are rapidly *distributed* and dispersed throughout their available distribution volumes, their slow *elimination* may give rise to cumulative effects if large doses are administered at frequent intervals.

Precise excretion and elimination studies are difficult to conduct in human subjects, and some products of drug metabolism may escape detection and therefore appear to be retained in the body (Reynolds, 1971). After breakdown in the liver the amide drugs and their products are excreted in the urine; wide species variations exist. Table 3–4 from data by Keenaghan and Boyes (1972) shows the percentage of lidocaine and lidocaine products excreted in the urine of animals and man during the first 24 hours after oral administration of lidocaine.

Radioactive tracer studies in animals show the time course of the distribution and elimination of local anesthetics more clearly than any other method. Figure 3–13, drawn from data by Goehl and associates (1973), shows the distribution and gradual disappearance of tritium-labeled bupivacaine from various organs in the monkey after a subcutaneous injection of 2 mg per kilogram body weight of bupivacaine. This amount is approximately equivalent

TABLE 3-4 Species Variation in the Metabolism and Excretion of Lidocaine 24 Hours After Oral Administration*

Species: / *Oral Dose of Lidocaine (mg/kg):*	*Rat* 20	*Guinea Pig* 10	*Dog* 20	*Man* 3
COMPOUND	% DOSE RECOVERED IN URINE			
Lidocaine	0.2	0.5	2.0	2.8
Monoethylglycinexylidide (Meg X)	0.7	14.9	2.3	3.7
Glycinexylidide	2.1	3.3	12.6	2.3
3-Hydroxylidocaine	31.2	0.5	6.7	1.1
3-Hydroxymonoethylglycinexylidide	36.9	2.0	3.1	0.3
2,6-Xylidine	1.5	16.2	1.6	1.0
4-Hydroxy-2,6-dimethylaniline	12.4	16.4	35.2	72.6
Total:	85.0	53.8	63.5	83.8

*Data from Keenaghan and Boyes (1962).

to a sizable clinical dose in a human subject. It can be seen that elimination is quite slow. Moderate amounts of the drug are present in highly perfused organs such as brain, liver and kidney at six hours, and small amounts are still present at the end of 24 hours.

In the presence of this slow rate of elimination, large and repeated doses of local anesthetic are likely to lead to progressive accumulation in the body (Moore et al., 1968). If administration of the drug in excessive dosage is continued long enough, a time will eventually arrive when the body's large

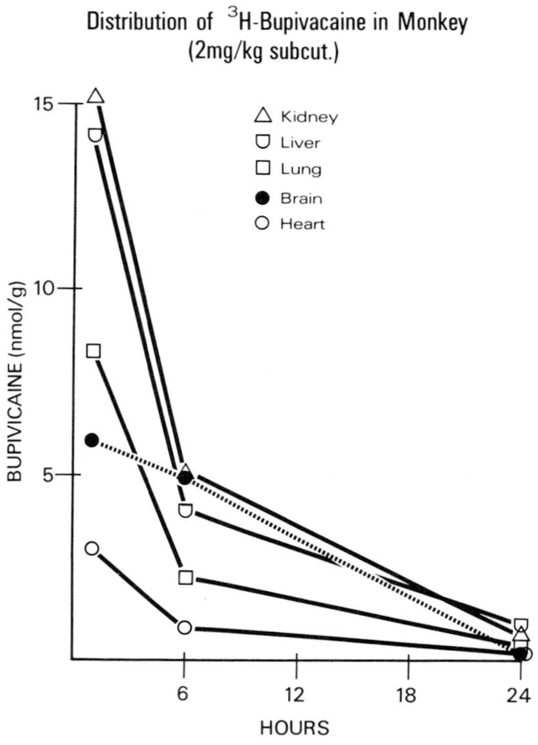

Figure 3-13. Distribution and slow elimination of tritium-labeled bupivacaine in the monkey, following subcutaneous injection of 2 mg/kg. (After Goehl, Davenport and Stanley, 1973.)

distribution volume of lipid stores becomes saturated. From then on, rapidly rising blood levels of unchanged drug and active metabolites will cause signs of overt toxicity if further dosage is continued. For this reason dosage schedules in continuous epidural blockade should always be as parsimonious as possible, and the tendency to drug accumulation should be kept in mind whenever prolonged therapeutic blockade is indicated. Toxic accumulation is not likely to occur with the ester-type anesthetics which are rapidly broken down in the blood stream. However, at the time of writing these agents are not among the most effective from a clinical point of view. When the more powerful amide agents are used, toxic accumulation is likely to occur faster with drugs having a relatively short duration and low lipid solubility (e.g., mepivacaine) than with the long-acting agents having a high lipid solubility, such as etidocaine. Long-acting and highly lipid-soluble drugs need to be injected less frequently than short-acting agents, and they are sequestered out of circulation more safely in the body's lipid stores (Henn and Brattsand, 1966).

TOXICITY

Toxic depression of excitable membranes in the central nervous system and the cardiovascular system depends on:

1. Net tissue levels resulting from the balance of uptake, distribution and elimination of the agent absorbed from the epidural space. Tissue levels will depend on the tissue/blood partition coefficient of the drug and the rate of tissue perfusion. Uptake is greatest in tissues with high perfusion rates, such as heart, liver and brain. Tissue concentrations in highly perfused organs may be 3 to 4 times greater than in the blood (Finster et al., 1972).

2. The state of receptor membranes at the time, determined by factors such as ionic concentrations and acid-base balance.

In order to avoid confusion, we will consider these two elements separately, but in practice they operate together. The apparently paradoxical effects of pH and pCO_2 on acute toxicity only make sense when it is appreciated that changes of acid-base balance affect both distribution of the drug *and* the receptor sites at the same time. Measurement of tissue concentration of drug by itself gives an incomplete picture of events at the membrane, as membrane permeability may be greatly affected by modifications of electrical charge in the membrane itself.

In practice, local anesthetics become much more toxic than usual under conditions of acidosis, and animals and men with respiratory acidosis are more prone to convulsions (Munson et al., 1970; Munson and Wagman, 1969) and cardiovascular depression (Andersson et al., 1970) than when hypercapnia is corrected. Considering the availability of cation and its distribution across lipid membranes, this seems to be a paradoxical situation, for one might expect that diffusion into the CNS and the cardiovascular tissues would be less and not greater than usual, on the basis of distribution of cationic and noncationic moieties and the fact that there should be more nondiffusible cation present in the circulation during acidosis, as Table 3–5 shows with values for bupivacaine, lidocaine and mepivacaine at normal pH and under conditions of slight acidosis at pH 7.0. However, this simple theoretical approach does not fit the observed

TABLE 3–5 Percentage of Local Anesthetic as Diffusible Nonionized Base and Nondiffusible Charged Cation at Normal and Slightly Acidotic pH

Drug	*Diffusible Nonionized Base (%)* *pH 7.4*	*pH 7.0*	*Nondiffusible Charged Cation (%)* *pH 7.4*	*pH 7.0*
Bupivacaine	18	8	82	92
Lidocaine	26	12	74	88
Mepivacaine	36	18	64	82

facts, either clinically or under controlled laboratory conditions, and one must conclude that some of the changes observed are due to alterations of tissue membranes under acidotic conditions.

Two very elegant studies from Uppsala, Sweden, have thrown some light on this problem. Sjöstrand and Widman (1973) carried out infusion experiments of tritium-labeled bupivacaine in rabbits under normal and acidotic conditions, and they found two very interesting things. First, blood concentrations of bupivacaine in the acidotic rabbits were about twice as high as in the normal rabbits, as shown in Figure 3–14, while the proportion of drug carried in the red cells rather than in the plasma rose from about 9 per cent to 14 per cent.

Second, the amount of drug taken up by rapidly perfused organs such as brain, heart, lungs, liver and kidneys rose by 28 per cent. Under these circumstances the proportion of active cationic form present in the brain and heart would be increased by the tissue acidosis, and therefore the drug would be proportionately more active and more toxic at membrane sites in the myocardium and central nervous system.

Englesson (1974) extended the earlier seizure threshold work of DeJong (1964) and Munson and his colleagues (1969, 1970) under rigorously controlled conditions of acute and chronic respiratory acidosis in cats, using a number of different local anesthetics. He showed that a complex helical relationship exists between toxicity and the plasma pH and pCO_2 of the animal, probably reflecting the intracellular pH changes brought about by differential mobilities of carbon dioxide, hydrogen ion and bicarbonate across cell membranes. This work confirmed earlier studies that had shown increasing toxicity

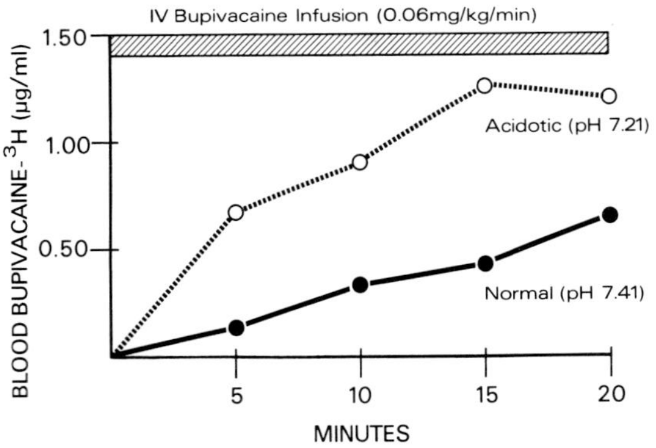

Figure 3–14. Toxicity of local anesthetic drugs: intravenous infusion of tritium-labeled bupivacaine in normal and acidotic rabbits. Note high blood concentrations of bupivacaine in acidotic animals. (After Sjöstrand and Widman, 1973.)

TABLE 3–6 Influence of pH on Central Nervous System Toxicity in the Cat*

	Seizure	*No Seizure*
Dose of lidocaine (mg/kg)	14.2	60
Blood concentration of lidocaine (μg/ml)	26.2	17.8
pH	7.30	7.43
pCO_2	31	21

*Data from Englesson (1974).

for lidocaine and prilocaine with rising pCO_2 (Englesson, Paymaster and Hill, 1965).

Englesson also confirmed the observations of Sjöstrand and Widman that higher and more toxic blood levels of local anesthetics are encountered in acidotic than in alkalotic situations (Table 3–6). In this study a cat convulsed with a small dose and a high blood level of lidocaine under acidotic conditions, while the same animal had a low blood concentration and failed to convulse after a much larger dose of lidocaine under alkalotic conditions.

The general pattern of the influence of carbon dioxide on local anesthetic mobility, activity and toxicity now begins to fall into place. The familiar concept of local anesthetic distribution across a cell membrane can be extended from a single cell or axon to encompass the idea of distribution volumes within the body as a whole (Boyes et al., 1971; Rowland et al., 1971; De Jong et al., 1972; Englesson, 1974).

Let us imagine that the sum of both the water phase and the lipid phase in the body is represented by two compartmental volumes. The initial volume available for distribution in the water phase will be quite small and approximately equal to the blood volume, before the drug has had time to diffuse out into the extracellular and intracellular water. The available lipid phase is relatively enormous and 40 to 1,000 times greater than the water phase, depending on the lipid solubility of the local anesthetic agent. The drug will distribute itself between the water and lipid phases according to its degree of ionization, with the possibilities shown in Figure 3–15.

These distribution patterns are reflected in the shape of decay curves of blood concentration after injection of a bolus intravenous dose of

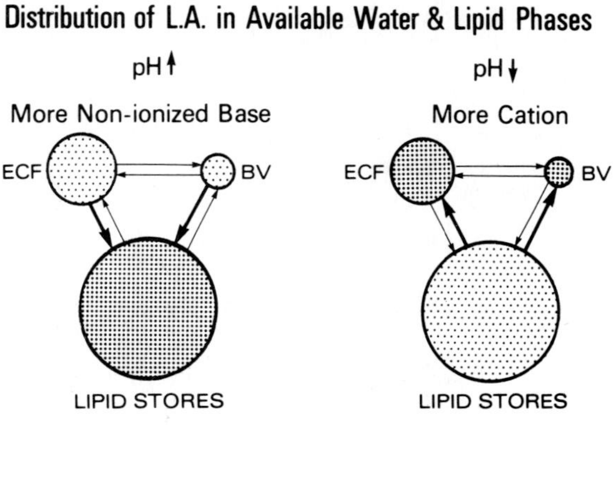

Figure 3–15. Relative distribution volumes for local anesthetic in body lipid and water phases. The water space is subdivided into the circulating blood volume (BV) and the extracellular fluid (ECF). Concentration of local anesthetic is represented by density of stipple. The *relative* lipid distribution is enlarged in alkalosis and contracted in acidosis.

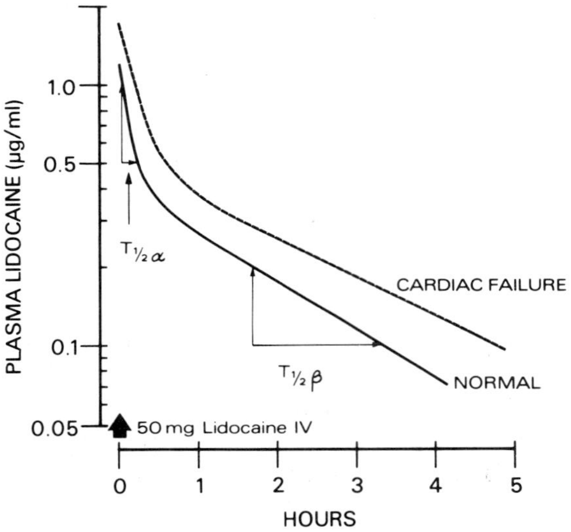

Figure 3–16. Plasma decay curves after IV bolus injection of 50 mg lidocaine in normal subjects and in heart failure.
$T_{1/2\alpha}$: initial distribution in blood, ECF and rapidly perfused tissues
$T_{1/2\beta}$: "steady-state" distribution to intracellular water and lipid stores
(After Thomson et al., 1973.)

local anesthetic (Rowland et al., 1971). Blood concentrations rise to a rapid peak and then decline in an exponential fashion, as shown in Figure 3–16 (Thomson et al., 1973). The curves are biexponential. That is to say, there is an initial very steep decline of blood concentration as the local anesthetic is quickly diluted in the blood volume, extracellular fluid and rapidly perfused tissues such as heart and lungs. A later "steady-state" distribution phase occurs as drug is taken up in total body water and in body lipids. The plasma half-life ($T\frac{1}{2}$) of the drug is readily measured by plotting these curves on semi-logarithmic paper and then reading off the time taken for the drug concentration to be reduced by one half. In patients with heart failure, peripheral blood flow is reduced and uptake into lipids is slower than normal, so that the plasma half-life is prolonged and the apparent volume of distribution is reduced (Stenson et al., 1971; Thomson et al., 1973). A similar slowing of distribution is seen in normal patients under general anesthesia (Adjepon-Yamoah et al., 1973) and in animals with reduced cardiac outputs from pretreatment with propranolol (Branch et al., 1973).

A third and ultrarapid distribution phase could be demonstrated if sampling methods were available and fast enough to measure the "slug of drug" effect that occurs while the initial bolus of drug is traveling in high concentration during its first transit through the circulation. This is an important distribution concentration that determines acute toxic effects during accidental and rapid intravenous injection, and it will be considered in more detail later in this chapter. Steady-state half-lives and apparent volumes of distribution for intravenous lidocaine, bupivacaine and etidocaine in normal subjects are shown in Table 3–7.

The highly lipid-soluble nature of etidocaine gives it an apparent distribution volume that is larger than that of the other two agents. Therefore, blood concentrations of etidocaine are generally much lower than those of lidocaine or bupivacaine, and the toxicity of etidocaine is also correspondingly low, *provided the speed of uptake is slow.* However, with a rapid bolus type of injection, as may occur with accidental intravenous injection into an epidural

TABLE 3–7 Steady-State Half-life and Distribution Volumes for Lidocaine, Bupivacaine and Etidocaine After Rapid Intravenous Infusions

Drug	*Steady-State Half-Life ($T_{\frac{1}{2}\beta}$) (minutes)*	*Steady-State Distribution Volume (V_{ss}) (liters)*
Lidocaine	98*	91*
Bupivacaine	76‡	72†
Etidocaine	57‡	133†

*Data from Thomson et al. (1973).
†Data from Tucker and Mather (1975).
‡Data from Scott et al. (1973).

vein, there is no time for the drug to distribute in the lipid phase, and then the toxicity of etidocaine rises dramatically.

The pathways for uptake, distribution and elimination of local anesthetics from the epidural space are summarized in Figure 3–17. Compared to the relatively simple uptake and distribution from an intravenous infusion, this situation is more complex, and different kinetic equations have been proposed (Tucker and Mather, 1975). Epidural fat and other lipid and protein sites in and around the spinal canal provide a depot for considerable quantities of local anesthetic drug, and these stores are gradually released into the circulation as if a slow intravenous infusion were taking place within the spinal canal. Attempts to express the relevant pharmacokinetics in mathematical terms through either biexponential or triexponential equations have resulted in a proliferation of Greek symbols that may be confusing to the average reader, so a short resumé is necessary. The following pharmacokinetic symbols will be encountered in the literature of epidural uptake and distribution:

$T_{\frac{1}{2}\alpha}$ Plasma half-life for rapid phase of local anesthetic distribution in blood volume (Belfrage et al., 1975; Magno et al., 1976)

$T_{\frac{1}{2}\beta}$ Plasma half-life for slow phase of elimination (Belfrage et al., 1975; Magno et al., 1976)

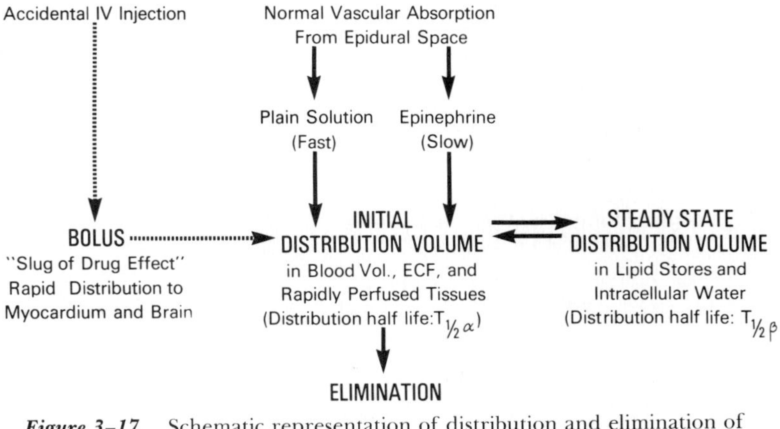

Figure 3–17. Schematic representation of distribution and elimination of local anesthetics injected into the epidural space (see text).

$T_{\frac{1}{2}\gamma}$ Plasma half-life for ultraslow phase of elimination in a triexponential equation (Tucker and Mather, 1975)

$T_{\frac{1}{2}\chi}$ A revised expression for the rapid phase of distribution in a biexponential equation (Stanton-Hicks et al., 1976; Mather et al., 1976a)

$T_{\frac{1}{2}\psi}$ A revised expression for the slow phase of elimination in a biexponential equation (Stanton-Hicks et al., 1976; Mather et al., 1976a)

For ease of interpreting and reconciling the data from several research groups, in Table 3–8 I have retained the earlier symbols for a biexponential curve; that is, $T_{\frac{1}{2}\alpha}$ represents the early phase of distribution, and $T_{\frac{1}{2}\beta}$ represents the later slow phase of elimination (Belfrage et al., 1975; Magno et al., 1976). In so doing I have taken the liberty of lumping together $T_{\frac{1}{2}\beta}$, $T_{\frac{1}{2}\gamma}$ and $T_{\frac{1}{2}\psi}$ under one single heading of $T_{\frac{1}{2}\beta}$. The enormous individual variations for "$T_{\frac{1}{2}\psi}$" reported by Stanton-Hicks and his colleagues (1976) suggest that this simplification may not be of any serious mathematical consequence.

Table 3–8 summarizes the data from several authors on the distribution and elimination half-lives for lidocaine, bupivacaine and etidocaine after epidural injection. The rapid phase of distribution ($T_{\frac{1}{2}\alpha}$) is practically identical for all three drugs (except in parturient women) and about twice as long as after intravenous infusion. However, the slow phase of elimination ($T_{\frac{1}{2}\beta}$) varies widely and unpredictably, even in healthy subjects. In the series

TABLE 3–8 Decay of Plasma Concentrations of Local Anesthetic After Epidural Injection—Rapid and Slow Distribution Half-Lives ($T_{\frac{1}{2}\alpha}$ and $T_{\frac{1}{2}\beta}$) for Lidocaine, Bupivacaine and Etidocaine

	Drug	*Rapid Elimination* $T_{\frac{1}{2}\alpha}$ *(minutes ± S.D.)*	*Slow Elimination* $T_{\frac{1}{2}\beta}$ *(minutes ± S.D.)*
Volunteers			
2%	Lidocaine		
	Plain	13*	426*
	+ 1/200,000 epinephrine	18*	162*
0.5%	Bupivacaine		
	Plain	–	–
	+ 1/200,000 epinephrine	19 ± 10†	440 ± 365†
1%	Etidocaine		
	Plain	24 ± 12‡	390 ± 210‡
	+ 1/200,000 epinephrine	20 ± 5†	497 ± 336†
Obstetrical Patients			
0.25%	Bupivacaine		
	+ 1/200,000 epinephrine	–	540 ± 36§
0.75%	Bupivacaine plain		
	Maternal	47 ± 15‖	564 ± 186‖
	Neonatal	28 ± 10‖	486 ± 150‖

*Tucker and Mather (1975).
†Stanton-Hicks et al. (1976).
‡Mather et al. (1976a).
§Belfrage et al. (1975).
‖Magno et al. (1976).

published by Stanton-Hicks et al. (1976), the experimental subjects were young, fit volunteers with an average weight of 83.9 ± 9.2 kg, yet their $T\frac{1}{2}\beta$ ranged between 3.7 hours and 17.8 hours for bupivacaine and between 3 hours and 16.3 hours for etidocaine. The precise cause of these wide individual differences in the slow elimination phase is unknown at the present time, but many variables are involved, including the characteristics of lipid and protein depots in the spinal canal, hepatic function and blood flow, and blood flow in the extradural space. Even a transient surge of blood flow from an IV injection of a vasopressor such as ephedrine will cause a measurable increase in vascular uptake of local anesthetic from the epidural space (Mather et al., 1976b). It is not surprising that the vector of all these variables expressed as $T\frac{1}{2}\beta$ should be such a very individual and unpredictable factor. The obstetrical data by Magno et al. (1976) is interesting in that the elimination characteristics of bupivacaine in the newborn seem to be surprisingly similar to those in the nonpregnant adult. This would suggest that both age groups are likely to recover from toxic concentrations of local anesthetic in roughly the same time.

Normally, analgesic potency and toxicity go hand in hand. The greater the potency of a local anesthetic on peripheral nerves, the more likely it is to be toxic at other excitable membranes in the central nervous system and cardiovascular system. A systemic rise of pH or pCO_2 is likely to make the agent more effective peripherally, but central toxicity will also increase in accordance with the model in Figure 3–15. The only way to break away from the normal association of potency and toxicity is through the use of carbonated local anesthetics. With these agents hypercapnia is confined to the injection site, and increased cation is available where it is intended, without decreasing lipid storage in the rest of the body.

The theoretical treatment of overdosage and systemic toxic reactions from local anesthetics is quite clear from Figure 3–15. Since alkalosis and hypocapnia favor lipid storage and remove cation from the blood and tissue fluids, it follows that hyperventilation and carbon dioxide elimination should be the first line of therapy, followed if necessary by intravenous administration of sodium bicarbonate. In practice the urgency of a convulsive toxic reaction does not allow time for management by manipulation of the acid-base status, and faster measures must be taken. Convulsions must be controlled by intravenous diazepam in doses of 2.5 to 10 mg, and vasopressors may be indicated if arterial hypotension occurs.

Factors Modifying Toxicity

Competitive binding

Positively charged drugs or biochemical products may compete with circulating local anesthetic and bind to tissue or plasma protein sites that would otherwise be available to "mop up" the cationic local anesthetic. Bilirubin in the newborn is the commonest example of this phenomenon. Serum bilirubin concentration in normal adults is about 0.3 to 0.7 mg/100 ml, but in the newborn this level may rise to 3.0 mg/100 ml, a four- to tenfold increase (Chignell et al., 1971). This phenomenon is shown schematically in Figure 3–18. In addition the binding capacity of fetal proteins is less than in the adult.

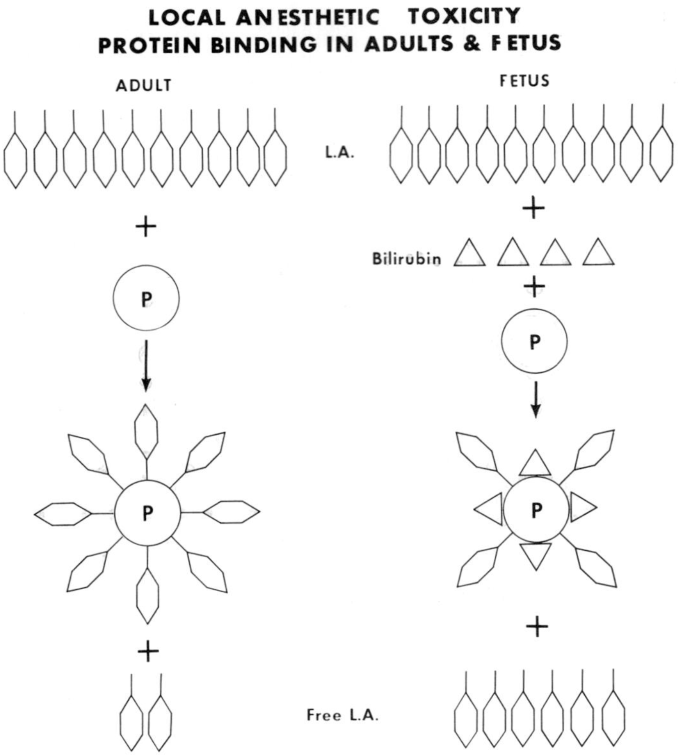

Figure 3–18. Competitive protein binding and local anesthetic toxicity. Bilirubin and certain positively charged drugs compete for protein binding sites, leaving more unbound local anesthetic free in the plasma to exert toxic effects.

Local anesthetic
Ⓟ Plasma protein
△ Bilirubin (or other competing substances)

From a clinical point of view, it follows that local anesthetic drugs are relatively more toxic in the fetus than in the adult, as more free cation is available at any given concentration of drug. Other agents such as meperidine, diphenylhydantoin, quinidine and desipramine may also compete for protein binding sites (Ghoneim and Pandya, 1974).

Renal failure

Patients with uremia and anemia secondary to renal failure have some degree of metabolic acidosis, and plasma proteins are often lower than normal. These patients are more prone to local anesthetic toxicity than the normal population, and they should be treated circumspectly. A hyperdynamic circulation goes along with the anemia, and cardiac output is raised (Mostert et al., 1970). Duration of action of local anesthetic is shortened proportionally, so maintenance injections may have to be given more frequently than usual in these patients, with the added hazard of large cumulative doses (Bromage and Gertel, 1969).

Temperature

Morishima et al. (1971) found that circulating concentrations of lidocaine were slow to decline in newborn puppies that were allowed to become chilled. Impaired excretion could be due to reduced microsomal activity in the liver. However, once again the question of acid-base balance arises, as the chilled puppies were more acidotic than warm ones, and plasma levels of local anesthetic therefore tended to remain high from retention of the water-soluble cationic form circulating in the plasma (Fig. 3–19).

Very definite and important clinical implications arise from these animal experiments. Babies must be protected from heat loss by being dried and placed in a warm environment as soon as possible after birth to prevent hypothermia and acidosis. Maintenance of a normal body temperature is particularly important if high drug levels are present in the fetus, in order to ensure a normal body pH and a large "distribution volume" for dispersion of circulating local anesthetic into lipid storage sites.

Circadian rhythm

Many species show differences in susceptibility to different drugs at different times of the day and night. Lutsch and Morris (1967) showed that

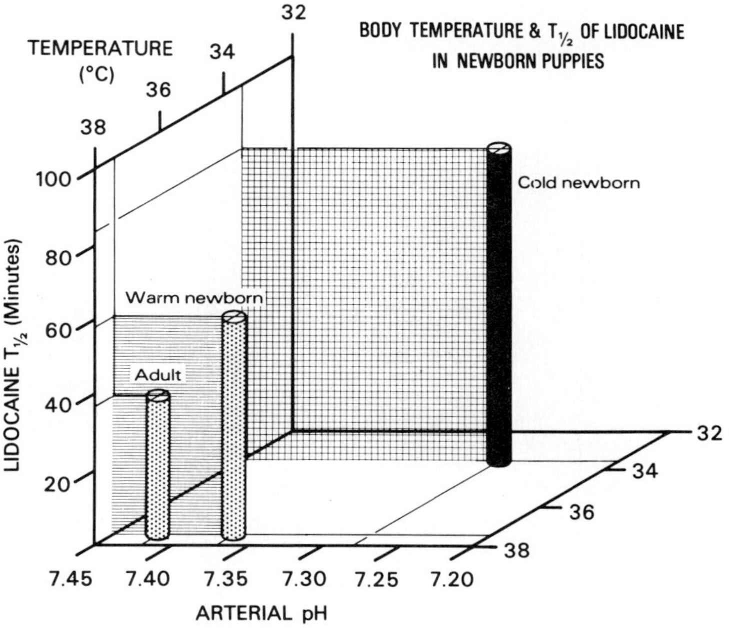

Figure 3–19. Influence of body temperature on arterial pH and rate of fall of plasma lidocaine concentration ($T_{1/2}$) in newborn puppies. The $T_{1/2}$ is 56 per cent longer in normal puppies than in adults and 124 per cent longer in hypothermic puppies. (After Morishima et al., 1971.)

mice have a very marked circadian periodicity in their susceptibility to lidocaine toxicity. This nocturnal animal was about ten times more susceptible to convulsions during the hours of its evening activities than during its siesta time in the middle of the day. No data exist for similar circadian susceptibility in man, but one might suppose that the cycle would be in opposite phase to the nocturnal mouse, with maximum susceptibility in daylight hours.

TACHYPHYLAXIS

Tachyphylaxis is a name of Greek origin for acute tolerance, and as is so often the case when a condition is given a long imposing name, its basis is ill understood. Repeated injections of local anesthetics produce successively diminishing effect in duration and in quality of blockade (Bromage et al., 1964; Bromage, 1967). Acute tolerance or tachyphylaxis is a nuisance in epidural analgesia, and although unavoidable, its effects can be reduced in ways which will be discussed in Chapter 7.

Tachyphylaxis, or acute tolerance to local anesthetic drugs, has been observed following topical applications (Régnier and Lambin, 1938) as well as after injection (Griffié and Brunel, 1959; Lechat et al., 1962), and its occurrence is well recognized in association with subarachnoid (Smith and Rees, 1948), caudal (Brown, 1948) and lumbar epidural anesthesia (Soehring et al., 1954; Bonica, 1957; Bryce-Smith and Williams, 1955; Cox and Spoerel, 1964; Bromage et al., 1964; Bromage, 1967; Bromage et al., 1969).

Bromage and his colleagues studied epidural tachyphylaxis in man by observing the changes in segmental spread and duration of blockade that occurred with successive doses of epidural local anesthetic, as shown in Figure

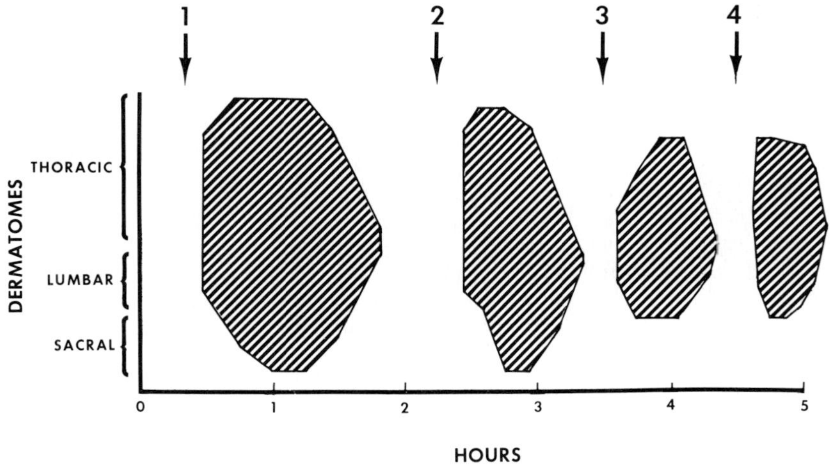

Figure 3–20. Example of acute tolerance to repeated epidural injections. Diminishing segment-minute diagrams of cutaneous analgesia in a 65-year-old woman after abdominal surgery; 150 mg plain lidocaine injected at each arrow. Considerable motor paralysis of the legs followed the first injection, but none followed the second, third and fourth doses. (From Bromage et al., J. Clin. Pharmacol., 1969.)

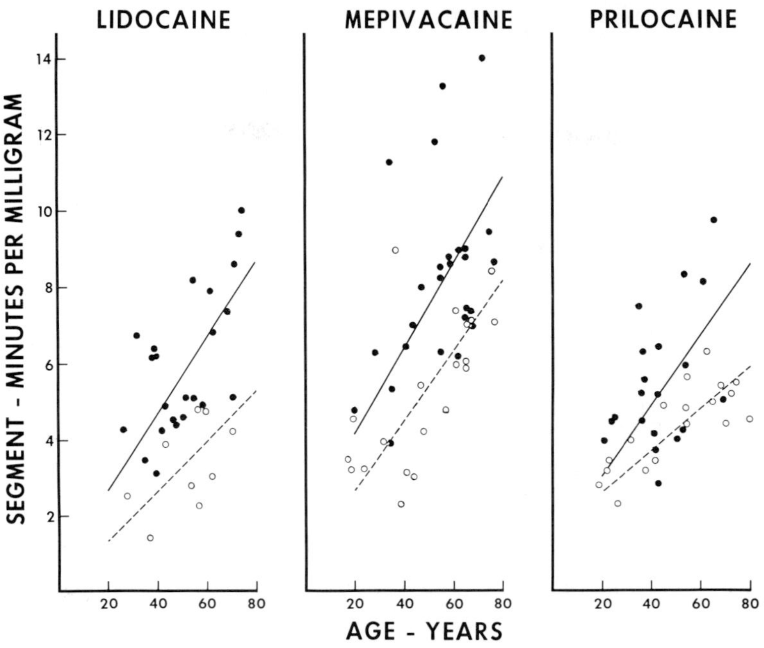

Figure 3–21. Comparative segment-minute responses to initial epidural injections related to age in 115 patients receiving 2 per cent solutions of lidocaine, mepivacaine or prilocaine. Calculated regression lines.
○ Plain solution
● With epinephrine 1/200,000
(From Bromage et al., J. Clin. Pharmacol., 1969.)

3–20. These results will be given in some detail, as they have important clinical implications in the management of continuous epidural analgesia. By plotting out the segmental spread and regression of each injection and computing each segment-time area, the effectiveness of each injection could be expressed numerically as so many "segment-minutes" per milligram of injected drug. The unit "segment-minutes per milligram" was then used as a quantitative basis for comparing the effectiveness of different agents, as well as their tendency to develop acute tolerance with successive injections. Figure 3–21 shows the segment-minutes per milligram calculated from the results of initial injections in 115 cases. There is a wide variation, but it can be seen that age is positively correlated with dose-response and that epinephrine causes a marked increase in the number of segment-minutes per milligram for each of the three drugs tested.

Figure 3–22 shows the raw data from a comparative study of lidocaine, mepivacaine and prilocaine in which 329 injections were given to 140 patients. In the figure, the segment-minutes per milligram for successive injections in each individual patient are joined by connecting lines. A general decay of effectiveness is apparent in the downward trend following successive injections of all three drugs tested. Clinically, the decay affected all measurable components of anesthesia. Fewer segments were anesthetized, the duration of action was shortened and motor and sensory blockade became less intense with each successive administration. Close inspection of Figure 3–22 reveals that

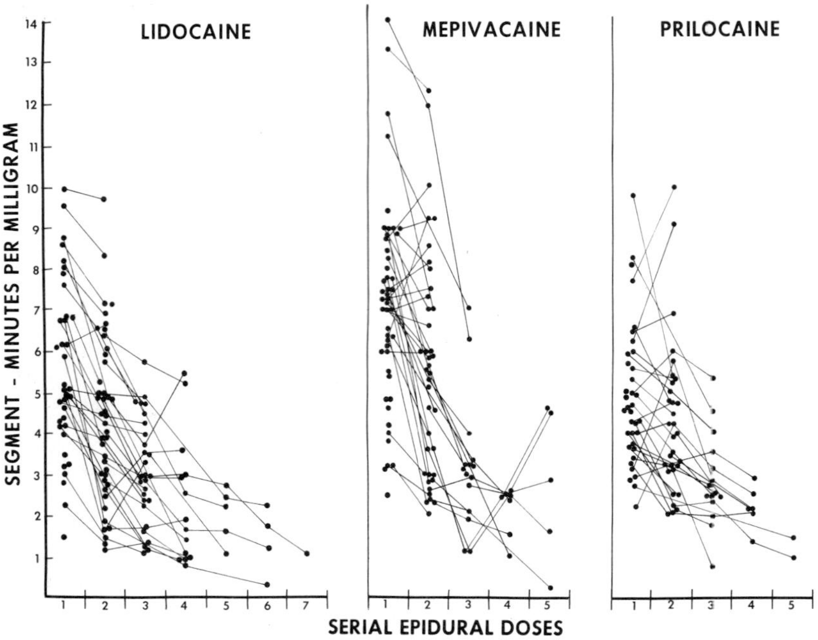

Figure 3–22. Segment-minute responses to 2 per cent solutions of lidocaine, mepivacaine or prilocaine with or without epinephrine 1/200,000 in 140 patients (329 injections). Connecting lines link successive doses in individual patients. (From Bromage et al., J. Clin. Pharmacol., 1969.)

some of the cases did not conform to the general downward trend but showed an augmented response instead of a decay.

Records of the cases showing augmentation of analgesic effectiveness were reexamined more closely for some explanation of their special behavior. In almost every instance it was found that an enhanced effect was associated with a relatively short interval between injections. It was therefore necessary to examine all the data for a possible relationship between change of response and the lapse of time between injections. The interval that appeared to be the most significant was the period between the disappearance of analgesia from the previous dose and the moment of the next injection, that is, the "interanalgesic interval." The mean changes of analgesic potency, in terms of segment-minutes per milligram, were grouped against duration of interanalgesic interval, as shown in Figure 3–23.

From Figure 3–23 it can be seen that analgesic potency tends to be augmented if the interanalgesic interval is short. However, augmentation declines and gives way to decay of effect and tachyphylaxis if the interval exceeds 10 minutes. Tachyphylaxis increases with the length of interanalgesic interval up to 60 minutes and is fairly constant thereafter. This relationship between tachyphylaxis and the timing of injection was not influenced by the number of injections given, for decay of effect could be prevented equally well at the second injection or the fifth, provided the interanalgesic interval was sufficiently short.

The tachyphylactic trends shown in the raw data of Figure 3–22 were now analyzed in greater detail, taking into account the previously unknown

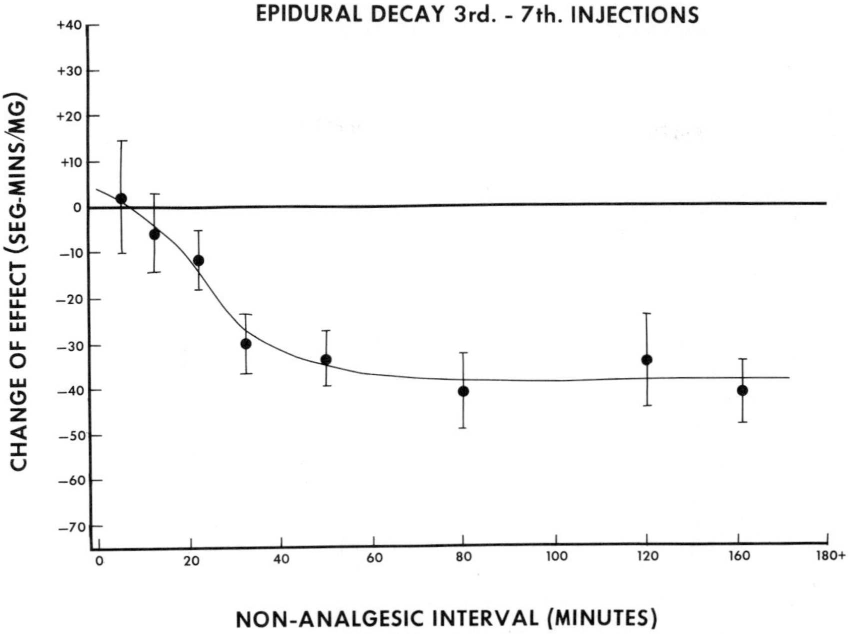

Figure 3–23. Augmentation or decay of analgesic effectiveness related to timing of administration of successive epidural injections. Influence of interanalgesic interval on response of one epidural injection in relation to that of its immediate predecessor. Mean ± SE. (From Bromage et al., J. Clin. Pharmacol., 1969.)

effects of the interanalgesic interval. The data were regrouped after all doses with an interanalgesic interval of less than 10 minutes were excluded, on the grounds that these were the ones that showed augmentation rather than decay and that it was these doses that were responsible for the small number of deviations from the general downward trend in Figure 3–22.

The regrouped observations are shown in Figure 3–24. The individual characteristics of the three drugs and the general trend with each successive injection can now be seen more clearly. Plain lidocaine has a relatively short action, but the duration is markedly prolonged by adding epinephrine. Plain mepivacaine has a longer action than either lidocaine or prilocaine, and the action of prilocaine is less affected by epinephrine than is that of the other two drugs.

All three local anesthetics showed the same ambivalent pattern of either augmentation or attenuation of effect, depending on the timing of succeeding doses, the crucial turning point being an interval of about 10 minutes after the preceding area of analgesia had disappeared (see Fig. 3–23). One may speculate that this time interval represents the period in which appreciable amounts of local anesthetic persist from the previous injection and that these residues probably combine with, or are activated by, the succeeding injection.

It is more difficult to find an explanation for the decay of effect that develops after a nonanalgesic interval of 10 minutes. The cause of tachyphylaxis is speculative, but several possibilities exist:

1. Local vasodilatation and edema at the injection site may cause progressively increased vascular uptake and disposal.

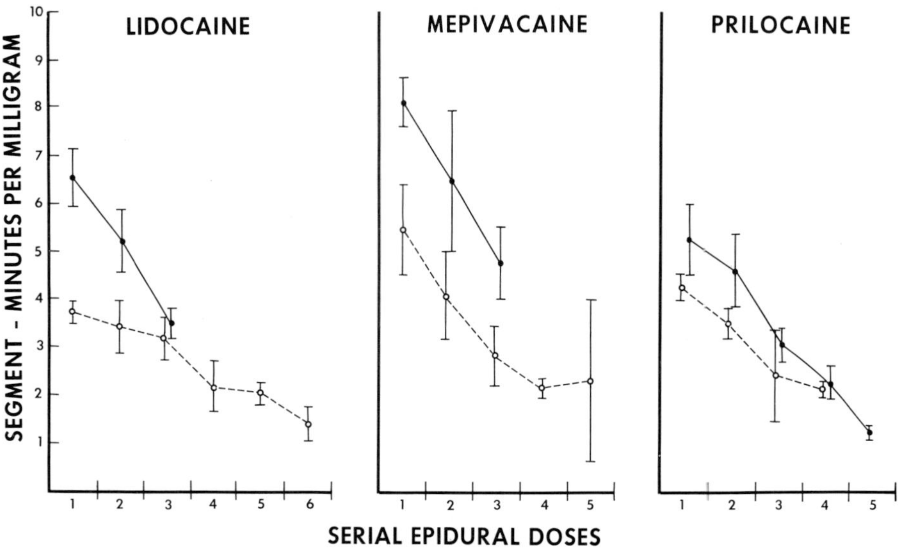

Figure 3–24. Epidural tachyphylaxis, or acute tolerance. Data from Figure 3–22 after all injections preceded by a nonanalgesic interval of less than 10 minutes are excluded. Means ± SE.

○------○ Plain solutions
●——● With 1/200,000 epinephrine

2. Local tissue reaction causes fibrin deposition and "walling off" of indwelling epidural catheters (Lebeaux, 1973). In chronic animal preparations with implanted catheters, the catheter tip becomes surrounded by a pocket of fibrin after a few days, and subsequent injections do not disperse readily.

3. Once again acid-base phenomena and concentrations of available local anesthetic may be invoked to explain obscure events. Ellis Cohen and his colleagues at Stanford have obtained data from subarachnoid injections suggesting that repeated doses of acid solutions reduce the pH of the surrounding tissue spaces, leading to persistence of nondiffusible cation in the injectant and therefore failure of penetration to target neurons. Cohen was able to show that repeated intrathecal injections of local anesthetics in dogs caused the pH of the cerebrospinal fluid to fall and the local anesthetic concentration in the cerebrospinal fluid to rise progressively, although the duration of analgesic blockade became shorter with each successive injection (Cohen et al., 1968).

"True" tachyphylaxis or desensitization of an active effector response (as in the case of angiotensin II and smooth vascular muscle) is not likely to be the cause of the diminished response that we are considering (Khairalhah et al., 1967), which is rather the result of *restored* activity of the effector mechanism at the excitable membrane in the face of a blocking agent and not diminished activity. However, it is conceivable that alterations of membrane configuration associated with blockade may expose more charged sites for capture and neutralization of local anesthetic molecules.

Certain important practical applications to the clinical management of epidural blockade arise from these studies:

1. In continuous epidural analgesia the timing of successive doses is quite critical. Premature reinjection may overcorrect the tendency to acute tolerance, but the resulting degree of blockade becomes more intense than

after the previous injection. This augmentation or "ripening" of analgesia may be an advantage in certain circumstances, such as the end of a long labor under epidural analgesia, when good perineal analgesia is required for painless episiotomy and delivery. On the other hand, it may be undesirable after major surgery if intensified motor blockade interferes with active postoperative exercises.

2. Tachyphylaxis will appear if intervals between injections are long enough to allow analgesia to wear off completely. Then it is likely that each delayed dose will have to be increased by 25 to 30 per cent above that of its immediate predecessor, in order to maintain a stable segmental level of analgesia.

3. The degree of tachyphylaxis that develops in a given time is a function of the number of reinjections that are required. Therefore, anything that reduces the need for frequent reinjection also reduces the number of occasions for tachyphylaxis to develop. Thus, long-acting agents and the addition of epinephrine to prolong their action further will both tend to postpone the effects of acute tolerance.

ALLERGY AND DRUG INTERACTIONS

Patients are commonly mislabeled as "allergic to local anesthetics" if they react unfavorably under local anesthesia. This can be an important and potentially dangerous label, for it may force an anesthesiologist to use general anesthesia under circumstances in which regional anesthesia might be the safer choice (Aldrete and Johnson, 1970).

Allergy to local anesthetics is very rare. There does not appear to be any well-documented case of allergy to the amide-type local anesthetics, and when allergy does occur, it is usually in response to the ester-type agents, with the *p*-aminobenzoic acid residue NH_2 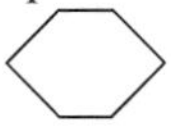 COOH forming a hapten with immunoglobulin E. Methylparaben, or methyl *p*-hydroxybenzoate, is

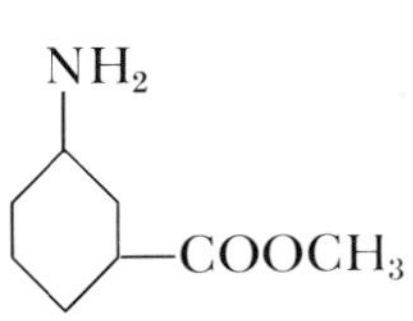

widely used as a preservative in local anesthetic solutions and other drug preparations, and it is another potential source of allergy, also through hapten formation (Figure 3–25).

Suspected cases of allergy should be tested by:

1. *Conjunctival test.* A drop of the local anesthetic solution is placed in the conjunctival sac, with normal saline as control in the opposite eye, and the eye is examined 10 minutes later (Adriani, 1966).

2. *Intracutaneous skin wheal.* A very small volume of the test solution (0.05 ml) is injected intracutaneously on the volar surface of the forearm, with normal saline as control. The test and control sites are examined for wheal diameter, flare and pseudopodia at 15 minutes and 30 minutes after injection.

3. *Basophil degranulation test.* Hapten formation with antibody-anti-

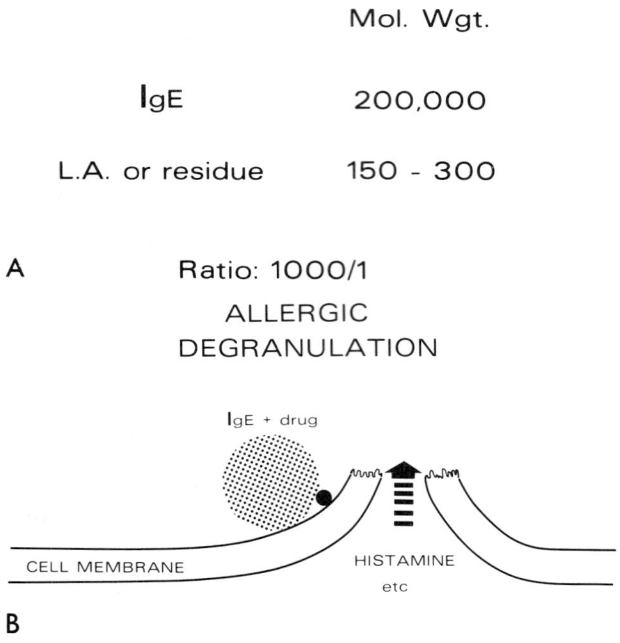

Figure 3–25. Allergic response to local anesthetics. *A*, Hapten formation between immunoglobulin E (IgE) and local anesthetic residue. *B*, Antibody-antigen reaction and disruption of intracellular granules.

gen reaction can be carried out safely and elegantly in a test tube. Briefly, fresh rabbit basophil cells are incubated with the human serum under test. This coats the basophils with any antibody that may be present. The coated basophils and a control uncoated sample are then challenged with a weak concentration of the suspected allergenic agent. The cells are then stained and the basophil granules counted in the two samples. An antigen-antibody reaction will lead to degranulation of affected cells and a lower count in the coated sample.

Reactions may arise from absorption of vasoconstrictor agents that have been added to the local anesthetic solution. These reactions may be particularly severe in patients being treated with tricyclic antidepressant drugs, and as an increasing proportion of the population is receiving antidepressant therapy, for one reason or another, this is a hazard to bear in mind. In these patients epinephrine as a vasoconstrictor should be avoided. Aellig et al. (1970) and Goldman et al. (1971) have suggested that a vasopressin derivative such as felypressin may be a suitable substitute for epinephrine in such cases.

CARDIOVASCULAR TOXICITY OF LOCAL ANESTHETICS

Local anesthetics depress excitable membranes in the cardiovascular system (Galindo and Sprouse, 1964) and depress intracardiac conduction and contractility (Lieberman et al., 1968) in a dose-related manner. Subconvulsive concentrations may produce circulatory embarrassment, particularly in the fetus and newborn in whom competitive binding phenomena and slow elimination will make the situation worse than in the adult. The determinants of toxicity in the central nervous system also operate in the cardiovascular system, and acidosis intensifies the effects of circulating anesthetic drugs.

Andersson and his colleagues (1970) have analyzed some of these variables in isolated fetal hearts obtained at elective hysterotomy. Figure 3–26 drawn from Andersson's data shows the effects of metabolic acidosis and mepivacaine (separately and combined) on maximum ventricular ejection [(dp/dt) max]. In this study the effects of acidosis and local anesthetic appear to be additive. Thus, the influence of acidosis on local anesthetic toxicity is similar in both the central nervous system and the cardiovascular system.

Most experimental preparations for testing the cardiovascular toxicity of local anesthetics have been concerned with establishing threshold concentrations that will cause cardiovascular depression or alterations of conduction in the heart. Unfortunately, none have sought to mimic the conditions that may arise if an accidental injection is made directly into an extradural vein while an epidural block is being induced or maintained. Good information exists on the cardiovascular response to systemic intravenous infusions. Quite large amounts of local anesthetic can be infused into normal adults without causing cardiovascular depression, provided the blood concentration is kept below convulsive levels and provided sympathetic activity is not impaired (Jordfelt et al., 1968; Bonica et al., 1970; Sjögren and Wright, 1972). Jordfelt and his colleagues infused local anesthetics intravenously in conscious human volunteers and obtained peak plasma concentrations in the range of 4 to 8 μg/ml for lidocaine and mepivacaine and 1.5 to 3.0 μg/ml for bupivacaine, without evidence of cardiovascular depression (Jordfelt et al., 1968). However, cardiovascular depression is more likely to become evident under general anesthesia, or during epidural block accompanied by sympathetic blockade or after a seizure. As an example of the depressive effects of general anesthesia combined with circulating local anesthetics, Scott and his associates (1971) gave 150 mg lidocaine intravenously over a period of 90 seconds to a series of patients under light halothane anesthesia. Plasma lidocaine rose to peak concentrations in the range of 4.9 to 8.7 μg/ml (mean 7.1 μg/ml), and in these anesthetized patients there was a brief negative inotropic effect, with a 16 per cent fall of cardiac output and a 30 per cent rise of central venous pressure lasting for about 5 to 10 minutes.

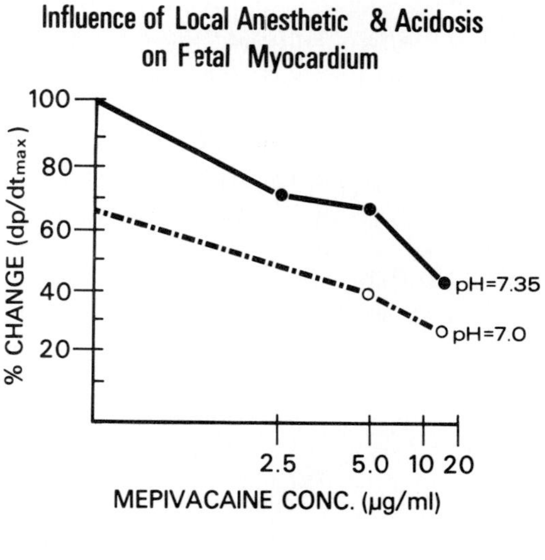

Figure 3–26. Influence of local anesthetic (mepivacaine) on contractility (dp/dt_{max}) of isolated human fetal hearts at normal and low pH (From Andersson et al., Acta Physiol. Scand., 1970.)

Thus, it seems that heightened sympathetic tone can maintain a normal circulation in the presence of quite high blood concentrations of local anesthetic, provided the patient is conscious and undepressed, but cardiac output falls when this compensatory mechanism is obtunded for any reason. Safe concentrations resulting from slow absorption can be exceeded if local anesthetic is injected in a bolus of concentrated solution rather than as a gradual infusion. De Jong and Heavner (1973) investigated the effects of bolus injections of lidocaine in cats. Although these doses were relatively large, they were given into a peripheral systemic vein, and therefore they may be indicative of the effects of somewhat smaller amounts given directly into the azygos system closer to the heart. In De Jong and Heavner's series, a brief bolus was injected about 12 times faster than in most other investigations, at the rate of 1 mg of lidocaine per kilogram per second for 5 seconds. This produced dramatic cardiovascular depression with ventricular tachycardia and a profound fall of blood pressure, requiring external cardiac massage in some animals.

Somewhat similar bolus effects can occur clinically if accidental injection of a much smaller amount is made into an extradural vein. Accidental intravascular placement of an epidural catheter happens very rarely in normal subjects, but in pregnant women at term it occurs more frequently, and the incidence may be as high as 1.0 to 1.25 per cent. If extradural venous cannulation goes undetected and a sizable bolus of local anesthetic is injected, then the concentration of drug reaching the heart may be suddenly but briefly elevated to levels far above the range encountered in slow infusion experiments, and the results may be very different and much more depressing. No measurements have been made of the actual concentration of drug that would reach the heart via the azygos vein under these circumstances. However, a rough estimate can be made.

The amount of local anesthetic arriving at the heart will be a function of concentration in the azygos blood and azygos flow. The immediate distribution volume in part of the extradural venous plexus can only be guessed at, but under conditions of high flow, as in pregnancy, little mixing probably occurs, and in the presence of streaming, dilution is likely to be slight, with an effective distribution volume that is proportionately small. Azygos flow measurements in nonpregnant dogs suggest that about 5 to 10 per cent of the venous return travels in the azygos vein (Burfoot and Bromage, 1971), and in man this will amount to 250 to 500 ml per minute or 4 to 8 ml per second.

Let us suppose that 4 ml of 2 per cent lidocaine (i.e., 80 mg) is injected accidentally into a lumbar extradural vein over a period of 10 seconds. Figure 3–27 represents the contrasting situations that are likely to prevail under conditions of low azygos flow and of high azygos flow as in pregnancy at term (see Chapter 12). Vascular streaming in the high flow state will reduce the effective distribution volume. If we assume an effective distribution volume of 100 ml for the low flow state and 50 ml for the high flow state, the amount of lidocaine reaching the heart in unit time will be given by the expression:

$$\frac{\text{Mass of drug injected}}{\text{Distribution volume}} \times \frac{\text{Azygos flow}}{\text{Infusion time}}$$

and with the values we have assumed, the respective rates will be:

Low Flow	High Flow
$\frac{80{,}000\ \mu g}{100\ ml} \times \frac{4\ ml/sec}{10\ sec}$	$\frac{80{,}000\ \mu g}{50\ ml} \times \frac{8\ ml/sec}{10\ sec}$
$= 320\ \mu g/sec$	$= 1{,}280\ \mu g/sec$

That is, the amount of drug reaching the heart per unit time is four times higher in the high flow state than in the low flow state.

When parturient patients are placed on their backs, the heavy uterus compresses the iliac veins as they cross the pelvic brim, and venous return from the pelvis and lower limbs is forced into the vertebral plexus (Kerr et al., 1964). This raises the pressure in the epidural space and at the same time lowers the central venous pressure (Galbert and Marx, 1974). Thus, patients lying supine will have high extradural venous flow rates, and "bolus" toxic effects from accidental intravenous injection are likely to be more severe than in patients lying on their sides, in whom flow in the inferior vena cava is unimpeded (see Chapter 12).

AXOPLASM AND NEURAL BLOCKADE

So far, discussion has centered around the effects of local anesthetics on impulse conduction along axon membranes and on distant cardiovascular and neurological toxicity that may arise from excessive systemic absorption. This section will consider the lesser known functions of the axoplasm and the effects that local anesthetics may exert on intra-axonal events. Much of this is relatively new knowledge, and some of the discussion will necessarily touch on areas that are still speculative and untested by experiment.

For the past 20 years evidence has gradually accumulated that local anesthetics not only block conduction of the nerve impulse but also have a

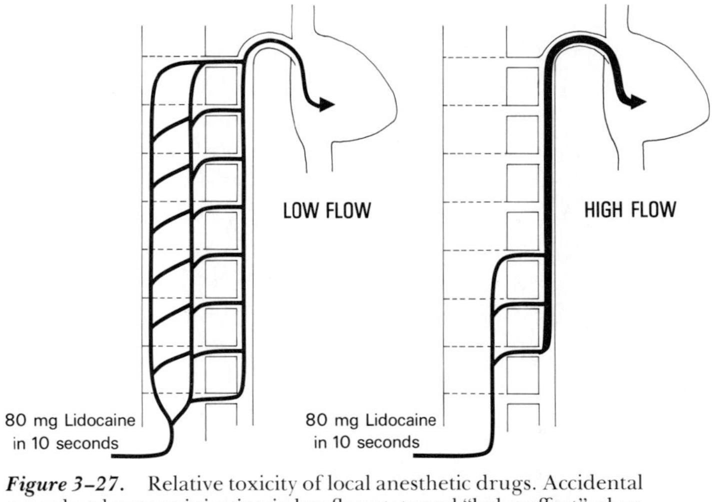

Figure 3–27. Relative toxicity of local anesthetic drugs. Accidental extradural venous injection in low flow state and "bolus effect" when inferior vena caval obstruction causes high extradural flow (see text).

reversibly depressant effect on the metabolism of the nerve itself and the oxidative processes that restore and sustain axonal function (Geddes and Quastel, 1956; Pietra, 1963). Local anesthetics arrest conduction along the axon membrane more easily than the metabolic processes going on within the nerve cell, and higher concentrations of drug are needed to block metabolism than to block conduction. Clinical concentrations of local anesthetics block nerve conduction in a fully reversible fashion, and of course, complete reversibility is fundamental to the safe use of these drugs. The question is being asked, however, does the same degree of reversibility hold for axoplasmic function, or may subtle but lasting changes be brought about by clinical doses of local anesthetics? Clearly, this is a question of fundamental importance on two counts. First, it challenges the basic assumption of reversibility that underlies the routine use of local anesthetics. Second, if irreversible changes do occur in the axoplasm under certain circumstances, can they be exploited in some way to produce permanent blockade for relief of intractable pain in cancer patients?

Axoplasmic Transport

Axons of motor and sensory nerves have very slender, extended lines of communication that require an efficient and reliable transport system to sustain functional activity. The magnitude of the transport problem can be appreciated by considering the relative length and size of a limb axon which may be more than 100,000 times longer than its diameter (Jeffrey and Austin, 1973; Dahlström, 1974).

In 1962, Droz and Leblond in the Department of Anatomy at McGill University obtained the first direct evidence of axoplasmic transport. They showed that tritium-labeled leucine flowed centrifugally along rat nerves at the rather slow rate of 1.5 mm per day. Since then, other amino acids have been shown to move at much faster rates of up to 430 mm per day. Movement is two-way. Metabolic supplies from the center (i.e., perikaryon of the nerve) are transported centrifugally down the axon, while chemical signals from the periphery are carried back centripetally to the cell body (Kristensson, Olsson and Sjöstrand, 1971).

The structural basis for this transport and humoral communication system is a series of microtubules and microfilaments running within the substance of the axoplasm along the length of the nerve (Smith et al., 1975). A brief description of the structure of axonal microtubules is necessary in order to understand the mechanisms under discussion. For a full review of the subject, the reader is referred to the collected papers of a conference on The Biology of Cytoplasmic Microtubules, published by the New York Academy of Sciences (Soifer, 1975).

Axoplasmic microtubules have a diameter of about 270Å, and they are formed from hollow bundles of 13 protofilaments made up of molecules of the protein tubulin (Fujiwara and Tilney, 1975). It is of interest that the same ultrastructural design is identical throughout all the animal phyla, from the cilia of paramecium to the flagellum of the human sperm. In organs concerned with locomotion, such as cilia or flagella, unity of design extends a step further to the spatial arrangement of the microtubules in the well-known "9 + 2"

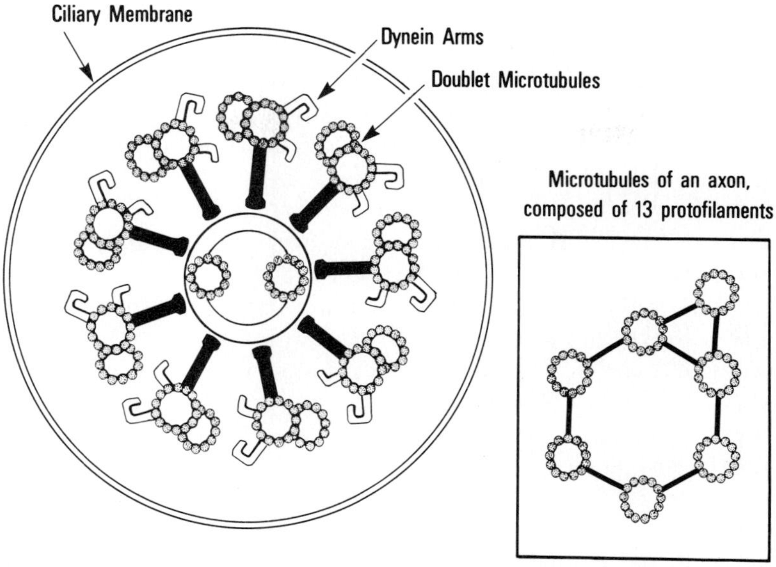

Figure 3–28. "9 + 2" design of microtubule doublets with dynein arms, present in cilia and in certain neural elements. *Inset:* Axoplasmic microtubules: archetypal arrangement of 13 protofilaments in tubule construction.

design, in which a halo of nine doublets of microtubules, interconnected by dynein arms, surrounds a central pair (Satir, 1974), as shown in Figure 3–28. Dynein arms form temporary cross bridges between adjacent microtubules and are believed to be responsible for generating movements of cilia and sperm tails. In the nervous system, this formal arrangement of microtubules is lost, with the exception of certain specialized neural organs (Bertiloni et al., 1970). Nevertheless, it has been suggested that dynein arms may be retained in axonal microtubules and perhaps be concerned with propulsion along the tubules (Edström and Mattsson, 1976). If this speculation is correct, then certain genetic diseases may impair the efficiency of axoplasmic transport and make the system more susceptible to injury. For example, in Kartagener's syndrome involving situs inversus, chronic bronchitis and sinusitis, and infertility, cilia and spermatozoa are devoid of dynein arms and incapable of movement. In this rare condition affecting about one person in 68,000, mucociliary and oviductal transport are at a standstill, secretions accumulate in the air passages and spermatozoa are immotile (Camner et al., 1975; Afzelius, 1976). At present it is not known whether a similar deficiency of dynein arms also exists in the axonal microtubular system of patients with Kartagener's syndrome, nor whether such a deficit would make the nerves unusually susceptible to drugs that affect axoplasmic transport.

Effect of Local Anesthetics on Axoplasmic Transport

Local anesthetics and antimitotic drugs, such as colchicine and the Vinca alkaloids, can interfere with axoplasmic transport when administered in high enough doses (Albuquerque et al., 1972; Aasheim et al., 1974; Bisby,

1975; Fink and Kish, 1976; Fernandez and Inestrosa, 1976). Natural neurotoxins, such as tetrodotoxin, stabilize the axon membrane selectively at the external surface, block impulse conduction in very high dilution but have no effect on axoplasmic transport. On the other hand, toxins that act on the inside of the membrane, such as batrachotoxin, produce irreversible block of axoplasmic flow in extremely low concentrations (Ochs and Worth, 1975). As we have seen earlier, local anesthetics do penetrate the axon membrane and arrive at the inside, so it might be expected that they would affect axoplasmic flow to some degree.

To interfere with axoplasmic transport, local anesthetics must reach the axoplasm in sufficient concentration to depress oxidative metabolism (Haschke and Fink, 1975) and to depolymerize the microtubules and disrupt their continuity. Within limits, this disruptive process is reversible. When the concentration of local anesthetic declines below a certain threshold, oxidative metabolism is restored, the microtubules reassemble themselves and axoplasmic transport is resumed in a normal fashion (Byers et al., 1973). There are formidable difficulties in arriving at an experimental estimate of this critical threshold in living animals. Qualitative estimates of the effects of prolonged blockade have been obtained by wrapping the sciatic nerve in a Silastic cuff containing high concentrations of local anesthetic in the range of 20 to 25 per cent lidocaine. This treatment causes complete paralysis and electromyographic silence of the innervated muscles while the cuff is in place. Robert and Oester (1970a, 1970b) reported complete neurological and EMG recovery within 4 to 18 hours after Silastic lidocaine cuffs that had been continuously in place for eight days were removed. However, others found that a two-day application of 25 per cent lidocaine in Silastic cuffs inhibited axonal transport acutely and delayed complete neurological recovery for a period of one to two weeks (Bisby, 1975). While these experiments showed that intimate and prolonged contact with local anesthetics was eventually reversible, they were not able to provide a quantitative estimate of the actual amounts of local anesthetic in the axoplasm at the time of paralysis, nor did they indicate any hypothetical danger level of drug that might damage the axoplasm irreversibly.

Fink and his colleagues at Seattle have come closest to providing this type of information in vivo by painstaking analysis of the acute effects of local anesthetic blockade of the rat's maxillary nerve. Using a double labeled technique, these workers were able to measure both rapid axoplasmic transport and neural uptake of local anesthetic simultaneously, and thus arrive at a figure for the concentration of local anesthetic in the nerve that was associated with inhibition of axoplasmic transport. They found that the minimal neural concentration of lidocaine required to inhibit rapid axoplasmic transport was in the range of 1.1 to 2.7 μg/g of nerve and about four to ten times the critical neural concentration required for blockade of sensory conduction (Fink et al., 1975; Fink and Kish, 1976). They also showed that the time interval for recovery of axoplasmic flow was prolonged by adding epinephrine 1/200,000 to the anesthetic solution and by increasing the concentration and mass of local anesthetic injected into the nerve. Thus, there are intra-axonal correlates of what is seen clinically when the same factors are employed to prolong and intensify blockade in human patients.

The picture that emerges from these diverse and elegant experiments is relatively reassuring. Part of the uneasy question that was posed about the effects of local anesthetics on axoplasmic flow has been answered. Yes, they do inhibit rapid axonal transport to some degree under conditions akin to clinical usage and profound conduction blockade, but they do so reversibly and with what seems to be a very wide margin of safety.

The other part of the question that remains unanswered at the present time is, what is the dangerous intra-axonal concentration of local anesthetic that will produce irreversible arrest of axoplasmic transport, and can this level be achieved with standard drugs in ordinary clinical practice? The available evidence seems reassuring on this point also, for the animal work discussed above shows that axoplasm has remarkable powers of recuperation in the face of intense and prolonged blockade. However, rare exceptions may possibly be encountered, for unusual genetic factors may modify normal response to drugs and introduce unexpected hazards, such as those seen with barbiturates in porphyria and with succinylcholine in malignant hyperpyrexia. As yet, we do not know whether ultrastructural abnormalities exist in the microtubules in genetic taints, such as Kartagener's syndrome, in which one may suspect that the lack of dynein arms in ciliary structures may perhaps be mirrored by a comparable deficit in the analogous design of the axonal microtubular transport system. Also, is the microtubular system unusually fragile in regenerating nerves that are recovering from injury, as has been tentatively suggested by Dahlström (1974)?

Future work will undoubtedly resolve these outstanding doubts, but in the meantime it seems extremely unlikely that local anesthetics in clinical dosage can be expected to cause irreversible damage to normal nerves. For the same reason, local anesthetics are not likely to provide permanent analgesia in cases of intractable pain, even when administered for very long periods of time.

This general survey of local anesthetics, their disposition and elimination and their interactions with axon membranes and submembrane structures, forms the basis for understanding some of the practical aspects of epidural blockade that will be discussed later. The clinical performance of individual local anesthetics will be considered in Chapter 9 on Drugs and Equipment.

REFERENCES

Aasheim, G., Fink, B. R., and Middaugh, M.: Inhibition of rapid axoplasmic transport by procaine hydrochloride. Anesthesiology *41*:549, 1974.

Aceves, J., and Machne, X.: The action of calcium and of local anesthetics on nerve cells and their interaction during excitation. J. Pharmacol. Exp. Ther. *140*:138, 1963.

Adjepon-Yamoah, K. K., Scott, D. B., and Prescott, L. F.: Impaired absorption and metabolism of oral lignocaine in patients undergoing laparoscopy. Brit. J. Anaesth. *45*:143, 1973.

Adriani, J.: Reactions to local anesthetics. J.A.M.A. *196*:405, 1966.

Aellig, W. H., O'Neill, R., Laurence, D. R., et al.: Cardiac effects of adrenaline and felypressin as vasoconstrictors in local anaesthesia for oral surgery under diazepam sedation. Brit. J. Anaesth. *42*:174, 1970.

Afzelius, B. A.: A human syndrome caused by immotile cilia. Science *193*:317, 1976.

Albuquerque, E. X., Warnick, J. E., Tasse, J. R., and Sansone, F. M.: Effects of vinblastine and colchicine on neural regulation of the fast and slow skeletal muscles of the rat. Exp. Neurol. *37*:607, 1972.

Aldrete, J. A., and Johnson, D. A.: Evaluation of intracutaneous testing for investigation of allergy to local anesthetic agents. Anesth. Analg. *49*:173, 1970.
Andersson, K.-E., Gennser, G., and Nilsson, E.: Influence of mepivacaine on isolated human foetal hearts at normal and low pH. Acta Physiol. Scand. *80*(Suppl. 353):34, 1970.
Anfinsen, C. F.: Principles that govern the folding of protein chains. Science *181*:223, 1973.
Armstrong, C. M., Bezanilla, F., and Rojos, E.: Destruction of sodium conductance inactivation in squid axons perfused with Pronase. J. Gen. Physiol. *62*:375, 1973.
Arvanitaki, A., and Chalazonitis, N.: Diffusibilité de l'anhydride carbonique dans l'axone géant, les effets sur les vitesses de l'activité biolélectrique. C. R. Soc. Biol. Paris *148*:952, 1954.
Beckett, A. H., Boyes, R. N., and Appleton, P. J.: The metabolism and excretion of lignocaine in man. J. Pharm. Pharmacol. *18*:76S, 1966.
Belfrage, P., Raabe, N., Thalme, B., and Berlin, A.: Lumbar epidural analgesia with bupivacaine in labor. Determination of drug concentrations and pH in fetal scalp blood, and continuous fetal heart rate monitoring. Amer. J. Obstet. Gynecol. *121*:360, 1975.
Bertolini, B., Monaco, G., and Rossi, A.: Ultrastructure of a regular arrangement of microtubules and neurofilaments. Ultrastruct. Res. *33*:173, 1970.
Bisby, M. A.: Inhibition of axonal transport in nerves chronically treated with local anesthetics. Exp. Neurol. *47*:481, 1975.
Blaustein, M. P., and Goldman, D. E.: Competitive action of calcium and procaine on lobster axon. A study of the mechanism of certain local anesthetics. J. Gen. Physiol. *49*:1043, 1966.
Bonica, J. J., Berges, P. U., and Morikawa, K.: Circulatory effects of peridural block. I. Effects of levels of analgesia and dose of lidocaine. Anesthesiology *33*:619, 1970.
Boyes, R. N., Scott, D. B., Jebson, P. J., Godman, M. J., and Julian, D. G.: Pharmacokinetics of lidocaine in man. Clin. Pharmacol. Ther. *12*:105, 1971.
Braid, D. P., and Scott, D. B.: The systemic absorption of local analgesic drugs. Brit. J. Anaesth. *37*:394, 1965.
Braid, D. P., and Scott, D. B.: Dosage of lignocaine in epidural block in relation to toxicity. Brit. J. Anaesth. *38*:596, 1966.
Branch, R. A., Shand, D. G., Wilkinson, G. R., and Nies, A. S.: The reduction of lidocaine clearance by dl-propranolol: an example of hemodynamic drug interaction. J. Pharmacol. Exp. Ther. *184*:515, 1973.
Bromage, P. R.: A comparison of the hydrochloride and carbon dioxide salts of lidocaine and prilocaine in epidural analgesia. Acta Anaesth. Scand. (Suppl.) *16*:55, 1965.
Bromage, P. R., and Burfoot, M. F.: Further studies in the distribution and site of action of extradural local anaesthetic drugs using 14 C-labelled lidocaine in dogs. 3rd Congr. Mund. Anaesth. Tom. 1, Sao Paulo, 1964, p. 371.
Bromage, P. R., and Burfoot, M. F.: Quality of epidural blockade. II. Influence of physicochemical factors; hyaluronidase and potassium. Brit. J. Anaesth. *38*:857, 1966.
Bromage, P. R., and Gertel, M.: Brachial plexus anesthesia in chronic renal failure. Anesthesiology *36*:488, 1972.
Bromage, P. R., and Robson, J. G.: Concentrations of lignocaine in the blood after intravenous, intramuscular, epidural and endotracheal administration. Anaesthesia *16*:461, 1961.
Bromage, P. R., Burfoot, M. F., Crowell, D. E., and Pettigrew, R. T.: Quality of epidural blockade. I. Influence of physical factors. Brit. J. Anaesth. *36*:342, 1964.
Bromage, P. R., Burfoot, M. F., Crowell, D. E., and Truant, A. P.: Quality of epidural blockade. III. Carbonated local anaesthetic solutions. Brit. J. Anaesth. *39*:197, 1967.
Bromage, P. R., Pettigrew, R. T., and Crowell, D. E.: Tachyphylaxis in epidural analgesia. 1. Augmentation and decay of local anesthesia. J. Clin. Pharmacol. *9*:30, 1969.
Büchi, J.: Chemische Konstitution, chemische Reaktivität und Wirkung in einigen homologen Lokalanästhetica-Reihen. Pharm. Acta Helv. *42*:534, 1967.
Burfoot, M. F., and Bromage, P. R.: The effects of epinephrine on mepivacaine absorption from the spinal epidural space. Anesthesiology *35*:488, 1971.
Byers, M. R., Fink, B. R., Kennedy, R. D., Middaugh, M. E., and Hendrickson, A. E.: Effects of lidocaine on axonal morphology, microtubules and rapid transport in rabbit vagus nerve *in vitro*. J. Neurobiol. *4*:125, 1973.
Caldwell, P. C.: Studies on the internal pH of large muscle and nerve fibres. J. Physiol. (Lond). *142*:22, 1958.
Camner, P., Mossberg, B., and Afzelius, B. A.: Evidence for congenitally nonfunctioning cilia in the tracheobronchial tract in two subjects. Amer. Rev. Resp. Dis. *112*:807, 1975.
Catchlove, R. F. H.: The influence of CO_2 and pH on local anaesthetic action. M. Sc. Thesis, McGill University, Montreal, Canada, 1971.
Catchlove, R. F. H.: The influence of CO_2 and pH on local anesthetic action. J. Pharmacol. Exp. Ther. *181*:298, 1972.

Catchlove, R. F. H.: Potentiation of two different local anaesthetics by carbon dioxide. Brit. J. Anaesth. *45*:471, 1973.
Cerbón, J.: NMR evidence for the hydrophobic interaction of local anaesthetics: Possible relation to their potency. Biochim. Biophys. Acta *290*:51, 1972.
Chignell, C. F., Vesell, E. S., Starkweather, D. T., et al.: The binding of sulfaphenazole to fetal, neonatal and adult plasma albumin. Clin. Pharmacol. Ther. *12*:897, 1971.
Clausen, T., Harving, H., and Dahl-Hansen, A. B.: The relationship between the transport of glucose and cations across cell membranes in isolated tissue. Biochim. Biophys. Acta *298*: 393, 1973.
Cohen, E. N., Levine, D. A., Coliss, J. E., and Gunther, R. E.: The role of pH in the development of tachyphylaxis to local anesthetic agents. Anesthesiology *29*:994, 1968.
Condouris, G. A.: A study on mechanism of action of cocaine on amphibian peripheral nerve. J. Pharmacol. *131*:243, 1961.
Condouris, G. A.: Conduction block by cocaine in sodium-depleted nerves with activity maintained by lithium, hydrazinium or guanidinium ions. J. Pharmacol. Exp. Ther. *141*:253, 1963.
Condouris, G. A., and Shakalis, A.: Potentiation of the nerve depressant effects of local anaesthetics by carbon dioxide. Nature *204*:57, 1964.
Dahlström, A.: "Axoplasmic transport"—The catering and communication system within nerve cells. Anesthesiology *41*:537, 1974.
de Jong, R. H.: Local Anesthetics. 2nd ed., Springfield, Ill. Charles C Thomas, Publisher, 1977.
de Jong, R. H., and Heavner, J. E.: Diazepam and lidocaine-induced cardiovascular changes. Anesthesiology *39*:633, 1973.
de Jong, R. H., Prince, D. A., and Wagman, I. H.: Effect of carbon dioxide on the cortical threshold to lidocaine. Exp. Neurol. *17*:221, 1967.
De Jong, R. H., Heavner, J. H., and de Oliveira, L.: Effects of nitrous oxide on the lidocaine seizure threshold and diazepam protection. Anesthesiology *37*:299, 1972.
Dettbarn, W-D.: Neuropoisons: Their pathophysiological actions. *In* Simpson, L. L. (ed.): Poisons of Animal Origin. New York, Plenum Press, 1971, pp. 169–186.
Droz, B., and Leblond, C. P.: Migration of proteins along the axons of the sciatic nerve. Science *137*:1047, 1962.
Edström, A., and Mattsson, H.: Inhibition and stimulation of rapid axonal transport *in vitro* by sulfhydryl blockers. Brain Res. *108*:381, 1976.
Englesson, S.: The influence of acid-base changes on central nervous system toxicity of local anaesthetic agents. I. An experimental study in cats. Acta Anaesth. Scand. *18*:79, 1974.
Englesson, S., Paymaster, N. J., and Hill, T. R.: Electrical seizure activity produced by Xylocaine and Citanest. Acta Anaesth. Scand. (Suppl.) *XVI*:47, 1965.
Eriksson, E., and Granberg, P-O.: Studies on the renal excretion of Citanest and Xylocaine. Acta Anaesth. Scand. (Suppl.) *XVI*:79, 1965.
Feinstein, M. B.: Reaction of local anesthetics with phospholipids. A possible chemical basis for anesthesia. J. Gen. Physiol. *48*:357, 1964.
Feinstein, M. B.: Inhibition of contraction and calcium exchangeability in rat uterus by local anaesthetics. J. Pharmacol. Exp. Ther. *152*:516, 1966.
Feinstein, M. B., and Paimre, M.: Specific reaction of local anesthetics with phosphodiester groups. Biochim. Biophys. Acta *115*:33, 1966.
Fernandez, H. L., and Inestrosa, N. C.: Role of axoplasmic transport in neurotrophic regulation of muscle end plate acetylcholinesterase. Nature *262*:55, 1976.
Fernandez, M. S., and Cerbón, J.: The importance of the hydrophobic interactions of local anesthetics in the displacement of polyvalent cations from artificial lipid membranes. Biochim. Biophys. Acta *298*:8, 1973.
Fink, B. R., and Kish, S. J.: Reversible inhibition of rapid axonal transport *in vivo* by lidocaine hydrochloride. Anesthesiology *44*:139, 1976.
Fink, B. R., Aasheim, G., Kish, S. J., and Croley, S.: Neurokinetics of lidocaine in the infraorbital nerve of the rat *in vivo:* Relation to sensory block. Anesthesiology *42*:731, 1975.
Finster, M., Morishima, H. O., Boyes, R. N., and Covino, B. G.: The placental transfer of lidocaine and its uptake by fetal tissues. Anesthesiology *36*:159, 1972.
Foldes, F. F., Davidson, G. M., Duncalf, D., and Kuwabara, S.: The intravenous toxicity of local anesthetic agents in man. Clin. Pharmacol. Ther. *6*:328, 1965.
Franz, D. N., and Perry, R. S.: Mechanisms for differential block among single myelinated and nonmyelinated axons by procaine. J. Physiol. *236*:193, 1974.
Fujiwara, K., and Tilney, L. G.: Substructural analysis of the microtubule and its polymorphic forms. Ann. N.Y. Acad. Sci. *253*:27, 1975.
Galbert, M. W., and Marx, G. F.: Extradural pressures in the parturient patient. Anesthesiology *40*:499, 1974.

Galindo, A., and Sprouse, J. H.: The influence of epidural analgesia on cardiac excitability in profound hypothermia. Canad. Anaesth. Soc. J. *11*:614, 1964.
Geddes, I. C.: Metabolism of local anesthetic agents. Int. Anesth. Clin. *5*:525, 1967.
Geddes, I. C., and Quastel, J. H.: Effects of local anesthetics on respiration of rat brain cortex in vitro. Anesthesiology *17*:666, 1956.
Ghoneim, M. M., and Pandya, H.: Plasma protein binding of bupivacaine and its interaction with other drugs in man. Brit. J. Anaesth. *46*:435, 1974.
Goehl, T., Davenport, J. B., and Stanley, M. J.: Distribution, biotransformation, and excretion of bupivacaine in the rat and the monkey. Xenobiotica *3*:761, 1973.
Goldman, V., Astrom, A., and Evers, H.: The effect of tricyclic antidepressant on the cardiovascular effects of local anaesthetic solutions containing different vasoconstrictors. Anaesthesia *26*:91, 1971.
Gorter, E., and Grendel, F.: On biomolecular layers of lipoids on the chromocytes of blood. J. Exp. Med. *41*:439, 1925.
Green, D. E. (ed.): Membrane structure and its biological applications. Ann. N.Y. Acad. Sci. *195*:5, 1972.
Halpern, B. N., and Binaghi, R.: Selective permeability of living tissues to carbonic acid. Nature *183*:1397, 1959.
Harley, J. D., and Celermajer, J. M.: Neonatal methaemoglobinaemia and the "red-brown" screening-test. Lancet *2*:1223, 1970.
Haschke, R. H., and Fink, B. R.: Lidocaine effects of brain mitochondrial metabolism *in vitro.* Anesthesiology *42*:737, 1975.
Henn, F., and Brattsand, R.: Some pharmacological and toxicological properties of a new long-acting local analgesic. LAC-43 (Marcaine), in comparison with mepivacaine and tetracaine. Acta Anaesth. Scand. (Suppl.) *21*:9, 1966.
Hille, B.: The permeability of the sodium channel to organic cations in myelinated nerve. J. Gen. Physiol. *58*:599, 1971.
Hille, B.: An essential ionized acid group in sodium channels. Fed. Proc. *34*:1318, 1975.
Hillman, D. E., and Llinás: Calcium-containing electron-dense structures in the axons of the squid gaint synapse. J. Cell Biol. *61*:146, 1974.
Hoffman, A., and Kochmann, M.: Verminderung der Novokainkonzentration durch Kaliumsulfat bie der Lokalanästhesie. Dtsch. Med. Wschr. *38*:2264, 1912.
Huxley, A. F., and Stämpfli, R.: Effect of potassium and sodium on resting and action potentials of single myelinated nerve fibers. J. Physiol. *112*:496, 1951.
Jeffrey, P. L., and Austin, L.: Axoplasmic transport. Progr. Neurobiol. *2*:207, 1973.
Jordfelt, L., Löfstrom, B., Pernow, B., Persson, P., Wahren, J., and Widman, B.: The effect of local anesthetics on the contral circulation and respiration in man and dog. Acta Anaesth. Scand. *12*:153, 1968.
Keenaghan, J. B., and Boyes, R. N.: The tissue distribution, metabolism and excretion of lidocaine in rats, guinea pigs, dogs and man. J. Pharmacol. Exp. Ther. *180*:454, 1972.
Kerr, M. G., Scott, D. B., and Samuel, E.: Studies of the inferior vena cava in late pregnancy. Brit. Med. J. *1*:532, 1964.
Keynes, R. D.: Excitable membranes. Nature *239*:29, 1972.
Keynes, R. D., Richie, J. M., and Rojas, E.: The binding of tetrodotoxin to nerve membranes. J. Physiol. *213*:235, 1971.
Khairalhah, P. A., Page, I. H., Bumpus, F. M., et al.: Angiotensin tachyphylaxis and its reversal. Circ. Res. *19*:247, 1966.
Kristensson, K., Olsson, Y., and Sjöstrand, J.: Axonal uptake and retrograde transport of exogenous proteins in the hypoglossal nerve. Brain Res. *32*:399, 1971.
Kwant, W. O., and Seeman, P.: The membrane concentration of local anesthetic (chlorpromazine). Biochim. Biophys. Acta *183*:530, 1969.
Landon, D. N., and Langley, O. K.: The local chemical environment of the nodes of Ranvier. A study of cation binding. J. Anat. *108*:419, 1971.
Langley, O. K.: Ion exchange at the node of Ranvier. Histochem. J. *1*:295, 1969.
Langley, O. K.: Local anaesthetics and nodal polyanions in peripheral nerve. Histochem. J. *5*:79, 1973.
Lebeaux, M. I.: Experimental epidural anaesthesia in the dog with lignocaine and bupivacaine. Brit. J. Anaesth. *45*:549, 1973.
Lechat, P., Deleau, D., and Griffié, R. A.: Influence de l'ion potassium sur l'activité des anesthésiques locaux. Med. Exp. (Basel) *11*:157, 1964.
Lee, A. G.: Model for action of local anaesthetics. Nature *262*:545, 1976.
Lettvin, J. Y., Pritchard, W. F., McCulloch, W. S., and Pitts, W.: A theory of passive ion flux through axon membranes. Nature *202*:1338, 1964.
Lieberman, N. A., Harris, R. S., Katz, R. I., Lipschutz, H. M., Dolgin, M., and Fischer, V. J.: The effects of lidocaine on the electrical and mechanical activity of the heart. Am. J. Cardiol. *22*:375, 1968.

Lutsch, E. F., and Morris, R. W.: Circadian periodicity in susceptibility to lidocaine hydrochloride. Science *156*:100, 1967.

Magno, R., Berlin, A., Karlsson, K., and Kjellmer, K.: Anesthesia for Cesarean section. IV. Placental transfer and neonatal elimination of bupivacaine following epidural analgesia for elective Cesarean section. Acta Anaesth. Scand. *20*:141, 1976.

Mather, L. E., Tucker, G. T., Murphy, T. M., Stanton-Hicks, M. d'A., and Bonica, J. J.: The effects of adding adrenaline to etidocaine and lignocaine in extradural anaesthesia. II. Pharmacokinetics. Brit. J. Anaesth. *48*:989, 1976a.

Mather, L. E., Tucker, G. T., Murphy, T. M., Stanton-Hicks, M. d'A., and Bonica, J. J.: Hemodynamic drug interaction: Peridural lidocaine and intravenous ephedrine. Acta Anaesth. Scand. *20*:207, 1976b.

Meecker, W. R.: The potentiation of novocaine solutions. J. Lab. Clin. Med. *11*:139, 1925.

Moore, D. C., Bridenbaugh, L. D., Bagdi, P. A., and Bridenbaugh, P. O.: Accumulation of mepivacaine hydrochloride during caudal block. Anesthesiology *29*:585, 1968.

Moore, J. W., Narahashi, T., and Shaw, T. I.: An upper limit to the number of sodium channels in nerve membrane? J. Physiol. *188*:99, 1967.

Morishima, H. O., Mueller-Heubach, E., and Shnider, S. M.: Body temperature and disappearance of lidocaine in newborn puppies. Anesth. Analg. *50*:938, 1971.

Mosher, H. S., Fuhrman, F. A., Buchwald, H. D., and Fischer, H. G.: Tarichatoxin-tetrodotoxin: A potent neurotoxin. Science *144*:1100, 1964.

Mostert, J. W., Evers, J. L., Hobika, G. H., Moore, R. H., Kenny, G. M., and Murphy, G. P.: The haemodynamic response to chronic renal failure as studied in the azotaemic state. Brit. J. Anaesth. *42*:397, 1970.

Munson, E. S., and Wagman, I. H.: Acid-base changes during lidocaine induced seizures in Macaca mulatta. Arch. Neurol. *20*:406, 1969.

Munson, E. S., Martucci, R. W., and Smith, A. E.: Circadian variations in anesthetic requirement and toxicity in rats. Anesthesiology *32*:507, 1970.

Mushin, W. W.: Intramuscular gallamine with hyaluronidase. Anaesthesia *11*:135, 1956.

Narahashi, T.: Drugs affecting axonal membranes. *In* Dikstein, S. (ed.): Fundamentals of Cell Pharmacology. Springfield, Ill., Charles C Thomas, Publisher, 1973, p. 395.

Narahashi, T., Frazier, D. T., and Yamada, M.: The site of action and active form of local anesthetics. I. Theory and pH experiments with tertiary compounds. J. Pharmacol. Exp. Ther. *171*:32, 1970.

Nash, H. A., and Tobias, J. M.: Phospholipid membrane model: Importance of phosphatidylserine and its cation exchanger nature. Proc. Nat. Acad. Sci. *51*:476, 1964.

Nathan, P. W., and Sears, T. A.: Differential block by sodium-free and sodium-deficient solutions. J. Physiol. *16*:375, 1962.

Ochs, S., and Worth, R.: Batrachotoxin block of fast axoplasmic transport in mammalian nerve fibers. Science *187*:1087, 1975.

Oschman, J. L., Hall, T. A., Peters, P. D., and Wall, B. J.: Association of calcium with membranes of squid giant axon. Ultrastructure and microprobe analysis. J. Cell Biol. *61*:156, 1974.

Perlia, X.: Chemische Konstitution, physikalisch-chemische Eigenschaften und Wirkung in einigen homologen Lokalanästhetica-Reihen. Pharm. Acta Helv. *42*:517, 1967.

Pietra, P.: The action of procaine on the conduction and oxygen consumption of the frog isolated nerve. Arc. Int. Pharmacodyn. *144*:522, 1963.

Reynolds, F.: A comparison of the potential toxicity of bupivacaine, lignocaine and mepivacaine during epidural blockade for surgery. Brit. J. Anaesth. *43*:567, 1971.

Reynolds, F., and Taylor, G.: Plasma concentrations of bupivacaine during continuous epidural analgesia in labour: The effect of adrenaline. Brit. J. Anaesth. *43*:436, 1971.

Ritchie, J. M.: Mechanism of action of local anaesthetic agents and biotoxins. Brit. J. Anaesth. *47*:191, 1975.

Ritchie, J. M., and Greengard, P.: On the active structure of local anesthetics. J. Pharmacol. Exp. Ther. *133*:241, 1961.

Ritchie, J. M., and Ritchie, B.: Local anesthetics: Effect of pH on activity. Science *162*:1394, 1968.

Ritchie, J. M., Ritchie, B., and Greengard, P.: The active structure of local anesthetics. J. Pharmacol. Exp. Ther. *150*:152, 1965a.

Ritchie, J. M., Ritchie, B., and Greengard, P.: The effect of the nerve sheath on the action of local anesthetics. J. Pharmacol. Exp. Ther. *150*:160, 1965b.

Robert, E. D., and Oester, Y. T.: Nerve impulses and trophic effect. Absence of fibrillation after prolonged and reversible conduction block. Arch. Neurol. *22*:57, 1970a.

Robert, E. D., and Oester, Y. T.: Absence of supersensitivity to acetylcholine in innervated muscle subjected to a prolonged pharmacologic nerve block. J. Pharmacol. Exp. Ther. *174*:133, 1970b.

Rowland, M., Thomson, P. D., Guichard, A., and Melmon, K. L.: Disposition of kinetics of lidocaine in normal subjects. Ann. N.Y. Acad. Sci. *179*:383, 1971.

Satir, P.: How cilia move. Sci. Amer. *231*:45, Oct., 1974.

Scott, D. B.: Hyaluronidase in epidural analgesia. Brit. J. Anaesth. *28*:187, 1956.
Scott, D. B., Davie, I. T., and Stephen, G. W.: Cardiovascular effects of intravenous lignocaine during nitrous oxide-halothane anaesthesia. Brit. J. Anaesth. *43*:595, 1971.
Scott, D. B., Jebson, P. J. R., Braid, D. P., Örtengren, B., and Frisch, P.: Factors affecting plasma levels of lignocaine and prilocaine. Brit. J. Anaesth. *44*:1040, 1972.
Scott, D. B., Jebson, P. J. R., and Boyes, R. N.: Pharmacokinetic study of the local anaesthetics bupivacaine (Marcaine) and etidocaine (Duranest) in man. Brit. J. Anaesth. *45*:1010, 1973.
Seeman, P.: The membrane action of anesthetics and tranquilizers. Pharmacol. Rev. *24*:583, 1972.
Seeman, P.: The membrane expansion theory of anesthesia: Direct evidence using ethanol and a high-precision density meter. Experientia *30*:759, 1974a.
Seeman, P.: Ultrastructure of membrane lesions in immune lysis, osmotic lysis and drug-induced lysis. Fed. Proc. *33*:2116, 1974b.
Seimiya, T., and Ohki, S.: Ionic structure of phospholipid membranes and binding of calcium ions. Biochim. Biophys. Acta *298*:546, 1973.
Shanes, A. M.: Drugs and nerve conduction. Ann. Rev. Pharmacol. *3*:185, 1963.
Singer, M. A.: Effects of amiloride and dibucaine on a model phospholipid membrane-structure-activity relationships. Biochem. Pharmacol. *23*:2939, 1974.
Singer, S. J., and Nicholson, G. L.: The fluid mosaic model of the structure of cell membranes. Science *175*:720, 1972.
Sjögren, S., and Wright, B.: Blood concentrations of lidocaine during continuous epidural blockade. Acta Anaesth. Scand. *16*:51, 1972.
Sjöstrand, U., and Widman, B.: Distribution of bupivacaine in the rabbit under normal and acidotic conditions. Acta Anaesth. Scand., Suppl. 50, 1973.
Skou, J. C.: The effect of drugs on cell membranes with special reference to local anaesthetics. J. Pharm. Pharmacol. *13*:204, 1961.
Smith, D. S., Järlfors, U., and Cameron, B. F.: Morphological evidence for the participation of microtubules in axonal transport. *In* Soifer, D. (ed.): The Biology of Cytoplasmic Microtubules. Ann. N.Y. Acad. Sci. *253*:472, 1975.
Soifer, D. (ed.): The Biology of Cytoplasmic Microtubules. Ann. N.Y. Acad. Sci. *253*, 1975.
Spyropoulos, C. S.: The effects of hydrostatic pressure upon the normal and narcotized nerve fiber. J. Gen. Physiol. *40*:849, 1957.
Stanton-Hicks, M. T., Murphy, T. M., Bonica, J. J., Mather, L., and Tucker, G. T.: Effects of extradural block: Comparison of the properties, circulatory effects and pharmacokinetics of etidocaine and bupivacaine. Brit. J. Anaesth. *48*:575, 1976.
Stenson, R. E., Constantino, R. T., and Harrison, D. C.: Interrelationships of hepatic blood flow, cardiac output, and blood levels of lidocaine in man. Circulation *43*:205, 1971.
Strichartz, G. R.: The inhibition of sodium currents in myelinated nerve by quaternary derivatives of lidocaine. J. Gen. Physiol. *62*:37, 1973.
Strobel, G. E., and Bianchi, C. P.: The effects of pH gradients on the action of procaine and lidocaine in intact desheathed sciatic nerve. J. Pharmacol. Exp. Ther. *172*:1, 1970.
Sung, C. Y., and Truant, A. P.: The physiological disposition of lidocaine and its comparison in some respects with procaine. J. Pharmacol. Exp. Ther. *112*:432, 1954.
Thomson, P. D., Melmon, K. L., Richardson, J. A., Cohn, K., Steinbrunn, W., Cudihee, R., and Rowland, M.: Lidocaine pharmacokinetics in advanced heart failure, liver disease, and renal failure in humans. Ann. Int. Med. *78*:499, 1973.
Tucker, G. T., and Mather, L. E.: Pharmacokinetics of local anaesthetic agents. Brit. J. Anaesth. *47*:213, 1975.
Tucker, G. T., Boyes, R. N., Bridenbaugh, P. O., and Moore, D. C.: Binding of anilide-type local anesthetics in human plasma. I. Relationships between binding, physicochemical properties, and anesthetic activity. Anesthesiology *33*:287, 1970a.
Tucker, G. T., Boyes, R. N., Bridenbaugh, P. O., et al.: Binding of anilide-type local anesthetics in human plasma. II. Implications *in vivo,* with special reference to transplacental distribution. Anesthesiology *33*:304, 1970b.
Urry, D. W.: Conformation of protein in biological membranes and a model transmembrane channel. Ann. N.Y. Acad. Sci. *195*:109, 1972.
Woodhull, A. M.: Ion blockade of sodium channels in nerve. J. Gen. Physiol. *61*:687, 1973.

chapter 4
Mechanism of Action

"The need for skepticism"
.... All that was required to overthrow a respectable and entrenched dogma was a few hours of effort and a germ of skepticism.... The great shortage in science now is not opportunity, manpower, money or laboratory space. What is really needed is more of that healthy skepticism which generates the key idea—the liberating concept

Editorial: P.H.A.
Science, October 12, 1962, p. 38

For over 50 years epidural anesthesia was practiced more as an art than as a science, in deep ignorance of its mechanisms. In fairness, one must appreciate that the mechanisms are extremely complex; they are difficult to study in living subjects, and conditions are so grossly altered by death that anatomical information alone is of limited value. It is only comparatively recently, in the last 20 years or so, that methods have become available to unravel the tangled chain of events from injection to neural uptake in this deceptively simple procedure. Even now many questions remain unanswered.

In 1885 Leonard Corning proposed that the spinal cord would absorb drugs injected close to it and that the cord could be medicated in this way. Little attention was paid to Corning's proposition, and it was never seriously considered as a mechanism of action in epidural blockade. Early investigations proceeded along more logical lines of enquiry into the physical boundaries of the epidural space and the diffusion characteristics of the meninges around the spinal cord.

In 1904, three years after caudal epidural analgesia was first described, Sicard and Cestan showed that India ink suspensions injected into the epidural space of dogs did not enter the subarachnoid space; instead, the ink particles spread out through the intervertebral foramina into the paravertebral spaces. Later, Sicard repeated this work with Forestier using Lipiodol in humans, and these experiments confirmed the ease with which solutions pass from the epidural space into the paravertebral space (Sicard and Forestier, 1921, 1926). Some other experiments by Bertocchi in 1932 on the dialyzing properties of postmortem dura mater suggested that the dura was almost impermeable to local anesthetics. These were the two principal pieces of evidence encouraging the firmly held view that an epidural block was really just a multiple paravertebral block caused by seepage through the intervertebral foramina and action on the mixed spinal nerves distal to the spinal canal (Gutierrez, 1939; Dogliotti, 1939; Säker and Schröder, 1954).

Belief in the impermeability of the dura gave rise to other notions that are now known to be dangerously incorrect. Since the dura is fused with vertebral periosteum at the base of the skull, it followed that an impermeable dura would be an assured safety barrier preventing entry of local anesthetics from the epidural space into the intracranial parts of the central nervous system, and one of the advantages claimed for epidural anesthesia was that even extreme overdosage could not result in cranial nerve involvement and a "total spinal" anesthetic. Unfortunately, this is not true, and experience with laboratory animals and clinical accidents has shown that in fact the dura is permeable in certain areas and that liberties cannot be taken with gross overdosage.

During the past two decades technical advances in laboratory measurements have made it possible to look at many of the factors influencing epidural anesthesia, and a rational view is emerging that was not available before. As long as the idea of dural impermeability had existed, there seemed almost no logical limit to the volume of solution that could be injected into the epidural space. Supposedly, epidural solutions could not pass the meningeal barriers, and excessive amounts would only leak out harmlessly through the intervertebral foramina. Two related beliefs dominated technique. First, segmental spread was thought to be dependent on the volume injected, with the area of analgesia controlled by the amount of solution instilled into the cylindrical epidural space. Second, intensity of blockade was held to be influenced by concentration, and it followed that a high concentration would give a more effective block than a low concentration. This latter idea found its logical expression in the German technique of "plombe" injections, first used by Denecke in 1937, in which concentrated anesthetic drugs were used in viscous solutions so that a powerful concentration of the agent would be confined to a limited number of segments. Some plombes or slugs contained concentrations of tetracaine as high as 1.5 per cent in 6 per cent polyvinylpyrrolidone, and up to 8 ml of this material would be injected at any one time (Buchholz and Lesse, 1951; Poppelbaum, 1954).

We now know that these beliefs were partially incorrect and incomplete, and technical practices have had to be altered accordingly.

The precise mode of action remains controversial. During the evolution of ideas about epidural analgesia over the past 50 years, theories of the mechanism of action have centered around one or more of the following sites of action:

1. The mixed spinal nerves in the paravertebral spaces, after passage of local anesthetic outward through the intervertebral foramina (Dogliotti, 1939; Gutierrez, 1939; Odom, 1940; Bryce-Smith, 1954; Foldes et al., 1956).

2. Dorsal root ganglia (Dawkins, 1945; Frumin et al., 1953a; Shantha and Evans, 1972).

3. Spinal roots within their dural root sleeves (Krönke, 1951; Rudin et al., 1951; Bromage et al., 1963; Usubiaga et al., 1964).

4. Periphery of the spinal cord (Bromage et al., 1963; Bromage, 1975).

The following section will examine these options in the light of the laboratory and clinical evidence that has led up to our present, but still incomplete, understanding of how epidural anesthesia works.

PASSAGE OF LOCAL ANESTHETICS FROM EPIDURAL SPACE INTO SUBARACHNOID SPACE AND NEURAXIS

In Chapter 2 evidence was presented that the dura mater varies in thickness and that it is breached by arachnoid villi and numerous blood vessels in the region of the spinal root cuffs. It is here that fine particulate matter, such as India ink or colloidal carbon, can find its way out of the subarachnoid space into neighboring lymph glands and the epidural space (Elman, 1923; Brierley and Field, 1948), and it is probably here too that local anesthetics can enter the subarachnoid space in the reverse direction, in spite of the relative impermeability that Bertocchi (1932) had found in the rest of the spinal dura.

Since the early 1940's, investigations in animals and man using chemical as well as radiant methods of drug assay have demonstrated conclusively that local anesthetics do pass quite rapidly from the epidural space into the cerebrospinal fluid, and in sufficient amounts to cause some degree of subarachnoid blockade (Foldes and Davis, 1954; Foldes et al., 1956; Frey and Soehring, 1954; Frumin et al., 1953b; Numans and Havinga, 1943; Onchi et al., 1956; Rudin et al., 1951; Usubiaga et al., 1961, 1964; Bromage et al., 1963; Bromage and Burfoot, 1964).

The first investigations of transdural spread in living animals were done by Numans and Havinga in 1943; they measured the concentration of procaine in bovine cerebrospinal fluid after injecting 1.5 per cent procaine into the sacral epidural space. In calves, peak concentrations of procaine in the cerebrospinal fluid rose to 200 to 240 μg/ml 10 minutes after volumes of 12 to 15 ml of 1.5 per cent procaine were injected. Unfortunately, this paper was published during wartime in a journal little read by medical men, and the importance of the investigation was not appreciated until eight years later, when Beecher and his colleagues at Harvard measured the passage of epidural procaine into cerebrospinal fluid by continuous perfusion of the subarachnoid space of dogs (Rudin et al., 1951). Their experimental methods necessarily introduced highly artificial conditions, so the results must be treated with some reserve. Nevertheless, they did reflect the diffusion properties of living meninges, and they showed that up to one-tenth of an epidural dose could be recovered from the cerebrospinal fluid in the first two hours after injection. A further lapse of ten years passed until 1961 when these experiments were repeated in Buenos Aires by Usubiaga and his colleagues, who used a large number of animals (51 dogs) and varying concentrations of procaine. They obtained a mean recovery rate of 7.3 per cent from the subarachnoid space, which agreed quite closely with the range of recovery of 3 to 10 per cent found by the Harvard group (Usubiaga et al., 1961, 1964). They also found that more procaine entered the cerebrospinal fluid with high epidural concentrations than with low ones.

These were the only formal studies of subarachnoid clearance, but in the meantime a number of other investigations of cerebrospinal fluid uptake were done in man and in animals, and these are summarized in Table 4–1. Partitioning of the original epidural dose across the dura varies widely in the different reports shown, and the ratio of epidural to cerebrospinal fluid concentration ranges from 139:1 to 14:1, with peak concentrations in the

TABLE 4–1 Diffusion of Local Anesthetics From Epidural Space To Subarachnoid Space

			Epidural Dosage		Cerebrospinal Fluid (CSF)				
							TOTAL CLEARANCE INTO PERFUSED SUBARACHNOID SPACE		
Authors	Animal Species	Analgesic Drug	CONCN. (%)	DOSE (mg)	TIME OF PEAK CONCN. (min)	PEAK CONCN. (mg/ml)	mg	% OF EPI-DURAL DOSE	SITE OF SAMPLING CSF
Numans and Havinga (1943)	Calf	Procaine	1.5	120–150	10	0.2–0.4			Lumbar
Numans and Havinga (1943)	Cow	Procaine	1.5	1500–2100	10	0.5			Lumbar
Rudin et al. (1951)	Dog	Procaine	2	200	4–8	0.8	8–24	3–10	Cisterna magna
Krönke (1951)	Man	Tetracaine	0.3	50	30–40	0.2–0.5			Lumbar
Buchholz and Körner (1952)	Man	Tetracaine	0.3	60	30–40	0.01–0.02			Lumbar
Frey and Soehring (1954)	Dog	Procaine	2		10	1.0–1.2			Lumbar
Foldes and Davis (1954)	Man	2-Chloro-procaine	3	1000	30	0.23			Lumbar
Frumin et al. (1953b)	Man	Procaine	2	400	20	0.15–0.2			Lumbar
Onchi et al. (1956)	Man	Lidocaine	0.8–2.0	280–400	15	0.1–0.25			Lumbar
Krumperman et al. (1960)	Man	2-Chloro-procaine	3	Varied	–	0.25			Lumbar
Usubiaga et al. (1964)	Dog	Procaine	2	5 mg/kg	5–25 (av. 15)	0.2–0.5 0.5–0.7*		7.3	Lumbar
Bromage and Burfoot (1964)	Dog	^{14}C-Lidocaine	2	100–200	5–10	1.4–2.2*			Lumbar via cisterna magna
Lund (1965)	Man	Lidocaine and prilocaine	2 & 3	600–900	30–45	0.09–0.27			Lumbar
Lund and Covino (1967)	Man	Lidocaine	2	300	20	0.24			Lumbar
Wilkinson and Lund (1970)	Man	Bupivacaine	0.5	150	30	0.036			Lumbar

*After second injection.

cerebrospinal fluid occurring 10 to 30 minutes after injection, depending on the diffusion characteristics of the drug.

Figure 4–1 represents a typical clinical experiment by Frumin and his colleagues (1953b). By using two spinal catheters simultaneously, one in the epidural space and the other in the subarachnoid space, these workers found that procaine appeared in the cerebrospinal fluid quite soon after epidural injection, and the rise and fall of concentration was associated with the waxing and waning of clinical analgesia. Skin analgesia was present when the concentration of procaine in the cerebrospinal fluid rose above 0.015 per cent (or 150 μg/ml).

The question arises, do these concentrations of local anesthetics have any clinical relevance? Are they strong enough to produce clinical spinal anesthesia, or are they just camp followers to some more important event? Available data suggest that they are relevant, but probably only marginally so. It is worthwhile reviewing the evidence at this point, because it is crucial to our understanding of the role that spinal root block plays in the total picture.

In the laboratory the results were complex and at first confusing, but

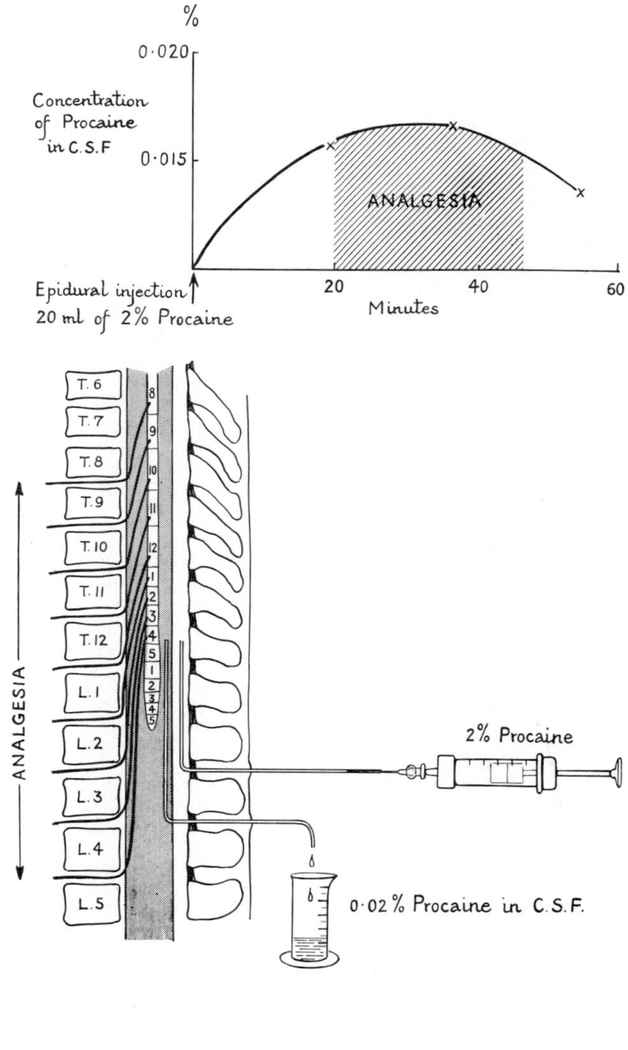

Figure 4–1. Recovery of procaine from cerebrospinal fluid after epidural injection. (Data from Frumin et al., 1953b.)

the evidence is now more precise; for a detailed discussion the reader is referred back to the section on Differential Blockade in Chapter 2. Briefly, the question of whether a given nerve fiber will be blocked or not depends on four variables: time, space, nerve species and concentration—that is, the duration of exposure to the anesthetic, the length of axon exposed, the type and site of axon and the concentration of anesthetic cation at the axon membrane. It will be recalled that unmyelinated C-fibers, thought to be heavily implicated in pain sensation, are quite resistant to very dilute solutions of local anesthetic and may continue to fire when most myelinated A-fibers are blocked. Nathan and Sears (1961) showed that 0.01 per cent procaine is sufficent to block small myelinated A-delta fibers in spinal roots, but twice the concentration (0.02 per cent procaine) will block all A-delta fibers and some C-fibers. The studies of Franz and Perry in 1974 confirmed that 0.02 per cent procaine would block even the largest *myelinated* A-fibers, provided at least 2 cm of axon was exposed to the local anesthetic for 37 minutes, but even then some unmyelinated C-fibers were still firing.

In the light of these findings and the data summarized in Table 4–1 it is clear that all the animal experiments, and most of the human ones, had peak spinal fluid levels high enough to cause partial if not complete spinal root blockade, at least in segments close to the sampling site.

In some of these investigations a possible artifact could have arisen from epidural solution leaking inward around a sampling subarachnoid catheter, as in the model shown in Figure 4–1 (Frumin et al., 1953b). This technical objection can be avoided by threading the intrathecal catheter downward from the cisterna magna (Rudin et al., 1951; Bromage and Burfoot, 1964), as shown in Figure 4–2. With this arrangement, repeated cycles of epidural injection and cerebrospinal fluid sampling can be made without fear of leakage artifacts arising. Figure 4–3 shows the pattern of cerebrospinal fluid concentration that is produced when a second epidural injection is given at a relatively short interval after the first (Bromage and Burfoot, 1964; Bromage et

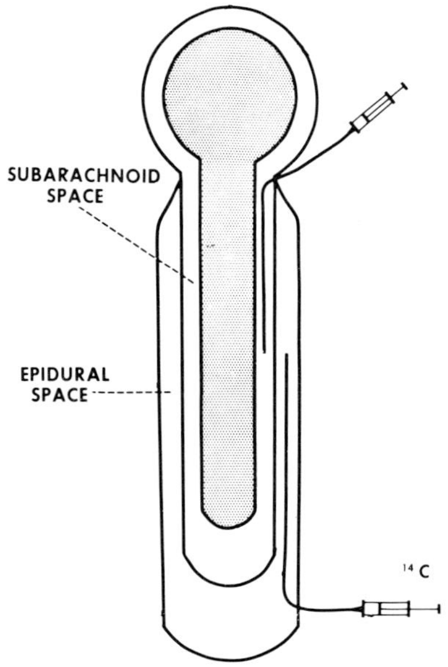

Figure 4–2. Penetration of local anesthetic through the spinal meninges. A sampling catheter is inserted downward in the subarachnoid space via the cisterna magna. A second catheter is threaded upward in the epidural space via a sacral bur hole until the tips of the two catheters lie opposite each other, separated only by the intact meninges. ^{14}C-labeled local anesthetic is injected through the epidural catheter, and serial cerebrospinal fluid samples are withdrawn through the upper catheter. (After Rudin et al., 1951, and Bromage, 1975.)

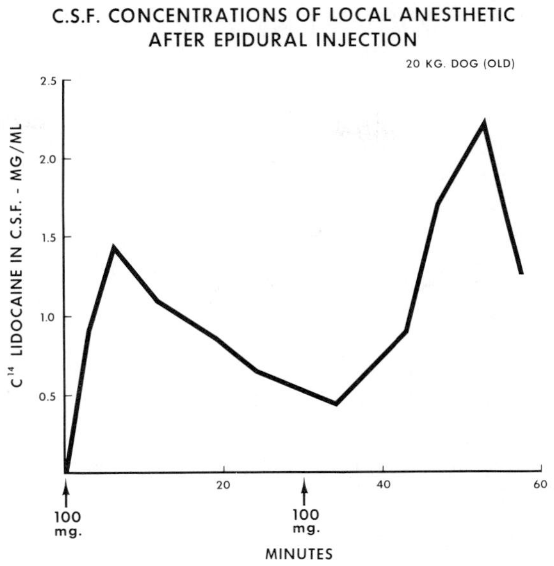

Figure 4–3. Cerebrospinal uptake of local anesthetic from the epidural space in dogs. Concentration of ^{14}C-lidocaine (expressed as mg lidocaine HCl per ml CSF) after extradural injection of 100 mg of 2 per cent ^{14}C-labeled lidocaine HCl (at arrows), using the experimental arrangement shown in Figure 4–2. (From Bromage, et al., 1964.)

al., 1964). The second curve summates with residues from the first, and the second peak is appreciably higher. A corollary of the second augmented peak is seen as intensified sensory and motor blockade in clinical practice, as shown in Figure 4–4. The results in Figure 4–4 are drawn from patients receiving either 2 per cent lidocaine or mepivacaine, and in each case half the initial dose was injected after an interval of 35 to 60 minutes following the original induction dose. It can be seen that the intensity of motor blockade is markedly increased by the second reinforcing dose. This augmented effect from a second reinforcing injection is the reverse of the phenomenon of tachyphylaxis discussed in the preceding chapter (Bromage et al., 1964).

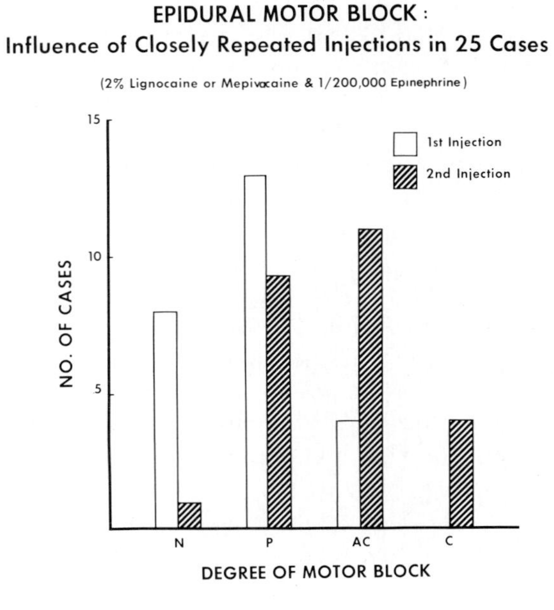

Figure 4–4. Epidural motor block: influence of closely repeated injections in 25 patients receiving 2 per cent lidocaine or 2 per cent mepivacaine with 1/200,000 epinephrine. Motor blockade is intensified by injecting a second epidural dose before the effects of the first have worn off. N = No motor block; P = partial block; AC = almost complete block; C = complete block. (See Figure 4–16 for criteria for measuring motor blockade.) (From Bromage, P. R., Burfoot, M. F., Crowell, D. E., and Pettigrew, R. T.: Quality of epidural blockade. I. Influence of physical factors. Brit. J. Anaesth. *36*:342, 1964.)

Neuraxis

For some reason investigators have been slow to acknowledge the spinal cord as a possible site of blockade in either subarachnoid or epidural analgesia. This is surprising in view of Corning's original intent of medicating the cord in his much quoted report of 1885.

In 1949, Frank Howarth at Cambridge approached this question in an original manner using autoradiographic and radioassay techniques to analyze the distribution of labeled local anesthetics from the subarachnoid space. Subsequent studies of cord uptake have been strongly influenced by this work. Although Howarth's measurements were done on subarachnoid rather than epidural solutions, his findings indicated the general pattern of uptake into the spinal roots and cord. Cerebrospinal fluid, spinal roots and the peripheral and central portions of the spinal cord of cats were assayed at intervals after 12 mg of radioactive dibromoprocaine were injected into the subarachnoid space. Within 5 minutes the labeled drug had reached a concentration of 3.9 μg/mg in the cerebrospinal fluid, 1.0 μg/mg in the spinal roots and 0.52 μg/mg in the peripheral parts of the cord. Twenty minutes later the ratio of cerebrospinal fluid to neural concentrations had changed, with more drug present in the neuraxis than in the cerebrospinal fluid bathing it, and the respective concentrations were then 0.2 μg/mg in the cerebrospinal fluid, 0.4 μg/mg in the roots and 0.3 μg/mg in the peripheral parts of the lumbar cord. This demonstrated a rapid redistribution of local anesthetic, with movement of drug out of the cerebrospinal fluid into the neighboring neural tissues, and pointed to the very incomplete information available from cerebrospinal fluid measurements alone.

Ellis Cohen repeated this work at Stanford in 1968 using ^{14}C-lidocaine in dogs and obtained similar results. Cohen paid more attention to detailed regional distribution, and it is interesting to see that he found the highest concentrations of labeled drug in the posterior and lateral columns of the cord (1.38 and 1.36 μg/mg), while only two-thirds of this amount was present in the dorsal roots and about one-tenth in the dorsal root ganglia.

In 1954 Frey and Soehring turned to the question of neuraxial distribution after epidural injection, and their findings were surprisingly similar to those obtained by the experiments of Howarth and Cohen with subarachnoid injection. Frey and Soehring injected 2 per cent procaine into the epidural space of dogs and then sampled cerebrospinal fluid, spinal roots and cord at various intervals afterwards. Within 10 minutes of epidural injection, the concentrations of procaine in the cerebrospinal fluid and spinal roots were equal and at a level of 1.0 μg/mg, while about half this amount was present in the spinal cord. During the next 20 minutes the cerebrospinal fluid concentration fell rapidly toward zero, while the concentration in the cord and roots declined relatively slowly (Frey and Soehring, 1954).

We carried out similar studies at McGill in 1963 using ^{14}C-labeled mepivacaine and lidocaine in anesthetized, ventilated dogs, with injection and cerebrospinal fluid sampling arrangements as shown diagrammatically in Figure 4–2. After a decay curve for cerebrospinal fluid concentration was obtained (see Figure 4–3), the epidural space was flushed with saline and then the dogs were killed and the spinal cords excised with the meninges intact. Scintillation assays

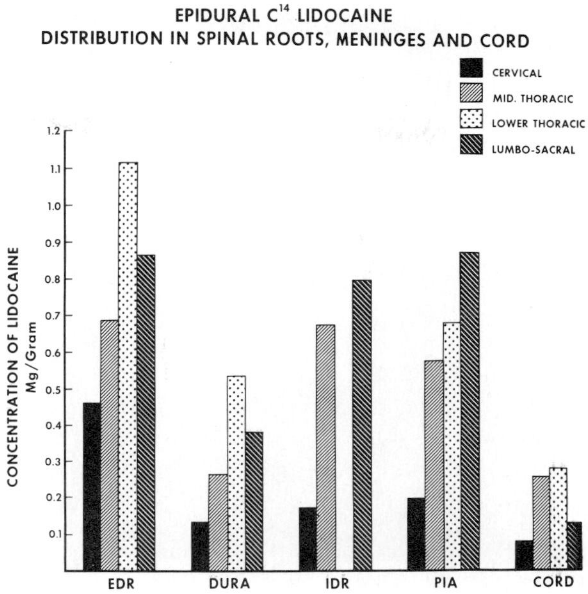

Figure 4–5. Concentration of ^{14}C-labeled lidocaine (expressed as mg/g wet tissue) in the neuraxis and its coverings after extradural injection of 2 per cent ^{14}C-labeled lidocaine in dogs. EDR = Extradural roots; IDR = intradural roots. (From Bromage, P. R.: Mechanism of action of extradural analgesia. Brit. J. Anaesth. *47*:199, 1975.)

were then done on extradural spinal nerves, the intradural spinal roots, the dura mater, the pia arachnoid stripped from the surface of the cord and segments of the whole stripped cord. The results after injection of 100 mg of ^{14}C-labeled lidocaine in five dogs are shown in Figure 4–5. It was almost as if the dura did not exist as a diffusion barrier. The concentration of local anesthetic was nearly as high in the intradural roots as in the extradural nerves, at about 1.0 to 1.5 μg/mg, and the pia mater also contained similar quantities, while about half this amount was present in the cord itself.

Autoradiograms of sections of frozen cord, illustrated in Figure 4–6, showed radioactivity distributed principally around the periphery, while sections of the brain showed that some radioactivity had extended as far as the medulla, and concentrations of up to 0.034 μg/mg were found in the cerebellum (Bromage et al., 1963; Bromage and Burfoot, 1964).

It is interesting to see that the distribution of local anesthetic in spinal roots and cord is very similar whether a small dose of local anesthetic is injected intrathecally or a larger one given extradurally. To illustrate this point, Table 4–2 compares the distribution of local anesthetics in the cerebrospinal fluid, spinal roots and cord from the independent studies by Howarth (1949), Cohen (1968) and Bromage and his colleagues (1963, 1964). Details of lidocaine concentrations after subarachnoid and epidural injection are also compared in Figure 4–7 to show the relationship of tissue concentrations to the minimum effective concentration, or C_m, of lidocaine. Note that in the subarachnoid study by Cohen, only very small amounts of drug were found in the dorsal root ganglia, in spite of the close proximity of the ganglia to the cul-de-sac draining the subarachnoid space. Also note that some of the lidocaine concentrations measured in the CSF and spinal cord were five times greater than the minimum effective concentration.

Thus, from available laboratory evidence it seems clear that epidural injections do reach the neuraxis and penetrate the peripheral parts of the cord

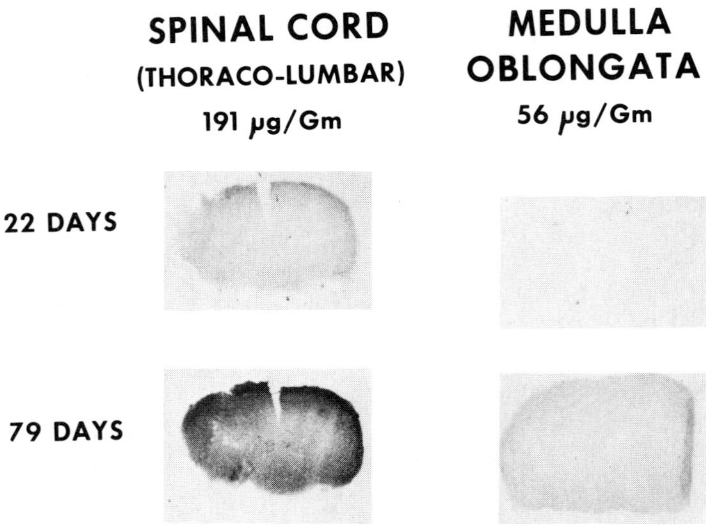

Figure 4–6. Autoradiograms of spinal cord and medulla oblongata of dog killed 45 minutes after epidural injection of ^{14}C-labeled lidocaine HCl. Sections exposed to photographic film for 22 days (top) and 79 days (bottom). Sections contain 191 µg/g and 56 µg/g of lidocaine, respectively. Dense line on right of medullary section is an artifact from folding of tissue. (From Bromage, P. R., Joyal, A. C., and Binney, J. C.: Local anesthetic drugs: Penetration from the spinal extradural space into the neuraxis. Science *140*:392, 1963.)

in appreciable quantities equal to the concentrations found in the spinal roots. Again the question arises, is this relevant to the clinical situation? The answer is probably yes, as we shall see when we come to consider the clinical evidence.

Dorsal Root Ganglion

The dorsal root ganglion has been a strong favorite in the list of speculative sites for epidural blockade. Since it is enclosed in the dural root

TABLE 4–2 Approximate Concentrations of Radioactive Local Anesthetic (µg/mg) in Lumbar Roots and Spinal Cords of Animals 30 Minutes after Intrathecal or Extradural Injection

	Subarachnoid Injection		*Epidural Injection*
	HOWARTH (1949)	*COHEN (1968)*	*BROMAGE ET AL. (1963, 1964)*
Sampling Site	Dibromoprocaine in Cats (µg/mg)	Lidocaine in Dogs* (µg/mg)	Lidocaine in Dogs (µg/mg)
Cerebrospinal fluid	0.2	0.83	1.5
Spinal roots	0.4	0.59	0.5–1.3
Whole cord	–	0.27	0.2–0.87
Peripheral cord	0.3	1.38	–
Central cord	0.049	0.34	–
Dorsal root ganglion	–	0.16	–

*C_m (lidocaine) = 1 mM/L ≡ 0.028 per cent ≡ 0.28 µg/mg.

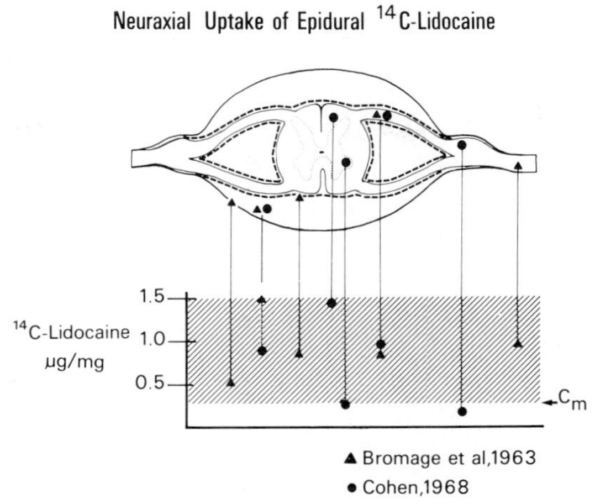

Figure 4–7. Neuraxial uptake of ^{14}C-labeled lidocaine after epidural (▲) or subarachnoid (●) injection. A minimum effective concentration (C_m) of 1 mM/L or 0.028 per cent is assumed. Hatched area covers range of CSF and tissue concentrations that exceed C_m. Note that the highest tissue concentrations are five times greater than the C_m.

sleeve where dural permeability is very high, it seemed self-evident that ganglion cells of afferent fibers lying in the funnel of these permeable sleeves should be particularly vulnerable to local anesthetics flowing past them. Frumin and his colleagues (1953a, 1954) suggested that the dorsal root ganglion was the primary site for subarachnoid and peridural anesthesia with threshold amounts of local anesthetic, and the idea has received fairly general acceptance (Shantha and Evans, 1972).

However, Cohen's figures for dorsal root ganglion uptake shown in Table 4–2 do not support this, as he found relatively small quantities of local anesthetic in the ganglion and only one-fifth of the amount that was present in the spinal roots. Moreover, local anesthetics are more likely to act upon the axonal extensions of afferent neurons at the nodes of Ranvier rather than on the soma of these monopolar cells. Although local anesthetics may penetrate the dural sleeve close to the ganglion, it does not follow that the ganglion is the prime target. In fact, available evidence suggests that it merely lies in the pathway of drugs penetrating to more absorptive sites in the roots and posterolateral portions of the spinal cord.

Extradural Nerves and Subperineural Spread

Since the early work of Sicard and Cestan in 1904, it has been known that epidural solutions escape readily through the intervertebral foramina into the paravertebral spaces. The areolar tissue around the exit of the intervertebral foramina varies in density according to age. In the young it is soft and tenuous, but with advancing age it undergoes increasing condensation and can form a definitely recognizable structure, tending to obstruct passage outward to the paravertebral spaces. Peridurograms from oily radiopaque injections in old people show less lateral spread than in the young (Bromage, 1954), but reports with water-soluble contrast media do not seem to demonstrate this difference so clearly (Luyendijk and van Voorthuisen, 1966; Burn et al., 1973).

The length of nerve exposed to local anesthetic in the paravertebral space is therefore quite variable and dependent on the volume of solution injected and the age of the subject. The degree of paravertebral spread is likely to be negligible when small volumes are used in old people, but in the young when volumes of 20 ml or more are used, the length of paravertebral nerve exposed may exceed 1 cm (Burn et al., 1973). Solutions reaching the paravertebral space are in a position to diffuse through the nerve coverings to the subperineural space, entering a pathway which in theory could take them centripetally into the contiguous subpial space of the cord, as discussed in Chapter 2 (Falk, 1936). This roundabout route is a theoretical option open to all major nerve blocks, but the amount of drug it carries to the cord is not likely to be of great practical importance in comparison with the alternate and more direct pathway in the region of the dural root cuff.

CORRELATION OF PHYSICAL AND ANALGESIC SPREAD: RADIOPAQUE AND RADIANT TRACER STUDIES IN THE EPIDURAL SPACE

Spread of radiopaque materials in the epidural space is strongly affected by pneumatic and hydrodynamic changes associated with respiratory movements; therefore, postmortem radiographic studies of epidural spread in the corpse have only limited relevance to events taking place in living subjects (Heile, 1913; Moore et al., 1958). However, it would clearly be of great interest if the physical spread of solutions in the epidural space could be correlated with the clinical spread of analgesics in living subjects. Numerous attempts have been made to do this using X-ray or radiant tracer materials, but with only partial success.

Sicard and Forestier's radiological studies of epidural spread in the 1920's were confined to X-ray diagnostic methods using Lipiodol, and this work eventually led to the development of intrathecal myelographic techniques (Sicard and Forestier, 1932). It is curious to note that Lipiodol must have been used in many thousands of extradural and intrathecal injections since 1921, yet no satisfactory method existed for sterilizing it (Ardley, 1954). Presumably, there must be enough free iodine present to suppress microbial growth.

Later, in 1940, Odom used emulsions of Lipiodol and 2 per cent procaine. Serial X-rays showed initial longitudinal spread in the epidural space, followed by lateral transforaminal spread 15 to 30 minutes later, so he assumed that the site of anesthetic action must also be transforaminal and at the spinal nerves in the paravertebral spaces. However, using a similar technique in elderly patients, Bromage (1954) found that in many instances when clinical anesthesia was complete and symmetrical, the radiopaque emulsion was almost entirely confined within the spinal canal. Contrary to Odom's findings, this suggested an intraspinal rather than a paraspinal site of action, at least in old subjects.

Other radiological studies done over the next 15 years showed little more than a general tendency for radiopaque solutions to travel upward in the spinal canal rather than downward in a caudal direction (Frumin et al., 1953a; Cheng, 1963; Usubiaga et al., 1967). Nishimura and his colleagues (1959) used a scintillation counting method with a mixture of lidocaine and ^{131}iodine, and they too confirmed a preferential cephalad spread of radioactive solution that roughly coincided with the segmental spread of analgesia.

Varella (1971) attempted to demonstrate a correlation between radiological and clinical spread by using a mixture of 2 per cent lidocaine with 50 per cent Hypaque. He found that while X-ray levels and analgesic levels coincided in some cases, in others there were marked differences, with a tendency for clinical anesthesia to spread further than the contrast medium. Burn et al. (1973) carried out similar studies, also without obtaining a very satisfactory correlation. Schulte-Steinberg (1976, Schulte-Steinberg and Rahlfs, 1977) used caudal injections of contrast material and 4 per cent lidocaine in children, and they confirmed Varella's impression that the segmental level of cutaneous analgesia extended further in a cephalad direction than the upper limit of contrast material within the epidural space. One of the difficulties with this sort of experiment is that a tracer solution, in this case a water-soluble contrast medium, and a local anesthetic are absorbed and distributed at different rates. Better correlation between radiographic and anesthetic spread might be obtained by reverting to emulsions of oily, nonabsorbable agents, such as Pantopaque.

As the matter stands, these studies have not done much more than provide a rather general impression that physical spread and analgesic spread are partially associated and that both tend to travel upward in a cranial direction more easily than downward to the caudal canal. Futhermore, clinical analgesia spreads beyond the upper segmental level of the radiographic indicator, whether injectiòn is made by the lumbar route or via the sacral hiatus.

CLINICAL STUDIES OF SPREAD OF EPIDURAL ANALGESIA

Clinical and laboratory observations complement one another, and each provides different opportunities for testing hypotheses. The clinical investigations that follow have been carried out slowly over a period of 25 years. The clues that they provide to the mechanism of action of epidural analgesia are often indirect and poorly susceptible to measurement, but taken together they constitute a reasonably plausible body of hints and guesses to yield a practical working hypothesis until more direct methods of analysis are applied to the problem. In my opinion these clinical studies have yielded as much, if not more, fundamental information than more glamorous laboratory experiments directed to the same questions, and I believe their efficiency as a research tool has been greater in terms of cost-effectiveness.

For a long time, clinical management of epidural blockade was based on three assumptions that seemed self-evident. First, the number of segments anesthetized would depend on the volume of the anesthetic injected. Second, since the epidural space is like a cylinder, a larger volume would be needed for tall patients with long backs than for short ones. Third, the quality or intensity of sensory and motor blockade would be governed by the concentration of the local anesthetic. In fact, each of these factors is poorly correlated with the practical outcome, so it is understandable that techniques based on the essential irrelevance of these premises should have given rise to the idea that epidural analgesia is inherently unpredictable (Morrow, 1959; Mostert, 1960). The clinical interrelationships of concentration, volume and effect are indeed surprising, as we shall see; nevertheless, they are predictable with considerable accuracy,

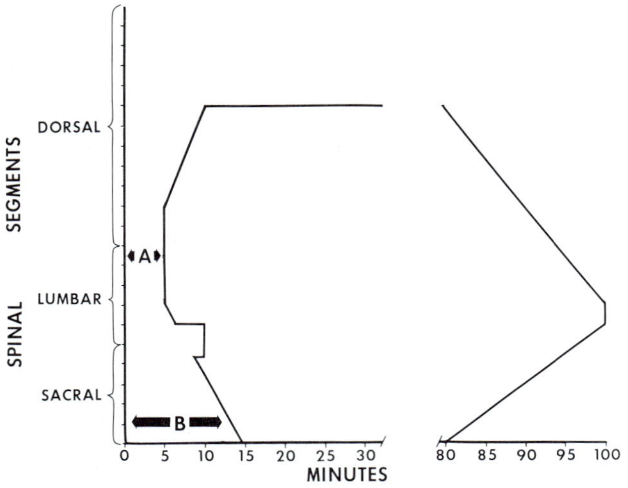

Figure 4–8. Segment-time diagram of spread and regression of epidural analgesia after injection at the second lumbar interspace. A = Latency of initial onset; B = latency of complete spread of analgesia.

and they add to the body of circumstantial evidence for the probable mode of action of epidural blockade.

By maintaining constant technical conditions in a large number of patients and altering one variable at a time, it has been possible to analyze the effects of several independent variables on the predictability and clinical outcome of epidural anesthesia. Every case of epidural analgesia was tested for the onset, spread and decay of blockade using pin-prick as a measurement of sensory blockade, and segment-time diagrams were constructed as shown in Figure 4–8. A diagram of this sort yields a considerable amount of basic information if it is constructed rigorously, with attention to detail and to accurate measurements on both sides of the body. The following components of the diagram are then susceptible to statistical analysis:

1. Speed of initial onset of analgesia. That is, the time from injection to the first appearance of analgesia.

2. Segmental profile of analgesic spread.

3. Symmetry or asymmetry of analgesic spread.

4. The number of segments anesthetized. The segmental spread of anesthesia is of major interest, and the relationship of the dose to the number of anesthetic segments expresses the average amount of anesthetic required per spinal segment, thus:

$$\text{Dose requirements per spinal segment} = \frac{\text{Dose injected}}{\text{Number of spinal segments anesthetized}}$$

For example, if it is supposed that 20 ml of 2 per cent lidocaine caused complete cutaneous analgesia of all segments up to and including the seventh thoracic dermatome on both sides of the body, the number of segments blocked would be five sacral, five lumbar and six thoracic, or a total of 16 on each side. The dose requirements in this case would be expressed as:

$$\frac{\text{Dose of local anesthetic}}{\text{Average number of spinal segments anesthetized}} = 20 \div (16 + 16)/2$$

$$= 1.25 \text{ ml per segment (or 25 mg lidocaine per segment)}$$

The expression "dose requirements" is not an accurate index of the amount of anesthetic required for each individual segment that is blocked, for some segments close to the site of injection take up more drug than others at the marginal extremes of segmental spread (Bromage et al., 1963). However, it gives a workable and relevant indication of the amount of drug that is needed for that particular individual, and it serves as a basis for predicting the needs of other cases under the same clinical circumstances. This statistic has been used extensively in our clinical investigations, and it has served well to clarify many points that were previously obscure.

5. Area of the segment-time diagram in Figure 4–8 expressed in terms of segment-minutes. The area of the segment-time diagram can be related to the epidural dose, and then it is expressed as so many segment-minutes per milligram of local anesthetic. This expression provides a quantitative basis for studying the phenomenon of acute tolerance, or tachyphylaxis, that accompanies repeated epidural injections, as outlined in the preceding chapter on Pharmacology.

6. Duration of action, from the time of complete spread of analgesia until the upper level of analgesia has receded two spinal dermatomes.

Segmental profile of analgesic spread

After injection of an epidural anesthetic, a latent period of 2 to 6 minutes follows before any clinical analgesia becomes apparent. Then cutaneous analgesia appears in two or three segments close to the site of injection and gradually spreads to involve neighboring segments. The onset and spread of anesthesia can be recorded as a segment-time diagram by plotting on graph paper the upper and lower limits of analgesia against time, as shown in Figure 4–8.

The profile of segmental spread depends on the site of injection, and the shape of the onset profile is different for the thoracic, lumbar and caudal regions. The characteristic shapes of the onset profiles at these three different injection sites are determined by the size of the underlying nerve roots, the thickness of their coverings and the distance the local anesthetic must travel to reach them, as well as by the intrathoracic pressures influencing physical spread within the spinal canal. The basic characteristics of thoracic, lumbar and caudal epidural spread are outlined in Figure 4–9.

Mid-thoracic profile

After injection in the mid-thoracic region, analgesia spreads upward and downward, as shown in Figure 4–9. The dose requirements, in terms of the amount of drug required to block one spinal segment, are least in the thoracic region. The amounts required are about seven-tenths the quantity needed in the lumbar region and about one-third the amount needed for caudal blockade. A relatively pure segmental block develops when small volumes of local anesthetic are injected in the thoracic region, and full sensation and motor power are retained in the legs. If larger volumes are injected, analgesia gradually spreads

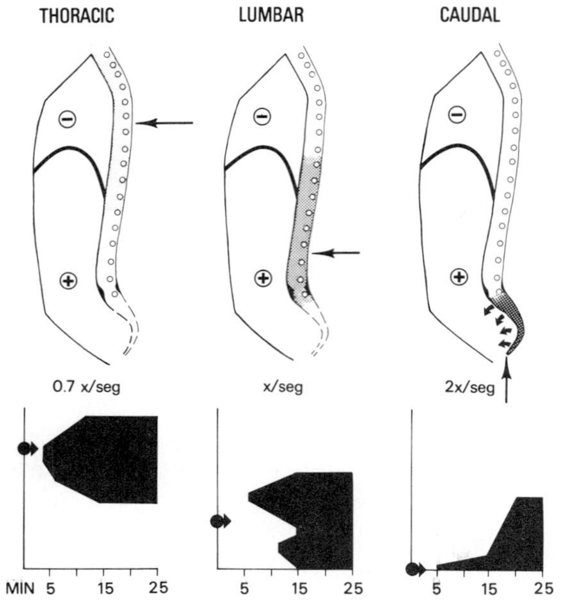

Figure 4–9. Pattern of fluid dispersion within the extradural space after injection in mid-thoracic, lumbar or caudal regions, with typical onset profiles of segmental analgesia for 2 per cent lidocaine.
⊖ = Negative intrathoracic pressure
⊕ = Positive intra-abdominal pressure
Relative dose requirements are shown as:
Thoracic 0.7x/seg
Lumbar x/seg
Caudal 2x/seg

downward to involve the lumbar and sacral segments, and voluntary control of the legs becomes impaired.

Lumbar profile

Epidural injection at the second lumbar interspace results in the characteristic shape of the onset profile shown in Figure 4–8. Initial spread of analgesia occurs fairly rapidly in the lower thoracic and upper lumbar segments, and the upward march of analgesia proceeds in a roughly linear fashion. However, downward spread is slowed at the fifth lumbar and first sacral segments. Analgesia jumps these two resistant segments and proceeds downward into the lower sacral segments. The salient of delay at L_5–S_1 is exaggerated when slowly penetrating local anesthetics, such as tetracaine or dibucaine, are used, and satisfactory analgesia often fails to develop at the outer aspect of the foot and calf. However, the salient of delay at L_5 and S_1 is virtually eliminated when powerfully penetrating agents, such as carbonated lidocaine, are used, and then satisfactory analgesia develops rapidly in all the lumbar and sacral segments (see Chapters 3 and 9). The phenomenon of delay at L_5 and S_1 is almost entirely due to the large size of the spinal roots and thickness of their dural coverings, as well as to the great number of neurons subserving these segments. In addition, the spinal cord reaches its largest girth at this segmental level, so any local anesthetic action at the periphery of the cord will reach to relatively shallow depths at this point (see Chapter 2).

Caudal profile

Analgesia is slow to develop after caudal injection. With lidocaine, 12 to 17 minutes usually elapse before the sacral segments develop surgical analgesia. However, the exaggerated delay at L_5 and S_1, so characteristic of lumbar blockade, is less obvious with the caudal approach. The reason for this clinical difference is not clear. Dose requirements (i.e., milligrams of drug per spinal segment) are very large by the caudal route compared to thoracic or lumbar blockade. Anatomical factors determine this difference (see Chapters 2 and 8). In adults, condensation of epidural fat at the lumbosacral junction hinders upward spread in the extradural space, while the large anterior sacral foramina allow local anesthetic solution to leak out of the sacral canal, to become lost in the retroperitoneal tissues.

Factors Affecting Physical Spread in the Spinal Cylinder: Height, Gravity and Speed of Injection

At first sight it seems self-evident that factors such as height, posture and speed of injection should play an important role in the physical spread of solutions within the epidural space and in the subsequent extent of clinical analgesia, yet these physical influences are rather poorly correlated with segmental spread of analgesia.

Height

The volume of the epidural space is proportional to its length, and this in turn is related to body height. To test the association of height with segmental spread, dose requirements were plotted against height in 155 normal subjects between the ages of 20 and 81 years. The results are shown in Figure 4–10. There is a general trend toward larger dose requirements with increasing

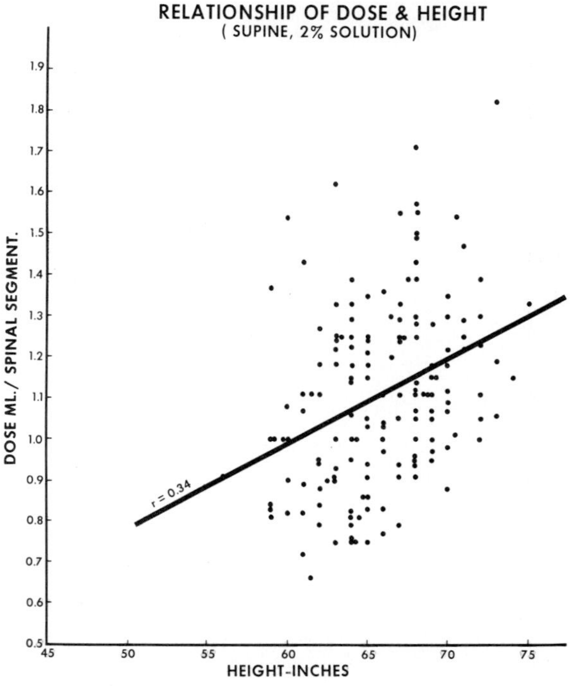

Figure 4–10. Relationship of lumbar epidural dose requirements to body height in 155 normal patients. Single injection at second lumbar interspace of 2 per cent solution of either lidocaine, mepivacaine or prilocaine. (From Bromage, P. R.: Spread of analgesic solutions in the epidural space and their site of action: A statistical study. Brit. J. Anaesth. *34*:161, 1962a.)

height, but the statistical association is weak, as shown by the low correlation coefficient ($r = 0.34$). Thus, while the length of the spinal cylinder may be taken into account when dose requirements are being computed, the actual predictive value of this measurement is relatively insignificant, and for all practical purposes it can be ignored except in extremely short or extremely tall individuals.

POSTURE

The effects of gravity on epidural spread have been rather poorly investigated, and there is still some difference of opinion about the influence of posture on caudal or cephalad spread of analgesia. Nishimura et al. (1959) used a radioactive tracer (^{131}I) to track the physical spread of epidural solutions in human subjects, and they came to the conclusion that posture had no appreciable influence. In a clinical study of 80 normal subjects induced in the sitting position, Bromage (1962a) found that there was a slight but significant difference between dose requirements in the supine and sitting positions. At 40 years of age about 20 per cent more solution was needed when patients were sitting up than when they were lying down (see Figure 4–11). This study suggested that gravity does in fact favor downward spread and hinder upward spread and that, from a clinical point of view, it is worthwhile exploiting gravity to favor spread in dependent parts of the epidural space. However, the magnitude of this physical influence is not great, and other factors are probably more important in determining segmental spread.

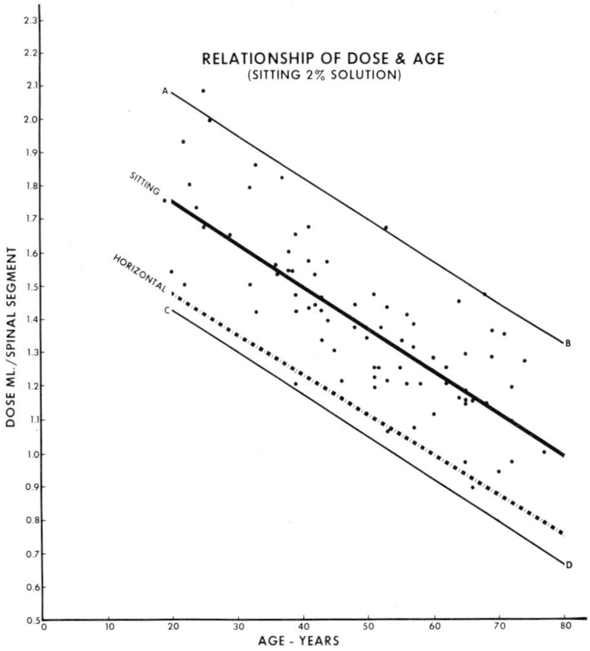

Figure 4–11. Effect of horizontal versus seated posture on lumbar epidural dose requirements. Regression lines for dose requirements (ml/spinal segment) related to age. Single-shot injections of 2 per cent lidocaine, mepivacaine or prilocaine in 80 normal subjects in sitting position (●) compared to mean for horizontal posture.

——— Mean regression line for 80 seated patients with 95 per cent confidence limits to the population (AB, CD)

■I■I■I Mean regression line for patients in horizontal position ($p < 0.001$)

(From Bromage, P. R.: Spread of analgesic solutions in the epidural space and their site of action: A statistical study. Brit. J. Anaesth. 34:161, 1962a.)

Speed of Injection

The anatomy and mechanics of the epidural space might lead one to suppose that a rapid forceful injection of local anesthetic would produce more effective spread of analgesia than a slow rate of injection. However, this is not so. Early investigators stressed that the best results followed slow injection rates in the range of 0.3 to 0.75 ml/sec, and this has been confirmed by comparative clinical measurements of slow and fast injection rates in human volunteers (Erdemir et al., 1965; see Chapter 6, Table 6–5).

Thus, the body of available data suggests that physical factors affecting anatomical spread of epidural anesthetic solutions have little relevance to the segmental analgesia that actually develops. The a priori assumption that segmental levels of analgesia should be determined by the physical extent of longitudinal spread in the epidural space is not in accordance with existing evidence. Therefore, other factors affecting segmental spread must be sought.

Dose Requirements and Age

The relationship between epidural dose requirements and age follows a pattern that is both unexpected and at the same time basic to many biological measurements. Schulte-Steinberg and Rahlfs (1970, 1972, 1977) have made a careful study of the alterations in segmental dose requirements with advancing age in babies and children receiving caudal anesthesia, and they found a linear and highly predictable increase in dose requirements up to the age of puberty.

My own studies of epidural spread and dose requirements in relation to age were obtained with a number of different local anesthetic agents in more than 2,000 patients between 4 and 102 years. Injection was made under standardized conditions at the second lumbar interspace (Bromage, 1954, 1962a, 1962b, 1965b, 1967, 1969a, 1969b; Bromage and Gertel, 1970). The association of segmental dose requirements with age for one single agent (2 per cent lidocaine) is shown in Figure 4–12. A computer search was made of the data from Figure 4–12, and lines of best fit were sought by polynomial and by linear regression. The closest fit was given by two straight lines intersecting with their apex between 18.25 and 18.5 years of age. In other words, the total data could be described more accurately as two independent populations represented by two discontinuous straight lines than as a single population described by a continuous polynomial.

This rather striking finding implies that some crucial event occurs at about 18½ years, converting the continuum of age into two quite distinct epochs. Dose requirements rise steeply during the period of growth and maturation, and then at 18½ years, when body growth has reached its limits, the opposing effects of senescence become unmasked and the inexorable march of decay from birth to grave is revealed as a linear downhill progression that declines predictably into the ninth decade at the rate of about one-tenth of the zenith value per decade. By that age the data become widely scattered, and acceleration of the slope becomes apparent as a second downward trend in the curve.

Again, what does this mean in terms of the process we are studying? First, one can recognize that the general pattern of relationship between dose

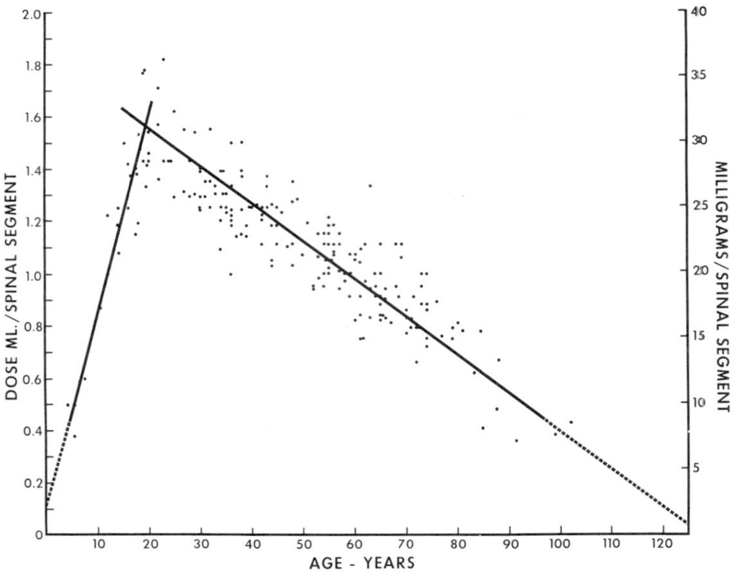

Figure 4–12. Dose requirements related to age for 2 per cent lidocaine with 1/200,000 epinephrine (supine position) in 210 surgical patients. Best fitting regression lines cross at 18¼ years of age. (From Bromage, P. R.: Ageing and epidural dose requirements. Brit. J. Anaesth. *41*:1016, 1969b.)

requirements and age is not unique to epidural analgesia but is common to many other biological measurements. For example, a curve of the same general shape is obtained by plotting vital capacity against age (Jouasset, 1960; Berglund et al., 1963; De Muth et al., 1965). The second part of the curve from 19 to 100 years is reflected by the downward slopes for such parameters as capillary resistance (Gough, 1962), nerve conduction velocity (Downie and Newell, 1961; Norris et al., 1953) and the population of nerve fibers in spinal roots (Corbin and Gardner, 1937; Semenowa-Tjan-Schanskaja, 1941; Shock, 1961, 1962).

It would seem that the first part of the curve before 18½ years is dominated by the simple physics of an expanding spinal cylinder. Dose requirements increase as the cylindrical space lengthens and enlarges and the binding sites increase within it. After growth ceases, neural barriers become less effective with age as mucopolysaccharides alter and condense within connective tissue and nerve coverings (Dyrbye, 1959; Ham and Leeson, 1961). The change in character of connective tissue is due to a gradual shift in the balance of fibroblast activity, with proportionately larger amounts of collagen formation and less production of the amorphous mucopolysaccharides that form the intercellular matrix between the collagen and elastic fibers (Lindner and Johannes, 1973). The proportion of mucopolysaccharide matrix to collagen (or the gel:fiber ratio) in connective tissue declines linearly with age (Clausen, 1963, 1966).

The nerve population of the neuraxis and spinal roots also declines with age, until by the ninth decade one-third of the neuronal population has disappeared (Corbin and Gardner, 1937; Hodge, 1894; Rexed, 1944). Thus, the pattern of changing dose requirements with age can probably be explained quite simply in terms of impaired tissue barriers, changing numbers of binding sites and a declining neuronal population.

If one were to take the absurd and statistically forbidden liberty of extrapolating beyond our data, the regression line for dose requirements would cut the abscissa somewhere between 110 and 135 years. At that point dose requirements would be zero, and the central nervous system would be so depleted from natural causes that communication with the external environment would be as effectively cut off as if a total epidural block were present all the time. With such a degree of deafferentation, there is reason to believe that respiration would cease spontaneously (Bromage, 1958; Salmoiraghi and Burns, 1960), and in the absence of extraordinary measures, death would be inevitable from this cause alone.

Arteriosclerosis

Dose requirements are reduced below the predicted chronological level when the natural aging process is accelerated by disease, as in diabetes or arteriosclerosis, and the spread of analgesia behaves as if the patients were 30 to 40 years older than their chronological ages (Bromage, 1962b). A trend toward diminished dose requirements is seen, even in early diabetes, before the occult effects of diabetic microangiopathy become evident in the cardiovascular system, reflecting the high incidence of subclinical neuropathy in diabetic patients (Skillman et al., 1961; Lawrence and Locke, 1963; Moore and Frew, 1965).

Spread of analgesia is affected both spatially and temporally by arteriosclerosis, for along with its tendency to spread abnormally far, analgesia also takes longer than usual to reach its furthest extent. In one series both parameters differed from normal by approximately the same degree, with a 40 to 50 per cent increase in the segmental spread of analgesia and a 35 per cent lengthening of latency (Bromage, 1962b).

Figure 4–13 shows the individual dose requirements for 2 per cent lidocaine, mepivacaine and prilocaine in arteriosclerotic patients, plotted against the average for a normal population, in the supine position (*A*) and in the sitting position (*B*). In Figure 4–13*B*, the abnormal arteriosclerotic data are superimposed on normal dose-age regression lines for 2, 3, 4 and 5 per cent lidocaine. If we refer the arteriosclerotic values to the normal 2 per cent regression lines, we can see that the arteriosclerotic dose requirements are reduced to the level of those of a normal subject who is 30 to 40 years older. To put it another way, in some of the arteriosclerotic patients 2 per cent lidocaine spreads equally as far as would 5 per cent lidocaine in a normal subject; segmental analgesia may spread up to 2½ times further than would be expected in normal subjects. Figure 4–14 summarizes the arteriosclerotic data in histogram form, showing the percentage reduction of epidural dosage below the calculated dose in a normal population (Bromage, 1962b).

Figure 4–15 shows the prolonged latency of analgesia with 2 per cent lidocaine in 48 arteriosclerotic patients compared to the onset and spread of analgesia in 126 normal patients. It can be seen that a delay of 30 minutes for complete spread of analgesia is not unusual in the presence of severe degenerative arterial disease. It is curious that this exaggerated spread takes

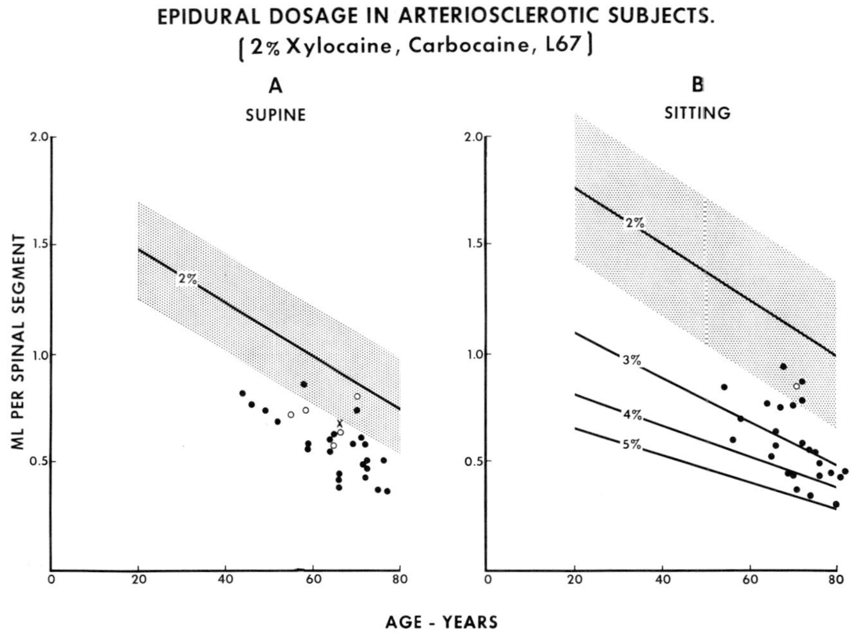

Figure 4–13. Relationship of age and epidural dose requirements (ml per spinal segment) in normal and arteriosclerotic patients. *A*, Horizontal position. Thirty arteriosclerotic subjects. *B*, Sitting position. Twenty-six arteriosclerotic subjects, superimposed on regression lines for, 2, 3, 4 and 5 per cent lidocaine in normal patients.

——— Mean regression lines and 95 per cent confidence limits of normal population (hatched area) for 2 per cent lidocaine

● 2 per cent lidocaine
○ 2 per cent mepivacaine
× 2 per cent prilocaine

(From Bromage, P. R.: Exaggerated spread of epidural analgesia in arteriosclerotic patients: Dosage in relation to biological and chronological ageing. Brit. Med. J. *2*:1634, 1962b.)

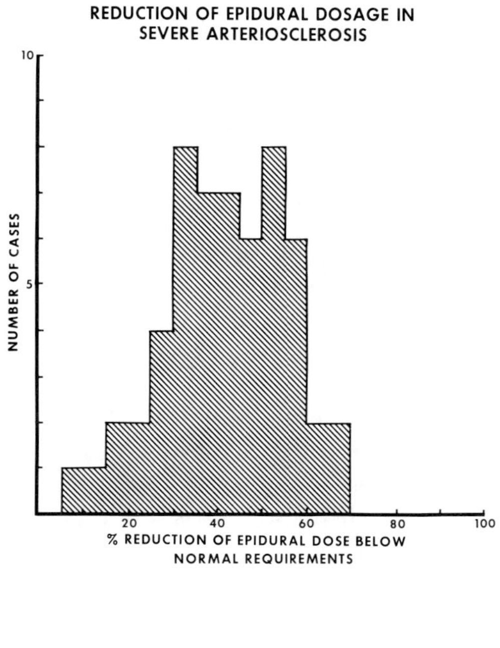

Figure 4–14. Distribution of epidural dose requirements in 53 arteriosclerotic patients, expressed as percentage reduction below normal dose requirements. (From Bromage, P. R.: Exaggerated spread of epidural analgesia in arteriosclerotic patients: Dosage in relation to biological and chronological ageing. Brit. Med. J. *2*:1634, 1962b.)

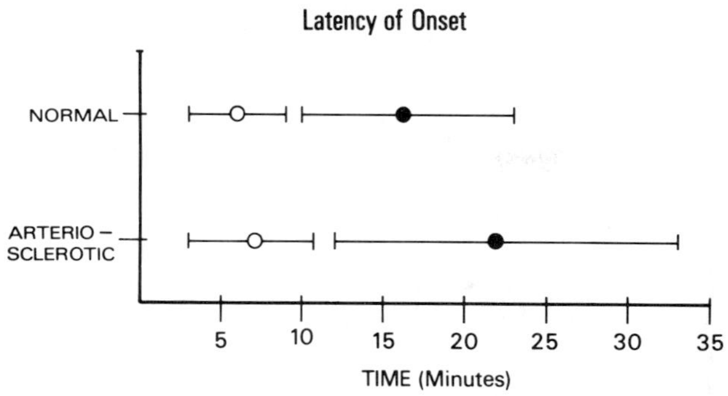

Figure 4–15. Latency of epidural analgesia induced at the second lumbar interspace in normal subjects (n = 126) and arteriosclerotic patients (n = 48). Means and range of observations.
○ = Latency of initial onset of analgesia
● = Latency for complete spread of analgesia
(After Bromage, 1962b.)

longer and not shorter than normal to reach its fullest extent. One would expect a shorter latency if some factors were favoring spread through the tissues. However, a slow latency would be compatible with a reduced and more widely dispersed number of target sites for local anesthetic absorption in neural and extraneural tissue, such as the loss of neurons (Greenbaum et al., 1964) and changes in ground substance of connective tissue (Dyrbye, 1959; Gough, 1962) that occur in diabetic neuropathy.

Thus, the abnormally slow spread and reduced dose requirements in arteriosclerosis present a caricature of the normal aging process, probably dependent upon a prematurely declining neural population.

Pregnancy

Another type of facilitated spread is observed in parturient women (see Chapters 10 and 12). In these subjects dose requirements are reduced by about one-third below normal values. However, latency of onset is shortened rather than prolonged in pregnant subjects, and the mechanism of facilitated spread is quite different from that seen in arteriosclerotic patients, two forces are at work: a cardiovascular component and an altered hormonal milieu.

At term the gravid uterus partially occludes the inferior vena cava, and a proportion of the venous return from the legs and pelvic structures is diverted into the internal vertebral venous plexus. The engorged vertebral veins reduce the effective volume of the epidural space and cause a rise in extradural pressure (Bromage, 1961; Kerr et al., 1964; Scott and Kerr, 1963; Galbert and Marx, 1974). These hemodynamic forces acting within the spinal canal tend to disperse fluids more widely than usual throughout the epidural and subarachnoid spaces, as shown radiographically by Hipona et al. (1966) and Barclay et al. (1968).

In addition, steroid hormonal influences probably contribute to the increased spread of epidural anesthetics in pregnant women (Walker and Balf, 1954; Salvatore, 1961), but the precise size and nature of this hormonal contribution are still unknown. However, evidence is accumulating that both neurons and their integuments are affected by the raised blood levels of cortisol and female reproductive steroids that accompany pregnancy.

Male and female hormones are taken up by motor and sensory cells to different degrees. Stumpf and his colleagues have shown that androgens are concentrated in motor cells (Sar and Stumpf, 1977), while estrogens are concentrated in sensory nuclei and in laminae I, II and III of the dorsal horn in the spinal cord (Stumpf et al., 1975). Stumpf (1975) has coined the term "hormone architectonics" to include this form of sexual discrimination exercised by the motor and sensory inhabitants of the central nervous system. At present there is no evidence that estrogens modulate the sensitivity of sensory neurons to local anesthetics. Nevertheless, it must be recognized that other hormones, such as thyroid and adrenal cortical hormones, do affect sensory performance (Henkin, 1975), and it is possible that some relationship may exist between the partiality of sensory neurons for estrogens and their increased susceptibility to spinal local anesthetics during pregnancy. Future work may shed light on this question.

The neural integuments acting as connective tissue barriers to local anesthetic diffusion are also targets for reproductive steroids during the altered endocrine "gestalt" that accompanies pregnancy (Schiff, 1966; Jeffrey et al., 1975). The intercellular matrix of connective tissue changes under the influence of progesterone and estrogen (Giannetti and Cerimele, 1970) and the collagen fibers become more widely dispersed, with increased quantities of ground substance between their interstices (Bryant et al., 1968).

The ease with which water and solutes such as local anesthetics diffuse through connective tissue ground substance depends on the relative amounts of free fluid and gel in the matrix, and this in turn is determined by the proportion of protein and long interlocking molecules of mucopolysaccharides in the system (Wiederhielm et al., 1976). The latter appears to be under hormonal control, and it is probable that the facilitated analgesic spread of pregnancy is at least partly due to an expanded volume of free fluid between the gel domains of the mucopolysaccharide meshwork in the intercellular ground substance.

VOLUME AND CONCENTRATION OF ANALGESIC SOLUTIONS

The effects of varying concentration and volume of local anesthetics on the spread and quality of epidural blockade seem unexpected and bizarre at first sight. However, underlying the oddity and the unexpectedness of these clinical effects lie some of the most important clues in arriving at a coherent idea about the basic mechanism of action of epidural analgesia.

The great popularizers of epidural anesthesia used large volumes of relatively weak local anesthetic to obtain adequate operating conditions (Dogliotti, 1939; Gutierrez, 1939; Dawkins, 1945). In the writings of Dogliotti and Gutierrez, volumes of 60 to 100 ml of 1.0 to 1.5 per cent procaine were recommended for extensive procedures. For more localized blocks, Dogliotti recommended small volumes of a more concentrated solution, of the order of 15 to 20 ml of 3 per cent procaine (Dogliotti, 1939). From this stemmed the generally accepted idea that a large *volume* ensured extensive segmental spread of analgesia, while *concentration* determined the quality and duration of blockade. More potent drugs such as dibucaine (Nupercaine) and tetracaine (Pontocaine) were used in slightly smaller volumes of 20 to 50 ml at concentrations of 0.15 to 0.2 per cent (Dawkins, 1945; Durrans, 1947). My own records from 1949 show doses as high as 48 ml of 1/600 (0.167 per cent) dibucaine given as a single injection in the lumbar region, with resultant analgesia reaching no higher than the fourth thoracic dermatome (Bromage, 1954).

Reports in the German literature between 1937 and 1955 gave support to the notion that highly concentrated solutions would produce intense and prolonged but restricted segmental analgesia. These writings developed from the assumption that a "plombe," or localized "slug," of a viscous solution containing up to 1.5 per cent tetracaine would restrict segmental spread, and highly complicated techniques were evolved on the basis of this idea (Denecke, 1937; Düttmann, 1941; Goepel, 1947; Buchholz and Lesse, 1951; Poppelbaum, 1954).

Doubts about the importance of volume in determining segmental spread began to emerge when lidocaine became available for clinical practice. Here was an agent that gave a more rapid and intense degree of analgesia than other established agents such as 1/600 Nupercaine. Analgesia spread excessively far with lidocaine in a concentration of 1.2 per cent compared to 1/600 Nupercaine, and the volume injected had to be reduced by 20 to 40 per cent below the accustomed amount in order to keep the segmental spread of blockade within acceptable limits (Bromage, 1954). Experience with lidocaine, and later mepivacaine, accumulated and eventually it was possible to construct dosage charts based on age and height that were highly predictable for 2 per cent solutions of these agents (Bromage, 1962a).

Prilocaine was introduced in 1960, and a study was designed to compare its performance with lidocaine in 2 per cent and 3 per cent concentrations. It was only then that we came to doubt seriously the relative roles of concentration and volume in determining the spread and quality of blockade. First, disappointment arose when it became obvious that the 3 per cent solutions of lidocaine and prilocaine did not produce more intense analgesia than the 2 per cent concentrations. Then confusion was added to disappointment when predicted volumes of the 3 per cent solutions, based on 2 per cent dosage requirements, were found to spread unpredictably far and to produce unexpectedly extensive segmental blockade. The confusion cleared when enough cases had been studied to draw a regression line of dose requirements against age. When this was done it could be seen that spread of analgesia with the 3 per cent solution was in fact completely predictable. Three per cent lidocaine spread predictably further than the 2 per cent solution, and simple arithmetic showed that, in calculating the dose for a particular number of segments at any given age, it was not the *volume* that was important but rather the *mass* of solute that determined the number of anesthetized segments (Bromage, 1962a, 1965a).

The concept of mass of drug rather than volume as the dominant factor in segmental spread of epidural analgesia was disturbingly at variance with accepted ideas about mechanism of action. How could volume not be the most important determinant of spread in the epidural space? Moreover, if volume was not the determinant, what model could one possibly propose to support the unlikely claim that mass of drug influenced segmental spread?

Before an attempt was made to answer these questions, it was necessary to see if the pattern could be repeated for other concentrations and for other agents. Accordingly, a large comparative series of lumbar epidural blocks was performed, and groups of patients were given 1, 2, 3, 4 or 5 per cent lidocaine, or 0.1, 0.2, 0.3, 0.4 or 0.5 per cent tetracaine. Each concentration was tested in populations of 20 to 40 patients between the ages of 18 and 85 years, and the groups were large enough to calculate regression lines for age and dose requirements for each test solution. In addition, an estimate of the quality of blockade was made by assessing the intensity of motor block in the legs according to the following simple criteria, as shown in Figure 4–16 (Bromage, 1965b):

Criteria	*Degree of Block*
Free movement of legs and feet	Nil (0%)
Just able to flex knees, with free movement of feet	Partial (33%)
Unable to flex knees, but with free movement of feet	Almost complete (66%)
Unable to move legs or feet	Complete (100%)

The patient was asked to move his legs and feet, and degrees of motor block were classed as nil, partial, almost complete or complete; for purposes of numerical comparison, these categories were given scores of 0 per cent, 33 per cent, 66 per cent and 100 per cent, respectively. Since the intensity of motor block is often asymmetrical in epidural analgesia, both legs were assessed and scored separately for each patient, and the total score was averaged for each test solution.

The results of these clinical measurements are shown in Figures 4–17 and 4–18 (Bromage et al., 1964; Bromage and Burfoot, 1966; Bromage, 1975). In Figure 4–17 it can be seen that the wide differences for volumetric dose requirements become resolved when expressed as mass of drug (i.e., volume × concentration). In terms of mass, the dose requirements for 2, 3, 4 and 5 per cent lidocaine are almost identical. A similar constancy of mass is seen with the lower dose requirements for the more potent agent tetracaine in concentrations of 0.2, 0.3 and 0.4 per cent. Within these ranges of concentration, the mass of drug required to block one spinal segment is almost constant at any given age,

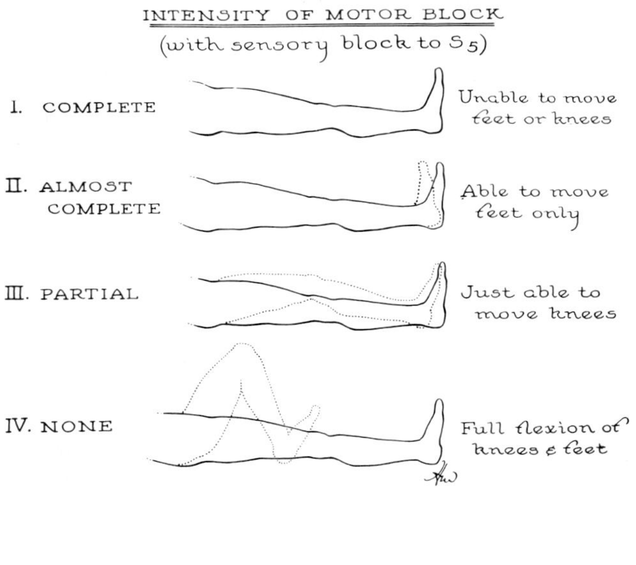

Figure 4–16. Assessment of motor block (see text). (From Bromage, P. R.: A comparison of the hydrochloride and carbon dioxide salts of lidocaine and prilocaine in epidural analgesia. Acta Anaesth. Scand. (Suppl.) *16*:55, 1965b.)

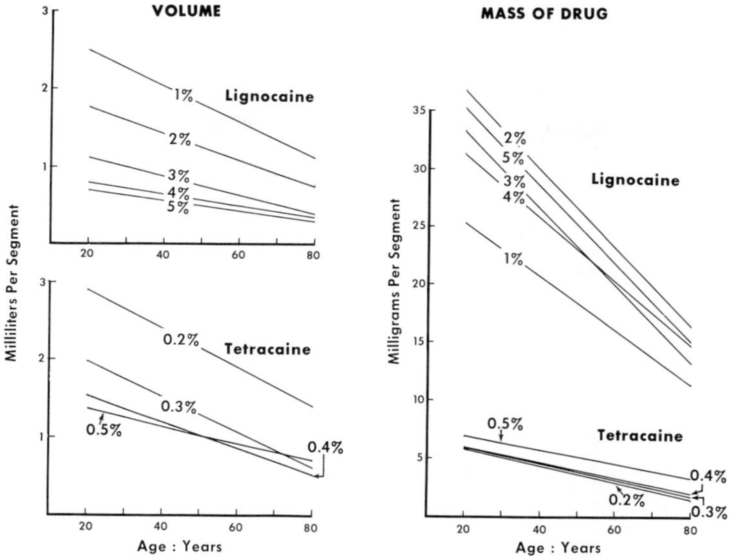

Figure 4–17. Mean segmental dose requirements for 1, 2, 3, 4 and 5 per cent lidocaine (lignocaine), and 0.2, 0.3, 0.4 and 0.5 per cent tetracaine. Results expressed volumetrically on left and gravimetrically on right. (From Bromage, P. R.: Mechanism of action of extradural analgesia. Brit. J. Anaesth. *47*:199, 1975.)

regardless of concentration and volume. Note that intensity of motor block with plain lidocaine is negligible, even at 5 per cent concentration. Increased concentration is also without effect in the 2 to 5 per cent range when epinephrine 1/200,000 is added, although the plateau of the motor block curve is raised very significantly by the vasoconstrictor action of epinephrine (see Figure 4–18).

The curves for intensity of motor block and for dose requirements

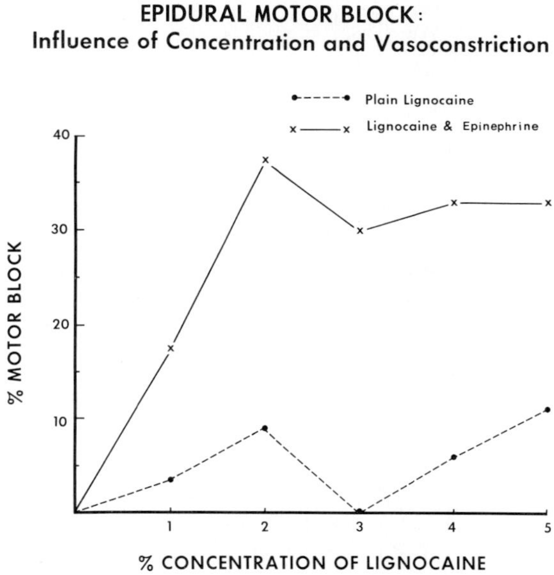

Figure 4–18. Intensity of motor blockade with epidural lidocaine (lignocaine). Influence of concentration and vasoconstriction. (From Bromage, P. R., Burfoot, M. F., Crowell, D. E., and Pittigrew, R. T.: Quality of epidural blockade. I. Influence of physical factors. Brit. J. Anaesth. *36*:342, 1964.)

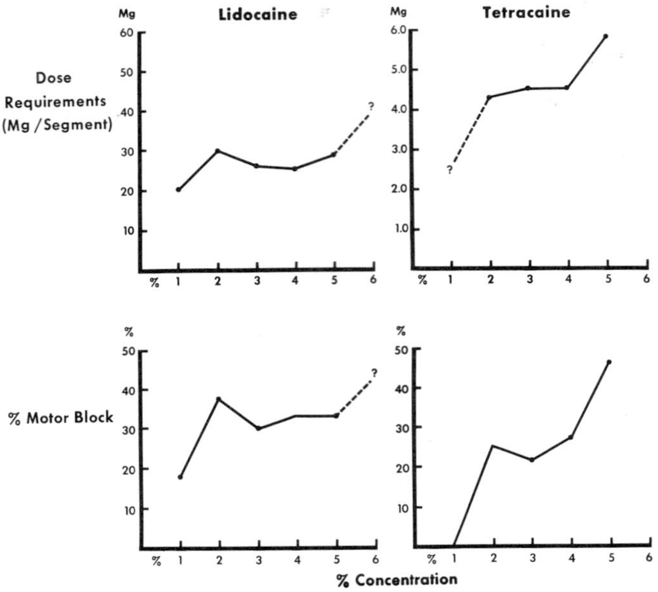

Figure 4–19. Mean segmental dose requirements and intensity of motor blockade at 40 years of age for 1, 2, 3, 4 and 5 per cent lidocaine, and 0.1, 0.2, 0.3, 0.4 and 0.5 per cent tetracaine. ? = Untested or inadequate data. Tetracaine, 0.1 per cent, gives inadequate analgesia for reliable sensory testing. (After Bromage et al. 1964; Bromage and Burfoot, 1966; and Bromage, 1975.)

follow a similar pattern in the case of lidocaine and tetracaine, as shown in Figure 4–19. Dose requirements and intensity for each drug remain on a plateau over a considerable range of concentration. However, beyond this range the curves leave the plateaus and adopt an "S" shape. Thus, 1 per cent lidocaine with epinephrine spreads further and requires about one-third less dosage than the other concentrations. At this low concentration there is a more obvious differential block, and the quality of motor block is halved in terms of clinical measurement. The other end of the curve for lidocaine was not tested with concentrations above 5 per cent, but tetracaine shows an upswing when concentration reaches 0.5 per cent. At that point there is a 30 per cent increase in dose requirements and in the degree of motor block. There is no apparent motor block in the legs with 0.1 per cent tetracaine, and sensory anesthesia is so patchy and tenuous that measurements of segmental spread cannot be made accurately.

Latency of onset does not show any consistent trend parallel with these alterations of dose requirements and intensity of motor blockade. A priori, one might expect that speed of onset would become faster with increasing concentration. This is not so, as shown by the two curves for onset and latency times of lidocaine in Figure 4–20. It is surprising that the time course of events for initial blockade and for complete spread of analgesia is almost identical with both 1 per cent and 5 per cent lidocaine. Onset time and spread for both of these concentrations are *slowed* by the addition of epinephrine 1/200,000 from 13.5 minutes for the plain solutions to 18 minutes for the epinephrine-containing solutions. Yet when epinephrine is added to the 2 and 3 per cent lidocaine solutions, the reverse effect is seen and latency is shortened. These curious observations are difficult to interpret, and one can only speculate that perhaps some vascular mechanism may be involved in the process of diffusion and penetration, and that vasoconstriction may delay this process at some stage in

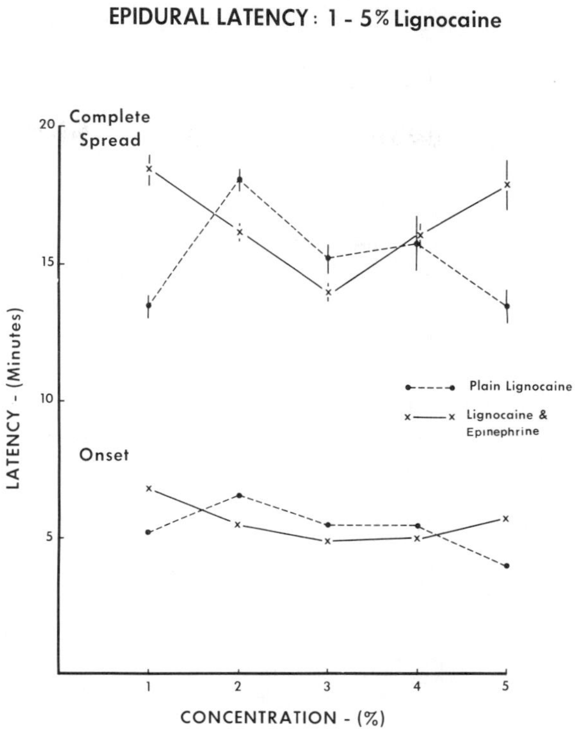

Figure 4–20. Latency of onset and complete spread of analgesia for 1 to 5 per cent lidocaine injected at the second lumbar interspace (means ± SE). (From Bromage, P. R., Burfoot, M. F., Crowell, D. E., and Pettigrew, R. T.: Quality of epidural blockade. I. Influence of physical factors. Brit. J. Anaesth. *36*:342, 1964.)

certain concentrations of local anesthetic. However, the final quality of blockade is superior when epinephrine is used as an adjuvant, regardless of the concentration of local anesthetic.

Sensory Dissociation and Reflex Changes

Three further bits of clinical information must be mentioned before we try to fit these apparently disjointed pieces together into a coherent whole.

First, the upper fringe of differential blockade that is so characteristic of established subarachnoid anesthesia is virtually absent in epidural analgesia. In subarachnoid block a zone of hypalgesia and thermoinsensitivity extends three to four segments cephalad beyond the upper limit of analgesia to pin-prick (Greene, 1958). This band of altered sensitivity is thought to be due to progressive dilution of local anesthetic in the cerebrospinal fluid, resulting in a zone in which only the smallest sensory fibers are blocked while the remainder escape. During induction of epidural blockade a similar but narrow and variable band of differential blockade may appear briefly for 5 to 10 minutes, but once the block is established, the upper level of insensitivity to cold coincides almost exactly with the segmental level for analgesia to pin-prick (Wugmeister and Hehre, 1967). The reason for this sensory difference between subarachnoid and epidural blockade is not immediately apparent, but it suggests that axial spread of epidural analgesia is more homogeneous than by the subarachnoid route, perhaps because the dilutional factors of the cerebrospinal fluid are bypassed by spread in some other space.

Second, some local anesthetic agents cause more sensory block than motor paresis, while others do the reverse. This dissociation of motor and sensory effect is seen most easily in obstetrical cases in which very small doses are used in patients who are temporarily more sensitive than usual to the action of epidural local anesthetics (see Chapter 12). For example, in parturient patients dilute bupivacaine (0.25 per cent) provides a good quality of sensory blockade with very little motor block, whereas 0.25 per cent tetracaine and etidocaine both produce relatively intense motor block with rather poor sensory anesthesia. This degree of dissociation of motor and sensory block is difficult to explain in terms of action on peripheral nerves, but it could be explicable if one were to envisage some degree of anesthetic action taking place within the spinal cord. Urban (1973) has found that the upper margin of cutaneous anesthesia follows a different pattern during induction and maintenance of analgesia than during regression. In his observations anesthesia spread upward in the classic pattern, following the familiar segmental contours. However, careful measurements during regression of analgesia on both the front and back of the body showed that the upper margin descended in a more even circumferential pattern in the sagittal plane. This is precisely the sort of pattern that might be expected from partial anesthetic section of the cord and is further supportive evidence that the spinal cord may be a significant site of action in epidural analgesia.

Finally, one other observation suggests involvement of the cord in epidural analgesia. During segmental epidural block carried out at the mid-thoracic level, reflex changes can be observed in the lower limbs that are normally interpreted as reflecting interruption of long descending pathways in the cord. Tendon jerks become more brisk, transient clonus may be seen and the Babinski reflex may become positive, with upgoing toes. These changes occur more frequently with etidocaine, which has very high lipid affinities, than with other agents (Bromage, 1974).

INTERPRETATION OF LABORATORY AND CLINICAL DATA

Now let us review all this clinical information and see if it can be interpreted in the light of the supporting laboratory data. The discussion that follows is only speculative, and it must not be taken in any way as a dogmatic representation of the mechanism of action, for much of the crucial laboratory evidence is still missing. However, enough hard data are available to put forward a working hypothesis with reasonable confidence that it will prove useful for a time.

The questions we are asking are (1) where is the spread of anesthetic drug occurring and (2) where is the drug acting? The cord and its coverings can be represented as a series of cylinders separated by spaces, as shown in Figure 4–2. Any of the spaces represented could be sites of dispersion and spread of the drug in its water-soluble cationic form, while any of the tissues, especially the peridural fat, could act as dispersion media and storage depots for the lipid-soluble, nonionized drug.

Figure 4–21 summarizes in diagrammatic form the clinical results of

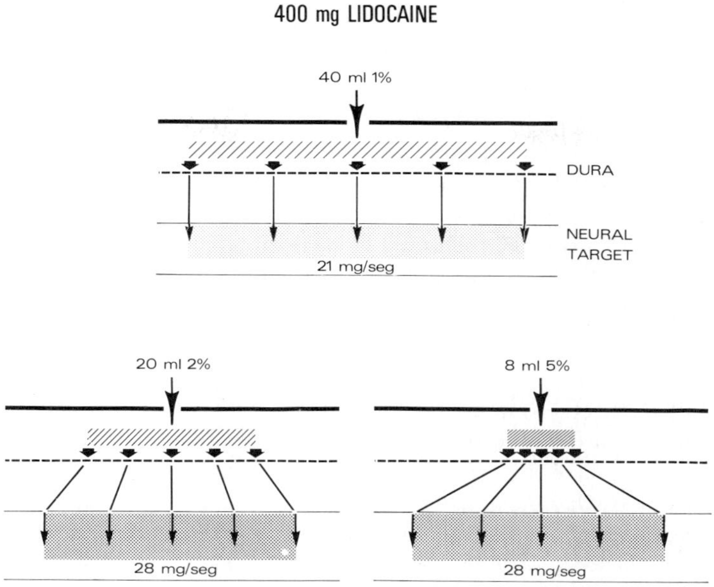

Figure 4–21. Schematic representation of segmental spread, dose requirements and intensity of motor blockade after epidural injection of 400 mg lidocaine in 1, 2 or 5 per cent concentrations. (From Bromage, P. R.: Mechanism of action of extradural analgesia. Brit. J. Anaesth. *47*:199, 1975.)

administering 400 mg of lidocaine to patients of comparable age (40 years) in concentrations of either 1 per cent, 2 per cent or 5 per cent, based on the data shown in Figure 4–19. The dilute 1 per cent solution produces a wide segmental spread but a rather feeble quality of blockade. The 2 per cent and 5 per cent solutions produce identical results, with about 35 per cent less segmental spread than the 1 per cent solution and about twice the intensity of blockade.

Immediately after injection, physical spread within the extradural space is presumably governed by the volume of solution injected. It is unlikely that osmotic dilution and volume expansion within the epidural space play a significant part in spreading the 5 per cent solution, as the osmotic strengths of all three solutions were adjusted to lie within the range of 200 to 300 milliosmoles/L. Similarly, it seems unlikely that dispersion by solution in the epidural fat could be the mode of spread in the short time available. Therefore, dispersion and spread of the concentrated 5 per cent solution probably occur *after* penetration of the dura and not within the epidural space. The observation that vasoconstriction prolongs the latency of both the 1 per cent and 5 per cent solutions to the same degree suggests that in both cases a vascular element may be involved in the mechanism of neural uptake. The pampiniform venous plexuses surrounding each nerve root have been cited as possible channels for uptake (Bromage, 1962a; Usubiaga et al., 1964). However, there is no experimental evidence that they indeed do perform a portal function and carry drug past tissue barriers into the nerve roots and spinal cord.

Whether or not a vascular element is involved, several possible diffusion pathways are available beneath the dura in the subdural, subarachnoid or subpial spaces, and at present the evidence is not strong enough to favor one more than any other. The high concentrations in the intradural roots found by radioactive tracer studies (see Figs. 4–5 and 4–7), suggest that the root sleeves with their arachnoid granulations are likely to be one of the principal sites of penetration through the dural barrier.

The next target and the site of greatest interest is in the cord itself, for here may lie an answer to some of the unresolved paradoxes of epidural analgesia. Pial concentrations of local anesthetic are high, almost as high as in the extradural and intradural roots. Beneath the pia there is a rich uptake at the surface of the cord, as shown in Figure 4–6, and local anesthetic penetrates inward for about one-third of the radius, so that actual values for local anesthetic concentrations in the periphery of the cord are probably about twice those for whole cord estimations and almost equal to the concentrations found in the spinal roots at the same segmental level. In our studies this would amount to concentrations of lidocaine in the range of 1.0 to 1.5 μg/mg in the outer third of the cord. This is equivalent to a 3 to 5 mM/L concentration and considerably in excess of the C_m (i.e., minimum effective concentration) of 2.5 mM/L lidocaine required to block a peripheral nerve in 10 minutes (Truant and Takman, 1959; De Jong, 1977). This concentration would be enough to cause significant blockade of some long pathways and modulation of inhibitory systems in the dorsal horn (Wall, 1967).

Figure 4–22 represents a cross section of the mid-thoracic cord showing the peripherally placed tracts involved by local anesthetic penetrating inward to a depth of 1 mm from the surface. Local anesthetics with high lipid-water solubility ratios will penetrate to greater depths than agents with low lipid solubility, and these differences in penetration could form the basis for the dissimilar clinical behavior of different local anesthetic drugs. It can be seen that the descending fibers of the sympathetic excitatory tracts lie just beneath the pia

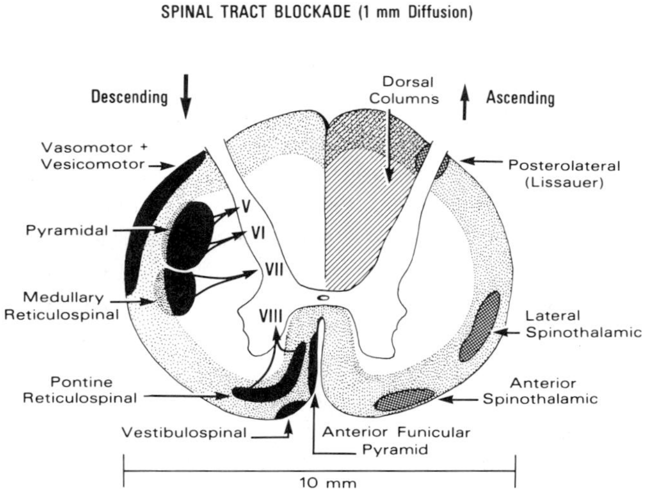

Figure 4–22. Local anesthetic penetration of mid-thoracic spinal cord from extradural space. Shallow penetration (light stippled area) affects peripheral ascending and descending pathways, but spares deeper descending pathways. Deep penetration affects excitatory and inhibitory functions of deep descending pathways. (After Bromage, 1975.)

(Kerr and Alexander, 1964; Foreman and Wurster, 1975) and in easy range of agents penetrating from the surface. This superficial anatomical location within the cord may partially explain the early onset of sympathetic blockade in epidural analgesia and the high incidence of Horner's syndrome during caudal blockade for obstetrical delivery (Mohan and Potter, 1975). The strange preponderance of motor blockade with the two highly lipid-soluble agents tetracaine and etidocaine also becomes intelligible in this light, as does the high incidence of upper motor neuron signs in the legs during a thoracic segmental block with etidocaine.

Progressive inward diffusion from the surface will affect successively deeper layers of cord. Superficially placed tracts will be bathed by blocking concentrations of local anesthetic before the deep ones, producing different patterns of inhibition and excitation depending on the proportion of ascending and descending pathways overtaken by the advancing circle of depression. In the mid-thoracic region where the cord is slimmest, with a lateral diameter of 9 to 10 mm, even shallow penetration will affect quite a large proportion of long pathways. At this level and at a depth of only 1 mm, as shown in Figure 4–22, a greater part of the anterior and lateral spinothalamic tracts will be blocked, together with some of the ascending tracts in the anterior funiculus, but the bulk of the more deeply placed lateral pyramidal tract will be spared. Consequently, most of the long afferent tracts subserving pain will be affected without any significant interruption of descending inhibitory pathways projecting to laminae V and VI from the pyramidal tract (Wall, 1967), and the net result will be a summation of analgesic influence suppressing the central projection of painful stimuli. The subject of sensory modulation in the spinal cord is discussed in Chapter 2 (see Fig. 2–27), and the reader is referred back to this section for a more detailed presentation of the relevant anatomy.

If cord blockade is indeed an important site of action in the overall picture of epidural analgesia, we may expect to find relative deficiencies of clinical analgesia at segmental levels where the girth of the cord is greatest. In fact, there does appear to be an inverse relationship between the diameter of the cord and the clinical efficacy of epidural analgesia at any given segmental level. Thus, in the mid-thoracic region where the cord is narrowest and the spinal roots are finest, blockade is rapid and intense. On the other hand, some of the segments subserved by the widest part of the lumbosacral enlargement are very resistant to blockade. The fifth lumbar and first sacral segments are notoriously difficult to block in lumbar epidural analgesia, particularly when poorly penetrating agents are used. This peculiar resistance may have a simple anatomical explanation in the large size of the spinal roots and in the very heavy girth of the spinal cord at that segmental level.

A paradoxical antianalgesic effect may be introduced by more powerful anesthetics penetrating to greater depths from the periphery of the cord. As increasing numbers of pyramidal fibers become affected, descending inhibitory influences on laminae V and VI will be weakened, allowing a heavier traffic of noxious stimuli to proceed along the few ascending tracts that still remain open, as represented in Figure 4–23. Many "gates" probably exist in the complex filtering system that colors the sensory images we form from the raw afferent input entering the cord, and it is quite likely that some of these gates concerned with pain sensation may lie in the deeper laminae VI, VII and

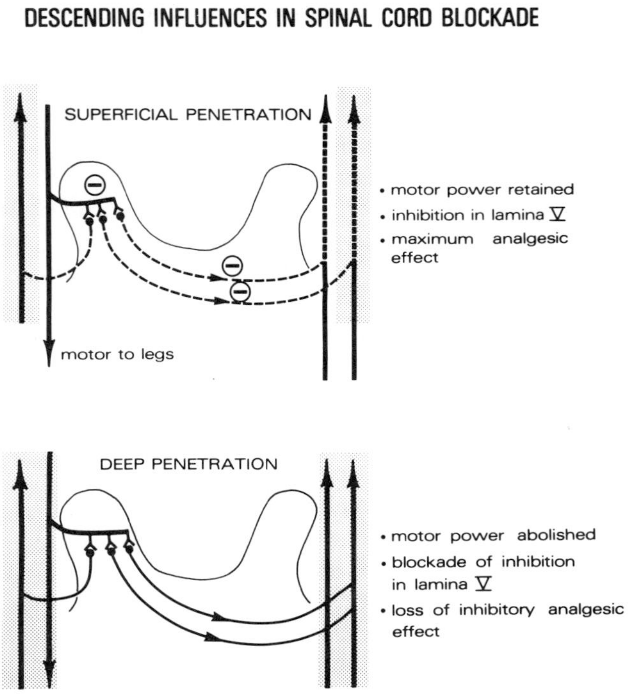

Figure 4–23. Diagrammatic representation of epidural blockade and modulation of sensory input in spinal cord. Effects of varying penetration of local anesthetic on peripheral sensory tracts, and on more deeply placed descending inhibitory pathways projecting to laminae V and VI.

Superficial penetration: Shallowly placed sensory tracts are blocked, but descending motor pathways and their inhibitory components are not blocked. Net result is maximal analgesia and minimal motor blockade.

Deep penetration: Superficial sensory tracts, deep motor pathways and inhibitory projections to laminae V and VI are all affected. Loss of inhibitory input to dorsal horn may allow some ascending sensory traffic to continue. Net result is maximal motor blockade and some anti-analgesic effect.

possibly VIII, acted upon by descending pathways traveling very superficially in the anterior sulcomarginal zone (see Fig. 4–24).

Therefore, suppression of facilitatory pathways would reinforce analgesia, whereas suppression of inhibitory pathways would have a contrary antalgesic effect. Variations in the balance of facilitatory and inhibitory blockade in the cord could account for the qualitative contrasts that we observe between different epidural anesthetics, such as tetracaine, etidocaine and bupivacaine, as shown in Figure 12–21 in Chapter 12 (Bromage, 1974; Bromage et al., 1974a, 1974b).

A more complex mechanism than the simple geometry of inward diffusion is suggested by the work of Cohen (1968) involving the use of radioactive tracers. Cohen's measurements of cord penetration in subarachnoid anesthesia showed greater uptake of procaine and lidocaine by the posterior and lateral parts of the cord than by the anterior funiculi, and he suggested that biochemical differences in various structures of the cord might account for these regional differences. If this idea is correct, then future research should be directed toward a better understanding of drug affinities within the neural and perineural elements of the cord, so that more accurate predictions can be made of the finer neurological responses to various epidural agents.

These subtle differences have some practical significance in the selection of drugs that are likely to be suitable for epidural analgesia. One of the most desirable features of epidural analgesia in the clinical field is the ability to provide sensory blockade without much loss of motor function. It would be most helpful if a reliable technique could be developed for quantitative examination of regional uptake in the cord as a prescreening test in animals before new agents are launched for clinical trial.

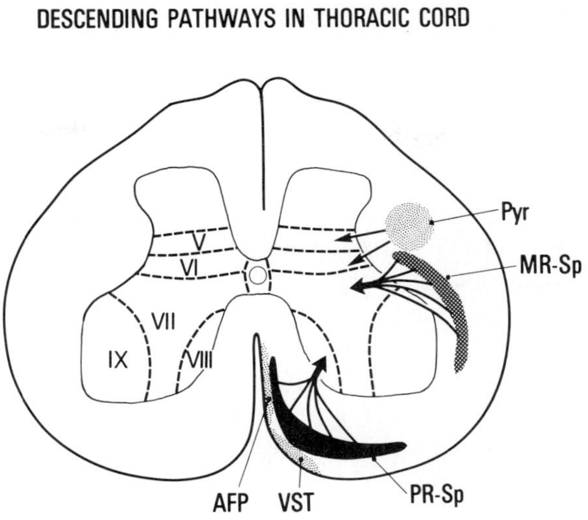

Figure 4–24. Descending pathways in spinal cord modulating sensory or motor activity. Proximity to the surface will determine the susceptibility of these tracts to blockade by local anesthetic penetration. Pyr = Pyramidal tract; MR-Sp = medullary reticulospinal fibers; VST = vestibulospinal tract; AFP = anterior funicular pyramid; RP-SP = pontine reticulospinal fibers. (After Nyberg-Hansen, 1965, 1969, and Kuypers, 1964.)

(From Bromage, P. R.: Lower limb reflex changes in segmental epidural analgesia. Brit. J. Anaesth. *46*:504, 1974.)

SUMMARY

In summary, then, the total weight of laboratory and clinical evidence reveals an unexpectedly complex, but to a degree predictable, interrelationship among the various factors involved in epidural blockade. We are left with the conclusion that epidural analgesia is not a simple matter of spinal root or ganglion blockade, but rather of action at several sites after passage through a labyrinth of diffusion pathways, both in series and in parallel, as outlined in Figure 4–25.

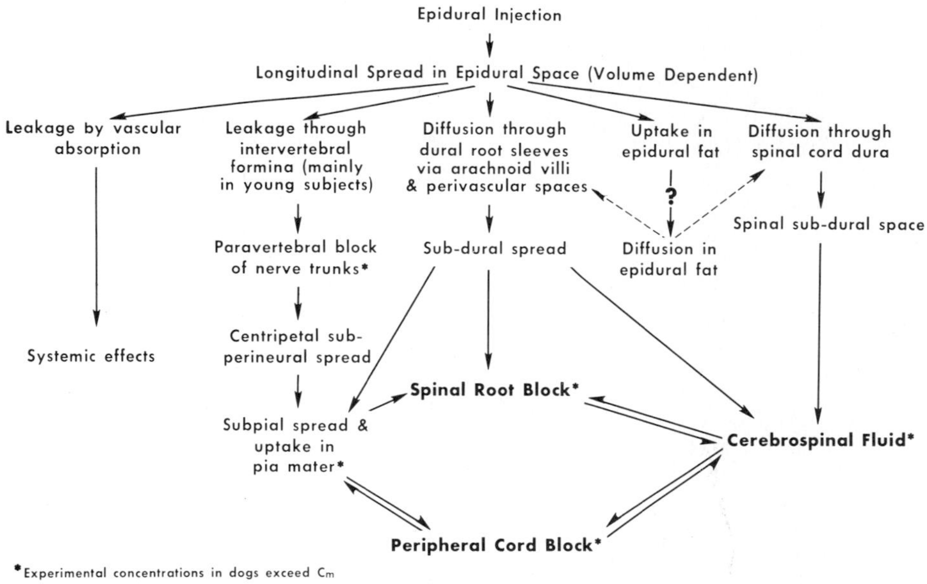

Figure 4–25. Fate of an extradural injection of local anesthetic. * = Sites where experimental measurement has demonstrated local anesthetic concentrations in excess of C_m. (From Bromage, P. R.: Mechanism of action of extradural analgesia. Brit. J. Anesth. *47*:199, 1975.)

Solutions spread longitudinally in the extradural space, and the distance they travel in this space will depend on the volume injected. Within the extradural space drug will be taken up and removed by blood flow, or it will be stored, and perhaps spread, in the extradural fat. In young subjects with freely patent intervertebral foramina, some solution will pass out of the spinal canal into the paravertebral spaces and along spinal nerves, producing a form of paravertebral block. From there, diffusion through the epineurium and perineurium into the subperineural space will allow some degree of centripetal spread backward toward the neuraxis, with subsequent access to the contiguous subpial space, and from there to the surface of the roots and the cord.

The most important portal of entry to the nervous system seems to lie in the region of the spinal root sleeves, where the arachnoid granulations and effluent spinal veins are concentrated in a small area. High extradural pressures probably favor passage through the root villi. Spread from this site can occur in the subdural space between the dura and the pia-arachnoid, or by further diffusion into the subpial space and subarachnoid space. From there, local anesthetic is taken up by the spinal roots and the surface of the cord, and the concentration of local anesthetic rises in the cerebrospinal fluid. In Figure 4–25, asterisks mark the sites where experimental measurements have demonstrated local anesthetic concentrations in excess of the C_m for lidocaine.

Given the present evidence, one cannot be dogmatic about the relative importance of the three principal sites of blockade. However, it is permissible to make a relatively enlightened guess.

1. Paravertebral block after foraminal escape is probably a nonessential and gratuitous feature confined to young subjects with freely patent intervertebral foramina. It is unlikely to occur to any significant extent in older subjects and with small volumes of solution.

2. The intradural spinal roots are probably the principal and essential site of blockade and the first elements to become anesthetized after an extradural injection. The concept of dorsal root ganglion block is appealing at first sight, but on reflection it is improbable. Local anesthetic agents have their principal action on nerve axons rather than on the soma of the nerve cell. Moreover, the little experimental evidence we have does not support ganglion block, and Cohen's figures showed only insignificant amounts of local anesthetic in the ganglia after subarachnoid blockade (Cohen, 1968).

3. Spinal cord block probably occurs after the roots are anesthetized, but involvement of incoming tracts (such as Lissauer's) and of the dorsal horn is likely to be an important and perhaps essential feature of extradural blockade. Penetration probably occurs to varying depths in the cord, depending on the local anesthetic agent and its physicochemical qualities. For example, one has the clinical impression that etidocaine penetrates the cord more effectively than lidocaine, as signs of upper motor neuron changes in the legs readily occur during segmental blockade after a single thoracic injection of etidocaine, but only rarely after lidocaine (Bromage, 1974).

The most interesting site of action is in the cord, for it is here that physicochemical differences of various local anesthetic agents will reveal their practical virtues and vices that normally become apparent only after prolonged clinical study. Future research should be directed toward developing an animal model for systematic study of regional uptake and distribution of local anesthetics in the spinal cord. The model should be designed to distinguish those agents that preferentially block facilitatory pathways and so reinforce analgesia rather than those which suppress inhibitory pathways, with resultant weakening of analgesic effect. Then, after the lapse of nearly a century, our system of ideas may return full circle, back again to a more sophisticated interpretation of Corning's original intention when in 1885 he proposed "spinal anaesthesia and local medication of the cord."

REFERENCES

Ardley, D. G.: Sterilization of Lipiodol. Personal communication in letter of 29 December 1954.

Barclay, D. L., Renegar, O. J., and Nelson, E. W.: The influence of inferior vena cava compression on the level of spinal anesthesia. Amer. J. Obstet. Gynecol. *101*:792, 1968.

Berglund, E., Birath, G., Bjure, J., Grimby, G., Kjellmer, I., Sandqvist, L., and Söderholm, B.: Spirometric studies in normal subjects. I. Forced expirograms in subjects between 7 and 70 years of age. Acta. Med. Scand. *173*:185, 1963.

Bertocchi, A.: Rilievi sulla tecnica dell' anestesia peridurale. Boll. Soc. Piemonte. Chir. *2*:163, 1932.

Brierley, J. B., and Field, E. J.: The connexions of the spinal subarachnoid space with the lymphatic system. J. Anat. *82*:153, 1948.

Bromage, P. R.: Spinal Epidural Analgesia. Edinburgh, E. & S. Livingstone, Ltd., 1954, pp. 17, 75, 77–83.

Bromage, P. R.: The phrenic reflex in epidural analgesia. Canad. Anaesth. Soc. J. *5*:29, 1958.

Bromage, P. R.: Continuous lumbar epidural analgesia for obstetrics. Canad. Med. Assoc. J. *85*:1136, 1961.

Bromage, P. R.: Spread of analgesic solutions in the epidural space and their site of action: A statistical study. Brit. J. Anaesth. *34*:161, 1962a.

Bromage, P. R.: Exaggerated spread of epidural analgesia in arteriosclerotic patients: Dosage in relation to biological and chronological ageing. Brit. Med. J. *2*:1634, 1962b.

Bromage, P. R.: A comparison of the hydrochloride salts of lignocaine and prilocaine for epidural analgesia. Brit. J. Anaesth. *37*:753, 1965a.

Bromage, P. R.: A comparison of the hydrochloride and carbon dioxide salts of lidocaine and prilocaine in epidural analgesia. Acta Anaesth. Scand. (Suppl.) *16*:55, 1965b.

Bromage, P. R.: Improved conduction blockade in surgery and obstetrics: Carbonated local anaesthetics. Canad. Med. Assoc. J. *97*:1377, 1967.

Bromage, P. R.: A comparison of bupivacaine and tetracaine in epidural analgesia for surgery. Canad. Anaesth. Soc. J. *16*:46, 1969a.

Bromage, P. R.: Ageing and epidural dose requirements. Brit. J. Anaesth. *41*:1016, 1969b.

Bromage, P. R.: Lower limb reflex changes in segmental epidural analgesia. Brit. J. Anaesth. *46*:504, 1974.

Bromage, P. R.: Mechanism of action of extradural analgesia. Brit. J. Anaesth. *47*:199, 1975.

Bromage, P. R., and Burfoot, M. F.: Further studies in the distribution and site of action of extradural local anaesthetic drugs using 14C-labelled lidocaine in dogs. 3rd Cong. Mund. Anaesth. Sao Paulo, 1964, Tom. *1*:371–372.

Bromage, P. R., and Burfoot, M. F.: Quality of epidural blockade. II. Influence of physico-chemical factors, hyaluronidase and potassium. Brit. J. Anaesth. *38*:857, 1966.

Bromage, P. R., and Gertel, M.: An evaluation of two new local anaesthetics for major conduction blockade: Canad. Anaesth. Soc. J. *17*:557, 1970.

Bromage, P. R., Joyal, A. C., and Binney, J. C.: Local anesthetic drugs: Penetration from the spinal extradural space into the neuraxis. Science *140*:392, 1963.

Bromage, P. R., Burfoot, M. F., Crowell, D. E., and Pettigrew, R. T.: Quality of epidural blockade. I. Influence of physical factors. Brit. J. Anaesth. *36*:342, 1964.

Bromage, P. R., Datta, S., and Dunford, L. A.: Etidocaine: An evaluation in epidural analgesia for obstetrics. Canad. Anaesth. Soc. J. *21*:535, 1974a.

Bromage, P. R., O'Beirn, P., and Dunford, L. A.: Etidocaine: A clinical evaluation for regional analgesia in surgery. Canad. Anaesth. Soc. J. *21*:523, 1974b.

Bryant, W. M., Greenwell, A. B., and Weeks, P. M.: Alterations in collagen organization during dilatation of the cervix uteri. Surg. Gynecol. Obstet. *126*:27, 1968.

Bryce-Smith, R.: The spread of solutions in the extradural space. Anaesthesia *9*:201, 1954.

Buchholz, H. W., and Körner, K. E.: Die Durchlassigkeit der Dura für Pantocainlösungen bei den verschiedenen Methoden der Periduralanaesthesie. Anaesthesist *33*:73, 1952.

Buchholz, H. W., and Lesse, K. T.: Die druckverhaltnisse im Periduralraum und im Liquorraum bei periduralen Injektionen. Chirurg *22*:102, 1951.

Burn, J. M., Guyer, P. B., and Langdon, L.: The spread of solutions injected into the epidural space: A study using epidurograms in patients with the lumbosciatic syndrome. Brit. J. Anaesth. *45*:338, 1973.

Cheng, P. A.: The anatomical and clinical aspects of epidural analgesia. Anesth. Analg. *42*:398, 1963.

Clausen, B.: Influence of age on chondroitin sulfates and hydroxyproline in human aorta, myocardium and skin. Lab. Invest. *12*:538, 1963.

Clausen, B.: Ageing of connective tissue. *In* Asboe-Hansen, G. (ed.): Hormones and Connective Tissue. Copenhagen, Munksgaard, 1966, pp. 396–422.

Cohen, E. N.: Distribution of local anesthetic agents in the neuraxis of the dog. Anesthesiology *29*:1002, 1968.

Corbin, K. B., and Gardner, E. D.: Decrease in number of myelinated fibers in human spinal roots with age. Anat. Rec. *68*:63, 1937.

Corning, J. L.: Spinal anaesthesia and local medication of the cord. N. Y. Med. J. *42*:483, 1885.

Dawkins, C. J. M.: Extradural spinal block. Proc. Roy. Soc. Med. *38*:299, 1945.

deJong, R. H.: Local Anesthetics. Springfield, Ill. 2nd ed. Charles C Thomas, Publishers, 1977, p. 52.

DeMuth, G. R., Howatt, W. F., and Hill, B. M.: The growth of lung function. Pediatrics *35*:162, 1965.

Denecke, K.: Die Periduralanästhesie in der Chirurgie. Zbl. Chir. *64*:130, 1937.

Dogliotti, A. M.: Anesthesia. Chicago, S. B. Debour, 1939, p. 537.

Downie, A. W., and Newell, D. J.: Sensory nerve conduction in patients with diabetes mellitus and controls. Neurology *11*:876, 1961.

Durrans, S. F.: High extradural segmental block. Anaesthesia *2*:106, 1947.

Düttmann, G.: Die peridurale segmentäre Anästhesie. Zbl. Chir. *68*:530, 1941.

Dyrbye, M. O.: Studies on the metabolism of the mucopolysaccharides of human arterial tissue by means of S^{35} with special reference to changes related to age. J. Gerontol. *14*:32, 1959.

Elman, R.: Spinal arachnoid granulations with especial reference to the cerebrospinal fluid. Bull. Johns Hopkins Hosp. *34*:99, 1923.

Erdemir, H. A., Soper, L. E., and Sweet, R. B.: Studies of factors affecting peridural anesthesia. Anesth. Analg. *44*:400, 1965.

Falk, P.: Gefahren der paravertebralen Leitungsanästhesie der Plexus cervicalis mit Versuchen an der Leiche dazu. Archiv. Ohren. Nasen Kehlkopfheilkunde *142*:254, 1936.

Foldes, F. F., and Davis, D. L.: The spinal fluid concentrations of 2-chloroprocaine. J. Pharmacol. Exp. Ther. *110*:18, 1954.

Foldes, F. F., Colavincenzo, J. W., and Birch, J. H.: Epidural anesthesia: A reappraisal. Current Researches in Anesth. Analg. *35*:33, 1956.

Foreman, R. D., and Wurster, R. D.: Conduction in descending spinal pathways initiated by somatosympathetic reflexes. Amer. J. Physiol. *228*:905, 1975.

Franz, D. N., and Perry, R. S.: Mechanisms for differential block among single myelinated and non-myelinated axons by procaine. J. Physiol. *236*:193, 1974.

Frey, H. H.,and Soehring, K.: Untersuchungen über die Durchlässigkeit der Dura mater des Hundes für Procain. Arch. Exp. Veterinaermed. *8*:804, 1954

Frumin, M. J., Schwarz, H., Burns, J. J., Brodie, B. B., and Papper, E. M.: Sites of sensory blockade during segmental spinal and segmental peridural anesthesia in man. Anesthesiology *14*:576, 1953a.

Frumin, M. J., Schwartz, H., Burns, J. J., Brodie, B. B., and Papper, E. M.: The appearance of procaine in the spinal fluid during peridural block in man. J. Pharmacol. Exp. Ther. *109*:102, 1953b.

Frumin, M. J.: Schwartz, H., Burns, J. J., Brodie, B. B., and Papper, E. M.: Dorsal root ganglion blockade during threshold segmental spinal anesthesia in man. J. Pharmacol. Exp. Ther. *112*:387, 1954.

Galbert, M. W., and Marx, G. F.: Extradural pressures in the parturient patient. Anesthesiology, *40*:499, 1974.

Giannetti, A., and Cerimele, D.: Effect of steroid hormones on the matrix of the dermis of the rat. *In* Balazs, E. A. (ed.): Chemistry and Molecular Biology of the Intercellular Matrix. Vol. III. London, Academic Press, Inc. Ltd., 1970, pp. 1821–1827.

Goepel, H.: Erfahrungsbericht über die Periduralanästhesie. Die Pantocain-Periston-Plombe zur segmentären Anästhesie. Zbl. Chir. *72*:467, 1947.

Gough, K. R.: Capillary resistance to suction in hypertension. Brit. Med. J. *1*:21, 1962.

Greenbaum, D., Richardson, P. C., Salmon, M. V., and Urich, H.: Pathological observations on six cases of diabetic neuropathy. Brain *87*:201, 1964.

Greene, N. M.: Area of differential block in spinal anesthesia with hyperbaric tetracaine. Anesthesiology *19*:45, 1958.
Gutierrez, A.: Anestesia Extradural. Buenos Aires, Rev. cirug. B. Aires 1939, p. 34.
Ham, A. W., and Leeson, T. S.: Histology. Philadelphia, J. B. Lippincott Company, 1961, p. 135.
Heile, B.: Der epidurale Raum. Arch. Klin. Chir. *101*:845, 1913.
Henkin, R. R.: Effects of ACTH, adrenocorticosteroids and thyroid hormone on sensory function. *In* Stumpf, W. E., and Grant, L. D. (eds.): Anatomical Neuroendocrinology. Basel, S. Karger, 1975, pp. 298–316.
Hipona, F. A., Yules, R., and Hehre, F. W.: Venous encroachment on the spinal peridural space due to experimental IVC occlusion: Possible clinical implications in late pregnancy. Invest. Radiol. *1*:157, 1966.
Hodge, C. F.: Changes in ganglion cells from birth to senile death. Observations on man and honey-bee. J. Physiol. (Lond). *17*:129, 1894.
Howarth, F.: Studies with a radioactive spinal anaesthetic. Brit. J. Pharmacol. *4*:333, 1949.
Jeffrey, J. J., Koob, T. J., and Eisen, A. Z.: Hormonal regulation of mammalian collagenases. *In* Burleigh, P. M. C., and Poole, A. R.: Dynamics of Connective Tissue Macromolecules. Amsterdam, North Holland/American Elsevier Publishing Company, Inc., 1975, pp. 147–158.
Jouasset, D.: Normalisation des épreuves fonctionelles respiratoires dans les pays de la Communauté Européenne du Charbon et de l'Acier. Poumon Coeur *10*:1145, 1960.
Kerr, F. W. L., and Alexander, S.: Descending autonomic pathways in the spinal cord. Arch. Neurol. *10*:249, 1964.
Kerr, M. G., Scott, D. B., and Samuel, E.: Studies of the inferior vena cava in late pregnancy. Brit. Med. J. *1*:532, 1964.
Krönke, E.: Der Wirkungsmechanismus der Periduralanästhesie. Chirurg *22*:321, 1951.
Krumperman, L. W., Meschter, S. C., Close, E. L., Wester, M. R., Erickson, J. C., and Strenge, H. J.: Transdural diffusion of 2-chloroprocaine hydrochloride in man. Anesth. Analg. *39*:55, 1960.
Kuypers, H. G. J. M.: The descending pathways of the spinal cord, and their anatomy and function. Progr. Brain Res. *11*:178, 1964.
Lawrence, D. G., and Locke, S.: Neuropathy in children with diabetes mellitus. Brit. Med. J. *1*;784, 1963.
Lindner, J., and Johannes, G.: Contribution on the ageing of arterial connective tissue. *In* Vogel, H. G. (ed.): Connective Tissue and Ageing. Amsterdam, Excerpta Medica, Int. Cong. Series 264, 1973, pp. 68–78.
Lund, P. C.: A correlation of venous blood concentrations and spinal fluid concentrations of Xylocaine and Citanest during peridural analgesia. Acta Anaesth. Scand. (Suppl.) *16*:97, 1965.
Lund, P. C., and Covino, B. G.: Distribution of local anesthetics in man following epidural anesthesia. J. Clin. Pharmacol. 7:324, 1967.
Luyendijk, W., and van Voorthuisen, A. E.: Contrast examination of the spinal epidural space. Acta. Radiol. Diag. *5*:1051, 1966.
Mohan, J., and Potter, J. M.: Pupillary constriction and ptosis following caudal epidural analgesia. Anaesthesia *30*:769, 1975.
Moore, D. C., Bridenbaugh, L. D., Van Ackeren, E. G., Belda, F. B., and Cole, F. V.: Spread of radiopaque solutions in the epidural space of the human adult corpse. Anesthesiology *19*:377, 1958.
Moore, J. M., and Frew, I. D. O.: Peripheral vascular lesion in diabetes mellitus. Brit. Med. J. *2*:19, 1965.
Morrow, W. F. K.: Unexplained spread of epidural anaesthesia. Brit. J. Anaesth. *31*:359, 1959.
Mostert, J. W.: The risk of epidural block in old people. Brit. J. Anaesth. *32*;613, 1960.
Nathan, P. W., and Sears, T. A.: Some factors concerned in differential nerve block by local anaesthetics. J. Physiol. (Lond.) *164*:565, 1961.
Nishimura, N., Kitahara, T., and Kusakabe, T.: The spread of lidocaine and I-131 solution in the epidural space. Anesthesiology *20*:785, 1959.
Norris, A. H., Shock, N. W., and Wagman, I. H.: Age changes in the maximum velocity of motor fibers of human ulnar nerve. J. Appl. Physiol. *5*:589, 1953.
Numans, S. R., and Havinga, E.: Die Wirkungsweise von Lokalanaesthetika bei der Epiduralinjektion. Rec. Trav. Chim. Pays-Bas. *62*:497, 1943.
Nyberg-Hansen, R.: Sites and modes of termination of reticulospinal fibers in the cat. J. Comp. Neurol. *124*:71, 1965.
Nyberg-Hansen, R.: Corticospinal fibres from the medial aspect of the cerebral hemisphere in the cat: An experimental study with the Nauta method. Exp. Brain Res. 7:120, 1969.
Odom, C. B.: Epidural anesthesia in resumé and prospect. Anesth. Analg. *19*:106, 1940.
Onchi, Y., Iwai, A., Mitzwani, K., and Ota, A.: Preliminary report on studies on permeability of Xylocaine through dura mater in man. Far East J. Anaesth. *1*:11, 1956.

Poppelbaum, F.: Sicherheitsmassnahmen bie der extraduralen spinalanaesthesie. Deutsch. Gesundh. *9*:499, 1954.

Rexed, B.: Contributions on the knowledge of the post-natal development of the peripheral nervous system in man. Acta Psychiat. Neurol. (Suppl.) *33*:1, 1944.

Rudin, D. O., Fremont-Smith, K., and Beecher, H. K.: Permeability of the dura mater to epidural procaine in dogs. J. Appl. Physiol. *3*:388, 1951.

Säker, G., and Schröder, G.: Grundlagenfragen der Periduralanaesthesie I. Durchlässigkeit der Dura? Anaesthesist *3*:259, 1954.

Salmoiraghi, G. C., and Burns, B. D.: Notes on the mechanism of rhythmic respiration. J. Neurophysiol. *23*:16, 1960.

Salvatore, C. A.: Capillary resistance during pregnancy. Obstet. Gynecol. *18*:96, 1961.

Sar, M., and Stumpf, W. E.: Androgen concentration in motor neurons of cranial nerves and spinal cord. Science *197*:77, 1977.

Schiff, M.: The influence of estrogens on connective tissue. *In* Asboe-Hansen, G. (ed.): Hormones and Connective Tissue. Copenhagen, Munksgaard, 1966, pp. 282–341.

Schulte-Steinberg, O.: Spread of local anesthetic solutions in caudal blocks in children. Sixth World Congress of Anesthesiology Abstracts, Mexico City, Excerpta Medica, Int. Cong. Series No. 387, 1976, p. 132.

Schulte-Steinberg, O., and Rahlfs, V. W.: Caudal anaesthesia in children and spread of 1 per cent lignocaine: A statistical study. Brit. J. Anaesth. *42*:1093, 1970.

Schulte-Steinberg, O., and Rahlfs, V. W.: Caudal-Anaesthesie bei Kindern und die Ausbreitung von 0.25% iger Bupivacain-Lösung. Eine statistische Untersuchung. Anaesthesist *21*:94, 1972.

Schulte-Steinberg, O., and Rahlfs, V. W.: Spread of extradural analgesia following caudal injection in children. A statistical study. Brit. J. Anaesth. *49*:1027, 1977.

Scott, D. B., and Kerr, M. G.: Inferior vena caval pressure in late pregnancy. J. Obstet. Gynaecol. Brit. Cwlth. *70*:1044, 1963.

Semenowa-Tjan-Schanskaja, W.: Die Morphologischen Veränderungen der peripheren Nerven beim Menschen im Greisenalter. Z. Neurol. Psychiat. *172*:587, 1941.

Shantha, T. R., and Evans, J. A.: The relationship of epidural anesthesia to neural membranes and arachnoid villi. Anesthesiology *37*:543, 1972.

Shock, N. W.: Physiological aspects of aging in man. Ann. Rev. Physiol. *23*:97, 1961.

Shock, N. W.: The physiology of aging. Sci. Amer. *206*:100, 1962.

Sicard, J. A., and Cestan, R.: Etude de la traversée méningo-radiculaire au niveau du trou de conjugaison—le nerf de conjugaison. Bull. Mém. Soc. Med. Hôp. Paris. *21*:715, 1904.

Sicard, J. A., and Forestier, J.: Radiographic method for exploration of the epidural space using lipiodol. Rev. Neurol. *28*:1264, 1921.

Sicard, J. A., and Forestier, J.: Roentgenologic exploration of the central nervous system with iodised oil (Lipiodol). Arch. Neurol. *16*:421, 1926.

Sicard, J. A., and Forestier, J.: The Use of Lipiodol in Diagnosis and Treatment. London, Oxford University Press, 1932, p. 178.

Skillman, T. G., Johnson, E. W., Hamwi, G. J., and Driskill, H. J.: Motor nerve conduction velocity in diabetes mellitus. Diabetes *10*:46, 1961.

Stumpf, W. E.: The brain: An endocrine gland and hormone target. *In* Stumpf, W. E., and Grant, L. D. (eds.): Anatomical Neuroendocrinology. Basel, S. Karger, 1975, pp. 2–8.

Stumpf, W. E., Sar, M., and Keefer, D. A.: Atlas of estrogen target cells in rat brain. *In* Stumpf, W. E., and Grant, L. D. (eds.): Anatomical Neuroendocrinology. Basel, S. Karger, 1975, pp. 104–119.

Truant, A. P., and Takman, F. K.: Differential physical-chemical and neuropharmacologic properties of local anesthetic agents. Anesth. Analg. *38*:478, 1959.

Urban, B. J.: Clinical observations suggesting a changing site of action during induction and recession of spinal and epidural anesthesia. Anesthesiology *39*:496, 1973.

Usubiaga, J. E., Wikinski, J. A., Wikinski, R. L., Usubiaga, L. E., Pontremoli, M., and Barrirer, M.: Permeabilidad de la duramadre a las soluciones anestheticas I. Pasaje de procaina en el perro in vivo y postmortem. Sem. Med. *119*:1845, 1961.

Usubiaga, J. E., Wikinski, J., Wikinski, R., Usubiaga, L. E., and Pontremoli, M.: Transfer of local anesthetics to the subarachnoid space and mechanisms of epidural block. Anesthesiology *25*:752, 1964.

Usubiaga, J. E., Wikinski, J. A., and Usubiaga, L. E.: Epidural pressure and its relation to spread of anesthetic solutions in the epidural space. Anesth. Analg. *46*:440, 1967.

Varella, A. L.: Hidrodinamica do espaço peridural: I. Rev. Bras. Anest. *21*:399, and 871, 1971.

Walker, C. H. M., and Balf, C. L.: Capillary resistance studies. Part II. Late pregnancy, labour and early puerperium. J. Obstet. Gynecol. Brit. Cwlth. *61*:17, 1954.

Wall, P. D.: The laminar organization of the dorsal horn and effects of descending impulses. J. Physiol. (Lond.) *188*:402, 1967.

Wiederhielm, C. A., Fox, J. R., and Lee, D. R.: Ground substance mucopolysaccharides and plasma proteins: Their role in capillary water balance. Amer. J. Physiol. *230*:1121, 1976.
Wilkinson, G. R., and Lund, P. C.: Bupivacaine levels in plasma and cerebrospinal fluid following peridural administration. Anesthesiology *33*:482, 1970.
Wugmeister, M., and Hehre, F. W.: The absence of differential blockade in peridural anaesthesia. Brit. J. Anaesth. *39*:953, 1967.

chapter 5
Epidural Pressures

... impelled of invisible tides ....
A. C. Swinburne, Hymn to Proserpine

GENESIS OF EPIDURAL PRESSURE

Much ink has been spilt in the protracted discussion centered around the problem of pressure differences in the epidural space. Is there a negative pressure in the space, and if so is it naturally occurring or is it an artifact caused by the recording devices used to explore the space? Some confusion has arisen from the assumption that pressure changes in the epidural space will be distributed uniformly throughout its length, and that what is found in the mid-thoracic region will also be present in the lumbar region. This uniformity does not exist, however, for the space is full of adipose and vascular dampers, and findings at one level cannot be translated to another.

Janzen stumbled across the problem accidentally in 1926 while undertaking careful manometric measurements of cerebrospinal fluid pressures. The manometer he used was filled with a mercuric iodide mixture of high specific gravity, so as to measure pressure changes with relatively little alteration of volume within the apparatus. Janzen was surprised to find that during the performance of lumbar puncture his manometer measured a *negative* pressure, and then after overcoming a slight elastic resistance, the negative pressure gave way to the expected positive pressure associated with subarachnoid tap, and cerebrospinal fluid flowed out of the needle. Janzen was intrigued by this curious phenomenon, and after investigating it in 39 patients and several cadavers he reached the following conclusions:

1. The degree of negative pressure obtainable depended upon the type of spinal needle used. Blunt needles gave greater negative pressure than sharp ones, and needles with side openings gave better readings than those with end openings.

2. Slow and careful introduction of the needle gave the greatest negative pressures. The negative pressure could be increased or diminished by advancing or withdrawing the needle.

3. Greater negative pressures were recorded with low cerebrospinal fluid pressures than with high ones (i.e., when the dura was less distended and resistant).

From these facts and his postmortem dissections, Janzen was satisfied that all his observations could be adequately explained by dimpling of the dura by the needle point, the negative pressure being an artifact arising in the epidural space as the advancing needle point dented a cone of resilient dura within the unyielding walls of the spinal canal (Fig. 5–1). This careful work and the logical conclusions drawn from it passed unnoticed, and two years later Heldt and Moloney (1928) rediscovered the phenomenon that Janzen had described earlier. The latter workers thought that two factors were at work in producing the epidural negative pressure. First, a "true" and normally existing negative pressure, which was somehow supposed to defy Nature's abhorrence of a vacuum, existed from early fetalhood. They claimed that the "true" pressure measured between −1 and −18 mmHg. Second, a "spurious" negative pressure was added to this, such as Janzen had described, caused by advancing the needle point, and the total negative pressure could amount to anything up to −30 mmHg or even higher. It was not made clear how the "true" and "spurious" pressures could be distinguished, and there is little doubt that it is impossible to do so. Heldt and Moloney made one significant observation which strongly suggests that the negative pressures they observed arose from small-volume sources, such as would be caused by local indentation of the dura within the spinal canal. By means of a two-way tap on the epidural needle, they were able to inject liquid into the epidural space and measure epidural pressures at the same time. They found that the injection of small amounts of saline (less than 6 ml) completely abolished the negative pressure.

Six years after Janzen's description of the creation of an artificial negative pressure in the epidural space, Gutierrez (1932), of Buenos Aires, turned the phenomenon to a practical account by using it as a landmark in performing epidural injections. Instead of using a manometer, Gutierrez placed a drop of fluid in the hub of the needle so that the hanging drop would be

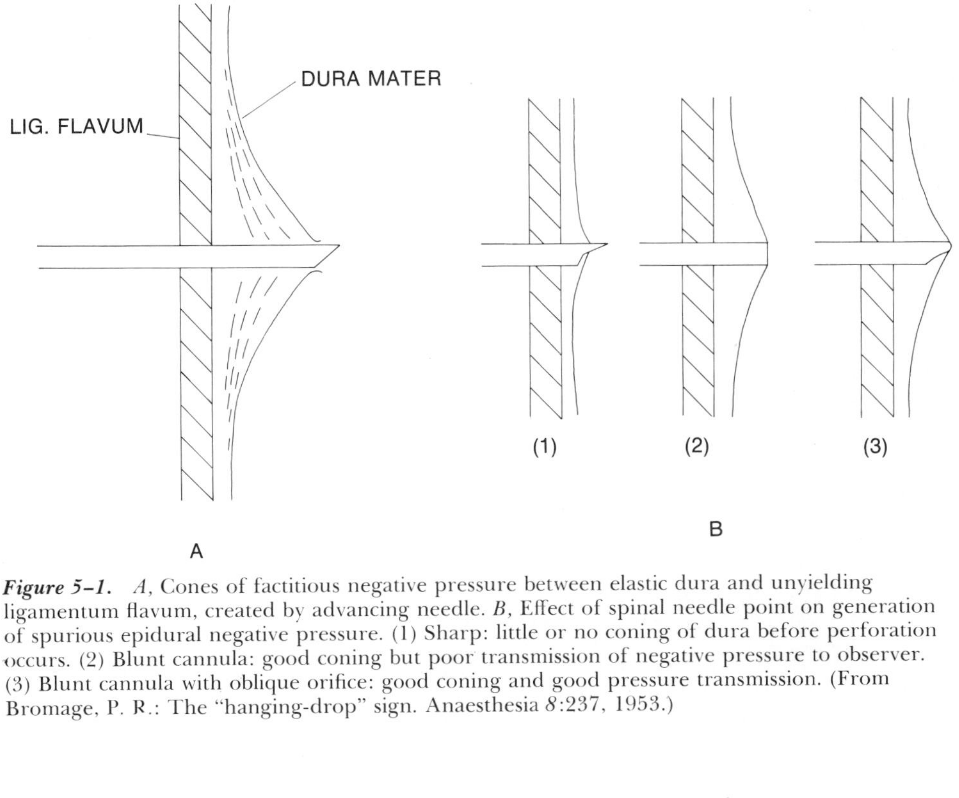

Figure 5–1. *A*, Cones of factitious negative pressure between elastic dura and unyielding ligamentum flavum, created by advancing needle. *B*, Effect of spinal needle point on generation of spurious epidural negative pressure. (1) Sharp: little or no coning of dura before perforation occurs. (2) Blunt cannula: good coning but poor transmission of negative pressure to observer. (3) Blunt cannula with oblique orifice: good coning and good pressure transmission. (From Bromage, P. R.: The "hanging-drop" sign. Anaesthesia *8*:237, 1953.)

sucked in when the space was entered. He called this the "seña de gota" or "sign of the drop," and the test became one of the most popular for identifying the epidural space, despite the admission of its originator that it could be elicited in only 82 per cent of cases.

Albert Bonniot (1934), of Grenoble, was the next to turn his attention to the question of epidural pressures, and he confirmed Janzen's finding that a decrease of cerebrospinal fluid pressure was associated with an increase of recordable negative pressure in the extradural space. These results were obtained when the position of the body was adjusted so that the site of puncture was at a higher level. than the rest of the body. For instance, upper thoracic punctures were done in the sitting position with the neck well flexed, and lumbar injections were done in the lateral or prone position with the head low. In the same year Houdard and his colleagues (1934) also used a water manometer to measure epidural pressure, and they concluded that the negative pressure they encountered was entirely an artifact.

The matter was not allowed to rest here, and further speculation, innocent of experimental backing but nevertheless quick with creative possibilities, followed. In 1936 Zorraquin suggested that the negative pressure observed was not an artifact but occurred naturally, and was induced by two forces transmitted to the epidural space via the intervertebral foramina. One, he suggested, was abdominal in origin and constant in nature, produced by the drag of viscera suspended from their mesentery; the other was variable and intermittent, produced by the transmitted intrathoracic negative pressure of inspiration. In the same year Odom (1936) suggested that the negative pressure was created by flexion of the spine. He claimed that bowing of the back lengthened the spinal canal and increased its volume, causing a temporary negative pressure in the epidural space. However, this hypothesis is not in accordance with the facts demonstrated by Reid and Sherrington in 1890, when they showed that flexing of the spines of cadavers produced a considerable diminution, and not an increase, in the volume of the spinal canal.

The next serious experimental work was done by Eaton of the Mayo Clinic in 1939, who used a water manometer in living subjects. He made three observations:

1. The negative pressure increases as the needle advances across the epidural space, until the moment when the dura is punctured, as Janzen had shown earlier.

2. If the needle is halted after a small negative pressure is recorded and the pressures are then equalized, further advance will produce a further fall in pressure.

3. An epidural puncture was done in the fourth lumbar interspace, then a second epidural puncture was made in the third interspace, and a blunt stylet was passed down the second needle. He found that by advancing the stylet, negative pressures up to -14 cmH_2O could be repeatedly obtained, the pressure returning to zero when the stylet was withdrawn (Fig. 5–2 and Table 5–2).

Eaton concluded that his observations were in agreement with those of Janzen, confirming that the epidural negative pressure is an artifact.

In 1947 one of Zorraquin's suggestions found an echo in some observations by Macintosh and Mushin at Oxford. By injection experiments and dissections they demonstrated the free connections that exist between adjacent

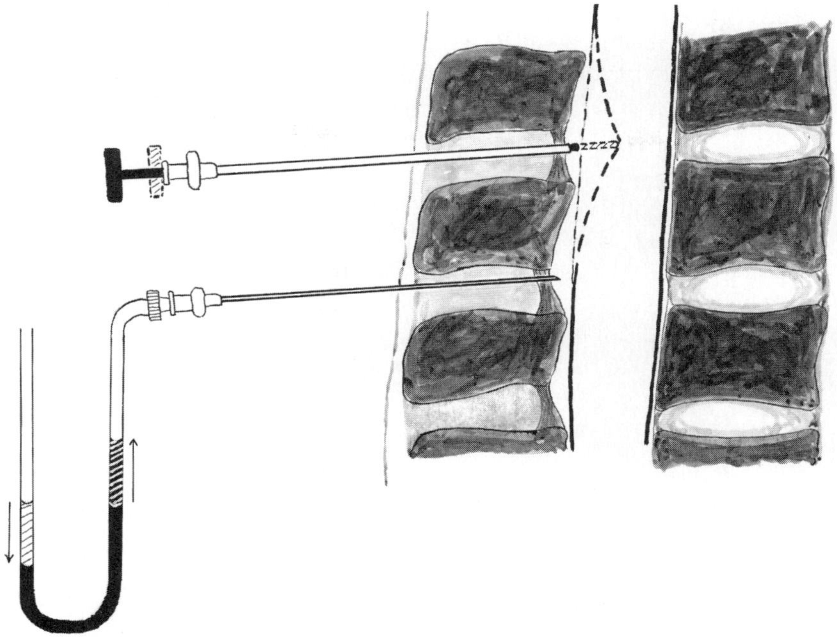

Figure 5–2. Artificial negative pressure at fourth lumbar interspace. Eaton's experiment of 1939, which demonstrates reversible tenting of the dura with a blunt stylet, creating a local reversible negative pressure in the lumbar epidural space.

and contralateral paravertebral spaces via the epidural space, and they restated Zorraquin's conclusion that the intermittent thoracic negative pressure of inspiration must therefore be transmitted to the epidural space. They pointed out, however, that this negative pressure would be quickly damped down by the fat and areolar tissue in the extradural space, so that the negative pressure wave would not be transmitted far from its site of origin. Later, Macintosh (1950) added further confirmation to this when he showed that after correct placement of the needle in the epidural space, his balloon indicator (see Chapter 6) could be partially reinflated by asking the patient to cough.

Another Oxford worker, Bryce-Smith (1950), carried out some important manometric observations in the same year. He took simultaneous manometer readings from two needles placed in the subarachnoid and epidural spaces at the same intervertebral level in the lumbar region and found that although coughing and jugular compression raised both CSF and extradural pressures, deep inspiration lowered the epidural pressure without changing the CSF pressure (Table 5–1).

REGIONAL AND POSTURAL INFLUENCES

While pressure in the subarachnoid space is uniformly distributed by a noncompressible fluid column in a semirigid container, pressure in the epidural space is not uniformly distributed. Epidural pressure is regionally affected by the local pneumatics and hydraulics of the thoracic and abdominal

TABLE 5-1 Effects of Coughing, Deep Breathing and Jugular Compression on Lumbar Epidural and Subarachnoid Pressures*

	At Rest (mmH_2O)	*Coughing (mmH_2O)*	*Jugular Compression (mmH_2O)*	*Deep Breathing (mmH_2O)*
Case One				
CSF pressure	65	+105	+260	No change
Epidural pressure	0	+ 7	+ 8	−4
Case Two				
CSF pressure	170	+178	–	No change
Epidural pressure	0	+ 3	–	−2
Case Three				
CSF pressure	25	+ 70	+245	No change
Epidural pressure	0	+ 9	+ 10	−8
Case Four				
CSF pressure	75	+ 85	+210	No change
Epidural pressure	0	+ 3	+ 2	−2

*From Bryce-Smith, R.: Pressures in the extradural space. Anaesthesia *5*:213, 1950.

cavities, separated by the moving piston of the diaphragm, as shown diagrammatically in Figure 5–3. The superior and inferior vena cava connect with the internal vertebral venous plexus and transmit local pressures on either side of the diaphragm. Intrapleural and intra-abdominal pressures are also transmitted to the spinal canal via the intervertebral foramina. Regional variations of pressure can occur in the vascular and compliant epidural space, but little or no compliance exists in the rigidly contained subarachnoid space where pressures are uniformly distributed. Within the thorax there is a balance of forces between the outward thrusts of the containing walls, formed by the rib cage and diaphragm, and the inward pull of the lung's elasticity. Under resting conditions there is a net negative pressure in the intrapleural space. However, below the diaphragm a slight positive pressure exists under resting conditions formed by the outward thrust from the bulk of the viscera and counteracted by the containing tension of the abdominal wall. In both cavities wide pressure swings can be generated by active or passive forces working through the muscles of the containing walls and through the hydraulic shifts of the major blood vessels within the thorax and abdomen.

Local conditions of epidural pressure in the thoracic region are different from those found caudally. The thoracic spinal canal is in immediate continuity with the thoracic cage via the intervertebral foramina, so negative intrapleural pressures are transmitted to the neighboring epidural space through these communicating channels with little or no attenuation. Further down the spinal canal, negative pressure falls off rapidly as the lumbar intervertebral foramina transmit a positive pressure from the abdominal cavity.

A negative pressure of −5 to −10 cmH_2O (mean −7 cmH_2O) usually exists in the pleural space, as well as in the esophagus, which makes it a convenient site for measuring intrathoracic pressures (Dornhorst and Leathart, 1952). As pointed out by Christie and Macintosh (1934) more than 40 years ago, the degree of intrapleural negative pressure tends to vary with the size of

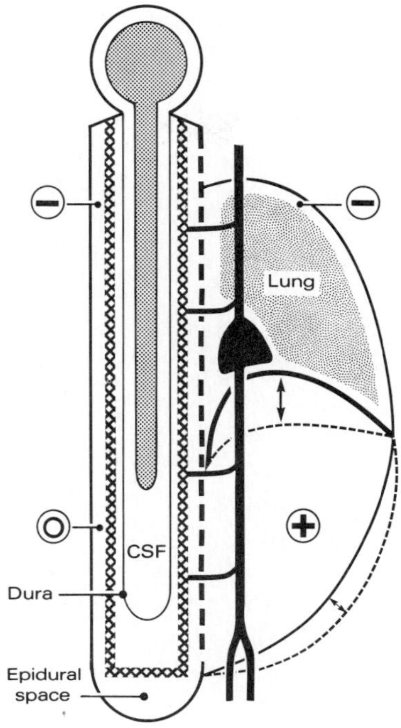

Figure 5–3. Determinants of epidural pressure. Diagram of extradural space and extradural vertebral venous plexus with collateral and azygos connections to caval venous system. Downward movements of diaphragm are transmitted to abdominal wall through abdominal contents. Lumbar extradural pressure varies with intra-abdominal pressure. Negative intrapleural pressure is transmitted to thoracic epidural space via intervertebral foramina. Symbols: XXX = internal vertebral venous plexus: (−), (0), (+) = negative, zero or positive pressure.

the functional residual capacity (FRC), and the FRC is larger in the sitting position than in the supine position. The intrapleural pressure falls when subjects move from the lying to the sitting position (Christie and Macintosh, 1934; McMichael and McGibbon, 1939). During quiet breathing Mead and Gaensler (1959) found that the average absolute intrapleural pressure was *4.0 cmH*$_2$*O lower in the sitting position than when the subjects were supine,* a discovery which is in agreement with Bonniot's independent observation that the lowest epidural pressures occur in the thoracic region when puncture is performed with the patient sitting up (Bonniot, 1934).

Processes of age and disease affecting the elasticity of the lung and the intrapleural pressure also affect the epidural pressure. Thus, in conditions such as asthma and emphysema, thoracic epidural negativity may be abnormally feeble and occasionally barely detectable (Frank, Mead and Ferris, 1957; Pierce and Ebert, 1958). Nevertheless, even in these conditions thoracic epidural negativity is more marked in the sitting position than when the subjects are lying down.

The inherent difficulties of recording undisturbed epidural pressures accurately have led to quite divergent views on the incidence of epidural negativity (Dawkins, 1963). Usubiaga and his colleagues performed a number of careful studies on epidural pressures in animals and man over a period of several years between 1962 and 1967, and their results will be drawn on quite heavily here to illustrate the relatively simple principles at work (Usubiaga et al., 1963a, 1963b; Usubiaga et al., 1967a, 1967b and 1967c). They performed several hundred epidural punctures at various spinal levels with a manometer attached to the advancing needle and noted the change of pressure at the moment of entering the extradural space. Figure 5–4 is adapted from their results (Usubiaga et al., 1967b).

It can be seen that negative pressure was most readily recorded in the cervical and thoracic region when the patients were sitting up, but negativity became less marked in the lumbar region and nonexistent in the sacrum. As might be expected, better negative pressure was obtained in the lumbar region when the patients were lying on their sides rather than sitting up in a flexed position, for the abdominal contents are more compressed and the intra-abdominal pressure is higher in the sitting position. A negative pressure was completely absent in the lumbar region in about 12 per cent of the cases.

The question arises, if positive intra-abdominal pressure is transmitted to the lumbar epidural space, why is a negative pressure found there at all, especially, in as high an incidence as 88 per cent, as shown in Figure 5–4?

First, it is clearly a question of degree. The phase change from negative inspiratory pressure in the thoracic epidural space to positive pressure in the lumbar region does not occur abruptly at the thoracolumbar junction but is gradually reversed over a distance of several segments, so that puncture in the upper lumbar region is more likely to encounter some degree of negative pressure than in the lower lumbar region (Usubiaga et al., 1963b). Second, there is the phenomenon of "tenting" of the dura, demonstrated in Eaton's experiments referred to earlier, caused by the advancing needle point pressing on the dura and forming a localized cone of spurious negative pressure. This mechanism is more likely to operate in the lumbar region, in which the needle is advanced squarely to the dural tube (unless an oblique approach is taken), than in the thoracic region, in which the approach is oblique and glancing. A head-down tilt reverses the pressure situation in the spinal canal to a slight extent, allowing the abdominal contents to slide upward against the diaphragm,

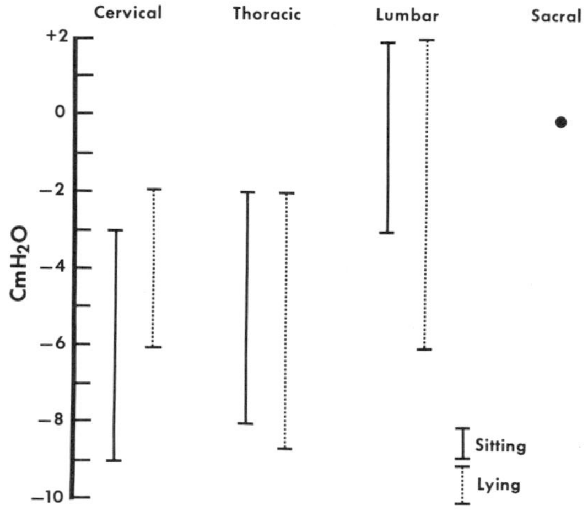

% Incidence of Negative Pressure

Puncture Site	Sitting	Lying
Cervical	100	98
Thoracic	100	98
Lumbar	87.5	88.3
Sacral	-	0

Figure 5–4. Influence of puncture site and posture on initial epidural pressure. Epidural pressure is most reliably negative in cervical and thoracic region with the patient sitting up. (After Usubiaga et al., 1967b.)

thus reducing the pressure in the lumbar extradural space and lessening the danger of dural puncture (Bonniot, 1934).

The belief has persisted that flexion of the spine will increase intraspinal volume and lower epidural pressure through the accordion-like effect of the laminae and yellow ligaments (Odom, 1936; Dawkins, 1963; Usubiaga et al., 1967a). As mentioned earlier in this chapter, Reid and Sherrington's postmortem studies showed that, on the contrary, the volume of the spinal canal is reduced rather than increased by flexion, at any rate in fresh corpses. It is doubtful whether the physical conditions associated with spinal flexion are very different during life. In any event, if an increment of negativity is produced by spinal movements, it is likely to be transient and annulled within a minute or two by influx of blood into the distensible epidural veins (Dawkins, 1963). These variables affecting epidural negative pressure are summarized in Figure 5–5.

Some simple observations of my own support the view that tenting of

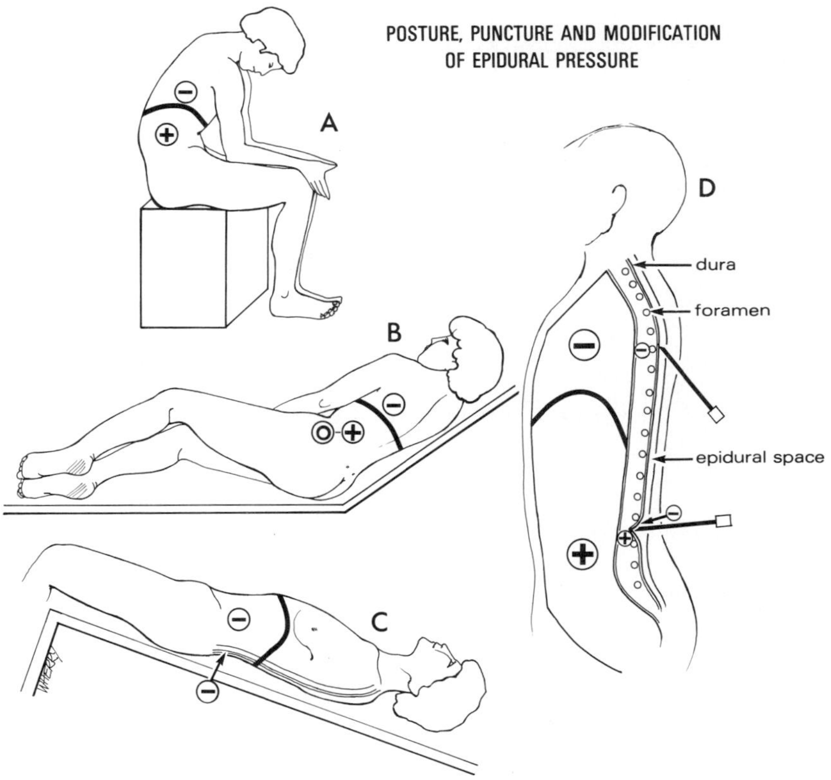

Figure 5–5. Summary of postural variables affecting pressure encountered during epidural puncture. *A*, In sitting position a true negative pressure exists above the diaphragm, transmitted through the intervertebral foramina, but pressure is positive in the abdominal cavity and lumbar epidural space. *B*, In lateral reclining position epidural pressure is still negative above the diaphragm, but intra-abdominal and lumbar epidural pressures are less positive than in sitting position. *C*, In head-down position the diaphragm rises, and intra-abdominal and lumbar epidural pressures may become negative. *D*, In upright position the needle encounters true epidural negative pressure in thoracic region. Lumbar epidural pressure is positive, but "coning" of dura by needle point causes a spurious negative pressure localized to the immediate zone of dural indentation.

the dura contributes significantly to any negative pressure that may be encountered in the lower lumbar region (Bromage, 1953). Lumbar epidural punctures using the hanging-drop technique with needles of varying sharpness were performed in 16 patients (see Chapter 6). The patients were sitting up for 4 or 5 minutes beforehand, so that the full hydrostatic effect of the column of cerebrospinal fluid would distend the dura as much as possible. The spine was kept as straight as was compatible with performing a lumbar puncture. The needle was introduced in the second or third lumbar interspace and advanced only during the expiratory phase of respiration, so that intrathoracic pressure would be positive rather than negative at the moment of entry into the epidural space. Despite these unfavorable conditions for producing a negative epidural pressure, a vigorous positive "drop" sign was obtained in 10 of the 16 cases. Moreover, after a positive sign was elicited, the needle was halted and the empty hub recharged with a second drop, and then a further advance was made. In eight of the cases the hanging-drop sign was positive a second time, and in one of these (using a moderately sharp needle) the sign was positive eight times in succession, before the needle point finally perforated the dura and cerebrospinal fluid flowed out (Bromage, 1953). There can be little doubt that in these cases the negative pressure effects were caused solely by dimpling of the dura.

Finally, having dealt with the manometric findings of several investigators, it is helpful to review them together for further evidence of the genesis and practical significance of *initial* negative pressures recorded in the lumbar epidural space. A glance at Table 5–2 reveals two interesting facts.

First, it will be noticed that the "Total Recorded Negative Pressures" can be arranged in two groups, those around 400 mmH_2O making one group and those between 110 and 170 mmH_2O falling into the other. The lower group

TABLE 5–2 Published Values for Extradural Pressure

Author	*Total Recorded Negative Pressure (cmH_2O)*	*Incremental Negative Pressure Caused by Deep Inspiration (cmH_2O)*	*Type of Manometer Used*
Janzen (1926)	0 – −40.0	–	Mercuric iodide, Sp. Grav.: 3.2
Heldt and Maloney (1928)	−1.0 – −40.8	–	Mercury, Sp. Grav.: 13.6
Bonniot (1934)	−6.0 – −16.0	–	Water
Eaton (1939)	0 – −14.0	–	Water
Lawrence (1948)	−2.0 – −17.0 (Depending on bluntness of needle)	–	Water
Bryce-Smith (1950)	0 – −11.0	−0.2 – −0.8	Water
Dawkins (1963)	−3.4 – −16.3	–	Electromanometer
Usubiaga et al. (1967b, 1967c)	Thoracic −1.0 – −9.0 Lumbar +2.0 – −30.0*	−1.0 – −4.0	Aneroid or electromanometer

*Just before dural puncture.

of readings was obtained with water-filled manometers (specific gravity = 1.0), while the manometers used in the higher group contained liquids of relatively high specific gravity. The latter type of manometer undergoes less volume change at a given pressure than the former, so that it is more suitable for recording true changes of pressure from small-volume sources. This suggests that the pressure changes being measured do in fact arise from a small-volume source, such as would be created by local dimpling of the resilent dura within the rigid walls of the spinal canal.

Second, if we look at Bryce-Smith's figures for pressure changes associated with deep inspiration, it will be seen that the values obtained in the lumbar region are insignificant when compared with the "Total Recorded Negative Pressures." Thus, even if the "hanging-drop" test in the lumbar region did depend upon puncturing the epidural space in phase with a *deep* inspiration, the amount of negative pressure obtained by respiratory movements would be slight and of little account compared with the negative pressure arising from coning of the dura.

Note that these last remarks apply to the genesis of negative pressure in the *lumbar* region. Clearly, in the thoracic region inspiratory negative pressure has a much greater influence on secondary pressure events in the adjacent epidural space.

To summarize, it may be concluded that although respiratory forces can cause a negative pressure in the *lumbar* epidural space, this effect will be slight or absent unless inspiratory effort is great, the puncture is in the upper lumbar region and the patient is lying on his side. In practice, during quiet respiration most negative pressure effects seen in the lower lumbar region are probably due to coning of the dura by the advancing needle point. Also, epidural pressure in the lumbar region will be at its lowest when the patient is relaxed and lying head-down in the lateral position (Bonniot, 1934; Cheng, 1963).

In the *thoracic* region, on the other hand, respiratory negative pressures are transmitted effectively to the local epidural space, especially in the sitting position. The existence of a genuine thoracic negative pressure explains why a positive "drop sign" is obtained more frequently by high thoracic puncture than by puncture in the lumbar region (Figueiredo, 1948). The practical aspects of these points will be developed in the next chapter on Identification of the Epidural Space.

CHANGE OF EPIDURAL PRESSURES FROM DISTURBANCE OF BODY CAVITY DYNAMICS

The normal distribution of pressure on the two sides of the diaphragm may be disturbed by obesity, pregnancy, disease or therapeutic procedures. The resulting pressure changes are all reflected in the corresponding region of the epidural space, either directly through the intervertebral foramina or indirectly by redistribution of blood within the hydraulic system of the caval-azygos-vertebral venous communications. Thus, abdominal compression, ascites, pneumoperitoneum or pregnancy at term all raise the intra-abdominal pressure and distend the lumbar portion of the internal vertebral venous plexuses, while causing very little alteration in the thoracocervical region (Usubiaga et al., 1967c).

Galbert and Marx (1974) have made careful measurements of lumbar epidural pressures throughout labor. Their study set out to analyze the factors that influence the various components of the type of pressure trace shown in Figure 12–3 (Bromage, 1961). They confirmed Bromage's earlier findings that peaks of epidural pressure occur synchronously with each uterine contraction, regardless of whether or not epidural blockade has been induced, and that bearing down efforts produce a Valsalva-like effect that augments the contraction peaks. These measurements confirmed the impression that a surge of inflow into the extradural plexus accompanies each uterine contraction during labor, distending the epidural veins and transmitting the extradural venous pressure to the epidural space through the walls of the epidural veins. Galbert and Marx's study also included measurements of baseline epidural pressures and central venous pressure during the course of labor, in both the lateral position and the dorsal position. These observations proved most interesting, and the results of the epidural baseline pressures are summarized in Figure 5–6. It can be seen that in the lateral position, lumbar epidural pressure rises progressively from a level of about 1 or 2 cmH_2O in early labor to about 11 or 12 cmH_2O near full dilatation. Turning the patient from the left lateral to the dorsal position results in a 40 per cent increase in baseline epidural pressure, and this is associated with a corresponding fall in central venous pressure, as discussed in Chapter 10. These changes reflect the additional degree of caval obstruction that occurs in the dorsal position during labor, resulting in further diversion of venous return to the extradural venous plexus and increased compression of the epidural space.

A Queckenstedt maneuver raises pressure throughout the subarachnoid space; however, in the epidural space pressure increases above the diaphragm but very little below the diaphragm. In a Valsalva maneuver or a cough, both body cavities are involved, and then increased pressure in the chest and abdomen forces blood into the entire length of the internal vertebral venous plexus, resulting in very high pressure peaks throughout the whole of the epidural space.

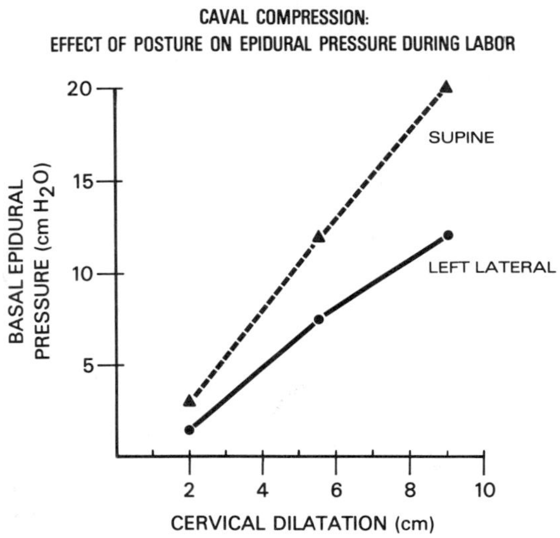

Figure 5–6. Epidural pressures during parturition in left lateral (●——●) and supine (▲– – –▲) positions. Note that epidural pressure rises during labor regardless of posture but that the greatest rise occurs when the mother lies in the supine position. (After Galbert and Marx, 1974.)

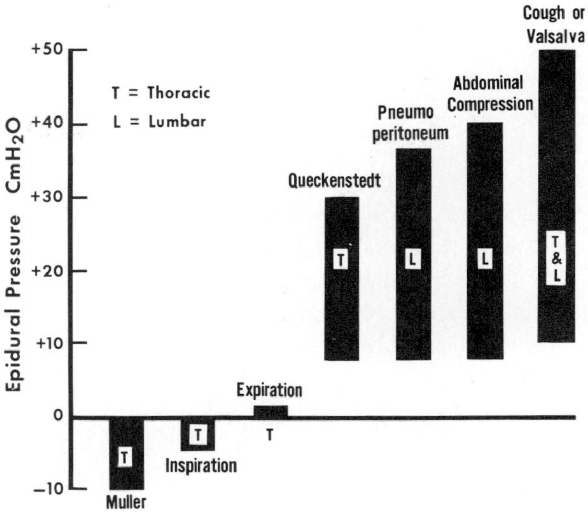

Figure 5–7. Circulatory and respiratory influences affecting epidural pressure in thoracic and lumbar regions. T = thoracic epidural pressure; L = lumbar epidural pressure. (After Usubiaga et al., 1963 and 1967.)

These factors and Usubiaga's data for resulting epidural pressure changes are summarized in Figure 5–7. Inevitably the massaging effects of these pressure changes will have profound effects on the spread of local anesthetic solutions in the epidural space. Normal respiratory negative pressures have a tendency to draw solutions upward toward the thoracic region of the spinal canal (Abajian, 1943; Frumin et al., 1953; Nishimura et al., 1959; Varella, 1971a, 1971b; Burn, Guyer and Langdon, 1973), and this tendency is exaggerated by inferior vena caval compression caused by an abdominal tumor or late pregnancy (Bromage, 1962; Hehre et al., 1966).

EPIDURAL COMPLIANCE

Sometimes the anesthesiologist sees a slight reflux of solution after an induction dose of local anesthetic is injected into the epidural space, and this may cause concern that the injection is wrongly placed or that the dura may have been accidentally punctured—a suspicion reinforced by the observation that in many of these patients blockade spreads unusually far (Bromage, 1962). However, the epidural space is not perfectly distensible, and a transient rise of pressure is bound to occur after injection of a moderate volume of solution. If this rise is exaggerated for any reason, then some degree of reflux is inevitable.

The compliance of the epidural space is of considerable practical interest because it has a direct effect on the physical spread of injected solutions in the space. The concept of compliance applied to the epidural space involves a number of elastic components in a partially rigid but leaky container, particularly the tissues abutting on the intervertebral foramina and the blood vessels within the space coursing through the intervertebral foramina. Pressure generated in the epidural space will obey the general physical rules that apply under these circumstances, and the normal expression for compliance—Compliance $= \frac{\text{Volume}}{\text{Pressure}}$—must be expanded to include the elements of resistance out of a leaky system, as well as the speed of injection or inflow into that system, so that:

$P \propto \frac{V}{C} + \frac{R}{T}$, where R is the resistance to outflow and T is the time taken for injection.

The earliest studies of epidural compliance were done by Evans in 1930 with caudal injections. He used forceful injections of local anesthetic into the sacral canal. With increments of 5 to 15 ml, the pressure rose steeply and then fell away again almost immediately. Successive injections caused incremental rises until a pressure of over 30 cmH_2O was reached (Evans, 1930). Evans used very large amounts of local anesthetic for therapeutic purposes, up to 140 ml at one time, and with these volumes patients usually became disorientated and anxious. Whether these symptoms were due to a transmitted rise of cerebrospinal fluid pressure or to toxic absorption is open to question. Some animals, such as sheep, appear to have a very low epidural compliance, and then even very small volumes of the order of 5 to 10 ml will cause transient syncope lasting 60 to 90 seconds (Lebeaux, 1974).

The idea of exploiting epidural resistance to limit segmental spread was developed by German workers between the 1930's and early 1950's (Denecke, 1937; Düttmann, 1941), especially by Buchholz and his colleagues, who used viscous "plombes" after filling the epidural space with saline (Buchholz and Lesse, 1951; Buchholz and Körner, 1952). Buchholz and Lesse noted that small-volume injections of 10 ml of saline produced only localized and transient rises of epidural pressure confined to three or four segments, and a sustained widespread rise of pressure did not occur until 50 to 60 ml of saline had been injected. With viscous plombes the pressure rise tended to be slower and more prolonged (Buchholz and Lesse, 1951). Many variables were involved in these studies, and quantitative conclusions of pressure-volume relationships were not obtained.

Controlled studies of epidural compliance were undertaken by Usubiaga and his colleagues in Buenos Aires in 1963 and later completed in Miami. The results were published in several papers in Spanish and English, and they are summarized here (Usubiaga et al., 1963a, 1963b; Usubiaga et al., 1967a, 1967b, 1967c). These investigations measured the rise and fall of epidural pressure over a 5-minute period after a standard volume (10 ml) of local anesthetic solution was injected at a constant rate (0.67 ml/sec). Pressure measurements were combined with observations of the resultant spread of analgesia to see if any correlation existed between epidural compliance and segmental spread. Peak pressures varied between 5 and 60 cmH_2O and were highest following injection in the sitting position and lowest after sacral injection. Changes of pressure were propagated over a relatively short length of the spinal canal, and they could not be detected at a distance of 10 or 12 vertebrae from the site of injection.

Pressure-volume changes fell into two extreme patterns, with gradations in between. In young subjects the epidural pressure rose sharply but slightly and then fell off equally steeply in a few seconds. In old patients the pattern was quite different, with a higher steep rise followed by a more gradual fall of pressure to a plateau which persisted for several minutes, as shown in Figure 5–8. The residual pressure was related to age, as shown in Figure 5–9.

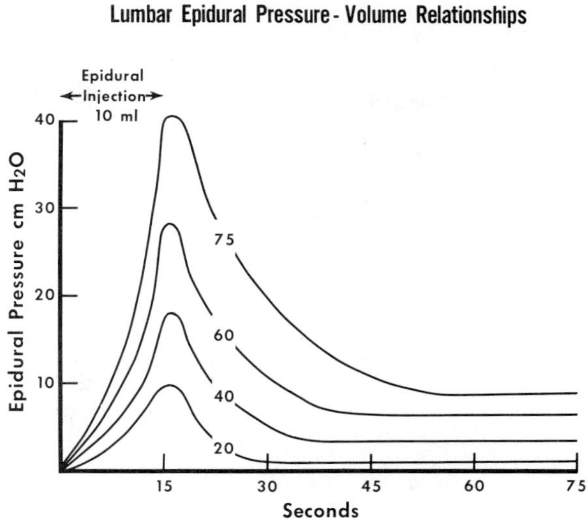

Figure 5–8. Reduction of epidural compliance with increasing age. Changes of epidural pressure after injection of 10 ml of solution over a period of 15 seconds in patients of 20, 40, 60 and 75 years of age. (After Usubiaga et al., 1967b.)

The clinical observations of analgesic spread in these studies demonstrated that residual epidural pressure is also positively correlated with segmental spread, as shown in Figure 5–10 in which the upper dermatome level of analgesia is plotted against residual pressure.

These findings confirmed what had been found by others, that the extent of epidural spread is dependent on age (Bromage, 1954, 1962, 1965; Bromage et al., 1964). In addition, however, they showed that not only age but also other factors causing extensive spread, such as pneumoperitoneum or pregnancy, probably have a common basis in a reduced epidural compliance. The common denominator of reduced compliance could be brought about through age blocking the leaks from the space by sealing off the intervertebral foramina, or by the space-occupying effect of distended extradural veins.

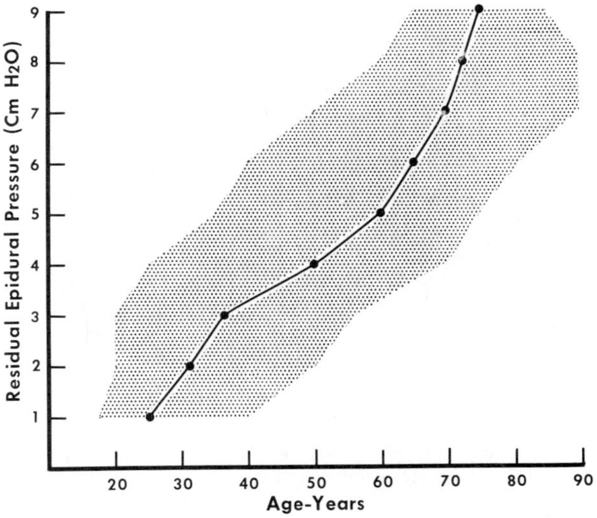

Figure 5–9. Residual increase of epidural pressure after injection of 10 ml of solution over a period of 15 seconds (see Fig. 5–8), related to age (mean ± range). (After Usubiaga et al., 1967b.)

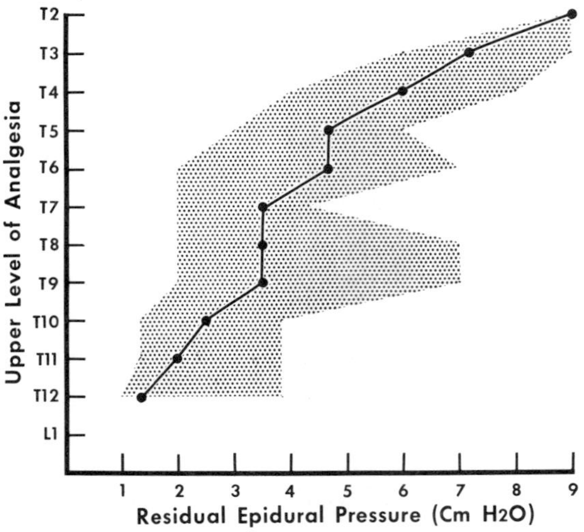

Figure 5–10. Correlation of segmental spread of analgesia with residual epidural pressure after injection of 10 ml of solution (see Figs. 5–8 and 5–9) (means ± range). (After Usubiaga et al., 1967b.)

Certain corollaries were also confirmed by these findings. In young patients, local anesthetics can flow freely through the patent intervertebral foramina into the paravertebral spaces under the influence of pressure or gravity, and little longitudinal spread occurs within the epidural space. By the same token, the gravitational effect of a lateral position is quite likely to cause predominant anesthesia on the underside in young patients. However, in old subjects the intervertebral foramina are less patent, and injected solutions are forced to spread longitudinally within the confines of the spinal canal (Sicard and Forestier, 1921; Nishimura et al., 1959).

The subject of epidural pressure has been dealt with at some length because of its fundamental importance in developing logical procedures for identifying the epidural space and for the general technical management of epidural blockade. These practical applications will be discussed in the succeeding chapter.

REFERENCES

Abajian, J.: Peridural segmental anesthesia with Intracaine. Anesthesiology *4*:372, 1943.

Bonniot, A.: Note sur la pression épidurale négative. Bull. Soc. Nat. Chir. *60*:124, 1934.

Bromage, P. R.: The "hanging-drop" sign. Anaesthesia *8*:237, 1953.

Bromage, P. R.: Spinal Epidural Analgesia. Edinburgh, E. & S. Livingston, 1954.

Bromage, P. R.: Continuous lumbar epidural analgesia for obstetrics. Canad. Med. Assoc. J. *85*:1136, 1961.

Bromage, P. R.: Spread of analgesic solutions in the epidural space and their site of action: A statistical study. Brit. J. Anaesth. *34*:161, 1962.

Bromage, P. R.: A comparison of the hydrochloride and carbon dioxide salts of lidocaine and prilocaine in epidural analgesia. Acta Anaesth. Scand. *16*:55, 1965.

Bromage, P. R., Burfoot, M. F., Crowell, D. E., and Pettigrew, R. T.: Quality of epidural blockade. I: Influence of physical factors. Brit. J. Anaesth. *36*:342, 1964.

Bryce-Smith, R.: Pressures in the extradural space. Anaesthesia *5*:213, 1950.

Buchholz, H. W., and Körner, K. F.: Die Durchlassigkeit der Dura für Pantocainlösungen bei den verschiedenen Methoden der Peridural anaesthesie. Der Anaesthesist *1*:73, 1952.

Buchholz, H. W., and Lesse, K. T.: Druckverhältnisse im Periduralraum und im Liquorraum bei periduralen Injektionen. Chirurg *22*:102, 1951.

Burn, J. M., Guyer, P. B., and Langdon, L.: The spread of solutions injected into the epidural space:

A study using epidurograms in patients with the lumbosciatic syndrome. Brit. J. Anaesth. *45*:338, 1973.
Cheng, P. A.: The anatomical and clinical aspects of epidural analgesia. Anesth. Analg. *42*:398, 1963.
Christie, R. V., and Macintosh, C. A.: The measurement of the intrapleural pressure in man, and its significance. J. Clin. Invest. *13*:279, 1934.
Dawkins, C. J. M.: The identification of the epidural space. Anaesthesia *18*:66, 1963.
Denecke, K.: Die Periduralanästhesie in der Chirurgie. Zbl. Chir. *64*:130, 1937.
Dogliotti, A. M.: Anesthesia. Chicago, S. B. Debour, 1939.
Dornhorst, A. C., and Leathart, G. L.: A method of assessing the mechanical properties of the lungs and air passages. Lancet *263*:109, 1952.
Düttmann, G.: Die peridurale segmentäre Anästhesie. Zbl. Chir. *68*:530, 1941.
Eaton, L. M.: Observations on the negative pressure in the epidural space. Proc. Mayo Clinic *14*:566, 1939.
Evans, W.: Intrasacral epidural injections in the treatment of sciatica. Lancet *ii*:1225, 1930.
Figueiredo, R. R.: Nossa experiência com 1,201 casos de anestesia extradural. Rev. Bras. de Cir. *17*:133, 1948.
Frank, N. R., Mead, J., and Ferris, B. G.: The mechanical properties of the lungs in healthy elderly persons. J. Clin. Invest. *36*:1680, 1957.
Frumin, M. J., Schwartz, H., Burns, J. J., Brodie, B. B., and Papper, E. M.: The appearance of procaine in the spinal fluid during peridural block in man. J. Pharmacol. *109*:102, 1953.
Galbert, M. W., and Marx, G. F.: Extradural pressures in the parturient patient. Anesthesiology *40*:499, 1974.
Gutierrez, A.: Anestesia metamerica peridural. Rev. Cir. Buenos Aires *12*:665, 1932.
Hehre, F. W., Yules, R. B., and Hipona, F. A.: Continuous peridural anesthesia in obstetrics. III: Attempts to produce spread of contrast media by acute vena cava obstruction in dogs. Anesth. Analg. *45*:551, 1966.
Heldt, H. J., and Moloney, J. C.: Negative pressure in the epidural space. Amer. J. Med. Sci. *175*:371, 1928.
Houdard, L., Judet, R., and Mathey: Sur l'anesthésie épidurale des racines dorsales, lombaires et sacrées. Bull. Mem. Soc. Nat. Chir. *60*:510, 1934.
Janzen, E.: Der negative Vorschlag bei Lumbalpunktion. Dtsch. Z. Nervenheilk. *94*:280, 1926.
Lawrence, E. D.: Spinal epidural block. Anesthesiology *9*:601, 1948.
Lebeaux, M.: Sheep syncope. Personal communication. Astra Pharmaceuticals, Inc., Worcester, Massachusetts, 1974.
Macintosh, R. R.: Extradural space indicator. Anaesthesia *5*:98, 1950.
Macintosh, R. R., and Mushin, W. W.: Observations on the epidural space. Anaesthesia *2*:100, 1947.
McMichael, J., and McGibbon, J. P.: Postural changes in the lung volume. Clin. Sci. *4*:175, 1939.
Mead, J., and Gaensler, E. A.: Esophageal and pleural pressures in man, upright and supine. J. Appl. Physiol. *14*:81, 1959.
Nishimura, N., Kitahara, T., and Kusakabe, T.: The spread of lidocaine and I-131 solution in the epidural space. Anesthesiology *20*:785, 1959.
Odom, C. B.: Epidural anesthesia. Amer. J. Surg. *34*:547, 1936.
Pierce, J. A., and Ebert, R. V.: The elastic properties of the lungs of the aged. J. Lab. Clin. Med. *51*:63, 1958.
Reid, R. W., and Sherrington, C. S.: The effect of movements of the human body on the size of the spinal canal. Brain *13*:449, 1890.
Sicard, J. A.,and Forestier, J.: Méthode radiographique d'exploration de la cavité épidurale par le Lipiodol. Rev. Neurol. *37*:1264, 1921.
Usubiaga, J. E., Wikinski, J. A., and Usubiaga, L. J.: La presion del espacio peridural tras la injeccion anestesica. Acta IX Congr. Arg. Anest. Buenos Aires, 79, 1963a.
Usubiaga, J. E., Wikinski, J. A., and Usubiaga, L. J.: La influencia de la circulacion y respiracion sobre la presion peridural. Acta IX Congr. Arg. Anest. Buenos Aires, 95, 1963b.
Usubiaga, J. E., Moya, F., and Usubiaga, L. E.: A note on the recording of epidural negative pressure. Canad. Anaesth. Soc. J. *14*:119, 1967a.
Usubiaga, J. E., Wikinski, J. A., and Usubiaga, L. E.: Epidural pressure and its relation to spread of anesthetic solutions in epidural space. Anesth. Analg. *46*:440, 1967b.
Usubiaga, J. E., Moya, F., and Usubiaga, L. E.: Effect of thoracic and abdominal pressure changes on the epidural space pressure. Brit. J. Anaesth. *39*:612, 1967c.
Varella, A. L.: Hidrodinamica do espaço peridural I. Rev. Bras. Anest. *21*:399, 1971a.
Varella, A. L.: Hidrodinamica do espaço peridural II. Rev. Bras. Anest. *21*:871, 1971b.
Zorraquin, G.: Anesthésie metamérique péridurale et physiologie chirurgicale de l'espace péridurale. Presse Méd. *44*:783, 1936.

chapter 6

Identification of the Epidural Space

Those beginners therefore, who go on well, do not rely on visible instruments, neither do they burden themselves with them. . . .

The Dark Night of the Soul
G. de S. Juan de la Cruz, 1619

The idea of passing a needle through 1¼ to 2½ inches of tissue and then halting the point accurately in a narrow space a few millimeters wide seems daunting to the beginner, yet the procedure is much less difficult than would appear at first sight. Most failures arise from two simple faults: poor control of the hands and lack of attention to detail. A steady hand and a willingness to take pains are essential to success. Without these basic ingredients, an otherwise admirable method may become discredited by careless practice or by poor psychomotor control.

This chapter will trace the development of techniques for epidural puncture, concluding with some practical instructions. Some of the latter may seem excessively detailed and elementary, but no apology is offered for this approach, as I am convinced that the majority of failures and mischances are rooted in sloppy or inadequate technique. I take the view, as a golfer would, that there is a right way, but many wrong ones, to handle the instruments. Mastery of correct detail will ensure a competitive score, while disregard of basic principles will result in wild inaccuracy.

Technical failures may arise occasionally from inadequate equipment or drugs, but inadvertent dural puncture should be a very rare occurrence. An incidence of dural tap of more than one in every hundred or two hundred cases should indicate to the anesthesiologist that there is probably something wrong with his technique and that he should set about correcting it.

The epidural space is a region of loosely bound tissue, presenting little resistance to the propagation of hydrostatic pressure changes, enclosed in tissues that are highly resistant to pressure changes. Methods of identifying the epidural space depend, in one way or another, upon the recognition of the passage of the needle tip from the tissues of high resistance to those of low resistance.

The lumbar approach to the epidural space was tried by Cathelin

(1901) and Tuffier (1901) at the beginning of the century and was abandoned as unreliable. In 1921 Fidel Pagés reexamined the problem and proposed some technical refinements for recognizing the space with greater precision. His chief sign was purely tactile in nature and depended on the sense of "give" that is felt by the operator when the point of the needle escapes from the tough ligamentum flavum and enters the epidural space. He also recommended making the puncture laterally, 1 to 1½ cm from the midline, with the bevel of the needle directed medially. In this way the bevel of the needle, the ligaments to be pierced and the surface of the dura mater are all parallel; Pagés claimed that recognition of the ligamentum flavum was facilitated, and puncture of the dura avoided, by the increased resistance presented by the flat of the bevel. However, this oblique approach has the disadvantage that the epidural space is narrower in its lateral parts than medially, and the vertebral veins running in the anterolateral parts of the epidural space are more liable to damage than in the median approach (Fig. 6–1). Once the needle was in place and no cerebrospinal fluid ran out, the position was confirmed by attaching a syringe of fluid and attempting injection. A lack of resistance indicated that the point of the needle was correctly placed and clear of the dense ligamentum flavum.

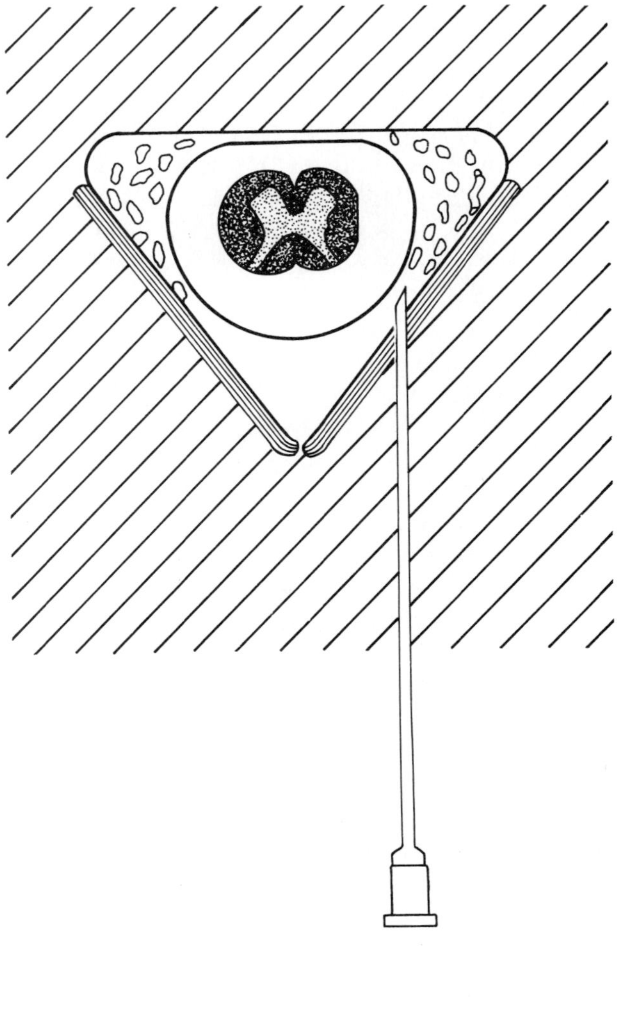

Figure 6–1. Pagés' approach. The needle is introduced 1 to 1.5 cm from the midline, with the bevel facing the median plane, parallel to the ligamentum flavum and the surface of the dura. Note that the epidural space is narrow at this point, and the epidural veins are liable to injury.

Pagés' confirmatory sign of lack of resistance to injection was later developed by others. In 1921, Sicard and Forestier applied epidural injections of radiopaque substances to the diagnosis of spinal canal abnormalities. They identified the epidural space by attaching a syringe of fluid to the needle and attempting injection continuously while advancing the needle through the ligaments (that is, *before* the ligamentum flavum was pierced) (Sicard and Forestier, 1921). In his thesis of 1922, Dr. Jacques Forestier described the sign thus: "On peut déduire que la pointe de l'aiguille est bien placée, si l'injection de la solution de cocaine à la seringue, qui était pénible, devient aussi aisée que si l'aiguille était dans la cavité sous-arachnoïdienne." (Translation: "It can be deduced that the needle point is well placed if injection of cocaine solution in the syringe, which was difficult, becomes as easy as if the needle were in the subarachnoid space.") In this technique the solution under pressure was functioning both as an indicator to the operator and as an atraumatic instrument to push the dura away from the advancing needle point, and Sicard aptly described it as "un mandrin liquide" ("fluid trocar"). The test was later popularized by Dogliotti in 1933 and is called the "loss-of-resistance" test. It will be considered in greater detail later in this chapter.

Another method of identifying the epidural space, mentioned only to be condemned, is that of puncturing the dura and then withdrawing the spinal needle into the extradural space until no more cerebrospinal fluid flows. Cathelin first attempted this technique in 1901 and abandoned it as unreliable. Later, the method found its way into works by Pagés (1921), Giordanengo (1931) and Dogliotti (1933), all of whom condoned breaching of the dura mater on the ground that a pressure gradient runs from the cerebrospinal fluid outward into the epidural space. It was thought that liquids in the epidural space are unlikely to find their way against the stream through a small dural puncture wound, which in any event quickly seals itself off. Bonniot (1934) and Gutierrez (1939) were very outspoken in their condemnation of this method, and there is little doubt that they were right. There is nothing to suggest that dural puncture wounds do seal quickly; in fact, all the evidence points to a slow repair over a period of days (Tuffier, 1901; Forestier, 1922; Pool, 1942; Franksson and Gordh, 1946). After epidural injection the local rise of pressure in the epidural space may temporarily exceed that of the cerebrospinal fluid and thus force a dangerous amount of analgesic fluid into the subarachnoid space, producing an extensive spinal block (Goepel, 1950).

It may happen that the dura is punctured accidentally during the induction of an epidural block. In such a case, if epidural analgesia is particularly preferred to a subarachnoid block, it may be justifiable to persist in attempting epidural block, provided the second puncture is performed one or more spinal interspaces away from the unsuccessful site, and provided that injection is made very slowly at the rate of 10 ml per minute. In this way an excess of pressure will be avoided in the immediate vicinity of the dural wound, and the injected analgesic solution will be less likely to force its way into the cerebrospinal fluid through the hole in the dura.

The existence of a real or apparent negative pressure in the epidural space has already been discussed (see Chapter 4). Gutierrez (1933) and Soresi (1932) were the first to apply internal pressure differences to the identification of the space, and they devised the "hanging-drop" sign. This simple test involves placing a drop of liquid in the open hub of the spinal needle during its introduction. As soon as the needle pierces the ligamentum flavum and enters the epidural space, the drop of liquid is sucked in. This sign is very startling and convincing when seen for the first time, but it is present in only 88 per cent of cases when the lumbar approach is used and therefore lacks reliability in the lumbar region (Usubiaga et al., 1967b).

Many ingenious devices have been designed to assist in locating the epidural space, and some of these will be described later in the chapter. However, if one looks at the failure rate associated with these mechanical devices, there is little doubt that simplicity wins (Dawkins, 1963). Mechanical indicators for locating the epidural space may have a limited place as teaching aids when pressure changes are being demonstrated to students under instruction, but in the long run they increase rather than reduce the possibilities of technical failure. The incidence of dural puncture is higher with their use than without them. The techniques that follow will be outlined in terms of the basic essential equipment—that is, a needle, a syringe and a gentle, steady pair of hands.

One mechanical aid must be conceded, and that is the superiority of the Tuohy needle with its ski-like Huber tip over straight beveled needles. In my hands I have found an irreducible incidence of 1.5 per cent dural punctures with straight beveled needles, but this failure rate is reduced tenfold to an incidence of less than 0.2 per cent when a Huber tip is used.

GENERAL PRINCIPLES OF TECHNIQUE IN EPIDURAL PUNCTURE

State of Consciousness

Twenty-five years ago it was commonplace to induce general anesthesia before inducing epidural blockade. The procedure was quickly performed, and the patient was pleasantly unaware of what was going on (Dawkins, 1945; Bromage, 1954). Since the knee jerk persists under very light general anesthesia, it can be used as a sign of onset of blockade in the lumbar segments in anesthetized patients (Dawkins, 1945). However, as a general rule it is safer to induce epidural blockade in a conscious patient than in one who is unconscious, especially when puncture is made above the termination of the cord. Pain, and particularly lancinating segmental pain, may be a warning signal that the needle point is dangerously close to nerve tissue. Reports of accidental neural damage from traumatic puncture usually include the observation that the patient complained of severe sharp pain at the time of injection. In addition to the safety of an awake patient, much useful information can be recorded, such as the precise segmental extent of blockade and the intensity of motor block (Mostert, 1958).

Occasionally, it may be necessary to induce blockade in unconscious or semiconscious patients. When this is done, care should be taken to perform the puncture below the conus medullaris. The caudal approach lends itself well to induction under general anesthesia, for the site of puncture is far removed from the cord. Nevertheless, short needles should be used in case the tip of the dural sac comes to an unusually low level.

Very rarely, there may be some therapeutic indication for performing a high-level epidural block in an obtunded patient. Then the procedure should be done with extreme care by a skilled epiduralist, and only after the relative risks of the procedure have been carefully weighed.

Epidural Technique

Before scrubbing, the anesthesiologist should survey the back and select the most appropriate interspinous space (Fig. 6–2). The midline should be identified by palpating the vertebral spines transversely, as shown in Figure 6–3. Midline puncture by the loss-of-resistance technique is easiest if made exactly in the midline at point **a** in Figure 6–3, not partially to one side at point **b** or **c.** It is helpful to mark the selected point with a cross, using a skin pencil, or preferably by simply applying thumbnail pressure in vertical and horizontal planes.

Scrupulous asepsis is essential because dural puncture is a possible hazard of the technique. The anesthesiologist should prepare as for a minor surgical procedure and don sterile gloves. A sterile epidural tray (see Chapter 9) is then opened by an assistant; the anesthesiologist lays out his own cart, thus avoiding the use of Cheattle's instrument forceps; and the assistant pours some 1 per cent iodine-in-spirit or povidone in the gallipot. The patient is then placed in position and the full length of the back exposed. After swabbing a generous area of skin with iodine, the anesthesiologist again identifies the spines above and below the chosen space (Fig. 6–4), marks the site of the puncture with his thumbnail and scrubs the site over with a second iodine swab.

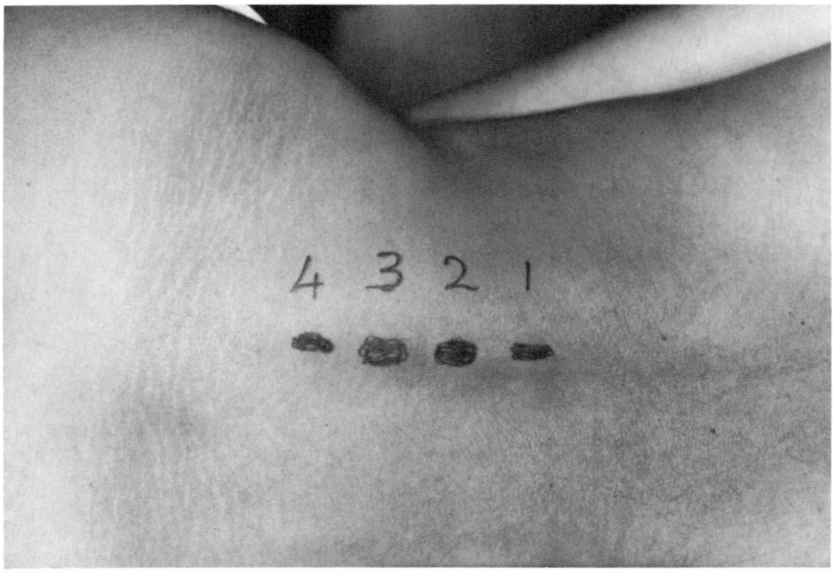

Figure 6–2. Preparation of patient for lumbar epidural puncture. Identification of vertebral spines and selection of suitable interspace for puncture site.

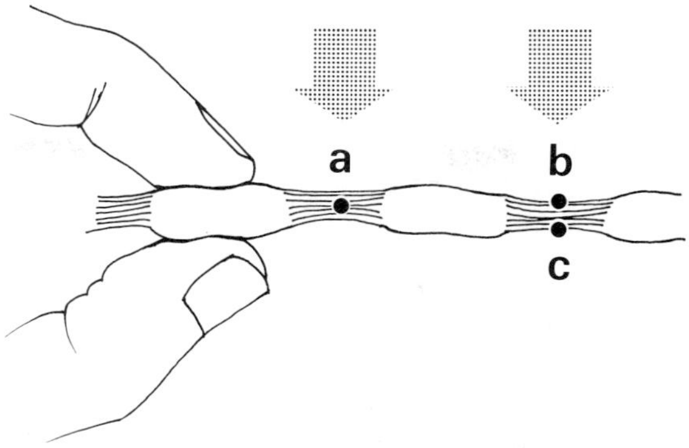

Figure 6–3. Midline approach for lumbar epidural puncture. Identification of interspinous space. Palpate spines *transversely*, above and below selected interspace to determine exact midline (*a*). Slight deviations from midline (*b*) and (*c*) increase technical difficulty by allowing needle to slide out of resistant interspinous ligament.

Do not waste time fussing about. Cultivate a combination of speed and gentleness. Administrative demands in a busy operating environment command despatch, while patient acceptance depends on a sympathetic, gentle touch. Cultivate a no-touch technique. Palpate and identify the puncture site after proper sterilization of the skin and mark it with a cruciform mark using thumbnail pressure. Then wipe the skin once again with an iodine swab. Palpation can still be done around the marked puncture site by gliding the skin over underlying bony landmarks, but there is no need to paw the point of needle entry repeatedly.

A skin wheal of local anesthetic is raised at the skin mark, using a fine 25-gauge needle. Never advance the needle right up to the hub. If needles are going to break, they break at the junction of shaft and hub. Buried broken needles are an embarrassment. Absence of palpable bony landmarks hidden by thick skin or obesity need not cause dismay, as they can be found easily by gentle exploration with the point of a longer needle. Change to a 1½ inch (5 cm) 22-gauge needle and infiltrate the deeper tissues in the line of the needle track,

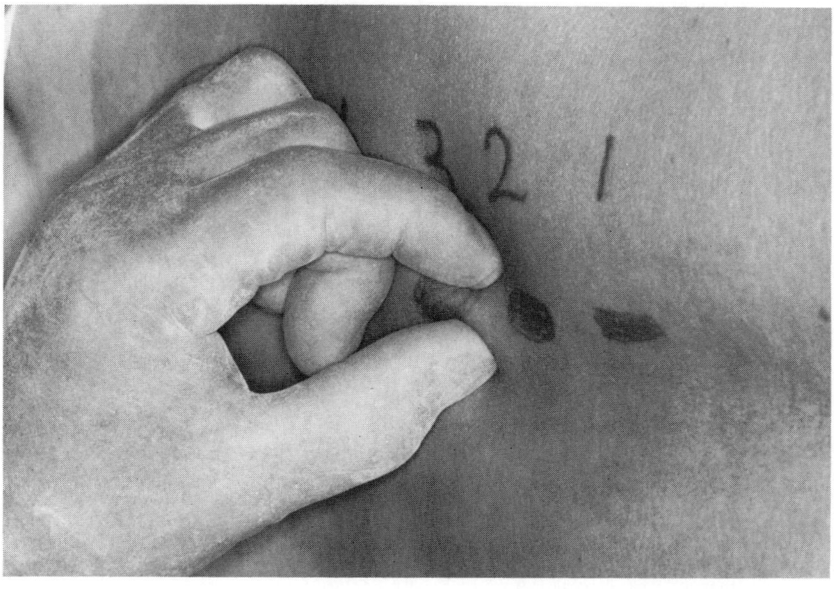

Figure 6–4. Identification of second lumbar interspace and midline. Transverse palpation of spines.

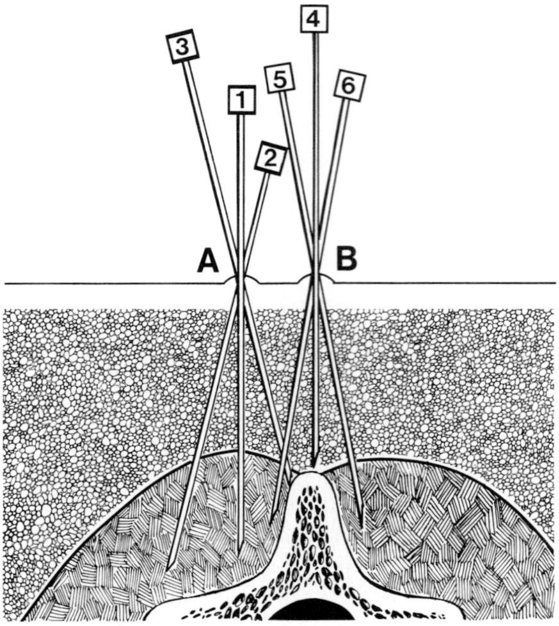

Figure 6–5. Identification of the midline in grossly obese patient. Diagram of transverse section of back. Trial skin wheal at *A*, and probes using local anesthetic infiltration. Infiltration probes 1 and 2 miss tip of spinous process. Probe 3 touches bony landmark, indicating that wheal *A* is placed too far laterally. A fresh wheal is made at *B*. Infiltration probes 4, 5, and 6 now confirm midline and lateral limits of spinous process. An epidural needle inserted along track 4 can be "walked" off the cephalad (or caudal) border of the spinous process and into the midline of the adjoining interspinous ligament.

probing for the hidden bony points. The lateral and anteroposterior limits of a hidden spinous process can then be determined systematically by gentle infiltration in the appropriate planes. If the original puncture site was miscalculated, it can be remade to one side or the other and the epidural needle inserted in the correct direction (Fig. 6–5). Handle all needles in such a way that the advancing point can be halted within a fraction of a millimeter. This means locking the needle in a viselike grip, with the hands braced securely against the patient's back. The grip should be such that there is no play or elasticity in it, and it should mimic all the rigidity and precision of a stereotactic instrument.

Textbook instructions are sometimes worded "advance the needle until you strike bone." This is a barbarous admonition and reveals that the writer himself has never had the experience of being at the receiving end of the regional block. Periosteum is sensitive and is not to be struck. Bony landmarks should be sought with a gossamer touch, local anesthetic being infiltrated as the needle advances, and once found, they should be bathed with a few drops of local anesthetic so that any subsequent encounters will be painless.

THE HANGING-DROP SIGN OF GUTIERREZ

The principles governing hydrodynamic changes in the epidural space were dealt with in the preceding chapter. It was pointed out that optimal conditions for negative pressure are found in the thoracic region when patients are sitting up and their abdominal muscles are relaxed. Under proper conditions a hanging-drop sign should be present in every case if puncture is made between C_7 and T_3 (Figueiredo, 1948). The poorest conditions for negative pressure are found in the lower lumbar region when patients are sitting, especially if they are crouched fully flexed in a posture that compresses the abdominal contents. In my view it is illogical to use the hanging-drop test in the lumbar region at all, and the technique should be confined to thoracic and cervicothoracic punctures. The loss-of-resistance technique, to be described later, is more appropriate in the lumbar region.

Good lighting is essential for the hanging-drop test. The anesthesiologist watches for indrawing of a drop of fluid in the needle hub, and he is utterly dependent on seeing a good light reflex to interpret the movements of the drop. A spotlight directed from one side is very helpful.

From a technical point of view the ideal posture for the patient is sitting up with the head and neck well flexed and the patient's shoulders steadied by an assistant standing in front (Fig. 6–6). This position brings the puncture site to a high point, and it provides the best conditions for generating an effective negative pressure. It also allows the anesthesiologist to align his needle without any distortion from lateral flexion or rotation of the spine. However, patients who are ill or heavily premedicated are best handled in the lateral recumbent position, with a steep head-up tilt as shown in Figure 5–5*B*.

When the hanging-drop sign is used, thumbs must be kept away from the opening of the hub, so as to avoid disturbing the meniscus of the hanging-drop, and at the same time the anesthesiologist must be able to keep an iron control on movements of the needle. This requires that the needle be designed with a large hub that is easy to grip, like the old Barker spinal needles, or with wing grips like the Labat or Macintosh needles. A combination of a Barker or Crawford hub with a Huber tip is ideally suited for this purpose.

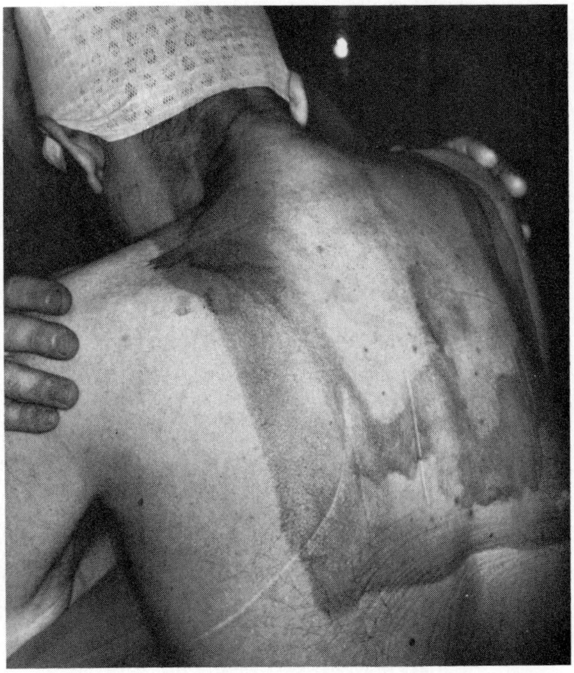

Figure 6–6. Sitting posture for epidural puncture and hanging-drop technique in upper thoracic region. Patient folds his arms across a pillow, and an assistant flexes the neck and steadies the shoulders.

Midline Approach

Conditions are most favorable in the cervical and upper thoracic region between the seventh cervical and fourth thoracic vertebrae. There the vertebral spines are readily palpable and less steeply inclined than in the mid-thoracic region, and the space between the spines is reasonably large when the neck is flexed. In this part of the back midline puncture is technically easy, but lower down between the fifth and ninth thoracic spines a paramedian approach is usually necessary in order to insinuate an epidural needle between the steeply inclined laminae.

The skin and subcutaneous tissues at the appropriate space are infiltrated with local anesthetic. The epidural needle, with stylet in place and with the orifice of the Huber tip pointing upward, is introduced strictly in the midline and in the sagittal plane, as for a subarachnoid puncture, to a depth of about 2 cm (Fig. 6–7). The stylet is then withdrawn, and a drop of analgesic solution is placed in the hub of the needle. The needle is now advanced very carefully and gradually through the ligaments with the hub and shaft held firmly by the thumb and first three fingers of both hands, while the little fingers and hypothenar eminences are steadied against the patient's back. In this way the operator can resist any tendency of the needle to jerk forward after the tough ligamentum flavum is pierced. Figures 6–8 and 6–9 show the grip used for the spool-type hub of a Crawford or a Bromage needle. A syringe of anesthetic solution tucked between the index and middle fingers is conveniently placed to replenish the hanging-drop if it becomes dislodged or sucked in. Figure 6–10 shows the grip for a winged epidural needle.

Since inspiratory movements transmit a further increment of negative pressure to the epidural space, albeit a small one, take advantage of the fact and

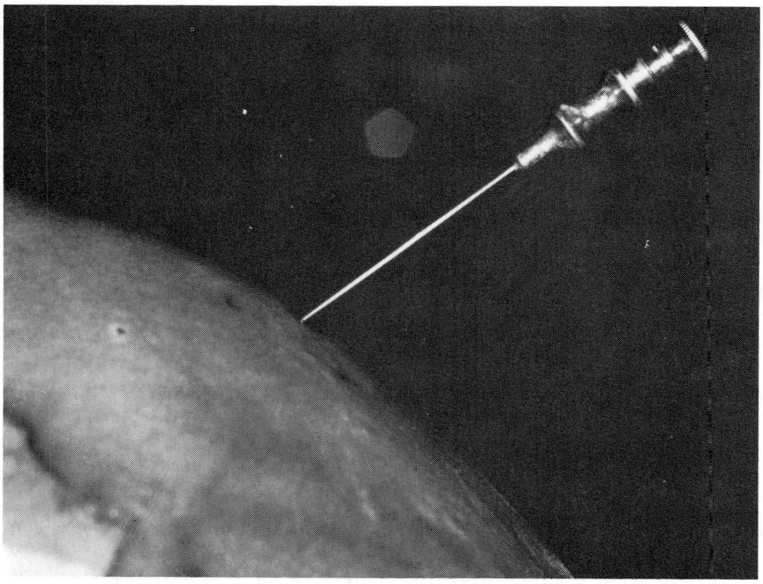

Figure 6–7. Thoracic epidural puncture at second thoracic interspace, using 18-gauge, thin-wall Bromage needle. Lateral view. Note angle of inclination of needle and stylet.

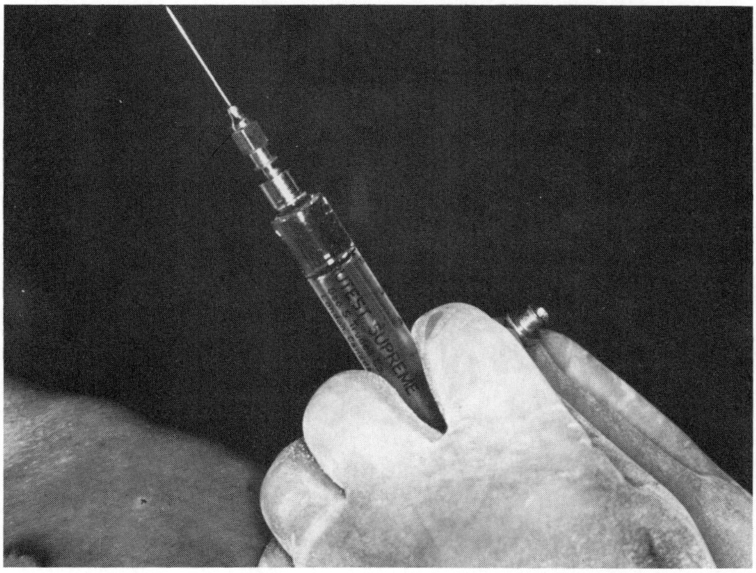

Figure 6–8. Hanging-drop technique. Introduction of epidural needle at second thoracic interspace. Lateral view. The stylet has been withdrawn, and a drop of anesthetic solution placed in the hub. A syringe of local anesthetic with a 22-gauge needle attached is tucked between the first and second fingers to replenish the hub when the drop is sucked in.

advance the needle only during the inspiratory phase of respiration, watching the hanging-drop keenly all the time. There is no need to distract one's gaze from the drop in order to watch the respiration, for the respiratory movements are felt by the operator's hands braced against the patient's back. A sudden sense of "give" is felt as soon as the needle point escapes from the resistant ligamentum

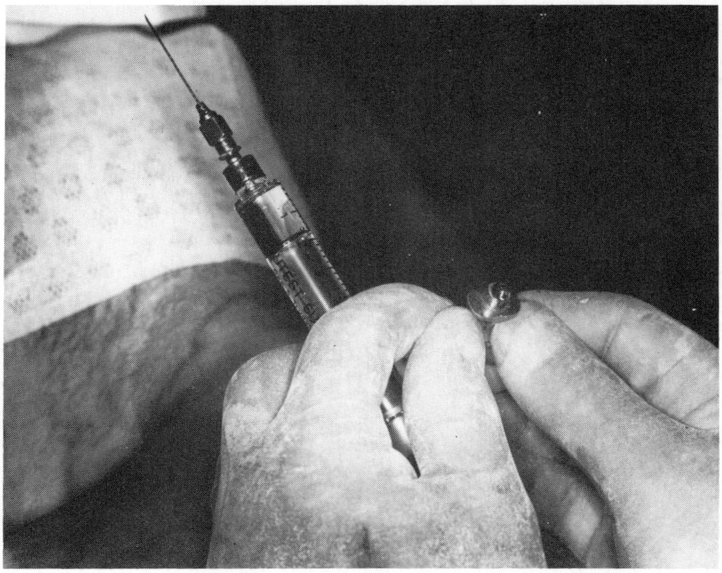

Figure 6–9. Hanging-drop technique at second thoracic interspace. Oblique posterior view. Note light reflex shining on the meniscus of the hanging drop.

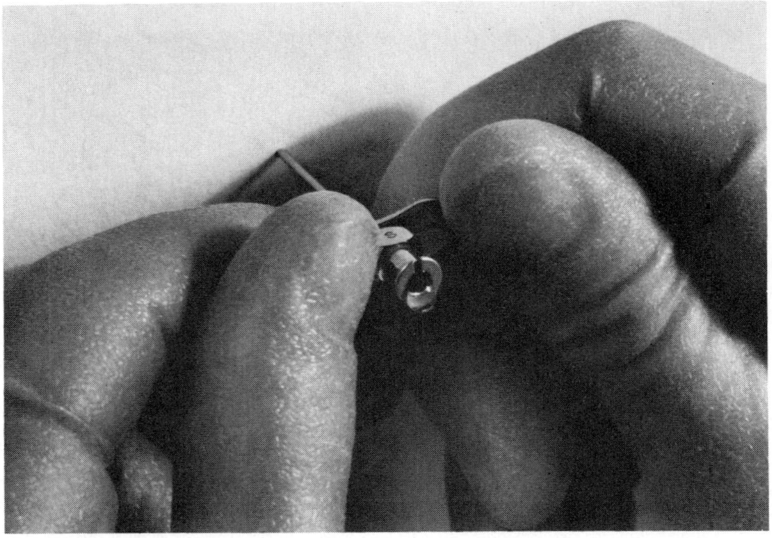

Figure 6–10. Hanging-drop technique of Gutierrez, using a winged Macintosh needle. Note the grip on the wings of the needle. The dorsa of the fourth and fifth fingers of both hands are firmly braced against the patient's back.

flavum into the epidural space, and the hanging-drop disappears into the shaft of the needle. It is essential to halt the advance of the needle instantly, as soon as these positive signs of epidural puncture are manifest, or the momentum of sudden release from resistant tissues may drive the needle onward through the dura into the subarachnoid space.

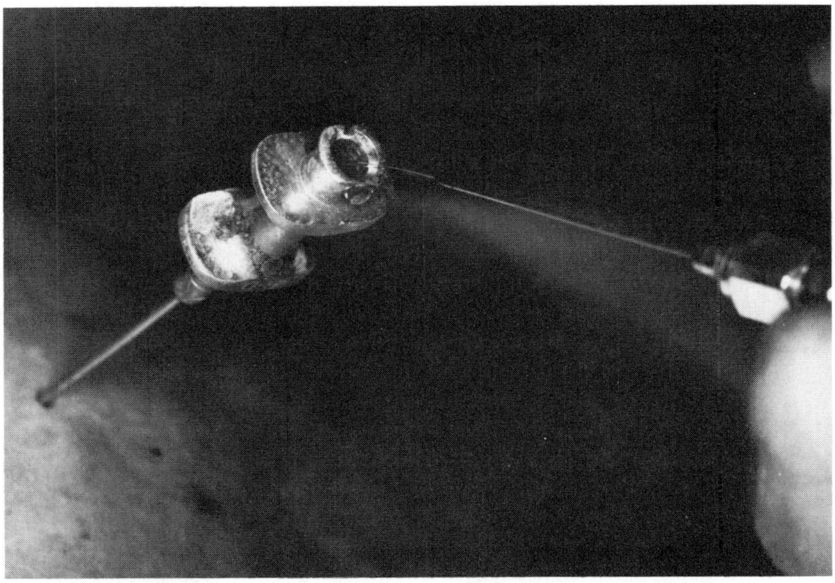

Figure 6–11. Hanging-drop technique at the second thoracic interspace. The epidural space has been successfully entered. A fine stream of anesthetic solution squirted from a syringe disappears down the hub, as if into an empty space. The hub should be kept filled with fluid or capped with a syringe to avoid the remote possibility of venous air embolism (see text).

In the midline and upper thoracic regions the negative pressure usually persists after the drop has been sucked in. If a fine stream of fluid is squirted into the hub, it too disappears rapidly into the epidural space, giving an elegant and convincing confirmatory sign that the needle is properly placed (Fig. 6–11). Vascular as well as respiratory pressures are reflected in the epidural space, and cardiac pulsations transmitted to the meniscus in the needle hub are an additional confirmatory sign that the tip of the needle is lying freely in the space, and not in some fascial plane superficial to the ligamentum flavum. This pulsation sign is particularly valuable when pleural negative pressure is enfeebled by trauma involving the chest wall, or by loss of pulmonary elasticity from emphysema.

Veins are richly distributed throughout the lateral parts of the epidural space, and on rare occasions the needle point may enter a vein. Under these circumstances the local hemodynamic conditions are similar to those in a craniotomy done in the sitting position, and air embolism could be caused by the presence of low intrathoracic and venous pressures if the needle is not kept filled with fluid or sealed by attaching a charged syringe. While I have never encountered this accident, the possibility should be kept in mind and the necessary steps taken to avoid it.

Paramedian Approach

Midline puncture is technically very difficult in the mid-thoracic region due to steep angulation and overlap of the vertebral spines and laminae, and a paramedian approach is indicated in this area to avoid the overhang of the spines. In this approach the needle is introduced at a slant and slightly to one side of the midline and directed medially toward the midline and on to one of the vertebral laminae. The tip is then "walked" upward along the medial extremity of the lamina until it slides off the cranial edge into the epidural space, close to the midline as shown in Figure 6–12.

A skin wheal of local anesthetic is raised 1.5 to 2 cm lateral to the tip of the vertebral spine. A 1½ inch 22-gauge needle is used to infiltrate the needle track and to locate the underlying lamina at the angle between the spinous

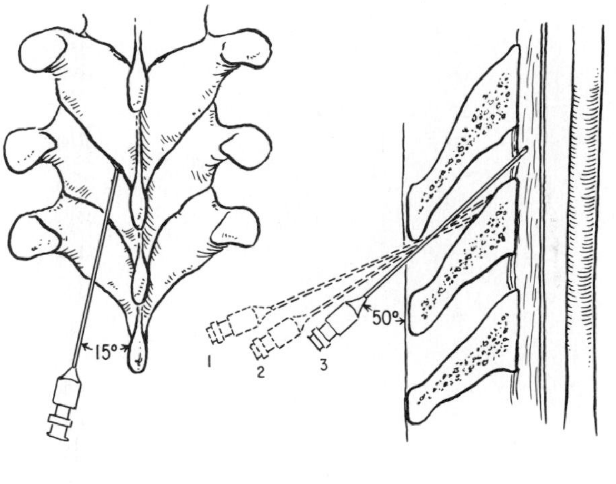

Figure 6–12. Paramedian approach.

process and the lamina. Two or 3 milliliters of local anesthetic are injected onto the lamina, and the Huber-tipped epidural needle with stylet in place is then advanced along the infiltrated track at an angle of about 120 to 130 degrees to the back until gentle contact is made with the lamina. The orifice of the needle faces upward toward the head, so that the rounded tip can slide forward like a ski over the upper surface of the lamina, and the shaft of the needle is angled toward the midline. The stylet is now removed. A drop of local anesthetic is placed in the hub and the needle gently "walked" along the bony surface of the lamina until it is felt to glide over the cranial edge and through the ligamentum flavum. Forward advances of the needle should be made synchronously with the patient's inspiratory movements in order to profit by the slight increment of negative pressure associated with inspiration. Once in the epidural space, the needle is halted.

The paramedian approach confers a very slanting direction to the epidural needle that makes the orifice of the Huber tip face directly along the axis of the spinal canal. This axial orientation of the Huber tip facilitates subsequent passage of an epidural catheter. A paramedian approach may also be used for the loss-of-resistance technique in the lumbar region, where the oblique angle of entry has the same advantage of easing the passage of an epidural catheter.

False Hanging-Drop Sign

A positive hanging-drop sign need not be an infallible index of correct extradural location; it may arise falsely from muscular movements, as shown by the following case:

A man of 76 was very restless during the insertion of a spinal needle on which a hanging-drop had been placed for demonstration purposes. During advance of the needle the patient moved continually and could not be induced to remain still. Suddenly the drop was sucked in with considerable vigor, and this was demonstrated to the onlookers as a sure sign that the epidural space had been entered. But, further advance toward the subarachnoid space was blocked by bony resistance, and on reinsertion of the needle it was evident that the first insertion had been arrested at a relatively shallow level by the dorsal surface of a vertebral lamina, and the epidural space had not in fact been entered.

Figueiredo (1948) reports that this spurious negative pressure sign is relatively frequent. It seems to be due to muscular movements associated with inspiration or with rotation of the spine, and the advancing needle sometimes enters a fascial plane where a small pocket of negative pressure appears briefly as the muscle groups slide one upon the other. In my experience the false drop sign arises in about 2 per cent of cases. Others have found about the same incidence (Castaños and Sagarnaga, 1971). It is troublesome and confusing, and the anesthesiologist must learn to distinguish it from the authoritative indrawing of true intrathoracic negative pressure. Characteristically, the false hanging-drop sign is usually feeble, hesitant and short-lived, in contrast to the brisk aspiration seen when the true space is entered. Also, it lacks vascular pulsations. Confusion in distinguishing between a true and a false hanging-drop sign is most likely to arise in cases of emphysema or

TABLE 6–1 Summary of Ancillary Signs to Differentiate the "False" (Superficial) Hanging-drop Sign from True Identification of the Epidural Space

Sign	*False*	*True*
Initial aspiration of drop	Feeble	Authoritative
Persistent negative pressure	Absent	Usually present
Cardiac pulsations	Absent	Present
Passage of epidural catheter	Difficult or impossible	Easy

trauma in which intrapleural pressure is less negative than usual, and then it may be difficult to decide on the precise origin of the faint negative pressure. Table 6–1 summarizes the main points to look for in differentiating the false and the true hanging-drop signs.

If any doubt remains about the exact position of the needle tip, the anesthesiologist should start again in a fresh adjacent space. The subarachnoid space and the underlying spinal cord are too close to permit tentative exploratory advances of the needle: safety demands prudence in this area of the spine.

Epidural Indicators for Negative Pressure

Gadgets tend to be forgotten and then rediscovered. The following indicating devices are mentioned for the sake of their ingenuity and historical interest, rather than for any encouragement to revive their use in practice. As stated earlier, these mechanical refinements have a certain esthetic and intellectual appeal as diverting examples of applied physics, but in clinical practice I have found that they are actually more of a hindrance than a help, and it is better to use the prosaic unadorned hanging-drop.

Visual aids

1. *U-tube manometers* (Janzen, 1926; Heldt and Moloney, 1928; Bonniot, 1934; and others).

2. *Aneroid manometer* (Ontenada, 1932).

3. *Zorraquin's bulb indicator* (1936), a small, spherical glass indicator containing a drop of liquid and bubble of air.

4. *Odom's indicator* (1936), a simple and quite practical accessory consisting of a short length of glass capillary tube ground to fit the hub of a spinal needle. A drop of liquid placed in the lumen gives a very sensitive indicator of pressure changes encountered by the needle point. However, a chipped or badly fitting indicator is worse than useless, since it may admit air around the taper-joint and so fail to register any change of pressure when the epidural space is entered (Fig. 6–13). Capillary tubes have been elaborated to include means of amplifying the movement of indicator bubbles by providing a slight vis a tergo, or push from behind, to the meniscus.

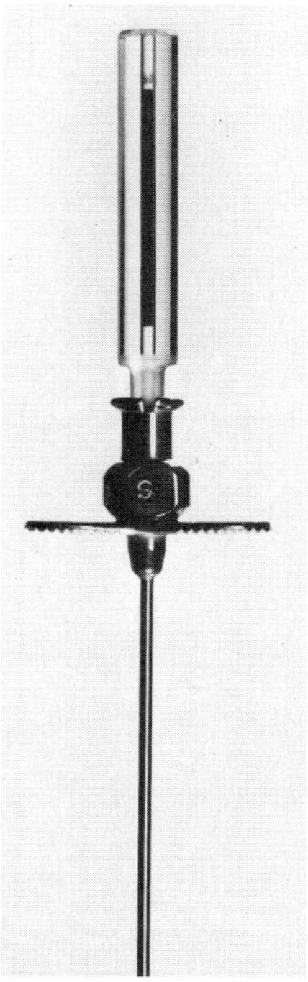

Figure 6–13. Odom's indicator.

5. *Zelenka balloon indicator* (1956), a small rubber balloon fixed at one end of a U-shaped tube with a small tap at the other (Fig. 6–14). The system is charged with 1 to 2 ml of air and a small amount of analgesic solution, and the tap is closed. When the epidural needle is deep in the tissues, the device is attached and the tap opened. As soon as the needle pierces the ligamentum flavum, the indicator discharges itself and the froth of bubbles is easily seen.

6. *Brooks' indicator* (1957), an Odom's indicator with a blown glass bulb on the end. A few drops of fluid are placed in the device, and after it is attached to the epidural needle, warmth is applied to the bulb, either by the operator's hand (a slow business if he has gloves on) or by an assistant holding a cigarette lighter under the bulb.

7. *Dawkins' gravity indicator* (1963), a vertical nylon tube of 3 mm internal bore fixed at right angles to the epidural needle. Gravity aids indrawing of a bubble placed in the indicator.

8. *Auditory devices.* A well-developed negative pressure can give rise to an audible hiss when the epidural space is entered. This sign was originally described by Bonniot in 1934, but others have rediscovered it independently (Sagarnaga, 1971; Mirakhur and Bandopadhyay, 1973). Sagarnaga designed a simple amplifying device to exploit this sign as a routine test, using a small plastic syringe covered with a rubber diaphragm and plugged into a stethoscope attachment. When the epidural space is entered, moving air is amplified

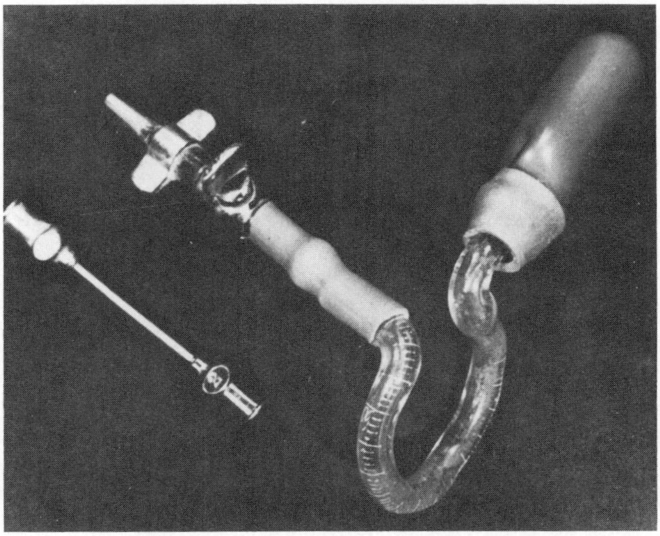

Figure 6–14. Zelenka's balloon indicator.

and "sounds like bursting bubbles." Castaños and Sagarnaga (1971) report a 95.4 per cent success rate with this instrument.

LOSS-OF-RESISTANCE TEST OF SICARD AND FORESTIER AND OF DOGLIOTTI

As the name implies, the test depends upon recognition of a sudden release of resistance to injection as the advancing needle emerges from the tough ligamentum flavum into the epidural space. The change is more readily experienced with a large-bore needle of low internal resistance than with a fine-bore needle of high internal resistance. Moreover, the needle should have a large enough internal diameter to admit passage of a suitable catheter for continuous techniques, and it should be rigid rather than flexible so that the shaft will advance in a straight line without any tendency to be deflected from its course. The most suitable sizes range between 16-gauge and 18-gauge thin-wall. A 16-gauge needle is unnecessarily large, while the 18-gauge thin-wall is just a little too flexible for routine use in the loss-of-resistance test. The 17-gauge Tuohy needle is a good compromise between the two sizes, having adequate rigidity without being needlessly traumatic. Needles of this size need cause no discomfort to the conscious patient if they are used carefully and with adequate local anesthetic infiltration. Fine needles with a higher internal resistance of their own increase the technical difficulties by being too flexible and by giving a less exact end point to the loss-of-resistance test.

As in the hanging-drop test, there is a choice between a midline puncture or the slanting paramedian approach. It is useful to learn both techniques, for each has its own advantages. Students should start with the midline approach. It is easier to master than the paramedian technique, since the directional coordinates are simple and rectilinear and the reassuring resistance of the interspinous ligament is encountered at a shallow depth. The paramedian approach is advantageous in older subjects with calcified interspinous ligaments, but the angled coordinates are more confusing to the beginner.

Midline Approach

The midline approach for the loss-of-resistance test is technically easiest in the lumbar region. The second or third lumbar interspaces are the sites of election, for there the resistant interspinous ligaments are broad and easily identified, and the ligaments provide a solid sense of resistance to the advancing epidural needle. Also, these spaces are safely below the conus medullaris, since the cord terminates at the lower border of the first lumbar vertebra in adults. In children the cord may extend further down the spinal canal, in which case it is wiser to make the puncture one or two spaces lower. Since technical success depends on sensing a *sudden* change of resistance, the method is easiest where the spinal ligaments are largest and toughest. Puncture becomes less easy as one moves away from the mid-lumbar region into areas where the interspinous ligaments are thinner and more tenuous. For example, at the lumbosacral junction the large L_5-S_1 space is often quite difficult owing to the very narrow interspinous ligament at that level.

After preliminary infiltration of the superficial tissues with local anesthetic, a Tuohy or Hustead needle is introduced exactly in the midline and advanced to a depth of 1½ to 2 cm, with the orifice of the Huber tip directed upward in a cephalad direction. A 5-ml or 10-ml syringe is filled with saline or local anesthetic and firmly attached to the hub of the needle. Constant pressure is now exerted on the plunger of the syringe and its incompressible contents, and syringe and needle are advanced together. As long as the needle point is in the ligaments, there is relative or absolute resistance to injection, but as the point emerges from the ligamentum flavum into the epidural space, resistance suddenly disappears. The plunger surges forward and injection becomes as easy as discharging the syringe into an empty space. A medium sized syringe of 5 ml or 10 ml is easier than a small one for this purpose. If a 2-ml syringe is used and the ligaments are at all diffuse, moderate pressure on the plunger may discharge the contents before the ligamentum flavum is reached, making repeated refills necessary.

Needless to say, a freely moving plunger is essential to this maneuver. If the syringe is sticky, then the loss of resistance in the tissues will be masked by the intrinsic resistance of the syringe, and dural puncture will be almost inevitable. From watching the difficulties of beginners, I believe that sticky syringes are one of the commonest causes of accidental dural puncture. If all-glass syringes are used, then the barrel must be well wetted and freely moving before the syringe is attached to the needle. Disposable plastic syringes are less likely to stick than all-glass syringes; however, they have a higher internal resistance than a well wetted all-glass syringe and are better suited to a fluid-filled system. Because the problem of a sticky plunger is frequent with all-glass syringes, it is preferable to use an air-filled system with this type of syringe.

FLUID-FILLED SYSTEM

A firm, braced grip on the needle and a slow, controlled advance are among the most essential conditions for the technique. All jerky movements must be avoided, and the needle must be halted instantly after the epidural space is entered. For this, the operator's stance and the position of the hands are crucially important and different from those adopted for ordinary lumbar puncture or the hanging-drop technique. Although the procedure can be carried out adequately from the sitting position, the standing position is more controlled. The operator should adopt the stance of a riveter at work, with his head and eyes over the work rather than behind it. The grip on the needle is all-important and is designed to reduce the natural compliance and elasticity in the operator's hand to a minimum, so that the needle is advanced steadily and evenly as if by a machine under micrometer control. The needle is grasped at the junction of the hub and shaft so that the grip exerts a three-point fixation, as shown in Figures 6–15 and 6–16. The needle is gripped between the thumb on top and the proximal and distal phalanges of the crooked forefinger below. The hand is supinated, with the wrist partially flexed and the back of the carpus braced against the patient's back. Forward motion is imparted to the needle by a gradual extension of the wrist, and the carpus and metacarpus roll in toward the back like an eccentric cam driving a piston (Fig. 6–17).

The hand must be rock-steady to supply a gradual, controlled forward movement to the needle, as well as an instantaneous braking force as soon

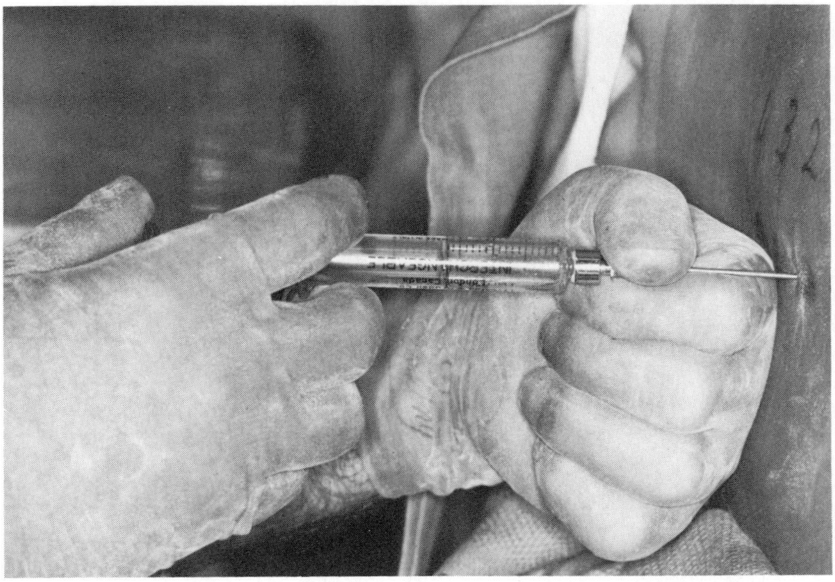

Figure 6–15. Loss of resistance test with an air-filled syringe at second lumbar interspace, right-handed grip. Note firm three-point grip of left hand, with needle hub and shaft locked between thumb and proximal and middle phalanges of index finger.

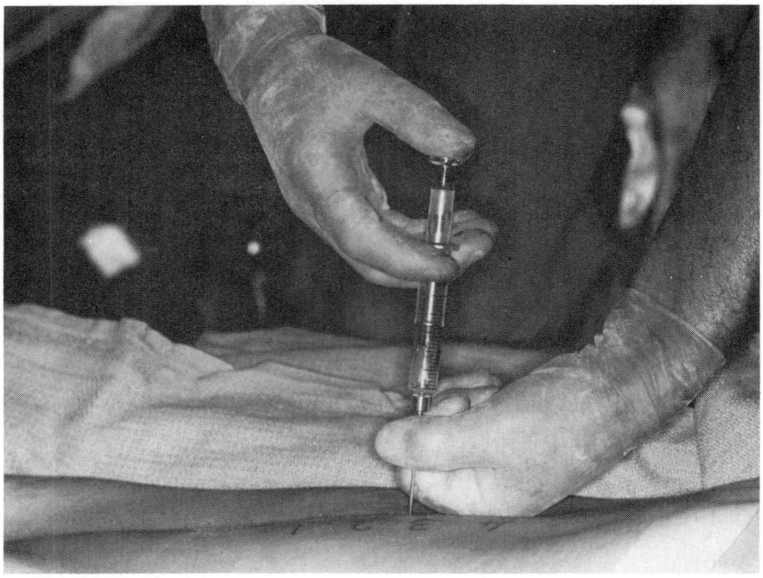

Figure 6–16. Loss of resistance, right-handed grip, viewed from above.

as the epidural space is entered. The forward movement should be gradual and continuous, never intermittent. The other hand holds the syringe, and the thumb exerts continuous firm pressure on the plunger, sensing the different resistances encountered during the advance of the needle. This hand is almost entirely concerned with supporting the syringe and interpreting the significance of changes in resistance to injection as the needle advances; the slight forward motion that it imparts to the needle is counterbalanced by the other hand braced against the patient's back. A 5-ml syringe is small enough to allow the backs of the fourth

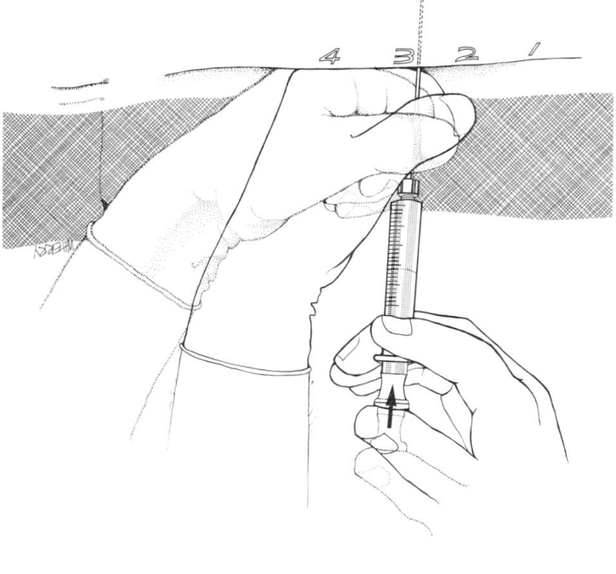

Figure 6–17. Loss of resistance test, right-handed grip. Diagram to illustrate extension of wrist and forward rocking movement on knuckle of right hand that drives the needle forward under rigid control. In air-filled system, thumb of left hand makes rapid tremolo movements on plunger of syringe.

and fifth fingers of both hands to remain in contact and braced against each other. The two hands move in concert like a slow exercise in isometric contraction. *Never advance the needle without simultaneous pressure on the plunger to tell you where you are.*

As soon as the needle point pierces the ligamentum flavum, the plunger surges forward. With proper control, forward movement of the needle is halted in a fraction of a millimeter. Once the space is entered, the syringe is disconnected by a gentle, rotary movement and confirmatory tests are carried out. At this point some authorities recommend that the needle be rotated through 180 to 360 degrees to ensure that the needle orifice lies cleanly in the epidural space. This maneuver is unnecessary and potentially traumatic, since the sharp tip may lacerate dura or veins as it arcs around within the epidural space. Once the needle orifice has entered the epidural space, all unnecessary and fussy adjustment of the needle position should be avoided. Very occasionally, difficulty may be encountered in passing an epidural catheter, and then a careful and slight rotation of the hub may be needed to advance the needle another half millimeter or so in order to free the entire orifice from the ligamentum flavum. However, the need for this very seldom arises and it should not be made a routine procedure.

AIR-FILLED SYSTEM

A rigid, fluid-filled system is theoretically ideal for a crisp and unequivocal end point to the loss-of-resistance test. Fluid is incompressible, and consequently the transition from complete resistance to loss of resistance is immediate and convincing. Unfortunately, the incidence of sticky syringes is high enough to introduce a significant source of error into this technique, and some method of monitoring the resistance of both the patient and the instrument is needed. Adoption of an air-filled system is an expedient compromise. Air is compressible, so theoretically it is a less ideal physical agent than fluid, but when used correctly it is more reliable than fluid if glass syringes are employed.

The procedure and position of the hands are exactly the same as for a fluid-filled system. The only difference lies in the way the plunger of the syringe is compressed by the thumb of the right hand (left hand in left-handed operators). The barrel and plunger of a 5-ml syringe are wetted and made freely moving. The syringe is filled with air and attached to the needle. Instead of firm, continuous pressure on the plunger, pressure is intermittent, with a rapid tremolo movement of the thumb alternately compressing and releasing the air in the syringe; the cushion of air confers a series of rebounding oscillations to the plunger. *Never advance the needle without simultaneously applying tremolo pressure to the plunger of the syringe.* As soon as the needle pierces the ligamentum flavum, the plunger snaps forward as the cushion of air empties itself into the epidural space. An aspiration test is now done to exclude blood or cerebrospinal fluid. The needle should not be rotated for fear that the sweeping point may lacerate one of the delicate epidural veins. Local anesthetic can now be injected once the anesthesiologist is certain that the needle lies cleanly in the epidural space and that it has not punctured the dura or a blood vessel.

Lumbar Paramedian Approach

The paramedian approach may be used in the lumbar region in a manner similar to the lateral approach for thoracic punctures. However, the relatively large lumbar spinous interspaces offer an extra hazard, for it is easy to miss the deep bony landmarks of the lamina and pass the needle straight through the interspinous space, with consequent inadvertent dural tap.

The technique is described by Bonica (1956) as follows: A skin wheal is made 1½ cm lateral to the caudal end of the spinous process of the vertebra, immediately below the chosen interspace. If the lumbosacral space is used (L_5–S_1), the wheal is made 1½ cm from the midline at the level of the posterior superior iliac spine. The subcutaneous tissue, muscle and periosteum of the lamina are infiltrated with dilute local anesthetic solution, using a sharp 22-gauge needle. The point of the needle is directed so that it will contact the medial extremity of the lamina. This maneuver serves to produce analgesia of the deep tissues and to explore the area prior to insertion of the epidural needle.

Some anesthesiologists like to prepare the track of the epidural needle by piercing the skin and underlying fascia with an 18-gauge needle or a Sise introducer, but this step is not necessary if a sharp Tuohy needle is used. The Tuohy needle with stylet in place is now introduced through the skin wheal with its orifice pointing upward, and its point is directed slightly medially so that its axis makes an angle of about 15 degrees with the mid-sagittal plane, and with a marked headward inclination of about 135 degrees to the long axis of the spinal canal. The needle is gently advanced through the paraspinal muscles until it touches the ipsilateral lamina at its junction with the spinous process. The needle is now "walked" upward along the lamina until the tip engages in the ligamentum flavum. The stylet is then removed, and the exploratory loss-of-resistance syringe is carefully attached. The needle point is now in resistant tissues for the first time, and further advance of the needle is carried out using the same loss-of-resistance technique as for the midline approach. The additional distance to be traveled is very slight—a matter of a few millimeters—and then the point emerges from the ligamentum flavum into the epidural space.

Depth of the Epidural Space

The depth at which the epidural space is encountered varies considerably, both at different parts of the spine in any one individual and at the same part of the spine in different individuals. The deepest levels are found at the lumbosacral space and at the thoracocervical junction.

Gutierrez kept extensive records of the distance between the skin and the mid-lumbar epidural space in 3,200 cases, and Figure 6–18 is a histogram drawn from his results. It can be seen that the commonest depth is about 4 cm from the surface. The shape of the distribution curve will of course depend on the type of population one is dealing with. In young children there will be a higher incidence of shallow spaces. We have used

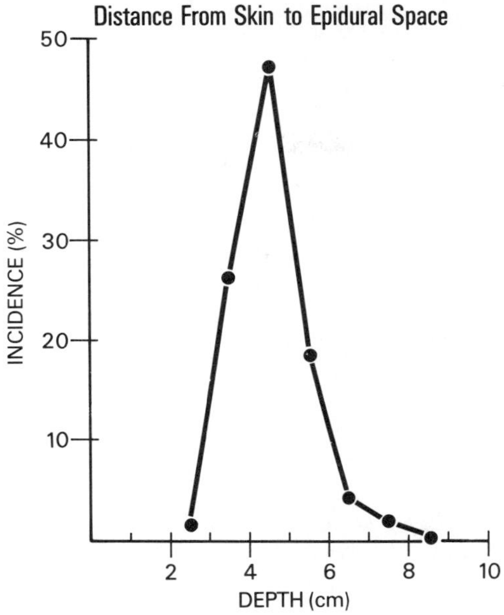

Figure 6–18. Distance between skin and epidural space in mid-lumbar region. Frequency distribution based on data from 3,200 observations by Gutierrez. (After Gutierrez, 1939.)

epidural analgesia in a number of grossly obese patients, and in these subjects it is sometimes scarcely possible to reach the epidural space even when the needle is inserted right up to the hub at a depth of 8 cm.

Epidural Indicators for the Loss-of-Resistance Test

Calibrated needles

Special calibrated needles have been designed with centimeter markings etched or scored on the shaft as an aid to both placing the needle (Lee, 1960) and judging the length of catheter passed through the needle (Doughty, 1974). These needles are excellent for collecting statistical data of depth, but I am in agreement with Lund (1966) that they may act as a distraction from the main task of attending to more important things while advancing the needle. The actual depth of the epidural space is variable, or unknown, in any given patient, so the precise depth is only of interest after the epidural space has been entered and not beforehand.

Mechanical stylets

The syringe full of fluid used in the loss-of-resistance test was originally described by Sicard as "un mandrin liquide," or liquid stylet. This very descriptive term describes exactly the jet action of the stream of fluid, or air, that tends to push the dura away from the advancing needle point like a delicate and insubstantial but effective stylet. Various mechanical contrivances have been designed to replace this tactile, atraumatic "mandrin liquide" by visible but rigid stylets of metal or plastic. Sicard used a blunt cannula within the epidural needle in order to diminish the risk of injuring the dura. Once the epidural space was entered by the loss-of-resistance test, the sharp needle was withdrawn and the cannula advanced a further 1 to 2 mm to ensure that its opening lay well within the space. Forestier, who worked with Sicard, also used the same principle, but he preferred to have a needle inside the cannula so that he was left with the larger cannula in place after the needle was withdrawn (Forestier, 1922).

In 1932 this principle was adapted by Ontenada. His cannula was about half a centimeter longer than the needle, and the needle and cannula were advanced together, with pressure applied to the cannula. As soon as the needle pierced the ligamentum flavum, the cannula, freed of resistance, jumped forward into the epidural space. The cannula, being blunt, pushed the dura away without piercing it (Gutierrez, 1932). Although this is an ingenious method, it must be regarded as a retrogression rather than an advance on Sicard's original technique, for the bland "mandrin liquide," or liquid stylet, formed by the stream of fluid in the loss-of-resistance test was replaced by a shaft of steel which, in spite of its bluntness, could injure the dura.

Goepel (1950) used a graduated blunt stylet to palpate the dura in difficult cases whenever a reflux of injected solution raised doubts that the dura might have been pierced. This graduated sound had a blunt, rounded end, and being delicately held between finger and thumb, it was probably a safe and effective means of confirming that the dura was intact.

Macintosh's extradural indicator is a further refinement of Ontenada's method (Macintosh, 1953) (Fig. 6–19). With this instrument the outer

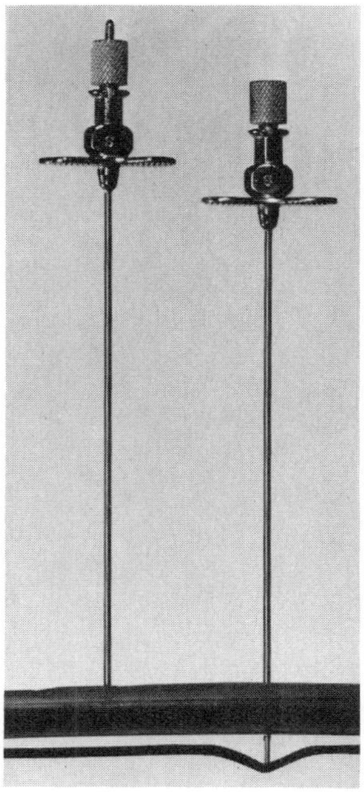

Figure 6–19. The Macintosh epidural needle. A blunt, spring-loaded indicator stylet is impelled forward when the needle passes from resistant ligaments into the epidural space. (From Macintosh, Brit. Med. J., 1953.)

needle is held by the winged finger grips and the blunt indicator-stylet is impelled forward by the action of a small spring when the epidural space is entered. In patients with well-defined ligaments, this gives a very convincing indication of correct epidural puncture, but in others in whom the ligaments vary in density, slight inward movements of the stylet may cause confusion and tempt the anesthesiologist to halt the needle at too shallow a depth.

Brunner and Iklé (1949) devised a spring-loaded syringe for use in the loss-of-resistance test, pressure being applied to the piston of the syringe by a spring instead of the operator's hand. The syringe discharges automatically when the needle enters the epidural space. In their original paper describing this instrument, they reported two failures in 105 cases; this is no improvement on the failure rate of less than 0.5 per cent that is to be expected after a little experience with the Sicard-Dogliotti method using a Tuohy needle and a simple syringe.

For those who prefer simplicity, a light and effective substitute for the Iklé syringe can be made by stretching an elastic band over the piston handle of an ordinary syringe, as shown in Figure 7–12 (Dawkins, 1954; Bromage, 1954).

Macintosh's balloon indicator (Macintosh, 1953) is a development of de Souza's epidural balloon (Figueiredo, 1948). A small air-filled balloon is mounted on a male adaptor. The balloon is constructed with a thick neck and a thin, distensible body. The needle is placed in the spinal ligaments and the balloon attached and inflated by injecting 2 ml of air through the thick part of the wall, using a fine needle. On entering the epidural space the balloon deflates (Fig. 6–20). Zelenka's U-tube and balloon indicator (1956) is another positive-pressure system that can be used to demonstrate a loss of resistance in the lumbar region (see Fig. 6–13).

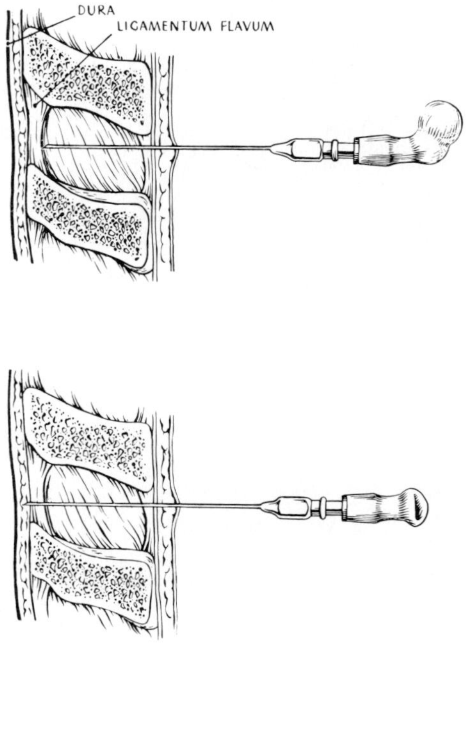

Figure 6–20. Macintosh balloon indicator.

With the possible exception of Goepel's sound, each of these devices has some peculiar disadvantage or weakness which all mechanical gadgets are heir to, and in my opinion these increase rather than decrease the difficulties of the method. Moreover, all these gadgets have the cardinal fault of substituting complexity for simplicity of technique, and they rely on a predetermined mechanical force instead of the delicacy of the human touch. On the other hand, with the Sicard-Dogliotti method a clear interpretation of the position of the needle can be made as slight changes of resistance in different parts of the ligament are transmitted to the thumb pressing on the plunger of the syringe. The operator feels the plunger surge forward and sees it move, and thus the sensation is tactile as well as visual and carries greater conviction than purely visual signals received from insentient apparatus.

CONFIRMATORY TESTS FOR EPIDURAL PUNCTURE

Once the needle has been placed correctly in the epidural space, its position must be confirmed by carrying out one or more of the following tests.

Aspiration Test

Aspiration is performed with a 2-ml syringe. Suction is greater with a small syringe than with a large one; and therefore, cerebrospinal fluid or blood is more easily detected if the dura or a vein has been punctured.

One to 2 ml of air is injected through the needle and aspiration is again performed. The air should go in easily, but nothing should return on aspiration.

Sterile Water Injection

Fluids that differ markedly from normal tonicity are painful in the epidural space. Lund recommends injecting a few milliliters of sterile water as a confirmatory test (Lund et al., 1956). This produces pain in the conscious subject or reflex movements if the patient is asleep. Because of its inherent unpleasantness, I have not used this test as evidence that the needle point is in the epidural space, but it would seem to be a reasonable procedure in unconscious patients, provided anesthesia is light enough to allow response to painful stimuli. Lund recommends that the test be used in conscious patients as an alternative safety measure if the "test dose" is omitted (Lund, 1966). However, the same reservations apply to its use as to the "test dose" (vide infra).

Rapid Injection of Saline or Local Anesthetic (in Unconscious Subjects)

Rapid forceful injection of saline into the epidural space causes a rise of cerebrospinal fluid pressure and feelings of discomfort and anxiety in the conscious subject, but without giving rise to any characteristic change of respiratory pattern. However, Durrans (1947) noticed that in the anesthetized subject there is an immediate increase in rate and depth of respiration. Dawkins recommends this respiratory sign as a useful confirmatory test in unconscious patients (Dawkins, 1963; Dawkins and Steel, 1971).

The Test Dose

The test dose is essentially a trial injection of 3 to 5 ml of local anesthetic solution through the epidural needle, followed by a waiting period of 5 minutes to ensure that injection has not been made into the subarachnoid space. The small test volume should be insufficient to cause noticeable analgesia in the epidural space, but it should cause quite appreciable block with paresis of the legs if accidentally placed in the subarachnoid space. If the test dose fails to show any evidence of intrathecal injection, then the main dose of anesthetic can be safely injected.

At first sight the idea of excluding subarachnoid puncture by a small test dose seems eminently sensible and prudent, but there are several practical criticisms.

1. Perforation of the dura is still possible after a test dose has been injected up the needle. The delay inherent in the test dose introduces fresh possibilities of inadvertent movements of the needle, either through the fidgety movements of a restless patient or by repeated handling of the needle while the syringe is attached and detached.

2. Even a small volume of 5 ml is a significant epidural dose in physiologically old patients, as explained in the previous chapter. In an elderly arteriosclerotic patient, 5 ml of 2 per cent lidocaine in the epidural space may be sufficient to block all the segments up to the umbilicus, and the test dose would have to be reduced to 1.5 ml to be meaningful in this type of patient.

3. There is a widely held clinical impression that injection of fluid into the epidural space separates tissue planes, making the subsequent passage of a catheter easier and less traumatic. Saline is not suitable for this purpose, as it disperses and dilutes the local anesthetic and attenuates its effect, so it is technically preferable to inject the major part of the induction dose through the needle before inserting the catheter.

4. The test dose is time-consuming. The waiting period is trying for the patient and irritating to the operating room staff who are standing by.

5. Finally, a test dose given through the needle is applicable only to a single-shot procedure. It is totally inappropriate if a catheter is used (Foldes et al., 1956), for in spite of a satisfactory test dose, the catheter may still pierce a vein or enter the dura, particularly if the epidural space has not been opened up by the prior injection of fluid.

A reasonable compromise is reached by giving the induction dose in three parts when a catheter is to be used. One-third is injected up the needle to open the epidural space, to initiate the block and to confirm the correct position of the needle. A few minutes now elapse in passing the catheter, taping it in place and performing an aspiration test through it. After that, if there are no signs of subarachnoid block and if the patient can move his feet freely, the second one-third of the calculated induction dose is injected up the catheter, and a further 5 minutes are allowed to pass before testing again. If signs of subarachnoid anesthesia are still absent, then the final one-third of the main induction dose is injected up the catheter. If the patient is heavily premedicated or is lightly asleep, the knee jerk may be used as a sign that subarachnoid block has not taken place (Dawkins, 1945).

With single-shot injections the anesthesiologist must make the choice whether to use a test dose up the needle or whether to inject the full calculated amount of local anesthetic without a prior test dose. While extremely hesitant in recommending others to abandon the use of a test dose under these circumstances, I must confess to having given it up after a very short acquaintance with the single-shot technique, and I have not yet had cause to regret this practice. For reasons already stated I believe a test dose through the needle is of doubtful value, except perhaps in the teaching of beginners when the need for vigilance must be stressed at all stages. However, a test dose does become a logical and appropriate step when a catheter is used, for then the test is applied under stable conditions with the catheter in place and after all the manual manipulations have been completed.

Drip-back Test

Occasionally, after injection of 10 to 15 ml of epidural solution, a few drops of fluid drip back from the needle, in spite of a negative aspiration test. The fluid may come from one of three possible sources:

1. The subarachnoid space has been entered, and the fluid is cerebrospinal fluid.

2. The needle has deviated from the midline into the extensor muscles of the spine, and a relative loss of resistance has been mistaken for the more marked loss of resistance to the epidural space. The injected solution has pocketed under pressure between tissue planes and is dripping back from there.

3. The epidural space has been entered correctly, but injection has been too rapid in relation to the compliance and distensibility of the epidural space. This has caused a temporary build-up of local epidural pressure and backflow of solution. A glance at Usubiaga's data on epidural compliance in relation to age, in the previous chapter, will show that this is most likely to happen in patients whose epidural spaces have become rigid with advancing years.

Three tests are described to decide the origin of the dripping liquid:

1. *Temperature.* Allow the drops to fall on the back of the bared wrist. Cerebrospinal fluid is warm; injected local anesthetic at room temperature will be cold.

2. *Chemical test for cerebrospinal fluid.* Normal cerebrospinal fluid contains between 45 and 65 mg per cent of glucose. This is sufficient to give a

positive color change to blue by the glucose oxidase test when a drop is allowed to fall on a reagent strip used for bedside testing of blood or urinary glucose (Berry, 1958; Gavin, 1965). Glucose oxidase reagent strips should be fresh, for a positive reaction may not be given if they are kept in opened containers for more than two or three weeks.

3. *Chemical tests for local anesthetic.* Practical tests should use reagents that are readily available.

The pH of the effluent fluid may provide a clue to its origin (Reisner, 1976). Cerebrospinal fluid has a pH above 7.0, whereas analgesic solutions containing epinephrine are manufactured with a pH in the range of 3.5 to 5.0. Some urine test strips include sensing zones that react to pH and protein, as well as to glucose. A markedly low pH would suggest that the refluxing fluid is analgesic solution and not cerebrospinal fluid. However, plain solutions of lidocaine and bupivacaine have their pH in the range of 6.2 to 6.8, and this is too close to the pH of cerebrospinal fluid for the reagent to be able to make a clear distinction between CSF and local anesthetic.

An engagingly simple test for distinguishing local anesthetic solution uses stock 2.5 per cent thiopental as the reagent (Catterberg, 1977). The pH of thiopental is high, about 10.6, and sufficiently alkaline to precipitate local anesthetics out of solution. The suspected drops are allowed to fall into a container holding a few milliliters of thiopental solution. An immediate precipitate indicates that the drops contain local anesthetic. However, this test, in common with all others that identify local anesthetic, does not rule out the possibility that the reflux may be a mixture of local anesthetic *and* cerebrospinal fluid. Specific tests exist for ester and amide types of local anesthetics, but they are too complicated for everyday use.

In practice, three simple tests are recommended:

1. The temperature test of Gutierrez, i.e., allowing the drops to fall on the bared wrist.

2. The glucose oxidase test for cerebrospinal fluid.

3. The precipitation test, allowing the drops to fall into the open barrel of a syringe of thiopental.

If dural puncture has been excluded and the cause of the reflux solution is either a misplaced intramuscular injection or a too rapid epidural injection, the puncture should be repeated in the same interspinous space, or an adjacent one, in the following way. The depth of the needle is noted and the needle is withdrawn until the point lies in the subcutaneous tissues. The shaft is then carefully realigned in relation to the sagittal plane and reinserted. A fresh loss of resistance at the same depth as before confirms correct placement in the epidural space.

A dye test has been described to confirm correct placement of the needle in cases in which there is still doubt whether the needle tip is properly positioned in the epidural space or whether it is superficial to the ligamentum flavum (Davidson, 1966). *This test is potentially dangerous, and it is mentioned now only to condemn it.* A second epidural needle is inserted at an adjacent space, and sterile methylene blue is injected up the first needle. If dye issues freely from the second needle, then both must be correctly placed in the epidural space. Unfortunately, methylene blue is neurotoxic and it may cause convulsions and permanent neurological damage if the dye comes in contact with the spinal cord, so methylene blue should *never* be used in any situation in which it might conceivably find its way into the subarachnoid space (Evans and Keegan, 1960; Arieff and Pyzik, 1960; Poppers et al., 1970).

If serious doubt exists about correct needle placement, it is best to start afresh and choose a new puncture site at an adjacent interspinous space.

SITE OF PUNCTURE

General Policy

In selecting the appropriate spinal level for epidural puncture a compromise must often be made between what is theoretically ideal and what is practically safe and feasible. The choice is sometimes difficult, and it should always be governed by common sense.

Ideally, the local anesthetic should be deposited as close as possible to the spinal roots of the operative area. In this way an efficient economical block is obtained. Dose is then minimal and concentrated around the target nerves, ensuring an effective quality of blockade in the segments concerned. Thus, for operations on the perineum or legs, a low puncture at L_5–S_1 would be logical, while a mid-thoracic puncture at T_7–T_8 would be indicated for upper abdominal surgery. Early writings set great store on this principle of selective segmental blockade, and there is no doubt that ideally they were right. However, the spinal cord ends at the first lumbar vertebra, and punctures above this level are potentially hazardous unless the anesthesiologist is sufficiently competent to reduce the dangers to vanishing point.

The hazard of cord damage can be obviated by deciding to restrict all punctures to a level below the second lumbar vertebra and by enlarging the dose of local anesthetic by whatever amount is necessary to reach the required segmental level. Injection in the lumbar region is easy and certain, owing to the favorable inclination of the vertebral spines, while the block can be carried up to any metameric level by increasing the quantity of local anesthetic. However, an exclusive policy of restricting all punctures to below the termination of the cord removes one danger at the expense of some serious disadvantages and therapeutic limitations. First, a policy of this nature eliminates the option of using therapeutic epidural analgesia for chronic pain in the upper part of the body and of acquiring the skill to do it. A department's responsibilities toward any Pain Clinic operation would be gravely hampered by such a restricted policy. Second, the doses required for high blocks in young patients are inordinately large when given by the lumbar route, and the mass of local anesthetic required may border on, or exceed, the prudent toxic limit. For example, imagine a young man of 20 years coming for upper abdominal exploration. Satisfactory operating conditions demand that analgesia should extend as far as T_5—that is, 18 spinal segments counting up from S_5. From the relationship of dose requirements to age, as shown in Chapter 4, Figure 4–12, it can be seen that the segmental dose requirements for 2 per cent lidocaine via the lumbar route are about 30 mg per segment at 20 years. Hence the induction dose would need to be 18 × 30

TABLE 6–2 Restricted Training Approach to Thoracic Epidural Puncture

Anatomical Region	*Ideal Puncture Site*	*Trainees and Occasional Anesthesiologist*	*Trained Staff and Selected Senior Residents*
Arm and shoulder	C_7–T_1	Exclude	Full discretion
Thorax	T_2–T_6	Exclude	↓
Upper abdomen	T_6–T_8	Exclude	↓
Lower abdomen	L_2–L_3	L_2–L_3 or	↓
Upper leg	L_2–L_3	L_3–L_4	↓
Lower leg and perineum	L_5–S_1 or Caudal	L_3–L_4 or Caudal	↓

= 540 mg of lidocaine, a dose that is considered by many to be slightly in excess of a safe maximum. This same individual receiving a mid-thoracic block would need only about 320 mg of lidocaine.

My own policy has been to restrict the performance of thoracic epidural block to trainees who have demonstrated their ability and dexterity with the lumbar approach, and then only under careful supervision until they have gained their own and their supervisor's confidence. The second and third lumbar interspaces are technically the easiest, and the main thrust of instruction should be directed toward obtaining as much versatility as possible from these two spaces. The lumbosacral space with its more tenuous interspinous ligament is technically more demanding, and residents are encouraged to master this space for lower level surgery after they have become proficient in the mid-lumbar region.

Dawkins and Steel (1971) have stressed that there is no logical justification for avoiding the mid-thoracic region while at the same time allowing trainees to use the T_{12}–L_1 space. The thoracolumbar space does not offer the advantage of being entirely free of danger to the cord, nor does it lie centrally over the relevant roots for upper abdominal surgery. Once the decision is made to teach puncture above the termination of the cord, it is preferable to take the logical step and teach the trainee to perform punctures at *all* appropriate levels.

This policy of cautious, partially restricted training is outlined in Table 6–2.

INJECTION OF EPIDURAL SOLUTION

Pressure in the epidural space rises appreciably during injection of solutions, and this change of extradural pressure is transmitted to the cerebrospinal fluid within the dural sac (Dogliotti, 1939; Buchholz and Lesse, 1951; Usubiaga et al., 1967b). In some animals, such as the sheep, the rise of pressure may be sufficient to cause transient syncope lasting 60 to 90 seconds (Hopcroft, 1967; Lebeaux, 1975). In man, uncomfortable feelings of vertigo and fullness in the head are caused unless the injection is made slowly. Even with slow injections at the rate of 0.5 ml per sec or less, slight dizziness lasting

TABLE 6–3 Speed of Epidural Injection—Comparison of Fast and Slow Rates of Injection in 17 Volunteers*

Speed of Injection	*n*	*Discomfort on Injection*	*Segmental Spread*	*Patchy Sacral Analgesia*	*Duration of Action*
Slow (0.33 ml/sec)	17	1 (6%)	0.7 more segments with fast injection	1 (6%)	Slightly longer with slow injection
Fast (1.0 ml/sec)	17	10 (59%)		5 (30%)	

*After Erdemir et al. (1965).

a minute or so may occur, and the patient should be warned of the possibility so that he will not be alarmed if it should arise. The presence of fluid tracking around the spinal roots may also give rise to transient slight paresthesiae in the legs, and the patient may experience a sensation of warmth or of water running down the legs. Solutions that are markedly hypertonic, or hypotonic, or of a low pH may cause transient local pain in the back, although most local anesthetic solutions are quite painless. In high thoracic or cervical punctures, forceful injection may cause sensations of pressure or aching in the shoulder and arms, and the patient must be warned to remain still and relaxed for a few moments until these feelings pass off.

If the likelihood of these sensations occurring is explained to the patient beforehand, they will cause him no worry should they arise, and they will confirm his confidence in the knowledge that the anesthesiologist has insight into his experiences and is with him all the way.

Early writers stressed that speed of injection should be slow rather than fast and in the range of 0.3 to 0.75 ml per sec. Clinical measurement has confirmed that there is no advantage to making a rapid, forceful injection. Erdemir and his colleagues (1965) carried out a careful comparative study of slow and fast injection rates in 17 conscious volunteers. Each subject received two lumbar epidural blocks on different occasions, one given at the rate of 0.33 ml per sec and the other three times faster at 1.0 ml per sec. Slow injection produced an even spread of analgesia, with discomfort in only one subject and incomplete sacral analgesia in two cases. Fast injection at the rate of 1.0 ml per sec was followed by a slightly more extensive segmental spread (averaging 0.7 additional segments), but 10 of the 17 subjects complained of discomfort, and sacral analgesia was incomplete in five cases. Duration of action was slightly longer in the slow injection series. These important results are summarized in Table 6–3, and they show that fast injection has tangible disadvantages. Injection rates should be kept slow and should be punctuated with appropriate pauses if the patient complains of any discomfort.

ACCIDENTAL DURAL PUNCTURE

Prevention

Accidental puncture of the dura should be a very rare occurrence, with an incidence of less than 0.5 per cent, when proper technique is used.

Unfortunately, the actual incidence of dural puncture is often higher than this, particularly in the hands of beginners, so an analysis of the commonest causes of "wet tap" is important. They fall under two headings: failures of technique and difficulties with the patient. Some failure of technique is the commoner cause of "wet tap."

TECHNICAL ERROR

Jerky Discontinuous Movements. The process of epidural puncture should emulate the smooth micrometer control of a machine. The habit of advancing the needle intermittently without continuously monitoring its progress is fundamentally unsound, and it is bound to lead to a high rate of dural puncture.

Sticky Syringes. This problem has been dealt with at length. Syringes must be well lubricated, and free movement of the plunger should be carefully checked before the loss-of-resistance test is begun.

Flabby Hands. All hands are flabby to a degree, but the amount of compliance and free play given to the needle depends on the way it is held in the hands. The firm grip described earlier reduces manual compliance to a minimum and ensures the greatest degree of control over the advancing needle.

PATIENT PROBLEMS

Moving Target. Restlessness from pain, discomfort or anxiety must be subdued. The best tranquilizer is empathy based on detailed and patient explanation of what is to be done, given *before* it is done. This is particularly important with children scheduled for elective surgery. Most children over the age of five years are amenable to sympathetic explanation, and a few minutes of friendly chat and careful instruction the evening before operation will be amply repaid by cheerful rapport and cooperation in the induction room the following day. Drugs must be used if verbal sedation is not enough. Diazepam is the first choice, because in addition to sedation it provides unique protection against toxic reactions to local anesthetics (De Jong, 1977).

Frightened parturient women in labor represent some of the most difficult moving targets. In this case depressant tranquilizing drugs must be avoided, and reliance must be placed on verbal communication, with whatever combination of gentle coaxing, firm commands and physical restraint necessary to keep the patient safely quiet and steady on the delivery bed. In difficult cases it is wise to make things as easy as possible for the operator by having the patient sitting up and supported by an assistant from in front. And of course, the puncture should be performed between contractions when the patient is least driven to wriggle about.

Obesity and Osteoarthritis. While presenting physical difficulties in reaching the epidural space, these conditions only increase the risk of dural puncture if the operator is sufficiently intimidated by them to forget the basic essentials of deliberate iron control in advancing the needle.

Obliterated Epidural Space. Congenital abnormalities or disease may obliterate part of the epidural space, making dural puncture almost inevitable at certain levels. This situation is rare, and enough warning signs are usually present to alert the anesthesiologist to choose another site. For example, spina bifida occulta disturbs bony landmarks and may obliterate the posterior epidural space at the level of the deficient laminal arch. A median tuft of hair or an unusually deep midline vertebral cleft should raise suspicions that a localized anomaly exists, and puncture should be made at a higher vertebral level. Previous laminectomy is a more common cause of local obliteration of the epidural space, and puncture should be made proximal or distal to the ends of the laminectomy scar.

Needles are not the only instruments that can puncture the dura. Epidural catheters may also find their way into the subarachnoid space on rare occasions (and more frequently into epidural veins). These problems will be dealt with in the next chapter on continuous epidural analgesia.

Treatment

Accidental puncture of the dura should be a rare event, with an incidence of less than 0.5 per cent, but when it does arise what should be done?

The rent made by a 17- or 16-gauge needle is large enough to allow fluids to pass through it with relative ease. Cerebrospinal fluid is able to leak out, or local anesthetic outside the dura can flow into the subarachnoid space if the epidural pressure is high enough. The hole will be slow to heal and will take at least 10 to 14 days to seal itself, and in some cases even longer (Jacobaeus and Frumerie, 1923; Solomon, 1924; Alpers, 1925; Nelson, 1930; Pool, 1942; Franksson and Gordh, 1946; Ahern, 1948).

There are four immediate options after inadvertent dural puncture:

1. Abandon the procedure.
2. Convert to a subarachnoid block.
3. Try again in the same space.
4. Try again in a different space.

I used to believe that the danger of injecting local anesthetic into the epidural space in the presence of a large hole was unjustifiable and that either the first or the second choice of the four options was the safest (Bromage, 1954). In the early 1950's this belief was probably correct. At that time it was still accepted practice to employ large volumes of dilute but potent agents, and induction doses of up to 45 ml of 1/600 dibucaine were commonplace. Studies of epidural compliance show that volumes of this magnitude will cause a sustained pressure over a large part of the epidural space for a period of several minutes, long enough to force an appreciable amount of local anesthetic into the subarachnoid space through the hole in the dura (Evans, 1930; Franksson and Gordh, 1946; Usubiaga et al., 1967b).

Today, more penetrating local anesthetics than dibucaine are used, and in volumes of about half the amount necessary for 1/600 dibucaine. Epidural pressure is not likely to rise as high, or to be sustained for so long, with these reduced volumes, so it seems reasonable to take a more lenient view of a second attempt at epidural puncture in the face of a dural rent.

Even so, the third option of trying again in the same space may be unwise. For one thing, resistance in the superficial tissues may well have been disturbed by the first attempt, and a second puncture in the same place is often more difficult than the first. Most importantly, the local cone of epidural positive pressure caused by the injected solution will be greatest immediately over the hole in the dura, and some degree of inward subarachnoid leak can be anticipated.

The fourth option of trying again in an adjacent space is reasonable, provided the induction dose is given slowly and the volume is small, as for example in obstetrical analgesia where volumes of 6 to 8 ml are sufficient for relief of pain in the first stage of labor. This appears to be a generally adopted policy that has proved to be safe in practice (Crawford, 1973). Safety is likely to be improved if the point of epidural injection is further removed from the dural hole by passing a catheter in a direction away from the original puncture site (Craft et al., 1973). It must be emphasized that the risk of extensive subarachnoid spread in the presence of a dural puncture is pressure-dependent and therefore dependent on the volume of local anesthetic that is injected into the epidural space. Epidural injections of small volume are likely to be safe, whereas large volumes are not, as illustrated by the following case report (Mesry, 1976):

> *An asthmatic woman of 37 years was scheduled for tuboplasty under epidural analgesia. Lidocaine, 24 ml of 1.5 per cent solution (i.e., 360 mg), was injected at T_{12}–L_1 after accidental dural puncture at L_2–L_3. Fourteen minutes later the systolic pressure fell to 40 mmHg, ventilation became inadequate and the patient lost consciousness. Routine management with artificial ventilation and vasopressor therapy was followed by recovery of consciousness in 15 minutes and return of normal sensation two hours after the epidural injection.*

The pupils remained small throughout the incident, and the author concluded that massive spread had occurred in the epidural space rather than the subarachnoid space. However, pupil size is an equivocal indicator of site of anesthetic action, depending as it does on the balance of blockade in the superficial sympathetic excitatory pathway and the somewhat deeper inhibitory pathway of the cord (Loewy et al., 1973; Foreman and Wurster, 1973). In this instance the profound sensory and motor blockade is suggestive of massive subarachnoid spread and action on the surface of the spinal cord and brain stem.

Headache Prophylaxis

Freedom from postpuncture headache is a vaunted claim of epidural analgesia that collapses miserably when the dura is accidentally pierced. The large size of epidural needles (18- to 16-gauge) almost guarantees that a low-pressure headache will follow from loss of cerebrospinal fluid. Typically, the headache starts on the following day and lasts five to eight days. It is worse on standing and sitting and is eased by recumbency, and it is often sufficiently incapacitating to require extended hospital stay until it passes.

Severe and crippling headache arises in about 20 per cent of large puncture holes, and Vandam and Dripps (1956) reported an incidence of 18 per cent after spinal puncture with a 16-gauge needle. However, minor headaches that are nevertheless severe enough to be a nuisance are more common and occur in 70 to 80 per cent of accidental dural punctures. Arner (1962) reported 72 per cent, Crawford (1972) 77.5 per cent with an 18-gauge needle and Craft and his colleagues (1973) 76.5 per cent after puncture with a 16-gauge Tuohy needle. Hence, accidental dural puncture should be taken seriously as a cause of morbidity and prolonged hospital stay, and the anesthesiologist should initiate treatment to prevent headache.

Prophylactic measures to prevent severe headache, or to treat it when it arises, are directed to restoring cerebrospinal fluid pressure that has been lowered by leakage through the puncture hole. Some methods are conservative and some are more aggressively active. There is a general acceptance of the conservative measures, although on the whole they are not dramatically effective, but there is some controversy about the active methods which are more effective than the conservative measures.

Conservative measures

1. Stimulation of cerebrospinal fluid formation by forced fluids.
2. Bed rest with feet elevated.
3. Abdominal binder to raise pressure in the epidural veins and so bolster a sagging dural tube.
4. Systemic analgesics.

Active measures

Cerebrospinal fluid pressure can be restored and headache relieved by plugging the dural leak, or by bolstering up the pressure from outside by injecting large volumes of saline into the epidural space.

Epidural Saline

Saline is rapidly absorbed from the epidural space, and the hydraulic supportive pressure exerted on the outside of the dural tube is relatively transient. Rice and Dabbs (1950) showed that injection of 30 to 100 ml of saline into the epidural space could relieve spinal headache temporarily, and Kaplan and Arrowood (1952) also found epidural saline to be an effective prophylactic against postpuncture headache.

A single epidural injection of 30 to 60 ml of saline tends to give temporary rather than permanent relief, and the procedure may have to be repeated, but this can easily be done without disturbing the patient if an epidural catheter is left in place.

Crawford (1972) advocated an epidural drip of 1 to 1.5 liters of Hartmann's solution, infused over a 24-hour period, in an effort to produce a constant and prolonged pressure in the lumbar epidural space. With this regimen the incidence of headache after dural puncture was reduced from 73 per cent to 21 per cent, and the headaches that did occur tended to be mild rather than severe. However, some of these patients complained of sharp interscapular pain while the drip was in progress, and this was sometimes severe enough to require narcotics for relief. The cause of this high back pain is not immediately apparent (Crawford, 1972, 1973).

Craft and his colleagues (1973) also left the catheter in place but took the simpler course of using two injections of 60 ml of normal saline. The first injection was given before the patient left the operating table, and the second 60 ml were injected the following morning. In this series the incidence of post–dural puncture headache was reduced from 76 per cent to 12 per cent.

Blood Patch

In 1960, Gormley demonstrated that postspinal headache could be relieved by an injection of autologous blood into the epidural space near the dural puncture hole. It was suggested that blood clot would both seal the hole and expedite healing of the dura.

DiGiovanni and his colleagues developed this procedure in a series of several hundred cases with excellent results, and the method has had a sufficient period of trial to appear safe and effective (DiGiovanni and Dunbar, 1970; DiGiovanni et al., 1972).

An epidural needle is inserted close to the site of dural puncture. Under fully sterile conditions 10 ml of venous blood are drawn from the patient's arm and immediately injected through the epidural needle. The needle is then withdrawn and the patient placed supine. DiGiovanni reports immediate and sustained relief of headache by this method in 92 per cent of cases. This dramatic relief is impressive, but doubts have been raised that the blood might lead to trouble through possible extradural or subarachnoid adhesions. However, animal experiments have not revealed any local sequelae, and in a large series of cases clinical complications do not seem to have arisen from the presence of the blood in the epidural space (DiGiovanni et al., 1972). Two cases of transient back pain and bilateral positive Lasègue's sign lasting a few days have been reported, but the process resolved in both patients within two weeks (Shantha et al., 1973; Cornwall and Dolan, 1975).

Epidural saline as a prophylactic measure appears to be effective and worthwhile, but the need for prolonged epidural catheterization is a nuisance, and even distressing in some patients receiving a continuous infusion. On the whole, the evidence appears to be in favor of the "blood patch" as a simple and practical therapeutic maneuver if headache develops. My personal preference as a patient with a large dural puncture would be to accept the sporting odds of 7:3 of suffering a headache and await events with conservative management, and then submit to a "blood patch" if the wager were lost and headache supervened. This expectant policy will avoid a number of unnecessary blood patches without undue morbidity, even in the presence of quite large puncture holes. For example, some years ago I received an accidental dural puncture with a 15-gauge Barker needle during the course of an experimental procedure. A prophylactic regime of copious oral fluids was followed, and there was no suspicion of headache in spite of ambulation the same day. Had an immediate blood patch been performed, the lack of symptoms would have been attributed to the aggressive form of treatment given at the time of puncture.

The long-term effects of the "blood patch" technique appear to be

TABLE 6–4 Results of Epidural Blood Patch in 185 Cases of Resistant Post–Lumbar Puncture Headache*

	Incidence of Success		*Incidence of Complications*		
	n	%	*DURATION*	*n*	%
Immediate and permanent relief	182	98.4	24–30 hours	4	2.16
Failure	5	1.6	10 days	1	0.54

*After Ostheimer et al. (1974).

quite innocuous. The Society for Obstetric Anesthesia and Perinatology undertook a prospective study of the efficacy and safety of epidural blood patch (EPL) for the treatment of post lumbar puncture headache; the results are outlined in Table 6–4 (Ostheimer et al., 1974). In all cases the headache was severe and had persisted for 3 to 4 days following dural puncture, in spite of conservative treatment with such measures as bed rest, analgesics, abdominal binders and epidural saline injections. The five complications reported at the end of one year's follow-up were all minor and transient. In this series the one case involving symptoms lasting ten days was attributed to nerve root compression or irritation; the other four patients complained of mild backache or "stiff back" lasting a day or so. Transient side effects were noticed by 15 patients, and these included backache, stiff neck or paresthesiae in the legs or abdomen that passed within a few minutes.

In an independent series of 118 epidural blood patches for postspinal headache (Abouleish et al., 1975a, 1975b), three of the patients underwent uncomplicated and successful epidural, caudal or subarachnoid blocks within a period of 13 months after the blood patch was performed. In these three cases analgesia developed normally, and there was no evidence that the injected epidural blood patch had caused any obliteration of the epidural space.

Thus, all the available evidence supports the epidural blood patch as effective and safe and probably the best treatment for refractory post–dural puncture headache.

REFERENCES

Abouleish, E., et al.: Long-term follow-up of epidural blood patch. Anesth. Analg. *54*:459, 1975a.

Abouleish, E., Wadhwa, R. K., de la Vega, S., Tan, R. N., and Lim Uy, N. T.: Regional analgesia following epidural blood patch. Anesth. Analg. *54*:634, 1975b.

Ahern, R. E.: Management of severe post lumbar puncture headaches. N.Y. J. Med. *48*:1495, 1948.

Alpers, B.: Lumbar puncture headache. Arch. Neurol. *14*:806, 1925.

Arieff, A. J., and Pyzik, S. W.: Quadriplegia after intrathecal injection of methylene blue. J.A.M.A. *173*:794, 1960.

Arner, O.: Complications following spinal anesthesia: Their significance and a technic to reduce their incidence. Acta Chir. Scand., Suppl. 167, 1962.

Berry, A.: Test for spinal fluid. Anaesthesia *13*:100, 1958.

Bonica, J. J.: Continuous peridural block. Anesthesiology *17*:626, 1956.

Bonniot, A.: Note sur la pression épidural négative. Bull. Soc. Chir. Paris *60*:124, 1934.

Bromage, P. R.: Spinal Epidural Analgesia. Edinburgh, E. & S. Livingston, Ltd., 1954, pp. 46, 55, 57, 116.

Brooks, W.: An epidural indicator. Anaesthesia *12*:227, 1957.

Brunner, C., and Ikle, F. A.: Beitrag zur peridural anästhesie. Scweiz. Med. Wschr. *79*:799, 1949.
Buchholz, H. W., and Lesse, K. T.: Die Druckverhaltnisse im Periduralraum und im Liquorraum bei periduralen Injektionen. Chirurg *22*:102, 1951.
Castanõs, C., and Sagarnaga, A.: Sinal acustico para identificação do espaço peridural. Rev. Bras. Anest. *21*:886, 1971.
Cathelin, F.: Mode d'action de la cocaine injectée dans l'espace épidurale par le procédé du canal sacré. C. R. Soc. Biol. Paris *53*:478, 1901.
Catterberg, J.: Local anesthetic vs. spinal fluid. Anesthesiology *46*:309, 1977.
Cornwall, R. D., and Dolan, W. M.: Radicular back pain following lumbar epidural blood patch. Anesthesiology *43*:692, 1975.
Craft, J. B., Epstein, B. S., and Coakley, C. S.: Prophylaxis of dural-puncture headache with epidural saline. Anesth. Analg. *52*:228, 1973.
Crawford, J. S.: The prevention of headache consequent upon dural puncture. Brit. J. Anaesth. *44*:598, 1972.
Crawford, J. S.: Epidural drip and post-spinal headache. Brit. J. Anaesth. *45*:1177, 1973.
Davidson, J. T.: Identification of the epidural space. Anesthesiology *27*:859, 1966.
Dawkins, C. J. M.: Discussion on extradural spinal block. Proc. Roy. Soc. Med. *38*:298, 1945.
Dawkins, C. J. M.: Personal communication, 1954.
Dawkins, C. J. M., and Steel, G. C.: Thoracic extradural (epidural) block for upper abdominal surgery. Anaesthesia *26*:41, 1971.
Dawkins, M.: The identification of the epidural space: A critical analysis of the various methods employed. Anaesthesia *18*:66, 1963.
De Jong, R. H.: Local Anesthetics. 2nd ed. Springfield, Ill. Charles C Thomas, Publishers, 1977, p. 109.
DiGiovanni, A. J., and Dunbar, B. S.: Epidural injections of autologous blood for postlumbar-puncture headache. Anesth. Analg. *49*:268, 1970.
DiGiovanni, A. J., Galbert, M. W., and Wahle, W. M.: Epidural injections of autologous blood for postlumbar-puncture headache. II. Additional clinical experiences and laboratory investigation. Anesth. Analg. *51*:226, 1972.
Dogliotti, A. M.: Segmental peridural anesthesia. Amer. J. Surg. *20*:107, 1933.
Dogliotti, A. M.: Anesthesia: Narcosis-Local-Regional-Spinal. Chicago, S. B. Debour, 1939, p. 528.
Doughty, A.: A precise method of cannulating the lumbar epidural space. Anaesthesia *29*:63, 1974.
Durrans, S. F.: High extradural segmental block. Anaesthesia *2*:106, 1947.
Erdemir, H. A., Soper, L. E., and Sweet, R. B.: Studies of factors affecting peridural anesthesia. Anesth. Analg. *44*:400, 1965.
Evans, J. P., and Keegan, H. R.: Danger in the use of intrathecal methylene blue. J.A.M.A. *174*:856, 1960.
Evans, W.: Intrasacral epidural injection in the treatment of sciatica. Lancet *2*:1225, 1930.
Figueiredo, R. R.: Nossa experiência com 1,201 casos de anestesia extradural. Rev. Bras. Cir. *17*:133, 1948.
Foldes, F. F., Colavincenzo, J. W., and Birch, J. H.: Epidural anesthesia: A reappraisal. Anesth. Analg. *35*:33, 1956.
Foreman, R. D., and Wurster, R. D.: Localization and functional characteristics of descending sympathetic spinal pathways. Amer. J. Physiol. *225*:212, 1973.
Forestier, J.: Le Trou de Conjugaison Vertebral. Paris, Jouve et Cie, 1922, p. 105.
Franksson, C., and Gordh, T.: Headache after spinal anesthesia and a technique for lessening its frequency. Acta Chir. Scand. *94*:443, 1946.
Gavin, R.: Continuous epidural analgesia, an unusual case of dural perforation during catheterization of the epidural space. New Zealand Med. J. *64*:280, 1965.
Giordanengo, M. G.: Segmental peridural anesthesia. Bull. Soc. Chir. Paris *23*:591, 1931.
Goepel, E.: Gefahren und Komplikationen in der Periduralanästhesie. Zbl. Chir. *75*:1622, 1950.
Gormley, J. B.: Treatment of postspinal headache. Anesthesiology *21*:565, 1960.
Gutierrez, A.: Anestesia metamerica peridural. Rev. Cir. Buenos Aires *12*:665, 1932.
Gutierrez, A.: Valor de la aspiracion liquida en el espacio peridural en la anestesia peridural. Rev. Cir. Buenos Aires *12*:225, 1933.
Gutierrez, A.: Anesthesia Extradural. Buenos Aires, Rev. cirug. B. Aires 1939, p. 52.
Heldt, H. J., and Moloney, J. C.: Negative pressure in the epidural space. Amer. J. Med. Sci. *175*:371, 1928.
Hopcroft, S. C.: Technique of epidural anaesthesia in experimental sheep. Aust. Vet. J. *43*:213, 1967.
Jacobaeus, H. D., and Frumerie, K.: About the leakage of spinal fluid after lumbar puncture and its treatment. Acta Med. Scand. *58*:102, 1923.
Janzen, E.: Der negative Vorschlag bei Lumbalpunktion. Dtsch. Z. Nervenheilk. *94*:280, 1926.
Kaplan, M. S., and Arrowood, J. G.: Prevention of headache following spinal anesthesia; use of epidural saline: A preliminary report. Anesthesiology *18*:103, 1952.

Lebeaux, M.: Sheep: A model for testing spinal and epidural anesthetic agents. Lab. Animal Sci. *25*:629, 1975.
Lee, J. A.: Specially marked needle to facilitate extradural block. Anaesthesia *15*:186, 1960.
Loewy, A. D., Araujo, J. C., and Kerr, F. W. L.: Pupillodilator pathways in the brainstem of the cat: Anatomical and electrophysiological identification of a central autonomic pathway. Brain Res. *60*:65, 1973.
Lund, P. C.: Peridural Analgesia and Anesthesia. Springfield, Ill., Charles C Thomas, 1966, pp. 71, 93.
Lund, P. C., Cwik, J. C., and Magaziner, R.: Epidural anesthesia in general surgery. Anesthesiology *17*:605, 1956.
Macintosh, R. R.: Extradural space indicator. Brit. Med. J. *1*:398, 1953.
Mesry, S.: Massive epidural spread of local analgesics. Anaesthesia *31*:576, 1976.
Mirakhur, R. K., and Bandopadhyay, A.: Auditory guide to the location of the extradural space. Anaesthesia *28*:707, 1973.
Moir, D. D.: Recent advances in pain relief in childbirth. II. Regional anaesthesia. Brit. J. Anaesth. *43*:849, 1971.
Mostert, J. W.: Coma contra-indicates spinal analgesia. Anaesthesia *13*:242, 1958.
Nelson, M. O.: Postpuncture headaches; a clinical and experimental study of the cause and prevention. Arch. Derm. Syph. *21*:615, 1930.
Odom, C. B.: Epidural anesthesia. Amer. J. Surg. *34*:547, 1936.
Ontenada, L. E.: Tension de espacio peridural su importancia practica en la anestesia epidural metamerica. Rev. Cir. Buenos Aires *11*:584, 1932.
Ostheimer, G. W., Palahniuk, R. J., and Shnider, S. M.: Epidural blood patch for post-lumbar puncture headache. Anesthesiology *41*:307, 1974.
Pagés, F.: Anestesia metamerica. Rev. Sanid. Mil. Madr. *11*:351, 1921.
Pool, J. L.: Myeloscopy: Intraspinal endoscopy. Surgery *11*:169, 1942.
Poppers, P. J., Mastri, A. R., Lebeaux, M., and Covino, B. G.: The effects of methylene blue on neural tissue. Anesthesiology *33*:335, 1970.
Reisner, L. S.: Epidural test solution or spinal fluid? Anesthesiology *44*:451, 1976.
Rice, G. G., and Dabbs, C. H.: The use of peridural and subarachnoid injections of saline solution in the treatment of severe postspinal headache. Anesthesiology *11*:17, 1950.
Sagarnaga, A.: Un sinal de identificaçao do espaço peridural. Rev. Bras. Anest. *21*:237, 1971.
Shantha, T. R., McWhirter, W. R., and Dunbar, R. W.: Complications following epidural "blood patch" for postlumbar-puncture headache. Anesth. Analg. *52*:67, 1973.
Sicard, J. A., and Forestier, J.: Radiographic method for exploration of the extradural space using Lipiodol. Rev. Neurol. *28*:1264, 1921.
Solomon, H. C.: Raising cerebrospinal fluid pressure. J.A.M.A. *82*:1512, 1924.
Soresi, A. L.: Preliminary report on epidural anesthesia. Med. Rec. N. Y. *135*:165, 1932.
Tuffier, T.: Analgésie cocaïnique par voie extradurale. C. R. Soc. Biol. Paris *53*:490, 1901.
Usubiaga, J. E., Moya, F., and Usubiaga, L. E.: Effect of thoracic and abdominal pressure changes on the epidural space pressure. Brit. J. Anaesth. *39*:612, 1967a.
Usubiaga, J. E., Wikinski, J. A., and Usubiaga, L. E.: Epidural pressure and its relation to spread of anesthetic solutions in epidural space. Anesth. Analg. *46*:440, 1967b.
Vandam, L. D., and Dripps, R. D.: Long term follow-up of patients who received 10,098 spinal anesthetics: Syndrome of decreased intracranial pressure (headache and auditory difficulties). J.A.M.A. *161*:586, 1956.
Zelenka, L.: A new indicator for spinal epidural analgesia. Anesthesiology *17*:210, 1956.
Zorraquin, G.: Anesthésie métamérique péridurale. Presse Méd. *44*:1, 783, 1936.

chapter 7
Continuous Epidural Analgesia

The present wide scope of epidural analgesia would be impossible without continuous catheter techniques for prolonging blockade. A single epidural injection creates a zone of analgesia lasting from one to four hours, depending on the agent chosen. Surgical tasks that extend beyond this period must be completed under general anesthesia unless some means are available to prolong blockade for as long as necessary. It is undesirable to change techniques during the course of an operation, and it is preferable to keep the duration and extent of analgesia under continuous control when difficult and lengthy procedures are planned. It is also a great advantage if effective analgesia can be prolonged into the postoperative period. These conditions can be provided by placing a plastic catheter in the epidural space. Then continuous analgesia may be prolonged for as long as necessary by intermittent injections through the catheter. For therapeutic blocks, in which the duration must be measured in days rather than hours, the catheter may be left in place for several days at a time so that the patient is spared the discomfort of repeated injections.

The idea of inserting an indwelling epidural catheter through a needle and then withdrawing the needle over the catheter stemmed from earlier applications of the same principle to other situations. Studies of the afferent pathways responsible for pain during labor led Aburel in Paris to the conclusion that prolonged blockade of the lumboaortic plexus would cause analgesia in the distribution of the eleventh or twelfth thoracic segments and provide effective pain relief during the first stage of labor (Aburel, 1930a, 1930b). At that time dibucaine (Percaine) was the longest acting local anesthetic available, but even doses as large as 30 ml of 1/1000 Percaine did not last for more than about four hours. To prolong analgesia even further during the first stage of labor, Aburel used a system of continuous lumbar paravertebral block by inserting a silk ureteral catheter through a long lumbar needle and then removing the needle over the catheter (Aburel, 1931). Aburel also suggested using the same technique in the caudal region, but this approach does not seem to have been followed up with any enthusiasm, perhaps because these earlier catheters were large and the needles of formidable size. The indwelling catheter technique was later adapted for treating meningitis, a No. 5 French catheter being inserted through a 13-gauge Barker spinal needle for continuous subarachnoid drainage (Love, 1935).

The first continuous caudal anesthetics in North America were administered through a malleable Lemmon spinal needle strapped in place with

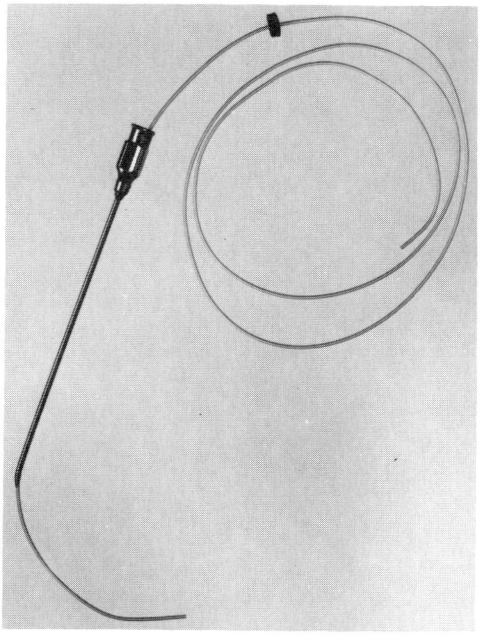

Figure 7–1. Tuohy needle and vinyl catheter. Note bias imparted to catheter by curved Huber tip. Depth markers may be printed on this catheter or may be external and adjustable, as shown in the illustration.

extension tubing attached to it (Hingson and Southworth, 1942). Shortly afterward, Manalan (1942) and Lundy and his colleagues (Adams et al., 1943) introduced the catheter technique as a safer and more practical method, using thinner needles and finer catheters than those Aburel originally used a decade earlier.

Straight needles with an orthodox oblique bevel have been accepted as technically suitable for introducing indwelling catheters through the sacral hiatus, for the catheter enters parallel to the axis of the dural tube, and the catheter tip is not likely to perforate the dura even if it is advanced beyond the termination of the dural sac at the second sacral vertebra. However, in the lumbar region the epidural space is so narrow that a semistiff catheter thrust straight across it impinges directly on the dura at right angles, with little chance of gliding harmlessly along the axis of the canal, and the possibility of dural perforation is greater. Tuohy (1945) designed a needle with a curved Huber tip for continuous subarachnoid anesthesia, and Curbelo (1949) adapted this needle for continuous lumbar epidural blockade. The curved directional point of the Tuohy needle imparts a bias to the epidural catheter and allows it to slide off the dura and travel up and down the spinal canal, according to the way the tip is orientated (Fig. 7–1). The Tuohy needle has become the prototype for a number of modifications that all have the common function of imparting a change of direction to the tip of the catheter as it emerges from the shaft of the needle into the epidural space.

TYPES AND QUALITIES OF CATHETERS

Various types of catheters have been used. Originally, lacquered gum elastic ureteric catheters were the only readily available material, but since the early 1940's a wide variety of materials have been introduced, including polyethylene, polyvinylchloride, nylon, and polytetrafluoroethylene (Teflon), and catheters have been made either radiolucent or radiopaque. They can be purchased either in bulk as rolls of uncut tubing, or prepackaged and gamma ray-sterilized.

Polyethylene tubing is unsatisfactory for epidural use since its caliber is altered by heat sterilization, and the catheter becomes swollen and too thick to pass down the needle. Vinyl, nylon and Teflon are the commonest materials in current use. Details of type, packaging and preparation will be dealt with in Chapter 9. At this point we need only consider the general qualities that are required of a catheter. The requisites of a good catheter are as follows:

1. The material must be of the right type, that is, inert, nonirritating and supple without being harsh and brittle. It should have good tensile strength so that it is not easily broken when traction is applied to it.

2. The question of radiopacity is controversial. Some anesthesiologists insist on using radiopaque catheters so that correct placement can be readily verified by X-ray. However, the visual density of currently available radiopaque catheters is so similar to that of bone that it is very difficult to identify the catheter in a radiograph or with an image intensifier. For accurate localization, the lumen of the catheter must be filled with contrast medium such as Pantopaque or Hypaque. Moreover, I believe it is not altogether wise to use radiopaque catheters in case of accidental breakage. A broken, sequestered piece of catheter is inert and unlikely to cause any harm or inconvenience, but if it is visible on X-ray, sooner or later a surgeon may be tempted to go and look for it with very slim chances indeed of finding the broken piece, and the patient may be subjected to an unnecessary and perhaps dangerous laminectomy to no avail.

3. The length of catheter should be sufficient to reach from above the shoulder to the lower lumbar region of a tall adult and still allow ample length to enter the epidural space.

4. The external diameter should be small enough to pass through a thin-walled 18-gauge Tuohy needle with ease.

5. The bore of the catheter must be large enough to allow injection of aqueous fluids through its lumen.

6. The wall of the catheter should be thick enough to ensure that kinking and obstruction do not occur when the catheter is bent sharply on itself. Some commercial catheters that are ideal in all other aspects fail in this important test.

7. The tip of the catheter should be smooth, even and as nontraumatic as possible. The end should be blunt rather than rounded or tapered in order to discourage perforation of veins or dura.

8. There should be an outlet hole at the tip of the catheter. An additional side hole close to the tip to provide an alternative exit in case the hole at the tip becomes obstructed by tissues is advantageous. This second hole should be sufficiently close to the tip to obviate kinking at the site of the lateral orifice.

9. Centimeter graduations should be marked at the distal end of the catheter, commencing 8 cm from the end, to indicate the point at which the catheter passes the tip of the needle, so that the anesthesiologist can advance the catheter to an accurate distance.

Once the Tuohy needle is in place and the usual confirmatory tests for correct placement have been carried out, preparations are made for inserting the catheter. Before doing so, one third of the calculated main dose of solution is injected directly up the needle. This serves four purposes.

First, it opens up the epidural tissue planes and facilitates passage of the catheter. Second, it saves time by initiating the block at the earliest possible moment rather than delaying until the catheter is in place a few minutes later. Third, it ensures that the lowest segmental parts of the epidural space are adequately bathed. For example, in abdominopelvic surgery it is important to provide adequate analgesia of the sacral segments as well as the lumbar and thoracic segments, and the former may partially escape if the catheter is passed too far cranially without an initial dose of local analgesic in the lower reaches of the epidural space. Fourth, the initial injection acts as a test dose for the needle, and any untoward sign from a subarachnoid or intravenous injection will become manifest during the ensuing minutes while the catheter is being secured in place.

INSERTION OF THE CATHETER

The catheter is now gently threaded through the needle with one hand while the other steadies the shaft of the needle with the knuckles braced against the patient's back (Fig. 7–2*A* and *B*). As the catheter tip passes from the

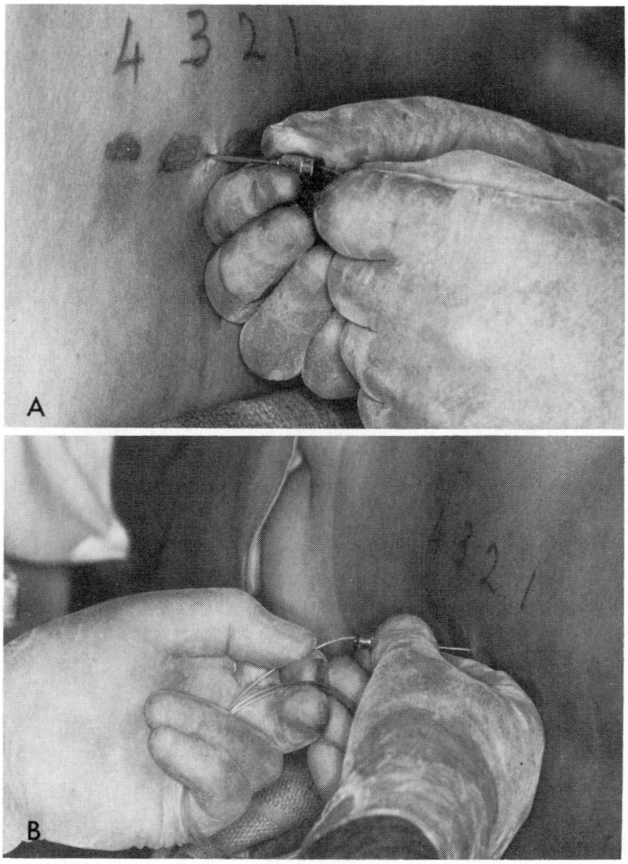

Figure 7–2. Insertion of epidural catheter at second lumbar interspace. *A*, Left view; *B*, right view. Note controlled grip of needle and catheter to forestall dislodgement by unexpected movements of patient. The right hand holds the needle braced in relation to the patient. The left hand is braced against the right hand while the catheter is fed into the needle. The coiled catheter is palmed in the left hand.

bevel of the needle into the epidural space, there may be a slight resistance if the bevel is insufficiently advanced into the space and partially occluded by the inner margin of the ligamentum flavum. A gentle rotation of the catheter, however, usually overcomes this, and from then on further advance is unimpeded. During advance of the catheter, the conscious patient may complain of paresthesia as the tip slides past the dural-covered nerve roots. If the patient complains of actual pain, the catheter should be halted and the needle withdrawn. Pain may be caused by pressure of the catheter on a nerve root or the cord itself, and it is unwise to persist in pushing the catheter onward in these circumstances.

Not more than 3 to 4 cm of catheter should be left in the epidural space (Iklé, 1952). This distance is sufficient for the catheter to remain securely in the epidural space during normal activity. It is permissible to insert a little more than this amount to ensure that a sufficient length is available in the tissues in case the needle should jam on the catheter while the needle is being withdrawn. Then, after the needle has been safely removed, the catheter can be gently pulled back until its marks indicate that 3 to 4 cm remain in the epidural space. Some authors have recommended inserting longer lengths of catheter on the assumption that the catheter will travel in a predictable direction along the axis of the spinal canal (Matouskova et al., 1975). Unfortunately, this is mistaken advice and quite contrary to X-ray evidence. Excessive lengths of catheter curl up in the lumbar region and sometimes pass outward through an intervertebral foramen into the paraspinal space.

An elegant variation of the "mandrin liquide" of Sicard and Forestier is used by some anesthesiologists to facilitate insertion of the catheter. A syringe is attached to the free end of the catheter, and an assistant injects a steady stream of saline while the catheter is being advanced within the epidural space. Theoretically, the jet of liquid issuing from the tip of the catheter should push its way through the epidural tissues with a minimum of trauma, like a gentle version of a high pressure hose clearing away rubble in a mine. This method is intuitively appealing, although it is dependent on an assistant being available. However, a radiological assessment by Muneyuki and his colleagues showed that while catheters could be inserted without resistance for twice as far with the catheter "mandrin liquide" than without it, the actual distance traveled by the catheter tip was no greater than usual. The facilitation of passage was more apparent than real, and the extra length of catheter was curled up near the site of injection (Muneyuki et al., 1970). The catheter "mandrin liquide" or hydraulic stylet will be considered in greater detail later in this section.

In the lumbar region the neurovascular bundles of the spinal roots and nerve trunks leave the intervertebral foramina in a downward-slanting direction, like the tiles of a roof. If an epidural catheter is introduced in a caudal direction and the tip encounters a neurovascular bundle, it will be likely to follow the same general run and find its way out of the spinal canal into the nearest paravertebral space. On the other hand, if it is directed upward, any tendency to deviate laterally will be corrected by the catheter being deflected off the neurovascular bundle and back into the spinal canal again (Fig. 7–3). For this reason catheters should always be directed upward toward the head, unless there is some special indication to pass the catheter downward, as in a "retrograde caudal" in which one attempts to enter the sacral canal via the

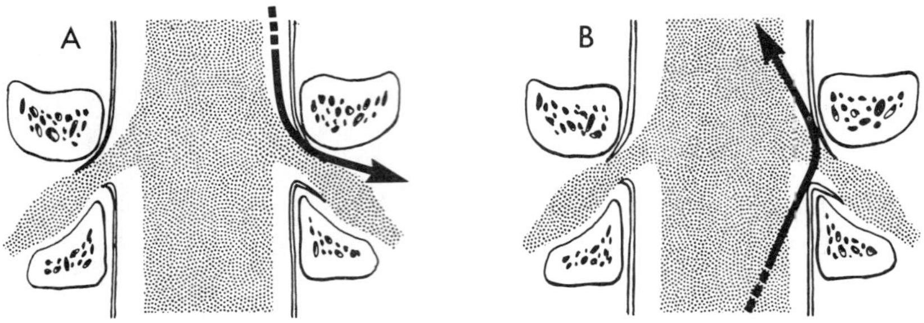

Figure 7–3. Catheter direction and transforaminal escape. *A*, Downward-directed catheter tends to follow downward slope of root sleeves and to exit via intervertebral foramen. *B*, Upward-directed catheter is deflected inward and returned to axis of spinal canal.

lumbosacral space. Moreover, the general slope of the vertebral spines is upward, and the natural trend of the needle and the catheter is in the same direction. It is inadvisable to rotate the needle once it is in the epidural space, in case the tip should lacerate an epidural vein or the dura as it sweeps around within the epidural space.

Figures 7–4 and 7–5 illustrate the tendency that catheters may have to stray beyond the confines of the epidural space when too much catheter has been inserted. The orifice of the Tuohy needle was directed upward in each of these cases, and the initial direction of the catheter was at an acute angle to the downward-sloping axes of the intervertebral foramina. If the catheters had been directed caudally, their line of travel would have been more nearly parallel to the steeply sloping axes of the foramina, and transforaminal escape would have been more likely.

It is not easy to predict the course a catheter will take once the epidural space has been penetrated. In the mid-thoracic region the steep inclination of the spines brings the axis of the Huber tip in line with the axis of the spinal canal, and catheters usually pass straight up the canal with very little deviation. In the lumbar area, however, their inclination is less favorable, and they tend to be deflected by the blood vessels and nerve roots that lie in their path, often doubling back in the reverse direction to that intended and even passing out through an intervertebral foramen. Figure 7–6*A* and B show an un-

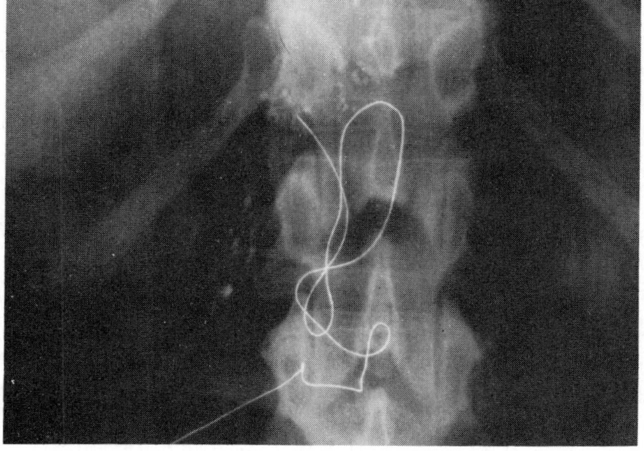

Figure 7–4. Excessive length of epidural catheter threaded upward at L_1–L_2. "Neohydriol (Fluid),," 0.4 ml, was injected to outline catheter. Tip of catheter has lodged at the T_{12}–L_1 intervertebral foramen on the right. Upward direction has avoided transforaminal passage, although some droplets of contrast medium have escaped into the right paravertebral space. The catheter has curled up behind the site of obstruction and has not advanced up the spinal canal.

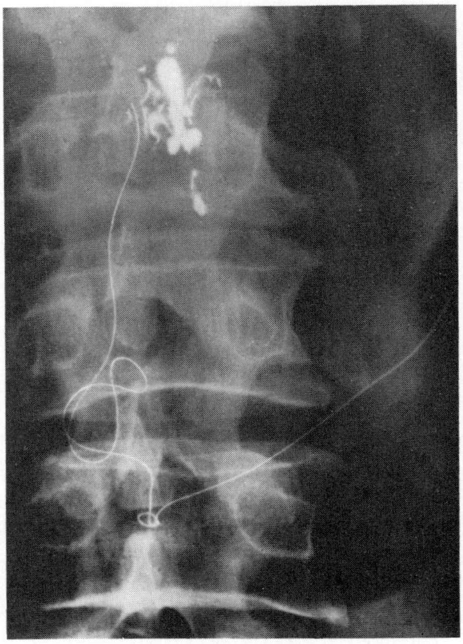

Figure 7–5. Excessive length of catheter inserted at third lumbar interspace. "Neohydriol (Fluid)," 0.4 ml, used as opaque medium. Note that the first few centimeters passed up the spinal canal, but the tip became arrested and further insertion caused the catheter to coil up within the epidural space.

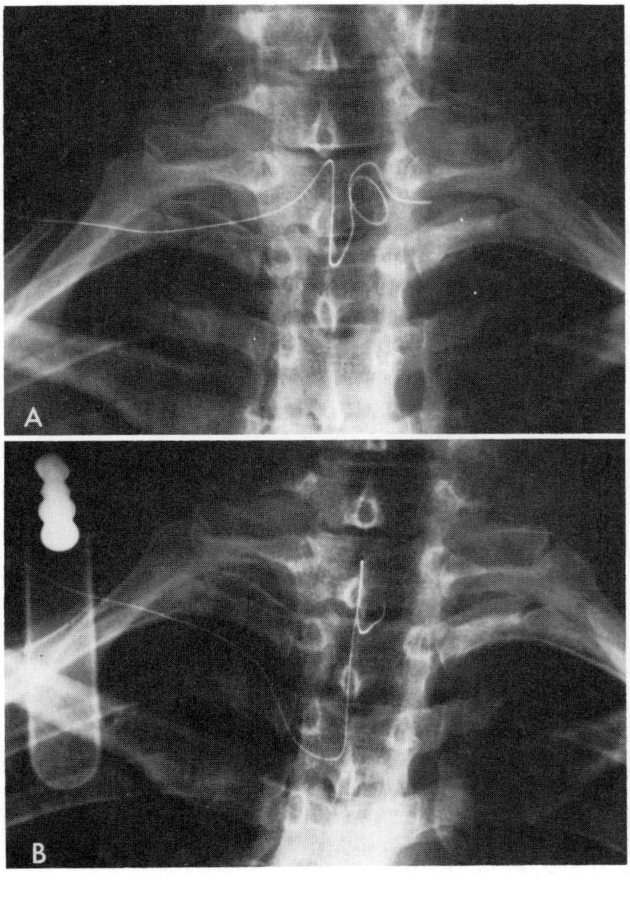

Figure 7–6. Transforaminal escape of epidural catheter: a cause of failure. *A*, Excessive length inserted at first thoracic interspace. Catheter curled up, with tip protruding under first rib. *B*, Catheter has been withdrawn 8 to 9 cm. The tip is now lying in the epidural space.

usual site of transforaminal escape at the first thoracic foramen. Here, as is so commonly the case, the basic technical fault lay in pushing too much catheter into the epidural space: 4 cm is quite enough; more than this may lead to misplacement of the catheter and technical failure (see below).

Sometimes difficulty is encountered in passing the catheter more than a short distance beyond the tip of the needle. This may be due to obstruction by local tissues or to partial rather than complete entry of the orifice into the epidural space, or it may indicate that the needle has failed to enter the epidural space and that the catheter is being inserted superficially to the ligamentum flavum, Whatever the cause, the catheter and needle should be removed and a fresh puncture attempted. *Always remove the needle and catheter together. Never remove the catheter with the needle still in place.* If the catheter is withdrawn while the needle is still in the back, the sharp chisel-like upper edge of the bevel may slice through the catheter and leave a portion sequestered in the epidural space (Fig. 7–7). Manufacturers are aware of this danger, and today most Tuohy needles are made with a rounded blunt upper edge to the orifice.

Some catheters are too soft and flexible to pass through a needle easily without a wire or nylon stylet to stiffen them. Personally, I prefer to avoid stylets if possible. They make the catheters whippy and awkward to handle; they uncoil themselves from their packages like an ebullient jack-in-the-box, and it is hard to prevent them from transgressing the bounds of the sterile field. Moreover, once the catheter is in the needle, it is very easy to forget that the stylet is there and hence to pass the catheter and stylet together into the epidural space. At one time this was done deliberately (Frumin and Schwartz, 1952), but the idea of a rigid catheter blundering its way blindly through the delicate labyrinth of epidural vessels is not an attractive one, courting as it does the likelihood of epidural hematoma and the intravenous absorption of injected local anesthetic solution through the open ends of torn blood vessels. Worse still, there is the possibility of perforating the dura and perhaps even the cord. In animal experiments I have been impressed by the ease with which stiff subarachnoid catheters can penetrate the spinal cord without any sense of resistance being imparted to the fingers advancing the catheter. At postmortem examination, after retrograde catheterization of the subarachnoid space from the cisterna magna, we found that in a number of dogs the plastic catheter had entered the cervical

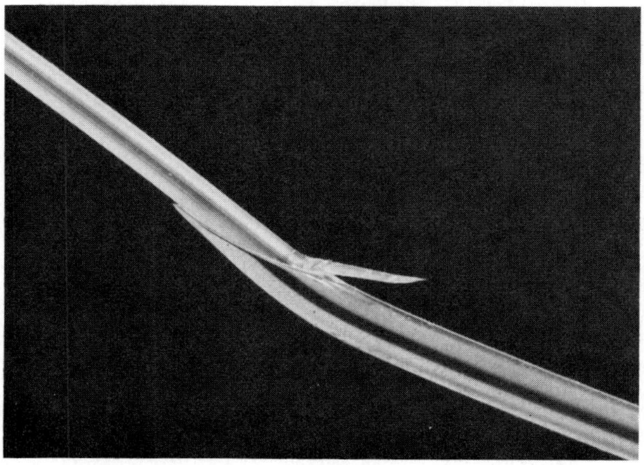

Figure 7–7. Consequence of attemping to withdraw epidural catheter while Tuohy needle is still in place. Catheter may be sliced and sheared off by sharp upper rim of needle orifice.

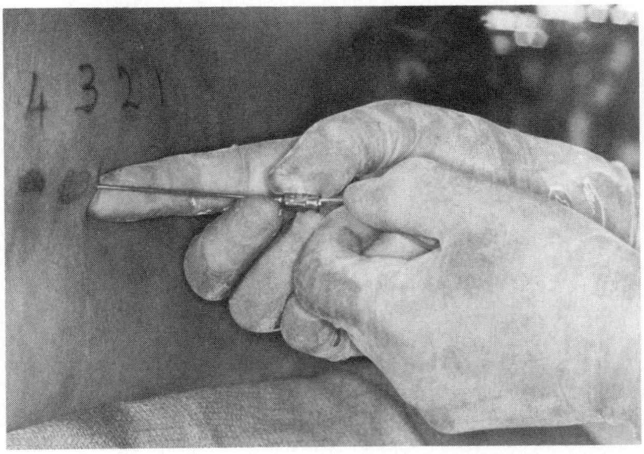

Figure 7–8. Removing needle over catheter. Slight forward pressure is exerted on the catheter with the left hand while the needle is withdrawn. Smooth, controlled extraction is obtained by extending the right forefinger against the patient's back.

and thoracic cord, traveled several centimeters in the substance of the cord and then emerged lower down in the subarachnoid space. If a stylet must be used, it should be withdrawn 2 cm from the tip of the catheter so that the advancing tip is soft, pliable and atraumatic.

Once the catheter is safely in place, the needle is removed by steady traction with the thumb and middle finger, while the extended forefinger exerts counterpressure against the back, as shown in Figure 7–8. A slight vis a tergo is applied to the catheter with the other hand so that the catheter is not pulled out as the needle is withdrawn.

A connecting syringe mount is now attached to the free end of the catheter. The Borst-Tuohy adaptor was specially designed for this purpose, but it is often difficult to obtain a satisfactory and secure fit. A simpler course is to use a 23-gauge hypodermic needle (blunt or sharp) and thread it into the open end of the catheter (Fig. 7–9).

An aspiration test is now carried out using an empty 2 ml syringe to exclude the presence of blood or cerebrospinal fluid and to confirm that the catheter tip is not lying in a blood vessel or in the subarachnoid space (Fig. 7–10).

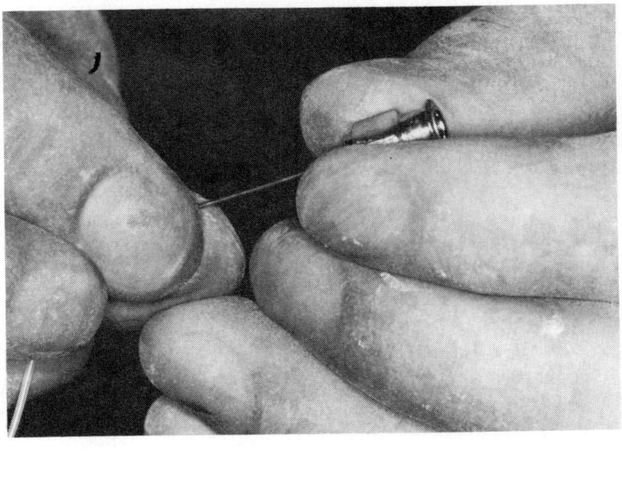

Figure 7–9. Insertion of 23-gauge connector needle into distal end of epidural catheter. Fingers of right hand hold the catheter and connector splinted while the connector is inserted with an axial rotary motion.

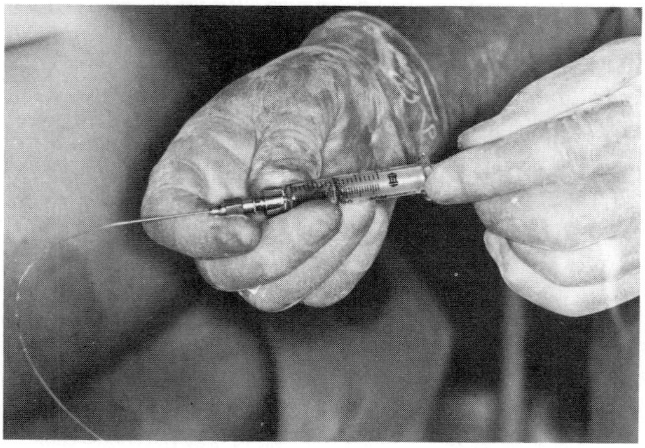

Figure 7–10. Aspiration test with 2-ml syringe to ensure that catheter tip is in the epidural space, not lying in a vein or in the subarachnoid space. This is an important safety check.

If the aspiration test is negative, one third of the calculated induction dose is injected up the catheter.

The catheter is taped in place using a rolled up 2 × 2 inch swab to prevent kinking at the site of puncture, and the catheter is brought up over one shoulder (Fig. 7–11). A special plastic shield 4½ inches in diameter has been designed to protect against kinking at the puncture site (Climie, 1960), but in practice a simple arrangement of well-anchored swabs is sufficient. Whatever system is chosen, care should be taken that it is not too bulky, in order to prevent pressure sores from developing in debilitated patients.

Some catheters tend to become softened by body heat and flattened by the weight of bony pressure points, so care should be taken to see that the catheter does not cross the midline while it is being taped in place.

The patient is placed in a supine position. If he can still move his legs after 3 to 4 minutes and if there is no evidence of subarachnoid puncture, the remaining one third of the induction dose is injected up the catheter. A charged syringe of local anesthetic is left attached to the catheter, protected in a sterile, folded towel or cloth bag ready for subsequent repeat doses. The supine position must be avoided in obstetrical patients, and pregnant women at term should be nursed on the side (see Chapter 12). In these patients symmetrical

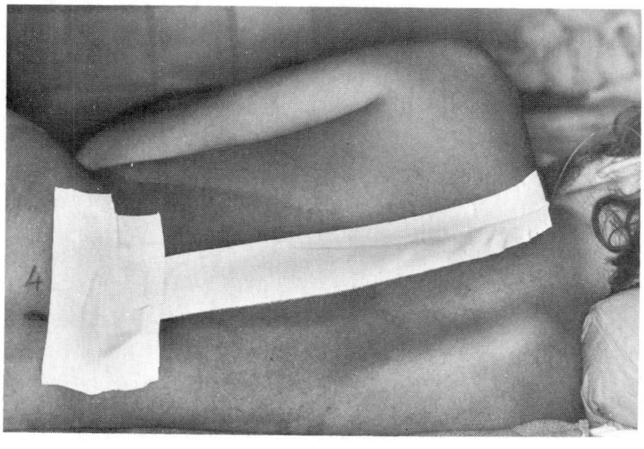

Figure 7–11. Catheter taped in place with sterile gauze dressing over puncture site.

analgesia is obtained by injecting small increments of anesthetic solution with the patient lying first on one side and then on the other.

Hydraulic Stylet

The use of a hydraulic stylet for gentle passage of the catheter was first reported by Thistlethwaite and his colleagues in 1953, and although the idea was adopted by a few individuals, it did not find wide appeal, probably because of the inherent awkwardness of the method and the need for a second pair of hands (Thistlethwaite et al., 1953; Brennecke, personal communication, 1966).

However, the general principle seems sound, and I have tried to overcome the manual objections by adapting it to a single-handed technique. Massey Dawkins' simple rubber band version of the Ilké syringe (see p. 199) can be used. The technique still adds an awkward and time-consuming extra maneuver to the process of passing an epidural catheter, and I suspect that the extra time and manipulations required may introduce fresh risks of misplacing the needle. Nevertheless, the method has worked well in over 100 cases without any incidence of epidural venous puncture, and it may be worth more attention than I have given it.

TECHNIQUE

A large broad rubber band, with a hole cut for a 5-ml or 10-ml syringe, is included in the sterile epidural tray. With the needle in the epidural space, the catheter is threaded to the tip of the needle but not beyond. A charged 5 ml or 10 ml syringe of saline is attached to the free end of the catheter with the nozzle of the syringe pushed through the hole in the rubber band. The syringe is now pressurized by slipping the rubber band over the end of the plunger, and the catheter is advanced 3 to 4 cm into the epidural space (Fig. 7–12). The syringe is then disconnected and the epidural needle withdrawn in the usual way.

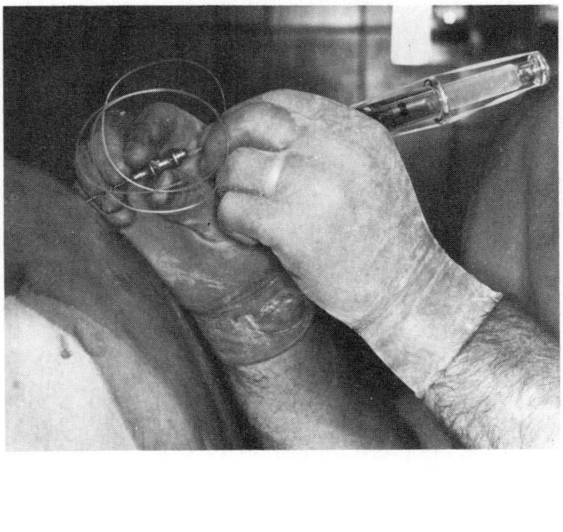

Figure 7–12. Hydraulic stylet for atraumatic catheter insertion. A rubber band is stretched over the piston of a 10-ml syringe filled with saline and attached to the epidural catheter. Pressure from the elastic band emits a jet of saline from the catheter tip. The jet stream is thought to cushion the advancing tip and to protect against inadvertent venous cannulation.

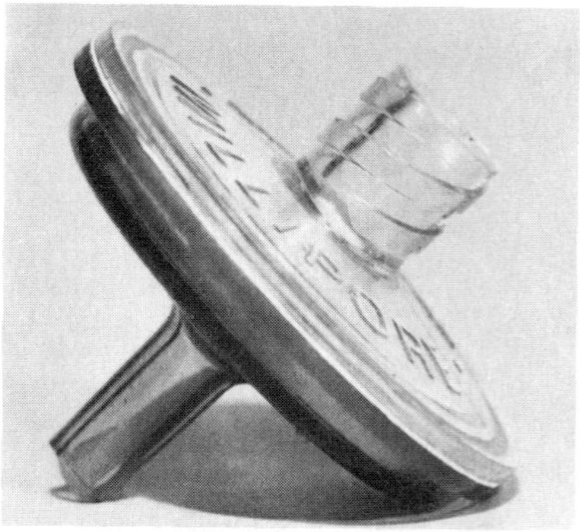

Figure 7–13. Disposable micropore (Millipore) filter provides protection against particulate contamination of the epidural space. A pore size of 0.2 microns or less is necessary to exclude bacteria.

A disposable bacterial filter of the Millipore type may be inserted between the syringe and the catheter, and in many centers this is considered to be obligatory practice (Fig. 7–13). At the Royal Victoria Hospital, Montreal, more than 30,000 continuous epidurals have been performed since 1956 without using antibacterial filters, and in many instances the catheters have remained in place for several days. To date we have not encountered any cases of epidural infection. Reported instances of epidural abscess have usually been metastatic, arising from a prime source elsewhere in the body (see Chapter 14).

Selwyn Crawford has pointed out that local anesthetic solutions prepared in sterile ampules may become contaminated by a shower of microscopic glass particles when the neck of the ampule is cracked open, and that some of these particles may find their way into the epidural space unless the solution is injected through a catheter system protected by a micropore filter (Crawford, et al., 1975).

TECHNICAL COMPLICATIONS OF EPIDURAL CATHETERS

Ideally, an epidural catheter should lie in the posterior part of the epidural space, close to the midline, so that diffusion of injected local anesthetic will be even and symmetrical. Every procedure can go wrong, however, and there are ample opportunities for a blindly placed catheter to stray from its intended path, either through available orifices or more rarely across forbidden tissue boundaries. With proper technique these problems should not arise very often, but there should be a clear understanding of their possibility and of what to do if they should occur.

Malposition

Most technical difficulties arise from the catheter being malpositioned. A few isolated reports of misplaced catheters were published before 1960 (Ilke, 1952; Bromage, 1954), but the first systematic study of catheter positions was done by Hehre and his colleagues at Yale (Hehre et al., 1960). These authors reported an incidence of 36 catheter failures in 1780 cases (2 per cent). Fourteen of these failures were easily corrected by partially withdrawing an excess of catheter from the epidural space, and analgesia was subsequently successful. Twenty-two cases were deliberately left uncorrected, and the position of the catheter tip was determined by radiological or clinical means. In six of these the tip was superficial to the space, presumably having been pulled out on withdrawing the needle. In the remaining 16 cases the tip had emerged through an intervertebral foramen into the paravertebral tissues. In about half of these cases of transforaminal passage a paresthesia from stimulation of a nerve root had been noted during insertion of the catheter.

Sanchez and his associates carried out a similar radiological study of 90 cases in which catheters had been inserted for lengths of 8 cm or 16 cm (Sanchez et al., 1967). In half of these cases the catheter curled up in tortuous patterns near the site of insertion, and transforaminal escape occurred in 6 per cent.

Bridenbaugh and his colleagues reported a similar type of study the following year. In this series in which catheters had been inserted for 5 cm or 10 cm in the epidural space, there was a 4.5 per cent incidence of inadequate analgesia from transforaminal escape or other misplacement (Bridenbaugh et al., 1968). The incidence of clinical failure from transforaminal escape is much lower than the radiological evidence from these series would suggest, and Moir and Willocks (1968) reported a clinical incidence of only 1 per cent in 300 obstetrical cases. These results are summarized in Table 7–1.

From these series one is left with the impression that transforaminal escape is the most frequent cause of failure, that it is normally due to passing too much catheter into the space and that it is often correctable by withdrawing some of the excess length of catheter.

Unilateral analgesia is an occasional form of failure that may arise after single injections or when a catheter is used (Singh, 1967). Some patients show consistent unilateral analgesia or patchy deficits in spite of repeated injections at different sites, and in these cases the cause is usually referable to local pathology related to previous back operations or subarachnoid adhesions. In other instances, however, unilateral analgesia may occur without any obvious cause.

Experiments with epidural catheters in dogs led Usubiaga and his associates to conclude that one-sided analgesia was caused by the catheter curling around the dural tube into the anterior portion of the epidural space where diffusion of local anesthetic is less symmetrical than posteriorly (Usubiaga et al., 1970). However, the picture is not simple, as there are well-documented cases of unilateral analgesia occurring in the presence of radiographs showing that contrast material has distributed itself evenly on both sides of the epidural space (Shanks, 1968).

TABLE 7–1 Incidence of Catheter Malposition in Lumbar Epidural Blockade

Author	*Number of Cases*	*Incidence of Transforaminal Escape (%)*
Ilké (1952)	145	1.4 – clinical incidence in obstetrical patients
Hehre et al. (1960)	1780	2.0 – radiological evidence
Sanchez et al. (1967)	90	6.0 – radiological evidence
Bridenbaugh et al. (1968)	198	4.5 – radiological evidence
Moir and Willocks (1968)	300	1.0 – clinical incidence in obstetrical patients

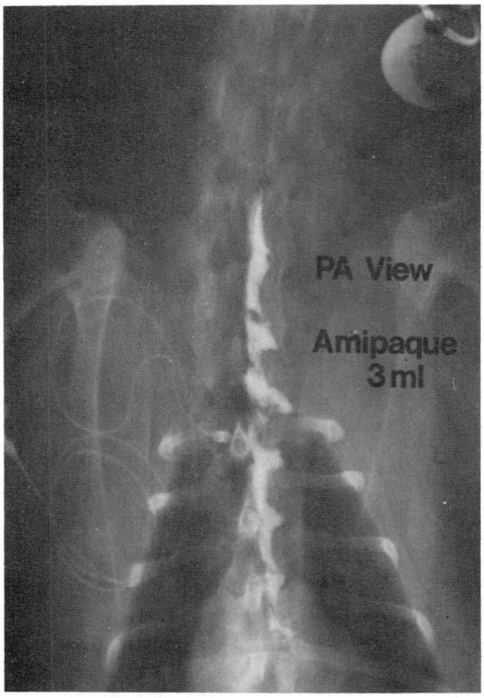

Figure 7–14 Unilateral cervicothoracic peridurogram of dog. Chronically implanted epidural catheter at T_1, with tip lying in left side of spinal canal.

In our laboratory we have consistently produced unilateral blockade of the forelimbs of dogs by implanting catheters to one side or the other of the epidural space at the level of the seventh cervical vertebra. Catheters were implanted through a bur hole in the lateral part of the lamina, using Lebeaux's technique, with about 1 mm of catheter protruding into the epidural space (Lebeaux, 1973). Small quantities of local anesthetic in the range of 1 to 2 ml of 2 per cent lidocaine injected through these laterally placed catheters produce discrete motor and sensory paresis of the ipsilateral forelimb without appreciable blockade elsewhere (Bromage et al., 1978). Peridurograms through these laterally placed catheters also show unilateral distribution of injected contrast medium, as shown in Figure 7–14.

While the true cause of unilateral epidural analgesia remains poorly understood, there are certain practical steps that can be taken to correct it:

1. On the assumption that the catheter is malpositioned, partially withdraw the catheter and inject a supplementary dose with the unanesthetized side downward.

2. If this fails, withdraw the catheter completely and insert a fresh one for a short distance (3 to 4 cm) in an adjacent space.

3. If this fails, try using a more penetrating type of local anesthetic such as carbonated lidocaine. In several obstetrical cases it has been possible to convert a unilateral block to symmetrical bilateral analgesia by this means alone.

Epidural Venous Cannulation

Inadvertent cannulation of an extradural vein is a rare cause of technical failure and of toxic reactions. The epidural veins are very prominent in diving mammals, such as the seal, and these animals customarily shunt a large proportion of their venous return through the extradural venous plexus when diving (Harrison and Tomlinson, 1956). Pregnant women, like the seal, also shunt a considerable proportion of their venous return through the extradural plexus, and at term the distended epidural veins form a more likely target for cannulation than at other times. Exact figures for the incidence of venous cannulation by epidural catheters is not available, but my own estimates for women at term are in the neighborhood of 1 per cent.

The danger of venous puncture has always been apparent (Bromage, 1954), but the actual occurrence of frank cannulation was first pointed out by Youngman in 1956. During studies of uptake of local anesthetics, Bromage and Robson (1961) found unusually high systemic concentrations of lidocaine in a patient in whom extradural venous cannulation was suspected. Further reports followed (Hylton et al., 1964; Duncalf and Foldes, 1964), and means were sought to make a positive diagnosis of venous cannulation. Blood is sometimes slow to travel up an epidural catheter, and its presence may be missed. Confirmation of venous cannulation may be obtained by injecting tracer substances. Duncalf and Foldes (1964) used radioactive albumen for this purpose. A more practical approach is to inject a small dose of some challenging drug and to watch for systemic effects. For example, injection of a small volume of an epinephrine-containing solution of local anesthetic (epinephrine 1/200,000) will be followed by a transient brisk rise of blood pressure if the catheter is in a vein. A more dramatic test that involves injecting 30 to 40 mg of succinylcholine up the catheter has also been suggested (Hylton, et al., 1964), but this is unnecessarily distressing to the conscious patient, and it should be reserved for patients who are already asleep under general anesthesia.

As with so many potential complications, the best cure is prevention through awareness of the possibility. The incidence of problems arising from intravenous cannulation will be virtually eliminated if the following steps are taken:

1. Gently insert catheters without using a stylet in the epidural space.
2. Avoid inserting unnecessarily long lengths of catheter: 3 to 4 cm is sufficient.
3. Perform an aspiration test up the catheter immediately after insertion.
4. Test a dose of local anesthetic with an epinephrine concentration of 1/200,000 through the catheter. If the catheter is in a vein, a brisk rise of blood pressure will follow, signaling the need to reposition the catheter.

Very rarely, a catheter may apparently find its way into a vein after previous injections were normal. Ryan reported a case of mild toxic reaction after a catheter dose of 50 mg bupivacaine, when a previous injection of the same quantity of bupivacaine through the same catheter had produced normal analgesic results 90 minutes earlier (Ryan, 1973).

Subarachnoid Cannulation

Continuous epidural analgesia was used widely for more than a decade before reports of inadvertent subarachnoid catheterization began to appear (Hamelberg et al., 1959). In a series of 3,132 surgical patients, Hehre reported 18 cases (0.57 per cent) in which the catheter had perforated the dura and entered the subarachnoid space (Carr and Hehre, 1962). Ten years later, in a larger series of 9,244 obstetrical patients, the incidence had fallen to 0.2 per cent (Kalas and Hehre, 1972). Other isolated cases have arisen from time to time (Moir and Hesson, 1965), and Moir reported an incidence of 0.7 per cent, also in obstetrical patients (Moir and Willocks, 1968).

This particular malplacement of the catheter is potentially dangerous if unrecognized, for a normal supplementary epidural dose accidentally injected into the subarachnoid space will be large enough to produce massive spinal blockade. The possibility of this accident should be borne in mind, and it provides a strong reason for injecting a small test dose of local anesthetic through the catheter before deciding that larger doses are safe.

Subdural Cannulation

Perforation of the dura alone without penetration of the pia-arachnoid is another rare possibility. The tip of the catheter will then lie in the true subdural space between the dura mater and the pia-arachnoid. Inadvertent subdural injection is a well-recognized difficulty of spinal subarachnoid anesthesia and of radiographic myelography (Schultz and Brogdon, 1962; Jones and Newton, 1963; Sechzer, 1963; Cohen and Kallos, 1972). It occurs more frequently than generally appreciated in myelography and in spinal anesthesia, and it probably arises as often as once in every 100 attempted subarachnoid punctures. An even higher incidence of about 5 per cent has been reported during contrast myelography (Jones and Newton, 1963). Contrast media injected into the subdural space do not move as freely as in the subarachnoid space, and a typical sausage-shaped shadow results from the material traveling up and down in the circumference of the thecal tube. Local anesthetic injected at this site produces bizarre results which are typical of neither subarachnoid block nor epidural analgesia, but may be patchy and markedly asymmetrical. Subdural block is almost impossible to diagnose except by exclusion or by radiological examination with contrast media, but it is probably a cause of some otherwise inexplicably bizarre types of analgesic spread after attempted epidural injection (Dawkins, 1969; Boys and Norman, 1975).

Knots

It seems almost ridiculous that epidural catheters should be able to tie themselves in knots, but given enough length they may do so. Three cases of knotted catheters have been reported in the literature, all in the caudal canal. In one case the catheter was safely removed in one piece by firm, manual traction (Nicholson, 1965), but in the other two cases it broke at the knot, and the distal knotted piece had to be removed by an incision into the sacrococcygeal membrane (Chun and Karp, 1966). Figure 7–15 shows a knotted lumbar catheter safely removed by manual traction. This case arose in my own department, and it represents a single instance of a knot in over 30,000 catheter insertions. These patients with knotted catheters were fortunate in that the

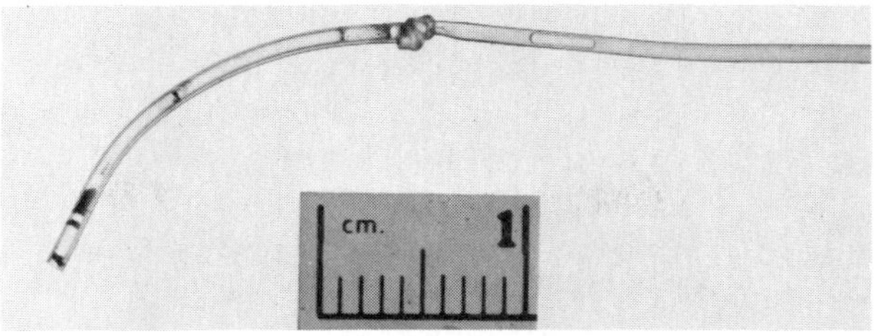

Figure 7–15. Knotted epidural catheter. A rare hazard from inserting an excessive length of catheter. This specimen was extracted intact by steady, gentle traction, without complications. (Courtesy of Dr. J. E. Wynands.)

loop did not lasso a nerve trunk before the knot tightened. Knots are preventable by ensuring that only a short length of catheter is passed into the epidural space.

Epidural Hematomas

Epidural needles or catheters may cause slight trauma to epidural veins from time to time, but the bleeding soon stops spontaneously. Complications arising from epidural hematomas in the presence of normal clotting mechanisms are extremely rare, and there were no recorded instances until 1973 when Lerner et al. reported a case of epidural hematoma and paralysis following numerous attempts at subarachnoid puncture with a 22-gauge needle. However, bleeding may persist if normal hemostasis is grossly disturbed through disease or anticoagulant therapy. Spontaneous epidural bleeding may also arise in the absence of spinal puncture during anticoagulant therapy, and a number of neurological sequelae have been reported following spontaneous intracranial or spinal extradural hemorrhage in patients receiving anticoagulant drugs (Winer, et al., 1959; Gold, 1963; Spurning, 1964; Jacobson et al., 1966; Sreerama et al., 1973).

Unfortunately, there are many instances in which both heparinization and epidural analgesia would seem to have their own particular indications at the same time. This is especially true in surgical cases of peripheral vascular insufficiency, in which systemic heparin may be necessary to prevent local thrombosis and in which prolonged sympathetic blockade would improve total limb blood flow (Cousins and Wright, 1971). A clear policy is needed to decide on wise therapeutic priorities under these circumstances, and the matter is discussed in detail at the end of this chapter.

Frumin reported the first case of peridural hematoma and paralysis associated with epidural catheterization and anticoagulation therapy in 1952 (Frumin and Schwartz, 1952). Two years later Bromage described a case of lumbar epidural hematoma without paralysis. This patient died of a sudden massive hemorrhage into a leg wound 36 hours after vascular surgery that had been followed by heparinization in the presence of continuous epidural blockade. No symptoms of cord compression or paralysis were present at any time ante mortem, but postmortem exploration revealed a large epidural hematoma (Bromage, 1954).

For some years a general opinion prevailed that although it was probably unwise to induce epidural analgesia in the presence of established heparinization, nevertheless the risk of starting anticoagulation therapy after a catheter was in place was negligible. However, more recently, other reports have appeared that throw considerable doubt on this assumption. These reports describe epidural hematoma formation and the occurrence of paralysis, although anticoagulation therapy was started after an appreciable interval of time following insertion of the epidural catheter (Gingrich, 1968; Butler and Green, 1970; De Angelis, 1972).

What, then, is reasonable advice for permitting epidural catheterization in the presence of heparinization or other forms of depression of the normal clotting mechanism? It is easy to take the exclusive stand that the two must never be combined under any circumstances (Cousins, 1973). However, figures for the degree of risk do not exist at the present time, and experience has shown that it is possible to combine both forms of therapy without untoward effects in a large number of cases, especially if coagulation is minimally affected, as it is in "low dose" heparin regimens. Personally, I incline toward the more liberal but cautious view that continuous peridural analgesia *may* be used in patients receiving anticoagulant therapy, but only after its advantage is weighed against the risk. The following precautionary measures should be taken if epidural analgesia is used under these circumstances:

1. Frequent aspiration (every hour or two) to ensure that the tip of the catheter has not eroded into a blood vessel.
2. Frequent flushing with saline and aspiration to diagnose bleeding, even when the tip of a catheter is not in a blood vessel.
3. Frequent neurological examination to promptly diagnose the development of hematoma in the epidural space.

To these precautions I would add:

1. Great gentleness in passing the catheter.
2. Introduction of the catheter to a minimum depth (i.e., 2 to 4 cm).
3. Immediate myelographic examination at the first complaint of pain in the back or legs, or weakness of the legs, followed by urgent laminectomy if there are any clinical or radiological signs of spinal cord compression. Neurological recovery is poor if decompression is delayed.

Thus, the decision to embark on a combination of epidural analgesia and heparinization should not be undertaken lightly, and it implies the adoption of a rigorous program of clinical vigilance and the willingness to proceed to urgent laminectomy the moment any suspicious signs of cord compression arise. Future refinements of methods for direct heparin assay may simplify the decision whether to administer epidural analgesia to a patient who is receiving low doses of prophylactic heparin (Yin et al., 1973; Denson and Bonnar, 1973).

Local Tissue Reaction

Catheters cannot be left in place indefinitely. A form of local tissue reaction occurs round the tip, and in the course of a few days the catheter is gradually sealed off from the rest of the epidural space. It is uncertain whether this reaction is due to the catheter or to the local anesthetic solution injected through it. In cats, chronically implanted catheters become almost completely enclosed in a fibrinous pocket within three weeks of insertion (Lebeaux,

1973; personal observations). This reaction has two effects in man. First, repeated doses become more difficult to inject and less effective (see Tachyphylaxis below); second, they may become painful, and then the patient complains of deep, sharp pain at the site of injection, presumably due to local stretching of the dural nerve endings near the end of the catheter.

To circumvent this problem during prolonged blockade, catheters should be changed every 72 hours, and a fresh catheter should be inserted in a neighboring interspinous space.

Tachyphylaxis

The phenomenon of acute tolerance or "tachyphylaxis" has been discussed already in Chapter 3 on Pharmacology. At this point we need only consider the practical aspects of acute tolerance. Analgesic effectiveness in terms of segment-minutes per milligram declines exponentially with each successive injection, as shown for lidocaine, mepivacaine and prilocaine in Figure 3–24 and on page 100 in Chapter 3 (Bromage et al., 1969). Other local anesthetics have not been tested in the same way, but there is every reason to suppose that their tachyphylactic behavior is essentially similar. Tachyphylaxis is a great practical handicap during prolonged epidural blockade, and there does not seem to be any really effective way to prevent it. All one can do is adjust technique to accommodate it, with the object of lessening the effects.

Tachyphylaxis is an exponential reduction of response, for which three practical steps can be taken. First, start with as small a dose as possible. This may imply using a thoracic segmental technique in abdominal cases in order to confine analgesia as economically as possible to the minimum number of essential segments. Second, choose a long-acting drug in order to keep the frequency of injection as low as possible; and third, increase the segment-minutes even further by adding epinephrine 1/200,000. In this way the effects of tachyphylaxis will be minimized but not prevented. Eventually, after several injections it will be necessary to increase the dose in order to maintain analgesia. There is a clinical impression that changing from one agent to another may diminish the effects of acute tolerance, but there is no experimental evidence to support this belief.

The opposite of tachyphylaxis is seen if reinjections are made at frequent intervals before analgesia has receded. Then an augmented response may be seen, with more extensive segmental spread and more intense sensory and motor blockade. This phenomenon of augmented analgesia is quite noticeable in obstetrical analgesia when very dilute solutions of bupivacaine are used. Then repeated injections of 0.125 per cent bupivacaine reveal a gradually intensifying quality of analgesia and sometimes an appreciable degree of motor blockade as well.

Management of the Indwelling Epidural Catheter

An indwelling catheter provides a convenient way to maintain intermittent or continuous analgesia for long periods of time. The block may be continued for many days, but because of local tissue reaction the catheter must be changed at the end of 72 hours and a fresh catheter inserted at an adjacent site.

In cases in which there is serious doubt about the correct placement of the catheter, an X-ray in two planes is helpful. The catheter can be seen clearly if it is filled with a strong contrast medium, such as Pantopaque (iophendylate); about 0.3 ml is usually sufficient to fill the catheter and leave a drop at the tip. X-ray visualization of the catheter should always be carried out in two planes and the position recorded if neurolytic agents are to be used (see Chapter 13 on Therapeutic Applications).

Sterility

Sterility must be maintained within the catheter system to avoid infection and the remote possibility of epidural abscess formation. This is a rare, but extremely serious, complication that will be discussed more fully in Chapter 14 on Complications.

Intrinsic infection

When epidural abscesses do occur, they are most commonly spontaneous and metastatic from infection elsewhere in the body (Baker et al., 1975). However, the presence of an epidural catheter may encourage a local metastatic focus, so it is wise to avoid the technique in the presence of septicemia. Also, the remote possibility of a metastatic abscess should be considered when infection exists in the pelvis or lower limb, and these cases should receive antibiotic protection (Grant, 1945).

Extrinsic infection

Infection may be introduced from improperly sterilized equipment or from contaminated solutions. Multidose vials are a potential source of infection unless used for one case only and then discarded. Rather than aspirate the contents via a needle inserted through the rubber bung, it is preferable to remove the top completely and draw up the contents into a sterile syringe or series of syringes. The filled syringes are then capped with sterile disposable needles with their sterile protective plastic covers in place. The charged syringes can be kept at hand in a sterile cloth bag or folded towel, ready for use.

The same all-glass syringe should never be refilled and used twice without resterilization, because the plunger may become contaminated and infect the barrel of the syringe. Atherley has designed a sterilizable metal sheath to enclose the plunger and allow repeated use of the same syringe without contamination of the plunger (Atherley, 1961). This apparatus may have some merit in situations in which a plentiful supply of sterile syringes is not available.

When syringes are being changed, the connecting parts of the syringe nozzle and the needle hub must be kept sterile. Provided this essential precaution is taken, the outer parts of the syringe may be handled with clean, but not necessarily sterile, hands. This has been the routine in my practice for the past 20 years, during which over 30,000 continuous epidural anesthetics have been given in this way without the occurrence of a single case of infection.

MICROPORE FILTERS

Sterile bacterial filters may be incorporated in the system between the syringe and the catheter mount, and some writers have stated categorically that these filters are an essential precaution (Crawford et al., 1975). This is a counsel of perfection, and experience shows that infection does not occur if sensible hygienic precautions are taken. Nevertheless, infection is not the only type of contamination that can reach the epidural space, and there are other good reasons for using a Millipore filter.

Every time a glass ampule is opened, a shower of microscopic glass particles is dispersed from the line of cleavage in the glass, and some of these particles fall back into the contents of the ampule, creating an unavoidable source of particulate contamination (Katz et al., 1973). These glass particles may range in size from less than 2 μ to 250 μ (Burke et al., 1972; Turco and Davis, 1972; Furgang, 1974), and they may become a potential cause of granulomatous reaction. The particles are filtered out by micropore filters, so it seems reasonable and advisable to place a micropore filter downstream of any syringe containing solutions that have been drawn up from a glass ampule. Disposable micropore filters are now mass-produced extremely cheaply, and their routine use is no longer precluded for economical reasons.

A number of rather obvious systems have been devised to reduce the risk of bacterial contamination: some are simple, some more complicated.

Sterile Bags. In 1952 I had sterile bags made of transparent plastic material in which to seal a large-volume syringe of 30 or 50 ml attached to the end of a catheter. The syringe could then be manipulated in a sterile fashion, fully isolated in its plastic container, and repeat injections could be given up to the volume of the attached syringe without infringing upon the sterile system.

Continuous and Intermittent Drip (Burn, 1963; Scott and Walker, 1963). Continuous or intermittent epidural injection can be maintained for long periods by means of an infusion apparatus, a dilute solution of local anesthetic being prepared under sterile conditions in the hospital pharmacy and dispensed in bottles or plastic bags. For example, 0.4 to 0.8 per cent lidocaine may be used in this way. The solution is then dripped in via an ordinary infusion set. The high resistance offered by the catheter does not usually allow rapid infusion rates, and this is quite a safe method provided the solution is not concentrated (Edmonds-Seal, 1964). There are two major disadvantages:

1. It is very difficult to adjust the drip rate to the exact speed that will maintain a constant metameric level of analgesia.

2. Active and inquisitive patients may be tempted to take a hand in their own treatment. One patient experienced a very high level of blockade and an inadvertent hypotensive episode after he had adjusted the drip himself to

run at a maximum speed. More concentrated solutions are particularly dangerous if they drip faster than intended (see Chapter 14, Complications and Contraindications).

In addition, continuous infusions of dilute solutions lead to very large cumulative doses of drug, while at the same time providing marginally satisfactory analgesia. For example, Holmdahl and his colleagues report dosages as high as 4.5 mg per kilo per hour with a 0.4 per cent concentration of lidocaine (Holmdahl et al., 1972; Sjögren and Wright, 1972). Thus, with such a regimen a 70-kg man would receive a total of 7.5 g of lidocaine in 24 hours, with significantly high blood levels of local anesthetic and central depressant effects.

From a practical point of view, it is necessary to incorporate a three-way tap in the infusion line, so that supplementary injections of more concentrated analgesic solution can be administered as a bolus injection if the segmental level of blockade sinks too low or the quality of blockade deteriorates. I have not been very impressed by the practicality of this method, and I no longer use it.

Intermittent or Constant Infusion Pumps (Cox and Spoerel, 1964). This is an elegant and expensive variant of the preceding method. A large syringe is charged with the required concentration of local anesthetic (e.g., 1.0 to 2.0 per cent lidocaine) and attached to an electrically driven pump timed to deliver a constant slow infusion or a preset intermittent injection of a given volume.

Griffiths and his associates (1975) have analyzed the respective advantages and disadvantages of intermittent injections compared with continuous infusion of bupivacaine for relief of pain in the first 48 hours after thoracic surgery. Their findings are summarized in Table 7–2. These figures support the general clinical impression that intermittent injections, while

TABLE 7–2 Advantages and Disadvantages of Intermittent Bupivacaine Injection Versus Continuous Epidural Infusion for Postoperative Thoracic Pain*

	Intermittent Injection (0.5%)	***Continuous Infusion (0.25–0.125%)***
Average cumulative dose after 48 hours (mg)	573.5	1054.6
Maximum plasma concentration at 48 hours (μg/ml)	–	0.95–3.76 (Toxicity level > 1.5 μg/ml)
Degree of pain relief	Very efficient	Less effective analgesia
Incidence of arterial hypotension	More frequent than by continuous infusion	Easily corrected by IV infusion of electrolyte solution
Incidence of urinary retention (in males only—did not occur in females)	37.5	100

*Data from Griffiths, D. P. G. et al.: Brit. J. Anaesth., *47*:48, 1975.

providing somewhat discontinuous pain relief, are more practical and more effective in the long run. After an extensive experience with bags and drips I have come to the conclusion, as Griffiths et al. have done, that in practice the simplest method is the best—that is, an intermittent technique using a series of sterile syringes filled with the required solution and changed under careful conditions to ensure that the connecting parts remain sterile at all times. The use of a disposable micropore filter is admirable but not essential, and its presence should not permit any relaxation of care and common sense in changing the syringes.

Wrong Solution

With an epidural catheter in place, the patient is at the mercy of human error, and it is possible that someone could inject the wrong solution through the catheter. Great care must be taken to identify all injected solutions correctly, and syringes or infusions attached to the catheter should be labeled with the nature and concentration of the contained drug.

Errors and wrongful injections have been reported, fortunately without lasting ill effects, and these will be discussed more fully in Chapter 14 on Complications and Contraindications.

Intermittent Dosage: Timing and Quantity

It is possible to administer any amount of analgesic solution once an epidural catheter is properly inserted. What guidelines can we propose for the right amount and the right time? The guidelines that do exist have been reached empirically by clinical trial and observation. The amount of local anesthetic needed to keep the segmental level of analgesia constant is about one half of the initial induction dose, and this "top-up" dose needs to be given when the upper level of analgesia has receded one or two dermatomes. During the normal course of an operation, two or three repeat injections of this magnitude do not seem to meet with serious degrees of tachyphylaxis, and it is seldom necessary to increase the size of the repeat dose while the patient is on the table.

Timing of the "Repeat Dose"

The need to keep a constant segmental level of analgesia during operation has focused attention on the factors that are important in maintaining this level. Since repeat injections need to be given when the upper segmental level has regressed two segments, it is necessary to be able to predict when this degree of regression is likely to occur. An estimate of this sort can only be obtained from observations on large numbers of conscious patients with each local anesthetic used. Figure 7–16 shows the way in which the data are collected. Segment-time diagrams are constructed for the onset and decay of analgesia in each patient, a pin-prick being used to determine the upper and lower margins of sensory analgesia.

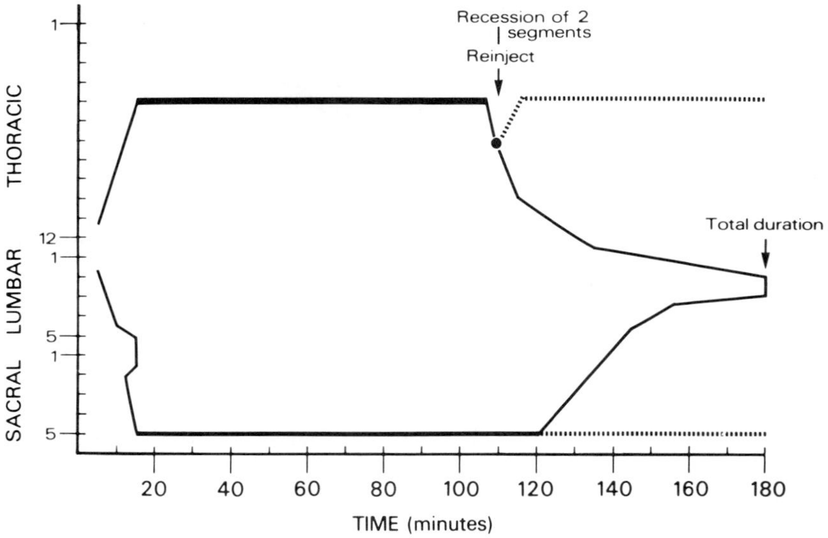

Figure 7–16. Timing of top-up dose in conscious patients. Segment-time diagram showing spread and regression of analgesia. A stable upper level of analgesia is maintained by injecting one-half of the induction dose when the upper level of analgesia has regressed two spinal segments.

Note that "total duration" is very much longer than the duration from the time of maximum spread until analgesia begins to recede. In the case illustrated in Figure 7–16, the total duration was three hours, but the upper level of analgesia began to recede at 90 minutes after the block was complete, and it had fallen two dermatomes 10 minutes later. This point, the point of "recession of two dermatomes," is the relevant clinical landmark at which a reinforcing dose of local anesthetic must be injected in order to maintain an effective level of surgical analgesia. The total duration of analgesia, confined at the end to just a few segments, is quite irrelevant to the clinical situation on the operating table (Bromage, 1965).

In the conscious patient there is no need to be able to predict the point of "recession of two dermatomes," for it can be determined by direct observation, and a top-up injection can be given at the first sign of segmental regression. However, some form of reliable prediction is necessary in patients who are asleep under light general anesthesia. A workable prediction can be obtained statistically.

If segment-minute diagrams of a sufficient number of comparable patients are made under standard conditions, it is possible to construct a distribution curve for duration of recession of two segments for each drug tested, as shown in Figure 7–17. From this distribution curve we obtain the mean duration and the standard deviation of the mean for predictive purposes (Bromage and Burfoot, 1966; Bromage et al., 1967).

Table 7–3 shows the average duration of recession of two segments for a number of local anesthetics we have tested, together with the standard deviation of the mean. The final column shows the average duration minus 1.5 × S.D., that is, the point at which reinjection should be made in order to maintain a predictably adequate level of analgesia in patients under light general

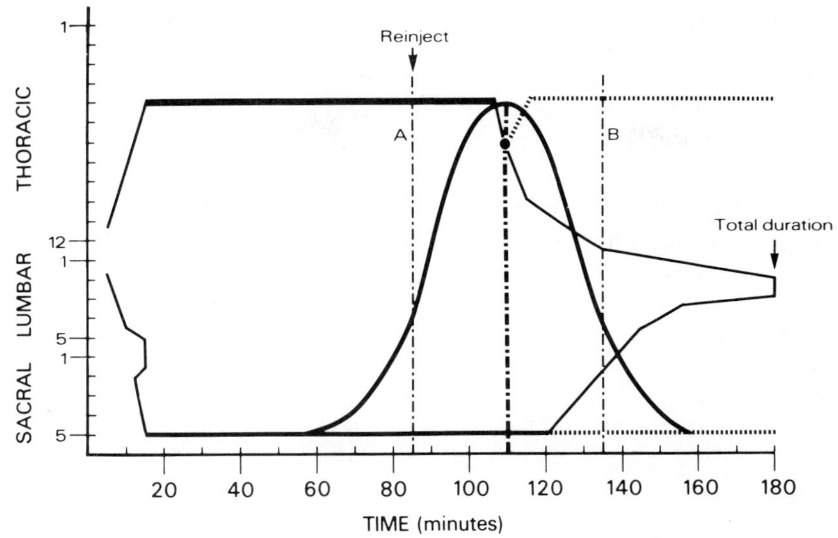

Figure 7–17. Timing of top-up dose in unconscious patients (see text). The bell-shaped curve represents the distribution about the mean for duration to recession of two spinal segments. Lines A and B represent ± 1.5 standard deviations (S.D.) on each side of the mean. Reinjection at A ensures that the upper level of analgesia will not drop in 90 per cent of patients.

anesthesia (Bromage and Burfoot, 1966; Bromage et al., 1967; Bromage, 1969; Bromage et al., 1974).

Removal of the Catheter

The catheter must be removed carefully and gently, and a small sterile dressing should be left over the puncture site for the next 24 hours. Vinyl catheters that have been in place for a long time may become brittle, and

TABLE 7–3 Duration of Lumbar Epidural Analgesia for Chloroprocaine, Lidocaine, Prilocaine, Tetracaine, Bupivacaine and Etidocaine with 1/200,000 Epinephrine

Drug	*Duration* (2-segment recession) (mins)*	*S.D.*	*Duration — (1.5 × S.D.) (mins)*
3% Chloroprocaine	57	7	47
2% Lidocaine	97.5	19	70
2% Prilocaine	97	10	82
3% Prilocaine	99	17	74
0.4% Tetracaine	135	23	100
0.5% Tetracaine	146	22	113
0.5% Bupivacaine	196	31	150
0.75% Bupivacaine	201	40	141
1% Etidocaine	170	57	85

*Duration is measured from the moment of complete spread until analgesia has regressed two spinal segments.

then special care is required (Bonica, 1959). This is one reason why it is important to change the catheter regularly at intervals of 72 hours in cases requiring prolonged blockade.

The overlying vertebral arches may grip the catheter and hinder withdrawal if the back is extended. The patient should be turned on the side with the back slightly, but not excessively, flexed; then gentle traction should be applied to the catheter close to the point of entry through the skin. After withdrawal, the catheter should be inspected, special attention being paid to the tip and the depth marks, to make sure that none has been cut or broken off. As mentioned earlier in this chapter, a sequestered piece of catheter should usually be left alone, as surgical exploration is unlikely to find it. However, if a catheter has broken off close to the skin, removal is usually a simple matter. Then it is reasonable to probe for the broken piece, using a small incision if necessary. Once the broken end is identified, it can be pulled out with the aid of a hemostat.

The very rare possibility of a knotted catheter has already been mentioned. This difficulty can only arise if an unnecessarily long length of catheter has been inserted into the epidural space. If a knot is suspected, great care and patience should be exercised in trying to coax the knot through the ligaments without breaking the catheter. It may be necessary to rotate the spine in different directions to relax the ligaments and to help the knot in its passage.

If pain is caused by traction on the catheter, the anesthesiologist should suspect that a loop may have become curled around a nerve root, with the possibility that avulsion might occur if persistent traction is applied. If this should happen, the position of the catheter would have to be checked by X-ray in two planes after the catheter lumen is filled with contrast medium (a volume of 0.3 ml will suffice for this), and if pain persists it would probably be wise to extract the catheter under direct vision by open surgical laminectomy. I do not know of any recorded instance of this unfortunate type of complication, but it is theoretically possible when excessive lengths of catheter are inserted into the epidural space.

CONTINUOUS EPIDURAL ANALGESIA AND THROMBOEMBOLISM PROPHYLAXIS

The death rate from postoperative pulmonary embolism has risen sharply over the past 30 years. Between 1947 and 1960 the incidence doubled from 1 per 1,000 operations to about 2 per 1,000 (Hodgson, 1964), and by 1969 it was about 3 per 1,000 (Roberts, 1971). As a result, a great deal of attention has been paid to the etiology and prevention of fatal thromboembolism, and within the past few years a strong movement has developed to introduce partial heparinization as a practical and routine method for protecting surgical patients against sudden death from postoperative pulmonary embolism.

This movement presents difficulties in the choice of continuous epidural analgesia for surgery, as most forms of regional anesthesia are contraindicated in the face of abnormal clotting mechanisms, since deeply placed and potentially dangerous hematomas are prone to develop in fully heparinized patients. While the prophylactic heparin regime that has been proposed barely affects the normal clotting process (Kakkar et al., 1975), nevertheless, individuals respond with such wide variability that the chances of deep hematoma formation are virtually unknown in any single patient receiving subclinical doses of heparin. Under these circumstances epidural analgesia may become a potential hazard that is unwarranted. Thus, a conflict of interest has arisen between the prudent conduct of regional anesthesia and the need for effective routine protection against postoperative thromboembolism. Continuous epidural blockade is of particular concern, since an epidural catheter may need to be left in place for relatively long periods, and during this time it poses a potential threat of mild trauma to the extradural veins, with the remote chance of persistent bleeding and extradural hematoma formation if hemostasis is disturbed by an unusually sensitive response to heparin.

It is most important that this issue be clearly understood, for without a rational approach to the subject, facile pressures of fashion and convenience are likely to displace regional anesthesia from a large part of surgical practice, for reasons that are shallow and illogical and to the ultimate detriment of sound anesthetic management. The following section will attempt to summarize the salient experimental work that has led to present methods of prophylaxis against thromboembolism, so that the reader can view the relevant options and arrive at a sensible compromise that will satisfy the need for protection against pulmonary embolism while permitting the use of continuous epidural blockade when indicated.

Pathogenesis of Thromboembolism

Pulmonary embolism usually arises from central extension of clots that have formed in deep veins of the calf or pelvis. The patient is relatively safe as long as the initial thrombosis remains confined to the deep veins and out of the main venous stream, but dangerous emboli are likely to be launched into the circulation when thrombi lengthen and protrude from the quiet backwaters of the calf sinusoids into the axes of the main veins where flow is faster.

Ninety per cent of deep vein thromboses (DVT) become apparent in the first four days after operation, and there is strong evidence that clotting begins during the actual course of surgical operation (Flanc et al., 1968). Therefore, preventive measures against DVT should start before or during surgery and continue throughout the operation and immediate postoperative period. Most DVT occurs in the lower calf.

Virchow (1856) proposed a triad of factors in the coagulation of blood, namely, changes in the vessel wall, in the flow of blood and in the nature of the blood itself. Each of these three basic elements proposed by Virchow has expanded to become a main heading for groups of factors that are important in the coagulation process (see below).

Virchow's Triad

Vessel Wall	***Rheology***	***Blood***
Damaged endothelial cells	Viscosity	Platelet adhesiveness
Irregularities of vessels	Turbulence	Coagulation factors
Valve cusps	Velocity	Fibrinolysis
	Obstruction to flow	

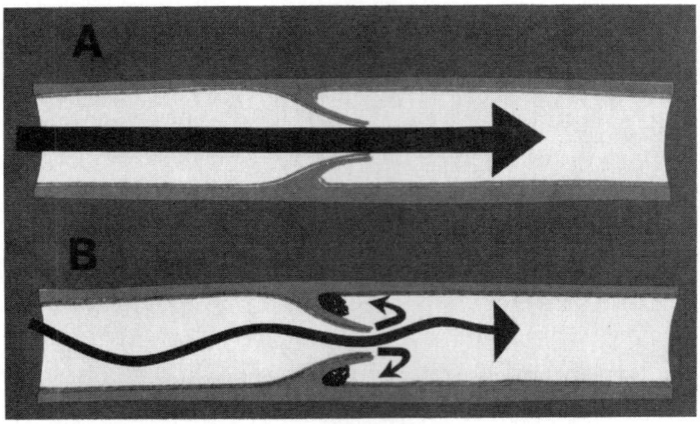

Figure 7–18. Deep vein thrombosis (DVT). *A*, Rapid flow in calf veins prevents clotting. *B*, Slow flow permits stasis and thrombus formation behind valve cusps.

The two principal factors affecting DVT are (1) slowing of blood flow and (2) changes of coagulability. Of these two, slowing of blood flow is the most important etiological factor in postoperative venous thrombosis (Paterson and McLaughlin, 1954; Mustard et al., 1962; Roberts and Cotton, 1974). Thrombi are especially prone to form in areas where flow is turbulent or out of the main stream. The cul-de-sac behind valve cusps is a favorite site for venous stagnation, and more than 30 per cent of all DVT originates at the apices of valve pockets in the walls of the veins (Paterson and McLaughlin, 1954; see Fig. 7–18). Therefore, logical methods of prophylaxis should be directed to the prime cause and should aim to promote venous blood flow in the calves and pelvis, where the trouble starts, rather than reduce the coagulability of the blood throughout the whole body.

However, there is evidence that certain factors in the blood do alter after operation and that these changes may predispose to clotting in regions of low flow. The plasma fibrinogen concentration is doubled and sometimes trebled after major surgery (Godal, 1962), and the rise of fibrinogen is associated with a 9 to 14 per cent increase in blood viscosity (Kemble and Hickman, 1972). This deterioration in rheological properties will tend to further impede the flow of blood in regions where the stream moves slowly, thus adding a systemic element to the local problem of sluggish flow.

In addition, a retrospective study by Gallus and his associates (1973a) has shown that patients who develop postoperative thromboembolism are more likely to have a low partial thromboplastin time (PTT) before surgery, whereas those with a longer preoperative PTT are less likely to suffer thrombosis. Thus, there is strongly suggestive evidence that a genuine "hypercoagulable state" may exist in certain patients and that they are at greater risk than the rest of the population. A number of predisposing factors are known to exist; some are extrinsic and related to surgical and anesthetic intervention, but others are intrinsic to the patient himself, and it is in these patients that systemic methods of prophylactic therapy may be indicated.

Influence of Anesthesia

Direct and indirect measurements of venous flow show that flow in the legs is reduced by 50 per cent after induction of general anesthesia (Browse,

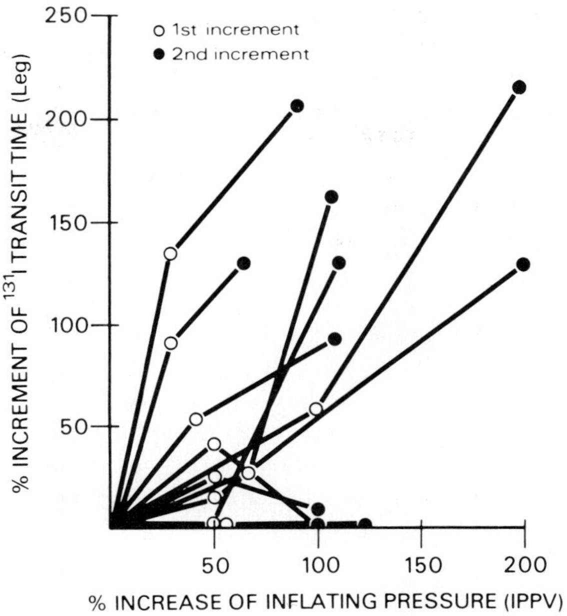

Figure 7–19. Respiration and DVT. Prolongation of venous transit time from legs by intermittent positive pressure ventilation (IPPV).
○ = first increment of airway inflating pressure
● = second increment of airway inflating pressure.
(Data from Dyde and Bethel, 1968.)

1962; Doran et al., 1964; Clark and Cotton, 1968). The widespread adoption of neuromuscular blockade combined with artificial ventilation during anesthesia in the early 1950's coincided with a brisk rise in the incidence of pulmonary embolism. Whether this is a true cause-and-effect relationship remains unproven, but the circumstantial evidence is suspicious. Change of respiratory dynamics from spontaneous respiration to intermittent positive-pressure ventilation (IPPV) alters the normal pattern of venous return from the lower leg and slows the transit time of blood within the leg veins. Hodgson (1964) found that under general anesthesia venographic emptying of leg veins was three times slower during IPPV than during spontaneous respiration. Dyde and Bethel (1968) used a modification of Helen Payling Wright's isotopic method to measure venous transit time (Wright et al., 1948; Osborn and Wright, 1949) and showed that there was a general tendency for transit times in the legs to lengthen proportionally with increased increments of inspiratory pressure under IPPV, as shown in Figure 7–19. An average increase of 121 per cent inflating pressure was associated with 108 per cent prolongation of venous transit time.

Duration of anesthesia appears to be related to the incidence of thrombosis, and DVT is more common after long operations (Sripad et al., 1971). However, this may merely reflect the greater severity of operations that require longer anesthesia time (Hills et al., 1972).

Obesity

Postmortem studies by Henderson (1927) and clinical evidence by Snell (1927) suggested that obesity was an important predisposing factor in death from pulmonary embolism. More recently, Kakkar and his colleagues

(1970) found a strong correlation between obesity and DVT using isotopic tracer methods to detect venous thrombosis in the leg.

Several interrelating factors are probably at work in predisposing the obese patient to postoperative deep vein thrombosis. Surgery in fat subjects tends to be more difficult and take longer than in thin subjects, and higher ventilating pressures are needed to overcome the reduced pulmonary compliance and increased work of breathing (Sharp et al., 1964), so venous slowing is more severe and lasts longer in these patients.

Site of Surgery

DVT is more likely to occur after upper abdominal and thoracic operations than after lower abdominal cases. Again, perhaps the difference may be linked to the greater inhibition of respiration and accompanying higher venous pressures associated with the more painful wounds close to the diaphragm and rib cage.

Malignant Disease

Patients with malignant disease are very prone to develop DVT (Sproul, 1938), and these patients seem to be more resistant to physical methods of prophylaxis aimed at increasing venous flow in the lower limb (Hills et al., 1972). Miller et al. (1967) have suggested that a hypercoagulable state exists in cancer patients due to release of thromboplastins from dead circulating tumor cells. This hypercoagulability is correctable by administration of small doses of heparin; then the incidence of DVT falls to a level comparable to that found in patients without malignant disease who received heparin prophylaxis (Kakkar et al., 1972).

Geography

A few studies supported by objective measurements have shown that DVT in the lower limbs is influenced by geographical location. The results of one such study are shown in Table 7–4 (Chumnikarakij and Poshyachinda, 1975). It is evident that the vital statistics of DVT show wide geographical variations, and it is difficult to draw conclusions from comparisons of prophylactic results in different parts of the world.

TABLE 7–4 Leg Vein Thrombosis After Major Pelvic Surgery in Women in England and Thailand

	Nonmalignant		*Malignant*	
	NUMBER OF CASES	*INCIDENCE OF DVT*	*NUMBER OF CASES*	*INCIDENCE OF DVT*
England (Oxford)	117	12%	45	35%
Thailand (Bangkok)	117	1.7%	52	3.8%

Detection of Deep Vein Thrombosis

The natural history and prevention of DVT only became intelligible after objective methods were developed to detect the presence of thrombosis. It is now clear that clinical methods of detecting DVT are insensitive and inaccurate. In many instances a silent peripheral thrombosis only becomes evident after a massive and fatal attack of pulmonary embolism (Coon and Coller, 1959; Sevitt, 1962). The classic signs of local calf tenderness, Homans' sign of pain on sharp dorsiflexion of the foot, and edema and swelling are present in only about one third of all proven cases (Flanc et al., 1968), and false positive findings are also common (Haeger, 1965). Thus, evaluation of DVT prophylaxis must be based on objective methods of thrombus detection. Unfortunately, current objective techniques are invasive, complicated and expensive, and limited to institutions with adequate investigational resources. In the future, noninvasive radiographic techniques based on the EMI scanner principle may attain sufficient resolution to reveal boundaries between fluid and clotted blood (Editorial, Brit. Med. J., 1975), but at the present time this goal has not yet been reached.

Phlebography

Radiographic techniques designed to outline the veins of the lower leg have been used for more than 20 years. In retrograde venography a large bolus of 30 to 40 ml of water-soluble contrast medium, such as 40 per cent Hypaque, is injected into a distal vein, and serial views of the leg are taken. Following a thrombotic episode, some of the deep veins cannot be filled and visualized (Nylander, 1968). Early and transient thrombi may be missed by phlebography.

Isotopic Scanning (Radioactive Fibrinogen)

Human fibrinogen labeled with ^{125}I is injected intravenously immediately before operation or shortly afterward. The circulating labeled fibrinogen is taken up by any developing thrombus, and the radioactivity overlying the site rises. The legs are scanned daily and the radioactivity recorded. Local rises of radioactivity denote an underlying clot (Negus et al., 1968; Flanc et al., 1968). This method of detection has proved to be the most sensitive and accurate index of deep vein thrombosis. It correlates well with phlebography, and it has become the most widely used method for studying the incidence and prophylaxis of DVT (Calnan and Allenby, 1975; Roberts, 1975).

Doppler Ultrasound

Transcutaneous Doppler ultrasound flowmeters have been adopted to measure slow-moving columns of blood in the leg veins. Patency of major veins can be demonstrated by squeezing the calf to produce a transient wave of augmented flow. Thrombosis extending into a main vein is indicated by the failure of this maneuver to augment the Doppler signal (Evans, 1970, 1971; Yao et al., 1972). This method is ineffective for detecting localized deep thromboses in the calf, but it does serve to demonstrate the presence of large and dangerous thrombi that have extended into popliteal or more proximal veins.

Electrical Impedance Plethysmography

Changes of calf blood volume can be measured by changes of electrical impedance. Essentially, the method entails passing a constant high frequency current of low amperage between two circumferential electrodes placed around the calf and measuring the resultant potential difference between a second pair of circumferential electrodes placed between the outer pair. Blood is a good conductor of electricity, and an increase of blood volume in the calf is reflected by a fall of electrical resistance.

Wheeler and his colleagues (1970, 1972) adopted electrical impedance plethysmography to diagnose DVT by observing the influence of fluctuations of the respiratory cycle on venous flow from the lower limb. Respiratory fluctuations of electrical resistance are reduced distal to the clot site when major veins are clotted. This method has limitations that are similar to those of Doppler ultrasound. While it is useful for detecting dangerous thrombi in the major veins, in which the incidence of embolization is as high as 50 per cent, it has poor sensitivity for detecting silent and relatively innocuous thrombi confined to the deep veins of the calf muscles (Johnston et al., 1974). Thus, although impedance plethysmography is a useful noninvasive clinical tool for detecting major thrombi, it fails to pick up the larger number of deep but limited thrombi.

METHODS OF PROPHYLAXIS AGAINST THROMBOEMBOLISM

Philosophically, the choices for preventing pathological clot formation are analogous to the choices for the relief of pain, and in both instances the forms of therapy selected will depend to a large degree upon the approach to basic problems—whether direct by frontal assault or indirect by devious means. Both pain and pathological clotting can be prevented either by general involvement of the whole body or by attacking the problem locally where it arises, while leaving the rest of the organism relatively unaffected. In this way the therapy of thromboembolism has become sharply divided into two distinct camps, with supporters of systemic anticoagulation on one side and devotees of augmentation of regional blood flow on the other. The therapeutic options must be examined in terms of their effectiveness and their compatibility with continuous epidural blockade, for some are effective and compatible, but others present serious difficulties.

Systemic Anticoagulation

The Dextrans. The dextrans were shown to have antithrombotic properties in 1959 (Borgström et al., 1959), but the precise mechanism of their

TABLE 7–5 Influence of Repeated Infusions of Dextran 70 on the Phlebographic Incidence of DVT in 52 Cases of Fractured Neck of Femur*

	Number of Cases	*Phlebographic Evidence of DVT*	*Incipient Pulmonary Edema*
Controls (no dextran)	25	52%	–
Repeated dextran IV infusions	27	4%	12%

*From Johnsson, S. R. et al., Acta Chir. Scand., Suppl. 387, 1968.

action is not clear. They do not appear to have a direct effect on the coagulation "cascade" but rather inhibit the initial platelet thrombi by lessening platelet adhesiveness. The clinical evidence in favor of dextran infusions is clouded and conflicting, and complicated by the fact that repeated dextran infusions may lead to overloading of the circulation and pulmonary edema.

Johnsson et al. (1968) produced phlebographic evidence confirming earlier clinical reports that repeated dextran infusions reduced the incidence of postoperative thrombotic complications, but at the cost of some cases of circulatory overload. Their regimen called for one infusion of 500 ml of 6 per cent dextran (mean MW 70,000) during operation, followed by 500 ml daily for two days and then 500 ml every third day until day 12. The results are summarized in Table 7–5.

However, other series using dextran prophylaxis in patients with fractured hips have not shown any significant reduction of thrombosis (Bronge et al., 1971; Bergquist et al., 1972). Whether the dextrans really work by a direct action in coating platelet and blood vessel endothelium, as has been suggested (Bloom et al., 1964), or whether their effects are due to blood volume expansion and increased flow is uncertain. In any event, dextran treatment does not appear to interfere with normal coagulation processes when used prophylactically in this way, and it is compatible with and safe in the presence of continuous epidural analgesia.

Aspirin, Rutin and Vitamin C. There is no objective support for the commonly held belief that aspirin protects against DVT, although doses in excess of 600 mg daily do appear to inhibit platelet aggregation to a degree. In a trial carried out by the British Medical Research Council, the incidence of postoperative isotopic DVT was 22 per cent in 150 controls and 27.5 per cent in 153 aspirin-treated patients (Butterfield et al., 1972). Similarly, claims for protection by rutin and large doses of vitamin C have not been substantiated (Calnan and Allenby, 1975).

Heparin. Heparin is a highly acidic mucopolysaccharide of large molecular weight (between 6,000 and 20,000) with a strong negative charge. These physicochemical attributes make for a very slow rate of vascular uptake from subcutaneous injection sites, so extremely low but significantly augmented concentrations of circulating heparin can be sustained for long periods of time after subcutaneous injections of small doses of the order of 5,000 units (Kakkar et al., 1972).

Very small doses of heparin in the range of 10 I.U. per kilogram IV have no effect on normal platelet clumping. However, platelet adhesiveness is increased after operation, and then these small doses produce a significant reduction in platelet stickiness, perhaps due to release of lipoprotein-lipase (Ham and Slack, 1968). In addition to inhibiting the formation of platelet thrombi, heparin has an important effect on the coagulation cascade. Activated factor X (i.e., Xa) occupies a key position in both the extrinsic and intrinsic coagulation pathways. A markedly increased activity of the Xa inhibitor occurs in plasma of patients receiving heparin (Yin et al., 1973). Other factors in the cascade are also affected by heparin, and activated factors IXa and XIa are rapidly inhibited (Rosenberg, 1974).

At the present time no simple but rigorous test exists for accurate adjustment of each stage of the coagulation cascade in individual patients. Therefore, current regimens of minidose heparin prophylaxis have been evolved from a combination of empiricism and statistics, and they are set at a level to produce the safest possible protection in the average patient. Under these circumstances the balance between effective protection from thrombosis and relative overdosage with consequent bleeding is held blindly, so individuals who are likely to bleed excessively from heparin will only be recognized by careful attention to the results of a partial thromboplastin test carried out before operation. Even then the results are not absolute, and they are no more than a qualitative index. Nevertheless, Wessler and Yin (1973) go so far as to say that a minidose heparin regimen essentially eliminates the risks of hemorrhage, except for human error in administering an overdose.

MINIDOSE HEPARIN PROPHYLAXIS. Heparin in small subcutaneous dosage was subjected to clinical trial by Sharnoff and his colleagues in 1962, with very promising results (Sharnoff et al., 1962; Sharnoff, 1966). Since that time a considerable number of well-designed trials have been carried out (Sharnoff and DeBlasio, 1970), some with both venographic and isotopic control, and dosage has been modified empirically to give the best compromise between effective prophylaxis on the one hand and excessive anticoagulation on the other (Kakkar et al., 1971, 1972; Williams, 1971; Gordon-Smith et al., 1972; Gallus et al., 1973b). The largest and most powerful investigation has been the International Multicentre Trial coordinated among 28 collaborating institutions in Europe, North America, South Africa and Australia, with a total of 4,121 patients (Kakkar et al., 1975).

The regimen proposed by Gallus et al. (1973b) has become the most commonly accepted dose schedule, 5,000 units of heparin being given *subcutaneously* two hours before operation, followed by 5,000 units subcutaneously every eight hours for seven days. New and highly sensitive methods of heparin assay show that this regimen accords well with the pattern of uptake of heparin from subcutaneous injection sites. A single subcutaneous dose of 5,000 units of heparin in normal adults produces a peak blood concentration of about 0.10 I.U./ml two to four hours after injection, and blood levels remain elevated for a period of five to eight hours (Kakkar et al., 1972; Yin et al., 1973). Thus, injections given every eight hours are likely to produce a very slightly raised and constant level of heparin in the blood stream.

The results of this schedule look convincing, especially when applied to large numbers of carefully controlled patients as in the International Multicentre Trial, in which the postoperative results in more than 2,000 nonheparinized controls were compared with those in a similar number of patients receiving the minidose heparin regimen (Table 7–6). This large study showed

TABLE 7–6 International Multicentre Trial of Small Doses of Heparin to Prevent Fatal Postoperative Thromboembolism*

	Total Number of Patients	*Deaths From Hemorrhage*	*Autopsies Done*	*Fatal Pulmonary Embolus Proven By Autopsy*	*DVT Diagnosis By ^{125}I-Fibrinogen* NUMBER TESTED	INCIDENCE
Controls (no heparin)	2,076	5	72	16 (0.7% of total)	667	24.6%
Small-dose	2,045	4	53	2 (0.09% of total)	625	7.7%

*Data from Kakkar, V. V., et al.: Lancet, *2*:45, 1975.

that minidose heparin resulted in a 66 per cent reduction in DVT and in a highly significant reduction in deaths from fatal pulmonary embolism. The study also showed that the technique is free from danger under the carefully controlled conditions of this trial. However, the range of blood heparin levels after subcutaneous administration is greater than generally appreciated, and peak concentrations are scattered widely about the ideal mean of 0.10 I.U./ml, with a range of 0.05 to 0.40 I.U./ml (Cooke et al., 1976). Nicoliades et al. (1975) pointed out that there is the ever present risk of heparin overdose and that the widespread use of the technique will probably fail to achieve a theoretically maximum effect because it cannot be made free of human error. These authors advise a cautious approach with selective restriction of heparin prophylaxis to patients at serious risk. Such a policy of selective choice is intuitively attractive and one that may lead to a working arrangement between the imperatives of thrombosis prophylaxis and the indications for continuous epidural analgesia.

Promotion of Venous Blood Flow

Venous blood flow in the lower legs during operation can be increased by passive or active means. Passive methods for promoting deep venous flow aim to collapse the superficial veins so that venous return is forced into the deep veins. These methods include leg bandaging, elastic stockings and elevation of the legs (Sigel et al., 1973). While these passive methods may improve venous transit time and *velocity* flow, they do not improve volume flow (Roberts, 1971), and they are ineffective in preventing DVT as measured by isotopic scanning (Rosengarten et al., 1970; Browse et al., 1974).

Active methods for promoting peroperative venous flow depend on the creation of alternating pressures in the leg to mimic the pumping effect of calf muscles during normal muscular activity. Active methods of augmenting venous flow appear to be much more promising than passive methods, and with proper technique volume flows approach values seen during physiological activity (Roberts and Cotton, 1972), and the prophylactic effects rival the best results of systemic heparinization (Roberts and Cotton, 1974, 1975).

Electrical Stimulation (Peroperative). Doran and his colleagues have used galvanic stimulation of the gastrocnemius-soleus muscle group to cause intermittent calf compression at the rate of about 12 contractions per minute

(Doran et al., 1964; Powley and Doran, 1973). This treatment has had encouraging clinical results (Doran et al., 1970), and isotopic scanning has confirmed that it reduces the incidence of DVT by about 50 to 60 per cent (Browse and Negus, 1970; Rosenberg et al., 1975).

Passive Foot Exercises (Peroperative). Roberts and his colleagues used a motorized foot exerciser to produce rhythmic flexion and extension of the ankles throughout surgical operations. Blood flow measurements with this device showed a 35 per cent increase in venous flow and a fourfold increase in pulsatile flow. The incidence of DVT using isotopic scanning criteria was reduced by 77 per cent (Sabri, et al., 1971a).

Intermittent Calf Compression. Intermittent external compression can be applied to the leg by a system of inflatable plastic boots and a suitable compression pump. Intermittent inflation pressure up to 40 to 50 mmHg produce a brief surge of venous flow in the leg, followed by a fall to below resting levels. It appears that this intermittent pattern of flow is beneficial in preventing deep vein stagnation. Two slightly different patterns of compression have been used, and there may be important functional differences between them, because one appears to be more effective than the other in preventing thrombosis in cancer patients.

Calnan and his associates (1970) have developed a machine (Flowtronaire) that produces a compression phase lasting 1 minute, followed by a relaxation phase of 1 minute (Hills et al., 1972). This machine reduced the incidence of DVT from 39 per cent in controls to 3 per cent in nonmalignant cases. There was no reduction of DVT in patients with malignant disease, although another group of investigators using the same device did find a lower incidence in a small group of cancer patients (Clark et al., 1974).

Roberts and his colleagues developed a slightly different pattern of compression based on careful in vivo flow studies (Roberts and Cotton, 1972). They emphasized the need for a sharp compression phase to produce maximum peaks of flow acceleration to the column of blood in the deep veins (Sabri et al., 1971b; Roberts and Cotton, 1972). The compression cycle of 1 minute started with a rapid acceleration phase of 8 mmHg/sec for 5 seconds, releasing abruptly to zero when the pressure reached 40 to 45 mmHg. This pattern of brief intermittent compression increased the peak pulsatile flow sevenfold and reduced the incidence of DVT from a control level of 26.0 per cent to 6.4 per cent in patient with and without malignancy (Roberts and Cotton, 1974).

When these results are compared with the figures from heparin prophylaxis, it can be seen that both methods provide equal degrees of protection against DVT. The results of augmented venous flow and minidose heparin prophylaxis are statistically indistinguishable. Therefore, the choice between the two should be determined not by matters of routine convenience and ward care but rather by wider considerations within the context of anesthetic and postanesthetic management. At our present state of knowledge, it would seem imprudent to promote a policy of combining minidose heparin with continuous epidural blockade. Although the small-dose regimen avoids gross changes in coagulation, the individual responses to heparin are too great, and the methods of monitoring these differences are too cumbersome for routine use and for assurance of absolute safety from intraspinal bleeding. Therefore, methods of augmenting venous flow for thrombosis prophylaxis would seem to be preferable to heparin whenever continuous epidural analgesia is indicated.

Voluntary Active Calf Compression (Active Exercise). One further but unassessed method of DVT prophylaxis remains to be considered, in which the epidural blockade alone is adapted to augmenting venous flow in the lower limb.

Active exercise is the most effective way to promote venous flow in muscle. Theoretically, there should be no better form of protection against thrombosis than to encourage voluntary calf exercises throughout the period of operation, with the patient analgesic under epidural blockade but awake and responsive to instructions. Clearly this approach has limited scope, for it is only practical in operations that lend themselves to these conditions. Moreover, the anesthetic technique and choice of analgesic solution are critical, for the right balance must be achieved between sensory and motor blockade so that a sufficient proportion of afferent fibers will be interrupted to provide acceptable analgesia while enough motor neurons are spared to ensure effective voluntary activity. This is not an easy technique to manage, but the required conditions can be met in a large proportion of suitable cases by choosing the right drugs and the right concentrations. The method is particularly applicable to lower abdominal and perineal operations in which the patient can remain awake and be encouraged to exercise his calf muscles at frequent intervals throughout the operation.

Unfortunately, individual responses to epidural solutions vary quite widely, and it is almost impossible to predict the precise amount of motor function that will persist in any one patient. The quality of motor blockade may range from zero to complete paresis of the legs. Of course, the latter is excessive and defeats the object of active calf exercises. The respective merits and potencies of various analgesic solutions are discussed in Chapter 9 on Drugs and Equipment. It will be seen that some agents are better suited than others to striking the delicate clinical balance between sensory blockade and persistent voluntary activity. With some solutions, such as 0.5 per cent bupivacaine, the distribution curve of motor blockade inclines to the left, with very few patients having significant degrees of motor paresis, although sensory blockade is satisfactory, if somewhat slow to develop. Other solutions such as 0.75 per cent bupivacaine, 1.0 per cent etidocaine and 2 per cent carbonated lidocaine produce intense motor blockade, and these solutions are quite unsuitable for active calf exercises, for while the patient is comfortably analgesic he may be completely incapable of moving his feet.

We have found an almost ideal solution for these purposes in a mixture of carbonated lidocaine and bupivacaine hydrochloride in the following concentrations:

1 per cent lidocaine – CO_2
0.25 per cent bupivacaine HCl
1/400,000 to 1/200,000 epinephrine

This mixture produces rapid spread of blockade in 8 to 12 minutes, excellent sensory analgesia lasting 2 to 3 hours and moderate motor blockade within an acceptable range that spares enough motor activity to permit active exercises of the calf during operation.

To date, no formal assessment with isotope scanning has been made

TABLE 7–7 Continuous Epidural Analgesia and Prophylaxis Against Postoperative Thromboembolism

Prophylactic Option	*Efficacy (% improvement)*	*Inherent Danger*	*Compatibility with Continuous Epidural Blockade*
Repeated dextran infusions	50–80% (variable data)	Fluid overload and right heart strain in 12% of cases	Compatible
Subcutaneous minidose heparin	66%	Excessive bleeding (extremely rare)	Doubtful. "Single shot" injection may be safe. Probably unwise to use indwelling catheter, but conclusions are speculative at present.
Electrical calf compression	60%	Burns of calf (very rare)	Compatible
Intermittent calf compression	75%	Nil	Compatible
Voluntary calf exercises	Unknown at present	Nil	Technically exacting

to evaluate active peroperative calf exercises as a practical method of protection against DVT. However, the method seems to be a logical step in the application of continuous epidural blockade to the overall management and protection of the surgical patient. If this form of active prophylaxis can be shown to work and to prevent DVT, it will do much to resolve the difficult choice between minidose heparin prophylaxis and continuous epidural blockade.

In the meantime the practicing anesthesiologist needs guidelines to choose the most appropriate combination of prophylaxis against thromboembolism, especially in situations in which multiple risks are present, as in grossly obese patients undergoing abdominal surgery. In these patients the risk of DVT is higher than in the normal population, yet segmental epidural analgesia is strongly indicated to preserve postoperative respiratory function. Table 7–7 summarizes the advantages and disadvantages of the various options that have just been discussed.

When continuous epidural analgesia is indicated, common sense should be used in choosing the most appropriate combination of prophylactic measures against thromboembolism. Ideally, an awake patient and the right choice of epidural solution will provide the best opportunity for peroperative calf exercises and for early postoperative mobilization. However, there will be many occasions when the patient cannot remain awake and when intermittent calf compression is indicated. At other times when calf compression is not feasible, it may be prudent to forego the advantages of continuous epidural analgesia in favor of minidose heparin.

REFERENCES

Aburel, E.: Contribution à l'étude des voies nerveuses sensitives de l'uterus. C. R. Soc. Biol. *105*:297, 1930a.

Aburel, E.: Anesthésie du plexus lombo-aortique en obstétrique. Bull. Soc. Obstet. Gynecol. *19*:616, 1930b.

Aburel, E.: L'anesthésie locale continue (prolongée) en obstétrique. Bull. Soc. Obstet. Gynecol. *20*:35, 1931.

Adams, R. C., Lundy, J. S., and Seldon, T. H.: Continuous caudal anesthesia or analgesia: A consideration of the technic, various uses and some possible dangers. J.A.M.A. *122*:152, 1943.

Atherley, D. W.: An apparatus for continuous epidural analgesia. Anaesthesia *16*:503, 1961.

Baker, A. S., Ojemann, R. J., Schwartz, M. N., and Richardson, E. P.: Spinal epidural abscess. New Eng. J. Med. *293*:463, 1975.

Bergquist, E., Bergqvist, D., Bronge, A., Dahlgren, S., and Lindquist, B.: An evaluation of early thrombosis prophylaxis following fracture of the femoral neck. Acta Chir. Scand. *138*:689, 1972.

Bloom, W. L., Harmer, D. S., Bryant, M. F., and Brewer, S. S.: Coating of vascular surfaces and cells. A new concept in prevention of intravascular thrombosis. Proc. Soc. Exp. Biol. Med. *115*:384, 1964.

Bonica, J. J.: Clinical Applications of Diagnostic and Therapeutic Nerve Blocks. Springfield, Ill., Charles C Thomas, 1959.

Borgström, S., Gelin, L.-E., and Zederfelt, T.: The formation of vein thrombi following tissue injury: An experimental study in rabbits. Acta Chir. Scand. (Suppl.) *247*:1, 1959.

Borgström, S., Greitz, T., van der Linden, W., Molin, J., and Rudics, I.: Anticoagulant prophylaxis of venous thrombosis in patients with fractured neck of the femur. A controlled clinical trial using venous phlebography. Acta Chir. Scand. *129*:500, 1965.

Boys, J. E., and Norman, P. F.: Accidental subdural analgesia. Brit. J. Anaesth. *47*:1111, 1975.

Brennecke, M. A.: Personal communication, 1966.

Bridenbaugh, L. D., Moore, D. C., Bagdi, P., and Bridenbaugh, P. O.: The position of plastic tubing in continous block-techniques: An X-ray study of 552 patients. Anesthesiology *29*:1047, 1968.

Bromage, P. R.: Spinal Epidural Analgesia. Edinburgh, E. & S. Livingstone, Ltd., 1954, pp. 92, 102, 117.

Bromage, P. R.: Concentrations of lignocaine in the blood after intravenous, intramuscular, epidural and endotracheal administration. Anaesthesia *16*:461, 1961.

Bromage, P. R.: A comparison of the hydrochloride and carbon dioxide salts of lidocaine and prilocaine in epidural analgesia. Acta Anaesth. Scand. (Suppl.) *16*:55, 1965.

Bromage, P. R.: A comparison of bupivacaine and tetracaine in epidural analgesia for surgery. Canad. Anaesth. Soc. J. *16*:37, 1969.

Bromage, P. R., and Burfoot, M. F.: Quality of epidural blockade. II. Influence of physico-chemical factors: Hyaluronidase and potassium. Brit. J. Anaesth. *38*:857, 1966.

Bromage, P. R., Burfoot, M. F., Crowell, D. E., and Truant, A. P.: Quality of epidural blockade. III. Carbonated local anaesthetic solutions. Brit. J. Anaesth. *39*:197, 1967.

Bromage, P. R., Pettigrew, R. T., and Crowell, D. E.: Tachyphylaxis in epidural analgesia. I. Augmentation and decay of local anesthesia. J. Clin. Pharmacol. *9*:30, 1969.

Bromage, P. R., O'Beirn, P., and Dunford, L. A.: Etidocaine: A clinical evaluation for regional analgesia in surgery. Canad. Anaesth. Soc. J. *21*:523, 1974.

Bronge, A., Dahlgren, S., and Lindquist, B.: Prophylaxis against thrombosis in femoral neck fractures: A comparison between dextran 70 and dicumarol. Acta Chir. Scand. *137*:29, 1971.

Browse, N. L.: Effect of surgery on resting calf blood flow. Brit. Med. J. *1*:1714, 1962.

Browse, N. L., and Negus, D.: Prevention of postoperative leg vein thrombosis by electrical muscle stimulation. An evaluation with ^{125}I-labelled fibrinogen. Brit. Med. J. *3*:615, 1970.

Browse, N. L., Jackson, B. T., Mayo, E., and Negus, D.: The value of mechanical methods of preventing postoperative calf vein thrombosis. Brit. J. Surg. *61*:219. 1974.

Burke, D. T., Porter, K. S., and Sansom, L. N.: A problem when ampoules are opened. Med. J. Aust. *2*:1128, 1972.

Burn, J. M. B.: A method of continuous epidural analgesia. Anaesthesia *18*:78, 1963.

Butler, A. E., and Green, C. D.: Haematoma following epidural anaesthesia. Canad. Anaesth. Soc. J. *17*:635, 1970.

Butterfield, W. I. H., et al.: Effect of aspirin on postoperative venous thrombosis. Report of the Steering Committee of a trial sponsored by the Medical Research Council. Lancet *2*:441, 1972.

Calnan, J. S., and Allenby, F.: The prevention of deep vein thrombosis after surgery. Brit. J. Anaesth. *47*:151, 1975.

Calnan, J. S., Pflug, J. J., and Mills, C. J.: Pneumatic intermittent-compression legging simulating calf-muscle pump. Lancet *2*:502, 1970.

Carr, M. F., and Hehre, F. W.: Complications of continuous lumbar peridural anesthesia. I. Inadvertent lumbar puncture. Anesth. Analg. *41*:349, 1962.

Chumnijarakij, T., and Poshyachinda, V.: Postoperative thrombosis in Thai women. Lancet *1*:1357, 1975.

Chun, L., and Karp, M.: Unusual complications from placement of catheters in caudal canal in obstetrical anesthesia. Anesthesiology *27*:96, 1966.

Clark, C., and Cotton, L. T.: Blood-flow in deep veins of leg. Recording technique and evaluation of methods to increase flow during operation. Brit. J. Surg. *55*:211, 1968.
Clark, W. B., MacGregor, A. B., Prescott, R. J., and Ruckley, C. V.: Pneumatic compression of the calf and postoperative deep-vein thrombosis. Lancet *2*:5, 1974.
Climie, C. R.: Shield for epidural catheters. Anaesthesia *15*:331, 1960.
Cohen, C. A., and Kallos, T.: Failure of spinal anesthesia due to subdural catheter placement. Anesthesiology *37*:352, 1972.
Cooke, E. D., Lloyd, M. J., Bowcock, S. A., and Pilcher, M. F.: Monitoring during low-dose heparin prophylaxis. New Eng. J. Med. *294*:1066, 1976.
Coon, W. W., and Coller, F. A.: Clinicopathologic correlation in thromboembolism. Surg. Gynecol. Obstet. *109*:259, 1959.
Cousins, M. J.: Hematoma following epidural block. Anesthesiology *37*:263, 1972.
Cousins, M. J., and Wright, C. J.: Graft, muscle, skin blood flow after epidural block in vascular surgical procedures. Surg. Gynecol. Obstet. *133*:59, 1971.
Cox, J. M. R., and Spoerel, W. E.: Continuous epidural analgesia—The use of an intermittent injection device. Canad. Med. Assoc. J. *11*:72, 1964.
Crawford, J. S., Williams, M. E., and Veales, S.: Particulate matter in the extradural space. Brit. J. Anaesth. *47*:807, 1975.
Curbelo, M. M.: Continuous peridural segmental anesthesia by means of a ureteral catheter. Curr. Res. Anesth. Analg. *28*:13, 1949.
Dawkins, C. J. M.: An analysis of the complications of extradural and caudal block. Anaesthesia *24*:554, 1969.
De Angelis, J.: Hazards of subdural and epidural anesthesia during anticoagulant therapy: A case report and review. Anesth. Analg. *51*:676, 1972.
Denson, K. W. E., and Bonnar, J.: The measurement of heparin. A method based on the potentiation of anti-factor Xa. Thrombos. Diathes. Haemorrh. (Stuttg.) *30*:471, 1973.
Doran, F. S. A., Drury, M., and Sivyer, A.: A simple way to combat the venous stasis which occurs in the lower limbs during surgical operations. Brit. J. Surg. *51*:486, 1964.
Doran, F. S. A., White, M., and Drury, M.: A clinical trial designed to test the relative value of two simple methods of reducing the risk of venous stasis in the lower limbs during surgical operations, the danger of thrombosis, and a subsequent pulmonary embolus, with a survey of the problem. Brit. J. Surg. *57*:20, 1970.
Duncalf, D., and Foldes, F. F.: The use of radio-iodinated serum albumin to confirm accidental intravascular insertion of epidural catheters. Anesthesiology *25*:564, 1964.
Dyde, J. A., and Bethel, A. N.: The effect of intermittent positive-pressure respiration on the speed of blood-flow in the deep veins of the lower limb. Brit. J. Surg. *55*:917, 1968.
Editorial: Low-dose heparin and the prevention of venous thromboembolic disease. Brit. Med. J. *2*:477, 1975.
Edmonds-Seal, J.: An overdose of lignocaine: A case report on epidural analgesia for post-operative pain. Anaesthesia *19*:222, 1964.
Evans, D. S.: The early diagnosis of deep-vein thrombosis by ultrasound. Brit. J. Surg. *57*:726, 1970.
Evans, D. S.: The early diagnosis of thrombo-embolism by ultrasound. Ann. Roy. Coll. Surg. Eng. *49*:225, 1971.
Flanc, C., Kakkar, V. V., and Clarke, M. B.: The detection of venous thrombosis of the legs using ^{125}I-labelled fibrinogen. Brit. J. Surg. *55*:742, 1968.
Frumin, M. J., and Schwartz, H.: Continuous segmental peridural anesthesia. Anesthesiology *13*:488, 1952.
Furgang, F. A.: Glass particles in ampoules. Anesthesiology *41*:525, 1974.
Gallus, A. S., Hirsh, J., and Gent, M.: Relevance of preoperative and postoperative blood tests to postoperative leg-vein thrombosis. Lancet *2*:805, 1973a.
Gallus, A. S., et al.: Small subcutaneous doses of heparin in prevention of venous thrombosis. New Eng. J. Med. *288*:545, 1973b.
Gingrich, T. F.: Spinal epidural hematoma following continuous epidural anesthesia. Anesthesiology *29*:162, 1968.
Godal, H. C.: Quantitative and qualitative changes in fibrinogen following major surgical operations. Acta Med. Scand. *171*:687, 1962.
Gold, M. E.: Spontaneous spinal epidural hematoma. Radiology *80*:823, 1963.
Gordon-Smith, J. C., Grundy, D. J., LeQuesne, L. P., Newcombe, J., and Bramble, F. J.: Controlled trial of two regimes of subcutaneous heparin in the prevention of postoperative deep vein thrombosis. Lancet *1*:1133, 1972.
Grant, F. C.: Epidural spinal abscess. J.A.M.A. *128*:509, 1945.
Griffiths, D. P. G., Diamond, A. W., and Cameron, J. D.: Postoperative extradural analgesia following thoracic surgery: A feasibility study. Brit. J. Anaesth. *47*:48, 1975.
Haeger, K.: Den klinska trombosdiagnosens (o) tillförlitlighet. Läkartidnningen *64*:1067, 1965.

Hamelberg, W., Siddall, J., and Claassen, L.: Perforation of dura by a plastic catheter during continuous caudal anesthesia. A.M.A. Arch. Surg. *78*:357, 1959.
Ham, J. M., and Slack, W. W.: The effect of small doses of heparin on platelet adhesiveness and lipoprotein-lipase activity before and after operation. Brit. J. Surg. *55*:227, 1968.
Harrison, R. J., and Tomlinson, J. D. W.: Observations on the venous system in certain Pinnipedia and Cetacea. Proc. Zool. Soc. Lond. *126*:205, 1956.
Hehre, F. W., Sayig, J. M., and Lowman, R. M.: Etiological aspects of failure of continuous lumbar peridural anesthesia. Anesth. Analg. *39*:511, 1960.
Henderson, E. F.: Fatal pulmonary embolism. A statistical review. Arch. Surg. *15*:231, 1927.
Hills, N. H., Pflug, J. J., Jeyasingh, K., Boardman, L., and Calnan, J. S.: Prevention of deep vein thrombosis by intermittent pneumatic compression of calf. Brit. Med. J. *1*:131, 1972.
Hingson, R. A., and Southworth, J. L.: Continuous caudal anesthesia. Amer. J. Surg. *58*:93, 1942.
Hodgson, D. C.: Venous stasis during surgery. Anaesthesia *19*:96, 1964.
Holmdahl, M., Sjögren, S., Ström, G., and Wright, B.: Clinical aspects of continuous epidural blockade for postoperative pain relief. Uppsala J. Med. Sci. *77*:47, 1972.
Hylton, R. R., Eger, E. I., and Rovno, S. H.: Intravascular placement of epidural catheters. Anesth. Analg. *43*:379, 1964.
Ilké, A.: L'anesthésie péridurale continue en obstétrique. Technique spéciale et expériences personelles. Rev. Franc. Gynecol. Obstet. *47*:185, 1952.
Jacobson, I., McCabe, J. J., Harris, P., and Dott, N. M.: Spontaneous spinal epidural haemorrhage during anticoagulant therapy. Brit. Med. J. *1*:522, 1966.
Johnsson, S. R., Bygdeman, S., and Eliasson, R.: Effect of dextran on postoperative thrombosis. Acta Chir. Scand. (Suppl.) *387*:80, 1968.
Johnston, K. W., Kakkar, V. V., Spindler, J. J., Corrigan, T. P., and Fossard, D. P.: A simple method for detecting deep vein thrombosis. An improved electrical impedance technic. Amer. J. Surg. *127*:349, 1974.
Jones, M. D., and Newton, T. H.: Inadvertent extra-arachnoid injections in myelography. Radiology *80*:818, 1963.
Kakkar, V. V., et al.: Deep vein thrombosis of the leg. Is there a "high risk" group? Amer. J. Surg. *120*:527, 1970.
Kakkar, V. V., Field, E. S., Nicolaides, A. N., and Flute, P. T.: Low doses of heparin in prevention of deep-vein thrombosis. Lancet *2*:669, 1971.
Kakkar, V. V., et al.: Efficacy of low doses of heparin in prevention of deep vein thrombosis after major surgery. A double-blind, randomised trial. Lancet *2*:101, 1972.
Kakkar, V. V., et al.: Prevention of fatal postoperative pulmonary embolism by low doses of heparin. An international multicentre trial. Lancet *2*:45, 1975.
Kalas, D. B., and Hehre, F. W.: Continuous lumbar peridural anesthesia in obstetrics. VIII. Further observations on inadvertent lumbar puncture. Anesth. Analg. *51*:192, 1972.
Katz, H., Borden, H., and Hirscher, D.: Glass-particle contamination of color-break ampoules. Anesthesiology *39*:354, 1973.
Kemble, J. V. H., and Hickman, J. A.: Postoperative changes in blood viscosity and the influence of haematocrit and plasma fibrinogen. Brit. J. Surg. *59*:629, 1972.
Lebeaux, M. I.: Experimental epidural anesthesia in the dog with lignocaine and bupivacaine. Brit. J. Anaesth. *45*:549, 1973.
Lerner, S., Gutterman, P., and Jenkins, F.: Epidural hematoma and paraplegia after numerous lumbar punctures. Anesthesiology *39*:550, 1973.
Love, J. G.: Continuous subarachnoid drainage for meningitis by means of a ureteral catheter. J.A.M.A. *104*:1595, 1935.
Manalan, S. A.: Caudal block anesthesia in obstetrics. J. Indiana Med. Assoc. *35*:564, 1942.
Matouskova, A., Dottori, O., Forssman, L., and Victorin, L.: An improved method of epidural analgesia with reduced instrumental delivery rate. Acta Obstet. Gynecol. Scand. *54*:231, 1975.
Miller, S. P., Sanchez-Avalos, J., Stefanski, T., and Zuckerman, L.: Coagulation disorders in cancer. I. Clinical and laboratory studies. Cancer *20*:1462, 1967.
Moir, D. D., and Hesson, W. R.: Dural puncture by an epidural catheter. Anaesthesia *20*:373, 1965.
Moir, D. D., and Willocks, J.: Epidural analgesia in British obstetrics. Brit. J. Anaesth. *40*:129, 1968.
Muneyuki, M., Shirai, K., and Inamoto, A.: Roentgenographic analysis of the positions of catheters in the epidural space. Anesthesiology *33*:19, 1970.
Mustard, J. F., Murphy, E. A., Rowsell, H. C., and Downie, H. G.: Factors influencing thrombus formation in vivo. Ann. J. Med. *33*:621, 1962.
Negus, D., Pinto, D. J., and Le Quesne, L. P.: ^{125}I-labelled fibrinogen in the diagnosis of deep-vein thrombosis and its correlation with phlebography. Brit. J. Surg. *55*:835, 1968.
Nicholson, M. J.: Complication associated with use of extradural catheter in obstetric anesthesia. Anesth. Analg. *44*:245, 1965.

Nicolaides, A. N., et al.: Small doses of subcutaneous sodium heparin in the prevention of deep vein thrombosis after elective hip operations. Brit. J. Surg. *62*:348, 1975.
Nylander, G.: Phlebographic diagnosis of acute deep leg thrombosis. Acta Chir. Scand. (Suppl.) *387*:30, 1968.
Osborn, S. B., and Wright, H. P.: Method of estimating time at which counting rate changes, using Geiger-Müller counter. Brit. J. Radiol. *22*:110, 1949.
Paterson, J. C., and McLachlin, J.: Precipitating factors in venous thrombosis. Surg. Gynecol. Obstet. *98*:96, 1954.
Powley, J. M., and Doran, F. S. A.: Galvanic stimulation to prevent deep-vein thrombosis. Lancet *1*:406, 1973.
Roberts, V. C.: Thrombosis and how to prevent it. New Scientist and Science Journal, 16 September 620, 1971.
Roberts, V. C.: Fibrinogen uptake scanning for diagnosis of deep vein thrombosis: A plea for standardization. Brit. Med. J. *3*:455, 1975.
Roberts, V. C., and Cotton, L.: Positive pressure circulatory assist devices for the leg. *In* Roberts, C. (ed.): Blood Flow Measurements. Baltimore, The Williams & Wilkins Company, 1972, p. 115.
Roberts, V. C., and Cotton, L. T.: Prevention of postoperative deep vein thrombosis in patients with malignant disease. Brit. Med. J. *1*:358, 1974.
Roberts, V. C., and Cotton, L. T.: Failure of low-dose heparin to improve efficacy of peroperative intermittent calf compression in preventing postoperative deep vein thrombosis. Brit. Med. J. *3*:458, 1975.
Rosenberg, I. L., Evans, M., and Pollock, A. V.: Prophylaxis of postoperative leg vein thrombosis by low dose subcutaneous heparin or peroperative calf muscle stimulation: A controlled clinical trial. Brit. Med. J. *1*:649, 1975.
Rosenberg, R. D.: Heparin action. Circulation *49*:603, 1974.
Rosengarten, D. S., Laird, J., Jeyasingh, K., and Martin, P.: The failure of compression stockings (Tubigrip) to prevent deep vein thrombosis after operation. Brit. J. Surg. *57*:296, 1970.
Ryan, D. W.: Accidental intravenous injection of bupivacaine: A complication of obstetrical anaesthesia. Brit. J. Anaesth. *45*:907, 1973.
Sabri, S., Roberts, V. C., and Cotton, L. T.: Prevention of early postoperative deep vein thrombosis by passive exercises of leg during surgery. Brit. Med. J. *3*:82, 1971a.
Sabri, S., Roberts, V. C., and Cotton, L. T.: Prevention of early postoperative deep vein thrombosis by intermittent compression of the leg during surgery. Brit. Med. J. *4*:394, 1971b.
Sanchez, A., Acũna, L., and Rocha, F.: An analysis of the radiological visualization of the catheters placed in the epidural space. Brit. J. Anaesth. *39*:485, 1967.
Schultz, E. H., and Brogdon, B. G.: The problem of subdural placement in myelography. Radiology *79*:91, 1962.
Scott, D. B., and Walker, L. R.: Administration of continuous epidural analgesia. Anaesthesia *18*:82, 1963.
Sechzer, P. H.: Subdural space in spinal anaesthesia. Anesthesiology *24*:869, 1963.
Sevitt, S.: Venous thrombosis and pulmonary embolism. Their prevention by oral anticoagulants. Am. J. Med. *33*:703, 1962.
Shanks, C. A.: Four cases of unilateral analgesia. Brit. J. Anaesth. *40*:999, 1968.
Sharnoff, J. G.: Results in the prophylaxis of postoperative thromboembolism. Surg. Gynecol. Obstet. *123*:303, 1966.
Sharnoff, J. G., and DeBlasio, G.: Prevention of fatal postoperative thromboembolism by heparin prophylaxis. Lancet *2*:1006, 1970.
Sharnoff, J. G., Kass, H. H., and Mistica, B. M.: A plan of heparinization of the surgical patient to prevent postoperative thromboembolism. Surg. Gynecol. Obstet. *115*:75, 1962.
Sharp, J. T., Henry, J. P., Sweany, S. K., Meadows, W. R., and Pietros, R. J.: The total work of breathing in normal and obese men. J. Clin. Invest. *43*:728, 1964.
Sigel, B., Edelstein, A. L., Felix, W. R., and Memhardt, C. R.: Compression of the deep venous system of the lower leg during inactive recumbency. Arch. Surg. *106*:38, 1973.
Singh, A.: Unilateral epidural analgesia: Case report. Anaesthesia *22*:147, 1967.
Sjögren, S., and Wright, B.: Circulation, respiration and lidocaine concentration during continuous epidural blockade. Acta Anaesth. Scand. *16* (Suppl. 46):5, 1972.
Snell, A. M.: Relation of obesity to fatal postoperative pulmonary embolism. Arch. Surg. *15*:237, 1927.
Sproul, E. E.: Carcinoma and venous thrombosis: Frequency of carcinoma in body or tail of pancreas with multiple venous thrombosis. Am. J. Cancer 34:566, 1938.
Spurning, O. M.: Spinal epidural hematoma—Two cases. Arch. Int. Med. *114*:103, 1964.
Sreerama, V., Ivan, L. P., Dennery, J. M., and Richard, M. T.: Neurosurgical complications of anticoagulant therapy. Canad. Med. Assoc. J. *108*:305, 1973.

Sripad, S., Antcliff, A. C., and Martin, P.: Deep-vein thrombosis in two district hospitals in Essex. Brit. J. Surg. *58*:563, 1971.

Thistlethwaite, R. J., Edison, T. G., Gruenwald, C., and Harrison, I.: Experiences with epidural analgesia for sympathetic block. Surgery *33*:818, 1953.

Tuohy, E. B.: Continuous spinal anesthesia: A new method of utilising a ureteral catheter. Surg. Clin. N. Amer. 25 August 1945, p. 834.

Turco, S. J., and Davis, N. M.: Glass particles in intravenous injections. New. Eng. J. Med. *287*:1204, 1972.

Usubiaga, J. E., Reis, A. D., and Usubiaga, L. E.: Epidural misplacement of catheters and mechanisms of unilateral blockade. Anesthesiology *32*:158, 1970.

Virchow, R. L. K.: Gesammelte Abhandlungen zur Wissenschaftlichen Medicin. von Meidinger Sohn u. Comp. Frankfurt a.M., 1856.

Wessler, S., and Yin, E. T.: Theory and practice of minidose heparin in surgical patients. Circulation *47*:671, 1973.

Wheeler, H. B., and Mullick, S. C.: Detection of venous obstruction in the leg by measurement of electrical impedance. Ann. N.Y. Acad. Sci. *170*:804, 1970.

Wheeler, H. B., Pearson, D., O'Connell, D., and Mullick, S. C.: Impedance phlebography. Technique, interpretation and results. Arch. Surg. *104*:164, 1972.

Williams, H. T.: Prevention of postoperative deep-vein thrombosis with perioperative subcutaneous heparin. Lancet *2*:950, 1971.

Winer, B. N., Horenstein, S., and Starr, A. M.: Spinal epidural hematoma during anticoagulant therapy. Circulation *19*:735, 1959.

Wright, H. P., Osborn, S. B., and Edmonds, D. G.: Rate of flow of venous blood in the legs measured with radioactive sodium. Lancet *2*:767, 1948.

Yao, S. T., Gourmos, G., and Hobbs, J. T.: Detection of proximal-vein thrombosis by Doppler ultrasound. Lancet *1*:1, 1972.

Yin, E. T., Wessler, S., and Butler, J. V.: Plasma heparin: A unique, practical, submicrogramsensitive assay. J. Lab. Clin. Med. *81*:298, 1973.

Youngman, H. R.: Toxic reactions in epidural anesthesia. Anesthesiology *17*:632, 1956.

chapter 8
Caudal Analgesia

. . . 'fatis accede deisque,' that men do not only turn with the occasions, but also run with the occasions, and not strain their credit or strength to over-hard or extreme points; but choose in their action that which is most passable: for this will preserve men from foil.

Sir Francis Bacon
Apophthegms, 1605

INTRODUCTION

The discovery of caudal epidural analgesia or sacral anesthesia antedated the lumbar approach by several years (Cathelin, 1901, 1903), but the technique has not enjoyed consistent popularity. Desultory articles on sacral anesthesia appeared during the first two decades of the century, mainly by authors in Germany and North America (Stoeckel, 1919; Läwen, 1910; Schlimpert, 1913; Lewis and Bartels, 1916; Thompson, 1917). Most of these early investigators concentrated on the clinical aspects of the technique without paying much attention to basic underlying principles, although Thompson (1917) pointed out the difficulties that arose from the bewildering variety of types and shapes of sacral bones encountered in an apparently normal population. Formal anatomical and injection studies with tracer substances did not develop until the third decade of this century. Then, a number of authors began to investigate the dispersion of colored and radiopaque solutions injected into the caudal canal, and all of them observed wide variations of spread (Brenner, 1924; Clay Shaw, 1926; Elliott, 1926; Grodinsky and Best, 1929). The technique seemed basically unpredictable, and little enthusiasm was generated during the next 15 years.

The greatest resurgence of caudal analgesia occurred in the early 1940's when Hingson and his colleagues (1943) popularized caudal blockade for pain relief in childbirth, but this renewal of interest was short-lived as the lumbar approach became more popular. Perhaps one of the most discouraging practical aspects of caudal analgesia is the frequent difficulty encountered in identifying the sacral hiatus and in performing a successful caudal puncture. Easy cases are very easy, but difficult cases can be impossible, and an overall technical failure rate of 5 to 10 per cent is to be expected in most hands. Such a high incidence of clinical unreliability is not acceptable in ordinary practice. To avoid disappointment, patients should be selected prudently, after careful examination and palpation of the sacral region to make sure that only the technically easy cases are chosen, while the difficult ones are rejected in favor of the lumbar approach.

As we have seen earlier in Chapter 4, lumbar epidural analgesia spreads upward more easily than downward, and reluctance to pass the lumbosacral junction is associated with relatively poor analgesia of the fifth lumbar and first sacral segments subserving the outer border of the foot and ankle, unless powerful local anesthetic agents are used. The alternative approach to the extradural space through the sacral hiatus has the advantage that it gives precedence to these obstinate segments and allows injected local anesthetic solutions to bathe the sacral nerves before extending upward to areas that are more easily reached by the lumbar epidural route.

Caudal analgesia is a useful option for relief of acute or chronic pain involving the lumbosacral segments, and it is sometimes a more appropriate choice than the lumbar approach. During the past 15 years interest has been renewed in pediatric caudal anesthesia by a group of Brazilian anesthesiologists, and their favorable reports have led to a more widespread use of the technique in children (Spiegel, 1962; Fortuna, 1967). In practice, the average anesthesiologist will probably find that he does not resort to caudal analgesia very often, but the following sections will outline the factors that influence his choice of technique. One important practical point has already been mentioned and it should be reemphasized. Because caudal analgesia is often technically difficult, the *overall* failure rate exceeds 5 per cent, even in the best hands. No procedure or practitioner can survive this inherent degree of inefficiency. The key to technical success is obvious, and that is to exercise unashamed common sense in selecting cases. The caudal approach should be avoided altogether unless the anatomy is easy or unless there are compelling clinical reasons for using it instead of the lumbar approach. With this very biased but practical method of selection, the failure rate can be reduced to less than 1 per cent.

ANATOMY

A stroll among the skeletons of any anatomy department will reveal the rich variety of contours surrounding the sacral hiatus. In childhood, sacral topography usually conforms to the ideal description found in anatomy textbooks. The cornua are neatly symmetrical in most cases, flanking a clearly defined hiatus, and during life the margins are easily palpated under tissues that are supple and thin. Overlying integuments thicken and blur the hiatal margins as age advances, however, and inequalities of growth may narrow, flatten or skew the original pattern. In fat or osteoarthritic patients, the hiatal margins often defy recognition by even the most skillful fingertips, and then luck must bolster judgment. With these inherent anatomical difficulties, it is really no surprise that the technical failure rate is so high.

The practical problems of caudal analgesia are mainly referable to the wide anatomical variations in size, shape and orientation of the sacral bone. These anatomical variations may be summarized as follows (from an extensive study by Doctor Mildred Trotter in 1947):

1. *Size and position of sacral hiatus.* The hiatus may be almost closed, asymmetrical or widely open owing to anomalies in the pattern of fusion of the

laminae of the sacral arches. Sacral spina bifida occurs in about 2 per cent of males and 0.3 per cent of females (Trotter, 1947). Figures 8–1 to 8–3 show a small sample of normal and abnormal sacral hiatuses.

2. *Anteroposterior depth of sacral canal.* This may vary from less than 2 mm to more than 1 cm. Differences of depth can be appreciated from the mid-line sections of sacral bones shown in Figure 8–4.

3. *Lateral width of sacral canal.* Lead casts of the sacral canal show that the lateral width varies widely (Trotter, 1947).

4. *Volume of sacral canal.* Since the depth and the width vary widely, it follows that the volume of the canal will also vary widely. Trotter (1947) found that sacral volumes varied fivefold, with a range between 12 ml and 65 ml (Table 8–1).

5. *Size and patency of sacral foramina.* The sacral foramina afford anatomical escape routes for injected solutions, and the size of these exits also varies over a large range. The posterior sacral foramina are effectively sealed by the multifidus and sacrospinal muscles, but the anterior foramina are unob-

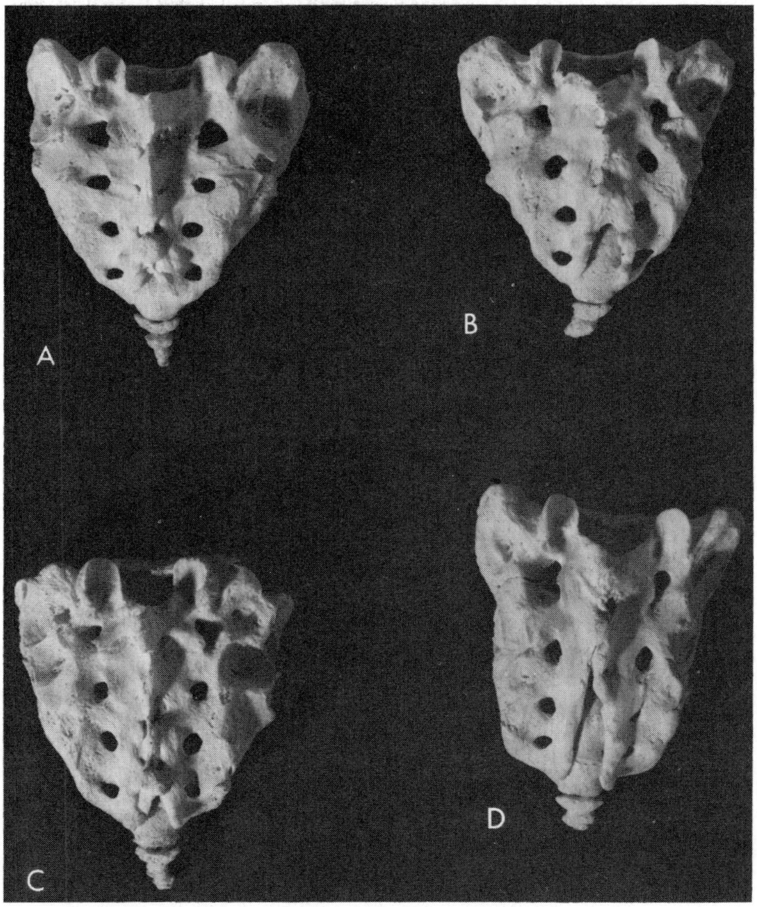

Figure 8–1. Four variations of sacral hiatus. *A*, Normal and symmetrical. *B*, Partial narrowing of hiatus. *C*, Spina bifida of S_4. *D*, Spina bifida of S_4 and S_3.

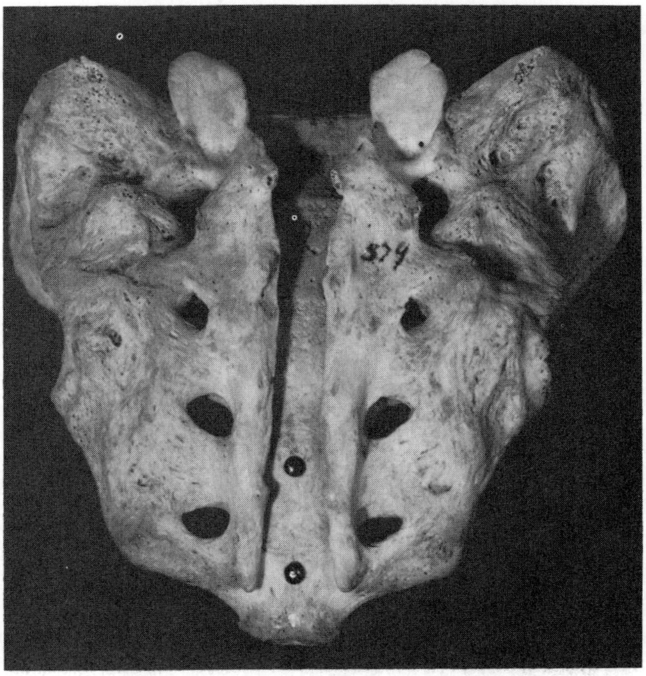

Figure 8–2. Spina bifida of all sacral laminae.

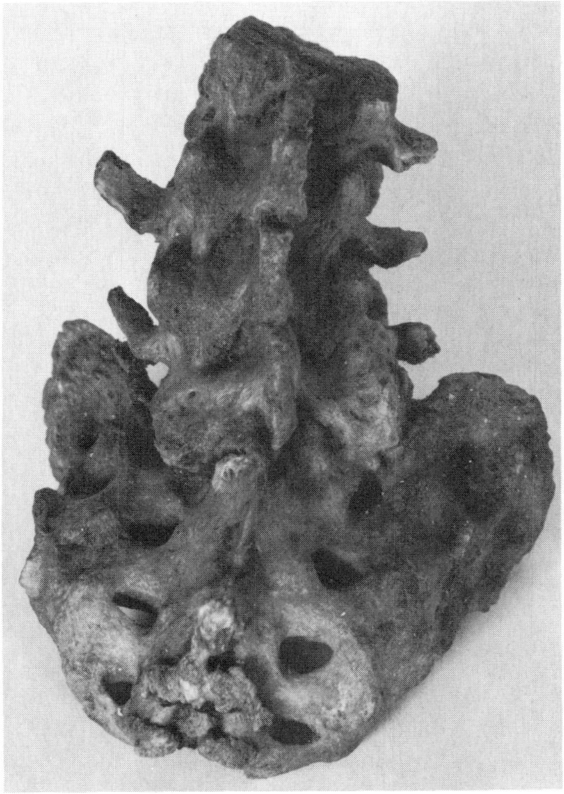

Figure 8–3. A difficult back. Stenosis of sacral hiatus combined with "kissing" vertebral spines, left-sided sacralization of the fifth lumbar vertebra and consequent scoliosis, and obliteration of the L_5–S_1 interspinous space.

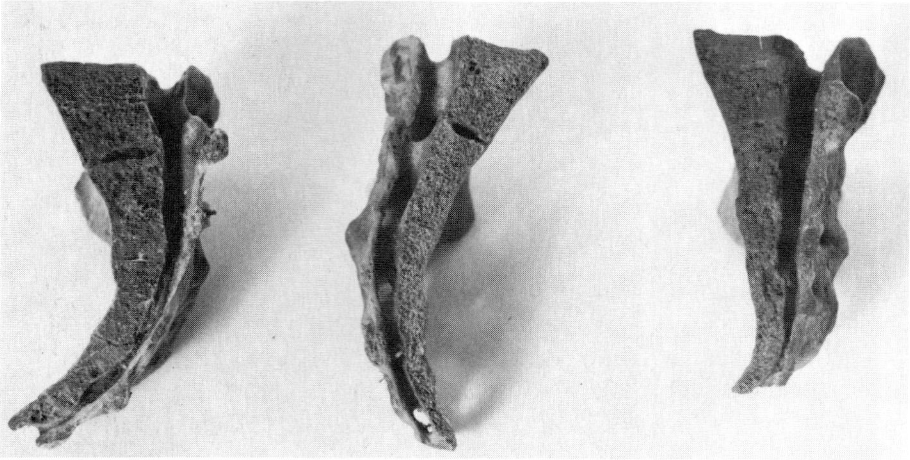

Figure 8–4. Sagittal sections of three sacral bones, showing differences of anteroposterior depth of the canal and variations of curvature.

structed by muscles and ligaments, and solutions may flow through them unhindered (Bryce-Smith, 1954).

6. *Curvature of the sacral canal.* The sacral curvature varies widely (Brenner, 1924) and tends to be more pronounced in males than in females. Hence, when a caudal puncture is being performed, a straight, rigid needle is more likely to pass easily along the canal in females than in males.

7. *Degree of lordosis and size of lumbosacral angle.* The angle between the axis of the lumbar canal and the sacral canal may vary between 7 degrees in subjects with very flat lumbosacral angles and 70 degrees in subjects with marked lordosis. Bryce-Smith (1954) has postulated that the cephalad flow of caudal solutions will tend to be more obstructed in lordotic patients with exaggerated lumbosacral angles than in patients with flatter lumbosacral angles, in whom the axes of the sacral and lumbar canals are more closely aligned.

TABLE 8–1 Sacral Canal: Range of Certain Measurements Relevant to Caudal Analgesia*

		Range	
Observation	***Mean***	*LOWER*	*UPPER*
Tip of dural sac (spinal level)	Midpoint of S_2	Midpoint of S_3	Midpoint of S_1
Upper rim of sacral hiatus (spinal level)	Lower third of S_4	Lower border of S_5	Unfused sacral arch in 1.1% of cases
Net distance between tip of dural sac and upper edge of sacral hiatus	45 mm	16 mm	75 mm
Anteroposterior diameter of sacral hiatus	5.5 mm	<2 mm in 5% of cases	–
Volume of sacral canal	33 ml	12 ml	65 ml

*From Trotter, M., Anesth. Analg. *26*:192, 1947.

8. *Character and consistency of epidural fat.* The character of epidural fat changes with age in animals and in man. During childhood the epidural fat has a loose and wide-meshed texture, but in adults it becomes more firmly packed and fibrous (Tretjakoff, 1926, von Lüdinghausen, 1967). Schulte-Steinberg (1976) has suggested that these changes may be partly responsible for the transition from the free and predictable mode of caudal spread that occurs in children to the limited and unpredictable segmental spread seen in adults.

The gross anatomy of the sacral region was reviewed by Trotter (1947), and a summary of her findings from 1,227 sacral bones is shown in Table 8–1. From a clinical point of view, one of the most important measurements is the distance between the bottom of the dural sac and the top of the sacral hiatus. The tip of the dura usually ends opposite the middle of the second sacral vertebra, on a level with the posterior inferior iliac spines, but it may end as high as the middle of the first sacral vertebra or as low as the third. In addition, the level of the upper edge of the sacral hiatus also varies widely. Thus, the net distance between the tip of the dura and the upper edge of the sacral hiatus is highly variable and not very predictable. It is this net distance that is of clinical importance in avoiding accidental dural puncture during caudal injection. In a series of 53 cadavers Trotter found that this distance between the upper edge of the sacral hiatus and the tip of the dura lay anywhere in the range of 16 mm to 75 mm—a fivefold difference between the shortest and longest extremes—as shown diagrammatically in Figure 8–5. In a larger series the range would be even wider, since complete spina bifida of the sacral canal has an incidence of 1 per cent, so the true range should run between 0 and 75 mm.

Two other measurements in Table 8–1 require comment. First, it can be seen that in about 5 per cent of the population the anteroposterior diameter of the sacral canal may be too small to admit anything larger than a 21-gauge needle. In these subjects a continuous technique would be impossible, and reliance must be placed on a single-shot injection with a small needle. Second, the wide range of capacity of the sacral canal between the extremes of 12 ml and 65 ml adds an important element of uncertainty to the physical spread of injected solutions within the adult sacral canal.

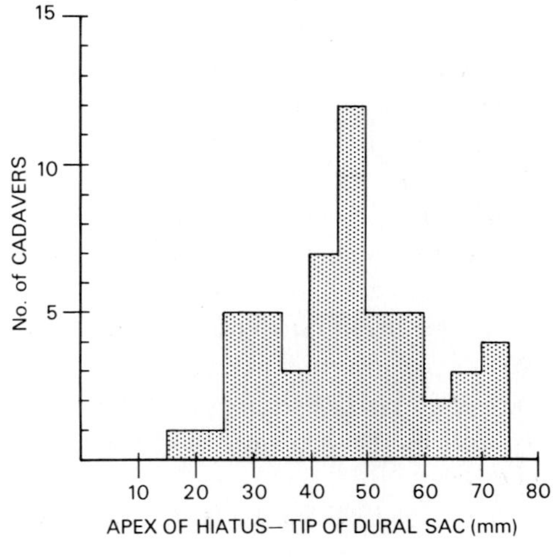

Figure 8–5. Variability of net distance between upper edge of sacral hiatus and caudal tip of dural sac in 53 cadavers. (Data from Trotter, 1947.)

Infants and young children before the age of puberty, and lean adults are usually very easy subjects for caudal puncture, and an acceptable success rate of 98 to 100 per cent can be expected if the method is confined to this selected and anatomically favored population. Unfortunately, clinical indications, and especially therapeutic indications for relief of chronic pain, often include patients with difficult caudal landmarks; then the lumbar approach to the extradural canal should be considered as a practical alternative.

PRACTICAL TECHNIQUE

Palpation, identification and puncture are most easily carried out with the patient lying prone, and a pillow placed under the pelvis to produce slight flexion of the hips. The toes should be turned inward to relax the gluteal muscles and simplify palpation. If, for clinical reasons, the patient cannot be placed prone, puncture may have to be performed in the lateral position with the hips fully flexed, but the procedure is technically more difficult and less certain to be successful when attempted in the lateral position.

Figure 8–6 shows a patient lying prone with the contours of the sacral hiatus marked with a skin pencil. The following clues are important for accurate identification of the hiatus:

1. *Surface markings.* Although skin folds are never completely reliable, the buttock skin folds provide a useful hint to the location of the underlying hiatus. In Figure 8–6 note that the two buttock folds lead medially toward the underlying hiatus, and the point where their extension crosses the midline is usually directly over the sacrococcygeal membrane. In the lateral postion, gravity drags the skin folds away to one side, and then this useful landmark becomes distorted and unreliable.

2. *The coccyx.* The left forefinger is placed on the tip of the coccyx in the natal cleft, while the thumb of the same hand feels for the two sacral cornua 3 to 4 cm more rostrally at the upper end of the natal cleft. The thumb should sink into the slight hollow between the two cornua as if between two knuckles of a fist. This point may be marked with a skin pencil before preparing to perform the block.

The skin is prepared with 0.5 per cent or 1 per cent iodine in spirit, taking care to avoid an excess of the solution running down onto the perineum, as tincture of iodine is painful on glabrous skin in the conscious patient. A sterile swab pushed well into the natal cleft from above will act as a satisfactory sponge to soak up any drips of iodine solution and prevent them from reaching the sensitive skin of the perineum. Iodophors such as povidone-iodine are favored antiseptics in this situation, as they are painless on sensitive skin and their antiseptic efficacy is almost as good as 1 per cent tincture of iodine.

A small skin wheal of local anesthetic is raised over the sacrococcygeal membrane, using a 25-gauge needle, and a few drops are infiltrated on the surface of the membrane. Generous infiltration should be avoided in this situation, as anything more than a few drops of local anesthetic may obscure anatomical landmarks and increase the technical difficulties of inserting the caudal needle.

The needle is directed through the sacral hiatus at an angle of about

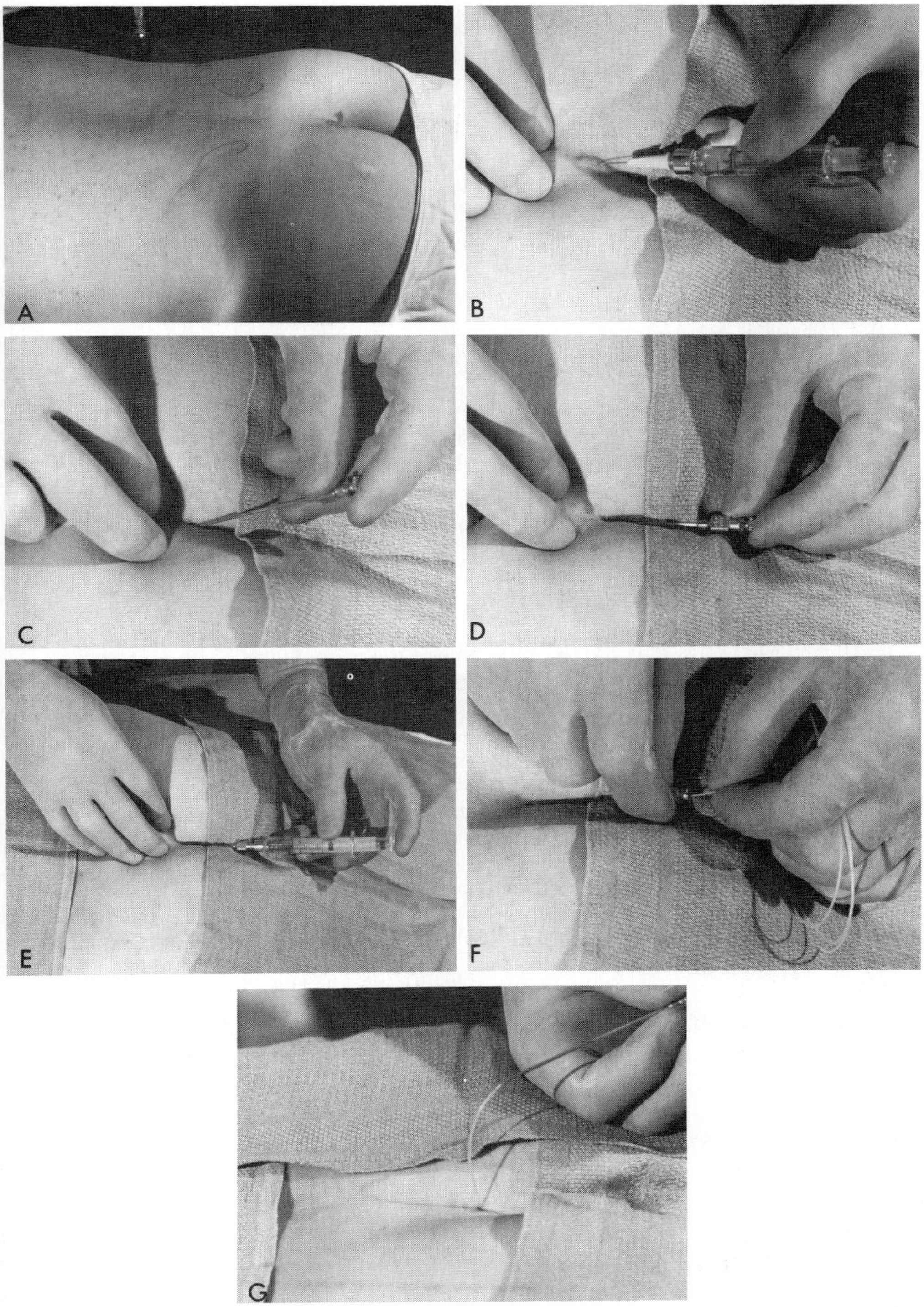

Figure 8–6. Steps in continuous caudal blockade. *A*, Patient prone. Contours of sacral hiatus and posterior superior iliac spines have been marked by skin pencil. (Scars are from previous laminectomy and spinal fusion.) *B*, Skin wheal over sacral hiatus. *C*, Insertion of Tuohy needle through sacrococcygeal membrane. *D*, Depression of needle shaft and advance into sacral canal. *E*, Test injection into caudal canal. *F*, Threading epidural catheter through Tuohy needle. *G*, Withdrawal of Tuohy needle, catheter being left in caudal canal.

120 degrees to the back. The needle tip can be felt to pierce the sacrococcygeal membrane with a slight snap, and the point then comes to lie in the sacral canal. The needle must now be depressed, both at the hub and at the point where it pierces the skin (by means of a finger pressing down on the shaft), and the shaft is advanced about 1.5 cm into the sacral canal.

If the needle has been introduced correctly, it is possible to swing the hub from side to side quite easily while the shaft is held like a fulcrum at the sacrococcygeal membrane, and the tip moves freely in the sacral canal. Injection through the needle is now as easy as into an empty space.

SINGLE INJECTION

There is no need to use a large needle for single injections. A 25-gauge needle is sufficient for infants, and a 23- or 22-gauge for adults.

As in any regional anesthetic technique, *never advance the needle to the full length of the shaft.* When needles break, they usually do so at the junction of the shaft and hub, and if the broken shaft is entirely buried in the tissues, a surgical operation becomes necessary to retrieve the broken piece.

Difficulties and Complications

MALPLACEMENT OF THE NEEDLE

The commonest malplacements of the needle are:

1. *Superficial to the sacrum.* The needle point slides over the posterior aspect of the sacrum and fails to enter the canal. Lateral movements of the needle tip can be felt through the skin over the sacrum, unless the needle is actually under the periosteum, in which case lateral movements are almost impossible owing to fixation of the needle.

2. *Under periosteum of sacral canal.* The needle tip may impinge on the periosteum of the posterior wall of the canal so that further advance or injection is impossible. The needle should be withdrawn slightly, rotated on its axis and gently reinserted in a slightly different direction.

3. *Anterior to sacrum.* Occasionally, the needle may be forced between the sacrum and the coccyx so that it lies anterior to the sacrum. It is then in danger of perforating the rectum—or, during parturition, the baby's head. In fact, this unlikely accident of fetal cranial puncture has been recorded on four occasions, with fatal results to the baby in two of them (Finster et al., 1965; Sinclair et al., 1965). The possibility of this grave accident makes caudal puncture a hazardous and unsuitable procedure for obstetrical pain relief, once the presenting part has descended to the perineum (Bonica, 1967).

INTRAVENOUS AND INTRAOSSEUS INJECTION

The sacral canal, like the rest of the epidural space, is rich in veins, and inadvertent venous puncture has been reported to occur in about 0.6 per cent of cases (Dawkins, 1969).

The cortical layer of sacral bone is often quite thin, especially in infants and in old subjects, and puncture of the cancellous bone is relatively easy in these patients, especially if a little force is used. The sensation of entering cancellous bone is not unlike that of penetrating the sacrococcygeal membrane and entering the sacral canal: a feeling of resistance is suddenly overcome and the needle advances more freely, and subsequent injection is unhampered. However, careful aspiration will produce some blood-stained aspirate which, on microscopy, will show immature blood cells. This hazard was described by DiGiovanni in 1971, and in the following year McGown (1972) reported four cases of accidental marrow puncture in 700 caudal injections (i.e., approximately 0.6 per cent). Injected solutions are absorbed extremely rapidly from bone marrow, and toxic reactions occur very readily if local anesthetic solutions are forced into the intramedullary cavity. Aspiration of viscous marrow fluid may be difficult through a narrow lumen, so the hazard of unrecognized intraosseous injection and toxic reaction is greatest when fine needles are used.

Aspiration tests are carried out with a 2-ml syringe once the correct position of the needle has been verified, and a test dose of solution is injected, followed by a waiting period of a few minutes. The full dose of local anesthetic is then injected if no signs of spinal anesthesia or toxic reaction have developed.

The needle is then withdrawn and the patient placed in a supine position; however, if the caudal is being given for pain relief in labor, the patient should be placed on her side (see Chapter 12). A sterile dressing is not usually necessary over the puncture site if a single-shot injection is made with a fine needle.

DURAL PUNCTURE

Care should be taken that the needle is not advanced more than 2 cm into the sacral canal so that the dura is not penetrated. As already stated, the dural sac usually ends at the lower border of the second sacral vertebra (the surface marking of this is about 1 cm below the posterior superior iliac spines). However, on rare occasions the dura extends lower than this, as illustrated by the following case of massive subarachnoid block.

A man of 68 years was given caudal analgesia for hemorrhoidectomy. The theca extended to an abnormally low position, and cerebrospinal fluid was tapped after the caudal needle had been advanced only 2 cm. The needle was withdrawn until cerebrospinal fluid ceased to flow (the point was then only just within the sacrococcygeal membrane), and 25 ml of 0.2 per cent tetracaine solution were injected slowly without a preliminary test dose. All the signs of a total spinal block followed. Blood pressure was maintained with a pressor drug, and ventilation was supported manually for 30 minutes until spontaneous respiration returned. The patient made an uninterrupted recovery.

This case illustrates two points. First, the need to be constantly aware that the dural sac *may* extend abnormally far down into the sacral canal. Second, that a test dose through the needle is prudent in single-shot injections, especially if there is any doubt at all about the correct placement of the needle.

CONTINUOUS CAUDAL

A straight-tipped, wide-bore needle or a Huber-tipped Tuohy needle may be used to pass a catheter into the caudal canal. Personally, I prefer a Tuohy needle for this purpose, as the ski-like tip finds its way into the caudal canal with less tendency to become snagged on the sacral periosteum. If a Tuohy needle is chosen, the tip is inserted with the shoulder anteriorly and its orifice dorsally. Once the tip has penetrated the sacrococcygeal membrane, the shaft is depressed and advanced with a rotary movement to turn the orifice through 180 degrees until it is facing anteriorly. The rounded tip then glides easily along the posterior wall of the caudal canal.

A catheter is inserted gently for 2 to 3 cm beyond the tip of the needle, and the needle is then withdrawn over the catheter. A 23-gauge needle is inserted into the free end of the catheter, and aspiration tests are performed to exclude the presence of blood or cerebrospinal fluid. A small test dose of 3 to 4 ml of local anesthetic is now injected up the catheter. A sterile gauze dressing is placed over the puncture site, and the catheter is sealed in place with adhesive tape. The catheter is taped along the back and over one shoulder for easy access and for repeated injections. The patient is then turned supine, and the remainder of the induction dose is injected through the catheter.

The following modification of the usual caudal technique has been described by Owens, Slater and Battit (1973), and it is recommended because it avoids some of the difficulties and dangers of the technique just outlined. After the usual landmarks are identified, caudal puncture is made with a standard 16-gauge intravascular 2.5-inch Teflon cannula and needle stylet instead of a regular epidural needle. The composite unit is advanced for about 1 to 1.5 cm into the sacral canal; the inner needle stylet is then withdrawn about 0.5 cm within the plastic cannula, and the assembly is then advanced again for about 3 cm with the blunt atraumatic tip of the plastic cannula leading. The inner stylet is then withdrawn completely (Fig. 8–7). A test dose of the appropriate anesthetic solution is given, followed by the full induction dose, after a suitable waiting period to evaluate the results of the test dose. The plastic cannula has an internal bore that is wide enough to accept a standard epidural catheter. If a continuous technique is planned, a sterile epidural catheter is threaded through the cannula for a distance of 2 to 3 cm beyond the tip, and the cannula is then removed over the epidural catheter, leaving the catheter in place in the usual way (Fig. 8–8).

This technique has several advantages:

1. The stylet-cannula assembly is advanced for a very short distance, and the main advance into the sacral canal is performed by the soft, blunt cannula, so that risks of dural puncture, or fetal scalp perforation in labor, are eliminated.

2. Perforation of sacral cortex and intracancellous injection is less likely than with a rigid needle.

3. Confirmation of correct placement is simplified. The Teflon cannula advances very easily and painlessly when properly placed within the sacral canal, but it is very difficult or impossible to advance if incorrectly placed in tissues overlying the sacrum.

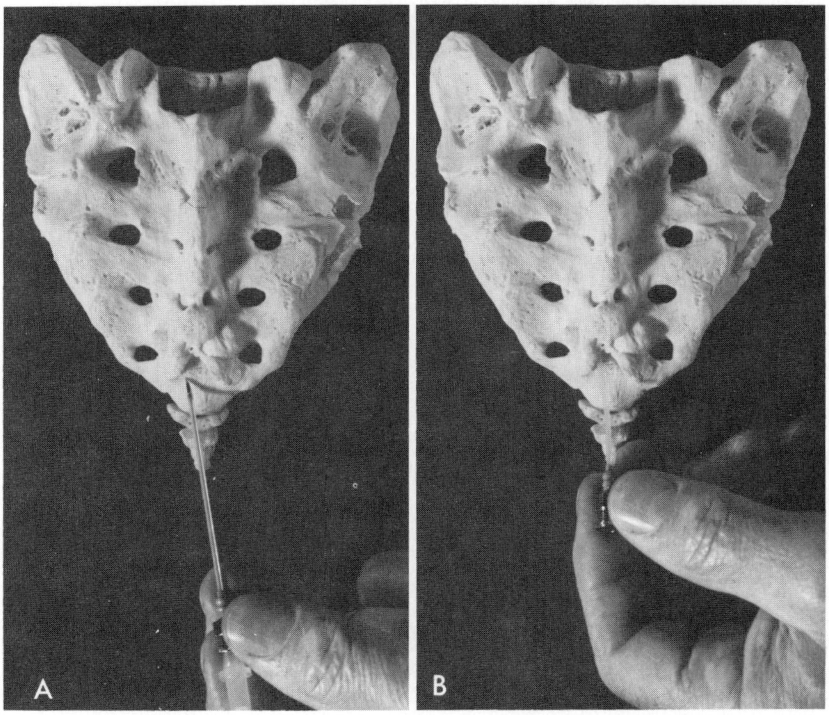

Figure 8–7. *A*, Plastic intravenous cannula and needle-stylet ready for insertion into the sacral hiatus. *B*, Teflon cannula inserted in caudal canal with needle-stylet withdrawn.

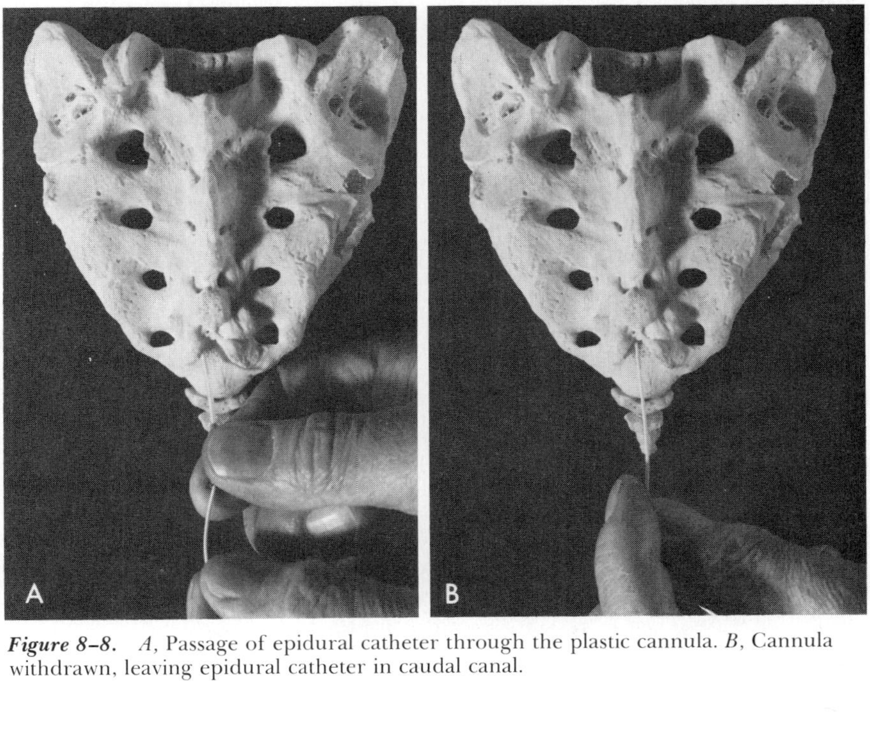

Figure 8–8. *A*, Passage of epidural catheter through the plastic cannula. *B*, Cannula withdrawn, leaving epidural catheter in caudal canal.

Dural Perforation by Caudal Catheter

Some authorities recommend threading a caudal catheter upward for 8 to 12 cm until the tip lies at the lumbosacral junction, in order to reduce the volume of solution required to produce a block to the umbilicus (Bonica, 1967). However, it must be remembered that this incurs a remote risk of perforating the dura, and a careful test dose should always be made through the catheter before the main dose is injected. The following case summary described by Hamelberg et al. (1959) illustrates this point:

A 60-year-old man received caudal analgesia for repair of bilateral inguinal hernia. Caudal puncture was performed with an 18-gauge thin-walled needle, and a test dose of 4 ml of 1 per cent lidocaine was injected through the needle. A blunt-ended plastic catheter was then inserted for 4 cm beyond the tip of the needle, and 10 ml of 1 per cent lidocaine were injected up the catheter. One minute later analgesia extended up to T_{10}. Thirty minutes later a second injection of 10 ml of 1 per cent lidocaine resulted in hypotension and respiratory insufficiency requiring resuscitation. Cerebrospinal fluid was aspirated from the catheter, and X-ray examination revealed the tip of the catheter lying in the subarachnoid space near the lumbosacral junction.

DOSE REQUIREMENTS AND SEGMENTAL SPREAD OF ANALGESIA IN CAUDAL BLOCKADE

At puberty the pelvis enlarges markedly, and the sacrum takes part in the general development that occurs. In addition, the epidural fat seems to undergo a form of compaction and increased fibrous content in the lumbosacral region that hinders the upward spread of solutions from the caudal part of the epidural space. Before puberty, segmental dose requirements are highly correlated with age and are very predictable (Schulte-Steinberg and Rahlfs, 1970, 1977). After puberty predictability is lost, and in contrast to lumbar epidural blockade, segmental spread of caudal analgesia varies widely in accordance with the great individual differences of sacral anatomy already discussed.

The large capacity of the sacral canal accommodates correspondingly large volumes of analgesic solution, varying amounts of which are lost through the wide anterior sacral foramina. Thus, extradural dose requirements via the sacral canal are inherently large compared with the relatively small volumes needed by the lumbar epidural route; as a rough guide, the doses for caudal analgesia in adults are about twice those for lumbar blockade.

Adults

The lack of correlation between dose requirements and age for single-dose caudal injections of lidocaine hydrochloride and carbonated lidocaine in a series of patients over 20 years of age is shown in Figure 8–9. The wide scatter around the means reflects the gross unpredictability of segmental spread in adults (Cousins and Bromage, 1971).

Table 8–2, based on clinical experience, gives an approximate indication of caudal dose requirements in adults, with the mean segmental dose for

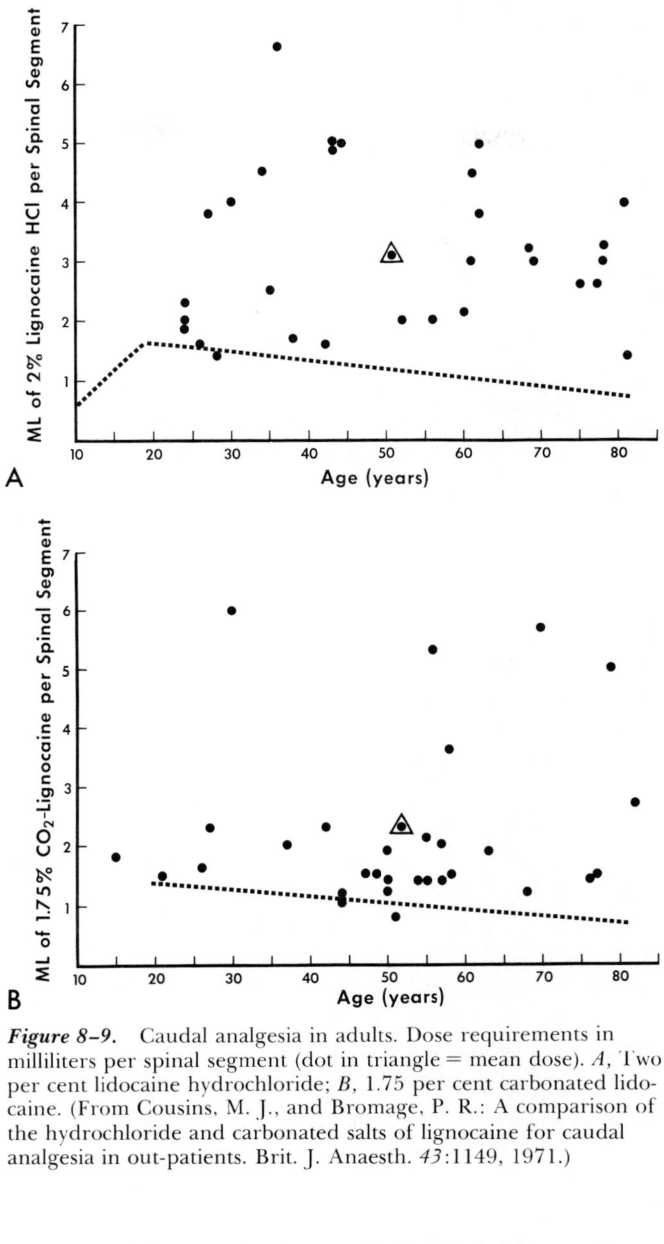

Figure 8–9. Caudal analgesia in adults. Dose requirements in milliliters per spinal segment (dot in triangle = mean dose). *A,* Two per cent lidocaine hydrochloride; *B,* 1.75 per cent carbonated lidocaine. (From Cousins, M. J., and Bromage, P. R.: A comparison of the hydrochloride and carbonated salts of lignocaine for caudal analgesia in out-patients. Brit. J. Anaesth. *43*:1149, 1971.)

TABLE 8–2 Caudal Analgesia in Adults: Approximate Dose Requirements and Range of Segmental Spread Following a Single-shot Injection of 20 ml

Solution	*Mean Segmental Dose Requirements (ml/segment)*	*Upper Limit of Analgesia*	
		AVERAGE	*RANGE*
2% Lidocaine HCl + epinephrine 1/200,000	3.1	L_4–L_5	S_2–T_8
1.75 CO_2-Lidocaine + epinephrine 1/200,000	2.3	L_2–L_3	S_1–T_4
0.5% Bupivacaine + epinephrine 1/200,000	3.0	L_4–L_5	S_2–T_8
1% Etidocaine + epinephrine 1/200,000	3.0	L_4–L_5	S_2–T_8
3% Plain prilocaine	2.2 (10 ml)	S_1–L_5	S_2–T_{10}

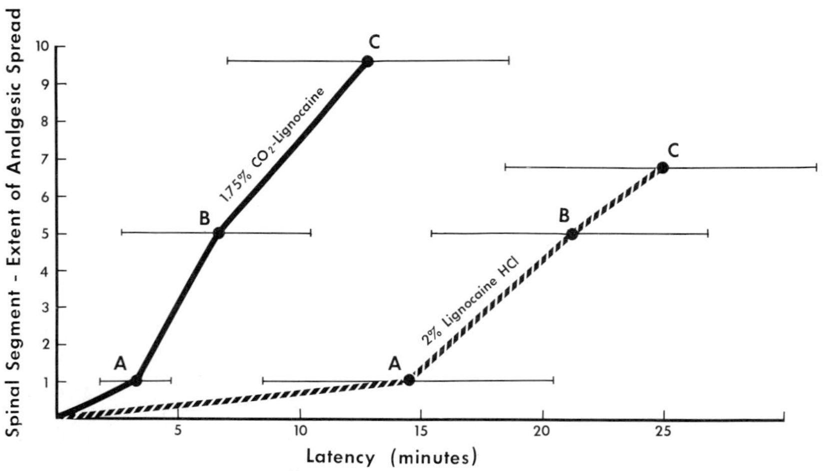

Figure 8–10. Latency of onset and spread of analgesia for hydrochloride and carbonated base salts of 2 per cent lidocaine; mean (min) ± S.D. (From Cousins, M. J., and Bromage, P. R.: A comparison of the hydrochloride and carbonated salts of lignocaine for caudal analgesia in out-patients. Brit. J. Anaesth. *43*:1149, 1971.)

lidocaine, prilocaine, bupivacaine and etidocaine. Since age is not correlated with caudal segmental spread in adults, the upper level of analgesia resulting from a 20-ml dose of any of these solutions will vary widely and may come to lie anywhere between the second sacral and the eighth thoracic dermatome.

Not only does the caudal route demand more drug than the lumbar route, but also analgesia takes longer to spread. Figure 8–10 shows the mean latency profiles for lidocaine hydrochloride and carbonated lidocaine by the caudal route. Both agents take appreciably longer to achieve full segmental spread than by the lumbar route. From these data one can appreciate that although caudal analgesia is admirably suited to produce effective block of the sacral and lower limb segments, it is not a logical way to obtain analgesia of more rostral segments supplying the abdomen *in adults*. The doses required for abdominal surgery are disproportionately large and their effects unpredictable, and the waiting time for full blockade is long compared with induction by the lumbar approach.

Children

Schulte-Steinberg and his colleagues have obtained consistent data for segmental spread of caudal analgesia in infants and children between the ages of 7 weeks and 12 years, using 1 per cent lidocaine with 1/100,000 epinephrine, or 0.25 per cent bupivacaine (Schulte-Steinberg and Rahlfs, 1970, 1972, 1977; Schulte-Steinberg, 1976). These authors examined the statistical influence of age, weight and height on caudal dose requirements before puberty and found that the relationship of spread to age was very different in children and adults. Instead of the unpredictable relationship to age that is seen in adults, the pattern of spread proved to be highly predictable in children. The relationship between age and dose requirements was strictly linear, with a high degree of

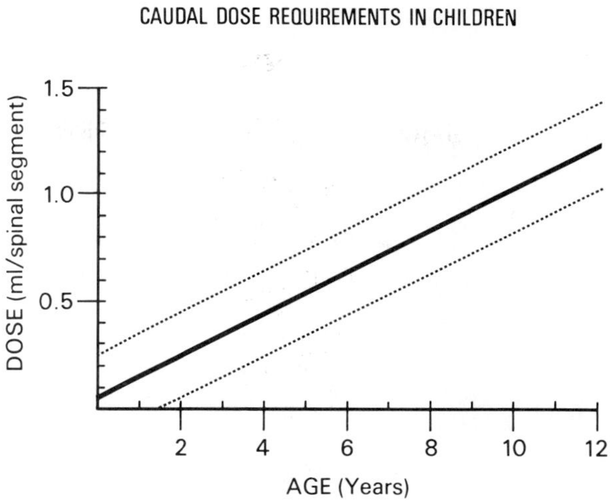

Figure 8–11. Caudal analgesia in children. Segmental dose requirements related to age for 1 per cent lidocaine or 0.25 per cent bupivacaine, showing mean ± 1.96 × S.D. (After Schulte-Steinberg and Rahlfs, 1970, and Schulte-Steinberg, 1976.)

correlation up to the age of 12 years. In these young patients the dose requirements were approximately 0.1 ml per segmental per year for 1 per cent lidocaine or for 0.25 per cent bupivacaine, as shown in Figure 8–11. On this scale the dose required to produce analgesia up to the umbilicus (i.e., 13 segments) in a 10-year-old child would be:

0.1 × 13 × 10 = 13 ml, 1 per cent lidocaine *or* 0.25 per cent bupivacaine

These findings suggest that the upward spread of caudal solutions in children is not hampered by the same anatomical constraints that develop from puberty onward. Before puberty, anatomical impedance at the lumbosacral junction has not yet developed to a marked degree, and caudal solutions can flow freely upward into the higher reaches of the spinal canal. As a consequence, rostral spread of caudal analgesia is more extensive and more predictable in children than in adults.

Table 8–3 summarizes Schulte-Steinberg's data for dose requirements in pediatric caudal analgesia, together with my own data for duration of action. The duration of action for both lidocaine and bupivacaine is relatively short in these young patients compared to adults. Total duration of action in the lower sacral segments is considerably longer than the duration to beginning of recession, and perineal analgesia may persist for four to five hours after caudal block with bupivacaine and epinephrine.

TABLE 8–3 Approximate Dose Range and Duration of Action of 1% Lidocaine and 0.25% Bupivacaine for Caudal Analgesia in Children

			Duration (minutes) to 2 Segments Recession	
Drug	***Dose Range (mg/kg/segment)***	***Maximum Single-shot Dose (mg/kg)***	*PLAIN*	*+ EPINEPHRINE 1/200,000*
1% Lidocaine	1.0	10	40–50	70–100
0.25% Bupivacaine	0.25	2.5	120	150

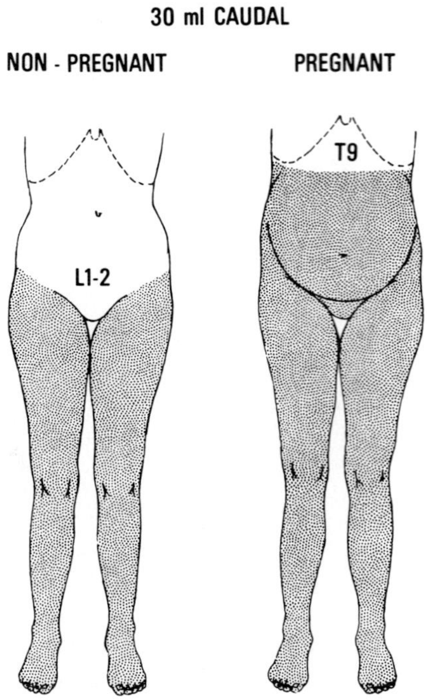

Figure 8–12. Segmental levels of analgesia in pregnant and nonpregnant patients. (After Crawford and Chester, 1949.)

Pregnancy

The sacral canal shares in the general engorgement of extradural veins that occurs during late pregnancy, and indeed in any other clinical condition in which the inferior vena cava is partially obstructed (see Chapter 5 on Epidural Pressures). Crawford and Chester (1949) observed that the effective volume of the caudal canal appears to be markedly diminished during later pregnancy, and they recommended that caudal dosage should be reduced proportionately in women at term. These authors reported a substantial increase of segmental analgesic spread in pregnant women at term. They found that 30 ml of caudal anesthetic seldom produced analgesia above the first lumbar segment in normal, nonpregnant patients, whereas in parturient patients the segmental level rose four or five segments higher, to the eighth or ninth thoracic segment (Fig. 8–12). This difference represented a 40 to 50 per cent increase in segmental spread, or, in other words, a 28 to 33 per cent decrease of dose requirements in pregnant women at term.*

Crawford and Chester's important observation escaped general notice at the time, and more than a decade passed before the principle of diminished dose requirements at term was confirmed for the lumbar approach to the epidural space (Bromage, 1961).

---

*In case these percentages appear incongruous, the reader is reminded that "segmental spread" as such is recorded independently of dosage, whereas "dose requirements" are expressed as the fraction: dose/segmental spread. Thus, in Crawford and Chester's series term pregnancy increased average segmental spread from 10 dermatomes to 14 or 15 dermatomes, that is, 40 to 50 per cent. However, dose requirements (ml/seg) were decreased from 30/10 or 3 ml/segment to 30/14 to 30/15, or 2.143 to 2 ml/segment, that is, 28.6 to 33.3 per cent.

Recently, attention has again been drawn to the very extensive segmental spread of some modalities of epidural blockade that must be anticipated in pregnant women at term when injection is made by either the lumbar route (Evans et al., 1975) or the caudal approach. Horner's syndrome has been noted as a fairly frequent occurrence when large doses of local anesthetic are injected into the caudal canal during labor. Kepes and his colleagues (1972) described a case of high unilateral spread of analgesia and Horner's syndrome on the dependent side after 22 ml of 3 per cent chloroprocaine were given for relief of labor pain. In this case the patient was turned on to her back immediately after the caudal injection was completed.

Epidural spread is likely to be most exaggerated if injection is made when the mother is lying on her back (see Chapters 2 and 12), for then obstruction of the inferior vena cava is greatest, and as a consequence the spinal epidural veins are maximally engorged. Mohan and Potter (1975) described 17 cases in which signs of unilateral or bilateral paralysis of the ophthalmic sympathetic arose in a consecutive series of 20 women receiving caudal anesthesia for labor. The doses of local anesthetic were large but not excessive, in the range of 12 to 20 ml of 0.5 per cent bupivacaine. However, in this series all the women were lying in the dorsal position when they received their caudal injections through indwelling catheters. Once again, this is an example of a lesson that must be emphasized: epidural dosage, whether by the lumbar or the caudal route, should be kept to a minimum in patients at term, and injections should *not* be made when the patient is in such a position that the inferior vena cava is likely to be occluded. Failure to observe these two simple rules will inevitably give rise to a significant incidence of very high segmental blocks.

CLINICAL APPLICATIONS OF CAUDAL ANALGESIA

Bearing in mind the inherent technical difficulties of the technique and its relative inefficiency in terms of large dose requirements, the practical applications of caudal analgesia are somewhat limited. Easy subjects or situations in which extensive segmental blockade is unimportant constitute the chief indications for its use. Pediatric surgery on the lower limb, perineal surgery in adults, if the sacral anatomy is easy, and therapeutic blocks for chronic lower limb or perineal pain compose the main repertoire. Caudal blockade is seldom the best choice for obstetrical analgesia, but occasionally it may be indicated in selected cases (see Chapter 12).

Adult Surgery

Perineal surgery provides the main indication for caudal analgesia in adults. Also, severe postoperative pain following perineal surgery under general anesthesia may be effectively relieved by a small caudal injection carried out in the recovery ward. Some patients emerging from general anesthesia after hemorrhoidectomy have severe pain, restlessness and hypotension. Centrally acting narcotics seem to have little effect on this distressing clinical situation, and male patients may become difficult to manage, particularly if they are powerfully built. Under these circumstances a quick single-shot caudal produces a dramatic change, and within 6 or 7 minutes the patient is calm, cooperative and resting comfortably, with his arterial blood pressure restored to normal.

Once again, I stress the admonition to avoid caudal analgesia in favor of the lumbar approach whenever possible, *unless the puncture is technically easy.* Single-shot caudal injections are suitable for short procedures, or to overcome the immediate reflex effects of overwhelming postoperative pain. An indwelling catheter inserted through an 18-gauge Tuohy needle or a 16-gauge Teflon intravenous cannula is more appropriate for long procedures.

Plain prilocaine (Citanest) in 3 per cent solution is a useful agent for single-shot postoperative caudal injections. It has a lower acute toxicity than lidocaine, and this advantage is well suited to a technique that requires relatively large doses for satisfactory clinical results.

Prolonged analgesia with an indwelling catheter in the caudal canal gives an opportunity to adjust dosage by adding successive increments of local anesthetic until the level of analgesia is brought up to the desired segment. Intermittent dosage is managed in the same way as for lumbar epidural block; that is, about half the original dose is injected at regular intervals of 75 minutes for lidocaine with epinephrine, and at intervals of 120 minutes for bupivacaine. Because of the large amounts of local anesthetic that are given with each caudal injection, particular attention should be paid to the possibility of toxic reactions. Blood concentrations rise to increasingly high peaks after each successive injection; cumulative doses are larger and peak blood concentrations higher than during continuous lumbar block (Moore et al., 1968).

Pediatric Surgery

Infants and children are technically ideal subjects for caudal analgesia (Spiegel, 1962, 1976; Fortuna, 1967; Touloukian, 1971; Lourey and McDonald, 1973; Kosaka, 1975). The hiatus is readily felt, and puncture is easily done with a small needle. By the age of four or five years the sacral canal is usually large enough to accept an 18-gauge thin-walled needle for passage of a catheter, if prolonged blockade is required.

Schulte-Steinberg's formula is a useful guide in calculating dosage, that is about 1.0 mg of lidocaine per segment per year of age, using 1 per cent lidocaine. A strength of 1/200,000 epinephrine appears to be adequate for a satisfactory quality of blockade in these cases, and it is recommended as preferable to the higher concentration of 1/100,000 used by Schulte-Steinberg. For longer lasting blocks, bupivacaine in a dose of 0.25 mg per segment per year may be used in 0.25 per cent concentration, with or without epinephrine.

Young children and infants do not take kindly to injections in their caudal region, and heavy premedication or a small dose of intravenous barbiturate or intramuscular ketamine may be needed to insert the needle under tranquil conditions. The needle point should not be advanced more than a few millimeters beyond the sacrococcygeal ligament, as the dural sac extends lower in children than in adults, and accidental subarachnoid injection may occur if the needle is pushed too far. The usual precautions of aspiration must be followed to exclude intravascular or subarachnoid injection, and the solution is then injected at a rate of about 0.5 to 1 ml per second.

It is wise to have an intravenous infusion running in case of accidents. My own practice is to give a small dose of intramuscular ketamine (about 2 mg/kg) when the child arrives in the induction room. Five minutes later when the patient is asleep, the intravenous infusion is set up before caudal analgesia is induced. Intelligent and well-disciplined children over six years of age will often cooperate remarkably well without premedication, provided the anesthesiologist has already won their confidence by a full and sympathetic explanation of everything the child will experience, and provided the technique is gentle and impeccable. There is no excuse for forcing regional anesthesia on a terrified struggling child, and it is better to resort to central sedation rather than physical force if the patient is frightened or reluctant.

The dose administered must be kept within the safe therapeutic limits of 10 mg/kg lidocaine or 2.5 mg/kg bupivacaine. The technique is not appropriate for upper abdominal surgery. It must be remembered that the dose required by caudal injection is twice that needed by the lumbar route, and attempts to extend analgesia upward beyond the fifth and sixth thoracic segments will almost inevitably involve quantities of drug that are likely to cause undesirably high blood concentrations of local anesthetic. Dose range and duration of action of lidocaine and bupivacaine for caudal analgesia in children are summarized in Table 8–3.

With these reservations, caudal analgesia has wide applications for general and orthopedic surgery below the diaphragm in children. Central venous pressure remains low under a combination of caudal block and light general anesthesia with spontaneous respiration, and operative bleeding is markedly reduced. For example, in surgery of the hip, such as innominate osteotomy, blood loss and transfusion requirements are about 50 per cent less than under general anesthesia with muscle relaxants and intermittent positive pressure ventilation. This advantage also makes caudal analgesia an excellent choice for major perineal operations in young children and infants. Anesthetic management is technically simple, while surgical bleeding is minimal and the patients are remarkably comfortable in the postoperative period (Touloukian et al., 1971; Kosaka, 1975).

Minor outpatient surgery, such as circumcision, is very well suited to a single-shot caudal block with bupivacaine. The patient leaves the hospital in a comfortable and cooperative state, and the lingering postoperative analgesia makes home management easy for the parents and pleasant for the patient (Kay, 1974).

Obstetrical Applications

Caudal analgesia is still used extensively in some centers for relief of pain in labor (Moore et al., 1971), but more and more evidence is accumulating that caudal analgesia, compared to the lumbar approach, is a poor choice in obstetrics. The basic objection is one of dosage. All drugs administered to the mother eventually cross the placenta and find their way into the fetus to a greater or lesser degree. High fetal concentrations of local anesthetic make for "floppy but alert" babies who may score relatively well on the Apgar scale, but who show a poorer reflex performance by more sophisticated criteria such as the Brazelton scale (Scanlon et al., 1974). The caudal route requires more than twice as much local anesthetic as does the lumbar route to achieve adequate analgesia in first and second stage labor, and this is poor economy from the baby's point of view, since fetal accumulation of local anesthetic will be proportionately higher under caudal blockade.

In addition, there are anatomical objections. First, as already pointed out, the technical difficulty of locating and identifying the caudal canal gives rise to an unacceptably high failure rate of more than 5 per cent. Second, puncture is made in an area that is prone to soiling by feces and meconium, and it is difficult to maintain the sterility of an indwelling catheter throughout labor. Lastly, a rare complication has been reported of misdirected caudal needles, with accidental injection of local anesthetic into the fetal head instead of into the caudal canal (Finster et al., 1965; Sinclair et al., 1965). This particular disaster can only occur after the baby's head has descended to the perineum, when the fetal scalp is just beneath the sacrum and the coccyx. So as a general rule, if caudal analgesia is to be used at all, it should be induced before the head has reached the perineum (Bonica, 1967).

TECHNIQUE

Puncture and insertion of the caudal catheter should be done early in labor, while the fetal head is high and before severe pain and restlessness hamper technique. In thin women the lateral position may be satisfactory, but in most cases the knee-elbow position gives clearer landmarks and more favorable conditions for caudal puncture.

The usual precautionary test dose of local anesthetic is given after the epidural catheter is inserted and before the main induction dose is injected. Large volumes are needed to reach as high as T_{10} and to give adequate relief of pain during the first stage of labor. About 25 to 30 ml of 1 per cent lidocaine or 0.375 per cent bupivacaine are required for the induction dose. A somewhat smaller volume of 20 ml may be sufficient if the catheter has been threaded upward so that the tip lies at the level of L_5 to S_1 (Bonica, 1967). However, this maneuver increases the risk of accidental dural puncture, so it is safer to halt the catheter below the tip of the dura, at the level of the third sacral vertebra (Hamelberg et al., 1959).

Repeat doses for maintenance of blockade are given every 60 to 75 minutes with lidocaine, and every 90 to 100 minutes with bupivacaine. Volumes of about one-third less than the induction dose are usually sufficient to maintain an adequate level of analgesia. With this technique perineal anesthesia is usually profound, and there is marked loss of motor power in the legs.

TWO-CATHETER TECHNIQUE

Undesirably large amounts of local anesthetic are required when caudal anesthesia alone is used for labor and delivery. However, a two-catheter technique described by Cleland (1949) reduces cumulative dosage to a minimum. With Cleland's method, one catheter is inserted in the upper lumbar region, and the second catheter is placed in the caudal canal. Test doses are given through both catheters, but only the upper (lumbar) catheter is used during the first stage of labor to provide analgesia in the segmental distribution of T_{10} to L_2. The second (caudal) catheter is held in reserve for the second stage and for delivery. When delivery is imminent, a small dose of local anesthetic—about 8 ml of 2 per cent lidocaine or 3 per cent chloroprocaine—is given through the lower catheter to produce a limited blockade of the sacral segments innervating the perineal area.

This technique is a logical approach to the problem of using minimal dosage to interrupt the required spinal segments at the most appropriate time, and at first sight it seems an ideal solution. However, the practical disadvantages are very real. Two continuous conduction techniques are required instead of one, and each must be technically impeccable to succeed in the primary aim of minimal dosage. Unfortunately, the inherent technical difficulties of caudal puncture still intrude upon this ideal concept, and in practice the chances of technical failure and associated hazards are doubled by using a double-catheter technique. In most instances a more reliable compromise can be reached by using a single lumbar epidural catheter, as described more fully in Chapter 12.

Caudal blockade can be adopted for cesarean section if large enough volumes of anesthetic are injected to force the upper level of analgesia as high as T_6. However, in the light of what has already been said about the effects of excessive dosage on the infant, this could clearly be an inappropriate tour de force and an abuse of the method. Caudal analgesia is not recommended as a primary technique for cesarean section.

Chronic Pain Relief

The caudal approach to the epidural space offers many advantages for the palliative treatment of low back pain and sciatica. Often, patients with this type of complaint have a history of one or more spinal explorations, and the presence of a laminectomy scar in the lumbosacral region makes lumbar epidural puncture difficult and inexact. In such patients caudal injections of large volumes of dilute local anesthetics, with or without steroids, give symptomatic relief and sometimes effect an apparent cure in long-standing lumbosacral pain of obscure origin (Cyriax, 1975).

The caudal route may also be used for extradural injection of neurolytic solutions for relief of malignant pain confined to the perineal nerves (see Chapter 13). As an example, Figure 8–13 shows a radiogram of a caudal catheter placed for instillation of absolute alcohol in a patient with intractable pain from carcinoma of the cervix and radiation necrosis of the bladder and rectum.

SUMMARY

Caudal analgesia is a valuable technique in special circumstances, particularly for surgery on the perineum, but a satisfactory success rate of 99 per cent can only be achieved by prudent selection of suitable patients. Dosage

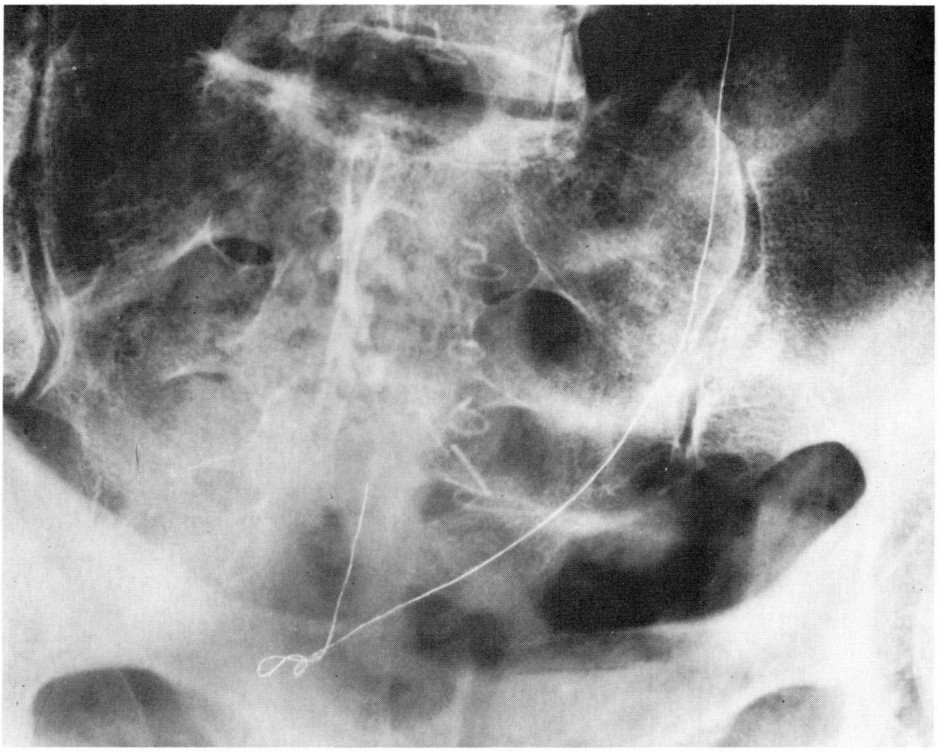

Figure 8–13. Sixty-year-old female with intractable pain from radiation necrosis of bladder and rectum. Caudal catheter inserted for instillation of absolute alcohol under general anesthesia.

requirements are 50 to 100 per cent greater than by the lumbar extradural approach, so the possibility of toxic effects from large doses of local anesthetic must be kept in mind. The technique in children is usually easy, predictable and very satisfactory for operations involving spinal segments below T_{10}, and it is an excellent choice for pediatric surgery below the umbilicus. On the other hand, caudal analgesia compared to the lumbar approach is a poor choice for obstetrics because of the relatively large quantities of local anesthetic that are needed and the correspondingly larger amounts that accumulate in the fetus. Caudal analgesia is useful for perineal surgery in adults and for palliative relief of chronic lumbosacral pain.

REFERENCES

Bonica, J. J.: Principles and Practice of Obstetric Analgesia and Anesthesia. Philadelphia, F. A. Davis Company, 1967, pp. 578, 718, 620, 586.

Brenner, E. C.: Sacral anesthesia. Ann. Surg. *79*:118, 1924.

Bromage, P. R.: Continuous lumbar epidural analgesia for obstetrics. Canad. Med. Assoc. J. *85*:1136, 1961.

Bryce-Smith, R.: The spread of solutions in the extradural space. Anaesthesia *9*:201, 1954.

Cathelin, M. F.: Une nouvelle voie d'injection rachidienne. Méthode des injections épidurales par le procédé du canal sacré. C. R. Soc. Biol. Paris *53*:452, 1901.

Cathelin, M. F.: Les Injections Epidurales. Paris. Baillière, 1903, pp. 1–231.

Cleland, J. G. P.: Continuous peridural and caudal analgesia in obstetrics. Anesth. Analg. *28*:61, 1949.

Cousins, M. J., and Bromage, P. R.: A comparison of the hydrochloride and carbonated salts of lignocaine for caudal analgesia in out-patients. Brit. J. Anaesth. *43*:1149, 1971.

Crawford, O. B., and Chester, R. V.: Caudal anesthesia in obstetrics: A combined procaine-pontocaine single injection technic. Anesthesiology *10*:473, 1949.

Cyriax, J. H.: Textbook of Orthopaedic Medicine. Vol. 1. Diagnosis of soft tissue lesions. London, Baillière Tindall, 1975, pp. 469–486.

Dawkins, C. M. J.: An analysis of the complications of extradural and caudal block. Anesthesia *24*:554, 1969.

DiGiovanni, A. J.: Inadvertent intraosseous injection—A hazard of caudal anesthesia. Anesthesiology *34*:92, 1971.

Elliott, D. C.: X-ray studies on caudal anesthesia and the intravenous absorption of substances injected into the spinal canal. Amer. J. Surg. *40*:139, 1926.

Evans, J. M., Gauci, C. A., and Watkins, G.: Horner's syndrome as a complication of lumbar epidural block. Anaesthesia *30*:774, 1975.

Finster, M., Poppers, P. J., Sinclair, J. C., et al.: Accidental intoxication of fetus with local anesthetic drug during caudal anesthesia. Amer. J. Obstet. Gynecol. *92*:922, 1965.

Fortuna, A.: Caudal analgesia: A simple and safe technique for paediatric surgery. Brit. J. Anaesth. *39*:165, 1967.

Grodinsky, M., and Best, R. R.: Sacral anesthesia. An experimental and clinical study. J. Urol. *22*:187, 1929.

Hamelberg, W., Siddall, J., and Claassen, L.: Perforation of dura by a plastic catheter during continuous caudal anesthesia. AMA Arch. Surg. *78*:357, 1959.

Hingson, R. A., and Edwards, W. B.: An analysis of the first ten thousand confinements managed with continuous caudal analgesia with a report of the authors' first one thousand cases. J.A.M.A. *123*:538, 1943.

Kay, B.: Caudal block for post-operative pain relief in children. Anaesthesia *29*:610, 1974.

Kepes, E. R., Martinez, L. R., Pantuck, E., and Stark, D. C. C.: Horner's syndrome following caudal anesthesia. N.Y. State J. Med. *72*:946, 1972.

Kosaka, Y., et al.: Caudal anesthesia in pediatric surgery. Jap. J. Anesth. *24*(12):1286, 1975.

Läwen, A.: Über die Vertwertung der Sakralanästhesie fur chirurgische Operationen. Zbl. Chir. *37*:708, 1910.

Lewis, B., and Bartels, L.: Caudal anesthesia in genito-urinary surgery. Surg. Gynecol. Obstet. *22*:262, 1916.

Lourey, C. J., and McDonald, I. H.: Caudal anesthesia in infants and children. Anaesth. Intens. Care *1*:547, 1973.

Mohan, J., and Potter, J. M.: Pupillary constriction and ptosis following caudal epidural analgesia. Anaesthesia *30*:769, 1975.

Moore, D. C., Bridenbaugh, L. D., Bagdi, P. A., and Bridenbaugh, P. O.: Accumulation of mepivacaine hydrochloride during caudal block. Anesthesiology *29*:585, 1968.

Moore, D. C., Bridenbaugh, L. D., Bridenbaugh, P. O., and Tucker, G. T.: Caudal and epidural blocks with bupivacaine for childbirth. Report of 657 parturients. Obstet Gynecol. *37*:667, 1971.

McGown, R. G.: Accidental marrow sampling during caudal anaesthesia. Brit. J. Anaesth. *44*:613, 1972.

Owens, W. D., Slater, E. M., and Battit, G. E.: A new technique of caudal anesthesia. Anesthesiology *39*:451, 1973.

Scanlon, J. W., Brown, W. U., Weiss, J. B., and Alper, M. H.: Neurobehavioural responses of newborn infants after maternal epidural anesthesia. Anesthesiology *40*:121, 1974.

Schlimpert, H.: Concerning sacral anesthesia. Surg. Gynecol. Obstet. *16*:488, 1913.

Schulte-Steinberg, O.: Spread of local anesthetic solutions in caudal blocks in children. Sixth World Congress of Anesthesiology Abstracts, Mexico City, 1976. Excerpta Medica, Int. Cong. Series No. 387, 1976, p. 132.

Schulte-Steinberg, O., and Rahlfs, V. W.: Caudal anaesthesia in children and spread of 1 per cent lignocaine: A statistical study. Brit. J. Anaesth. *42*:1093, 1970.

Schulte-Steinberg, O., and Rahlfs, V. W.: Caudal-Anaesthesie bei Kindern und die Ausbreitung von 0.25% iger Bupivacain-Lösung. Eine statistische Untersuchung. Anaesthesist *21*:94, 1972.

Shaw, E. C.: Epidural anesthesia for perineal prostatectomy. J. Urol. *15*:219, 1926.

Sinclair, J. C., Fox, H. A., and Lentz, J. F.: Intoxication of the fetus by a local anesthetic. A newly recognized complication of maternal caudal anesthesia. New Eng. J. Med. *273*:1173, 1975.

Spiegel, P.: Caudal anesthesia in pediatric surgery: A preliminary report. Anesth. Analg. *41*:218, 1962.

Spiegel, P. A.: Anestesia peridural sacra em pacientes pediatricos. Panorama atual. Rev. Bras. Anest. *26*:566, 1976.

Stoeckel, W.: Über sakrale Anästhesie. Z. Gynäk. *33*:1, 1909.
Thompson, J. E.: An anatomical and experimental study of sacral anaesthesia. Ann. Surg. *66*:718, 1917.
Touloukian, R. J., Wugmeister, M., Pickett, L. K., and Hehre, F. W.: Caudal anesthesia for neonatal anoperineal and rectal operations. Anesth. Analg. *50*:565, 1971.
Tretjakoff, D.: Das epidural Fettgewebe. Zeit. f. Anat. *79*:100, 1926.
Trotter, M.: Variations of the sacral canal: Their significance in the administration of caudal analgesia. Anesth. Analg. *26*:192, 1947.
Von Lüdinghausen, M.: Die Bänder und das Fettgewebe des Epiduralraumes. Anat. Anz. Bd. *121*:294, 1967.

chapter 9
Drugs and Equipment

Give us the tools, and we will finish the job.
Winston Churchill
Radio Address to President
Roosevelt, 9 February 1941

We shall die of the absolute paternal care that will not leave us, but prevents us everywhere.

T. S. Eliot
East Coker

Chapter 3 outlined the general principles of uptake, site of action and disposition of local anesthetics. This chapter will deal with the clinical attributes and selection of individual agents, together with the equipment available for performing epidural blockade. A large number of local anesthetic agents have been used for epidural blockade with varying degrees of success. The following limited selection is confined to those drugs that have been tested by the author under standardized conditions outlined in Chapter 4, Mechanism of Action. The description of each drug will include a brief summary of its pharmacology, followed by a clinical description of its practical performance in epidural analgesia under standardized conditions. Observed values for latency, segmental dose requirements, intensity of motor block and duration of action are summarized in Table 9–1, showing the arithmetic means and in some instances the standard deviation of the mean. Where the author has not made direct observations of a particular aspect, data from other sources will be identified in the text.

DRUGS

The list of drugs described is not complete, but it is intended to be reasonably practical. A number of agents, such as piperocaine, hexylcaine and primacaine, have been omitted for various reasons of unsuitability. Perhaps some other drugs, such as procaine and dibucaine, could also have been omitted, but they have been retained mainly for historical reasons and to evaluate their potential for possible resurgence of interest in the future.

We have entered an era when North American anesthesiologists are unlikely to see many new drugs specifically designed for epidural analgesia. The introduction of new anesthetic agents has become increasingly difficult since the

TABLE 9–1 Summary of Epidural Performance of Various Local Anesthetic Solutions in Normal, Nonpregnant Subjects: Injection Site L_2–L_3*

Analgesic Solution	*Latency* INITIAL (min)	*Latency* COMPLETE (min)	*Dose Requirements* (mg/seg at 40 yr)	*Motor Block* (%)	*Duration* (to recession of two segments—min)
Lidocaine plain 1%	5.2	13.5	—	3.6	37±5
2%	6.6	18.1	27	9.2±18	46±5
3%	5.5	14.8	25	4.5	46±12
4%	5.5	15.8	25	6.5	52
5%	4.0	13.5	28	12.0	50
Lidocaine + epinephrine 1%	6.8	18.5	20	17.5	—
2%	5.0	16.2	28	37.5±20	97±19
3%	4.9	14.0	26	30.0	98±10
4%	5.0	16.1	25	33.0	100
5%	5.9	17.9	28	33.0	98
Prilocaine plain 2%	7.5	20.6	24	25.5	77±20
3%	6.9	17.3	34	31.2	85±16
Prilocaine + epinephrine 2%	7.3	19.5	28	36.2	97±10
3%	5.1	16.5	26	34.6	99±17
Mepivacaine + epinephrine 2%	6.2	17.5	28	30	117
2-Chloroprocaine + epinephrine 3%	4.9	12.3	37	40.2±21	56.8±7
Lidocaine–CO_2 plain 1.73%	4.9	11.75	22.5	38.3±33	—
Lidocaine–CO_2 + epinephrine 1.73%	3.4	9.9	20	52.3±20.5	108±13
Prilocaine–CO_2 + epinephrine 1.71%	4.1	13.1	20	48.3	113±17
Tetracaine + epinephrine 0.1%	—	—	—	—	—
0.2%	8.1	24.9	4.25	21.5±25	135
0.3%	6.2	19.8	4.5	22.0±25	145
0.4%	6.7	20.6	4.5	27.0±23	135
0.5%	6.6	18.3	5.8	46.4±30	145.7±22
Dibucaine + epinephrine 0.167%	8.0	25.0	3.75	Slight	>180
Etidocaine plain 1%	5.0	18.1	12.0	50.4±18.6	128±43
Etidocaine + epinephrine 1%	3.6	10.8	12.5	60.0±28	170±57
Bupivacaine + epinephrine 0.5%	5.8	18.2	5.8	28.9±29	196±31
Bupivacaine plain 0.75%	5.0	17.0	7.4	30.5±30	164.5±46
Bupivacaine + epinephrine 0.75%	5.0	16.8	7.4	54.0±29	201±40

*From data collected by Bromage and colleagues.

thalidomide tragedy of 1957–1961, which involved the birth of 8,000 malformed children throughout the world. Government machinery set up to protect the North American public from further pharmacological misfortune has created a formidable set of regulations to ensure that any new drug is tested extremely thoroughly for short-term and long-term side effects. The resulting cost to the pharmaceutical industry of introducing new drugs in North America is so high that specialty agents for limited aspects of regional anesthesia are not likely to reach the general public. As a consequence, the anesthesiologist will find himself faced with a restricted number of well-tried agents to choose from, but sometimes the range of choice will be less than ideal.

Epinephrine

Epinephrine holds a special place as an adjuvant for local anesthetic solutions, and it is listed first in order to reemphasize its clinical importance in epidural analgesia. The chapters on Pharmacology, Mechanism of Action and Physiology discuss various aspects of the marked improvement in quality of blockade that is brought about by the influence of epinephrine in competition for local anesthetic uptake between vascular and neural elements in the spinal canal. In this chapter the difference in clinical performance between plain and epinephrine-containing solutions will become even more apparent from the behavior of local anesthetics in the list that follows.

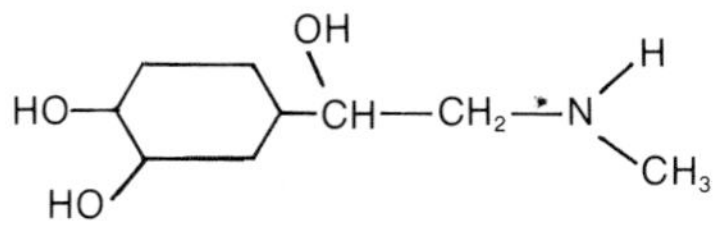

Epinephrine is available as a 0.1 per cent solution (1:1,000) of epinephrine hydrochloride. A 1-ml ampule contains 1 mg of epinephrine hydrochloride. Ampules may be autoclaved once or twice without appreciable loss of potency (Berry and West, 1944; Thomas, 1956). Epinephrine-containing solutions are prone to oxidation and loss of potency, a process that is hastened by heat and sunlight. Commercially prepared local anesthetics with epinephrine usually have an antioxidant, such as 0.1 per cent sodium bisulfite, added to them, and the pH is adjusted to a lower level than the plain solutions. This increased acidity tends to make the solution more irritating and painful on injection. In addition, onset of blockade is slowed due to increased ionization of the local anesthetic.

Many anesthesiologists prefer to add small measured amounts of epinephrine to the plain solution immediately before use. In this way the pH is kept high, the solution is more comfortable on injection and onset of blockade is faster. All unnecessary variables must be eliminated when clinical trials of new agents are conducted; then it is essential to use freshly added epinephrine in order to ensure that the pH of the epinephrine-containing solution and of the plain solution remain the same. A concentration of 1/200,000 (i.e., 5μg/ml) is prepared by adding 0.2 ml of 1:1,000 epinephrine to 40 ml of plain anesthetic solution. Concentrations of epinephrine between 1/200,000 and 1/400,000 are clinically useful. Beyond this range the concentration is either unnecessarily powerful or too dilute to be effective in the epidural space.

Epinephrine is rapidly broken down in the body, first by catechol-o-methyl transferase (COMT) to metanephrine, and then by monoamine oxidase (MAO) in the liver and blood stream. Patients receiving antidepressant medication with MAO inhibitors, such as Nardil or Parnate, may show exaggerated and prolonged pressor responses to injected catecholamines. Caution should be exercised against this type of drug interaction, and it is probably wise to avoid epinephrine-containing solutions in patients under treatment with MAO inhibitors.

Accidental intravenous injection of epinephrine-containing analgesic solutions is characterized by the bolus effect of the catecholamine. Blood pressure rises sharply and falls back to normal levels in a few minutes. If the dose is large, headache and transient signs of acute left ventricular failure may be apparent.

All drugs injected into the epidural space undergo some degree of systemic absorption. Since epinephrine has powerful stimulating effects on both beta-adrenergic and alpha-adrenergic receptors, it is probably wise to use extremely small doses, or to avoid the use of epinephrine altogether in situations in which activation of the adrenergic system is contraindicated. Omission of epinephrine from epidural analgesic solutions should be considered in the following conditions:

1. Thyrotoxicosis.
2. Patients receiving therapy with MAO inhibiting drugs.
3. Cardiac pathology in which cardiac output is fixed and on the brink of failure.
4. Malignant hyperpyrexia (see Chapter 3).
5. Severe arteriosclerosis. The severely arteriosclerotic patient is always at risk of suffering spinal stroke from inadequate perfusion of the spinal cord (see Chapters 3 and 14). It has been suggested that epidural epinephrine in a clinical concentration of 1/200,000 may reduce blood flow to the spinal cord, and so increase the hazard of spinal stroke. At the present time there is very little objective evidence to support this assertion. My own practice has been to add epinephrine 1/200,000 even in arteriosclerotic patients, but to reduce the volume of local anesthetic injected, as explained in Chapter 4.
6. Obstetrics. The controversy over epinephrine-containing solutions in obstetrics is discussed in Chapter 10 on Physiology and Chapter 12 on obstetrical indications. In these chapters data are assembled to show that the newborn is exposed to lower concentrations of local anesthetic when maternal epidural solutions contain small amounts of epinephrine. However, there is also good evidence that epinephrine does slow the progress of labor, and this has led to a widespread reluctance to use epinephrine-containing solutions in child-birth. The effects of epinephrine on labor are dose-dependent; large doses slow labor, while small ones do not. In one series of nearly 2,000 patients Gunther and Bellville (1972) showed very convincingly that the first stage of labor under caudal analgesia was appreciably longer when epinephrine 1/200,000 was added to the local anesthetic. However, in that study an initial dose of 125 μg of epinephrine was used, and an average cumulative dose of 205

μg was given over a period of less than 2½ hours. These are generous doses inherent in the caudal technique, which demands large volumes to be effective. Much smaller quantities are needed when the lumbar approach is used, and then with proper dosage the effect on the progress of labor is negligible. Used in this way the balance of advantages to mother and child is in favor of epinephrine as an adjuvant, and my own practice has been to employ analgesic solutions containing 1/400,000 to 1/200,000 epinephrine for obstetrical analgesia by the lumbar route.

7. Procedures of short duration. In short outpatient procedures on the lower limbs and pelvis, it is convenient for the patient to be able to walk within an hour or so of surgery, and then it is appropriate to use a powerful short-acting agent without epinephrine added. However, omission of epinephrine inevitably leads to greater systemic absorption of local anesthetic drug and to a less intense degree of analgesia.

Hyaluronidase

At one time hyaluronidase was used to increase vascular uptake of drugs and solutions from extravascular injection sites (Mushin, 1956). The idea that hyaluronidase might also augment neural uptake of local anesthetics has been investigated. Scott (1956) reported that the onset of epidural blockade was shortened by adding hyaluronidase to the local anesthetic solution, but he did not comment on any alteration in the quality of sensory and motor blockade. In contrast, Bromage and Burfoot (1966) found that the general effect of hyaluronidase on the quality of analgesia was disappointing, and a series of 26 epidural blocks with hyaluronidase as an adjuvant was terminated prematurely because of unsatisfactory clinical conditions. Scott's earlier finding of shortened latency was partially confirmed, as shown in Figure 9–1, but the change of latency was not significantly different from control values. The quality of blockade was impaired rather than enhanced, presumably due to loss of local anesthetic from increased vascular uptake, and the intensity of motor and sensory blockade was markedly reduced. It was concluded that hyaluronidase has no place as an adjuvant in epidural analgesia.

Potassium

The conductive properties of nerves may be altered markedly by manipulation of the extracellular ionic environment (see Chapter 3). An increased concentration of potassium outside nerves lowers the electrochemical gradient across the axon membrane according to the Donnan equilibrium, where

$$E_m \propto \log \frac{[K^+]\text{ inside}}{[K^+]\text{ outside}}$$

The membrane potential, E_m, will decrease as the potassium concentration outside the cell, $[K^+]_o$, increases. The lowered membrane potential implies an

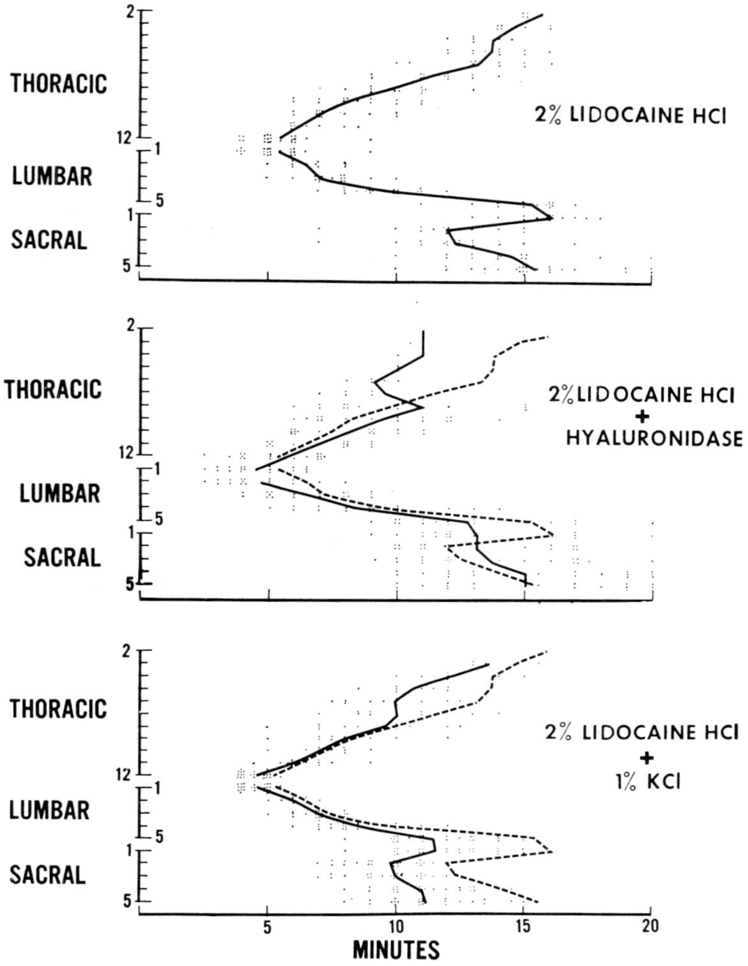

Figure 9–1. Epidural onset profiles to show influence of hyaluronidase and potassium on latency of onset and segmental spread (injection at second lumbar interspace).

Top: 2 per cent lidocaine HCl + 1/200,000 epinephrine.

Middle: 2 per cent lidocaine HCl + 1/200,000 epinephrine + hyaluronidase 5 USP units/ml.

Bottom: 2 per cent lidocaine HCl + 1/200,000 epinephrine + 1 per cent KCl.

(———) Mean latency profile for each solution.

(- - - -) Mean profile of 2 per cent lidocaine HCl for comparison.

(From Bromage, P. R., and Burfoot, M. F.: Quality of epidural blockade. II. Influence of physico-chemical factors; hyaluronidase and potassium. Brit. J. Anaesth. *38*:857, 1966.)

equivalent degree of depolarization and possibly a heightened susceptibility to local anesthetic agents.

Potassium salts have long been used as adjuvants to local anesthetics (Hoffmann and Kochmann, 1912; Meeker, 1925). Lechat and his colleagues (1964) reported that the duration of action of procaine was doubled and the blocking activity heightened by adding KCl in concentrations of 135 to 150 mM, that is, approximately the same strength as the normal intracellular concentration of potassium.

Bromage and Burfoot (1966) examined the effects of 1 per cent KCl as an adjuvant to 2 per cent lidocaine hydrochloride in 50 epidural blocks and found encouraging results. The latency of onset was shortened, particularly in the resistant segments L_5 and S_1 and in the lower sacral segments, as shown in Figure 9–1. Intensity of motor block was not appreciably affected, but the quality of sensory anesthesia appeared to be improved in the sacral segments. Duration of action was prolonged by about 20 per cent.

Since the remote possibility of accidental subarachnoid injection is always present in epidural blockade, the effects of intrathecal KCl were tested in dogs. Injection of 1 per cent KCl by itself into the cisterna magna induced strong muscle spasms and twitches which lasted more than 1 hour. The spasms were masked by the addition of local anesthetic, which of course produced flaccid paralysis during its period of action. However, on recovery from the local anesthetic, the dogs experienced spasms for a short period while the effects of the potassium still lingered. The animals recovered fully, and there was no histological evidence of neural or meningeal abnormality when the animals were killed seven days later.

While the results of the clinical study were favorable, the animal experiments sounded a note of caution. Accidental injection of potassium-containing solutions into the CSF would be undesirable under clinical conditions. Although 1 per cent KCl was apparently harmless in the dogs, the occurrence of potassium-induced spasms during regression of blockade would be temporarily painful and alarming in human subjects. This possibility is borne out by a case of accidental epidural injection of a stronger potassium mixture, described in Chapter 14, in which painful muscle spasms were indeed an unpleasant after-effect. In the face of this evidence, potassium salts cannot be recommended as adjuvants for local anesthetic solutions in the epidural space.

Procaine

para-aminobenzoic diethylaminoethanol,
molecular weight = 273, pKa = 8.92

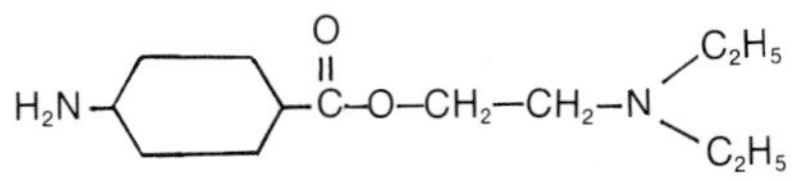

Procaine is hydrolyzed by pseudocholinesterase to the breakdown products:

para-aminobenzoic acid diethylaminoethanol

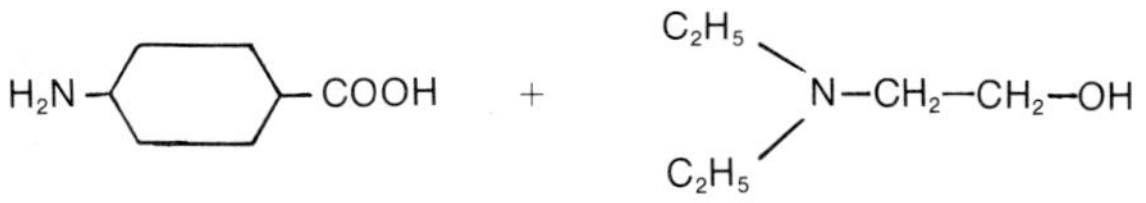

Para-aminobenzoic acid is a potential allergen in sensitive patients, with cross sensitivity to other agents containing p-aminobenzoic groupings, such as the sulfonamides and certain suntan lotions.

The rapid hydrolysis of procaine makes it one of the safest local anesthetics and one of the least likely to cause toxic effects if accidentally injected into the blood stream. Doses up to 1 g can be given into the epidural space without causing toxic effects from vascular absorption (Odom, 1936).

Unfortunately, procaine does not have intensely penetrating properties, and the quality of analgesia produced is inferior to that of lidocaine. Procaine must be used in quite high concentration to be effective in the epidural space. Although the drug was widely used prior to 1948, good statistical studies of epidural dose requirements have not been carried out, and there is a need for reinvestigation of this well-established agent, especially in the concentration range of 3 to 5 per cent. Rough estimates from earlier work suggest that epidural dose requirements range between about 60 mg per segment at 20 years down to about half that amount at 80 years, with a maximum safe dosage of about 1000 mg given as a single injection. Ansbro and his colleagues (1953) pointed out that a 5 per cent concentration was necessary for satisfactory clinical results, and they published a series of 700 cases using an induction dose of 20 ml of 5 per cent procaine (i.e., 1 g of procaine), with only a 1 per cent failure rate from technical inadequacies.

Rapid breakdown of procaine makes it short-acting as well as clinically safe. There may still be a useful place for the drug in certain applications of epidural analgesia after its behavior in the 3 to 5 per cent concentration range has been more fully documented.

Chloroprocaine (Nesacaine)

β-diethylaminoethyl 2-chloro-4-aminobenzoate hydrochloride, molecular weight = 307

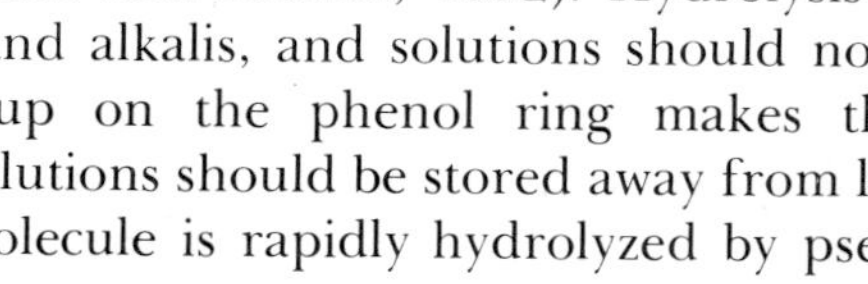

Chloroprocaine is a rapidly acting ester-type agent with a short duration and very low toxicity. The toxicity in mice appears to be about one-half that of procaine (Foldes and McNall, 1952). Hydrolysis at the ester bond is accelerated by heat and alkalis, and solutions should not be autoclaved. The aromatic amine group on the phenol ring makes the molecule slightly photosensitive, and solutions should be stored away from light in order to avoid discoloration. The molecule is rapidly hydrolyzed by pseudocholinesterase as shown:

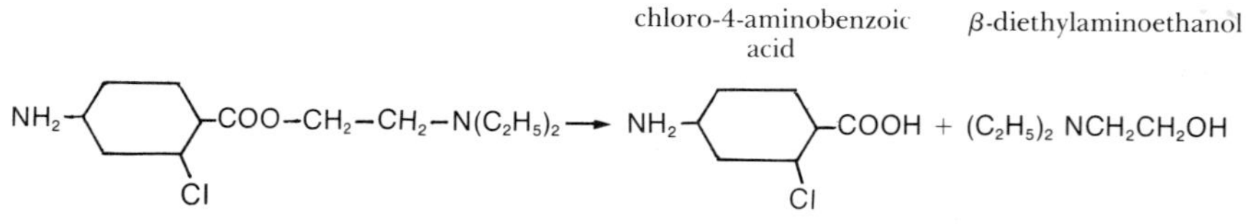

2-Chloroprocaine is one of the least toxic local anesthetics available for epidural use, and it appears to be an outstandingly safe agent. However, its duration is very short, and epidural analgesia begins to wear off after 45 to 65 minutes, even when epinephrine is added to the solution. Foldes and Davis (1954) found that epidural doses of 1 g of 3 per cent chloroprocaine (i.e., 33 ml) produce cerebrospinal fluid concentrations of about 235 μg per ml.

It must be pointed out that the safety of chloroprocaine depends largely on a normal mechanism of hydrolysis in the plasma. In patients with a normal pseudocholinesterase, the drug is remarkably safe, and in obstetrical patients very little unchanged drug is apparent in the fetus. However, in patients with atypical pseudocholinesterase, the situation is analogous to that of prolonged suxamethonium paralysis, and hydrolysis of chloroprocaine proceeds very slowly. The incidence of seriously atypical pseudocholinesterase is about 1 in 2,400 patients (Wylie and Churchill-Davidson, 1972), and one may expect to see toxic effects with large doses of chloroprocaine in these abnormal subjects. Raj and his colleagues (1977) have shown that an epidural dose of 450 mg of chloroprocaine may be followed by signs of toxicity and an elevated plasma level of chloroprocaine lasting for over 45 minutes in patients with atypical pseudocholinesterase.

A 3 per cent solution of chloroprocaine is necessary to provide adequate epidural analgesia for surgical operations, but a weaker concentration in the range of 1.5 to 2.0 per cent is adequate for control of pain in labor. A small personal series has confirmed the short duration of the agent. The latency of initial onset of blockade is rapid; however, total latency is not found to be as short as had been claimed by earlier reports (Foldes et al., 1956; Colavincenzo et al., 1956), and the average waiting time for complete segmental spread of blockade is 12.3 minutes (range 10 to 18 minutes). The quality of analgesia is inferior to that of carbonated lidocaine, with a relatively high incidence of poor analgesia in segments L_5 and S_1. The mean latency profile for 3 per cent chloroprocaine with 1/200,000 epinephrine is shown in Figure 9–2, and dose requirements between the ages of 20 to 76 years are shown in Figure 9–3. It can be seen that rather large amounts of the drug, of the order of 45 mg per segment, are required for patients in their early twenties, so volumes in excess of 25 ml may be needed to achieve blockade up to T_5 in this young age group. A rather heavy degree of motor block is observed in the legs, with an average

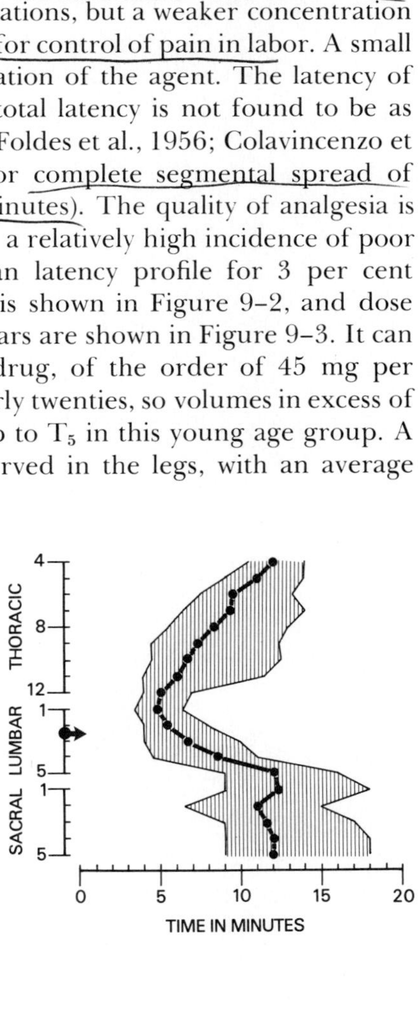

Figure 9–2. Mean latency profile of 25 patients receiving epidural analgesia with 3 per cent chloroprocaine and 1/200,000 epinephrine injected at the second lumbar interspace. Stippled area shows the standard deviation.

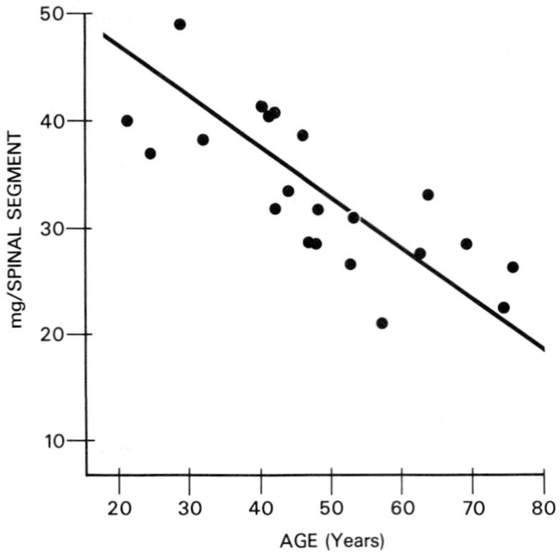

Figure 9–3. Segmental dose requirements for 3 per cent chloroprocaine plus 1/200,000 epinephrine injected at the second lumbar interspace.

intensity of 40.2 ± 21 per cent. Sensory and motor block regress rapidly, and the upper level of blockade recedes two segments in 56.8 ± 7.0 minutes (range 40 to 65 minutes). Mixtures of chloroprocaine with long-acting amide-type drugs offer the advantage of rapid onset with prolonged duration (Cunningham and Kaplan, 1974). The advantages and potential dangers of such mixtures will be discussed at the end of this section.

In summary, chloroprocaine has a rapid initial onset, but latency of analgesia in the fifth lumbar and first sacral segments is not remarkably quick. The intensity of motor blockade is high in comparison to the quality of sensory blockade. Duration to recession of two segments is less than one hour. The agent is rapidly acting, and it appears to have a place for use in short surgical procedures and in vaginal delivery, when its low toxicity is an advantage from the point of view of the fetus.

Tetracaine (Pontocaine, Amethocaine)

parabutylaminobenzoyl-dimethylaminoethanol hydrochloride,
molecular weight = 300, pKa = 8.49

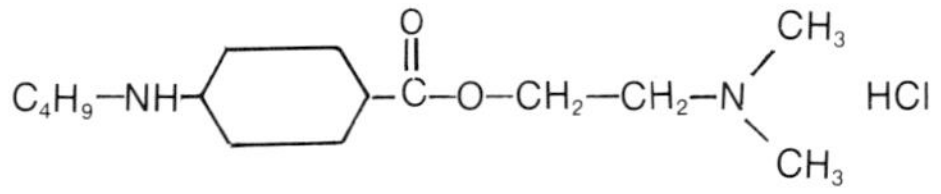

The structural formula is very similar to that of procaine, but in addition there is a long butyl side chain attached to the lipophilic phenolic portion of the molecule that confers additional lipid solubility and protein binding ability. The agent is about eight times as potent and as toxic as procaine. Hydrolysis occurs at the ester linkage, but at a much slower rate than with procaine. Solutions of tetracaine tend to deteriorate on repeated autoclaving (Whittet, 1954), and they are best prepared freshly for clinical use by adding 100 mg of sterile niphanoid crystals to the required amount of physiological saline at the time of administration.

Tetracaine was commonly used for epidural blockade in the 1940's before lidocaine was introduced into clinical anesthesia. At that time a 0.2 per cent solution was the popular concentration, and 50 ml, or 100 mg, of the drug was the generally accepted safe maximum dose. Unfortunately, the agent has rather poor penetrating qualities in the 0.2 per cent dilution, and the latency is very slow, with a waiting time of 20 to 30 minutes before satisfactory analgesia is complete. At weaker dilutions skin analgesia is patchy and incomplete, and with a 0.1 per cent solution patients frequently complain of bizarre sensations and dysesthesia in the legs. Latency shortens progressively with increasing concentration, as shown in Figure 9–4, in which latency profiles of 0.2, 0.3, 0.4 and 0.5 per cent tetracaine from a series of 116 cases are shown for comparison (Bromage, 1969a; Bromage and Burfoot, 1966). Note the prolonged salient of delay at L_5–S_1 with 0.2 per cent tetracaine. This waiting time is too long for practical purposes in a busy clinical environment. The 0.5 per cent solution has a latency profile that is almost identical to that of 0.5 per cent bupivacaine and an average waiting time of 18.3 minutes for complete spread of analgesia.

Dose requirements and intensity of motor block also vary with concentration. Accurate data for dose requirements of 0.1 per cent tetracaine are difficult to obtain, since this concentration is barely sufficient to provide sensory analgesia of the skin, and no appreciable amount of motor block is achieved. The 0.2, 0.3 and 0.4 per cent concentrations have roughly similar dose requirements and potency of motor blockade, but the 0.5 per cent concentration has sharply increased dose requirements and potency of motor blockade, as shown in Figures 4–17 and 4–19 in the chapter on Mechanism of Action. From Figure 4–17 it can be seen that segmental dose requirements for the 0.5 per cent solution decline from 7.0 mg per segment at 20 years to 3.5 mg per segment at 80 years. These amounts are approximately one-fifth of the segmental dose requirements for lidocaine (vide infra), and they appear to be proportional to the relative toxicity of tetracaine.

While the speed of onset of 0.5 per cent tetracaine is acceptable for clinical use, the quality of blockade leaves much to be desired. The 0.5 per cent solution causes a marked degree of motor block in the legs (46.4 per cent), but

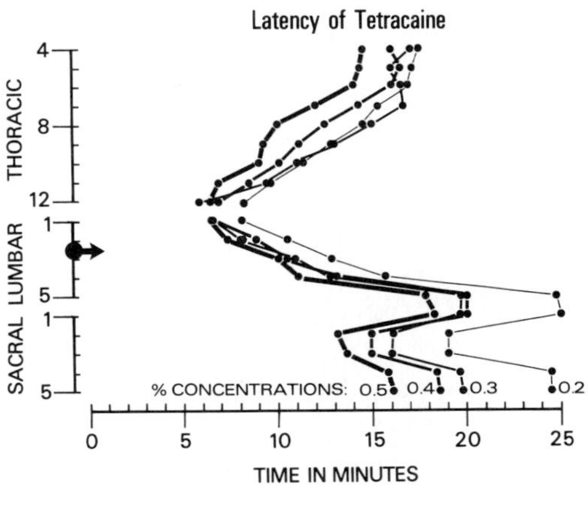

Figure 9–4. Mean latency profiles for 0.2, 0.3, 0.4 and 0.5 per cent tetracaine injected epidurally at the second lumbar interspace. (From Bromage, P. R.: The physiology and pharmacology of epidural blockade. *In* Bonica, J. J.: Clinical Anesthesia. 2. Regional Anesthesia: Recent Advances and Current Status. Philadelphia, F. A. Davis Company, 1969.)

strangely enough the quality of sensory analgesia is disproportionately poor. When 0.5 per cent tetracaine is used for pain relief after abdominal surgery, it is not uncommon for a patient to complain of severe pain at a time when the upper level of cutaneous analgesia is still above the seventh thoracic dermatome. When postoperative pain does return, it tends to strike with brutal suddenness, in contrast to a more gradual and gentle appearance when bupivacaine is used (Bromage, 1969b).

The duration of action for the 0.5 per cent solution, in terms of recession of two segments, is 145.7 ± 22.4 minutes. This length of action puts the drug in the class of long-acting agents, together with etidocaine, bupivacaine and dibucaine.

Tetracaine is not well suited for epidural use in relief of postoperative pain or for relief of pain in labor. The characteristics of profound motor block with marginally satisfactory sensory block are the antithesis of what is required clinically. In both the postoperative situation and in obstetrical labor the patient should be active, with mobile limbs, and should be capable of muscular control although free of pain. Unfortunately, tetracaine produces conditions that are the reverse of these requirements, with an excessive degree of motor block but without a comparably intense analgesia. The possible mechanisms underlying this dissociation of sensory and motor blockade have been discussed in a preceding chapter (p. 148). Here we need only reiterate the facts and place tetracaine low down on the list of priorities when a suitable drug for epidural analgesia is chosen.

Although tetracaine by itself is a poor agent for epidural analgesia, some authors have had extensive and favorable experience with mixtures of tetracaine and other agents that were faster acting. Moore and his colleagues (1972) reported on 9,535 cases in which tetracaine had been used in 0.2 per cent concentration with other agents, such as lidocaine or chloroprocaine. These authors found that the duration of caudal or epidural block was approximately doubled when 0.2 per cent tetracaine was added to lidocaine, mepivacaine or chloroprocaine.

Dibucaine (Cinchocaine, Nupercaine)

a-butyloxycinchoninic diethyl ethylene diamide,
molecular weight = 380, pKa = 8.54

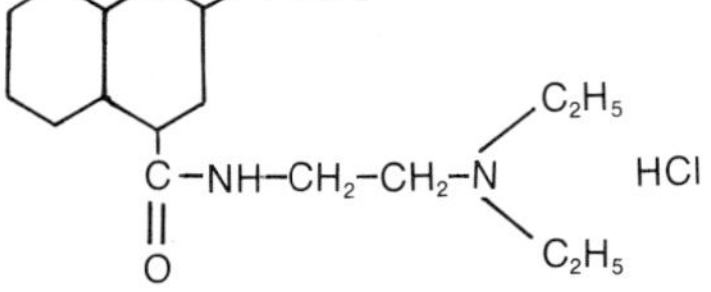

Dibucaine is about 12 to 15 times as potent and as toxic as procaine, and it has a very high degree of lipid solubility and protein binding (Truant and Takman, 1959). The molecule is not hydrolyzed by plasma pseudocholinesterase, but it is broken down slowly in the liver. Solutions are stable and can be sterilized by autoclaving (Whittet, 1954). The maximum recommended safe dose

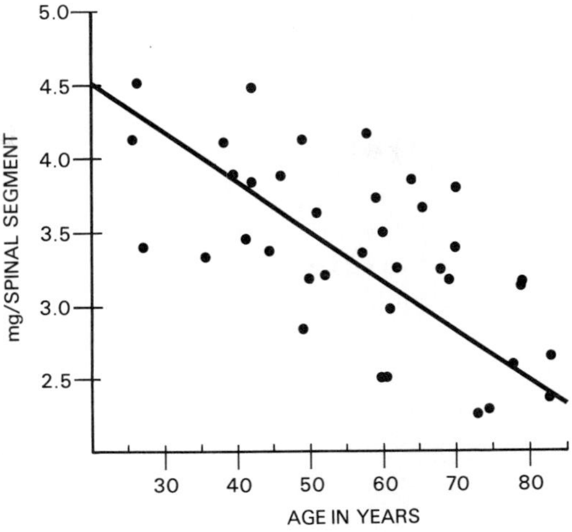

Figure 9–5. Epidural dose requirements related to age for 1/600 dibucaine (i.e., 0.167 per cent dibucaine) with 1/200,000 epinephrine injected at the first or second lumbar interspace. (From Bromage, P. R. Spinal Epidural Analgesia. Edinburgh, E. & S. Livingstone Ltd., 1954.)

by the epidural route lies in the range of 75 to 85 mg, although epidural doses of up to 100 mg of a 0.33 per cent solution have been reported (Stout, 1957).

Clinically, dibucaine has poor tissue penetrating power, and it has a very slow epidural latency of about 30 to 40 minutes but a long duration of three to four hours. Accurate figures for latency profiles and intensity of motor block have not been obtained. Data for segmental dose requirements collected in 1954 confirm that the dose needed per spinal segment is approximately in proportion to the known potency and toxicity of the agent. Figure 9–5 shows the segmental dose requirements for 1/600 dibucaine related to age. The maximum dose requirements are approximately 4.5 mg per spinal segment at age 20 years, declining to 2.5 mg per segment at 80 years.

The quality of analgesia obtained with 1/600 dibucaine is relatively poor compared with lidocaine, and patients frequently require sedation or general anesthesia as supplementation. Stout (1957) made a very thorough comparison of dibucaine and other local anesthetics in reference to epidural analgesia in surgery; he concluded that the quality of analgesia with dibucaine in concentrations of 0.167 to 0.33 per cent compared unfavorably to the effects of similar concentrations of tetracaine. Stout found that 1/600 dibucaine gave an intensity of blockade that was approximately equivalent to 1 per cent procaine.

The slow latency of onset of dibucaine is a serious practical disadvantage. However, this can be overcome by adding a short-acting and rapidly detoxified ester-type agent, such as chloroprocaine, in order to obtain a reasonably short latency combined with long duration.

Dibucaine for Epidural Analgesia in Obstetrics. Dibucaine 1/1500 (i.e., 0.067 per cent) has been proposed as a suitable epidural solution for relief of pain in the first stage of labor (Shykoff, 1969). As a rule, quite weak solutions of local anesthetics are sufficient to relieve the low abdominal and lumbosacral pain of the first stage of labor. However, my own experience with dibucaine in concentrations between 0.067 and 0.2 per cent has not been promising, and a trial obstetrical series was abandoned after a high incidence of unsatisfactory analgesia.

The 0.067 per cent solution in a dose of 15 ml (i.e., 10 mg) may produce adequate pain relief in early first stage labor, but no skin analgesia is apparent, and it is impossible to obtain objective measurements of segmental spread. Moreover, the analgesia is inconsistent, and first stage pain may not be completely relieved. The 0.1 per cent solution in doses of 12 to 15 mg produces mild cutaneous hypalgesia without any apparent motor blockade, but perineal analgesia tends to be inadequate for episiotomy and forceps delivery, even when dosage is increased to 30 mg. The 0.2 per cent solution was no more impressive, and doses in excess of 30 mg failed to provide adequate analgesia for forceps delivery without nitrous oxide–oxygen supplements. In view of the marked systemic toxicity of dibucaine, there seems little advantage in pushing the dosage to a level that can provide adequate analgesia at the expense of disproportionate toxicity when other agents such as lidocaine or bupivacaine can achieve better clinical results with less danger to the mother and fetus.

Dibucaine has been surpassed by less toxic and more effective drugs. In spite of its widespread use in the past, at present there does not seem to be any strong reason for using dibucaine in epidural blockade.

Lidocaine (Lignocaine, Xylocaine)

diethylamino-2,6-aceto-xylidide hydrochloride,

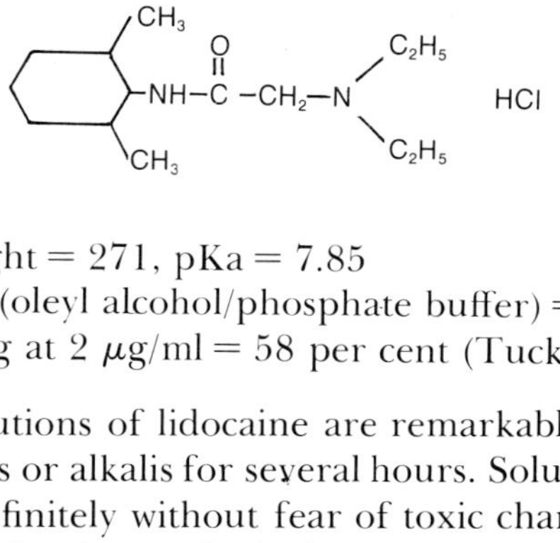

molecular weight = 271, pKa = 7.85
lipid solubility (oleyl alcohol/phosphate buffer) = 28:1
protein binding at 2 μg/ml = 58 per cent (Tucker et al., 1970)

Aqueous solutions of lidocaine are remarkably stable and withstand boiling with strong acids or alkalis for several hours. Solutions can be stored and resterilized almost indefinitely without fear of toxic changes or loss of potency (Whittet, 1954). Lidocaine is not hydrolyzed by pseudocholinesterase in the blood, but in man the molecule is broken down at the amide bond by amidase in the liver (Keenaghan and Boyes, 1972), mainly to the product *p*-hydroxy xylidine.

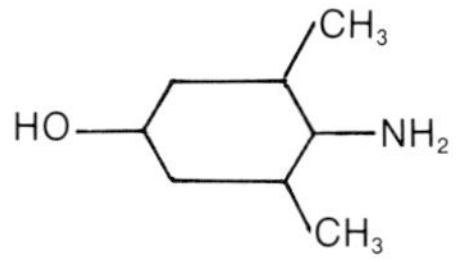

Under normal conditions of hepatic blood flow, the half-life of intravenous lidocaine is about 1.5 hours in conscious volunteers (Rowland et al., 1971; Tucker and Mather, 1975), but elimination is considerably slowed under conditions of general anesthesia and reduced splanchnic blood flow (Adjepon-

Yamoah et al., 1973; Thomson et al., 1973). Vascular uptake of lidocaine from the epidural space is markedly slowed by the addition of epinephrine, 5 μg per ml (Scott et al., 1972; Tucker and Mather, 1975; Mather et al., 1976).

Lidocaine was introduced into clinical practice by Löfgren in 1948 as the first of a series of amide-type local anesthetics. From the outset it was clear that the agent had properties that placed it above the other local anesthetics, such as procaine, tetracaine, dibucaine and piperocaine, that were available at that time. It has a fast onset and great dependability; it is a durable compound with a long shelf life; and it can be resterilized by heat without loss of potency. Lidocaine is the most thoroughly studied and widely used of all the local anesthetics, and it has supplanted procaine as the standard against which the performance and toxicity of other drugs are measured. Its potency is about twice that of procaine, and its toxicity is also approximately twice as great.

Acute toxicity depends on the circulating blood concentration of lidocaine, and this in turn depends on whether or not epinephrine has been added to the epidural solution. In adults subjective toxic effects become apparent at blood lidocaine concentrations of 5 μg per ml, while objective signs of toxicity appear when the blood concentration is in the region of 10 μg per ml. Vascular uptake of lidocaine from the epidural space is markedly reduced by adding epinephrine to the analgesic solution, and plasma levels are lowered about 40 per cent by the presence of epinephrine in a concentration of 5 μg per ml (Bromage and Robson, 1961). Figure 9–6 from more recent data by Scott and his colleagues (1972) summarizes the differences in plasma concentrations of lidocaine that are found with varying epidural doses between 200 mg and 600 mg, with and without epinephrine. Values from an earlier investigation by Bromage and Robson (1961) are shown for comparison, and it can be seen that there is close agreement between the two studies at a dose level of 400 mg of lidocaine. As explained in Chapter 3, the benefits of epinephrine are twofold: less drug is absorbed into the blood stream, while more is left available in the spinal canal to perform the task of neural blockade, and the quality of analgesia is greatly enhanced.

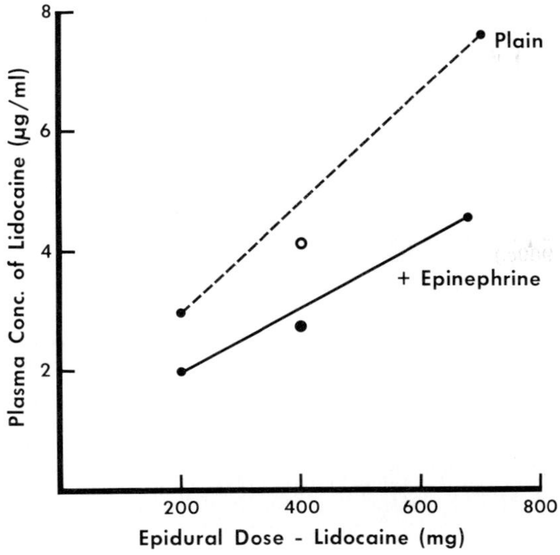

Figure 9–6. Vascular uptake of epidural lidocaine. Peak plasma concentrations of lidocaine related to dose after epidural injection of 2 per cent lidocaine in plain solution and with epinephrine 1/200,000 added.

Symbols:

Plain Lidocaine	Lidocaine + 1/200,000 epinephrine
Data by Scott et al. (1972): ●------●	Data by Bromage and Robson (1961): ●——●
○	●

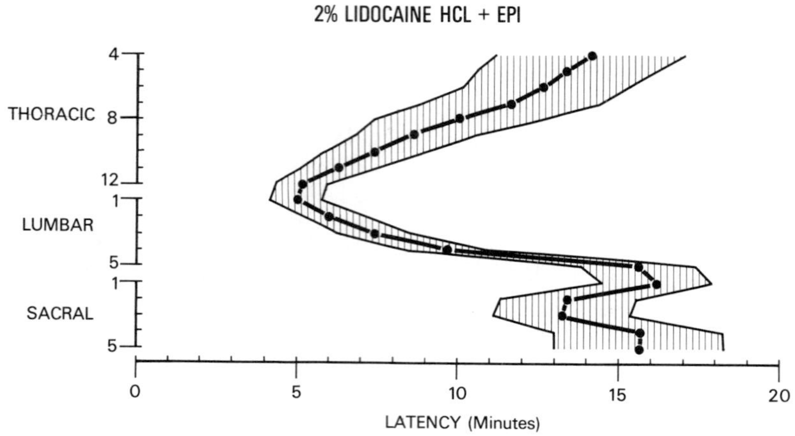

Figure 9–7. Mean latency profile for 2 per cent lidocaine with 1/200,000 epinephrine injected at second lumbar interspace.

The mean latency profile for 2 per cent lidocaine hydrochloride with 1/200,000 epinephrine is shown in Figure 9–7. The average time for initial onset of analgesia is 5.0 ± 1.1 minutes, and for complete segmental spread 16.2 ± 2.6 minutes.

Epidural dose requirements in relation to age are shown in Figure 9–8. Maximum dose requirements at the second lumbar interspace are approximately 31 mg lidocaine per segment at 18½ years of age, declining to 15 mg per segment at 80 years.

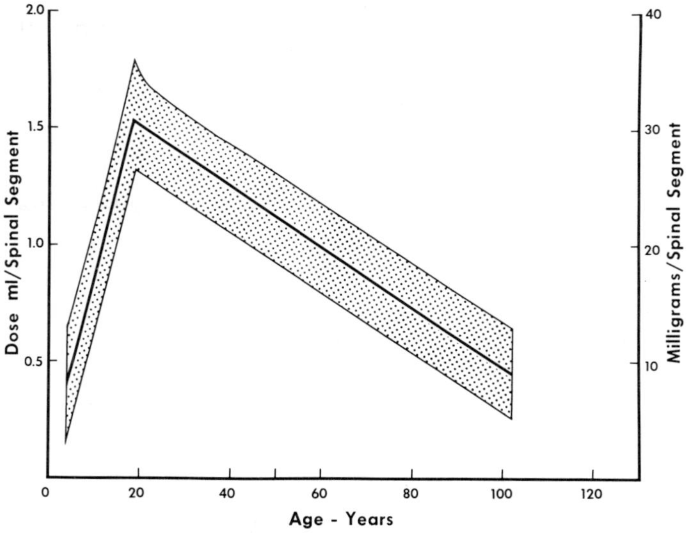

Figure 9–8. Relationship of epidural dose requirements to age for 2 per cent lidocaine hydrochloride injected at the second lumbar interspace with patients in the supine position, showing mean and 90 per cent confidence bands for the population. (After Bromage, 1969c.)

Intensity of motor blockade, as measured by the criteria outlined in Chapter 4, is approximately 38 per cent when epinephrine is added to the solution. However, when plain lidocaine is used, the degree of motor block is scarcely appreciable, with a numerical average of only 9 per cent.

Duration of action to recession of two segments is 46 ± 5.0 minutes with plain lidocaine and 97 ± 19 minutes with the epinephrine-containing solution.

Concentration. The peculiar relationship between concentration and intensity of blockade is discussed in Chapter 4. Little or no advantage is obtained by increasing the concentration of lidocaine to 5 per cent. Dose requirements, in milligrams per spinal segment, are almost identical for the 2, 3, 4 and 5 per cent solutions, and intensity and duration of block are also very similar. However, at low concentrations, e.g., 1 per cent lidocaine, there is a departure from this constant relationship of dose, segmental spread and quality of blockade. With 1 per cent lidocaine about 20 to 40 per cent less drug is required per spinal segment, and the intensity of motor blockade is about one-half that found with the 2 per cent solution (Bromage et al., 1964; Erdemir et al., 1965). Thus, the 1 per cent concentration is well suited for situations in which motor block is not required, as for postoperative analgesia and for relief of pain in labor.

Prilocaine (Citanest, Propitocaine)

n-propylamino-2-methylpropionanilide hydrochloride,
molecular weight = 257, pKa = 7.9

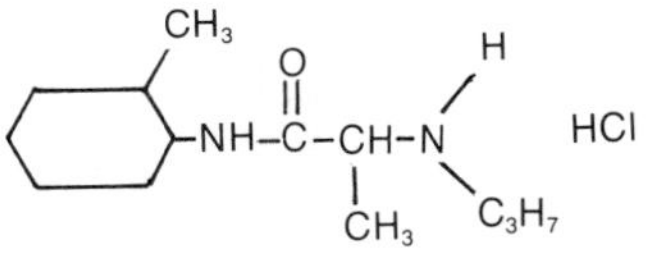

The structure is very similar to that of lidocaine, but the propyl chain on the hydrophilic part of the molecule confers longer duration. Also, there is a single methyl group instead of two on the phenol ring, and this detracts from the stability of the neighboring amide linkage, —NH—CO, so that the molecule is more easily split into its component halves, one of which is o-toluidine. By virtue of this increased ease of destruction, the drug is less acutely toxic than lidocaine. Initially, investigations in animals and man showed that prilocaine had about the same potency as lidocaine, whereas its duration of action was longer and its toxicity about 40 per cent less than that of lidocaine (Wiedling, 1960; Aström and Persson, 1961; Englesson et al., 1962). Thus the drug seemed well suited for all forms of regional analgesia, and especially for epidural analgesia in which large doses of local anesthetics are commonly required.

Comparative trials of lidocaine and prilocaine for epidural analgesia were begun at the Royal Victoria Hospital, Montreal, in 1959, and the results from 317 patients are summarized in Table 9–1. As can be seen from Table 9–1, prilocaine has a slower latency than lidocaine, and the 3 per cent solution is approximately equivalent to 2 per cent lidocaine with epinephrine in terms of speed of onset and efficiency of blockade. Moreover, 3 per cent prilocaine without epinephrine has the important advantage of being almost as effective as 2 per cent lidocaine with epinephrine. Therefore, 3 per cent prilocaine is a suitable substitute for lidocaine in some situations in which epinephrine is contraindicated, as in cases of thyrotoxicosis. Although the 3 per cent plain solution of prilocaine requires about 25 to 30 per cent larger doses than the other solutions, particularly in young patients, the need for more drug is offset by the lower acute toxicity of the agent.

Methemoglobinemia. Unfortunately, one of the breakdown products of prilocaine, orthotoluidine, causes methemoglobinemia by inhibiting the reducing mechanism of red cells and allowing hemoglobin to become oxidized to methemoglobin, a form that is incapable of transporting oxygen. Less oxygen is carried in the blood, and at the same time oxygen unloading in the tissues is impaired by a shift of the oxygen dissociation curve to the left at methemoglobin levels above 0.8 g per 100 ml of blood (Harris et al., 1968). Daly et al. (1964) reported an 11 per cent incidence of cyanosis in 82 patients receiving epidural blocks for pain relief in labor, seven of whom had proven methemoglobinemia. One per cent prilocaine was used, and cumulative doses ranged between 400 and 1520 mg. Methemoglobinemia cannot usually be appreciated clinically when doses are kept below 600 mg of prilocaine. However, beyond this amount methemoglobin formation rises steeply with increased dosage (Lund and Cwik, 1965; Climie et al., 1967). Doses of 800 mg regularly produce methemoglobinemia to the extent of 1 to 3 g per 100 ml, three to seven hours after administration (Fujimori et al., 1964). Blood concentrations of methemoglobin in excess of 1.5 g per 100 ml are sufficient to produce cyanosis (Joseph, 1962), and this may confuse the clinical picture of a difficult case in the postoperative period.

Methylene blue given intravenously in a dose of 1 mg per kg body weight is a specific antidote to methemoglobinemia, but its action is transient, and it should not be repeated, for in larger doses it acts as a hemoglobin oxidant in its own right and so may actually worsen the situation.

Any impairment of the normal oxygen transport system is clearly undesirable in cases in which oxygen supplies may be jeopardized from other causes, as in anemia or cardiac failure. The fetus at birth is especially vulnerable to any diminution of its tenuous oxygen supplies, and it would therefore seem wise to avoid the use of prilocaine for relief of pain in labor (Scott, 1965; Arens and Carrera, 1970).

Mepivacaine (Carbocaine)

1-methyl pipecolic 2,6-dimethyl xylidide hydrochloride, molecular weight = 285, pKa = 7.65

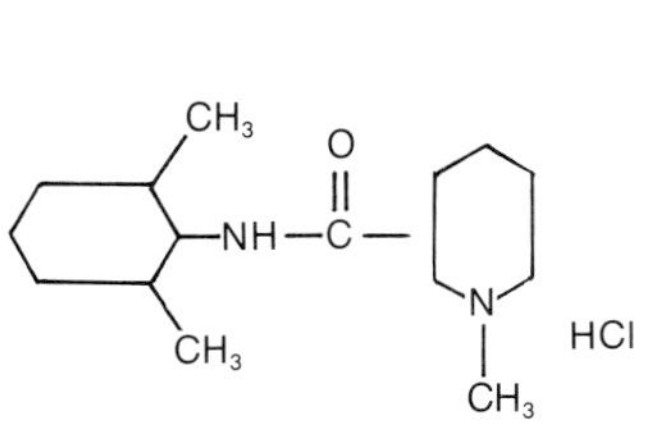

In many respects the clinical performance of 2 per cent mepivacaine with 1/200,000 epinephrine in the epidural space is very similar to that of lidocaine, but there are a few significant differences.

Latency. Onset of blockade is slightly slower than with lidocaine, being 6.2 minutes for initial onset and 17.5 minutes for complete segmental spread of analgesia.

Dose Requirements and Intensity of Motor Blockade. These qualities are almost identical to those of lidocaine.

Duration of Action. Duration of action to recession of two segments is 117 minutes and 20 per cent longer than that of lidocaine with 1/200,000 epinephrine. Duration of action of the plain solution is also longer than that of lidocaine. The idea that mepivacaine can achieve equally satisfactory results with or without added epinephrine is incorrect (Henn, 1960; Gordon et al., 1960). Duration of action is appreciably shorter and blockade is less intense when epinephrine is omitted. Also, vascular absorption is markedly reduced when epinephrine 1/200,000 is added (Dhuner et al., 1965; Burfoot and Bromage, 1971; Tucker et al., 1972; Brown et al., 1975).

Mepivacaine has a pKa (7.65) that is closer to physiological pH than the other local anesthetics in common use. Therefore, proportionally more uncharged lipid-soluble base is present after injection into body tissues, and this gives rise to blood concentrations that are about 50 per cent higher than when lidocaine is used (Reynolds, 1971a). Unfortunately, this tendency to high blood concentrations and accumulation in the maternal circulation makes mepivacaine ill-suited to obstetrical applications (Crawford, 1972). Placental transfer of mepivacaine is rapid, and high maternal concentrations inevitably lead to proportionately high fetal levels with a fetal/maternal ratio of about 0.65 to 0.7 (Morishima et al., 1966; Brown et al., 1975).

In summary, mepivacaine is similar to lidocaine but is somewhat longer-acting. The drug accumulates in the blood stream more rapidly than lidocaine, and mepivacaine is therefore a relatively poor choice for obstetrical analgesia.

Bupivacaine (Marcaine)

N-butyl pipecolic 2,6 dimethyl xylidide hydrochloride,
molecular weight = 324, pKa = 8.05

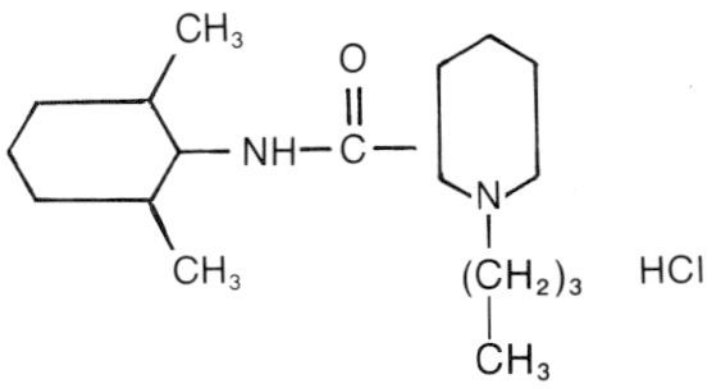

This important agent was introduced by Telivuo in 1963, and early favorable impressions were confirmed by other European investigators. In North America similar work was delayed for a further six years by governmental precautions and restrictions surrounding the use of new drugs. At present bupivacaine is acknowledged as one of the most suitable agents for epidural use in postoperative pain and for relief of pain in labor. It can be used in a sixfold range of concentration between 0.125 per cent and 0.75 per cent, depending on the clinical indications.

The structure of bupivacaine is identical to that of mepivacaine, except for the longer side chain of three extra methyl groups on the piperidine ring. This small addition to mepivacaine's structure increases lipid solubility and protein binding and transforms the clinical properties in a striking manner. Metabolic breakdown of the molecule is similar to that of mepivacaine and commences with removal of the piperidine side chain. The product pipecolyl xylidine (PPX) is approximately one-eighth as toxic as bupivacaine. PPX and unchanged bupivacaine are slowly excreted in about equal proportions in the urine (Reynolds, 1971b). The slow-phase half-life ($T^{1/2}\beta$) is about eight hours in normal subjects (Stanton-Hicks et al., 1976) and nine hours in newborn babies (Magno et al., 1976).

Toxic blood concentrations of bupivacaine are not definitely established. Jordfeldt et al. (1968) used intravenous doses in humans that achieved blood levels of 1.5 to 3.0 μg per ml without evidence of cardiovascular depression. However, as pointed out earlier in the chapter on Pharmacology, toxicity is largely a function of speed of injection, and relatively small doses given as an intravenous bolus are likely to be much more toxic than larger doses absorbed more gradually from the epidural space. Data by Scott (1975) suggest that a venous concentration of 2 μg per ml may give rise to toxic effects when the drug is administered rapidly.

Uptake of bupivacaine from the epidural space of adults has been studied by a number of investigators (Fujimori et al., 1967; Wilkinson and Lund, 1970; Reynolds, 1971a, 1971b; Lund et al., 1973), and the combined data from these authors show that vascular absorption is largely dose-dependent, as shown

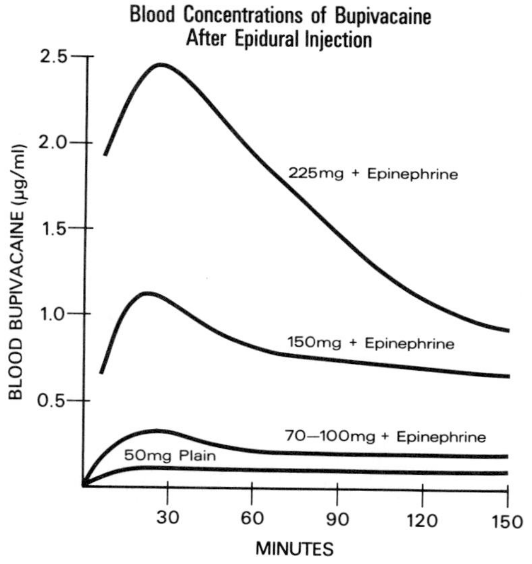

Figure 9–9. Vascular uptake of bupivacaine from the epidural space. Blood concentration/time curves in relation to dosage. (Data from Fujimori et al., 1967; Wilkinson and Lund, 1970; Reynolds, 1971a, 1971b; Lund et al., 1973.)

in Figure 9–9. Vascular uptake from the epidural space appears to be accelerated in pregnant women at term, and higher blood levels of bupivacaine are found in parturients than in the normal population (Thomas et al., 1969a, 1969b). These findings suggest that blood concentrations of bupivacaine in adult patients are likely to remain well within safe limits if epidural induction doses are restricted to 150 mg or less.

The question of whether or not epinephrine is a necessary adjuvant to bupivacaine solutions has been hotly debated. In this debate it must be clear that two quite different points are at issue. One is the question of clinical effectiveness, and the other is the matter of vascular uptake and systemic toxicity. The clinical efficiency of bupivacaine is said to be relatively little affected by the presence or absence of epinephrine, in contrast to lidocaine with which epinephrine 1/200,000 increases performance markedly. However, in my experience there are significant differences in the quality of blockade with and without epinephrine, as shown in Figure 9–13, and in the matter of vascular uptake epinephrine provides a very important advantage. Marked increases of blood levels of bupivacaine have been observed after other types of regional blockade when epinephrine is omitted (Yoshikawa et al., 1968; Hollmén et al., 1969).

Reynolds and her colleagues have shown that in continuous epidural block during labor with intermittent doses of 0.5 per cent bupivacaine, incremental concentrations of the drug in maternal blood rose about 50 per cent higher when the plain solution was used than when epinephrine 1/200,000 was added to the analgesic solution (Reynolds and Taylor, 1971; Reynolds et al., 1973). A similar reduction of maternal plasma bupivacaine by epidural epinephrine was found after single-shot injections (Hyman and Shnider, 1971). From the point of view of placental transfer to the fetus, this difference of maternal vascular uptake is most likely to be significant following the final epidural dose just prior to delivery, for the fetus will be exposed to appreciably higher maternal concentrations of bupivacaine if plain bupivacaine is used instead of the epinephrine-containing solution.

Bupivacaine disperses rapidly in the newborn, and plasma concentrations fall to low levels within a few hours of delivery. The slow-phase elimination time ($T\frac{1}{2}\beta$) is about nine hours, being approximately the same for both mother and neonate, and about 10 per cent slower than in normal adults. Measurable concentrations of the drug are present in fetal plasma up to 24 hours after delivery (Belfrage et al., 1975b; Magno et al., 1976). These findings reflect very rapid solution of bupivacaine in body lipids, followed by a slightly slower rate of breakdown and elimination than in nonparturient adults.

Neonatal blood concentrations depend on maternal blood levels. Small maternal doses of bupivacaine give rise to very low fetal and neonatal levels of the order of 40 to 60 nanograms (ng) per ml (Belfrage et al., 1975a, 1975b), whereas large maternal doses are followed by peak neonatal levels that may be five to ten times higher and of the order of 200 to 400 ng per ml. Figure 9–10, drawn from data by Magno and his associates (1976), shows that single maternal injections of 100 to 120 mg plain 0.75 per cent bupivacaine give rise to peak neonatal levels in excess of 200 ng per ml. Clinical impressions indicate that babies born after bupivacaine epidural analgesia do extremely well, and the drug appears to have little or no depressing effect on the neonate in carefully conducted

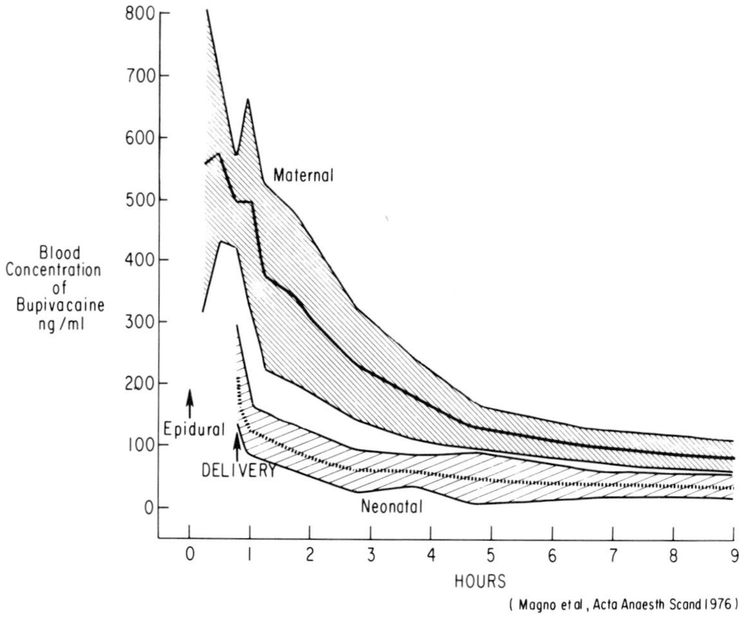

Figure 9–10. Plain bupivacaine, 0.75 per cent, for cesarean section. Maternal and neonatal blood concentrations of bupivacaine (mean ± S.D.) after average maternal dose of 103 mg (range 90 to 120 mg). (Redrawn from data by Magno et al., 1976.)

labors. Neurobehavioral studies carried out at two to four hours of age have confirmed these impressions. Scanlon and his colleagues (1976) found no evidence of neurobehavioral depression associated with peak neonatal concentrations up to 100 ng per ml. However, at the time of writing it has not been demonstrated that levels of the order shown in Figure 9–10 are entirely innocuous. In the absence of clear proof to the contrary, it is prudent to retain the cautious view that low neonatal concentrations of a *potentially* depressant drug such as bupivacaine are better than high ones, and to adopt the same restrained and parsimonious approach toward maternal dosage that one would with any other local anesthetic, as outlined in Chapter 12.

Uptake of epidural bupivacaine into the cerebrospinal fluid of humans has been studied by Wilkinson and Lund (1970). These investigators found peak cerebrospinal fluid concentrations of 30.6 μg per ml one half-hour after epidural injection of 150 mg bupivacaine (30 ml of 0.5 per cent solution) with 1/200,000 epinephrine. Cerebrospinal fluid concentrations of this order (i.e., 0.03 mg per ml) are relatively low compared to the levels of other agents found in the cerebrospinal fluid after epidural injection, as shown in Table 4–1 in Chapter 4. However, the very high lipid solubility and protein affinity of bupivacaine suggest that a considerable proportion of the drug will distribute itself rapidly out of the CSF phase into the neuraxis and that CSF concentrations will not necessarily reflect the actual degree of neural uptake that is taking place.

Clinical preparations

Bupivacaine is thermostable, and plain solutions may be reautoclaved almost indefinitely. However, solutions manufactured with epinephrine already added should not be resterilized by heat. Epinephrine-containing solutions are manufactured with the following additives as antioxidants: sodium bisulfite, thioglycerol, ascorbic acid and calcium sodium edetate. These epinephrine-containing solutions of bupivacaine are reported to turn light yellow after heat sterilization and to emit a foul odor that has been attributed to the breakdown of thioglycerol (DeLeo et al., 1974). As with all local anesthetics, ideal practice should avoid solutions of low pH premixed with epinephrine, and instead the epinephrine should be added freshly in accurately measured amounts to produce a concentration of 5 μg per ml just prior to use. In this way the pH is usually several units more alkaline than the premixed solution and therefore more likely to have a faster onset from the greater proportion of nonionized lipid-soluble base.

Bupivacaine is manufactured in concentrations of 0.25, 0.5 and 0.75 per cent for epidural use. Each of these solutions has its own special indications and limits of usefulness.

0.25 Per Cent Bupivacaine. Latency is slow, motor block is negligible and the quality of surgical analgesia in adults is barely adequate for satisfactory operating conditions. However, this dilute solution with epinephrine 1/200,000 to 1/300,000 is ideally suited for relief of pain in labor (see Chapter 12) and for postoperative pain relief (Downing, 1969). The 0.25 per cent solution with epinephrine provides good analgesia for labor pains and for episiotomy and vaginal delivery, provided the progress of labor is carefully supervised and provided dosage is titrated to the changing requirements of the individual case. As might be expected, this dilute solution is somewhat less satisfactory under conditions of desultory supervision.

0.5 Per cent Bupivacaine. A large amount of data has been collected relating to the clinical performance of 0.5 per cent bupivacaine. This was the strength originally selected for surgical analgesia, and the drug performs reasonably well in this concentration (Ekblom and Widman, 1966; Korkeila, 1966; Hollmén, 1966; Steel and Dawkins, 1968; Watt et al., 1968; Bromage, 1969b; Bromage and Gertel, 1970; Swerdlow and Jones, 1970; Moore et al., 1970; Stanton-Hicks, 1971, Peebles and Slack, 1971).

Clinical measurements made under standardized conditions have provided the following data (Bromage, 1969).

LATENCY. Figure 9–11 shows the latency profile for 0.5 per cent bupivacaine compared to 0.5 per cent tetracaine. It can be seen that the two profiles are almost identical, with a rather long waiting time of 18 minutes for complete spread to S_1.

DOSE REQUIREMENTS. Segmental dose requirements in terms of milligrams of bupivacaine hydrochloride per spinal segment are compared with those of tetracaine in Figure 9–12. Dose requirements decline from about 6.75 mg per segment at 20 years to 3.8 mg per segment at 80 years.

QUALITY OF BLOCKADE. The quality of motor blockade is characteristically slight compared to the relatively effective sensory analgesia. However, intensity of sensory block in L_5 and S_1 is unimpressive, and the quality of analgesia in these segments is not usually sufficient for comfort during operations on the lower leg and ankle in conscious patients. Motor blockade is relatively slight, being only 28.9 per cent compared to 46.4 per cent with the same strength of tetracaine.

In obstetrics the quality of sensory blockade is quite profound for

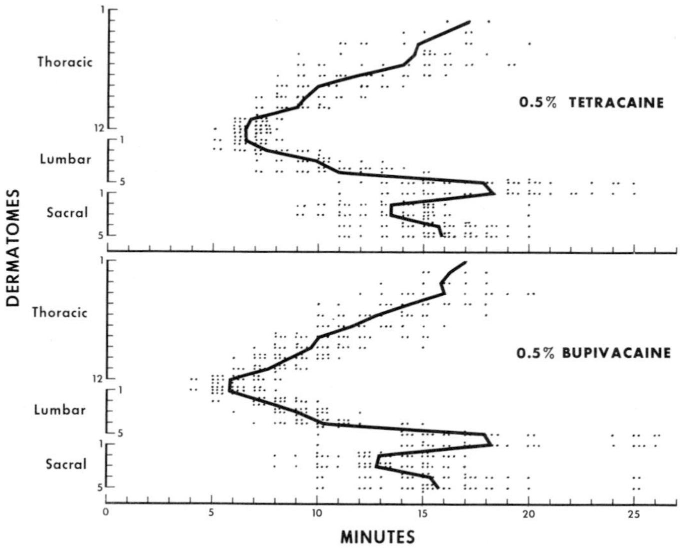

Figure 9-11. Latency of onset and segmental spread of epidural analgesia for 0.5 per cent tetracaine and 0.5 per cent bupivacaine injected at the second lumbar interspace. Each dot represents one observation of the advancing margin of skin analgesia to pin-prick. Mean latency profiles are shown by heavy lines. (From Bromage, P. R.: A comparison of bupivacaine and tetracaine in epidural analgesia for surgery. Canad. Anaesth. Soc. J. *16*:37, 1969b.)

vaginal delivery, and analgesia is adequate with or without epinephrine. This dissociation of capability for sensory and motor blockade is particularly desirable in obstetrical practice for relief of pain in labor, as shown in Figure 12-21 in the chapter on obstetrical applications. Satisfactory analgesia for abdominal section requires the 0.75 per cent concentration or a more intensely penetrating agent, such as etidocaine or carbonated lidocaine.

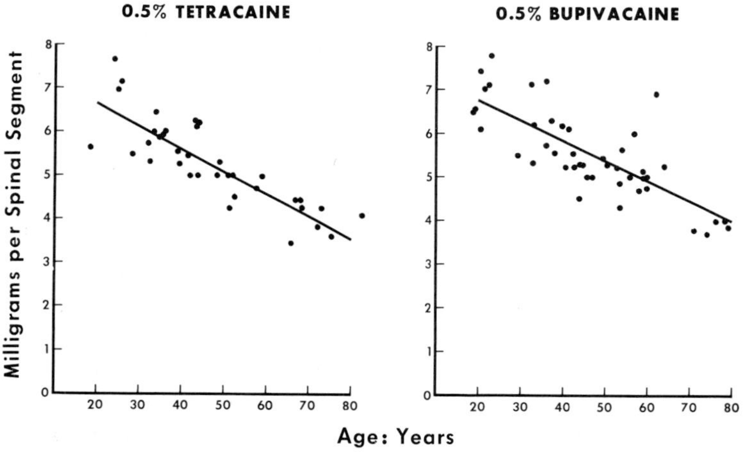

Figure 9-12. Dose requirements of 0.5 per cent tetracaine (n = 36) and 0.5 per cent bupivacaine (n = 44) in terms of milligrams per spinal segment related to age. Injection site: second lumbar interspace in sitting position. (From Bromage, P. R.: A comparison of bupivacaine and tetracaine in epidural analgesia for surgery. Canad. Anaesth. Soc. J. *16*:37, 1969b.)

DURATION OF ACTION. Next to dibucaine, bupivacaine is the longest acting drug available for epidural blockade at the present time. Duration of analgesia from the time of complete spread to recession of two segments is 196±31 minutes when epinephrine 1/200,000 is added to the solution. We have not obtained accurate comparative figures for the plain 0.5 per cent solution, but in a similar type of study, Waters et al. (1970) found that duration with plain bupivacaine was about 20 per cent shorter than with the epinephrine-containing solution.

After induction in the mid-thoracic region, where dose requirements are 40 per cent less than in the lumbar region, the length of action is appreciably shorter than after lumbar induction, and duration to recession of two segments is reduced to approximately 145 minutes.

0.75 Per Cent Bupivacaine. The 0.75 per cent concentration was introduced into clinical practice to correct the practical shortcomings of the weaker solutions of bupivacaine, and particularly to shorten latency and improve the quality of surgical analgesia (Moore et al., 1974; Nolte et al., 1974). These goals have been partially fulfilled, as can be seen by the data summarized in Table 9–1.

Latency is shortened somewhat from 18.2 minutes to 16.8 minutes, but there is still a marked salient of delay at L_5 and S_1, and analgesia often remains poor in these segments. Duration of action and degree of motor block vary widely and unpredictably, as shown in Figure 9–13, and motor block is more intense than with the 0.5 per cent solution when epinephrine is added.

Segmental dose requirements are highly predictable and are not influenced by the presence or absence of epinephrine. Dose requirements show an interesting relationship with age. In the third decade segmental dose requirements for the 0.75 per cent solution are about 40 per cent greater than for the 0.5 per cent concentration. However, the regression lines converge with advancing age, and by 80 years they have reached identical values (Fig. 9–14). At first sight this pattern suggests that the 0.75 per cent solution may be associated with a greater uptake of drug by neural tissues in the young age groups. However, intensity of motor block and duration of action are not correlated with dose requirements or with age, so one must conclude that the difference is probably not due to increased neural uptake but rather to increased vascular and *non-neural* uptake in the younger age groups.

The 0.75 per cent solution of bupivacaine has several practical advantages, as well as some disadvantages. Although it is long-acting, the precise duration is rather unpredictable, as can be seen in Figure 9–13; however, the solution can usually be relied on to provide 2½ hours of stable analgesia before the block begins to regress. The high intensity of motor blockade makes the epinephrine-containing solution unsuited to early postoperative movements. Motor block is profound, and the patients often remain with immobile legs for long periods of time after the operation is over. This degree of immobility is an undesirable feature that defeats the basic objective of early functional restoration, since it may set the stage for deep vein thrombosis.

The plain 0.75 per cent solution produces less motor block but good sensory analgesia, except in the resistant segments of L_5 and S_1, and it appears to produce excellent conditions for pelvic surgery in elderly patients. Needless to

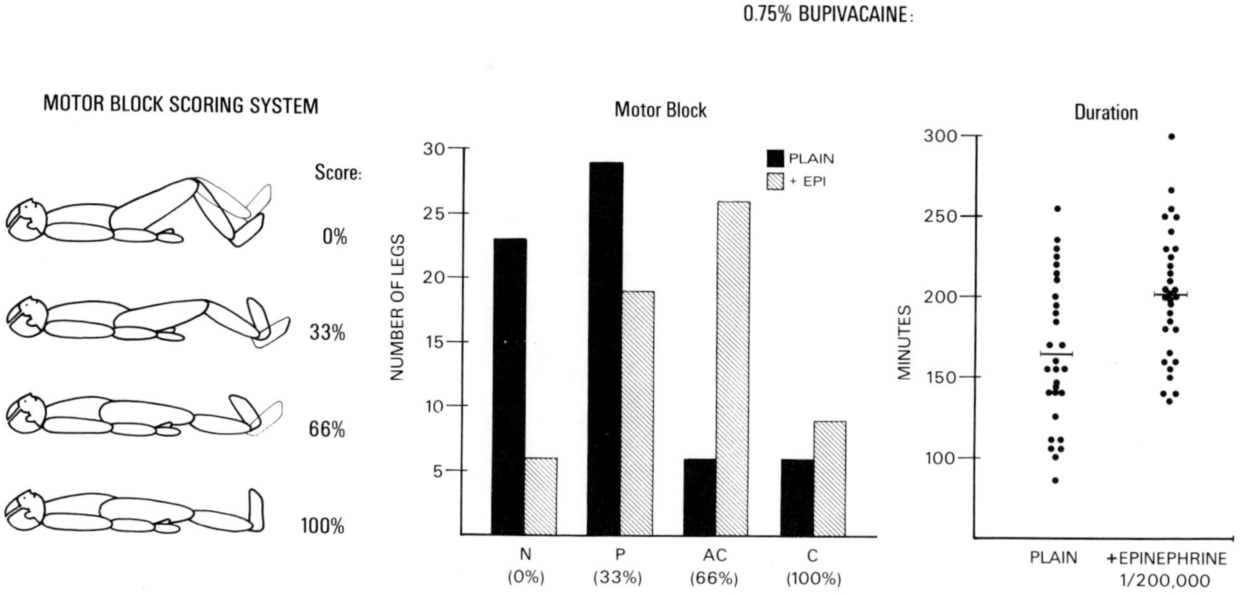

Figure 9–13. Bupivacaine, 0.75 per cent, plain and with 1/200,000 epinephrine, showing motor blockade and duration of action (to recession of two segments).

Motor Block Histogram

■ 0.75 per cent bupivacaine plain. Average motor block score: 30.5 ± 30 per cent.

□ 0.75 per cent bupivacaine with 1/200,000 epinephrine. Average motor block score: 54 ± 29 per cent.

(See Chapter 4 for explanation of method of motor score.)

Duration Scattergram

Plain solution, average duration: 164.5 ± 46 minutes.

Epinephrine solution, average duration: 201 ± 40 minutes.

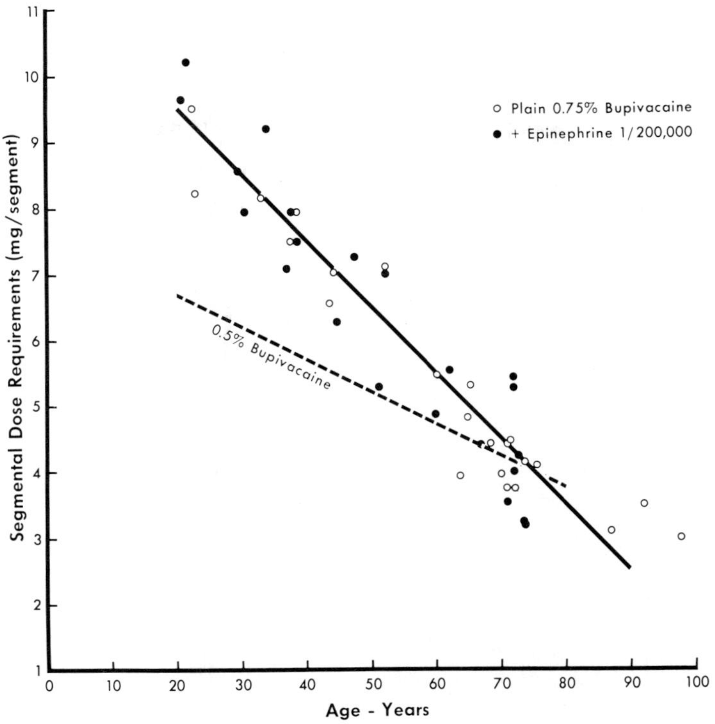

Figure 9–14. Epidural dose requirements for 0.75 per cent bupivacaine related to age in 45 patients.
○ = Plain solution
● = With Epinephrine 1/200,000
The regression line for 0.5 per cent bupivacaine (- - - - - -) is shown for comparison.

say the great intensity of motor block makes the 0.75 per cent solution entirely unsuitable for postoperative analgesia or for relief of pain in labor.

0.125 Per Cent Bupivacaine. Van Steenberge and his colleagues reported the use of 0.125 per cent bupivacaine with 1/400,000 epinephrine for relief of pain in labor and delivery in 500 patients, using relatively large volumes of anesthetic solution to compensate for the very weak concentration (Vanderick et al., 1974; Geerinckx et al., 1974). This is an old principle using a new drug and it recalls the early days of epidural technique when large volumes of dilute procaine or tetracaine were used to achieve a quality of analgesia that was marginally satisfactory for surgical pain relief (Odom, 1936). However, in pregnant women at term, effective epidural blockade can be achieved with appreciably smaller doses of local anesthetic than in the nonpregnant state (Bromage, 1961a), and the principle of striving for minimal dosage in obstetrics is sound and clearly in the best interests of the fetus.

An induction dose of 15 ml of 0.125 per cent bupivacaine (18.75 mg) is given when labor is established, followed by 10 ml (12.5 mg) at intervals of 45 to 90 minutes. A final dose of 15 ml is given in the sitting position for effective perineal analgesia at the time of delivery. With this regimen satisfactory results have been reported in over 500 oxytocin-driven labors, and maternal and fetal

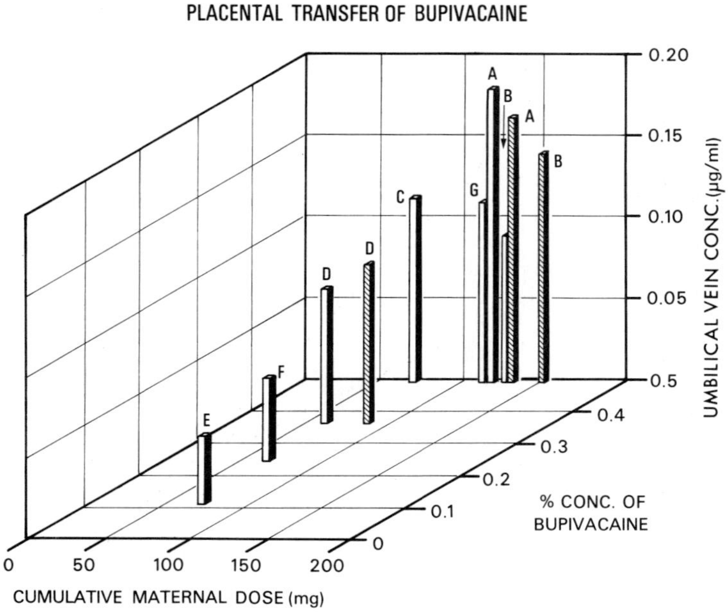

Figure 9–15. Summary of published data on fetal uptake of bupivacaine after epidural blockade for labor and delivery. Three-dimensional representation of relationship between concentration of bupivacaine administered, cumulative maternal dose, and umbilical vein concentration at birth.

Hatched columns: Plain bupivacaine
Clear columns: Bupivacaine with epinephrine

A. Reynolds and Taylor, Brit. J. Anaesth. 1971; B. Reynolds et al., Brit. J. Anaesth. 1973; C. Thomas et al., Brit. J. Anaesth. 1969b; D. Hyman and Shnider (average of 0.25 and 0.5 per cent bupivacaine), Anesthesiol. 1971; E. Geerinckx et al., Brit. J. Anaesth. 1974; F. Belfrage et al., Amer. J. Obstet. Gynecol. 1975b; G. Scanlon et al., Anesthesiol. 1976.

blood levels of local anesthetic have been kept lower than in any other reported series, as shown in Table 12–3 in Chapter 12 and in Figure 9–15.

Inspection of the measurements summarized in Figure 9–15 confirms what might be expected intuitively. Increasing concentrations of bupivacaine are accompanied by a steady upward trend toward higher cumulative dosage in the mother and higher blood levels in the fetus. Also, there is a tendency for fetal blood concentrations to be higher when epinephrine is omitted from the epidural solution. Our own experience with 0.125 per cent bupivacaine for obstetrics has been in almost complete accord with that of Van Steenberge's group. Pain is relieved within 5 minutes of injection, but skin analgesia is slow to develop, and 15 to 20 minutes usually elapse before a definite dermatome distribution can be mapped out. Repeat doses may not have to be given quite so frequently as Van Steenberge's group recommends, and intervals as long as two hours have occasionally been encountered without loss of control of the analgesic situation. However, small supplemental doses may have to be administered with the patient lying on her side in order to augment the patchy segmental escape that occasionally occurs at T_{12} or L_1. Perineal analgesia is surprisingly satisfactory, considering the extreme dilution and the very small mass of bupivacaine that is required.

The secret of success with this solution depends on two things. First, the analgesic situation must be watched closely throughout labor because of the rather wide individual differences in duration encountered between patients: "remote control" supervision is not appropriate. Second, analgesia is very tenuous at first, but it steadily deepens and creeps caudally with each successive injection. Therefore, labor must be long enough to require several top-up doses so that sacral anesthesia can ripen by the time delivery takes place. Short labors requiring only one or two injections are not suited to the technique, as satisfactory analgesia does not have time to develop in the sacral segments, and then a supplementary dose of a fast-acting agent such as chloroprocaine or carbonated lidocaine must be given to ensure good perineal analgesia.

In our initial series of 50 cases using 0.125 per cent bupivacaine and 1/400,000 epinephrine, perineal analgesia was satisfactory for episiotomy and low forceps delivery without any other analgesic supplementation. Cumulative dose requirements were also lower than with 0.5 per cent or 0.25 per cent bupivacaine, as shown in Figure 12–25 (Bramwell and Bromage, unpublished data, 1976).

Etidocaine (Duranest)

2-(N-ethyl propylamino)-2′,6′-butyroxylidide hydrochloride
molecular weight = 312, pKa = 7.74

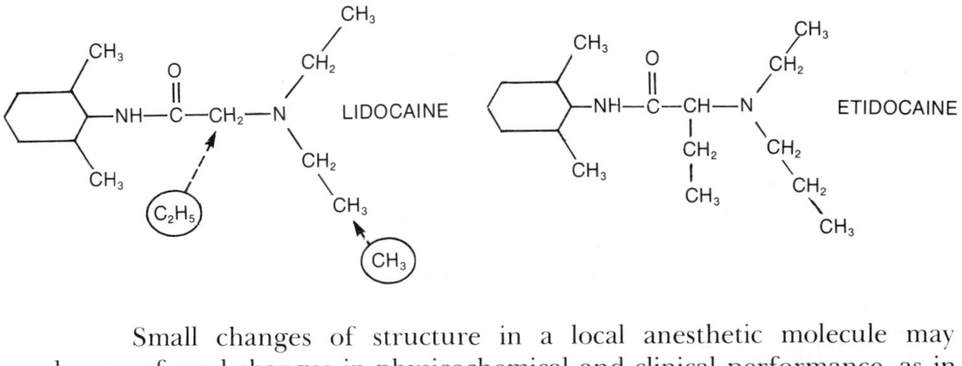

Small changes of structure in a local anesthetic molecule may produce profound changes in physicochemical and clinical performance, as in the case of carbocaine and bupivacaine. The addition of an ethyl and a methyl group to lidocaine, as shown above, confers a 50 per cent increase in protein binding power and a fiftyfold increase in lipid solubility, creating a local anesthetic agent with the unusual properties of both very rapid onset and long duration.

Etidocaine was introduced for clinical trial in 1973, and details of pharmacokinetics in man are now well understood. The toxicity of etidocaine seems to be largely dependent on its speed of uptake. The drug is about twice as toxic as lidocaine when absorbed slowly from subcutaneous sites, but about four times as toxic as lidocaine when given by rapid intravenous injection (Adams et al., 1972; Scott, 1975; Munson et al., 1975; Malagodi et al., 1977). Concentrations of 0.25 to 1.5 per cent etidocaine have been used for epidural analgesia (Lund et al., 1973; Bridenbaugh et al., 1973, 1974; Bromage et al., 1974a, 1974b; Stanton-Hicks et al., 1976). Lund and his colleagues have made extensive measurements of blood concentrations after a wide range of epidural doses between 100 and 450 mg with 1/200,000 epinephrine. Peak blood concentrations varied between 0.5 and 3.0 μg per ml according to the size of dose, and no toxic reactions were reported in this series (Lund et al., 1973).

Disagreement has existed over the role of epinephrine as a useful adjuvant for etidocaine. Some investigators concluded that epinephrine made no difference to the clinical performance of etidocaine apart from a more rapid onset of motor blockade (Bridenbaugh et al., 1974; Lund, 1976). However, others have found that epinephrine 1/200,000 improves the quality of analgesia markedly (Bromage et al., 1974a, 1974b; Murphy et al., 1976). Pharmacokinetic studies in unpremedicated volunteers by Mather and his colleagues (1976) support the view that epinephrine is likely to improve the quality of blockade. These workers have shown that the rapid phase of vascular uptake of etidocaine from the epidural space is significantly reduced by epinephrine 1/200,000, although the difference is not so marked as the reduction of vascular uptake that occurs when epinephrine is added to lidocaine.

Clinical experience with etidocaine for epidural analgesia at the Royal Victoria Hospital, Montreal, may be summarized as follows (Bromage et al., 1974a, 1974b).

SURGICAL SERIES

Etidocaine 1.0 per cent with 1/200,000 epinephrine was used in 171 cases, 1.0 per cent plain etidocaine was used in 20 cases. Transient local discomfort or mild pain accompanied the induction dose in many cases. This was attributed to local irritation caused by the rather marked acidity of etidocaine solutions (pH = 3.0 to 4.5). A similar observation has been made by others (Raksamani and Edelist, 1977).

Latency. Figure 9–16 shows latency profiles after mid-thoracic and mid-lumbar injection. Initial onset occurred in 4 minutes, and segmental spread was complete in an average time of 10.85 minutes. The usual salient of delay at L_5 and S_1 was almost eliminated. The onset and spread of analgesia with plain etidocaine was markedly slower than with the epinephrine-containing solution, and the mean time for complete segmental spread was 18 minutes.

Dose Requirements. Dose requirements per spinal segment are approximately one-half the amount required for lidocaine hydrochloride, as shown in Figure 9–17. Thus, the clinical potency of the 1.0 per cent solution is roughly twice that of lidocaine.

Quality of Blockade. Motor blockade was remarkably profound. An average score of 60 per cent was obtained with the epinephrine-containing solution and 50 per cent with the plain solution. This is the most intense degree of motor blockade encountered among all the epidural agents that I have tested, and other authors have reported the same observation (Bridenbaugh et al., 1973; Engberg et al., 1974; Gitschmann and Nolte, 1975; Murphy et al., 1976; Littlewood et al., 1977). However, the quality of sensory analgesia with etidocaine was less impressive than the degree of motor block, and traction on viscera

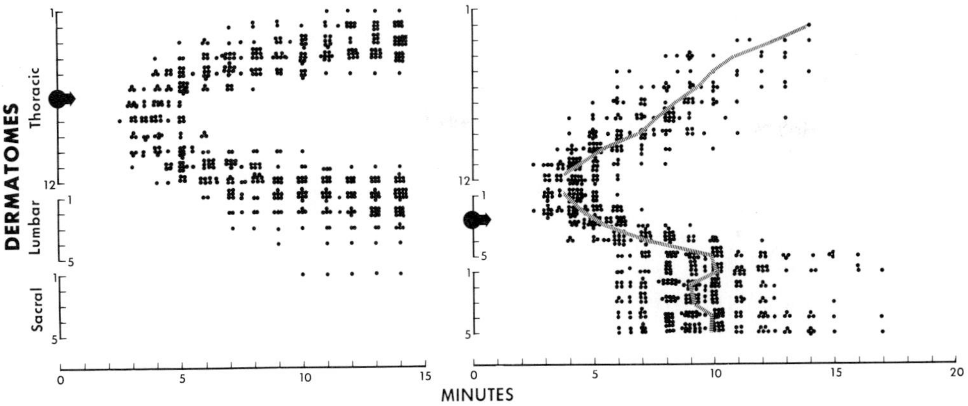

Figure 9–16. Epidural latency profiles for 1 per cent etidocaine with 1/200,000 epinephrine injected at the sixth thoracic or second lumbar interspaces. Each dot represents a single observation of the segmental spread of cutaneous analgesia to pin-prick.

(------) Mean latency profiles for lumbar block. Note relatively rapid onset of analgesia in the sacral segments.

(From Bromage, P. R., et al.: Etidocaine: A clinical evaluation for regional analgesia in surgery. Canad. Anaesth. Soc. J. *21*:523, 1974a.)

elicited complaints of pain and discomfort more frequently than under blocks with bupivacaine. Bridenbaugh and his colleagues (1973) have also reported on this rather unexpected dissociation between profoundly heavy motor block and disproportionately light sensory analgesia.

Duration of Sensory Blockade. Duration to recession of two segments varied widely. With the epinephrine-containing solution the average duration for the lumbar epidural blocks was 170±57 minutes and 147±44 minutes for the thoracic blocks. The shorter duration of the thoracic blocks has been noted with other agents and is probably related to the small mass of drug needed to block the slender roots and cord in this narrow portion of the spine. Lumbar epidural blocks were performed with plain 1 per cent etidocaine in 20 patients, and it was clear that adequate clinical performance is highly dependent on the addition of

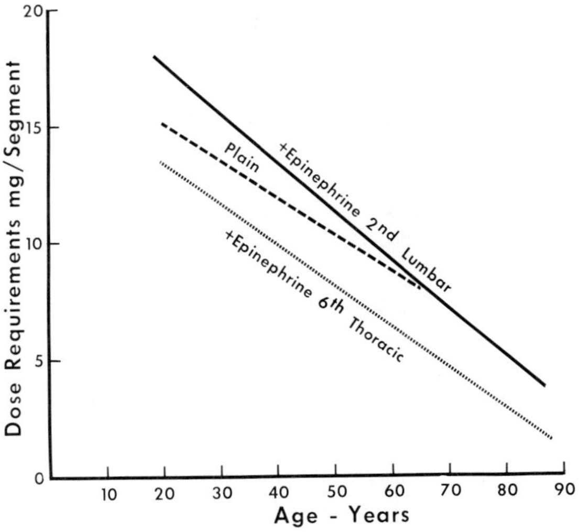

Figure 9–17. Epidural dose requirements for 1 per cent etidocaine related to age.

(———) + 1/200,000 epinephrine, injection at second lumbar interspace (n = 60).

(---------) Plain etidocaine, injection at second lumbar interspace (n = 18).

(''''''''') + 1/200,000 epinephrine, injection at sixth thoracic interspace (n = 35).

(From Bromage, P. R., et al.: Etidocaine: A clinical evaluation for regional analgesia in surgery. Canad. Anaesth. Soc. J. *21*:523, 1974a.)

epinephrine. With the plain solution, latency of complete spread slowed to 18 minutes and duration was shortened to 128 minutes. Analgesia tended to be asymmetrical and patchy, although motor blockade was still intense and only slightly less than in the epinephrine-containing series, with an average score of 50 per cent.

OBSTETRICAL SERIES

Etidocaine was used in 0.25 and 0.5 per cent concentrations in plain solution and with epinephrine 1/200,000 for pain relief in labor and in vaginal delivery with episiotomy and repair in 95 patients. The cumulative dose requirements and the success rate for these solutions are summarized in Figure 12–23 in the chapter on obstetrical applications. Again, it can be seen that etidocaine is highly dependent on added epinephrine for successful analgesia. The plain solutions gave unacceptably poor scores, whereas the epinephrine-containing solutions produced adequate results. Intense motor blockade was a serious disadvantage, hampering maternal movements and expulsive efforts. The marked dissociation of sensory and motor performance is summarized in Figure 12–21 and contrasted with the very different and more desirable characteristics of bupivacaine.

During cesarean section carried out under 1 per cent etidocaine with epinephrine 1/200,000 (dose range 140 to 225 mg), maternal blood concentrations were low, with a mean value of 0.45 μg etidocaine per ml, and umbilical vein concentrations were lower still, with an average of 0.16 μg per ml. Thus, the maternal-umbilical vein ratio is about the same as for bupivacaine, that is, approximately 3:1.

In summary, etidocaine has some strangely paradoxical qualities that make it an interesting agent from a research point of view. In our experience adequate clinical performance is heavily dependent on the presence of epinephrine in the epidural solution. However, this finding is at variance with a report by Bridenbaugh et al. (1974), in which epinephrine was found to make no difference to the clinical performance of etidocaine. Onset is remarkably rapid and duration long, but motor block is disproportionately severe compared to the more tenuous quality of sensory blockade, and repeated epidural doses may give rise to very prolonged blockade (Tucker et al., 1977). Thus, the drug is not suited to a situation in which muscular activity is required, such as postoperative pain relief or vaginal delivery. However, it is suitable for intraoperative use in abdominal surgery when profound muscular relaxation is an advantage.

Carbonated Local Anesthetics

The principle underlying carbonation of local anesthetics has been discussed in Chapter 3. This principle, discovered almost accidentally by a pharmaceutical engineer, represents one of the greatest practical advances in the history of local anesthetic drugs. The mere change of salt from a hydrochloride to a carbonated base can convert a mediocre drug to a star performer, with vivid action and commanding intensity. Unfortunately, the manufacturing process is relatively difficult and expensive, and at the time of writing, Canada is the only country where a carbonated local anesthetic is commercially available.* Two agents, carbonated prilocaine and carbonated lidocaine, have been studied at the Royal Victoria Hospital, Montreal, since 1963, and a third, carbonated bupivacaine, has been studied more recently in Britain (Appleyard et al., 1974) and in Germany (Schulte-Steinberg, 1976).

During the early comparative studies it was convenient to express the concentration of carbonated solutions in terms of the quantity of base per 100 ml in order to ensure strictly comparable amounts of analgesic base in solutions of the hydrochloride and the carbonated salts under comparison. Since 2 per cent lidocaine hydrochloride contains 20 mg of the salt per ml but only 17.3 mg of the base, it was necessary to prepare a 1.73 per cent solution of lidocaine base in carbonic acid for precise comparison. Thus, when carbonated solutions of lidocaine are described, it is pharmacologically correct to speak of a 1.73 per cent solution or a 0.87 per cent solution, but it is more convenient and more in accordance with custom to round these numbers out to 2 per cent and 1 per cent, respectively.

Carbonated prilocaine

Carbonated prilocaine is not commercially available at the present time, and its performance in the epidural space is summarized only as an example of the improved efficiency of the carbonated solutions (Bromage, 1965; Bromage et al., 1967). The following data relate to solutions containing 1/200,000 epinephrine.

Latency. Figure 9–18 shows the latency profile for 2 per cent prilocaine hydrochloride compared with the equivalent concentration of prilocaine CO_2-base. Latency of initial onset is shortened by 45 per cent and latency of complete spread by 25 per cent.

Quality of Blockade. The quality of sensory blockade is superior to that of the hydrochloride solution, and the intensity of motor blockade is 33 per cent greater.

Duration. Carbonated prilocaine has a slightly longer action than the hydrochloride salt.

Carbonated lidocaine

Carbonated lidocaine is prepared in an equivalent concentration to the 2 per cent hydrochloride solution, with 17.3 mg of lidocaine base per milliliter. The pH is approximately 6.5, and the pCO_2 is in the range of 600 to 700 mmHg. The solution is packaged in glass ampules of heavy gauge to resist pressure changes resulting from high ambient temperatures.

Carbonated lidocaine base is more difficult to produce than gassed solutions of the hydrochloride salt. During the initial investigations of carbonated solutions, trials were made of 2 per cent lidocaine HCl equilibrated with CO_2 at various partial pressures to see if the performance of these gassed hydrochloride solutions would match the carbonated base. However, it was soon apparent that the carbonated base was superior to the gassed hydrochloride salts

*Manufactured by Astra Chemicals, Inc., Mississauga, Ontario.

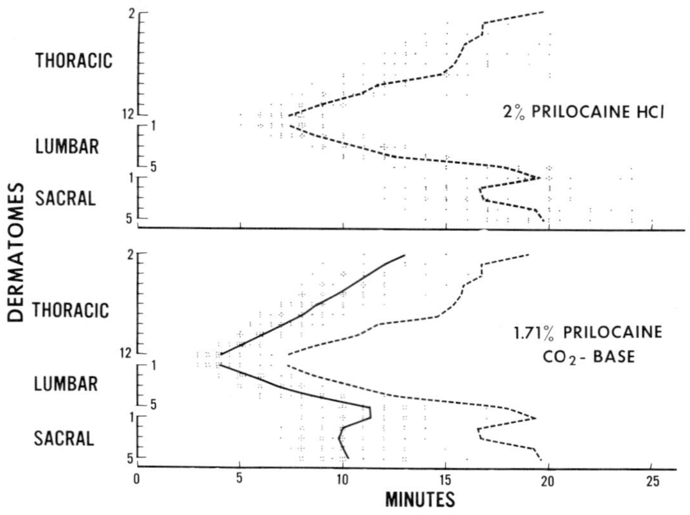

Figure 9–18. Latency profiles for 2 per cent prilocaine HCl (----) and 1.71 per cent prilocaine CO_2-base (——). Average profiles are drawn through the data points. (From Bromage, P. R., et al.: Quality of epidural blockade. III. Carbonated local anaesthetic solutions. Brit. J. Anaesth. *39*:197, 1967.)

in both speed of onset and quality of blockade and that its outstanding performance merited extended clinical trials.

Latency. Figure 9–19 shows latency profiles for carbonated lidocaine base compared with 2 per cent lidocaine HCl, both ungassed and gassed with CO_2 at approximately one-half atmosphere and at one atmosphere pressure. It can be seen that the latency of the HCl salt is shortened in the presence of a pCO_2 of 350 mmHg, and even more reduced with a pCO_2 of 700 mmHg, but most reduced when the carbon dioxide base solution was administered in association with a pCO_2 of 700 mmHg.

Figure 9–20 shows comparative latency profiles for two groups of outpatients who received caudal blockade for minor anorectal surgery with either 2 per cent lidocaine hydrochloride or the equivalent concentration of carbonated lidocaine base. It can be seen that the carbonated solution by the caudal route shortened the time of onset and spread of analgesia just as effectively as by the lumbar route. The lumbar latency profile for carbonated lidocaine is the quickest of all the local anesthetic solutions we have tested. Figure 9–21 contrasts the latency profile of 1.73 per cent carbonated lidocaine with a number of more familiar agents, and it can be seen that the usual salient of delay at L_5–S_1 is virtually abolished by carbonated lidocaine, as analgesia spreads rapidly downward through all the lumbar and sacral segments.

Dose Requirements. The carbonated solutions spread over more spinal segments than the hydrochloride solutions, so dosage must be reduced about 10 to 15 per cent below requirements for the orthodox hydrochloride solutions. Cumulative dose requirements are reduced in comparable amounts.

Quality of Blockade. The quality of sensory blockade with carbonated lidocaine is better than with any other agent we have tested. The resistant segments L_5 and S_1 are solidly anesthetized, and operations on the ankle and lower leg can be undertaken with confidence that analgesia will be satisfactory and that

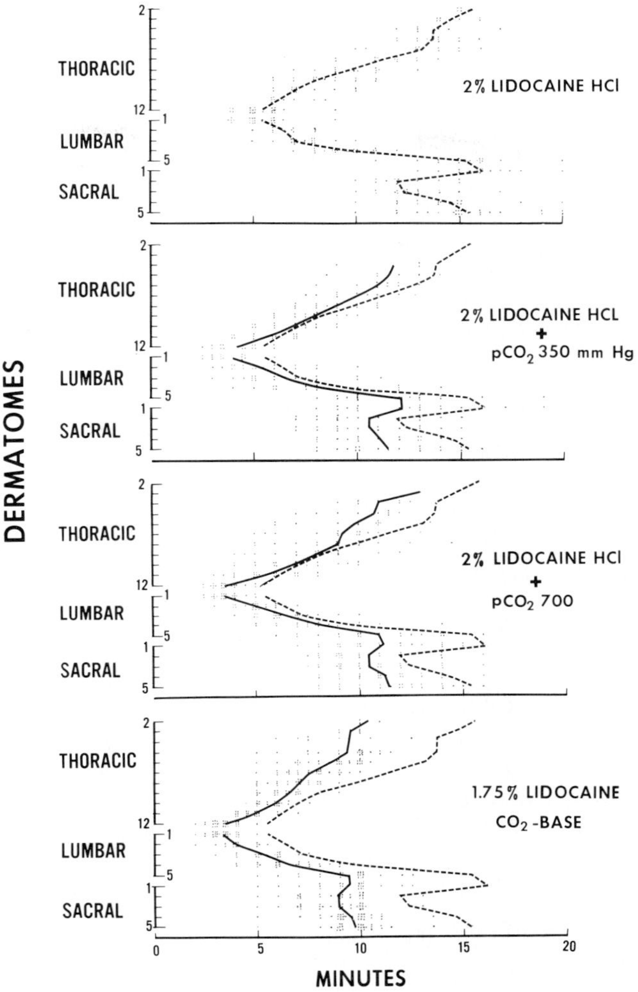

Figure 9–19. Mean latency profiles for epidural blockade at second lumbar interspace, comparing:

2 per cent lidocaine hydrochloride, ungassed (n = 22)

2 per cent lidocaine hydrochloride at pCO_2, 350 mmHg (n = 20)

2 per cent lidocaine hydrochloride at pCO_2, 700 mmHg (n = 24)

Carbonated lidocaine base, 2 per cent equivalent (n = 34)

(------) Control latency for lidocaine HCl at zero pCO_2

(——) Mean latencies for solutions under test

(After Bromage et al., 1967.)

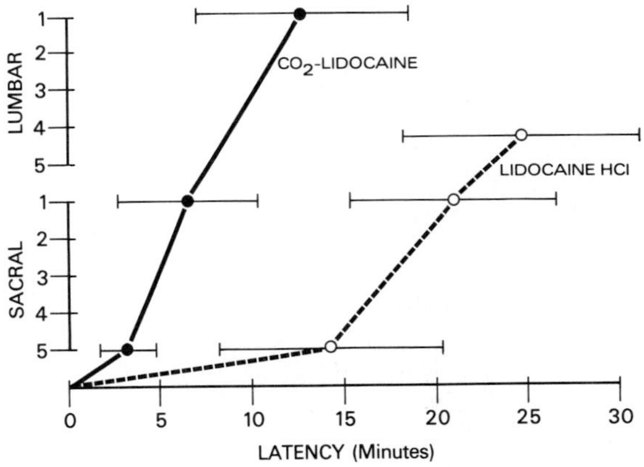

Figure 9–20. Latency and onset of spread of caudal analgesia with equivalent plain solutions (no epinephrine) of 2 per cent lidocaine hydrochloride and lidocaine CO_2-base. (Mean times ± S.D.) (From Cousins, M. J., and Bromage, P. R.: A comparison of the hydrochloride and carbonated salts of lignocaine for caudal analgesia in out-patients. Brit. J. Anaesth. *43*: 1149, 1971.)

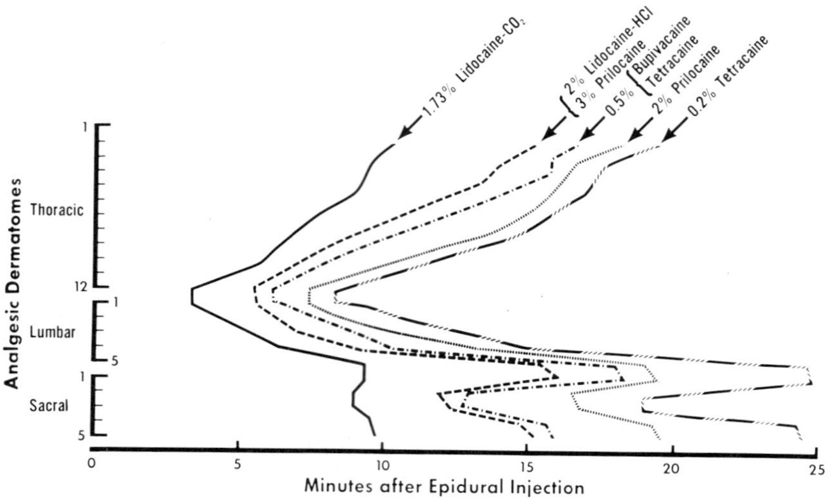

Figure 9–21. Mean latency profile of 1.73 per cent carbonated lidocaine contrasted with 2 per cent lidocaine HCl, 2 and 3 per cent prilocaine, 0.5 per cent bupivacaine and 0.2 per cent tetracaine. All solutions contained 1/200,000 epinephrine. Injection at the second lumbar interspace.

general supplementation will not be required. Patients who have received epidural blocks with other agents are quick to comment on the profound intensity of sensory analgesia produced by carbonated lidocaine.

Intensity of motor blockade is also more profound than with the hydrochloride salt of comparable concentration. Carbonated lidocaine 1.73 per cent with epinephrine produces an average motor block of more than 52 per cent compared to 36 per cent with the 2 per cent hydrochloride salt.

Carbonated lidocaine is a valuable asset for pain relief in obstetrics. The incidence of "missed segments" (see Chapter 12) is lower than with any other agent (Bromage, 1972), the cumulative dose requirements are less than with the hydrochloride salt and the quality of analgesia is more effective and reliable. However, the profound degree of motor block with the 1.73 per cent carbonated solution is too intense for routine vaginal delivery, and the 0.87 per cent solution is a better choice in normal labor. Figure 9–22 summarizes the saving in cumulative dose requirements and the increased analgesic success rate obtained with the carbonated solutions of prilocaine and lidocaine in labor, compared to the performance of their hydrochloride counterparts.

Duration. In peripheral plexus blocks carbonated lidocaine is slightly shorter-acting than the hydrochloride solution (Bromage and Gertel, 1970, 1972). However, in the epidural space the carbonated solution seems to be slightly longer-acting, but the difference is not great, as shown in Table 9–1.

Carbonated bupivacaine

Theoretically, bupivacaine would seem an ideal agent to use in the carbonated form. Bupivacaine has several desirable qualities that are marred only by slow onset of action. These include long duration, good quality of

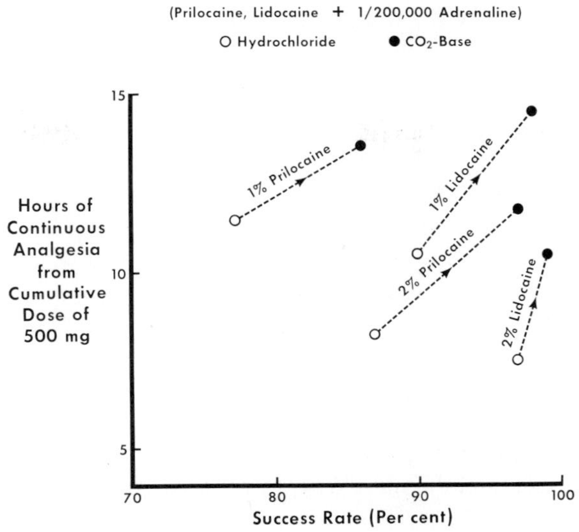

Figure 9–22. Improved performance of carbonated local anesthetics. Comparison of efficiency of carbonated and hydrochloride salts of prilocaine and lidocaine for relief of pain in labor.
○ Hydrochloride
● CO_2-base
All solutions with 1/200,000 epinephrine added.
(Data from Bromage, 1967.)

blockade in terms of sensory-motor dissociation and a low ratio of fetal-maternal uptake in obstetrical use. All that bupivacaine lacks is rapid onset and perhaps more profound analgesia—qualities that might be conferred by employing the carbonated salt.

Unfortunately, the limited trials that have been performed with carbonated bupivacaine have not shown the same dramatic improvement over the hydrochloride salt that was found with the carbonated solutions of prilocaine and lidocaine (Schulte-Steinberg, 1976). A small trial of my own using 0.5 per cent carbonated bupivacaine supplied through the courtesy of Dr. Schulte-Steinberg has been equally disappointing; the results are summarized in Table 9–2.

The slightly shorter latency of carbonated bupivacaine is too variable to be of practical consequence in epidural blockade, and this small advantage is bought at the cost of shortened duration. Carbonated bupivacaine is absorbed into the blood stream faster than the hydrochloride salt (Appleyard et al., 1974), and the increased vascular uptake is reflected in larger dose requirements and a shorter duration of action. Further work needs to be done to confirm these preliminary findings with carbonated bupivacaine. At present, it is not clear why

TABLE 9–2* **Comparison of Hydrochloride and Carbonated Salts of Bupivacaine in Lumbar Epidural Blockade**

	Bupivacaine Hydrochloride	*Bupivacaine-CO_2*
Latency of initial onset (minutes)	5.8	4.9 ± 0.6
Latency of complete spread (minutes)	18.2	14.2 ± 4.3
Segmental dose requirements at age 40 (mg/segment)	5.8	6.6
Intensity of motor block (%)	29 ± 29	20 ± 23
Duration to recession of two segments (minutes)	196±31	162 ± 26

*Data from Bromage (1969b).

carbonation confers such a poor advantage on bupivacaine compared to prilocaine and lidocaine.

Local Anesthetic Mixtures

No single local anesthetic can meet all clinical requirements for all occasions, since qualities that may be appropriate for one set of circumstances may be inappropriate for another. Mixtures of two or more agents have been used to combine the most desirable properties of each ingredient. Before the amide-type drugs were introduced, it was common practice to use mixtures of procaine with tetracaine or dibucaine in order to obtain a reasonably rapid onset from the procaine and a long duration from the slower-acting but more persistent companion drug. Techniques for continuous catheter administration arrived on the clinical scene almost simultaneously with the amide-type agents, so the need for mixtures of short- and long-acting drugs became less pressing. However, tetracaine in concentrations of 0.1 to 0.2 per cent has remained a favorite adjuvant with some authorities to prolong single-shot epidural injections of lidocaine (Moore et al., 1972).

The basic principles of mixing local anesthetic agents must be carefully considered, as some disagreement has existed over the possible dangers of mixing or "compounding" two local anesthetic agents. Experiments with small animals have indicated that the toxicity of amide- and ester-type drugs may be additive (Daos et al., 1962). However, other authors have denied that this danger exists in clinical practice, since the pharmacokinetics and mechanism of breakdown of the ester- and amide-types of local anesthetic are so different (Moore et al., 1972). Difficulty arises over the ever-present possibility of accidental intravenous injection. The safety of appropriate ester-amide mixtures would be assured if one could be absolutely certain that injection would be made accurately into the epidural space and that absorption of the mixture of agents would follow the usual pattern of slow vascular uptake from the space. However, the danger of toxicity becomes serious if accidental intravenous injection should occur. Using macaque monkeys as experimental animals, Munson and his colleagues (1977) have shown that the toxicity of lidocaine and tetracaine are indeed additive when the drugs are infused intravenously, for then the rapidly acting cholinesterase system of detoxification is overwhelmed by the speed of administration into the vascular compartment. In practice it is prudent to assume that accidental intravenous injection *may* occur on rare occasions. Therefore, a single injection of a "compounded" mixture of local anesthetics should be treated as a potentially toxic dose if the volume is large enough to exceed the safe limits of the sum of the ingredients. Then the induction dose should be given more slowly than usual and in divided amounts, with a pause of a minute or two between each increment in order to slow the speed of vascular uptake.

Ester-amide mixtures

Under normal circumstances ester-amide mixtures are likely to be less toxic than mixtures of two amide-type drugs since different detoxification pathways are involved. The ester drugs are rapidly broken down by pseudocholinesterase in the blood, while the amide types are split by the slower amidase system in the liver.

Moore and his colleagues (1972) report favorable results from a very large experience using mixtures of 0.2 per cent tetracaine as the long-acting ester component and 1.5 per cent lidocaine or 2 per cent chloroprocaine as the fast-acting companion drug for rapid onset. Experience at the Royal Victoria Hospital, Montreal, with 0.2 per cent tetracaine and 1/200,000 epinephrine as a single agent has shown a mean duration for recession to two segments of 135 ± 19 minutes, compared to 97 ± 19 minutes for lidocaine, which represents a useful, but not a dramatic, prolongation.

Mixtures of lidocaine with 0.1 per cent tetracaine have proved unsatisfactory in our hands, as a significant number of patients complained of unpleasant dyesthesias in the legs after the effects of the lidocaine had worn off while the weak tetracaine component was still active.

AMIDE-AMIDE MIXTURES

While ester and amide mixtures and amide-amide mixtures are equally toxic when accidental intravenous injection exerts a "bolus effect," the ester-amide mixtures are less toxic under normal conditions of slow absorption from the epidural space. Nevertheless, certain combinations of amide agents seemed likely to produce very desirable conditions of blockade that would be worth examining. Mixtures of carbonated lidocaine and bupivacaine give almost ideal conditions of extremely fast onset and predictably prolonged blockade in brachial plexus anesthesia (Bromage and Gertel, 1972), and the same qualities would be useful if they could be transplanted to the epidural context. Furthermore, bupivacaine blockade has a very favorable ratio of sensory to motor block, as described earlier, and of all the available agents it seems the one most suited to provide good sensory analgesia while sparing motor activity. This constellation of analgesic properties could bring the theoretical goal of epidural analgesia within reach at last, that is, profound analgesia in the presence of effective motor function. Accordingly, a clinical trial was conducted using 1 per cent carbonated lidocaine (0.87 per cent lidocaine base) combined with bupivacaine in two different concentrations of 0.25 or 0.375 per cent for patients with lower abdominal or lower limb operations. Latency, dose requirements, motor blockade and duration were measured as in earlier studies. The patients were lightly premedicated. Sensory analgesia was scored as either 100 per cent if no anesthetic supplementation was required, or zero if any supplementation was needed. The results of this trial are summarized in Table 9–3.

It can be seen that results did not reach expectations. Although latency was short with both solutions, the 0.25 per cent bupivacaine mixture gave imperfect analgesia, and 4 out of the 20 cases needed some anesthesia supplementation. However, the degree of motor block was not severe, and all 20 patients were able to move their feet during operation. The small increase of bupivacaine concentration from 0.25 to 0.375 per cent produced marked changes in the quality of blockade. Sensory block was more satisfactory in patients receiving the 0.375 per cent solution, and only 1 patient out of 24

TABLE 9–3 Epidural Performance of 1 Per Cent Lidocaine-CO_2 (0.87 Per Cent Base) + 0.25 Per Cent Bupivacaine HCl, Compared to 1 Per Cent Lidocaine-CO_2 + 0.375 Per Cent Bupivacaine (both solutions with 1/200,000 epinephrine; injection at $L_2 - L_3$)

		Latency (min)		*Segmental Dose Requirements at 40 yr*						
Analgesic Solution	***n***	*INITIAL*	*COMPLETE*	*VOLUME (ML)*	*LIDOCAINE BASE (MG)*	*BUPIVACAINE BASE (MG)*	*LIDOCAINE HCl EQUIVALENT DOSE (MG)**	***Sensory Success (%)***	***Motor Block (%)***	***Duration of Recession of Two Segments (min)***
1% Lidocaine-CO_2 + 0.25% Bupivacaine HCl	20	3.77 ±0.6	11.65 ±1.9	1.24	10.79	2.76	24.5	80	27.7	137 ± 30
1% Lidocaine-CO_2 + 0.375% Bupivacaine HCl	24	3.9 ±0.6	11.7 ±2.3	1.24	10.79	4.14	31.5	95.8	49.7	151 ± 19

*Lidocaine HCl equivalent dose is calculated from the sum of lidocaine base and bupivacaine base present in the volume dose required per segment at age 40 (i.e., 1.24 ml), assuming that bupivacaine is four times as potent as lidocaine.

required any supplementation for inadequate analgesia. However, the improved quality of analgesia was accompanied by a correspondingly profound degree of motor block, and 5 out of the 24 patients experienced complete immobility of one or both legs.

The segmental dose requirements in terms of volume (i.e., ml per spinal segment) was the same for both mixtures, so the anesthetic content has been converted into "lidocaine hydrochloride equivalents" in Table 9–3, on the assumption that bupivacaine is four times as potent and as toxic as lidocaine. Note that the "lidocaine equivalent" dose requirements of the 0.375 per cent mixture are somewhat higher than those for 2 per cent lidocaine HCl listed in Table 9–3. Therefore the relatively large quantities needed to produce a high level of segmental blockade in young subjects must be administered cautiously.

Adjuvants

Viscous solutions ("plombes")

The low viscosity of water allows aqueous solutions to disperse freely throughout the epidural space. Anesthetic solutions with a higher viscosity might be expected to stay closer to the site of injection, acting as a depot from which the anesthetic solute would be slowly leached out, providing both a localized segmental type of blockade as well as a more prolonged duration of anesthesia. This theoretical approach was applied extensively by German workers over a 20-year period from 1937 onward. Denecke (1937) was the first to apply the idea of prolonged segmental blockade using serum, and later gelatine, as the viscous agent and tetracaine as the local anesthetic. Concentrations of 0.3 or 0.4 per cent tetracaine were given in volumes of up to 15 ml, and with this technique Denecke obtained analgesia lasting five to seven hours and limited in extent to three segments on each side of the injection site.

In 1941 German chemists synthesized the macromolecular polymer "Periston" (polyvinylpyrrolidone or PVP) as a plasma substitute in wound shock, and Düttmann made use of this substance as a viscous vehicle instead of gelatine, since it was more easily stored and sterilized and gelatine was in short supply during wartime. Düttmann's results were similar to those of Denecke, and doses of 14 to 20 ml of 0.3 per cent tetracaine provided segmental analgesia for five to six hours (Düttmann, 1941). Further modifications of the technique were made by other workers. Goepel (1947) increased the concentration of tetracaine to 0.5 per cent in a 6 per cent solution of "Periston" and reduced the volume to 6 to 12 ml. Buchholz and Lesse (1950a, 1950b, 1951) modified the technique by preceding the injection of viscous solution (or "plombe," as it was called) by introducing about 30 ml of saline into the epidural space, in order to open up the tissue spaces ahead of the viscous mass. Later, the concentration of tetracaine was increased to 1.5 per cent in 6 per cent polyvinylpyrrolidone (Poppelbaum, 1954).

The total experience of these German writers and others using similar viscous solutions, runs into many thousands of cases, so their findings demand considerable respect; nevertheless, the principles involved deserve careful scrutiny. First, the viscous solutions are hyperosmolar, with an osmolality in the range of 450 to 500 mOsmol per L (normal = 280 to 300 mOsmol per L); therefore, they are likely to cause tissue irritation. Second, the epidural kinetics of small volumes of concentrated local anesthetic solutions are poorly understood, as discussed in Chapter 4. We do know that small volumes of concentrated aqueous solutions spread rather inexplicably over a large number of segments, and it is likely that a concentrated viscous "plombe" will behave somewhat in the same manner, especially when the "plombe" is introduced into a water-filled epidural space already primed with a prior injection of 30 ml of saline. Third, clinical measurements of my own with weaker solutions of local anesthetic in concentrated PVP failed to show the limitation of segmental blockade or the prolongation of analgesia that might be expected if the local anesthetic had been held in a restricted part of the epidural space by the viscous solvent. Observations with 1.4 per cent lidocaine in 7.5 per cent PVP with 1/150,000 epinephrine showed the following salient points (Bromage, 1954):

1. Speed of onset: slowed.

2. Segmental spread of analgesia: slowed, but the ultimate segmental spread was as extensive as predicted for an equal volume and concentration of an aqueous solution.

3. Duration: prolonged slightly (15 to 30 per cent), but not to the extent reported by the German workers.

At the time of writing, viscous solutions appear to have little to offer from the practical point of view. However, careful laboratory studies of uptake and distribution from concentrated plombes might throw additional light on the principles underlying the spreading characteristics and mechanisms of action of epidural local anesthetics.

ADRENOCORTICOSTEROIDS

Epidural corticoid injections are widely used for relief of chronic back pain and for immediate treatment of acutely prolapsed intervertebral discs (see Chapter 13). Injection of corticosteroid suspensions into the epidural space seems to reduce local edema and to improve symptoms arising from pressure on nerves and nerve integuments. Water-soluble solutions of corticosteroids should not be used, as they are taken up and eliminated from the epidural space too rapidly. Instead, suspensions of poorly soluble acetate salts are injected to provide a local depot site from which uptake occurs very gradually over a period of 10 to 20 days.

Corticoid suspensions do not cause pain when injected into the epidural space, and they may be injected alone without any local anesthetic added to them. However, most physicians prefer to mix the corticoid suspension with local anesthetic solution in order to provide immediate symptomatic relief and to give some tangible evidence of the probable degree of segmental spread within the epidural space. The preparations most commonly used are:

1. Hydrocortisone acetate in doses of 100 to 200 mg.
2. Methylprednisolone acetate (Depo-Medrol) in doses of 40 to 100 mg.

A mixture of the insoluble suspension is freshly prepared and evenly dispersed in the syringe by vigorous shaking immediately prior to injection.

The long-term effects of repeated intraspinal corticosteroids have not been established, but it is prudent to assume that destructive changes analogous to those found in joints may follow excessive administration (Smyth et al., 1963). Corticosteroid administration should therefore be limited to courses of three or four injections given three to ten days apart, with intervals of three to six months between courses. It is noteworthy that methylprednisolone acetate is suspended in a carrier solution containing 2.9 per cent polyethylene glycol. Wood and Arguelles (1977) report microscopic evidence of neurolysis in sciatic nerves of rats after perineural injection of the carrier solution. These authors make the intriguing suggestion that perhaps some of the symptomatic benefits of methylprednisolone injections in painful states may be caused by local injury of small nerve fibers independently of any anti-inflammatory effects of the corticoid suspension.

Summary

Table 9–1 summarizes the performance of various local anesthetic solutions for lumbar epidural blockade. Of all the local anesthetics available, only an elite few stand out as having the exceptional qualities necessary for daily use. Each of these elite has individual abilities that make it better fitted for some clinical tasks than for others, as outlined in Table 9–4.

Rapid latency of onset is confined to three agents—etidocaine, chloroprocaine and carbonated lidocaine—the latter being the fastest acting agent available at the present time. There is a distinctive range of sensory-motor dissociation among the agents tested. Bupivacaine in medium concentration (0.25 to 0.5 per cent) produces less motor block than most other agents in comparable concentration. Conversely, tetracaine and etidocaine produce disproportionately profound motor blockade in relation to their quality of sensory analgesia. The resistant spinal segments L_5 and S_1 offer the most rigorous test of analgesic potency, and very few local anesthetic agents can be relied upon to produce really effective analgesia in the distribution of these two segments along the outer calf, ankle and lateral border of the foot. Carbonated lidocaine with epinephrine stands in a class by itself as passing this test most consistently.

Contemporary views on the genesis of deep vein thrombosis have forced a more sophisticated approach to the quality of surgical anesthesia than formerly. Early postoperative movement and calf exercises even during the course of operation seem to be important prophylactic factors, as discussed in Chapter 7. Therefore, it is no longer appropriate to induce intense, long-lasting motor blockade that persists after operation and prevents early postoperative movements. The need to search for an ideal local anesthetic agent with distinctive differentiation between sensory and motor block has become more obvious and more urgent. Although a range of differentiation between motor and sensory capabilities does exist among agents, as shown in Figure 12–21, the degree of separation is not sufficient to ensure effective surgical analgesia while sparing motor activity. However, there is enough choice to approach close to the ideal by intelligent selection and combination of the agents that are available. Combinations of short- and long-acting drugs can be tailored to the needs of each individual operation with a fair degree of assurance that the patient will be

TABLE 9–4 Practical Attributes of Six Local Anesthetics for Clinical Use in Epidural Blockade

Local Anesthetic	*Surgery*	*Postoperative Relief of Pain*	*Obstetrics*	*Therapeutic Applications*
Chloroprocaine	Useful for fast onset, but intensity not outstanding; evanescent	Poor (too evanescent)	Safe; useful for fast onset, but very short acting	Useful for short-acting diagnostic blocks
Lidocaine HCl	A well-tried workhorse in 1.5–3.0 per cent solution	Satisfactory in 1 per cent solution	Satisfactory in 1 per cent solution	Useful for diagnostic and therapeutic blocks
Lidocaine-CO_2	Outstanding in speed and quality of blockade; the best available agent	Satisfactory in 1 per cent solution; no special advantage over the hydrochloride salt	Fast and intense action for quick perineal dose; too powerful for continuous use in labor; outstanding for cesarean section	Little or no advantage over the hydrochloride salt
Mepivacaine HCl	Similar to lidocaine HCl, but slightly longer-acting (the 3 per cent solution has not been tried)	Satisfactory in 1 per cent solution	A poor choice because of excessive fetal uptake (pKa is too close to physiological pH)	Useful for diagnostic and therapeutic blocks
Etidocaine HCl	Excellent; fast onset and intense motor block	Unsatisfactory; excessive motor block	Excellent for cesarean section, but excessive motor block makes it a poor choice for vaginal delivery	Long action occasionally useful, but excessive motor block a disadvantage
Bupivacaine HCl	Excellent in 0.75 per cent concentration, with moderately fast onset and powerful motor block; adequate in 0.5 per cent concentration; 0.25 per cent adequate in pediatric cases	Excellent in 0.5 per cent solution or with larger volumes of 0.25 per cent	Outstanding choice; excellent in 0.25 per cent or 0.125 per cent solution; 0.75 per cent solution for cesarean section causes prolonged postoperative motor blockade	Useful for long-acting therapeutic blocks; the 0.25 per cent solution gives good pain relief with minimal motor blockade

pain-free in the postoperative period and capable of greater activity than after a general anesthetic with muscle relaxants and narcotic supplementation.

The choice of appropriate agent is most critical in obstetrics, for there the effects on fetal well-being are of even greater concern than the quality of analgesic blockade. Many different agents and many different concentrations and techniques have been used for relief of pain in labor. In order to make the right choice, the question should be asked: Of all the agents that are available, which is the most efficient and at the same time least likely to be toxic to the baby? This question is difficult to answer because the literature is quite confusing and full of different experimental protocols. Therefore, in answering the question it is necessary to scan the published data for those authors who have made a deliberate and determined effort to reduce epidural dosage to the minimum compatible with effective pain relief, and then to use the blood concentrations achieved by these authors as a legitimate standard against which to compare other results. This has been done in Table 9–5, using data from Hehre and his colleagues (1965) and from the Royal Victoria Hospital, Montreal (Fox et al., 1971), two groups with rigid standards of minimal dosage as the basis for comparison. Both groups had the same goal—minimal dosage compatible with efficiency—and the findings from both groups are remarkably close to each other. It can be seen that several published figures exceed the ideal standard set by the careful minimal dosage regimens of Hehre and Fox and expressed as unity in the last column of Table 9–5. Use of large doses and stronger concentrations than actually needed for the task in hand lead to unnecessarily high concentrations of local anesthetic in the umbilical vein, with relative toxicities above the norm set as unity in the scale of comparative toxicity. From Table 9–5 it can be seen that among the amide-linked agents bupivacaine is the best, and 0.125 per cent bupivacaine with 1/400,000 epinephrine is the safest solution for pain relief in labor. However, repeated injections and very close supervision are required for satisfactory results with 0.125 per cent bupivacaine, and the majority of anesthesiologists will probably find the 0.25 per cent concentration a better compromise between the ideal and the practical in labor and delivery.

EQUIPMENT

The equipment necessary for epidural injection is basically simple. The essential ingredients are a needle of the right length and caliber, a syringe

TABLE 9–5 Epidural Analgesia in Obstetrics; Comparative Fetal Toxicity Related to Analgesic Agent and Concentration of Epidural Solution

Authors	*Epidural Solution*	*Toxicity Relative To Lidocaine*	*Umbilical Vein (UV) Concentration (μg/ml)*	*Fetal Toxicity Relative to Minimal Standard Low-Dose Regimen of Lidocaine HCl*
STANDARD LOW-DOSE REGIMEN				
Hehre et al. (1965)	1% Lidocaine HCl + Epi	1	0.80	= Av. 0.82 ≡ 1.0 Relative toxicity
Fox et al. (1971)	1% Lidocaine HCl + Epi	1	0.84	
Reynolds and Taylor (1970)	1.5% Lidocaine + Epi	1	1.0	1.22
Thomas et al. (1968)	1% Lidocaine + Epi	1	1.72	2.1
Scanlon et al. (1974)	1% Plain Mepivacaine	1	1.68	2.05
Reynolds and Taylor (1970)	0.5% Bupivacaine + Epi	4	0.077	0.375
Reynolds and Taylor (1971)	0.5% Plain Bupivacaine	4	0.161	0.785
Reynolds and Taylor (1971)	0.5% Bupivacaine + Epi	4	0.18	0.88
Reynolds et al. (1973)	0.5% Plain Bupivacaine	4	0.14	0.684
Reynolds et al. (1973)	0.5% Bupivacaine + Epi	4	0.088	0.439
Scanlon et al. (1976)	0.5% Plain Bupivacaine	4	0.11	0.539
Belfrage et al. (1975b)	0.25% Bupivacaine + Epi	4	0.051	0.249
Geerinckx et al. (1974)	0.125% Bupivacaine + Epi	4	0.04	0.195
Magno et al. (1976) (cesarean section)	0.75% Plain Bupivacaine	4	0.214	1.04
Bromage et al. (1974b) (cesarean section)	1% Etidocaine + Epi	2–4	0.16	0.39–0.78
Lund et al. (1977) (cesarean section)	1% Plain Etidocaine	2–4	0.38	0.93–1.85
	1% Etidocaine + Epi	2–4	0.28	0.68–1.36
CONTINUOUS CAUDAL				
Moore et al. (1968)	1% Plain Mepivacaine	1	4.9	5.98
Moore et al. (1971)	0.5% Plain Bupivacaine	4	0.215	1.05

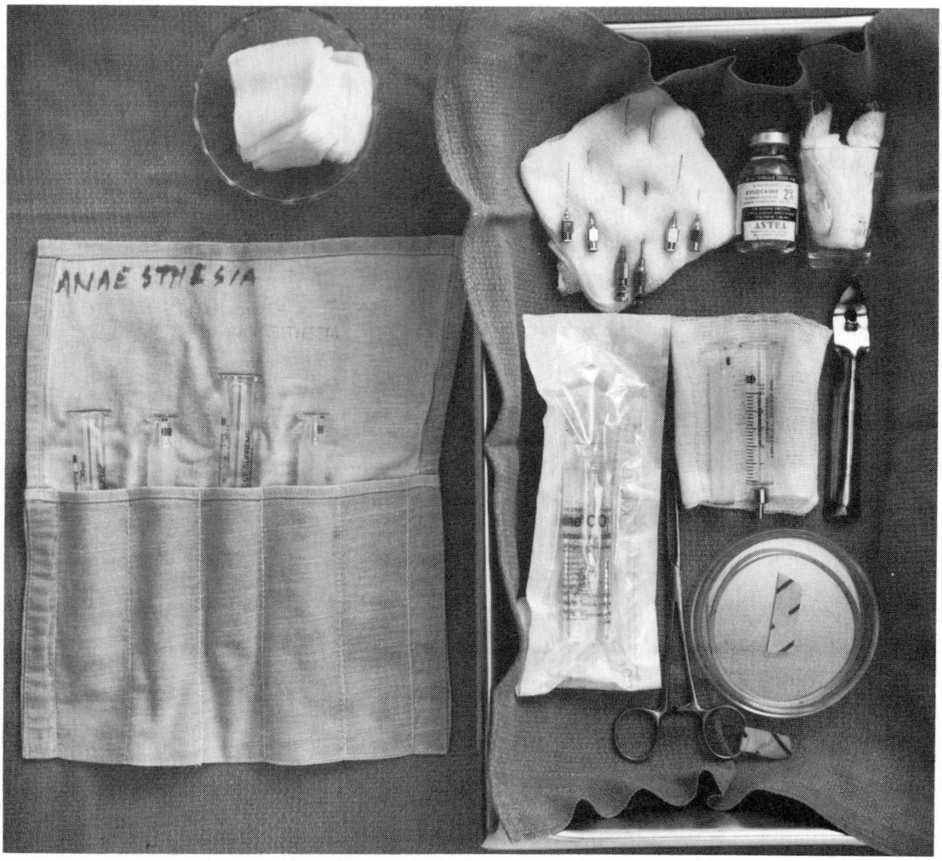

Figure 9–23. Epidural tray: hospital-packaged and reusable. Individual preferences can be indulged and favorite items included, e.g., a beer can opener for removing vial tops and special anesthetic solutions, such as carbonated lidocaine.

and some local anesthetic. Additional items such as fine needles for skin analgesia, swabs and so forth make up a standard tray for routine clinical purposes, and a wide range of choice exists to suit personal needs and preferences.

The following articles should be included in each sterile epidural set, as shown in Figure 9–23.

1. Instrument tray, 8″ × 12″, wrapped in sterile towels and containing the injection equipment.
2. Sterile towels to drape the injection field.
3. Syringes: (a) 1 × 2.0-ml syringe.
   (b) 1 × 5.0-ml all-glass syringe.
   (c) 2 × 10-ml syringes or 1 × 20-ml syringe.

These syringes should be standard, simple types without a Luer-Lok connection, which requires unnecessary rotation and manipulation of the syringes on the epidural needles and increases the hazards of accidental dural puncture. The syringes are either wrapped in gauze to protect them from damage or are slipped into the pocket of a canvas syringe holder (see Fig. 9–23).

Needles

1. 1 × ¾-inch 25-gauge needle for skin analgesia.
2. 1 × 1½-inch 22-gauge needle for infiltrating deep tissues.
3. 1 × 1-inch 23-gauge needle for insertion into the free end of the epidural catheter.
4. 1 × 18-gauge needle for piercing the skin prior to insertion of the epidural needle.
5. Two Huber-tipped 3½-inch Tuohy needles, 1 × 17-gauge and 1 × 16-gauge.
6. Epidural catheter coiled in protecting Petri dish.
7. 40-ml medicine glass to hold anesthetic solution.
8. Glass bowl to hold antiseptic solution.
9. Gauze swabs: (a) 2 × 2-inch.
   (b) 4 × 4-inch.
10. Swab-holding forceps.
11. Sterilizer indicating tape to indicate adequate sterilization of tray contents.
12. 20-ml vial of normal saline without added preservative (optional).
13. 2 × 20-ml vials of local anesthetic solution (e.g., 2 per cent lidocaine or 0.5 per cent bupivacaine).
14. Bottle opener for ease of opening vials (optional).
15. Millipore filter (optional).

Epidural Needles

During his experiments on epidural pressures, Janzen (1926) noted that needles with lateral openings were better suited to accurate pressure measurements than needles with end openings. This observation related to the physical constraints of recording pressures in a narrow space: terminal orifices are more likely to become occluded by tissue cores, or by the dura mater acting as a screen to block the end of the needle. In my experience the incidence of accidental dural puncture is also markedly influenced by the type of needle used. Needles with lateral openings have a lower incidence of puncture than those with terminal orifices, although it is doubtful whether the same forces that aroused Janzen's observation can be invoked to explain the clinical superiority of a Huber tip over an orthodox straight beveled needle. Whatever the explanation, and presumably it must have some hydrodynamic basis, in my hands the difference is tenfold, that is, a 1.5 per cent incidence of accidental dural puncture with an orthodox blunt beveled needle, but only 0.15 per cent with a standard 17-gauge Tuohy needle. I do not think that this is a personal idiosyncrasy, but as yet no well-controlled study has been done to confirm or refute the greater safety of the Tuohy needle.

If a straight beveled needle is to be used, it is best to choose one with a very obtuse bevel and with rounded edges, such as the Crawford needle, the orifice of which is designed to be as atraumatic as possible. It is important that the stylet should fit snugly at the orifice so that no gaps exist between the level of the stylet and the rim of the needle bevel. Ill-fitting stylets may allow the sharp edges of the needle point to core out microscopic fragments of skin, which are then carried inward on the needle point and implanted in the deep tissues (Gibson and Norris, 1958). A number of cases of intraspinal epidermoid tumors have been attributed to coring of skin at lumbar puncture and to subsequent slow growth of the implanted skin fragments (Manno et al., 1962; Shaywitz, 1972; Batnitzky et al., 1977). Needles with well-fitting stylets and those with side openings are not likely to implant skin fragments.

Large-bore needles, such as the 16-gauge size, are somewhat traumatic but technically easy to guide during insertion, whereas thin, fine-bore needles are more prone to bend and stray from their original course. A good compromise is found in the 18-gauge thin-walled needle or the 17-gauge size. Both of these sizes have internal diameters that will accommodate most epidural catheters in current use.

Tuohy Needle. The Tuohy needle (Fig. 9–24) was originally designed for continuous subarachnoid analgesia (Tuohy, 1945), and Curbelo adapted it for epidural use in 1949. The gentle curve of the Huber tip imparts a bias to an epidural catheter, tending to direct it obliquely into the axis of the spinal canal without impinging direcly on the dural tube.

In its original form the upper inside edge of the orifice was chisel-sharp, and this created a real danger of slicing the catheter and sequestering a piece in the epidural space if attempts were made to withdraw the catheter while the needle was still in place (see Fig. 7–7). Tuohy needles are now manufactured with a blunted upper rim (Lund, 1966), and these needles are much less likely to shear a catheter. Nevertheless, the possibility of damage to the epidural catheter should be borne in mind, and attempts should not be made to withdraw a catheter while the needle is still in place unless very great care is used. If there is reason to take out the catheter, it is better to remove both needle and catheter together.

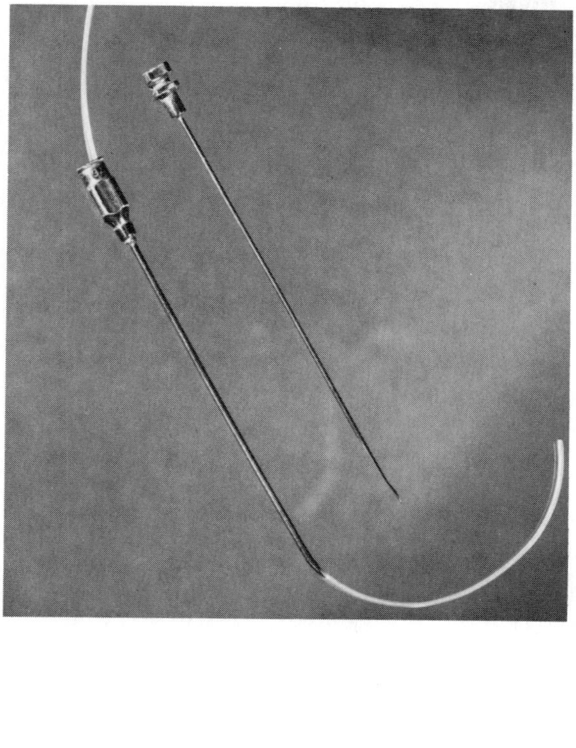

Figure 9–24. Standard Tuohy needle with stylet removed and catheter inserted.

Tuohy needles have been designed with depth marks etched on their surface. These provide a simple and direct way of recording the distance that the epidural space lies below the skin. The Lee needle has alternate black and metallic markings of 1 cm width (Lee, 1960). The Doughty needle has an 8-cm shaft with five marks at centimeter intervals from the base of the hub, the last mark being 3 cm from the proximal edge of the bevel (Doughty, 1974).

Cheng Needle. This is a heavy 16-gauge needle with an 8 cm-shaft marked in centimeter distances (Cheng, 1958). The end has a blunt unidirectional tip with an oval-shaped lateral orifice. A detachable winged grip is supplied to aid insertion. A sharp 15-gauge needle must be used to puncture the skin and subcutaneous tissues so that the blunt Cheng needle can be introduced into the deeper tissues.

The blunt tip is most unlikely to penetrate the dura, and accidental dural puncture is said to be very uncommon, with an incidence of only 0.3 per cent in one series of over 1,000 cases (Sheehan et al., 1962). However, the needle has two disadvantages. First, the blunt tip makes insertion quite a strenuous and sometimes jerky maneuver, especially in elderly patients with resistant calcified ligaments. Second, the incidence of backache is rather high following its use, presumably due to the blunt trauma caused by passage of the rounded tip.

Crawley Needle. The Crawley needle is similar in principle to the Cheng needle, having a blunt tip and a smooth-edged orifice set back 2 to 3 mm from the tip (Crawley, 1968). The advancing catheter is able to emerge from the orifice at less of an acute angle than from the standard Tuohy needle, with less chance of becoming kinked or sheared if the catheter is pulled back.

Wagner Needle. This needle is designed for single-shot epidural blockade (Wagner, 1957). The fine shaft has a 20- or 22-gauge, and the internal diameter is too narrow to accommodate standard epidural tubing. The tip is blunt and rounded with a unidirectional lateral orifice. This design of tip is relatively atraumatic and unlikely to penetrate the dura.

Hub Grips. Design of the needle hub is not critical when the standard loss-of-resistance technique is used, and both small hubs and the larger type of Barker spool hub are equally convenient. However, when the hanging-drop technique is used, it is important to have some form of grip firmly attached to the hub of the needle so that the operator's thumbs and fingers are placed well away from the hub orifice to avoid disturbing the meniscus of the hanging drop.

A number of modern adaptations of the old Barker type of spool hub or the Labat winged needle have been designed for this purpose. Examples are the Oxford-Tuohy needle, which is essentially a Tuohy needle with a winged grip, and the Bromage needle (1961b), which is a Tuohy needle with a large Barker spool-type hub (see Fig. 9–25). While the winged grip is excellent for the hanging-drop test, it is not well suited for the loss-of-resistance test, as the large protruding wings prevent a proper single-handed grip on the needle. On the other hand, the large spool-type hub is a good all-purpose design, and it can be gripped securely in either test.

Detachable winged grips made of metal (Bolpe, 1962) or of plastic (Winnie, 1971) have also been designed for use with the Tuohy needles of standard size. However, these detachable grips give a less solid and less controlled feel than the specially designed needles.

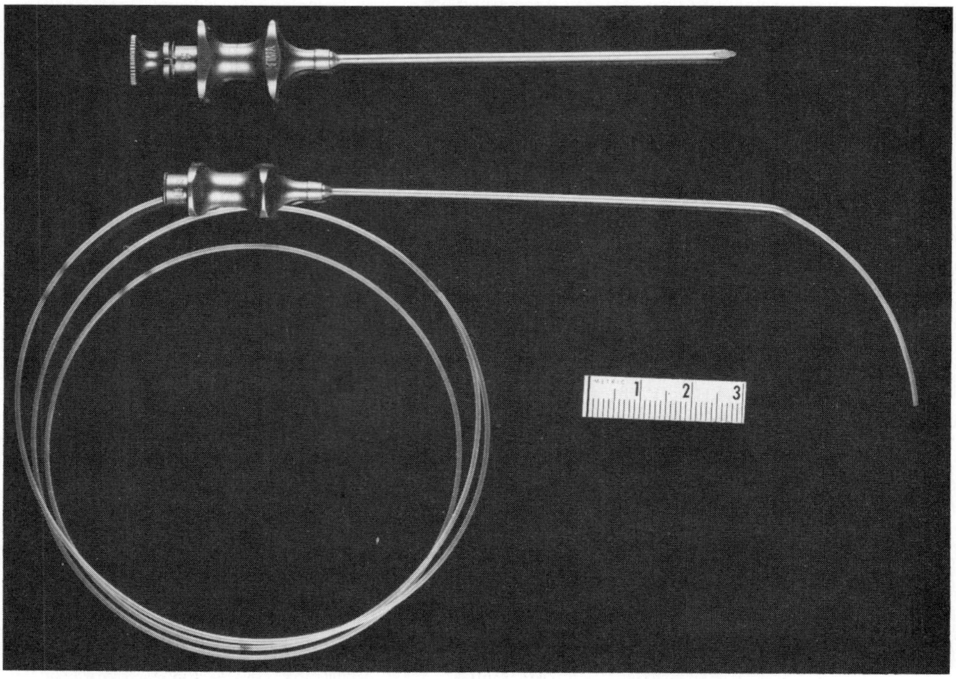

Figure 9–25. Bromage needle for use with hanging-drop technique in thoracic epidural punctures. (From Bromage, P. R.: Epidural needle. Anesthesiology *22*:1018, 1961b.)

Epidural Catheters

Early techniques of continuous extradural analgesia were made popular by Hingson and Southworth (1942), who used the malleable Lemmon needle and the caudal approach. Shortly afterward Manalan (1942) and Lundy and his associates (Adams et al., 1943) independently developed the method of continuous caudal analgesia with an indwelling catheter. The first catheters to be used were ureteral lacquered silk catheters, as they were already in established use in neurosurgical practice for prolonged drainage of cerebrospinal fluid (Love, 1935). Tuohy (1945) later employed the same type of catheter for continuous subarachnoid block, and four years later Curbelo (1949) adopted the method for continuous lumbar epidural blockade.

Silk and lacquered gum elastic catheters are difficult to sterilize by heat, and sepsis was relatively common in the early series. Manalan reported one case of staphylococcal meningitis following the insertion of a silk catheter in the first series of 46 cases (Manalan, 1942). Thus, gum elastic catheters were quickly superseded by more durable plastic materials as suitable plastic tubing became commercially available.

Various plastic materials have been used to manufacture epidural catheters. Polyethylene was among the first with the formula $-\overset{\displaystyle H}{\underset{\displaystyle H}{\overset{|}{\underset{|}{C}}}}-\overset{\displaystyle H}{\underset{\displaystyle H}{\overset{|}{\underset{|}{C}}}}-$, but this is an unsuitable material as it has a low melting point (85 to 110° C), it swells and thickens at autoclave heat and it is easily softened and deformed at body temperature.

Polyvinylchloride, with the formula $-CH_2-\underset{\displaystyle Cl}{\underset{|}{CH}}-CH_2-\underset{\displaystyle Cl\ (n)}{\underset{|}{CH}}-$ was the next, and this material has stood the test of time very well. When manufactured with the right dimensions of internal diameter and wall thickness, catheters of polyvinylchloride have many of the necessary characteristics. They are rigid enough to be threaded through a needle with ease and without kinking. However, their intrinsic stiffness tends to make them slightly more traumatic than nylon.

Nylon, with the formula $-\underset{\displaystyle O}{\underset{\|}{C}}(CH_2)_4-\underset{\displaystyle O}{\underset{\|}{C}}-NH-(CH_2)_6NH-_{(n)}$, has a melting point of 215° C, and it is less thermolabile than polyvinylchloride. Hence, it is less prone to become softened and flattened by pressure at body temperature. It can be autoclaved and is strong, tending to stretch rather than break under tensile loads. Prepackaged nylon catheters are very popular, and they have tended to supersede polyvinylchloride.

Polytetrafluroethylene (PTFE, or Teflon), with the formula $\overset{\displaystyle F}{\overset{|}{\underset{\displaystyle F}{\underset{|}{-C}}}}\overset{\displaystyle F}{\overset{|}{\underset{\displaystyle F\ (n)}{\underset{|}{-C-}}}}$, has a higher melting point at 325° C, and it is strong and stretches without breaking. It is also nonwettable, and it has an extremely low coefficient of friction. However, catheters of this material are prone to kink or fracture if the walls are thin. Abouleish (1974) has described three cases in which kinking of a Teflon catheter led to a localized breach in the wall. Subsequent injections through the catheter leaked out from the hole, and epidural analgesia failed to develop. The type of manufacture of these faulty Teflon catheters was not specified.

REQUIRED CHARACTERISTICS

There is no perfect epidural catheter. Choice of the best is a compromise between a number of desirable but sometimes mutually exclusive properties. Ideally, an epidural catheter should possess the following characteristics.

Biochemical Inertness. This is perhaps the most important feature. The catheter should be able to remain in the epidural space for long periods of time without causing any chemical irritation or provoking any local tissue reaction. All the plastic materials mentioned above are inert in this way. However, my own observations of chronically implanted preparations in cats show that the catheter tip tends to become walled off by a local fibrin reaction in the surrounding epidural tissues after a period of two or three weeks. Whether this reaction is due to the plastic catheter itself, to irritation from repeated injections of local anesthetic made through it or to infection introduced at the time of surgical implantation is debatable. Nevertheless, clinical signs suggest that a similar type of reaction occurs in human subjects if epidural catheters are left in place for more than 72 hours (see Chapter 7 on Continuous Epidural Analgesia).

Low Coefficient of Friction. Catheters should glide through the tissues easily without frictional resistance. Teflon, a material widely used for mechanical bearings, is the best substance from this point of view.

High Tensile Strength. Rarely, catheters may prove difficult to remove by becoming gripped between adjacent laminae, particularly if there is difficulty in flexing the spine to relieve the pincer-like grip exerted by the laminae. Catheters should be strong enough to resist breaking under the moderate tensile force that may be necessary to extract them under these circumstances. Nylon and Teflon are very strong and well-suited to resisting this type of stress. Polyvinylchloride is less rugged and requires greater care. Polyethylene is very weak and should be avoided.

Maneuverable Rigidity. Catheters must be rigid enough to be passed through an epidural needle, but not so rigid that damage will be caused to delicate tissues in the epidural space. Very compliant catheters may be given adequate rigidity for insertion by passing a stylet of wire, nylon or Teflon inside the lumen. However, this internal splinting makes them very springy and wayward and prone to leap beyond the sterile bounds of the field of operations while they are being inserted.

Kink Resistance. An epidural catheter is worse than useless if it becomes obstructed from kinking or torsional strangulation at some stage after insertion. Unfortunately, certain prepackaged catheters are especially prone to this nuisance, particularly those with thin walls in relation to their internal diameter. Lateral holes set back from the catheter tip also weaken resistance to buckling forces and increase the likelihood of kinking and obstruction (Skinner, 1966). Vinyl plastic tubing of 1 mm external diameter, manufactured by Becton-Dickinson,* seldom displays this fault, and catheters made from this material retain reliable patency under routine clinical conditions.

Atraumatic Tip. Catheter tips should be blunt to avoid trauma to dura or epidural veins. Sharply rounded ends are more likely to penetrate a vein than obtuse or square-ended catheters.

Depth Indicators. Some system of measured marks should be printed on the catheter to provide a readily visible indication of the length that has been inserted.

Radiopacity. There is a choice of radiolucent or radiopaque catheters. The radiopaque variety has advantages in certain types of research projects, especially in small animals in which the density of bone shadow is not too heavy to obscure the position of the catheter. However, for reasons outlined in Chapter 7, in routine clinical use my personal preference leans toward radiolucent catheters that are invisible to X-rays.

TYPES OF CATHETER

A variety of prepackaged epidural catheters embodying some or all of the above features are on the market. After trying a number of them, we re-

*Becton-Dickinson and Company, Rutherford, N.J. 07070.

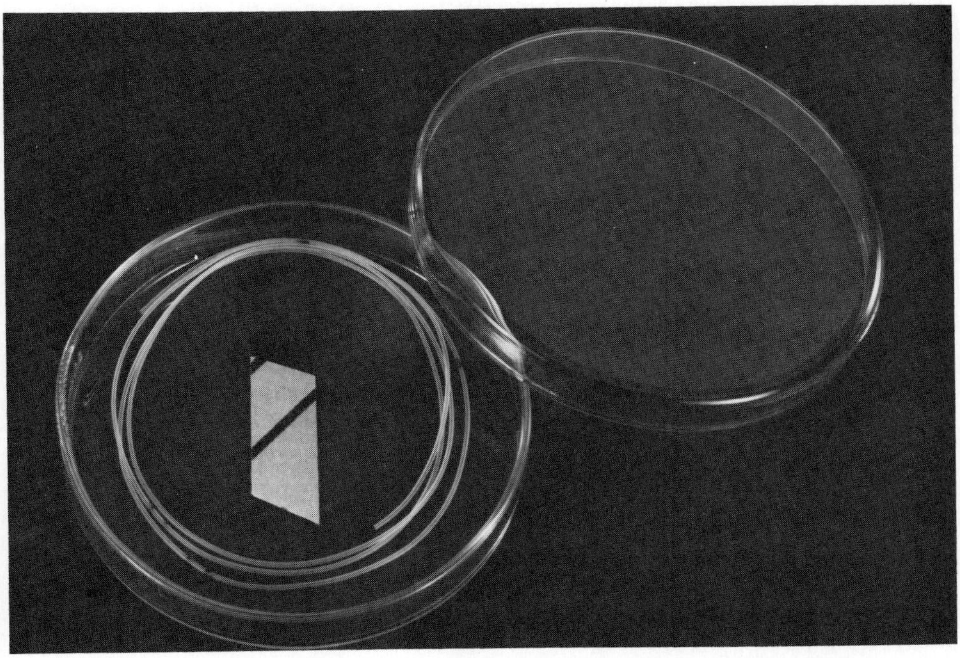

Figure 9–26. Marked vinyl plastic catheter coiled inside a glass Petri dish and sterilized by autoclaving.

turned to using our original if rather primitive method, which nevertheless carries the lowest incidence of technical failures in our hands.

Vinyl plastic tubing of 1 mm external diameter (Becton-Dickinson) is purchased in 100 foot rolls. The tubing is cut into meter lengths, care being taken to cut the tubing cleanly at right angles to its axis to avoid leaving an oblique sharp end. The tubing is then marked with an indelible pen at one or two needle lengths from each end (3½ inches and 7 inches from the end). Vinyl tubing softens at high temperatures, so it must be protected against compression and kinking by heavy objects pressing on it during the autoclaving process. Protection is afforded by coiling each catheter inside a glass Petri dish covered with a glass lid and marked with a strip of autoclaving indicator tape as an additional check on sterility (Fig. 9–26).

These catheters are simple and cheap to produce, and their physical characteristics seem to strike a reasonable balance between excessive stiffness and kink-prone compliance. They have been in almost continuous use at the Royal Victoria Hospital, Montreal, for more than 20 years and have retained their popularity over a number of more sophisticated newcomers.

Prepackaged catheters have much to recommend them for use in small clinical units where relatively few blocks are performed and where trained personnel are not available to prepare the homemade variety. The following represent examples of popular makes.

Lee Nylon Catheter (1962). This has a sealed end with a round, hard point and two lateral holes, one close to the end and one set back about 9 mm from the tip. Depth markings are placed at 5, 10 and 15 cm from the end. This catheter is somewhat prone to kinking and obstruction 1 cm from the end, at the weak point of the second lateral hole.

Skinner Nylon Catheter (1966). This design has proved most satisfactory. The end is square-cut and open, and a second lateral opening is placed 3 mm from the tip. With the lateral hole so close to the tip, kinking is virtually impossible under the stresses involved in normal use. Depth marks are placed at 7, 8, 9 and 10 cm from the end, providing easy reference marks to ensure that the catheter is not inserted unnecessarily far into the epidural space.

Deseret Teflon Catheter. This is supplied with a nylon stylet for ease of insertion. The catheter is square-cut and open-ended, without lateral holes. Depth markers are printed on the catheter. The catheter is easy to insert and to extract. This catheter is also rather prone to kinking and obstruction, as shown in Figure 9–27.

Epidural Cannulas

Orthodox epidural catheters are introduced through a large Tuohy needle of suitable bore. An alternative approach lies in a modified intravenous type of cannula, in which a tapered Teflon sleeve lies outside a removable metal needle. The two are inserted together, and when the epidural space is entered, the metal needle is withdrawn while the large, blunt Teflon cannula is advanced more deeply into the epidural space. This technique would seem to have the advantage of diminishing the danger of accidental venous or dural cannulation

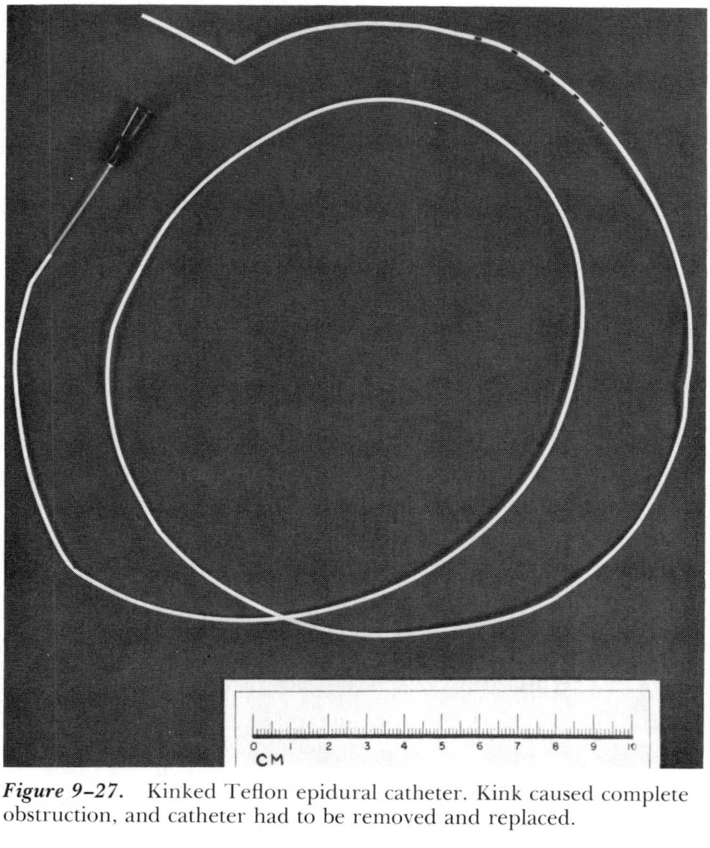

Figure 9–27. Kinked Teflon epidural catheter. Kink caused complete obstruction, and catheter had to be removed and replaced.

that exists when fine, small-bore catheters are used. However, there are three inherent drawbacks. First, existing design has not produced a combination of external cannula and Tuohy needle, and a straight beveled internal needle must be used instead. As pointed out earlier, for reasons that are not altogether clear dural puncture occurs more frequently with straight beveled needles than with the Huber-tipped Tuohy needle. Therefore, a relatively high incidence of dural puncture may be expected with the straight-tipped needle-cannula combination. Second, the short external plastic cannula must be attached to suitable extension tubing close to the point of entry, and this junction may become accidentally disconnected. Third, a short and slippery Teflon cannula is easily retracted and displaced from the epidural space by active body movements.

Two epidural cannulas have been designed, both with a precurved chordee-like tip to the cannula, so that when the cannula is advanced into the epidural space, its open end will veer away to one side and tend to lie in the long axis of the spinal canal.

Winnie-Jelco Cannula. Figure 9–28 shows the Winnie-Jelco unit, with its precurved Teflon cannula, straight inner needle and special extension

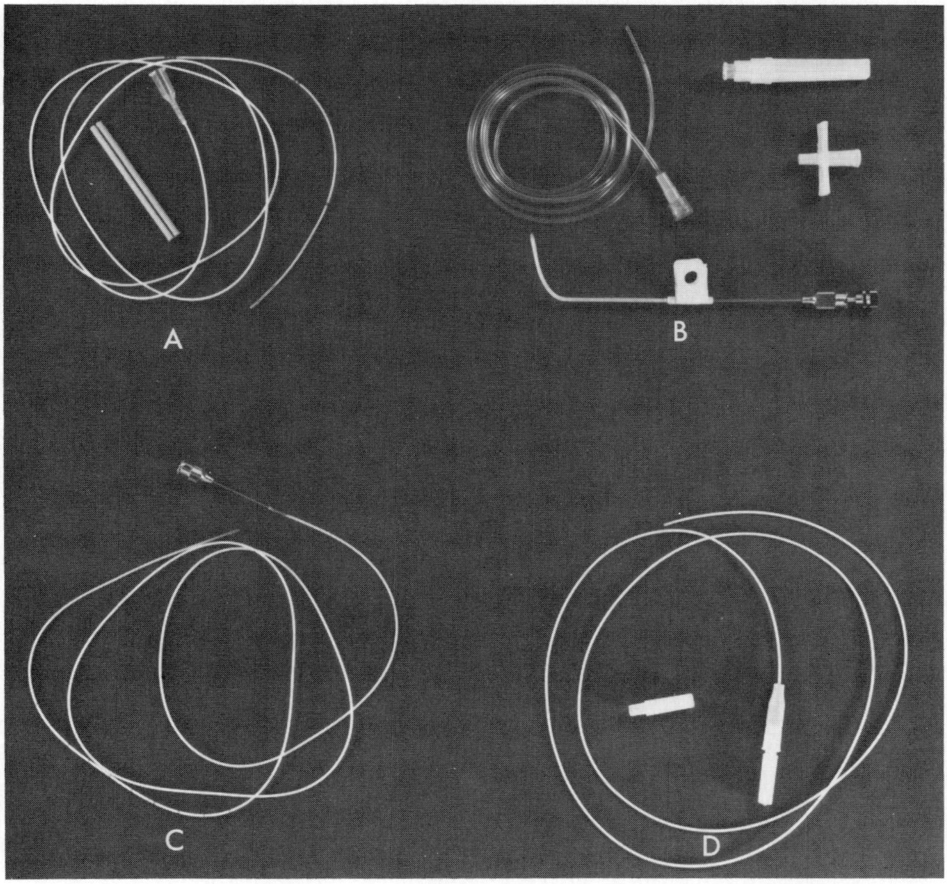

Figure 9–28. Four epidural catheters: *A*, Lee: *B*, Winnie-Jelco needle-cannula assembly with precurved plastic cannula and internal metal needle; disposable Winnie winged grip and extension tubing; *C*, Sinner; *D*, Deseret.

tubing for attachment to the cannula after satisfactory insertion. A detachable plastic winged Winnie grip is also supplied for use with the hanging-drop test.

After the epidural space is identified, the metal needle is held firmly in one hand while the Teflon cannula is advanced to its full extent beyond the metal needle and into the epidural space. The special extension tubing is then attached, padded with sterile sponges and taped in place.

Henkin-Bard Cannula (1970). This cannula is a more sophisticated version of the preceding design. A helical groove is placed in a special plastic hub. Withdrawal of the internal needle is effected by rotating it through 180 degrees, and this automatically retracts the needle in a single smooth movement. After the metal needle is withdrawn, the outer precurved Teflon cannula is advanced 1 or 2 cm into the epidural space, the sterile extension tubing is attached and the unit is taped in place.

Mechanical Aids to Epidural Puncture

Mechanical aids to identification of the epidural space have been discussed in Chapter 6. It is my personal view that while many of these devices are attractively ingenious, they are unnecessary and tend to complicate an otherwise simple procedure. While some of these gadgets were developed with considerable ingenuity, each has its own intrinsic weakness, and in my own experience accidental dural puncture occurs more frequently with mechanical aids than without them. The most reliable system is a well-trained pair of hands, and in the long run most anesthesiologists will find that their success rate is higher if they rely on their own hands rather than on accessory apparatus. A representative list of mechanical aids to epidural puncture with original reference sources is given in Chapter 6 for readers who wish to pursue them further.

PACKAGING

Sterile epidural sets may be prepared individually by hand and reused almost indefinitely, or they may be purchased as once-only packs.

Reusable Sets

There are certain major advantages to hand-prepared epidural sets that are processed and sterilized in the hospital central supplies department. The contents of the tray can be varied to suit changing individual requirements, and vials of favorite local anesthetic solutions can be conveniently included in the same sterile set. Trays of this nature are also very convenient for the anesthesiologist and quicker to set up at the time of induction than disposable trays with each individual item separately packaged inside.

Strict attention to mechanical cleanliness and safe, efficient sterilization is of paramount importance when reusable trays are employed. All reusable articles such as needles and syringes should be cleaned by scrubbing and by

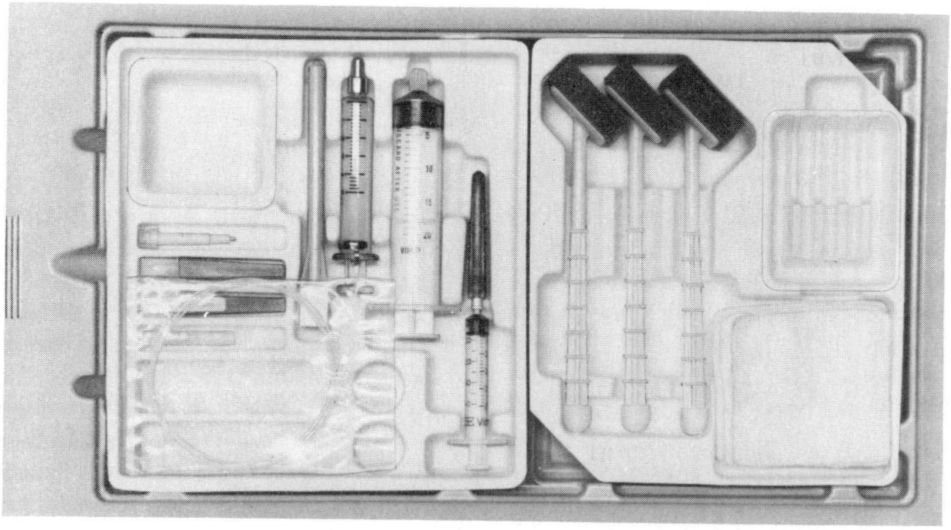

Figure 9–29. A prepackaged disposable epidural anesthesia set.

agitation in soap and water, followed by rinsing in an alcohol solution and finally a thorough rinse in distilled water. Commercial detergents should be avoided, as cases of myelitis following subarachnoid block have been reported, which may possibly have been caused by traces of detergents remaining in the syringes (Winkelman, 1952). More recent work with dogs suggests that this particular danger may have been overemphasized and that traces of detergents in extreme dilution are not likely to be hazardous (Smith and Connor, 1962). However, the suspicion remains, and since the possible sequelae are so grave, it is wise to avoid detergents at any point in the cleaning process.

Wrapped epidural trays should be marked with a sterilizer indicator outside and inside the tray to provide visible evidence that the contents have been sterilized. Trays are steam-autoclaved at 225 to 260° F at 18 to 20 pounds pressure for 20 to 30 minutes and then vacuum-dried. Trays are marked with the date of sterilization and stored in a dry place. All trays are reautoclaved if not used within 14 days of sterilization.

Disposable Sets

Disposable epidural sets are available with high quality materials and reliable sterilization control (Fig. 9–29). Although prodigal waste is offensive to the frugal minded, any thoughts of preventing waste should be pushed aside by the legal implications of the manufacturer's label stating "USE ONCE AND DESTROY."

The logic of disposable sets hinges around quality control, economics and medicolegal fear. In North America mass-produced disposable kits cost between $7.00 and 13.00 at current prices. The kits contain well-machined articles, some of which could be reused with safety if proper sterilization precautions were taken. The kits are neatly packaged, if somewhat less conveniently than reusable hand-prepared trays, and sterility is guaranteed. The internal hospital costs of preparing, packaging and sterilizing reusable kits are avoided, and the medicolegal risks of imperfect sterilization are transferred to the manufacturer. It can be appreciated that these wares have strong administrative appeal. However, it should be noted that in one bacteriological study of indwelling epidural catheters, after extraction there was no statistically significant difference between the incidence of contaminated catheters from hospital-prepared trays or from commercially prepared disposable trays (Hunt et al., 1977).

However, reports have been published of serious imperfections in these kits (DiGiovanni, 1971; Seltzer et al., 1977). Medicine cups designed to contain local anesthetic solutions in epidural trays from three prominent manufacturers were found to contain a significant number of loose plastic particles of visible size. These plastic contaminants were easily drawn into a syringe through an 18-gauge needle. The possible consequences of injecting showers of plastic particles into the epidural space are unknown but sufficiently disquieting to suggest more rigorous standards of quality control than obtain at the time of writing.

As with all mass-produced goods, disposable trays demand that individuality be sacrificed to uniformity in order to produce an economical product. The physician must accept what has been provided for him by the manufacturers, who in turn have taken advice upon a package most likely to satisfy the requirements of the majority. Special individual preferences can only be satisfied by separate packaging and sterilization within the organization of the hospital operating room or central supply department, thus defeating one of the prime objectives of disposable kits, that is, a unified and totally indemnified sterilization system. There would be a way around this dilemma if all conceivable varieties of drugs, needles and catheters could be sterilized and marketed separately, but the demand is too low to justify mass production of individual items, and the user of disposable kits must surrender his individual preferences to the uniformity imposed by a prepackaged disposable system.

Micropore Filters

The possibility that epidural solutions may become contaminated by bacteria or microscopic glass or plastic particles is mentioned in Chapters 7 and 14. With proper technique the chance of pathological effects arising from these sources seems to be extremely remote, for very large series of cases have been recorded without associated complications of this nature (Lund, 1966). When epidural infection does occur, it usually arises by metastatic spread from a primary source elsewhere in the body. Nevertheless, the fear still lingers that as long as a possibility exists, no matter how remote, sooner or later a rare case of infection may occur from extrinsic contamination (Hunt et al., 1977).

Protection is said to be afforded by using micropore bacterial filters as a routine. Disposable bacterial filters are available with a pore size of 0.22 μm, and these micropore units have been recommended for regular use whenever injections are made through an indwelling catheter (see Fig. 7–13).* James and

*Millex disposable filter unit.

his colleagues (1976) have shown that these filters are extremely effective in protecting epidural catheters from infection, even when imperfect technique allows heavy contamination of the interior of the syringes used for epidural injection. The micropore filter is mounted on the distal end of the catheter connection and is kept closed with a clean cap between injections.

Bacterial infection is not the only source of contamination, and nonmicrobial particulate matter appears to be more common than generally appreciated (Ho, 1967). A shower of microscopic glass particles may be released when a snap-neck ampule is opened (Groves, 1973; Somerville and Gibson, 1973). It has been suggested that microscopic glass foreign bodies of this nature may give rise to granulomatous reactions from time to time unless they are excluded by some reliable device such as a millipore filter (Katz et al., 1973; Crawford et al., 1975). Logically, complete protection from particulate contamination would only be assured if *all* injections were made through the micropore filter, including the loss-of-resistance test and the primary test dose given through the epidural needle before passage of the catheter (Crawford et al., 1975). At the time of writing, many anesthesiologists remain unconvinced by the logic of the plea to use micropore filters as a routine for single-shot as well as catheter injections, provided strict standards of sterility and care are maintained. However, the present trend toward more defensive practices will probably lead to a wider use of these inexpensive little filter units in the future.

REFERENCES

Abouleish, E.: Preventing and detecting leakage in epidural catheters. Anesth. Analg. *53*:474, 1974.

Adams, H. J., Kronberg, G. H., and Takman, B. G.: Local anesthetic activity and acute toxicity of (±)-2-N-ethylpropylamino)-2′6′ butyroxylidide, a new long-acting agent. J. Pharm. Sci. *61*:1829, 1972.

Adams, R. C., Lundy, J. S., and Seldon, T. H.: Continuous caudal anesthesia or analgesia: A consideration of the technic, various uses and some possible dangers. J.A.M.A. *122*:152, 1943.

Adjepon-Yamoah, K. K., Scott, D. B., and Prescott, L. F.: Impaired absorption and metabolism of oral lignocaine in patients undergoing laparoscopy. Brit. J. Anaesth. *45*:143, 1973.

Ansbro, F. P., Latteri, F. S., and Bodell, B.: Continuous segmental thoracolumbar epidural block. Curr. Res. Anesth. Analg. *32*:73, 1953.

Appleyard, T. N., Witt, A., Atkinson, R. E., and Nicholas, A. D. G.: Bupivacaine carbonate and bupivacaine hydrochloride: A comparison of blood concentrations during epidural blockade for vaginal surgery. Brit. J. Anaesth. *46*:530, 1974.

Arens, J. F., and Carrera, A. E.: Methemoglobin levels following peridural anesthesia with prilocaine for vaginal deliveries. Anesth. Analg. *49*:219, 1970.

Aström, A., and Persson, N. H.: Some pharmacological properties of O-methyl-alpha-propylamino-propionanilide—a new local anesthetic. Brit. J. Pharmacol. *16*:32, 1961.

Batnitzky, S., Keucher, T. R., Mealey, J., and Campbell, R. L.: Iatrogenic intraspinal epidermoid tumors. J.A.M.A. *237*:148, 1977.

Belfrage, P., Irestedt, L., and Berlin, A.: Bupivacaine concentration in arterial and venous plasma. Acta Anaesth. Scand. *19*:85, 1975a.

Belfrage, P., Berlin, A., Raabe, N., and Thalme, B.: Lumbar epidural analgesia with bupivacaine in labor. Drug concentration in maternal and neonatal blood at birth and during the first day of life. Amer. J. Obstet. Gynecol. *123*:839, 1975b.

Berry, H., and West, G. B.: The stability of adrenaline solutions. Quart. J. Pharm. *17*:242, 1944.

Bolpe, O.: Holder for epidural needle. Anesthesiology *26*:6, 1962.

Bridenbaugh, P. O., Tucker, G. T., Moore, D. C., Bridenbaugh, L. D., and Thompson, G. E.: Etidocaine: Clinical evaluation for intercostal nerve block and lumbar epidural block. Anesth. Analg. *52*:407, 1973.

Bridenbaugh, P. O., Tucker, G. T., Moore, D. C., Bridenbaugh, L. D., Thompson, G. E., and Balfour, R. I.: Role of epinephrine in regional block anesthesia with etidocaine: A double-blind study. Anesth. Analg. *53*:430, 1974.

Bromage, P. R.: Continuous lumbar epidural analgesia for obstetrics. Canad. Med. Assoc. J. *85*:1136, 1961a.

Bromage, P. R.: Epidural needle. Anesthesiology *22*:1018, 1961b.

Bromage, P. R.: A comparison of the hydrochloride and carbon dioxide salts of lidocaine and prilocaine in epidural analgesia. Acta Anaesth. Scand. (Suppl.) *16*:55, 1965a.

Bromage, P. R.: A comparison of the hydrochloride salts of lignocaine and prilocaine for epidural analgesia. Brit. J. Anaesth., *37*:753, 1965b.

Bromage, P. R.: Improved conduction blockade in surgery and obstetrics: Carbonated local anesthetics. Canad. Med. Assoc. J. *97*:1377, 1967.

Bromage, P. R.: The physiology and pharmacology of epidural blockade. *In* Bonica, J. J.: Clinical Anesthesia. 2. Regional Anesthesia: Recent Advances and Current Status. Philadelphia, F. A. Davis Company, 1969a.

Bromage, P. R.: A comparison of bupivacaine and tetracaine in epidural analgesia for surgery. Canad. Anaesth. Soc. J. *16*:37, 1969b.

Bromage, P. R.: Ageing and epidural dose requirements. Brit. J. Anaesth. *41*:1016, 1969c.

Bromage, P. R.: Unblocked segments in epidural analgesia for relief of pain in labour. Brit. J. Anaesth. *44*:676, 1972.

Bromage, P. R., and Burfoot, M. F.: Quality of epidural blockade. II. Influence of physico-chemical factors; hyaluronidase and potassium. Brit. J. Anaesth. *38*:857, 1966.

Bromage, P. R., and Gertel, M.: An evaluation of two new local anaesthetics for major conduction blockade. Canad. Anaesth. Soc. J. *17*:557, 1970.

Bromage, P. R., and Gertel, M.: Improved brachial plexus blockade with bupivacaine hydrochloride and carbonated lidocaine. Anesthesiology *36*:479, 1972.

Bromage, P. R., and Robson, J. G.: Concentrations of lignocaine in the blood after intravenous, intramuscular, epidural, and endotracheal administration. Anaesthesia *16*:461, 1961.

Bromage, P. R., Burfoot, M. F., Crowell, D. E., and Pettigrew, R. T.: Quality of epidural blockade. I. Influence of physical factors. Brit. J. Anaesth. *36*:342, 1964.

Bromage, P. R., Burfoot, M. F., Crowell, D. E., and Truant, A. P.: Quality of epidural blockade. III. Carbonated local anaesthetic solutions. Brit. J. Anaesth. *39*:197, 1967.

Bromage, P. R., O'Beirn, P., and Dunford, L. A.: Etidocaine: A clinical evaluation for regional analgesia in surgery. Canad. Anaesth. Soc. J. *21*:523, 1974a.

Bromage, P. R., Datta, S., and Dunford, L. A.: Etidocaine: An evaluation in epidural analgesia for obstetrics. Canad. Anaesth. Soc. J. *21*:535, 1974b.

Brown, W. U., Bell, G. C., Lurie, A. O., Weiss, J. B., Scanlon, J. W., and Alper, M. H.: Newborn blood levels of lidocaine and mepivacaine in the first postnatal day following maternal epidural anesthesia. Anesthesiology *42*:698, 1975.

Buchholz, H. W., and Lesse, K. T.: Anatomisch-physikalische Untersuchungen des Periduralraums. Chirurg *21*:135, 1950a.

Buchholz, H. W., and Lesse, K. T.: Die extradurale spinalanästhesie. Chirurg *21*:202, 1950b.

Buchholz, H. W., and Lesse, K. T.: Druckverhaltnisse im Periduralraum und im Liquorraum bei peridural Injektionen. Chirurg *22*:102, 1951.

Burfoot, M. F., and Bromage, P. R.: The effects of epinephrine on mepivacaine absorption from the spinal epidural space. Anesthesiology *35*:488, 1971.

Cheng, P. A.: Blunt-tip needle for epidural anesthesia. Anesthesiology *19*:556, 1958.

Climie, C. R., McLean, S., Starmer, G. A., and Thomas, J.: Methaemoglobinaemia in mother and foetus following continuous epidural analgesia with prilocaine. Brit. J. Anaesth. *39*:155, 1967.

Colavincenzo, J. W., Foldes, F. F., McNall, P. G., and Friday, R. H.: The use of 2-chloroprocaine hydrochloride for epidural block in outpatients. Pennsylvania Med. J. *59*:338, 1956.

Cousins, M. J., and Bromage, P. R.: A comparison of the hydrochloride and carbonated salts of lignocaine for caudal analgesia in out-patients. Brit. J. Anaesth. *43*:1149, 1971.

Crawford, J. S.: Principles and Practice of Obstetric Anaesthesia. 3d ed. Oxford, Blackwell Scientific Publications, 1972, p. 88.

Crawford, J. S., Williams, M. E., and Veales, S.: Particulate matter in the extradural space. Brit. J. Anaesth. *47*:807, 1975.

Crawley, B. E.: Catheter sequestration. A complication of epidural analgesia. Anaesthesia *23*:270, 1968.

Cunningham, N. L., and Kaplan, J. A.: A rapid-onset, long-acting regional anesthetic technique. Anesthesiology *41*:509, 1974.

Curbelo, M. M.: Continuous peridural segmental anesthesia by means of a ureteral catheter. Anesth. Analg. *28*:13, 1949.

Daly, D. J., Davenport, J., and Newland, M. C.: Methaemoglobinaemia following the use of prilocaine (Citanest). Brit. J. Anaesth. *36*:737, 1964.

Daos, F. G., Lopez, L., and Virtue, R. W.: Local anesthetic toxicity modified by oxygen and by combination of agents. Anesthesiology *23*:755, 1962.

DeLeo, B. E., Hamelberg, W., Stauffer, G. L., and Krause, S.: Instability of steam-autoclaved bupivacaine with epinephrine. Anesthesiology *40*:297, 1974.

Denecke, K.: Die Periduralanästhesie in der Chirurgie. Zbl. Chir. *64*:130, 1937.

Dhuner, K-G., Harthon, J. G. L., Herbring, B-G., and Lie, T.: Blood levels of mepivacaine after regional anaesthesia. Brit. J. Anaesth. *27*:746, 1965.

DiGiovanni, A. J.: A critical evaluation of disposable spinal anesthesia needles. Anesthesiology *34*:88, 1971.

Doughty, A.: A precise method of cannulating the lumbar epidural space. Anaesthesia *29*:63, 1974.

Downing, J. W.: Bupivacaine: A clinical assessment in lumbar extradural block. Brit. J. Anaesth. *41*:427, 1969.

Düttmann, G.: Die peridurale segmentäre Anästhesie. Zbl. Chir. *68*:530, 1941.

Ekblom, L., and Widman, B.: A comparison of the properties of LAC-43, prilocaine and mepivacaine in extradural anaesthesia. Acta Anaesth. Scand. (Suppl.) *21*:33, 1966.

Engberg, G., Holmdahl, M. H., and Edström, H. H.: A comparison of the local anesthetic properties of bupivacaine and two new long-acting agents, HS 37 and etidocaine, in epidural analgesia. Acta Anaesth. Scand. *18*:277, 1974.

Englesson, S., Eriksson, E., Wahlqvist, S., and Örtengren, B.: Difference in tolerance to intravenous Xylocaine and Citanest (L-67), a new local anesthetic. A double blind study in man. First European Congress of Anesthesiology Proc. *2*:1962, No. 206.

Erdemir, H. A., Soper, L. E., and Sweet, R. B.: Studies of factors affecting peridural anesthesia. Anesth. Analg. *44*:400, 1965.

Foldes, F. F., and Davis, D. L.: The spinal fluid concentrations of 2-chloroprocaine following its epidural administration in man. J. Pharmacol. Exp. Ther. *110*:18, 1954.

Foldes, F. F., and McNall, P. G.: 2-Chloroprocaine: A new local anesthetic agent. Anesthesiology *13*:287, 1952.

Foldes, F. F., Colavincenzo, J. W., and Birch, J. H.: Epidural anesthesia: A reappraisal. Curr. Res. Anesth. Analg. *35*:33, 89, 1956.

Fox, G. S., Houle, G. L., Desjardins, P. D., and Mercier, G.: Intrauterine fetal lidocaine concentrations during continuous epidural anesthesia. Amer. J. Obstet. Gynecol. *110*:896, 1971.

Fujimori, M., Kato, M., and Nishimura, S.: Use of LAC-43 for epidural anesthesia, and its blood concentration. Jap. J. Anesth. *16*:307, 1967.

Fujimori, M., Nishimura, K., and Goto, E.: Methemoglobinemia due to local anesthetics (A preliminary report). Far East J. Anesth. *4*:22, 1964.

Geerinckx, K., Vanderick, G., Van Steenberge, A. L., Bouche, R., and De Muylder, E.: Bupivacaine 0.125% in epidural block analgesia during childbirth: Maternal and foetal plasma concentrations. Brit. J. Anaesth. *46*:937, 1974.

Gibson, T., and Norris, W.: Skin fragments removed by injection needles. Lancet *2*:983, 1958.

Gitschmann, J., and Nolte, H.: Comparative study with etidocaine and bupivacaine in epidural block. Acta Anaesth. Scand. (Suppl.) *60*:55, 1975.

Goepel, H.: Erfahrungsbericht über die Periduralanästhesie. Die Pantocain-Periston-Plombe zur segmentaren Anästhesie. Zbl. Chir. *72*:467, 1947.

Gordon, R. A., Kerr, J. H., and Taylor, R.: A laboratory and clinical evaluation of mepivacaine (Carbocaine). Canad. Anaesth. Soc. J. *7*:290, 1960.

Groves, M. J.: Particulate contamination in intravenous fluids. I. Nature, origin and hazard. Pharmaceutical J. *210*:185, 1973.

Gunther, R. E., and Bellville, J. W.: Obstetrical caudal anesthesia. II. A randomized study comparing 1 per cent mepivacaine with 1 per cent mepivacaine plus epinephrine. Anesthesiology *37*:288, 1972.

Harris, W. H., Cole, D. W., Mital, M., and Laver, M. B.: Methemoglobin formation and oxygen transport following intravenous regional anesthesia using prilocaine. Anesthesiology *29*:65, 1968.

Hehre, F. W., Moyes, A. Z., Senfield, R. M., and Lilly, E. J.: Continuous lumbar peridural anesthesia in obstetrics. II. Use of minimal amounts of local anesthetics during labor. Anesth. Analg. *44*:89, 1965.

Henkin, M. L., Cohen, D. D., and Sadin, E. B.: An improved continuous epidural anesthesia technique. Anesthesiology *32*:151, 1970.

Henn, F.: Determination of the toxicological and pharmacological properties of Carbocaine, Lidocaine and Procaine by means of simultaneous experiments. Acta Anaesth. Scand. *4*:125, 1960.

Hingson, R. A., and Southworth, J. L.: Continuous caudal anesthesia. Amer. J. Surg. *58*:93, 1942.

Ho, N. F. H.: Particulate matter in parenteral solutions. I. A review of the literature. Drug Intelligence *1*:7, 1967.
Hoffmann, A., and Kochmann, M.: Verminderung der Novokainkonzentration durch Kaliumsulfat bie der Lokalanästhesie. Dtsch. Med. Wschr. *38*:2264, 1912.
Hollmén, A.: Experience with LAC-43, a new anaesthetic with prolonged action, in operative and therapeutic epidural and regional anaesthesia. Ann. Chir. Gynaecol. *55*:322, 1966.
Hollmén, A., Korhonen, M., and Ojala, A.: Bupivacaine in paracervical block—Plasma levels and changes in maternal and foetal acid-base balance. Brit. J. Anaesth. *41*:603, 1969.
Hunt, J. R., Rigor, B. M., and Collins, J. R.: The potential for contamination of continuous epidural catheters. Anesth. Analg. *56*:222, 1977.
Hyman, M. D., and Shnider, S. M.: Maternal and neonatal blood concentrations of bupivacaine associated with obstetrical conduction anesthesia. Anesthesiology *34*:81, 1971.
James, F. M., George, R. H., Naiem, H., and White, G. J.: Bacteriologic aspects of epidural analgesia. Anesth. Analg. *55*:187, 1976.
Janzen, E.: Der negative Vorschlag bei Lumbalpunktion. Dtsch. Z. Nervenheilk. *94*:280, 1926.
Jordfeldt, L., Löfström, B., Pernow, B., Persson, B., Wahren, J., and Widman, B.: The effect of local anaesthetics on the central circulation and respiration in man and dog. Acta Anaesth. Scand. *12*:153, 1968.
Joseph, D.: Methaemoglobinaemia and anaesthesia. Brit. J. Anaesth. *34*:309, 1962.
Katz, H., Borden, H., and Hirscher, D.: Glass-particle contamination of color-break ampules. Anesthesiology *39*:354, 1973.
Keenaghan, J. B., and Boyes, R. N.: The tissue distribution, metabolism and excretion of lidocaine in rats, guinea pigs, dogs and man. J. Pharmacol. Exp. Ther. *180*:454, 1972.
Korkeila, J.: LAC-43-clinical experiences with a new long-acting local anaesthetic agent in epidural anaesthesia. Acta Anaesth. Scand. (Suppl.) *23*:453, 1966.
Lechat, P., Deleau, D., and Griffié, R. A.: Influence de l'ion potassium sur l'activité des anesthésiques locaux. Med. Exp. (Basel) *11*:157, 1964.
Lee, J. A.: Specially marked needle to facilitate extradural block. Anaesthesia *15*:186, 1960.
Lee, J. A.: A new catheter for continuous extradural analgesia. Anaesthesia *17*:248, 1962.
Littlewood, D. G., Scott, D. B., Wilson, J., and Covino, B. G.: Comparative anaesthetic properties of various local anaesthetic agents in extradural block for labour. Brit. J. Anaesth. *49*:75, 1977.
Löfgren, N.: Studies on Local Anaesthetics. Xylocaine, a New Synthetic Drug. Stockholm, Haeggströms, 1948.
Love, J. C.: Continuous subarachnoid drainage for meningitis by means of a ureteral catheter. J.A.M.A. *104*:1595, 1935.
Lund, P. C.: Peridural Analgesia and Anesthesia. Springfield, Ill., Charles C Thomas, 1966, pp. 150, 309.
Lund, P. C.: Double blind peridural study of 1.0 per cent Duranest with and without epinephrine. Worcester, Massachusetts, Astra Pharmaceutical Products, Inc. Product Monograph on Duranest (Etidocaine) HC1, 1976, p. 23.
Lund, P. C., and Cwik, J. C.: Citanest—A clinical and laboratory study. Anesth. Analg. *44*:712, 1965.
Lund, P. C., Cwik, J. C., and Pagdanganan, R. T.: Etidocaine—A new long-acting local anesthetic agent: A clinical evaluation. Anesth. Analg. *52*:482, 1973.
Lund, P. C., Cwik, J. C., Gannon, R. T., and Vassallo, H. G.: Etidocaine for caesarean section—Effects on mother and baby. Brit. J. Anaesth. *49*:457, 1977.
Magno, R., Berlin, A., Karlsson, K., and Kjellmer, I.: Anesthesia for cesarean section. IV. Placental transfer and neonatal elimination of bupivacaine following epidural analgesia for elective cesarean section. Acta Anaesth. Scand. *20*:141, 1976.
Malagodi, M. H., Munson, E. S., and Embro, W. J.: Relation of etidocaine and bupivacaine toxicity to rate of infusion in rhesus monkeys. Brit. J. Anaesth. *49*:121, 1977.
Manalan, S. A.: Caudal block anaesthesia in obstetrics. J. Indiana Med. Assoc. *35*:564, 1942.
Manno, N. J., Uihlein, A., and Kernohan, J. W.: Intraspinal epidermoids. J. Neurosurg. *19*:754, 1962.
Mather, L. E., Tucker, G. T., Murphy, T. M., Stanton-Hicks, M. d'A., and Bonica, J. J.: The effects of adding adrenaline to etidocaine and lignocaine in extradural anaesthesia. II. Pharmacokinetics. Brit. J. Anaesth. *48*:989, 1976.
Meeker, W. R.: The potentiation of novocaine solutions. J. Lab. Clin. Med. *11*:139, 1925.
Moore, D. C., Bridenbaugh, L. D., Bagdi, P. A., and Bridenbaugh, P. O.: Accumulation of mepivacaine hydrochloride during caudal block. Anesthesiology *29*:585, 1968.
Moore, D. C., Bridenbaugh, D., Bridenbaugh, P. O., and Tucker, G. T.: Bupivacaine—A review of 2,077 cases. J.A.M.A. *214*:713, 1970.
Moore, D. C., Bridenbaugh, L. D., Bridenbaugh, P. O., and Tucker, G. T.: Caudal and epidural blocks with bupivacaine for childbirth: Report of 657 parturients. Obstet. Gynecol. *37*:667, 1971.

Moore, D. C., Bridenbaugh, L. D., Bridenbaugh, P. O., Thompson, G. E., and Tucker, G. T.: Does compounding of local anesthetic agents increase their toxicity in humans? Anesth. Analg. *51*:579, 1972.

Moore, D. C., Bridenbaugh, P. O., Bridenbaugh, L. D., Thompson, G. E., Balfour, R. I., and Lysons, D. F.: A double-blind study of bupivacaine and etidocaine for epidural (peridural) block. Anesth. Analg. *53*:690, 1974.

Morishima, H. O., Daniel, S. S., Finster, M:, Poppers, P. J., and James, L. S.: Transmission of mepivacaine hydrochloride (Carbocaine) across the human placenta. Anesthesiology *27*:147, 1966.

Munson, E. S., Tucker, W. K., Ausinsch, B., and Malagodi, M. J.: Etidocaine, bupivacaine and lidocaine seizure thresholds in monkeys. Anesthesiology *42*:471, 1975.

Munson, E. S., Paul, W. L., and Embro, W. J.: Central nervous system toxicity of local anesthetic mixtures in monkeys. Anesthesiology *46*:179, 1977.

Murphy, T. M., Mather, L. E., Stanton-Hicks, M. d'A., Bonica, J. J., and Tucker, G. T.: The effects of adding adrenaline to etidocaine and lignocaine in extradural anaesthesia. I. Block characteristics and cardiovascular effects. Brit. J. Anaesth. *48*:893, 1976.

Mushin, W. W.: Intramuscular gallamine with hyaluronidase. Anaesthesia *11*:135, 1956.

Nølte, H., Meyer, J., Köpf, B., and Zenz, M.: Klinische und elektrophysiologische Parameter zur Differenzierung der Wirkung von Lokalanaesthetica. Anaesthesist *23*:165, 1974.

Odom, C. B.: Epidural anesthesia. Amer. J. Surg. *34*:547, 1936.

Peebles, D. J., and Slack, W. K.: Extradural analgesia. A controlled trial of plain solutions of bupivacaine and lignocaine. Anaesthesia *26*:441, 1971.

Poppelbaum, F.: Sicherheitsmassnahmen bei der extraduralen spinalanaesthesie. Dtsch. Gesundheitswesen *9*:499, 1954.

Raj, P. P., Rosenblatt, R., Miller, J., Katz, R. L., and Carden, E.: Dynamics of local-anesthetic compounds in regional anesthesia. Anesth. Analg. *56*:110, 1977.

Raksamani, A., and Edelist, G.: A comparison of etidocaine and lidocaine in epidural analgesia for surgery. Canad. Anaesth. Soc. J. *24*:70, 1977.

Reynolds, F.: A comparison of the potential toxicity of bupivacaine, lignocaine, mepivacaine during epidural blockade for surgery. Brit. J. Anaesth. *43*:567, 1971a.

Reynolds, F.: Metabolism and excretion of bupivacaine in man: A comparison with mepivacaine. Brit. J. Anaesth. *43*:33, 1971b.

Reynolds, F., and Taylor, G.: Maternal and neonatal blood concentrations of bupivacaine. Anaesthesia *25*:14, 1970.

Reynolds, F., and Taylor, G.: Plasma concentrations of bupivacaine during continuous epidural analgesia in labour: The effect of adrenaline. Brit. J. Anaesth. *43*:436, 1971.

Reynolds, F., Hargrove, R. L., and Wyman, J. B.: Maternal and foetal plasma concentrations of bupivacaine after epidural block. Brit. J. Anaesth. *45*:1049, 1973.

Rowland, M., Thomson, P. D., Guichard, A., and Melmon, K. L.: Disposition kinetics of lidocaine in normal subjects. N. Y. Acad. Sci. *179*:383, 1971.

Scanlon, J. W., Brown, W. U., Weiss, J. B., et al.: Neurobehavioural responses of newborn infants after maternal epidural anesthesia. Anesthesiology *40*:121, 1974.

Scanlon, J. W., Ostheimer, G. W., Lurie, A. O., Brown, W. U., Weiss, J. B., and Alper, M. H.: Neurobehavioural responses and drug concentrations in newborns after maternal epidural anesthesia with bupivacaine. Anesthesiology *45*:400, 1976.

Schulte-Steinberg, O.: Spread of local anesthetic solutions in caudal blocks in children. Sixth World Congress of Anesthesiology Abstracts, Mexico City, Excerpta Medica, Int. Congr. Series No. 387, 1976, p. 132.

Scott, D. B.: Hyaluronidase in epidural analgesia. Brit. J. Anaesth. *28*:187, 1956.

Scott, D. B.: Methaemoglobinaemia due to prilocaine (discussion). Acta Anaesth. Scand. (Suppl.) *16*:199, 1965.

Scott, D. B.: Evaluation of the toxicity of local anaesthetic agents in man. Brit. J. Anaesth. *47*:56, 1975.

Scott, D. B., Jebson, P. J. R., Braid, D. P., Örtengren, B., and Frisch, P.: Factors affecting plasma levels of lignocaine and prilocaine. Brit. J. Anaesth. *44*:1040, 1972.

Seltzer, J. L., Porretta, J. C., and Jackson, B. G.: Plastic particulate contaminants in the medicine cups of disposable non-spinal regional anesthesia sets. Anesthesiology *47*:378, 1977.

Shaywitz, B. A.: Epidermoid spinal cord tumors and previous lumbar punctures. J. Pediat. *80*:638, 1972.

Sheehan, J. M., Wright, I. V., and Shepard, B. M.: An evaluation of the Cheng needle in the administration of 1002 single-dose lumbar epidural anesthetics. Anesth. Analg. *41*:552, 1962.

Shykoff, H. J.: Control of pain during labour. Canad. Anaesth. Soc. J. *16*:144, 1969.

Skinner, B. S.: A new epidural cannula. Canad. Anaesth. Soc. J. *13*:622, 1966.

Smith, R. A., and Connor, E. H.: Experimental study of intrathecal detergents. Anesthesiology *26*:5, 1962.

Smyth, C. J., et al.: Rheumatism and arthritis: Review of American and English literature of recent years. Ann. Int. Med. *59* (Suppl. 4):1, 1963.

Somerville, T. G., and Gibson, M.: Particulate contamination in ampoules: A comparative study. Pharmaceutical J. *211*:128, 1973.

Stanton-Hicks, M. d'A.: A study using bupivacaine for continuous peridural analgesia in patients undergoing surgery of the hip. Acta Anaesth. Scand. *15*:65, 1971.

Stanton-Hicks, M., Murphy, T. M., Bonica, J. J., Mather, L., and Tucker, G. T.: Effects of extradural block: Comparison of the properties, circulatory effects and pharmacokinetics of etidocaine and bupivacaine. Brit. J. Anaesth. *48*:575, 1976.

Steel, G. C., and Dawkins, C. J. M.: Extradural lumbar block with bupivacaine (Marcain: LAC-43). A clinical trial in lower abdominal and perineal surgery. Anaesthesia *23*:14, 1968.

Stout, R. J.: Anaesthetic potency in epidural analgesia. Brit. J. Anaesth. *29*:495, 1957.

Swerdlow, M., and Jones, R.: The duration of action of bupivacaine, prilocaine and lignocaine. Brit. J. Anaesth. *42*:335, 1970.

Telivuo, L.: A new long-acting local anaesthetic solution for pain relief after thoracotomy. Ann. Chir. et Gynaec. Fenniae *52*:513, 1963.

Thomas, D. V.: Sterilization of epinephrine. Anesthesiology *17*:752, 1956.

Thomas, J., Climie, C. R., and Mather, L. E.: Placental transfer of lignocaine following lumbar epidural administration. Brit. J. Anaesth. *40*:965, 1968.

Thomas, J., Climie, C. R., Long, G., and Nighjoy, L. E.: The influence of adrenaline on the maternal plasma levels and placental transfer of lignocaine following lumbar epidural administration. Brit. J. Anaesth. *41*:1029, 1969a.

Thomas, J., Climie, C. R., and Mather, L. E.: The maternal plasma levels and placental transfer of bupivacaine following epidural analgesia. Brit. J. Anaesth. *41*:1035, 1969b.

Thomson, P. T., Melmon, K. L., Richardson, J. A., Cohn, K., Steinbrunn, W., Cudihee, R., and Rowland, M.: Lidocaine pharmacokinetics in advanced heart failure, liver disease, and renal failure in humans. Ann. Int. Med. *78*:499, 1973.

Truant, A. P., and Takman, B.: Differential physical, chemical and neuropharmacologic properties of local anesthetic agents. Anesth. Analg. *38*:478, 1959.

Tucker, G. T., and Mather, L. E.: Pharmacokinetics of local anaesthetic agents. Brit. J. Anaesth. *47*:213, 1975.

Tucker, G. T., Morishima, H. O., Finster, M., et al.: Binding of anilide-type local anesthetics in human plasma. I. Relationships between binding, physicochemical properties and anesthetic activity. Anesthesiology *33*:287, 1970.

Tucker, G. T., Moore, D. C., Bridenbaugh, P. O., Bridenbaugh, L. D., and Thompson, G. E.: Systemic absorption of mepivacaine in commonly used regional block procedures. Anesthesiology *37*:277, 1972.

Tucker, G. T., Cooper, S., Littlewood, D., Buckley, F. P., Covino, B. G., and Scott, D. B.: Observed and predicted accumulation of local anaesthetic agents during continuous extradural analgesia. Brit. J. Anaesth. *49*:237, 1977.

Tuohy, E. B.: Continuous spinal anesthesia: A new method of utilising a ureteral catheter. Surg. Clin. N. Amer. *25*:834, 1945.

Vanderick, G., Geerinckx, K., Van Steenberge, A. L., and De Muylder, E.: Bupivacaine 0.125% in epidural block analgesia during childbirth: Clinical evaluation. Brit. J. Anaesth. *46*:838, 1974.

Wagner, R. S.: A needle for single-dose peridural anesthesia. Anesth. Analg. *36*(3):31, 1957.

Waters, H. R., Rosen, N., and Perkins, D. H.: Extradural blockade with bupivacaine. A double blind trial of bupivacaine with adrenaline 1/200,000 and bupivacaine plain. Anaesthesia *25*:184, 1970.

Watt, M. J., Ross, D. M., and Atkinson, R. S.: A double-blind trial of bupivacaine and lignocaine. Latency and duration in extradural blockade. Anaesthesia *23*:331, 1968.

Whittet, T. D.: The effect of autoclaving on ampoules of local analgesics. Anaesthesia *9*:271, 1954.

Wiedling, S.: Studies on α-n-propylamino-2-methylpropionanilide—A new local anaesthetic. Acta Pharmacol. (Kbh.) *17*:233, 1960.

Wilkinson, G. R., and Lund, P. C.: Bupivacaine levels in plasma and cerebrospinal fluid following peridural administration. Anesthesiology *33*:482, 1970.

Winkelman, N. W.: Neurologic symptoms following accidental intraspinal detergent injection. Neurology *2*:284, 1952.

Winnie, A. P.: A grip to facilitate the insertion of epidural needles. Anesth. Analg. *50*:23, 1971.

Wood, K. M., and Arguelles, J. E.: A study of the effect of methylprednisolone acetate, in sterile aqueous suspension, on peripheral nerves. 1977 ASA Annual Meeting. Abstracts of Scientific Papers, New Orleans, p. 631.

Wylie, W. D., and Churchill-Davidson, H. C.: A Practice of Anaesthesia. Chicago, Year Book Medical Publishers Inc., 1972, pp. 860–65.

Yoshikawa, K., Mima, T., and Egawa, J.: Blood level of Marcaine (LAC-43) in axillary plexus blocks, intercostal nerve blocks and epidural anaesthesia. Acta Anaesth. Scand. *12*:1, 1968.

chapter 10
Physiology

Thus the long war, from everlasting waged,
With equal strife among the elements
Goes on and on. Now here, now there, prevail
The vital forces of the world—or fall.

De Rerum Natura: *Lucretius*
(Translation by W. E. Leonard)

INTRODUCTION

This chapter is mainly concerned with the physiological alterations that follow somatic and autonomic neural blockade caused by epidural analgesia, especially in the realms of the cardiovascular, respiratory and metabolic control systems. The direct neural effects of epidural blockade have been dealt with in the chapters on Anatomy, Pharmacology and Mechanism of Action. Here, neural blockade will be discussed only in relation to structures and systems under neural control.

One essential aspect of epidural blockade, namely its protean and yet controllable nature, must be clearly understood and constantly kept in mind so that the rich variety of physiological and clinical results, and the apparent confusion that often arises in relating animal experiments to man, may be interpreted. As discussed in Chapter 4, epidural blockade is not the absolute anatomical event that some earlier workers supposed. The neurological consequences of epidural blockade are impure and occur at many different neural addresses, some metropolitan within the cord and others farther out in the suburbia of the spinal roots. At all these places blockade is partial. Some neural traffic lanes remain open for the execution of urgent commands initiated at higher centers—commands that may never be issued if the patient is asleep under general anesthesia. A wide range of neural blockade and of neural escape is possible in epidural analgesia, depending on the potency of the drugs and the dosage chosen. Clinically, epidural analgesia is not a single option in the business of neural isolation but rather encompasses a wide range of potential, from a barely perceptible effect to an intense blockade of the majority of segmental fibers, depending on the choice of local anesthetic drug and the way it is used. The later chapters on clinical applications will provide practical examples of this.

Although epidural analgesia can never aspire to the rigorous purity of surgical neural ablation that is possible in animal experiments, nevertheless there are experimental models that provide clues to the qualitative changes in organ systems that accompany epidural blockade, and it may be helpful to consider some of these models in the succeeding sections.

CARDIOVASCULAR SYSTEM

Neural control of the heart and circulation is extremely complex (Levy, 1971; Abboud, 1972), and no attempt will be made to give a detailed analysis of cardiovascular control in this section. Instead, emphasis will be placed on the relevant questions: what does epidural denervation do to the cardiovascular system, and how can its effects be modified to maintain acceptable pressure-flow states in vital organs?

In the past, opinions have differed widely over the clinical effects of epidural blockade on the cardiovascular system. Some authorities claimed that epidural analgesia, unlike subarachnoid block, spared the vasomotor nerves in some way so that blood pressure was altered very little, even in the presence of a high segmental block (Pagés, 1921; Odom, 1936; Gutierrez, 1939; Dogliotti, 1939; Dawkins, 1945; Figueredo, 1948), and a relative cardiovascular stability was claimed to be one of the characteristic advantages of the technique. However, others observed falls in blood pressure comparable to those found with subarachnoid analgesia and determined by the segmental extent of blockade (Shaw, 1926; Denecke, 1937; Düttmann, 1941; Goepel, 1943; Abajian, 1943; Goffen et al., 1950; Bromage, 1951; Havers, 1956; Defalque, 1962).

In a series of 120 cases of lumbar epidural analgesia combined with light general anesthesia, Bromage (1951, 1954) found that the diastolic pressure fell before the systolic pressure and that the final level of mean arterial blood pressure bore a linear relationship to the segmental height of blockade between T_1 and T_{10}. Under these conditions of epidural blockade with light general anesthesia, the degree of arterial hypotension depended entirely on the number of spinal segments involved and not on the initial height of blood pressure, as shown in Figure 10–1.

With this type of technique combining general anesthesia with high segmental blockade, other hypotensive influences are added to the effects of segmental neural blockade, and the net results are due to the summation of several different factors. Thus, general anesthesia suppresses reflex sympathetic recruitment, while vascular absorption of powerful local anesthetics from the extradural space may produce some degree of systemic cardiovascular depression. From a practical point of view, the combination of extensive epidural blockade with general anesthesia or heavy sedation came to be accepted as a reliable means of inducing controlled vascular hypotension to reduce surgical hemorrhage (Goffen, Fitzpatrick and Wood, 1950; Bromage, 1951; Havers, 1956; Morris and Candy, 1957). Blood pressure, being easy to measure, was the sole and sometimes misleading guide to cardiovascular status (Bendixen et al., 1964). At that time, the proportional roles of the various components contributing to overall cardiovascular function were not adequately understood, and a great deal of laboratory and clinical investigation was needed to unravel their complex interactions.

Epidural analgesia may influence cardiovascular dynamics in at least four different ways, and attempts to explain the net results of blockade in terms

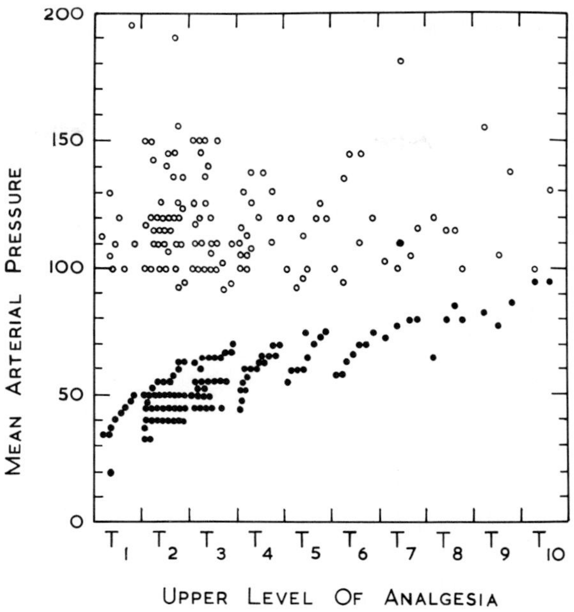

Figure 10–1. Relation between blood pressure and segmental involvement of the epidural block in 120 patients under light general anesthesia (thiopental, nitrous oxide, oxygen). The "mean arterial pressure" is expressed as the arithmetic mean of the systolic and diastolic pressures.
○ = Preoperative resting level
● = Lowest level of MAP after induction of epidural analgesia
Epidural analgesic solution: 1/600 Nupercaine (dibucaine) + 1.6 per cent procaine and 1/200,000 epinephrine in volumes of 15 to 50 ml, depending on age and required segmental spread. (From Bromage, P. R.: Spinal Epidural Analgesia. Edinburgh, E. & S. Livingstone, 1954.)

of any one of these effects alone does not give an accurate description of events. The possible cardiovascular influences may be classified according to the following schema.

Neural

1. Segmental sympathetic efferent blockade with resulting dilatation of resistance and capacitance vessels (Guyton et al., 1959; Mellander, 1960; Shimosati and Etsten, 1969).

2. Paralysis of cardiac sympathetic fibers from the upper four or five thoracic segments, with loss of chronotropic and inotropic drive to the myocardium, resulting in bradycardia and reduction of ejection force (Glick and Braunwald, 1965; Otton and Wilson, 1966; Randall and McNally, 1960; Woods and Richardson, 1959; McLean et al., 1967).

The sympathetic pathways affecting cardiovascular status are shown diagrammatically in Figure 10–2.

Pharmacological

1. From vascular absorption of local anesthetic from the epidural space, leading to significant concentrations of local anesthetic in the circulation and consequent distant effects on smooth muscle. Sufficiently high concentrations of local anesthetic may lead to smooth muscle depression and a fall in cardiac output from beta-receptor blockade (Defalque, 1962; Goldberg, 1949; Morales-Aguilerá and Vaughan Williams, 1965; Steinhaus, 1957; Stewart et al., 1963). The depressant effects of circulating local anesthetic are pH-dependent and are likely to be most severe in the presence of renal or respiratory acidosis (Andersson et al., 1970).

2. From beta-receptor stimulation as a result of vascular absorption of epinephrine, if this is present in the epidural solution, leading to a rise in cardiac output and a fall in peripheral resistance (Ahlquist, 1949; Ward et al., 1965; Bonica et al., 1971, 1972).

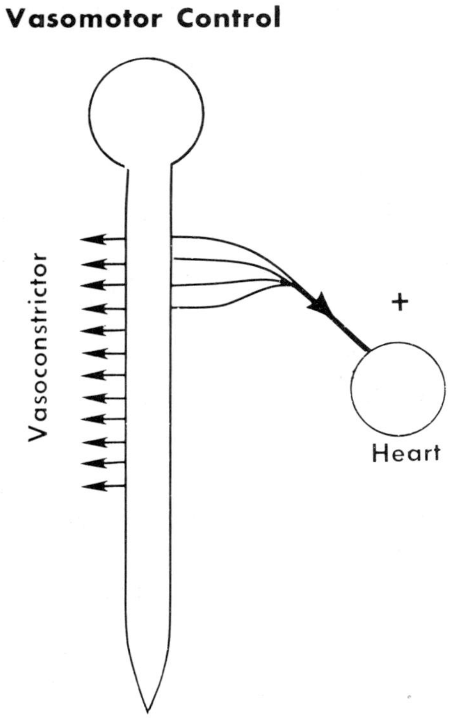

Figure 10–2. Segmental and cardiac distribution of the sympathetic outflow.

An additional cardiovascular influence was thought to arise from the increase in cerebrospinal fluid pressure following rapid epidural injection. However, this possibility has been investigated by Bonica's group, and they found that rapid epidural injection had no significant effect on cardiovascular dynamics, at least in elderly subjects (Akamatsu et al., 1967).

The neural effects of epidural analgesia and the systemic consequences of drug absorption are inseparable. With small epidural doses the systemic effects of absorbed local anesthetic may be negligible in comparison to the effects of neural blockade. Nevertheless, in practice, these two forces operate together to a greater or lesser extent, depending on technique and dosage, and any realistic analysis of the effects of epidural analgesia must consider both of them. In the succeeding paragraphs it will be necessary to dissect these two influences for the sake of clarity, but this is an artificial separation for descriptive purposes only.

NEURAL INFLUENCES OF EPIDURAL BLOCKADE

"Differential Blockade" and Central Recruitment

The physiological effects of epidural blockade are often confusing and difficult to understand unless one remembers the central fact stressed earlier that the process of blockade is not an absolute event. It does not fully live up to what its name claims; usually it is not a complete block but merely a reduction in neural traffic that is adequate for clinical purposes. Confusion over the physiological effects has arisen from failure to appreciate this essentially relative and partial nature of epidural "blockade." Many nerve fibers are interrupted within the territory of the block, but as we have seen earlier, and as anyone can see for himself clinically, not all the fibers are affected, and an appreciable number of motor fibers usually escape. It has always been assumed that because sympathetic efferent fibers are smaller than somatic efferents, they will all be blocked before the larger ones, as part of the phenomenon of "differential blockade." This is not necessarily so; powerful local anesthetic agents will produce more sympathetic block than weak ones, and the addition of epinephrine, by intensifying the block, will also have the same effect (Cousins and Wright, 1971).

The efferent sympathetic fibers that escape have a choice. They can either rest or work, depending on the compulsion of central recruitment. A low level of central activity, such as may exist under light general anesthesia, will lead to little or no central recruitment and leave the surviving fibers idle, with low vasomotor activity and almost complete vasodilatation within the area of blockade. On the other hand, a high level of central activity in a young, anxious and vigorous patient will fully recruit all available pathways that have escaped blockade, and the resulting traffic of vasomotor activity may so completely compensate for the blocked sympathetic fibers that no change of cardiovascular status is apparent.

Opportunities exist for interplay between blockade and recruitment both at the level of the spinal roots and within the peripheral pathways of the spinal cord, as explained in Chapter 4 on Mechanism of Action, so a rich variety of response is possible, depending on the balance of the two opposing factors: the effectiveness of blockade and the vigor of central recruitment.

Figure 10–3 shows a common example of this balance in practice. In this case, segmental blockade to T_7 was accompanied by a blood pressure of 125/70 mmHg. Induction of very light general anesthesia was followed by an immediate drop of pulse rate from 85 to 60 per minute and of blood pressure to 90/60 mmHg, at which levels they remained stable until the face mask was removed 45 minutes later, when the patient awoke and pulse and blood pressure quickly regained their former levels. These abrupt changes accompanying altered levels of consciousness are almost certainly attributable to altered degrees of central recruitment of vasomotor activity within the CNS, finding expression both in segments beyond the area of blockade and in sympathetic efferents that have escaped within the segmental territory of sensory analgesia.

Control of Resistance and Capacitance Vessels

The venous capacitance vessels contain about 80 per cent of the regional blood volume, and changes of smooth muscle tone in these vessels can produce very significant shifts of blood volume and alterations of venous return (Wiedeman, 1963). Distension of the venous compartment and a rising right auricular pressure lead to reflex vasoconstriction and a compensatory elevation of pressure on the arteriolar side of the capillary bed, to ensure that an adequate flow is maintained across the capillary bed. Disturbances of this mechanism by sympathetic blockade may lead to undesirable effects under certain combina-

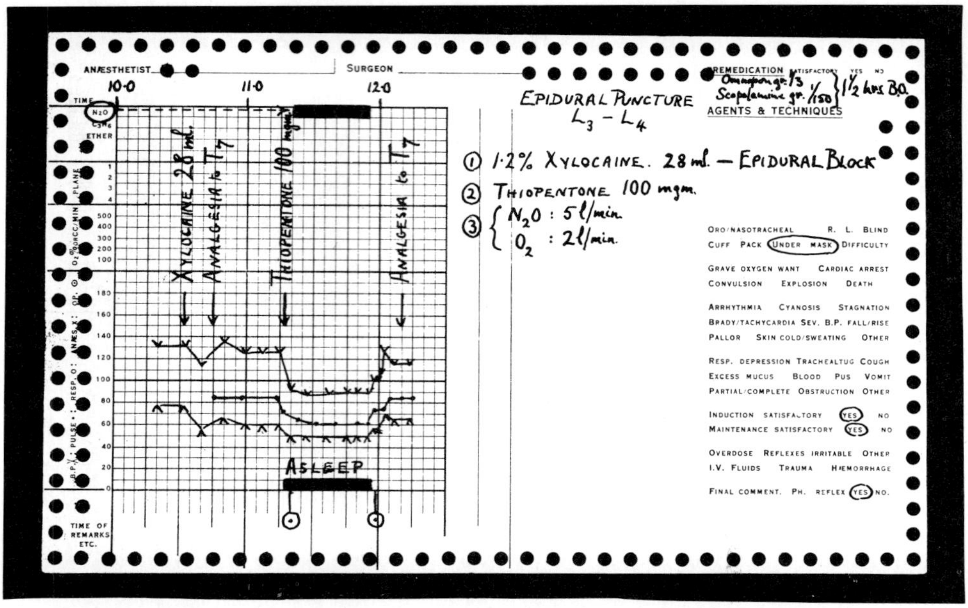

Figure 10–3. Consciousness and vasomotor recruitment as a pressor factor. Blood pressure chart of a woman aged 56 undergoing vulvectomy. Epidural block to T_7. Note that the blood pressure starts to fall after induction of epidural analgesia, but a compensatory rise maintains the blood pressure at its former level. Light sleep, induced with a small dose of thiopental and nitrous oxide and oxygen, is accompanied by an abrupt fall in blood pressure. An equally abrupt rise occurs when the patient regains consciousness. (From Bromage, P. R.: Spinal Epidural Analgesia, Edinburgh, E. & S., Livingstone, 1954.)

tions of circumstances. For example, if venous engorgement occurs in the extradural venous plexus following inferior vena caval occlusion, and if at the same time arterial pressure is abnormally low, then the stage may be set for the occurrence of venous stasis and infarction in the cord, with subsequent paralysis. Examples of this type of circulatory disaster will be given in Chapter 14.

Figure 10–4 shows the very wide range of blood flow that may exist in various organs at maximum dilatation and at rest. In the presence of sympathetic blockade these proportions may be altered, possibly to the detriment of the more important organs such as CNS, heart, liver and kidney, especially if the blood volume is reduced to a point where it fails to fill the available capacitance.

The control of peripheral vascular tone is mediated directly by segmental innervation of alpha and beta adrenergic receptors, and indirectly by circulating catecholamines released from the adrenal medulla (Mellander and Johansson, 1968). Vascular responsiveness to nerve stimulation in vessels and organs depends on the density of sympathetic innervation at any given point. For example, the renal arteriolar bed is about twice as responsive to neural stimulation as the limbs, and this greater reactivity is thought to be due to the larger number of sympathetic nerve endings in the kidney (Abboud, 1972). In the limbs small arteriolar and venous vessels close to the capillary bed are most sensitive to circulating norepinephrine, while larger vessels further away from the capillary bed and with a greater density of innervation are more sensitive to neural stimuli. The precapillary sphincters as final guardians of the capillary

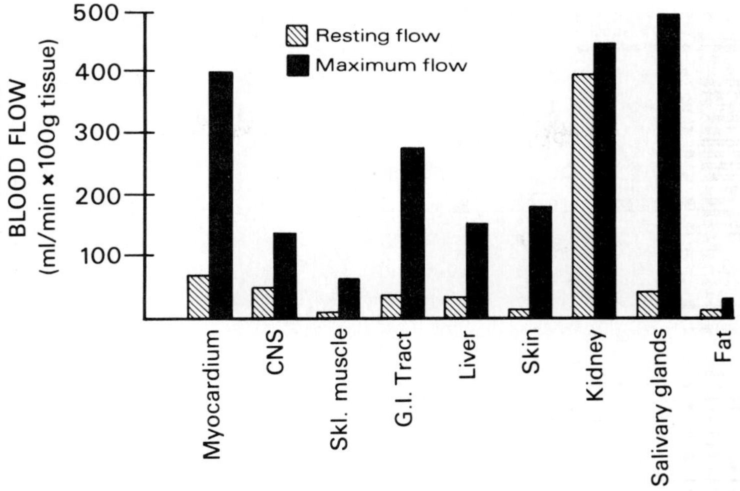

Figure 10–4. Approximate blood flows of different organs at maximum vasodilatation and at rest in man. (From Mellander & Johansson, Pharmacol. Rev. *20*:117, 1968.)

bed are responsible for vasomotor and autoregulation, probably under the influence of local oxygen tension (Granger and Guyton, 1969). These control systems are summarized in Figure 10–5.

Guyton has demonstrated the role of autoregulation in the total

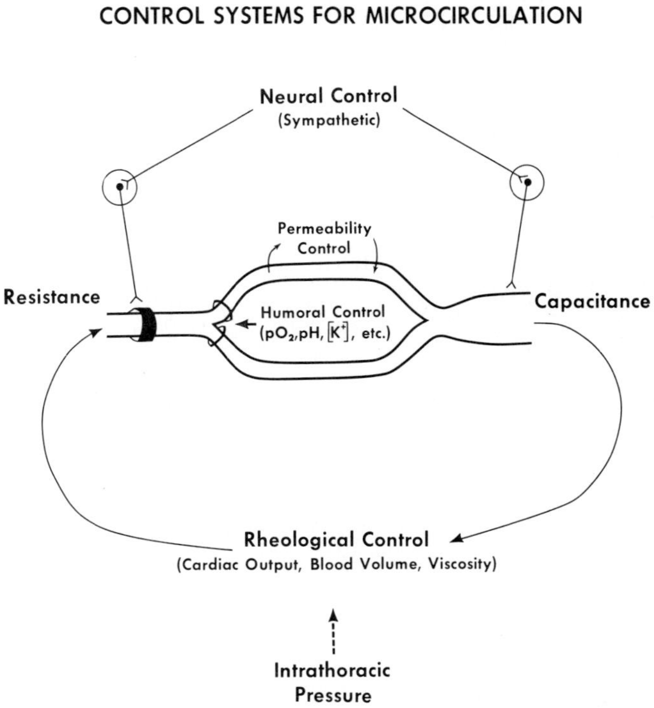

Figure 10–5. Control of the peripheral vasculature: neural (resistance vessels 0.5 to 2.0 mm diameter), humoral (resistance vessels > 0.5 mm diameter) and autoregulatory (at precapillary sphincters).

systemic circulation after complete ablation of the central nervous system in dogs by alcoholic neurolysis of the spinal cord followed by bloodless decapitation (Granger and Guyton, 1969). In this rigorously pure preparation, autoregulation readjusted peripheral flow after a relatively short time (average 35 minutes). Guyton concludes that autoregulation should rank along with cardiac output, arterial pressure and total peripheral resistance as one of the primary factors always to be considered in an analysis of long-term changes in circulatory function. The relatively slow course of onset of epidural analgesia compared to that of subarachnoid block may provide time for this type of readjustment to occur to a certain extent. A complete analysis of epidural action on the cardiovascular system may therefore have to include some consideration of autoregulation. However, its role in the overall picture is likely to be small compared to the more immediate effects of segmental neural blockade.

The adrenomedullary system, activated through the splanchnic sympathetic outflow between segments T_5 and L_1, contributes to cardiovascular control over a wide range. In the cat, Celander (1954) found that catecholamine output could increase more than 20-fold under conditions of strong sympathetic stimulation, as shown in Table 10–1.

This powerful potential for disturbance of vascular perfusion is uncontrolled during surgery under general anesthesia, but epidural blockade to T_5 ensures that the output of adrenal catecholamines remains at or below normal levels.

Interruption of sympathetic activity is followed by relaxation of arterioles, with reduction of precapillary resistance and increased capillary flow, together with a reduction of afterload to the heart and hence a reduction of cardiac work. However, the capacitance vessels also lose tone and the available venous capacitance increases, reducing venous return, so cardiac output falls. Under these circumstances the effects of any physical obstruction to venous return become magnified, and a slight degree of obstruction that might have gone unnoticed in the presence of normal capacitance tone and normal venous pressure may lead to almost total interruption of venous flow and a precipitous fall in cardiac output.

A classic example of the effects of obstructed venous return in the face of lowered capacitance tone is seen in late pregnancy. In the supine position, the heavy uterus falls back and blocks the thin-walled, low pressure inferior vena cava, and blood is forced to return to the heart through the vertebral venous plexuses and the azygos collecting system. Venous pressure rises

TABLE 10–1 Catecholamine Output from Adrenal Medulla of Cat at Rest and During Splanchnic Nerve Stimulation*

	Catecholamine Output (μg/kg/min)	***Circulating Concentration of Catecholamines (ng/ml)***
Resting	0.1	1–2
Splanchnic stimulation	2–3 (maximum 5.0)	25–50

*After Celander (1954).

in the legs and pelvic veins distal to the site of inferior vena caval obstruction. Provided the head of venous pressure is maintained at normal or slightly elevated levels, blood flows through collateral vertebral pathways to the azygos vein and back to the heart in adequate amounts. However, if sympathetic tone to the legs is diminished by general anesthesia or by blockade of the lower thoracic and lumbar segments, the capacitance vessels in the legs distend and the essential vis a tergo necessary to force blood back to the heart is lost. Then, cardiac output falls dramatically and death may occur unless something is done to overcome the venous obstruction. This phenomenon and the general question of "the supine hypotensive syndrome" are dealt with in greater detail in Chapter 12.

Neural Control of Cardiac Function

During the past six years it has become evident that medullary vasomotor centers have less of a monopoly on the neural control of cardiac output than had been supposed (Smith, 1974). Studies in tetraplegic patients (Corbett et al., 1971a, 1971b, 1971c) and in animals with high cord transections (Malliani et al., 1972, 1973) have shown that a significant part of the chronotropic and ionotropic control of the heart is mediated by afferent and efferent fibers carried through reflex arcs in the upper four or five thoracic spinal segments, quite independent of supraspinal influences. The independent potential for inotropic augmentation through the upper thoracic segments lies in the range of 13 to 21 per cent above control resting values (Malliani et al., 1972), although this cord reflex remains subservient to commands from above when the cord is intact, and it is overridden by parasympathetic influences (Levy, 1971).

Clearly this spinal reflex control of cardiac function will be attenuated or abolished by epidural blocks that extend above T_1 and at those points where the analgesic solution is powerful enough to interrupt a significant proportion of the spinal cord's afferent or efferent cardiac sympathetic pathways. The neural effect of high epidural blockade on cardiovascular function is therefore the sum of three separate components: segmental vasodilatation, adrenomedullary suppression and inhibition of segmental inotropic drive. The potential range of depressant effect from epidural blockade within the T_1–T_5 outflow will be quite broad, depending on the effectiveness of deafferentation within these five important segments. Modulation of spinal cardiac control is effected from higher centers, either positively by recruitment and facilitation of higher sympathetic motor pathways, as seen in conscious, anxious subjects, or negatively by overriding inhibition through vagal influences.

Randall's group at Loyola University has carried out detailed studies of the neural control of myocardial contractility in the dog, using simultaneous recordings from multiple strain gauge arches sutured to a number of different sites on the right and left ventricles (Norris et al., 1974; Randall and Armour, 1974). Their findings are unique in demonstrating specialized roles of the individual upper thoracic ventral roots on each side, and it is no longer possible to consider the upper four or five thoracic segments as equipotent influences in the control of cardiac function. Stimulation of the left side produced somewhat greater inotropic responses than stimulation of the right side, whereas chronotropic responses were dominated by the first three ventral roots on the right side. The blood pressure response to ventral root stimulation was asymmetrical, and the greatest increase of pressure was obtained by stimulating the upper four thoracic roots on the left side, with T_1 giving the greatest response, followed fairly closely by T_2, T_3 and T_4 on the left. T_5 on the left gave an insignificant response, while the same segment on the right side gave a very marked increase in pressure.

If these important findings are assumed to operate in man, it may be expected that the cardiovascular responses to high epidural block will not be directly proportional to the number of spinal segments involved, but they will be modified to a different extent as the upper level of blockade approaches the most potent segments at T_1 and T_2, and the greatest suppression of contractility and blood pressure may be expected to occur when the upper two thoracic segments become involved, especially on the left side.

Vagal Inhibition

Bradycardia and syncope are common accompaniments of diminished venous return to the heart (Jarisch, 1941; Jarisch and Zotterman, 1948; Sharpey-Schafer, 1956). In conscious subjects this mechanism is usually transient and self-correcting, unless the subject is forcibly held erect in the head-up position. However, under high subarachnoid or epidural blockade, it may not be self-correcting, and death may follow from ischemic cardiac arrest. Bradycardia and syncope may steal upon a patient quite suddenly and unexpectedly during high spinal epidural blockade, especially if venous return is physically impeded by inferior vena caval obstruction, as in the dorsal position during late pregnancy. A number of fatalities have occurred from this cause. The bradycardiac reflex follows vagal pathways through the medulla, and the receptors responsible for triggering it appear to lie in the cardiac ventricles. Electrophysiological recordings from vagal afferents arising in the ventricles show a characteristic pattern in response to a graded reduction of venous return (Öberg and Thorén, 1972a, 1972b). These inhibitory afferents show a gradual suppression of activity during bleeding and reduction of venous return, but then, at a certain point, their activity suddenly increases, accompanied by an abrupt slowing of the heart. Öberg and Thorén postulate that this is basically a protective reflex designed to prevent mechanical damage to the endocardium, arising from a strong sympathetic inotropic drive flogging the empty ventricles to contract in the face of inadequate venous return. With the onset of bradycardia, better diastolic filling occurs and pumping efficiency is increased. However, if diastolic filling cannot improve because venous return remains persistently low, then the vicious circle is completed and bradycardia proceeds inexorably to myocardial ischemia and arrest. On the operating table the onset of bradycardia during arterial hypotension is a signal for urgent treatment. Unless corrected, cardiac output and coronary perfusion will fall to dangerously low levels. The logical steps to follow are:

1. Increase venous return in order to allow proper filling of the heart. This may involve simple correction of mechanical obstruction to the vena

cava by change of posture, as in the supine hypotensive syndrome, or rapid filling of the capacitance in the presence of hypovolemia.

2. Suppress bradycardia by parasympathetic blockade with atropine (1.0 to 2.0 mg).

3. Diminish the capacitance and increase inotropic drive with an appropriate vasopressor.

Humoral Effects from Absorption of Epidural Drugs

The pharmacological effects of absorbed local anesthetics have been discussed in Chapter 3. The literature on the effects of local anesthetics on the cardiovascular system is confusing, because a large number of variables are involved, and controlled studies are difficult in the human. For example, the effects of lidocaine in normal volunteers may be quite different from the effects on a circulation compromised by hypovolemia or by sympathetic blockade.

Epidural injections of lidocaine in the range of 5 to 10 mg/kg give rise to peak plasma concentrations of 4 to 8 μg/ml (Bromage and Robson, 1961; Scott et al., 1972). Blood lidocaine levels of this order do not cause evidence of cardiovascular depression in normal conscious adults (Jordfeldt et al., 1968). However, ventricular contractility may be depressed by this level of lidocaine if the patient is asleep under general anesthesia, or if sympathetic blockade or hypovolemia or acidosis is present at the same time (Scott et al., 1971; Bonica et al., 1972). This question will be considered in more detail when the influence of hypovolemia is discussed.

Influence of Epinephrine on Cardiovascular Effects of Epidural Blockade

A great deal of discussion has centered on the cardiovascular effects of epinephrine in epidural solutions. Bonica's group in Seattle has studied the subject extensively and has come to the conclusion that cardiovascular differences observed between plain and epinephrine-containing solutions are due to the beta-stimulating effects of epinephrine absorbed from the extradural space (Ward et al., 1965; Bonica et al., 1971, 1972). However, there is an additional neural explanation that has been overlooked.

In epidural analgesia we are accustomed to thinking of sympathetic and somatic blockade as two distinct events occurring at different concentrations, with sympathetic blockade being complete using weak dilutions below the concentration necessary to affect sensory and motor fibers. This belief in the qualities of differential blockade is implicit in the practice of using diagnostic and therapeutic blocks with dilute solutions of local anesthetics. However, there is evidence that this view is not strictly correct (Cousins and Wright, 1971) and that instead there is a continuous development of blockade of fiber populations in all modalities, and that although sympathetic and sensory fibers are more susceptible than motor nerves, their available populations are seldom *completely* blocked at the concentrations normally used in clinical epidural analgesia for surgery. Indeed, it is readily apparent that, as far as sensory and motor blockade are concerned, epidural analgesia causes considerably less blockade than subarachnoid analgesia. The intensity of epidural analgesia increases with concentration and with the addition of epinephrine.

Objective measurements of flow and skin temperature in limbs show that sympathetic blockade also becomes functionally more complete with increasing concentrations of epidural anesthetic. Cousins and Wright (1971) found that 1 per cent lidocaine caused less vasodilatation in the leg than 2 per cent lidocaine, suggesting that a significant proportion of those vasoconstrictor fibers escaping blockade at the lower concentration did not escape blockade when the concentration was doubled. A comparable intensification of local anesthetic effect can be achieved without changing the concentration if epinephrine 1/200,000 is added to the plain solution. It is hard to quantitate this augmented effect precisely, but in the case of lidocaine the motor blocking potential of the 1 per cent solution with epinephrine is slightly superior to that of the 2 per cent plain solution (Bromage et al., 1964), and the 2 per cent concentration with epinephrine is markedly superior to the plain solution (see page 145, Figure 4–18, for a summary of these differences).

Thus, it is reasonable to assume that the intensity of sympathetic denervation following epinephrine-containing epidurals is likely to be appreciably greater than after administration of plain solutions, and this difference is likely to be apparent in terms of the amount of cardiovascular disturbance arising from the blockade.

Discussions of the cardiovascular effects of peridural epinephrine have centered on the beta-stimulating effects of absorbed catecholamines and have overlooked the fact that plain and epinephrine-containing solutions operate on different scales of effectiveness. Bonica and his colleagues, in a series of beautifully detailed experiments, found that epinephrine-containing epidurals gave rise to more peripheral vasodilatation than the sum of plain lidocaine blocks and peridural epinephrine administered separately. However, they did not offer a satisfactory explanation for this difference (Bonica et al., 1970, 1971). The data in their series of papers are immensely valuable, and it is worthwhile reviewing some of the facts, to interpret them anew in the light of a possible complementary neural component in addition to the exclusively humoral explanation offered by the authors. These studies by Bonica's group revealed the following important facts:

1. High peridural blockade accompanied by cutaneous analgesia in all segments below T_1 failed to produce evidence of sympathetic blockade in two out of ten subjects *when plain lidocaine was used* (Bonica et al., 1970).

The authors speculated that this observation might be due to a possible inotropic effect of absorbed lidocaine arising from large epidural dosage and subsequent blood concentrations of lidocaine in the range of 4 to 7 μg/ml. However, this explanation seems unlikely, particularly as the argument for the vasopressor effects of circulating lidocaine was reversed in a subsequent paper in which the same circulating levels of lidocaine were invoked to explain cardiovascular collapse occurring from a combination of epidural blockade and hypovolemia (Bonica et al., 1972). Indeed, the latter assessment of circulating lidocaine as a cardiovascular depressant seems more in accordance with general laboratory and clinical experience.

2. Peridural injection of plain lidocaine with blockade to T_5 caused

very slight cardiovascular changes, with only a 10 per cent fall of total peripheral resistance for approximately 60 minutes and a 10 per cent rise of heart rate for about 30 minutes. Heart rate and cardiac output were not significantly altered.

The authors attribute the absence of cardiovascular changes with plain lidocaine to the absence of a beta-stimulating drug, not to any possible inadequacy of neural blockade.

3. Peridural injections of epinephrine 1/200,000 alone (in saline without any local anesthetic) caused cardiovascular changes that were dose-dependent. With 100 μg of epinephrine, that is, the amount of epinephrine in 20 ml of a 1/200,000 solution, a 20 per cent fall of total peripheral resistance and a similar rise of cardiac output lasted about 55 minutes. Pulse rate rose about 10 per cent for approximately 30 minutes, but there were no changes of mean arterial blood pressure or of leg blood flow.

It should be noted that these cardiovascular effects of epinephrine alone were quite transient, although longer lasting than had been formerly supposed by Bromage (1967a).

4. Peridural blockade with epinephrine-containing lidocaine produced large falls of peripheral resistance, accompanied by an equivalent rise of cardiac output, in the range of 30 to 50 per cent that persisted for more than two hours, together with a fall of diastolic pressure and mean arterial pressure and a 175 per cent increase in leg blood flow for the same period of time. A 15 per cent increase in pulse rate lasted about 30 minutes.

The different cardiovascular performances of the plain lidocaine and epinephrine-containing lidocaine epidural solutions were attributed exclusively by these authors to the beta-stimulating effects of absorbed epinephrine. It should be noted that their data with peridural epinephrine alone in item 3 show a less intense effect and a much shorter time course than their data with lidocaine-epinephrine epidurals in item 4. It appears most unlikely that the latter is due to the former, as can be seen from a summary of some of their data in Figure 10–6. The beta-stimulating effects of epinephrine are relatively short-lived, compared to the much more prolonged cardiovascular consequences of a peridural block with lidocaine plus epinephrine.

The sum of evidence seems to favor a neural explanation for these findings, and the following mechanism is suggested. With plain lidocaine, blockade is short-lived and incomplete, and a significant proportion of sympathetic fibers escape with the capability of compensating for their blocked companions by carrying a heavier traffic of activity than in their resting state. On the other hand, with lidocaine plus epinephrine, penetration is more complete and a larger number of fibers are affected, approaching the profound autonomic and cardiovascular changes seen with subarachnoid block (Bonica et al., 1966). Careful hemodynamic studies under general anesthesia by Scott and his colleagues (1977) confirm the impression that epinephrine-containing epidural solutions cause more profound sympathetic blockade than plain analgesic solutions. These investigators found that total peripheral resistance fell significantly further when epinephrine 1/200,000 was added to the epidural anesthetic solution than when plain lidocaine was used.

The practical corollary of this is clear and is borne out by clinical experience. Blockade with plain solutions is likely to avoid heavy involvement

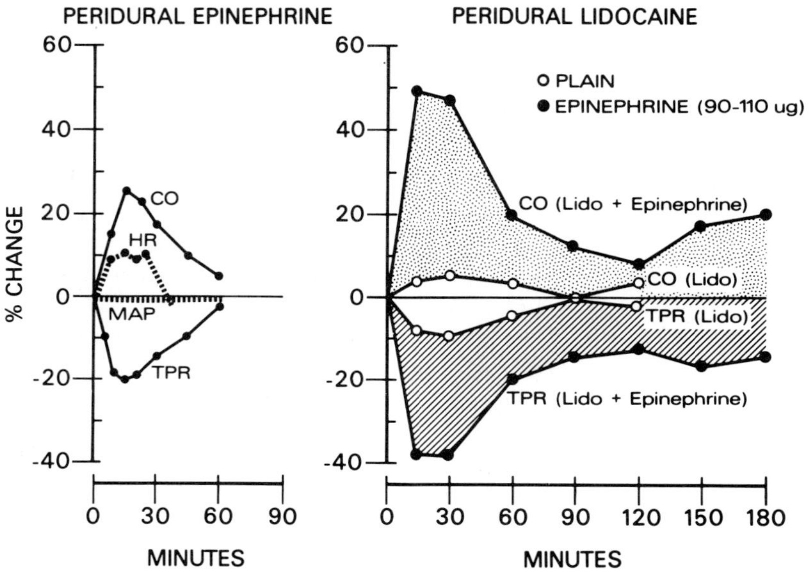

Figure 10–6. Circulatory effects of epidural blockade in human volunteers, summarized from data by Bonica and colleagues (1971). *Left,* Circulatory changes resulting from peridural injection of 20 ml 1/200,000 epinephrine in saline (100 μg epinephrine). *Right,* Circulatory changes resulting from peridural injection of 18 to 22 ml of 2 per cent lidocaine, with and without epinephrine 5 μg/ml. Segmental analgesia to T_5.

CO = Cardiac output; HR = heart rate; MAP = mean arterial pressure; TPR = total peripheral resistance.

Note short time course of cardiovascular changes following administration of epidural epinephrine in saline and long time course of changes following neural blockade with lidocaine and epinephrine (see text). (After Bonica et al., 1971.)

of sympathetic nerves, and the cardiovascular consequences will be relatively slight (Ueland et al., 1972); by the same token, however, the intensity of somatic sensory blockade will also be slight, and analgesia is likely to be marginal, patchy and unsatisfactory. On the other hand, epinephrine-containing analgesic solutions will provide more satisfactory clinical analgesia, but with the inescapable accompaniment of more intense sympathetic blockade and a cardiovascular outcome more nearly approaching that of subarachnoid blockade. Beta-stimulating effects from absorbed epinephrine may cause additional peripheral vasodilatation and provide transient inotropic support for 30 to 60 minutes, but after that time the influence of absorbed epinephrine will have passed, and all autonomic effects will be the result of sympathetic denervation accompanying the epidural blockade.

Having dealt with the individual humoral and neural influences of epidural analgesia on cardiovascular function, we are now in a position to put them together and see what actually happens in the component parts of the cardiovascular system during high and low segmental blockade. Three carefully planned studies have been done in man in an attempt to synthesize an intelligible picture of the cardiovascular effects of epidural analgesia, and to assess the respective sympathetic influence of peripheral vasodilatation and central cardiac drive.

The first of these investigations was carried out at McGill by Otton and his colleagues (Otton and Wilson, 1966; McLean et al., 1967), and it was specifically designed to answer the questions, what are the respective roles of the peripheral and central components of the sympathetic outflow in maintaining a normal cardiovascular status, and what happens if the upper thoracic segments containing the cardiac sympathetics are interrupted while the rest of the sympathetic system is spared? This study was crisply free of many unwanted variables. The subjects were unpremedicated, fit patients in ASA category one, undergoing upper abdominal surgery.

Minimal doses of weak local anesthetic were used in order to avoid significant vascular uptake, and epidural catheters were placed at C_7–T_1 and L_3–L_4 so that blockade of the upper thoracic segments could be aimed with great precision and assessed separately before the remainder of the sympathetic outflow was blocked through the lower catheter (Fig. 10–7). Tachyphylaxis and its attenuating effects on neural blockade were avoided by confining all observations to the results of a single injection through each catheter in turn.

The second study was from Seattle, as part of a major investigation into the cardiovascular effects of epidural analgesia on several body systems (Bonica et al., 1970). Here, the experimental set-up was similar to Otton's but different in several important aspects. The subjects were large, very fit volunteers from a neighboring prison population. Two epidural catheters were inserted as in Otton's study, but instead of starting blockade in the upper thoracic region and then proceeding to the lower catheter, the sequence was reversed, and incremental doses of 2 per cent plain lidocaine were injected through the lumbar catheter to raise segmental blockade in a stepwise fashion to the level of T_3–T_4, and then finally the upper catheter was used to establish

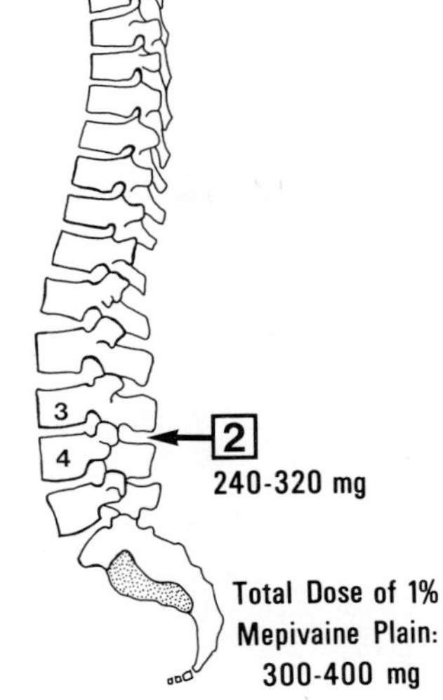

Figure 10–7. Experimental set-up in Otton's series. (1) Epidural catheter at C_7–T_1; initial dose of 1 mg/kg of 1 per cent plain mepivacaine. (2) Epidural catheter at L_3–L_4 used to establish total sympathetic blockade with a subsequent dose of 4 mg/kg of 1 per cent plain mepivacaine.

blockade in the remaining upper thoracic segments (Fig. 10–8). This sequence required large doses of lidocaine up to total amounts of 880 to 1,860 mg (mean = 1,586 mg), causing peak blood levels of lidocaine in the range of 4.0 to 6.65 μg/ml. Moreover, tachyphylaxis developed in response to the repeated injections, in some cases shortening the duration of the final block to less than 20 minutes, thus complicating the collection and interpretation of data.

The third study came from Uppsala and was a simple comparison of the effects of mid-thoracic and lumbar epidurals in two separate groups, using modest amounts of 2 per cent plain lidocaine, as shown in Figure 10–9 (Sjögren and Wright, 1972).

The results of these studies are summarized in Table 10–2. Starting with the simplest study it can be seen that Sjögren and Wright found very little alteration of cardiovascular function with either the thoracic or the lumbar blocks. The only significant changes were a 12 per cent fall of mean arterial pressure with the thoracic blocks and a 13 per cent fall of total peripheral resistance with the lumbar blocks. In the thoracic blocks the skin temperature rose in the hand and fell slightly in the foot, reflecting some degree of compensatory vasoconstriction in the lower limb when vasodilatation occurred in the upper limb. In the lumbar blocks the reverse occurred, and skin temperature and blood flow rose in the foot and fell in the hand, indicating compensatory vasoconstriction in the unblocked upper limbs.

Bonica's group found very little change in the various cardiovascular components as blockade was gradually extended upward to the third thoracic segment. Compensatory vasoconstriction occurred in the upper limb, counter-

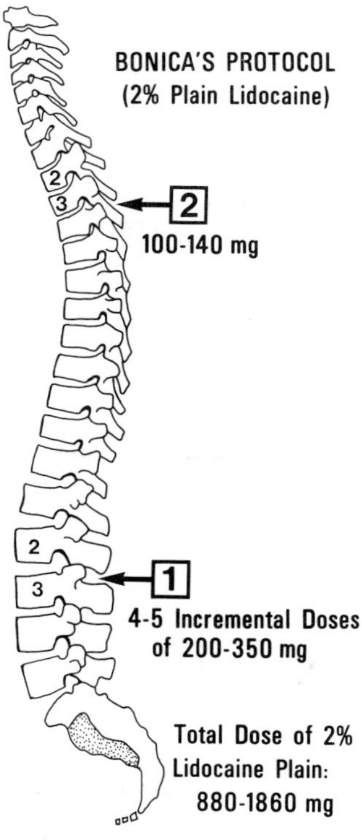

Figure 10–8. Experimental set-up in Bonica's series. (1) Lumbar epidural catheter with tip at L_2. Initial dose of 10 ml of 2 per cent plain lidocaine, followed by three to five progressively larger increments. (2) Thoracic epidural catheter with tip at level of T_2; final dose of 100 to 140 mg of 2 per cent plain lidocaine injected through the catheter to extend blockade above the first thoracic segment.

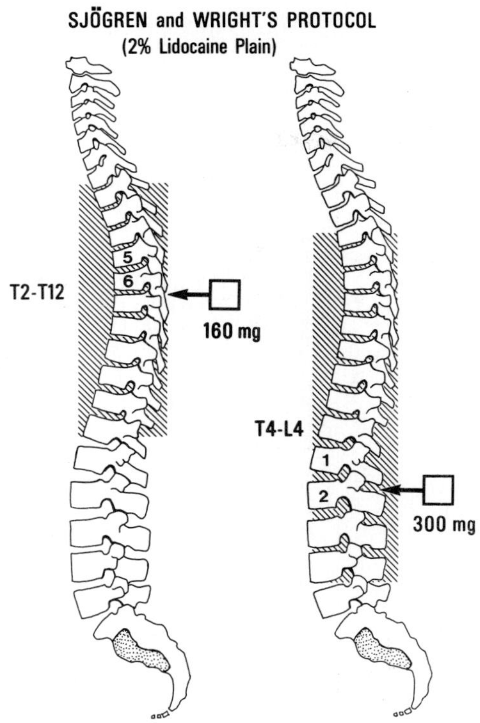

Figure 10–9. Experimental set-up in Sjögren and Wright's series. Patients with thoracic epidurals at T_5–T_6 received 8 ml of 2 per cent plain lidocaine, and blockade extended from T_2 (sometimes T_1) to T_{12}. Patients with lumbar epidurals at the second lumbar interspace received 15 ml of 2 per cent plain lidocaine, and blockade extended from about T_4–L_4.

balancing the vasodilatation in the lower limb, and heart rate increased by 21 per cent. Total peripheral resistance and cardiac output remained virtually unchanged. However, when the ascending segmental blockade reached T_1, the compensatory mechanisms that had maintained the cardiovascular status almost unchanged suddenly lost their control. Compensatory vasoconstriction in the upper limb failed, and upper limb blood flow increased while the resulting redistribution of blood caused a relative fall of blood flow in the legs. At the same time, cardiac sympathetic activity that had been increasing in a compensatory manner suddenly showed signs of failing. Heart rate showed a *relative* fall of 15 per cent, accompanied by a marked relative fall of dp/dt_{max}, and central venous pressure rose by 13 per cent. In discussing their data, the authors did not interpret these findings as signs of impending peripheral and central decompensation but stated that the circulation was well maintained. If one looks carefully at the extracted data in Table 10–2, it can be seen that the evidence of a sudden *relative* decompensation was unmistakable once blockade had reached the crucial upper thoracic segments, and the sympathetic defenses of peripheral vasoconstriction and chronotropic and ionotropic cardiac drive had fallen owing to the advancing neural blockade. The actual magnitude of these changes is not great, but it should be recalled that the quality of neural blockade with 2 per cent plain lidocaine is also relatively incomplete, and in these cases local anesthetic potency was further attenuated by tachyphylaxis arising from repeated incremental injections, so that by the time the final dose was given, its effects were slight and very transient and likely to have left a fair proportion of sympathetic fibers untouched.

TABLE 10–2 Influence of Segmental Level of Epidural Blockade on Cardiovascular Function (Data from Three Studies at McGill, University of Washington, Seattle, and Uppsala)

			Percentage Change From Preblock Control								
Investigators	*Extent of Segmental Block*	*Local Anesthetic Dose*	CARDIAC INDEX OR OUTPUT	HEART RATE	CVP	STROKE VOLUME	MEAN ARTERIAL BLOOD PRESSURE	TPR	dp/dt_{max}	ARM BLOOD FLOW	LEG BLOOD FLOW
McGill											
Otton and Wilson (1966)	C_5–T_4	60–80 mg Mep	−16.5	−16.5	+45	–	− 7.5	+ 7.7			
McLean et al. (1967)	C_5–T_4	60–80 mg Mep	−16.2	− 9.6	+41	− 6.6	− 9.2	+ 5.9			
	C_5–S_5	240–320 mg Mep increment	−18.9	− 8.2	−26.5	−13.2	−19.6	− 5.8			
Net increase	T_5–S_5		− 2.7	+ 1.4	−67.5	− 6.6	−10.4	−11.7			
Seattle											
Bonica et al. (1970)	T_3–S_5	780–1720 mg Lid	+20.5	+21.5	+13	+ 0.6	+ 5.2	−17.3	+23.2	−51 (at T_4–T_5)	+287
	C_8–S_5	100–140 mg Lid increment	+ 1.6	+ 6	+26	− 3.0	−16.7	−20.8	−11.6	+ 90.5	+177
Net increase	T_3–C_8		−18.9	−15.5	+13	− 3.6	−21.9	− 3.5	−34.8	+141.5	−110
Uppsala											
Sjögren and Wright (1972)	T_2–T_{12}	160 mg Lid	− 1	− 7	− 3	+10	−12	− 3	–	+ 46.5	+ 21.4
	T_4–L_4	300 mg Lid	+ 7	+ 3	+ 6	+ 6	− 9	−13	–	− 34.5	+510

Mep = mepivacaine
Lid = lidocaine
CVP = central venous pressure (cmH_2O)
TPR = total peripheral resistance (dynes/sec/cm^{-5})
dp/dt_{max} = maximum ventricular pressure rise

The original studies of Otton's group were designed to give the most precise analysis of epidural blockade on cardiac sympathetic action, uncomplicated by tachyphylaxis or by high levels of circulating local anesthetic. By restricting one small injection of local anesthetic to the upper four or five thoracic segments, the effects were limited to cardiac sympathectomy plus vasodilatation in the head, arms and upper thorax. Table 10–2 shows that the results were due almost entirely to direct cardiac depression reflected by a 16 per cent fall of cardiac index and heart rate and a rise of central venous pressure as the myocardium settled down to a lower level of cardiac function (Guyton, 1963). Expansion of segmental blockade to include the entire sympathetic outflow produced the expected signs arising from peripheral vasodilatation, with an increase of capacitance and a fall of peripheral resistance and central venous pressure, together with a further slight fall of cardiac output and an appreciable (20 per cent) fall of mean arterial pressure.

Plain solutions of local anesthetics were used in all three of these investigations, and while absence of epinephrine ensured freedom from beta-adrenergic stimulating effects, it also condemned the studies to somewhat inconclusive results, since the quality of neural blockade was probably insufficient to ensure interruption of all sympathetic fibers within the segmental distribution of cutaneous hypalgesia. The experimental difficulties and limitations in experiments of this nature have been emphasized by Shimosato and Etsten (1969), for as well as all the other variables, speed of onset of blockade appears to be an additional factor influencing compensatory recruitment. These workers found that slow onset of blockade was characterized by relatively effective vasoconstriction in unblocked segments, whereas with fast onset compensatory vasoconstriction was less effectively mobilized above the upper level of blockade (Shimosato and Etsten, 1969).

Hypovolemia and Sympathetic Blockade

The cardiovascular effects of sympathetic blockade become more obvious when venous return is restricted by loss of effective blood volume from hemorrhage or postural pooling in regions of vasodilatation. Then, filling pressure to the heart falls off, and as mentioned earlier in the section, a point is reached when parasympathetic tone suddenly increases to produce bradycardia and inhibition of vasoconstriction, with a resulting precipitous fall of cardiac output. This phenomenon was well analyzed by Sharpey-Schafer and his group 25 years ago, and it is the mechanism underlying the common faint (Brigden et al., 1950; Pugh and Wyndham, 1950). This sudden burst of parasympathetic activity is only seen in conscious man, and it is prevented by general anesthesia; it is not known to occur in species other than man (Sharpey-Schafer, 1956). Some degree of bradycardia frequently occurs with high epidural blocks under general anesthesia, but it is usually slower to develop and less dramatic in its consequences.

The depressant effects of circulating local anesthetic are likely to be exaggerated in hypovolemic states for several reasons. First, the effective distribution volume is diminished (see Chapter 3), so the drug will be relatively more concentrated. Second, compensated increased cardiac activity and raised coronary flow will divert a disproportionately large amount of circulating drug to the heart. Third, metabolic acidosis may arise from peripheral low blood flow, and this will increase the amount of effective ionized local anesthetic in the myocardium.

A series of four important papers by Bonica's group sought to differentiate the effects of epidural blockade to T_5 in normovolemic and in hypovolemic states. The first two of these papers (Bonica et al., 1970, 1971) dealt with the effects of varying heights of segmental blockade and the influence of added epinephrine on the cardiovascular system, and some of the results have been referred to already in the section on the effects of absorbed epinephrine. The third paper described the results of an arduous investigation into the cardiovascular changes in conscious volunteers, each subject acting as his own control under normal conditions and then being bled of 13 per cent of his blood volume (Bonica et al., 1972). In this study the catastrophic effects of parasympathetic overaction described by Sharpey-Schafer were well demonstrated, and some of the cardiovascular measurements were incomplete because of dangerous hypotension occurring in hypovolemic subjects who had received plain lidocaine. In this investigation the cardiovascular system remained acceptably stable when epinephrine 1/200,000 was added to the epidural anesthetic solution, presumably owing to the inotropic effects of the absorbed epinephrine. The fourth paper (Morikawa et al., 1974) concerned a similar study in anesthetized dogs in which parasympathetic reaction and sudden profound hypotension could not occur because of species difference and the presence of general anesthesia.

Some of the parameters measured in these papers are shown in Figure 10–10. The marked inotropic effect of epinephrine 1/200,000 is apparent in the studies on conscious volunteers before and after bleeding, and the lack of inotropic drive is obvious in the profound cardiovascular collapse that occurred after epidural blockade with plain lidocaine when subjects were hypovolemic.

These studies emphasize the care that must be used if high epidural analgesia is induced in the presence of hypovolemia, and they point out the advantage of using a solution with epinephrine 1/200,000 added to it. However, it would be unwise to assume that this amount of epinephrine can always be relied upon to counteract the cardiovascular depressant effects of high epidural blockade.

Control of Blood Pressure in Total Epidural Blockade

Some consideration must be given to the practical question of blood pressure control in total epidural blockade, for there are clinical situations in which a normal blood pressure and cardiac output should be preserved during high epidural analgesia. Technically, ideal vasopressor therapy would restore the cardiovascular system to exactly the same state that it was in before epidural blockade took effect. Clinically, this is impossible, and indeed probably undesirable. There are often advantages in the redistribution of blood flow that accompanies blockade, for the effects of pain or disease may have led to an inappropriate maldistribution of flow which the block may correct. All that

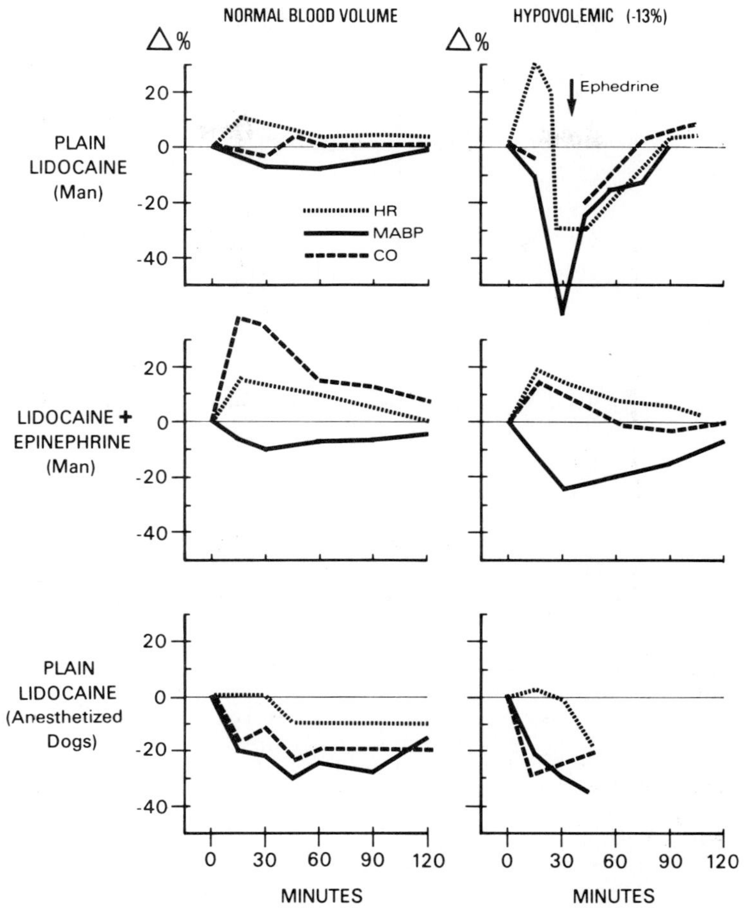

Figure 10–10. Effects of epidural blockade to T_5 in conscious man after administration of 2 per cent lidocaine with and without 1/200,000 epinephrine in normovolemia and after hemorrhagic loss of 13 per cent blood volume. Blockade without epinephrine in hypovolemic subjects led to collapse requiring vasopressor treatment in five out of seven cases. Note that dogs under general anesthesia did not show a similar pattern of parasympathetic discharge. (Data from Bonica et al., 1970, 1971; Morikawa et al., 1974.)

systemic vasopressor therapy need accomplish is a gross restoration of cardiac output and blood pressure to levels that are physiologically acceptable, so that all vital organs receive their sufficient share. To do this, a proper balance of alpha and beta adrenergic effects is required, and the secret lies in finding the right proportion of the two effects. At one time it appeared that simple replacement of norepinephrine by very dilute infusion would be a logical way to counteract diminished adrenergic activity in total spinal blockade (Bromage, 1960, 1967a). The normal catecholamine output in man has been calculated as approximately 0.05 μg/kg/minute (or 3 to 4 μg/min in a 70-kg man); of this, four-fifths is norepinephrine (Cohen et al., 1959), so replacement dosage of this order should be required to restore overall vascular tone in the presence of total sympathetic blockade.

However, studies by McLean and his colleagues (1967), using Otton's

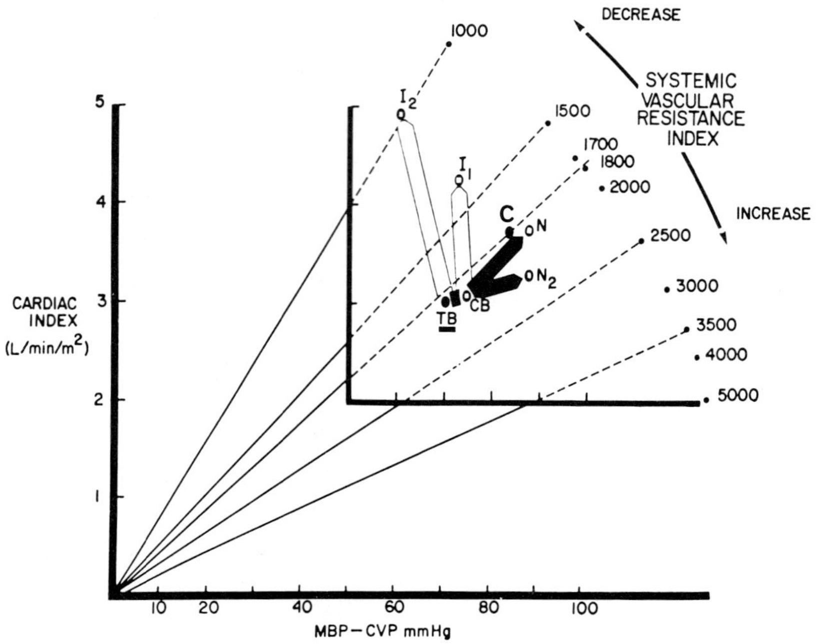

Figure 10–11. Graph shows the systemic vascular resistance index as a function of cardiac index plotted against the driving pressure (mean blood pressure minus central venous pressure). The lines from zero are resistance isopleths (each line is of constant resistance as the cardiac index and the driving pressure change).

C = Control; CB = upper thoracic epidural; TB = total epidural; I_1 = upper thoracic epidural with isoproterenol; I_2 = total epidural with isoproterenol; N = upper thoracic epidural with norepinephrine; N_2 = total epidural with norepinephrine.

With upper epidural block there is a fall in blood pressure and cardiac index, with a slight increase in systemic resistance. The addition of total epidural decreases the systemic resistance in a direction toward control but produces a further fall in cardiac index and blood pressure. Isoproterenol with either block enhances cardiac performance and diminishes systemic resistance. Norepinephrine in either block enhances cardiac performance mainly through increasing systemic resistance. (From McLean et al.: Surgery *62*:79, 1967.)

protocol, on subjects with upper thoracic and total epidural blockade showed that norepinephrine alone does not restore overall cardiovascular dynamics to the precise control point that existed before blockade. The predominant effect is vasoconstrictive, lacking the vasodilator beta adrenergic influence of epinephrine that is seen in a normal physiological adrenergic response.

The results shown in Figures 10–11 and 10–12 were obtained from Otton's protocol outlined in Figure 10–7, using two epidural catheters with a discrete upper thoracic block, followed later by total epidural blockade.

It can be seen that norepinephrine restores cardiovascular status with a bias toward a net vasoconstrictive situation, whereas isoproterenol, an almost pure beta adrenergic stimulator, produces a much wider bias in the opposite direction of increased cardiac performance combined with reduced peripheral resistance. The ideal vasoconstrictor therefore lies somewhere between the two, closer to the balance of alpha and beta effects found in the natural mixture of epinephrine and norepinephrine output in a normal

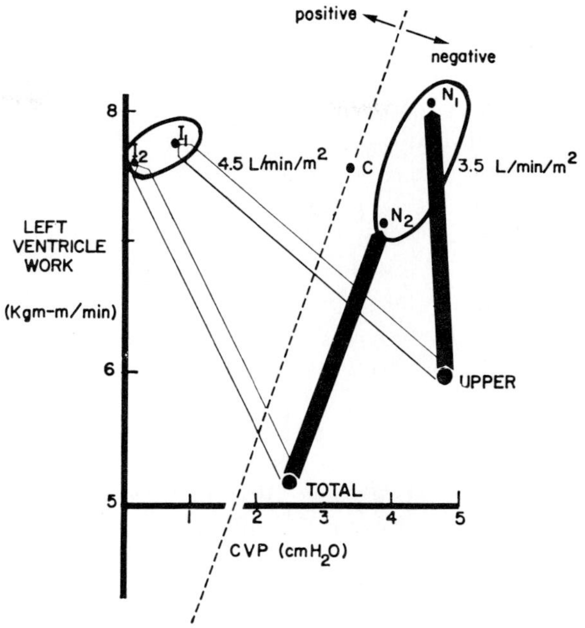

Figure 10–12. Graph of left ventricular work plotted against central venous pressure demonstrates the external energy expended in upper and total epidural analgesia and the effects of the vasopressors isoproterenol and norepinephrine at each level.

C = control; Upper = upper thoracic block; Total = upper plus lumbar thoracic block; I_1 = isoproterenol plus upper thoracic block; N_1 = norepinephrine plus upper thoracic block; N_2 = norepinephrine plus total thoracic block.

The approximate cardiac index produced with each drug is entered beside each drug zone of energy expenditure. All effects to the left of the line from control to zero represent a positive inotropic response and to the right a negative inotropic response. Isoproterenol produces a higher flow than norepinephrine with equivalent expenditure of energy.

Work = CO × BP. LVW = CO × MABP × 0.0144 (kg/m/min).

(From McLean et al.: Surgery *62*:79, 1967.)

adrenergic response of the intact organism. Substitution therapy with synthetic vasopressors can be satisfactory, provided the chosen drug closely mimics the mixed alpha and beta adrenergic effects of the natural epinephrine-norepinephrine response. For example, methamphetamine (Methedrine) or ephedrine is appropriate provided catecholamine stores in blood vessel walls have not been depleted by a drug such as reserpine (Burn and Rand, 1959). On the other hand, methoxamine (Vasoxyl), being a pure alpha stimulator with overriding vasoconstrictor effects, is an inappropriate choice, since it produces peripheral vasoconstriction and increases afterload and cardiac work without any direct improvement of cardiac contractility.

Cardiac Sympathectomy and Ventricular Irritability

Sympatholysis by drugs or denervation makes the myocardium less prone to fibrillation during deep hypothermia (Schumacker et al., 1956). Galindo and Sprouse (1964) showed that total epidural blockade with 5 mg/kg of 1 per cent lidocaine reduced the incidence of fibrillation in dogs cooled below 24° C. Part of this antiarrhythmic effect may be due to vascular absorption from the epidural space producing therapeutic levels of local anesthetic in the blood stream. However, with the dosage used, vascular uptake is not likely to have caused peripheral blood concentrations of lidocaine in excess of 2 μg/ml (Burfoot and Bromage, 1971). Peripheral vasodilation accompanying total spinal blockade facilitates peripheral heat exchange (Bromage, 1954), so the technique of high epidural block can be usefully applied to induce hypothermia by surface cooling (Stolar and Wynands, 1963).

Compression of Great Vessels Within the Abdomen

The inferior vena cava and aorta are vulnerable to compression within their long course through the abdomen. The commonest cause of obstruction is pressure from a heavy uterus in pregnant women at term (Runge, 1924; Burwell et al., 1938; McLennan, 1943). Other causes include certain unfavorable postures (Bull, 1949; Brigden et al., 1950) and pressure due to intestinal obstruction (Bellis and Wangensteen, 1939) or ascites (Ranniger and Switz, 1965; Doppman et al., 1966; Rubinson et al., 1967). During caval obstruction the vertebral plexus and azygos system provide an alternative route for venous return, and the epidural veins become distended and turgid, encroaching on the epidural space (Bromage, 1961; Kerr et al., 1964; Hipona et al., 1966). Compensatory vasomotor adjustments take place, especially in the legs and pelvis, and increased vasomotor tone maintains a raised pressure to free venous return through the collateral vertebral and paravertebral pathways. The degree of compensation may range all the way from complete adjustment to total inadequacy and death. Loss of vasomotor tone in the legs due to epidural blockade or any other vasodilatory influence may upset the finely balanced compensation, and a normally insignificant degree of vasodilatation may be enough to tip the scales and precipitate profound cardiovascular collapse. To prevent collapse either caval occlusion must be relieved or venous tone must be maintained in the legs by use of a suitable vasopressor drug.

Figure 10–13 shows the caval venous system and its collateral pathway in diagrammatic form, with the common sites of caval obstruction that may be involved. The following causes of obstruction may be commonly encountered.

Intestinal obstruction

Unrelieved intestinal obstruction distends the abdomen and compresses the inferior vena cava just below the diaphragm. Bellis and Wangensteen (1939) showed that experimental distension of the gut impedes venous return from the pelvis, causing a rise of venous pressure in the legs. Abdominal decompression relieves the venous obstruction and restores flow. Clearly, it would be unwise to use any anesthetic technique that caused significant vasodilatation of the lower limbs in the face of severe peritoneal distension. Intra-abdominal pressure should first be relieved by intestinal drainage; if that is impossible,

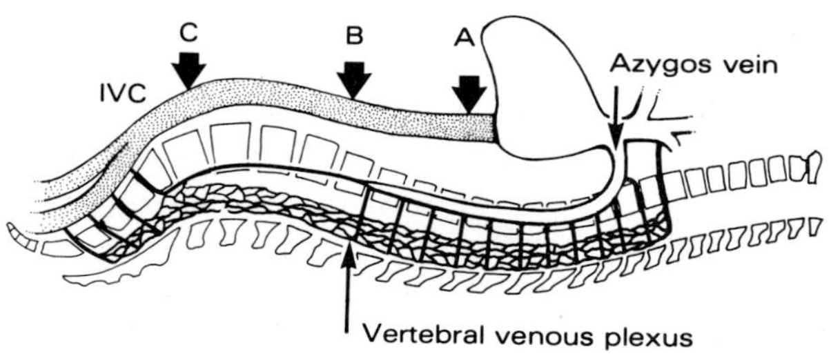

Figure 10–13. Diagram of the caval venous system and its connections with the vertebral and azygos systems. Commonest sites of compression of the IVC are: (A) suprahepatic, in lordotic position or ascites (Bull, 1949; Ranniger and Switz, 1965); (B) uterus at term (Bieniarz et al., 1968); (C) pressure at pelvic brim in exaggerated lordosis and term pregnancy.

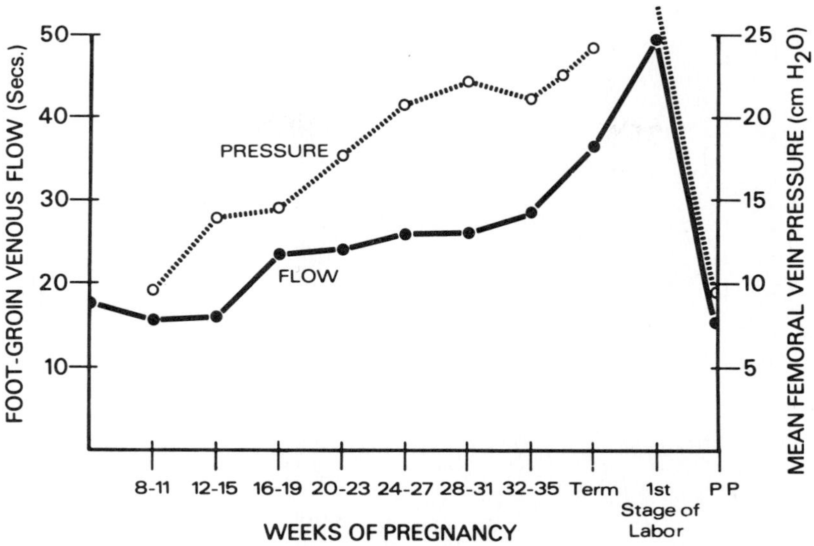

Figure 10–14. Compression of the inferior vena cava in the supine position during pregnancy. Femoral vein pressure and flow. (Data from McLennan, 1943, and Payling Wright et al., 1950.)

vasopressor therapy may be necessary to maintain adequate venous return in the face of continuing caval obstruction.

Intra-abdominal tumors and pregnancy

Pregnancy is the commonest cause of a large intra-abdominal mass, and the obstructing effects of the uterus on the inferior vena cava have been studied since 1924 when Runge made measurements of femoral and arm vein pressures during pregnancy. Other authors have confirmed that an elevation of femoral venous pressure is encountered in the supine position (Burwell et al., 1939; Hansen, 1942; McLennan, 1943). Payling Wright and her colleagues (1950) found a corresponding decrease in lower limb blood flow using an isotope counting method. The results of McLennan's pressure measurements and Payling Wright's observations of flow are shown together in Figure 10–14. The marked increase of caval obstruction near term is clearly reflected by the peak of pressure and flow times as labor approaches, followed by an immediate fall to normal nonpregnant values once the uterus is emptied.

Compression of the inferior vena cava occurs in the supine position, and it is almost completely relieved by turning the pregnant patient on her side. About 30 per cent of women near term manage to achieve an *apparent* circulatory compensation for caval obstruction, with little or no change of blood pressure or heart rate in the supine position, but the majority show significant falls of pressure when supine, and a very small minority suffer complete collapse if forced to remain flat on their backs. Figure 10–15, drawn from data in Holmes' classic study of sudden maternal death during cesarean section under spinal anesthesia, shows the incidence of systolic blood pressure changes caused by adopting the supine position near term (Holmes, 1957).

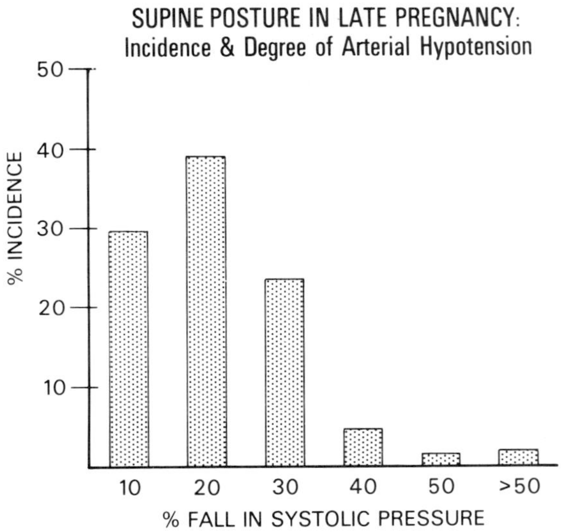

Figure 10–15. Blood pressure changes associated with the supine position in late pregnancy (between 38 weeks and term) in 500 patients. (Data from Holmes, 1957.)

Compensatory vasoconstriction can maintain a deceptively stable blood pressure in the face of quite large falls of cardiac output, and the true consequences of the dorsal posture are only revealed by direct measurement of cardiac output and peripheral resistance. Turning from the supine to the lateral position relieves caval compression, and the cardiac output rises about 20 per cent, while peripheral resistance falls by a comparable amount, with only slight changes of blood pressure and pulse in most cases (Ueland and Hansen, 1969a; Scott, 1973). Delivery in the supine position is also followed by a considerable rise in cardiac output as the uterus empties and weight is taken off the inferior vena cava (Lees et al., 1970). The earliest cardiac output studies of labor by Zimmerman (1950) showed very large increases of about 2.5 l/min after delivery under subarachnoid anesthesia, but more recent measurements in the supine position show a somewhat smaller rise in cardiac output of about 20 to 25 per cent, or about 1.5 l/min. Uterine contractions in the supine position give a paradoxical appearance of improved circulatory status, known as the Poseiro effect. The contracting uterus partially occludes the abdominal aorta, and cardiac output rises along with arterial pressure above the level of occlusion, while pressure falls in the lower half of the body (Bieniarz et al., 1968).

Figure 10–16 summarizes the various modifications of blood flow and pressure that accompany aortocaval compression arising from changes of posture and uterine contraction. In the supine position the combination of vascular obstruction and vasodilatation may result in a dangerous degree of hypotension. In the lateral position flow is unobstructed and venous return is safely maintained, even in the presence of extensive vasodilatation from either general anesthesia or spinal blockade.

Posture

For the sake of surgical access, patients are often subjected to unphysiological postures or to packing and retracting maneuvers that may place

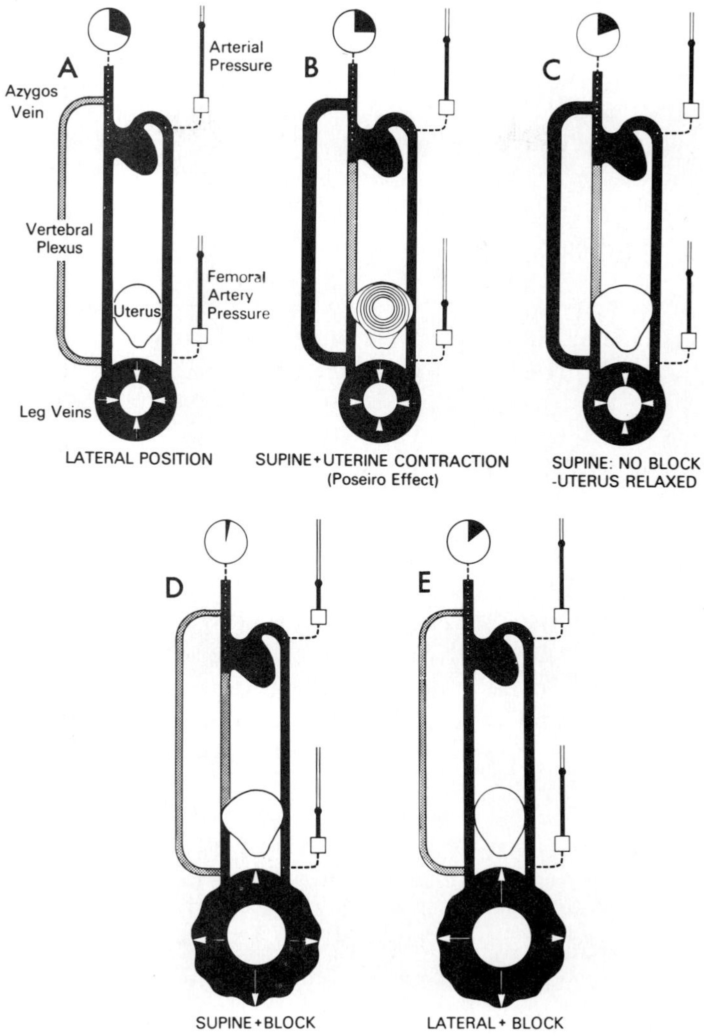

Figure 10–16. Aortocaval compression in labor. Diagram of effects on central venous pressure and arterial pressure in upper and lower limbs, and vertebral plexus flow.

A, Lateral position. Flow is unimpeded in aorta and inferior vena cava. Cardiac output, arterial pressure and CVP are all normal. Low flow through vertebral venous plexus.

B, Uterine contraction in the supine position. Aorta and IVC are both compressed. Reactive vascular tone in legs forces venous return through vertebral plexus. CVP falls slightly. Coarctation effect of aortic obstruction maintains arterial pressure in arms, but BP falls in legs (Poseiro effect).

C, Relaxed uterus in supine position. IVC severely compressed. Little or no aortic obstruction. CVP falls, but arterial pressure is maintained in upper and lower limbs. High flow through vertebral venous plexus.

D, Epidural block with loss of vasomotor tone in legs. In supine position IVC is compressed. CVP, cardiac output and arterial pressure all fall.

E, Epidural block and lateral position. Free flow in aorta and IVC. Slight reduction of CVP, but arterial pressure normal in upper and lower limbs. Low flow in vertebral venous plexus.

pressure on vessels and nerves. Extensive vascular obstruction arising from these causes usually gives immediate warning signs of hypotension and collapse that alert the anesthesiologist to correct the faulty posture. However, more subtle forms of obstruction in special circulations may cause few or no overt signs until the damage has been done. Normal sympathetic tone often maintains an adequate circulation in spite of severe obstruction to venous return, but in the presence of vasodilatation from high epidural blockade, venous pressure may be inadequate to force a passage back to the heart.

Examples of postures requiring special surveillance are the lateral jackknife position, the extended back from a raised gallbladder bridge and the hyperflexed lithotomy position (Young's position). These are all examples of postural stress that may partially, or sometimes completely, occlude major vessels and lead to a profound fall of cardiac output or cause compression of nerves with subsequent neurological deficits (Scott, 1963; Britt and Gordon, 1964; Courington and Little, 1968; Malatinsky and Kadlic, 1974).

The extended lordotic posture is a potent cause of high obstruction to the inferior vena cava in a proportion of patients (Brigden et al., 1950). In this situation the kidneys are exposed to a raised venous pressure, and proteinuria is commonly seen (Bull, 1949). As in ascites and intestinal obstruction, the primary site of venous obstruction lies in the collapsible subphrenic portion of the IVC (Ranniger and Switz, 1965; Doppman et al., 1966). A secondary site of venous obstruction may lie at the pelvic brim as the iliac vessels are stretched by the backward-tilting pelvis. This posture is likely to impair vascular exchange in the lower parts of the spinal cord, especially if combined with arterial hypotension, when the following hemodynamic handicaps are involved:

1. Low arterial inflow pressure
2. Impaired venous return from caval obstruction
3. Engorged extradural veins (collaterals) increasing pressure within the spinal canal

The possibility of spinal cord infarction or "spinal stroke" (Silver and Buxton, 1974) arising from the exaggerated lordotic posture will be discussed in Chapter 14.

As with all ischemic pathology, the injurious effects of bad posture on vessels and nerves are partly a function of time. A very fast and skilled surgeon may be able to trespass on dangerous ground with impunity if he can complete his task before vascular collapse or infarction occurs. A slow plodder, however, is likely to increase iatrogenic morbidity unless posture is faultless and blood flow adequate in all indispensable organs throughout the length of the operation.

Practical considerations

The interplay of major vascular obstruction and compensatory vasoconstriction imposes important constraints on the choice of priorities of management during induction of anesthesia in the presence of IVC obstruction. Three decisions are open; one is bad, one is good and the third is indifferent if expediency demands it.

1. The physician may decide to ignore the consequences of the prime anatomical obstruction and to rely on the body's compensatory devices to over-

come the circulatory embarrassment. For example, surgery may be pressed in the face of unrelieved intestinal obstruction inadequately prepared by decompression, or exploration of a large abdominal tumor may be attempted without a lateral tilt. In either case any vasodilatory influence, whether due to general anesthesia or epidural blockade, is likely to be followed by a severe fall of cardiac output and arterial blood pressure.

2. The physician may act logically and decide to correct the prime anatomical embarrassment as a preliminary step. Then, in the presence of a restored circulatory status, the choice of anesthetic technique and the speed of surgery become less crucial.

An interesting example of this is the introduction of the lateral tilt into obstetrical practice for cesarean section and vaginal delivery. Ignorance of the importance of caval compression had led to the belief that time was of the essence in cesarean section and in the second stage of labor, as indeed it was with the baby's gas exchange throttled by aortocaval compression. In both instances the baby's condition deteriorated steadily as time elapsed with the mother in the dorsal position (Lumley et al., 1970; Humphrey et al., 1973). However, with the pelvis tilted laterally by a wedge or sandbag placed under one hip, the uterus slides to one side away from direct pressure on the major vessels, and placental flow is restored. In this posture delay is no longer critical, and the fetus does not become increasingly acidotic and hypoxic with the passage of time (Crawford et al., 1972; Humphrey et al., 1974).

3. A third choice may be necessary if caval compression cannot be relieved. Then, expediency demands that vasoconstriction be maintained throughout the period of continued obstruction until the vascular embarrassment is relieved. Under these circumstances vasopressor therapy is indicated to maintain an adequate vis a tergo distal to the site of obstruction until the source of occlusion is removed. Then, sudden restoration of caval flow will be accompanied by an equally sudden increase of cardiac output and an abrupt surge of pressure within a constricted vascular bed. Hence, it is very important to use minimal amounts of vasopressor agents administered by carefully controlled intravenous drip, to avoid the disastrous possibilities of a cerebrovascular accident or pulmonary edema from persistent vasoconstriction and rebound hypertension (Scott and Kerr, 1963).

Effects of Epidural Block on Organ Blood Flow

Heart

The effects of acute hypotension on organ blood flow can be reduced to simple terms. Organ failure occurs when capillary flow no longer matches tissue requirements. However, the circulation of the heart is more subtle, for the heart is the one organ that is dependent on itself for its own blood supply. Myocardial blood flow and oxygen demands are determined by a complicated balance of forces that include not only preload, afterload and intramural pressure, but also the ratio of these forces during systole and diastole. It is during systole that work is performed, oxygen consumed and the necessary head of pressure generated to feed the coronary tree, but it is the diastolic phase that allows blood to flow to the myocardial cells. Normally, this balance operates over a very wide range, but in a damaged heart this balance between demand and supply is extremely fine, and hypertension may be just as dangerous as hypotension.

The normal myocardium tolerates induced falls of blood pressure to very low levels of 40 to 50 mmHg systolic without apparent ill effect. However, in the presence of coronary artery disease or ventricular hypertrophy, a systolic pressure of 75 to 85 mmHg may be associated with electrical signs of ischemia, such as ST segment depression or flattened or inverted T waves, especially in lead V_5 (Kaplan and King, 1976).

Hypertension exerts two unfavorable effects upon the heart. High peripheral vascular resistance imposes a heavy afterload and increases the oxygen needs of the myocardium. At the same time a raised intramural pressure during diastole impairs the inflow of coronary blood to the deeper layers of the muscle. With increasing hypertension a point is reached when the contractile demands of the myocardium exceed the available blood supply of diastole; then relative coronary vascular resistance increases (Mudge et al., 1976) and subendocardial ischemia results (Kirk and Honig, 1964). The concept of transmural variations in myocardial perfusion is discussed very thoroughly by Hoffman and Buckberg in Progress in Cardiology, 1976, Chapter III, and the interested reader will find this an excellent reference source. Buckberg and his associates have expressed the balance between systolic demands and diastolic supply in terms of the systolic pressure time index (SPTI) and the diastolic pressure time index (DPTI), measured from the systolic and diastolic areas under the arterial pressure tracing, as shown in Figure 10–17.

Wide ranges of supply and demand can be tolerated by normal hearts, and the DPTI/SPTI ratio can fall to quite low values without accompanying signs of subendocardial ischemia. The critical ischemic level is not

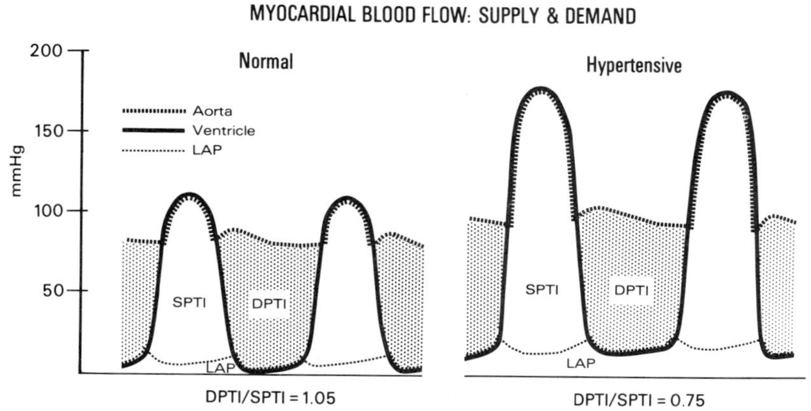

Figure 10–17. Theoretical supply/demand relationship of the subendocardial layer of the left ventricle derived from arterial pressure trace.

SPTI: Estimate of myocardial oxygen demand measured by area under systolic portion of the systemic arterial pressure tracing, from onset of systole to the closure of aortic valve at beginning of diastole (dicrotic notch).

DPTI: Estimate of myocardial supply measured by area between commencement of diastole (dicrotic notch) to onset of next systole minus the filling pressure from the left atrium (LAP).

precisely known in man, but a value of 0.5 has been suggested (Buckberg et al., 1972; Barnard et al., 1973). In abnormal hearts with coronary artery disease, the critical DPTI/SPTI ratio for ischemia is considerably higher at about 0.9 (Wisehart et al., 1974). A high blood pressure increases the SPTI, especially in the presence of tachycardia, and reduces the DPTI/SPTI ratio. Thus, hypertension in the operative and postoperative period may lead to severe degrees of subendocardial ischemia, and the anesthesiologist should strive to control the blood pressure within a safe range by appropriate manipulation of vascular tone, intravascular fluid volume and cardiac output.

The beneficial effects of vasodilator therapy to reduce peripheral vascular resistance have become increasingly recognized over the past 30 years, both in acute left ventricular failure (Sarnoff and Farr, 1944; Sarnoff and Berglund, 1952) and in chronic congestive failure (Davies et al., 1954; Miller et al., 1975, 1976). Reduction of afterload leads to a higher DPTI/SPTI ratio and a better balance of systolic demands and diastolic nourishment. Elevated left ventricular end diastolic pressure and pulmonary artery pressure fall toward normal levels and efficiency increases.

Many forms of vasodilator therapy have been employed to reduce abnormally elevated systemic and pulmonary arterial pressures, including high spinal or epidural analgesia, ganglion blocking drugs and alpha-receptor blockers, such as phentolamine. The latter has some direct cardiac stimulating action, and the claim that it has superior qualities of predominantly arteriolar rather than venodilator effects (Miller et al., 1976) should be regarded with caution. From among the available vasodilators, sodium nitroprusside has emerged as a popular choice after a long dormant period since its introduction in 1955 (Page et al., 1955). Nitroprusside infusions act rapidly and allow easy control of acute hypertensive crises. However, sodium nitroprusside has certain disadvantages that include resistance in young subjects, the danger of intracellular anoxia from cyanide, a relatively narrow therapeutic index and the absence of an effective antidote (McDowell et al., 1974). In addition, sodium nitroprusside is a powerful inhibitor of platelet aggregation in proportion to the dose given (Saxon and Kattlove, 1976), and interference with the clotting mechanism may be undesirable in the presence of hypertension after major vascular surgery.

Recently, interest has returned to epidural blockade as a useful therapeutic procedure in the management of acute hypertensive episodes, especially after major surgery on the trunk, when the advantages of blood pressure control are combined with effective analgesia free from respiratory depression. Hemodynamic measurements during reactive postoperative hypertension have shown that thoracic epidural blockade lowers peripheral resistance, central venous pressure and left atrial pressure, and improves the DPTI/SPTI ratio by more than 35 per cent (Hoar et al., 1976).

The practical application of epidural blockade in the treatment of reactive hypertension will be discussed in Chapter 12 on Surgical Applications and in Chapter 13 on Diagnostic and Therapeutic Applications.

Neuraxial circulation

Of all the tissues in the body the brain is least able to withstand anoxia. In recent years, the spinal cord has received increasing attention as a vulnerable target for anoxia, second only in importance to the brain, and the syndrome of "spinal stroke" has become more widely recognized as an infarctive process similar to cerebral stroke, with a common pathological background (Silver and Buxton, 1974).

Maintenance of adequate blood flow and gas exchange in the brain and spinal cord is of vital concern during anesthesia and afterward in the postoperative period. The factors that may lead to neuraxial hypoxia must be understood, so that clinical practice can be directed toward providing adequate tissue oxygenation at all times. The two major variables affecting tissue flow are blood pressure and the vascular resistance to that pressure (Betz, 1972).

Normal cerebral blood flow in man and primates is in the range of 42 to 60 ml/100 g/min, with a mean of 52 ml/100 g/min at a pCO_2 of 40 mmHg (Lassen, 1959; Reivich, 1964). Circulation time in the spinal cord is about twice as long as in the brain (Margolis et al., 1957); consequently, spinal cord blood flow is considerably lower in those animals in which it has been measured. In dogs, the normal flow for spinal white matter varies between 13.7 and 15.7 ml/100 g/min, depending on whether hydrogen or xenon clearance techniques are used (Griffiths, 1973a; Griffiths et al., 1975), and in goats the average flow in white and gray matter is slightly higher at 16.2 ml/100 g/min (Smith et al., 1969). Using the hydrogen clearance method, Kobrine et al. (1974) found even higher flows in the lateral white matter of monkeys, with a mean flow rate of 17.5 ± 0.35 ml/100 g/min at a pCO_2 of 30 to 35 mmHg. Blood flow throughout the various parts of the neuraxis is altered by three important variables: (1) arterial blood pressure, (2) venous pressure and (3) vascular resistance.

Arterial Blood Pressure. Normally, autoregulation maintains cerebral and cord blood flows at constant levels over a wide range of blood pressure, but if perfusion drops below a certain critical point, blood flow falls off sharply (Kobrine et al., 1976). Figure 10–18, constructed from data from several sources (Kety et al., 1950; McCall, 1953; Finnerty et al., 1954; Lassen, 1959; Griffiths, 1973c; Kobrine et al., 1976), shows the parallel behavior of cerebral and spinal cord blood flows related to mean arterial pressure in normal man and animals with normal respiratory gas exchange.

Cerebral and spinal oxygenation are likely to be adequate in normal subjects when the mean arterial pressure is kept *above* 50 mmHg, provided the hemoglobin concentration is normal, the arterial blood is completely saturated and perfusion is not impaired by a raised venous pressure (Harp and Wollman, 1973). Thus, in young, fit subjects, an arterial pressure of 70/40 mmHg is likely to be adequate under ideal conditions of respiration and oxygenation. However, in hypertensive and arteriosclerotic patients, cerebral blood flow deteriorates at a higher perfusion pressure, and in these subjects the blood pressure should not be permitted to run at marginally low levels for any appreciable length of time.

Venous Pressure. It is important to appreciate that tissue blood flow is determined not only by the inflow pressure from the arterial side of the capillary network, but also by the outflow pressure on the venous side. That is to say:

$$\text{Cerebral Blood Flow} \propto \text{Mean Arterial Pressure (MABP)} - \text{Mean Central Venous Pressure (MCVP)}$$

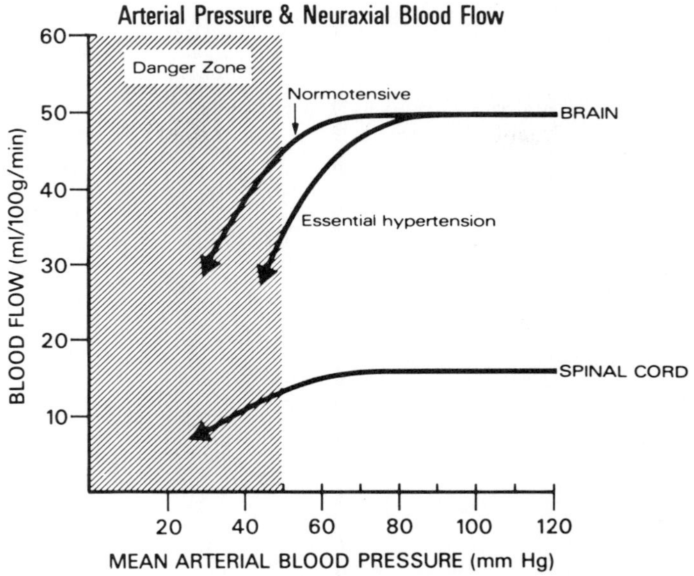

Figure 10–18. Cerebral and spinal cord blood flow and blood pressure curves constructed from several sources (see text). Note that cerebral flow becomes inadequate when it falls below 60 per cent of normal. This occurs at a MABP of about 50 mmHg in a patient with essential hypertension and at a somewhat lower figure in normal fit subjects. (Data from Reivich, 1964, Smith et al., 1969, and Griffiths, 1973c.)

Marked changes of venous pressure in the presence of a low arterial pressure will make a critical difference between survival and death of neuronal tissue. The mean arterial pressure curves shown in the previous figure are drawn to represent perfusion pressure on the assumption that the central venous pressure is zero or close to it. However, if the venous pressure rises to 25 cmH_2O (i.e., 18.4 mmHg), then the effective perfusion pressure is reduced accordingly, and the mean arterial pressure must be raised by a corresponding amount to keep capillary perfusion constant, as shown in Figure 10–19.

A raised venous pressure during arterial hypotension may obstruct capillary flow sufficiently to produce ischemic anoxia at a level of blood pressure that would otherwise be safe and sufficient for metabolic requirements. For example, a raised intrathoracic pressure from high inspiratory pressures during IPPV will raise the CVP. Under high epidural blockade the normal compensatory vasopressor response is abolished, and compensatory vasoconstriction cannot take place. Under these circumstances cerebral or cord ischemia may occur in the presence of a low but normally adequate blood pressure.

An occult form of venous obstruction to capillary flow may also operate at the level of the spinal cord and may be a factor in the genesis of "spinal stroke" or venous infarction of the cord. This is most likely to arise when low arterial blood pressure is accompanied by obstruction to the inferior vena cava from any cause. In the presence of caval obstruction, venous return from the lower limbs and pelvis is forced to take the vertebral venous pathway, and the extradural veins become engorged and distended, raising the pressure in the spinal canal and impairing venous drainage from the cord. Local spinal engorgement is not reflected by central venous pressure measurements (Gal-

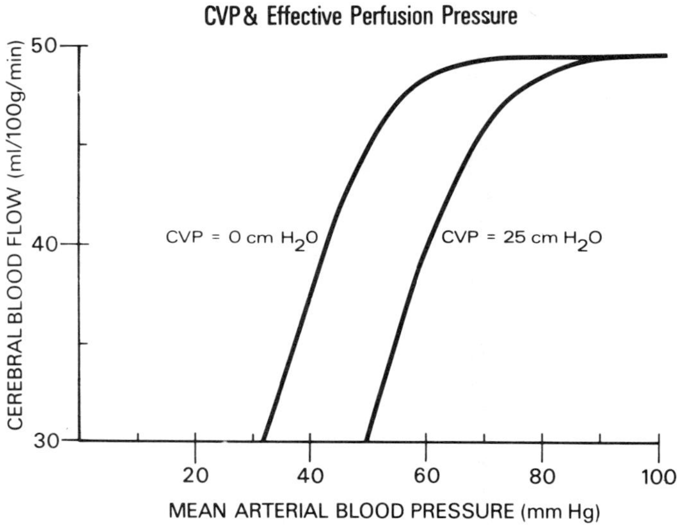

Figure 10–19. Effective perfusion pressure. At low levels of arterial pressure, a rise of central venous pressure must be balanced by a corresponding rise of arterial pressure in order for adequate cerebral perfusion to be maintained.

bert and Marx, 1974), and there is no warning to the anesthetist of the narrowed margin of safety in the circulation of the cord. Frank ischemia of the cord is likely to result if a high local venous pressure is allowed to persist in the presence of a critically low arterial pressure (Bromage, 1974). This mechanism of venous infarction is discussed further in Chapter 14.

Vascular Resistance. Carbon dioxide is one of the most potent regulators of vascular resistance within the neuraxis, and vascular tone varies inversely with P_{CO_2} in an almost linear fashion; the qualitative effects of P_{CO_2} still operate in parts of the brain where arterial inflow is mechanically reduced (Yamamoto et al., 1969). Figure 10–20, constructed from animal data by Reivich (1964), Smith et al. (1969) and Griffiths (1973b), shows the relationship between blood flow and P_{CO_2} in the brain and spinal cord. Flow rises with carbon dioxide retention but falls with hypocapnia. Cord blood flow is likely to be highest in the presence of a high arterial pressure, a raised P_{CO_2} and a low azygos venous pressure. Flow will be at its worst in the presence of a low arterial pressure, vasoconstriction from hypocapnia and a raised vertebral venous pressure. Afferent neural input also affects spinal cord blood flow. Neural stimulation produces a marked increase of flow in the central gray matter on the stimulated side of the cord. Using a multiple microsphere technique, Marcus et al. (1977) found that blood flow increased by 50 per cent in the gray matter of the lumbosacral enlargement of lambs when the sciatic nerve was stimulated, and they interpreted this as a local vasodilator response to increased metabolic demands in the stimulated cord. If this explanation is correct it would suggest that anesthetic blockade of afferent pathways may confer some degree of protection against cord anoxia at critically low levels of blood pressure by reducing segmental neural activity and local oxygen requirements within the spinal cord.

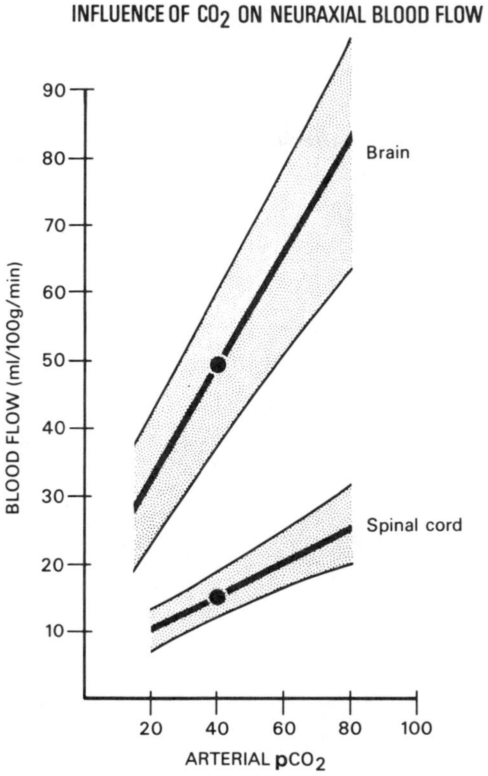

Figure 10–20. Influence of carbon dioxide on neuraxial blood flow. Regression lines constructed from data by Reivich (1964) on cerebral flow in monkeys, by Smith et al. (1969) on cord flow in goats and by Griffiths (1973b) on cord flow in dogs. Stippled area shows approximate range of variation. ● = Normocapnia.

The practice of adding epinephrine to epidural anesthetic solutions in order to prolong their action has been proposed as an obvious cause of cord ischemia (Catterberg and Insausti, 1964; Urquhart-Hay, 1969). However, no conclusive experimental proof exists that this is so (Bromage, 1974), and no investigations have been carried out to estimate the balance of vasoconstrictive and vasodilatory actions of epidural epinephrine and local anesthetics respectively on cord blood flow. One of the few relevant studies on this subject was begun by Dr. José Usubiaga and his colleagues in 1969, but unfortunately a full account of their preliminary work was prevented by Dr. Usubiaga's untimely death in 1970 (Usubiaga et al., 1969). The arteries supplying the spinal cord are less reactive to vasopressor agents than neighboring arteries supplying other tissues (Abraham et al., 1966), and it is quite possible that extradural vasoconstrictive solutions may cause a relative shift of blood flow from extraneural tissues to the substance of the cord. This important point needs to be settled, and radioactive tracer techniques, such as xenon 133 washout, appear to be the most sensitive methods for this type of investigation at the present time (Smith et al., 1969; Griffiths, 1973a). From a clinical standpoint, the danger of cord thrombosis in elderly arteriosclerotic patients will be lessened by the following precautions:

1. Maintain a mean arterial pressure above 80 mmHg. This implies a lower limit of about 100/70 mmHg during maintenance of anesthesia.

2. Avoid hyperventilation and hypocapnia. At first sight hypercapnia might appear to be a desirable safeguard, but there is no good evidence that

it will afford clinical protection in arteriosclerotic vessels that have lost their ability to vasodilate. It is more logical to seek normocapnia for each individual patient (i.e., the preoperative P_{CO_2} that he has been accustomed to). For example, emphysematous patients with a resting P_{CO_2} in the range of 45 to 55 mmHg should have their carbon dioxide maintained at that level. No attempt should be made to lower this value to the accepted "normal" of 40 mmHg, for that would represent a *relative* hypocapnia, and it would induce a corresponding degree of neuraxial vasoconstriction.

3. Avoid high intrathoracic pressure. A high airway pressure causes a raised central venous pressure, and this in turn will diminish the net perfusion pressure across capillary beds throughout the body.

4. Avoid posture that may lead to compression and occlusion of the inferior vena cava, such as the lateral jackknife position or extreme lordosis (Bull, 1949; Sharpey-Schafer, 1950), with consequent engorgement of the vertebral venous plexuses.

LIVER

Sympathetic nerve stimulation reduces hepatic blood flow (Green et al., 1959; Shoemaker, 1964) and depletes glycogen (Shimazu and Fukuda, 1965) and norepinephrine stores in the liver and spleen (Dahlström and Zetterstrom, 1965; Gillespie and Kirpekar, 1966). Interruption of the splanchnic nerves protects the liver against these effects during trauma, toxic insults and surgical operation (Brody et al., 1961; Bauer, 1963; Palmeiro et al., 1963), and prolonged splanchnic blockade with continuous epidural analgesia prevents the normal hyperglycemic response to abdominal or thoracic surgery (Bromage et al., 1971; Brandt et al., 1976a).

Hepatic blood flow is largely dependent on mean systemic blood pressure (Papper et al., 1950; Bauer, 1963; Galindo, 1965a, 1965b), so net liver flow is reduced if the blood pressure is allowed to drop significantly during high segmental blockade. Under epidural analgesia, the effect of diminished hepatic blood flow becomes startlingly apparent if the systolic pressure is allowed to fall below 60 to 70 mmHg. At this point the liver becomes darker and more turgid to the touch, but the normal consistency and appearance are restored when the blood pressure is elevated by administration of a suitable vasopressor (Bromage, 1952). These changes have been interpreted as being due to release of vasodilator substances in the liver during low flow states (Shorr et al., 1945; Bromage, 1952).

Kennedy and his colleagues at Seattle (1970, 1971) carried out studies of hepatic blood flow and splanchnic resistance in man using indocyanine green to compare the effects of subarachnoid block and epidural block carried to the level of T_5. Epidural blocks were performed with either plain 2 per cent lidocaine or lidocaine with 1/200,000 epinephrine. The results of these experiments are summarized in Figure 10–21. It can be seen that all three types of blockade reduced hepatic blood flow to almost exactly the same degree, with a maximum fall of 22 to 23 per cent. After subarachnoid block and epidural analgesia with lidocaine and epinephrine, splanchnic flow fell parallel with arterial pressure as expected. However, plain lidocaine was associated with less

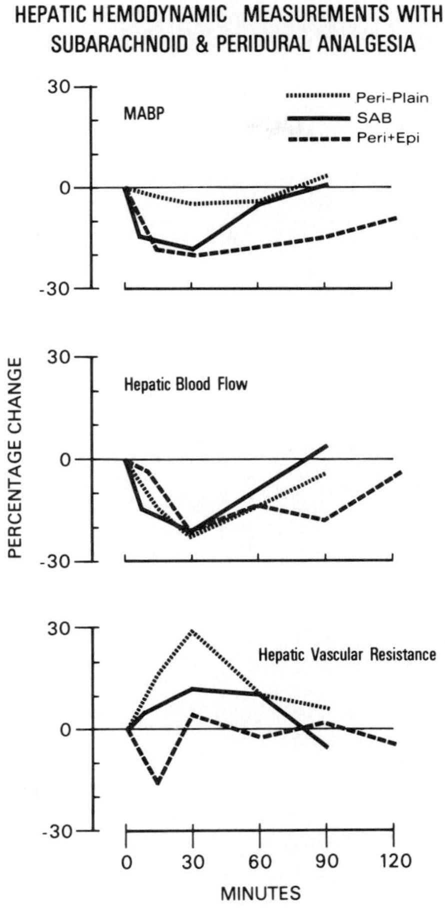

Figure 10–21. Systemic and hepatic hemodynamic changes during subarachnoid and epidural block to T_5 in man.
——— Subarachnoid block
,,,,,,,,, Epidural block with plain 2 per cent lidocaine
--------- Epidural block with 2 per cent lidocaine and 1/200,000 epinephrine
(After Kennedy et al., 1970, 1971.)

vasodilatation in peripheral and splanchnic beds, so that systemic arterial pressure was maintained. The investigators speculated that the relatively greater but transient splanchnic resistance was due to higher levels of absorbed lidocaine in the range of 2 to 3 μg/ml associated with the plain epidural solution.

The same technique of measuring hepatic blood flow with indocyanine green has been used by Price's group in Philadelphia to investigate the effects of general anesthesia (Price et al., 1965, 1966; Epstein et al., 1966; Cooperman et al., 1968; Libonati et al., 1973). The results from the two groups in Philadelphia and Seattle are summarized in Table 10–3. Note that all the general anesthetic regimens tested, except halothane, cause a greater disturbance of splanchnic hemodynamics than spinal or epidural analgesia. Although epidural block lowers splanchnic flow by about 20 to 25 per cent, very little change of splanchnic resistance occurs when epinephrine 1/200,000 is added to the analgesic solution. These findings suggest that epidural blockade with epinephrine 1/200,000 provides very stable hepatic hemodynamic conditions, provided cardiac output and systemic blood pressure are not allowed to fall unduly low.

TABLE 10–3 Changes of Splanchnic Blood Flow and Resistance After Induction of Subarachnoid Anesthesia, Epidural Block and General Anesthesia

		% Change	
Authors	*Anesthetic*	*SPLANCHNIC BLOOD FLOW*	*SPLANCHNIC VASCULAR RESISTANCE*
Regional anesthesia			
Kennedy et al. (1970)	Subarachnoid block to T_5	−22	+12
Kennedy et al. (1971)	Epidural block (plain lidocaine) to T_5	−23	+30
	Epidural block (lidocaine-epinephrine 1/200,000) to T_5	−22	0 (brief initial fall to −16)
General anesthesia			
Price et al. (1965)	Cyclopropane 16–20%	−33	+87
Price et al. (1966)	Cyclopropane 16–20%	−28	+66
	Halothane 1.5%	−24	−5
Epstein et al. (1966)	Halothane 1.5%	−30	0
	Halothane-hypercapnia (pCO_2 = 56.6 mmHg)	+40	−31
Cooperman et al. (1968)	$N_2O + O_2$ + curare: normocapnia	−46	+118
	$N_2O + O_2$ + curare: hypocapnia (pCO_2 = 18 mmHg)	−32	+75
Libonati et al. (1973)	Methoxyflurane (end expiratory conc'n = 0.2%)	−53	Significantly increased (exact figures not given)

Kidneys

The renal and adrenal response to injury are among the major mechanisms that seem designed for survival in a hostile environment. The kidney responds to trauma by conserving salt and water, the most vital elements of the "milieu intérieur." The mechanism of this antidiuretic response is partly humoral and partly neural (Moore, 1959; Zimmerman, 1965). This discussion will be limited to the neural elements of the response that may be modified by epidural blockade.

During the past few years there has been a reawakening of interest in the neural and vascular factors affecting the control of sodium and water by the kidney. A number of new isotope techniques have made it possible to study the distribution of intrarenal blood flow in much greater detail than before. These new methods include gas washout techniques with radioactive xenon (^{133}Xe) or krypton (^{85}Kr) and studies of the anatomical distribution of injected radioactive microspheres in postmortem kidney slices. Sometimes there are apparent discrepancies between the results of gas washout and microsphere injections, since the two methods do not measure precisely the same thing, and this may add to difficulties of interpretation (Stein et al., 1973). Nevertheless, these new methods of measuring renal blood flow have provided a clearer impression of the influences of neural stimulation and neural blockade on the distribution of blood flow and on the different functions of the nephron.

It is well known that both acute and chronic denervation of the kidney are followed by a moderate increase of water and sodium excretion, known as "denervation diuresis and natriuresis" (Sartorius and Burlington, 1956). The underlying mechanism has been the subject of considerable controversy (Nomura et al., 1972). An early opinion held that denervation increased salt and water excretion by increasing overall renal blood flow and glomerular filtration rate (Berne, 1952; Surtshin et al., 1952; Bricker et al., 1958; Kamm and Levinsky, 1965). More recent work has suggested a neural control of tubular transport of sodium and water by shifts of intrarenal blood flow (Blake and Jurf, 1968; Pomeranz et al., 1968; Nomura et al., 1972; Bonjour et al., 1969).

Thirty years ago the beautiful experiments of Trueta and his colleagues (1947) demonstrated that "tourniquet shock" shunted blood from the renal cortex to the medulla and that this was prevented by division of the splanchnic nerves. Pomeranz et al. (1968) have pointed out that the redistribution of intrarenal flow will increase sodium retention by diverting blood to nephrons with the longest loops of Henle and therefore the greatest capacity for reabsorbing sodium. Outer cortical nephrons have relatively short loops of Henle. The deeper juxtamedullary nephrons have long loops reaching deep into the renal medulla, and these have a greater capacity for reabsorbing sodium in the long ascending part of the loop.

Using xenon washout methods, Hollenberg and his colleagues (1970, 1972) have shown that intravenous infusion of a salt load is followed by increased blood flow to the cortex. This accords with a control mechanism designed to switch preferential cortical flow to nephrons that are appropriate to the needs of the moment. With a high salt load, blood is diverted to the outer cortical nephrons with short loops of Henle and relatively limited capabilities for reabsorbing sodium, so salt is lost in the urine. In salt or volume deprivation, or splanchnic nerve stimulation, preferential distribution is switched to the juxtamedullary nephrons and salt is effectively reabsorbed in their long ascending loops.

It must be admitted that this mechanism of redistribution of intrarenal blood flow has not been confirmed by microsphere injection techniques (Nomura et al., 1976). Stein and his colleagues (1973) found that moderately intense splanchnic nerve stimulation reduced renal blood flow by 40 per cent, but with the microsphere technique blood flow was found to be reduced equally in all zones of the cortex. Nomura et al. (1972, 1976) have suggested that there may be direct neural control of peritubular blood flow and sodium excretion, and such a mechanism acting directly at the tubular level might help to reconcile the apparent contradictions of the gas washout and the microsphere techniques. In any event, the effects of acute renal denervation on salt and water excretion are quite evident, even though the precise mechanism may still be debatable.

Normally, surgical trauma is followed by retention of salt and water, even in the presence of adequate fluid and electrolyte replacement. Salt and water balance studies by Bevan (1971, 1973) have shown that this mechanism is markedly altered by effective splanchnic blockade maintained for a period of

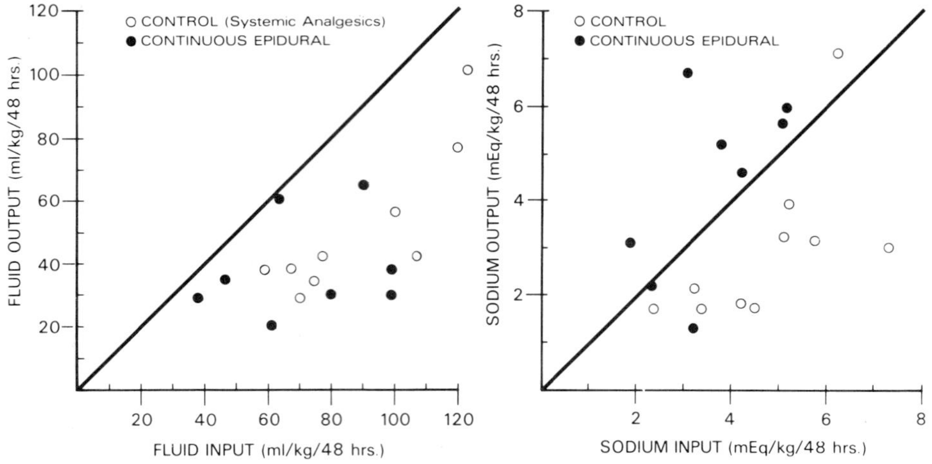

Figure 10–22. Postoperative water and sodium balance in two groups of patients after upper abdominal surgery.

○ = Control group: general anesthesia and postoperative narcotic analgesia

● = Epidural group: continuous epidural analgesia for 48 hours postoperatively with 0.5 per cent bupivacaine (epidural catheter at T_6–T_7 or T_7–T_8)

Note that water is retained after both general anesthesia and continuous epidural block, but salt is excreted freely during epidural blockade. (After Bevan, 1971.)

48 hours after abdominal surgery. Bevan found that although epidural blockade of the splanchnic outflow does not affect the normal postoperative retention of water, it does prevent sodium retention, as shown in Figure 10–22. This suggests that postoperative water and sodium retention act through different, unrelated mechanisms. Reflex distribution of intrarenal blood flow is prevented by blockade of splanchnic efferent impulses to the kidney, so normal sodium excretion continues as if nothing had happened. However, postoperative water retention is mediated through reflex release of antidiuretic hormone. Since some of the afferent pathways for this reflex run in the vagus and spinal blockade is incapable of interrupting the vagal input caused by upper abdominal surgery, water retention is not prevented by epidural analgesia. The difference between the effects of epidural blockade on salt and water excretion is analogous to the different effects of epidural blockade on postoperative cortisol and glucose responses, to be discussed a little later in this chapter. In both instances, vagal afferent input appears to play a major role in triggering one response that has its reflex center in the hypothalamus rather than at a spinal level, while the other response is prevented by splanchnic blockade, as outlined in Figure 10–25.

Trauma and splanchnic nerve stimulation reduce total renal blood flow and urine output (Cort, 1951, 1953; Folkow and Langston, 1964; Johannson and Langston, 1964). Similarly, reduction of renal blood flow is caused by bladder and ureteral distension (Mukherjee, 1957; Hix, 1958). In all these conditions reduction of renal blood flow is abolished by spinal blockade. Renal vasoconstriction is also markedly intense in acute pancreatitis, in which renal vascular resistance may increase to more than twice its normal value (Werner et al., 1974). Although epidural analgesia is frequently used as a therapeutic measure in acute pancreatitis, detailed studies of changes of renal function and blood flow have not been done under these circumstances.

EPIDURAL ANALGESIA AND CONTROL OF THE BLADDER

Spinal control of bladder function resides mainly in the second, third and fourth sacral segments. Classically, neurological deficits fall into upper motor neuron and lower motor neuron types. Upper motor neuron lesions that transect the cord and leave the conus medullaris intact allow sacral segmental reflexes to persist, but their action on detrusor and sphincter muscle is incoordinate, resulting in functional obstruction at the pelvic floor, with small volumes of residual urine at high pressure (Yeates, 1972). Lower motor neuron lesions result in an atonic bladder with a large residual volume.

The effects of epidural analgesia on bladder control will depend on the segmental level of blockade and the presence or absence of an intact spinal reflex arc through the conus. Thoracic epidural analgesia, confined to a few thoracic segments, usually produces very little disturbance of bladder function. On the other hand, lumbar blockade involves the sacral segments and results in an analgesic bladder of the tabetic and lower motor neuron type, with distension usually accompanied by functional obstruction. Therefore, during prolonged lumbar blockade it is necessary to observe the height of the bladder fundus by palpation and to drain the bladder by catheterization if distension becomes severe.

METABOLIC EFFECTS

The Adrenal Gland

Medulla

The influence of nervous stimulation on catecholamine output has been known for a long time. In the cat, splanchnic nerve stimulation increases the output of catecholamines from the adrenal medulla about five to ten times above the resting rate of production, and at the same time it increases the rate of methylation of norepinephrine to epinephrine (Holland and Schumann, 1956; Marley and Paton, 1961). In man, surgery, trauma and pain also cause a rise of circulating catecholamines (Miller and Morris, 1961; McDonald et al., 1969), and plasma concentrations of epinephrine and norepinephrine are approximately doubled after abdominal operations (Nikki et al., 1972). The analgesic drug pentazocine also causes a release of catecholamines (Tammisto et al., 1971), and this response is partially blocked by high epidural blockade (Takki et al., 1973).

The true magnitude of these changes has been difficult to estimate precisely because of the limited sensitivity of the methods of measurement (Ngai, 1974). Within the past few years, however, new techniques have improved the sensitivity of assay more than 16 times, while reducing the very large quantities of blood that were needed previously (Table 10–4). This spectacular advance in technology has made it possible to measure significant changes in plasma catecholamine concentrations that were hidden by the limits of resolution of earlier methods (Roizen et al., 1974).

TABLE 10–4 Methods of Catecholamine Assay: Limits of Accuracy

Method of Assay	*Volume of Blood Required (ml)*	*Limits of Accuracy**	*References*
Trihydroxyindole: fluorometric	25	0.4 nanogram/ml	Lund (1949), Euler and Floding (1955), Woods et al. (1956)
Modified trihydroxyindole: fluorometric	25	0.1 nanogram/ml	Häggendal (1963), Valori et al. (1970), Perry et al. (1974)
Radioisotopic enzymatic	0.5–1.0	25 picograms/ml	Coyle and Henry (1973), Iverson and Jarrott (1970), Roizen et al. (1974)

*Système Internationale (SI) nomenclature:
1 microgram (μg) = 1×10^{-6} gram
1 nanogram (ng) = 1×10^{-9} gram
1 picogram (pg) = 1×10^{-12} gram

Using these new methods of measurement in the rat, Roizen and his colleagues (1974) found that the normal concentration of total catecholamines is approximately 12 ng/ml, of which about 83 per cent is norepinephrine and 17 per cent epinephrine. Under light halothane anesthesia, total catecholamines fall about 90 per cent, mainly by a profound fall of norepinephrine. Under deepening anesthesia, epinephrine undergoes a further fall. Dreyer et al. (1974) have found similar changes with methoxyflurane anesthesia.

The available evidence shows that although excessive catecholamine release during operation may be effectively prevented by light general anesthesia, as soon as anesthesia is terminated there is a marked outpouring of catecholamines, with widespread effect on circulatory beds throughout the body. This postoperative flood of catecholamines can probably be brought under control by effective epidural blockade. However, further work with these new methods of assay will be needed to analyze the exact capabilities of epidural blockade for controlling catecholamine balance in postsurgical and traumatic states.

Cortex

The adrenal cortex responds to trauma by an increased output of hydrocortisone (cortisol) (Steenberg et al., 1956; Lefemine et al., 1957; Estabrooks et al., 1959; Goldenberg et al., 1959; Thomasson, 1959). The magnitude of this response is quite large and greater than reflected by measurements made in systemic venous blood. Prolonged adrenal vein catheterization in man has shown a tenfold increase in cortisol output from a basal rate of 3.1 μg/min to a rate of 30 to 50 μg/min after abdominal operations (Hume et al., 1962).

A considerable amount of work has been done to see if this response is neurally mediated, and if so, whether it can be modified under clinical conditions by appropriate neural blockade. Early measurements of the eosinopenic response to abdominal surgery suggested that the adrenocortical response did not operate in the face of complete deafferentation, as shown in Figure 10–23 (Bromage, 1954; Thorne et al., 1954; Hume and Egdahl, 1959). Virtue et al.

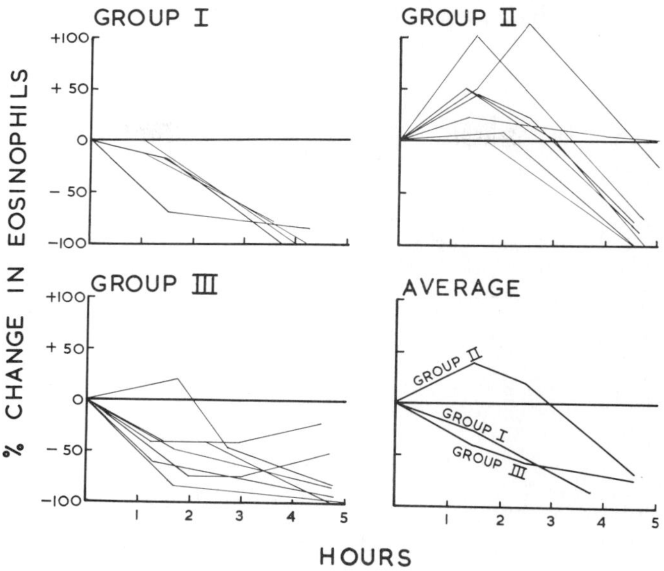

Figure 10–23. Eosinophil responses to laparotomy modified by afferent blockade.

Group I. Controls. Five patients under general anesthesia. Normal eosinopenic response to stress, commencing after one hour and almost complete after four hours.

Group II. Eight patients. Lower laparotomy under epidural block and light general anesthesia (complete afferent blockade). Note delay in fall of circulating eosinophils until the block wears off.

Group III. Seven patients. Upper laparotomy under epidural block and light general anesthesia (partial afferent blockade). The eosinophil responses are comparable to those in Group I.

(From Bromage, P. R.: Spinal Epidural Analgesia. Edinburgh, E. & S. Livingstone, 1954.)

(1957) and Hammond et al. (1958) also found that subarachnoid anesthesia delayed the rise in 17-hydroxycorticosteroids that normally occurs after abdominal operations.

Subsequent investigations with more precise methods of measurement have tended to confirm these earlier findings, but they have also underlined the difficulty of ensuring complete deafferentation during major abdominal surgery, and they suggest that a significant proportion of upper abdominal afferent traffic travels in vagal pathways. In five studies of patients undergoing surgery limited to the lower abdomen (hysterectomy), a slight to complete delay in the normal cortisol response occurred under epidural blockade (Lush et al., 1972; Gordon et al., 1973; Cosgrove and Jenkins, 1974; Brandt et al., 1976b; Enquist et al., 1977). However, in more stimulating procedures involving the abdomen and thorax, prolonged epidural blockade had no influence on either the operative or the postoperative phase of the cortisol response (Bromage et al., 1971; Lines et al., 1971; Brandt et al., 1976a).

Major abdominal surgery is normally followed by a four- or fivefold rise of plasma cortisol from a resting level of about 10 to 15 μg/100 ml to a peak of 40 to 60 μg/100 ml by the fourth postoperative hour, and then a gradual decline to preoperative levels about 24 to 36 hours after surgery (Bromage et al., 1971; Brandt et al., 1976a). Figure 10–24 shows the compara-

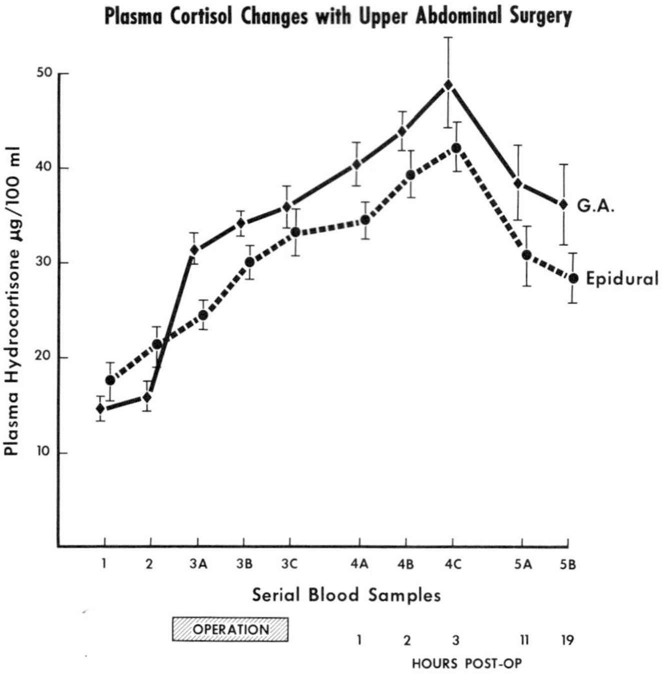

Figure 10–24. The mean and standard errors of blood cortisol changes associated with upper abdominal and thoracic operations in 44 patients.
◆———◆ Thiopental, nitrous oxide and curare followed by postoperative narcotics in 22 patients
●------● Thiopental, nitrous oxide and continuous epidural blockade maintained for 19 hours in 22 patients
(From Bromage et al.: Surg. Gynecol. Obstet., 1971.)

tive concentrations of blood cortisol obtained in a series of 44 patients undergoing upper abdominal or thoracic surgery, half of whom received general anesthesia followed by systemic postoperative analgesia and half of whom received continuous epidural blockade during operation. The epidural block was then carefully maintained for a further period of 19 hours to ensure that the upper level of analgesia never fell below T_4 in the abdominal cases or below T_1 in the thoracic cases. It can be seen that the plasma cortisol curves are almost indistinguishable in the two groups (Bromage et al., 1971).

These results suggest that if the adrenocortical response to trauma is under neural control, then unlike the adrenal medullary response, the reflex arc must involve pathways outside the range of high segmental analgesia, probably through afferent impulses traveling along the vagus nerves. The suggested pathways of the adrenal medullary and adrenal cortical responses are outlined in Figure 10–25.

One study of obstetrical patients has shown that epidural blockade may suppress the normal rise of plasma cortisol that occurs in labor. Plasma cortisol increases during pregnancy, and at term plasma levels are three to four times higher than in nonpregnant subjects. Buchan and his colleagues (1973) have shown that these high levels are increased further during childbirth and are doubled during the first stage and quadrupled during the second stage of labor. Effective epidural blockade reduces this terminal acute rise of plasma cortisol by about 50 per cent. The question arises, does this artificial reduction in the peak maternal cortisol during labor deprive the fetus of a supplementary supply of cortisol that might be important in the final maturation of the fetal lung and in the prevention of hyaline membrane disease (Avery, 1975)? Does it rob the fetus of a kind of viaticum necessary for the journey from dependent to independent life? At the present time there is no clear answer to this hypothetical question, but it seems unlikely that a partial reduction of the relatively brief surge of cortisol output is of serious consequence, coming as it does on top of a much longer period of augmented basal output. If suppression of the cortisol peak at delivery does prove to be important, then substitution therapy with betamethasone would be a logical step whenever regional anesthesia is used to abolish pain in childbirth or whenever elective cesarean section is undertaken.

Blood Sugar and the Endocrine Pancreas

Blood sugar rises sharply after major surgery, as part of the general reaction to trauma (Mackay, 1928; Mackay and Dyke, 1928). The curve of this hyperglycemic response has almost exactly the same shape and duration as the cortisol response described in the previous section. However, the two responses differ markedly in the way they are modified by spinal blockade. Whereas the cortisol response persists virtually unchanged in the presence of prolonged spinal analgesia, hyperglycemia can be completely suppressed by effective splanchnic blockade. This section will review some of the published work related to the control of blood sugar during surgery, in order to provide an

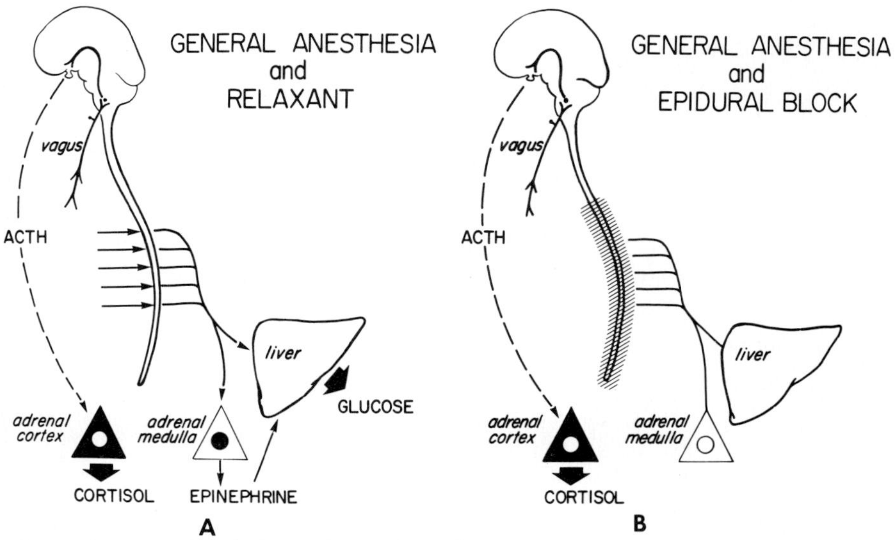

Figure 10–25. Reflex pathways involved in adrenal medullary and cortical responses to operations upon the upper abdomen and thorax, and the influence of segmental epidural blockade extending above T_6. *A*, General anesthesia and muscle relaxants. *B*, General anesthesia and continuous epidural blockade. (From Bromage et al.: Surg. Gynecol. Obstet., 1971.)

understanding of the role that epidural analgesia can play in modifying this segment of the alarm system.

The blood sugar response is proportional to the degree of stress. Minor surface operations usually elicit very little response (Griffiths, 1953), but in major abdominal surgery the blood sugar begins to rise within the first hour, reaches a peak 60 to 90 per cent above control levels about four hours after the operation has finished and then gradually returns to normal after 36 to 48 hours. Some papers have suggested that racial differences exist in the degree of hyperglycemic response, with Asiatics and Africans showing a more florid response than Caucasians (Keating, 1958; Cullingford, 1966). However, subsequent investigations taken together have failed to confirm any marked association between geographical ancestry and degree of response (Clarke, 1970; Oyama et al., 1971; Bromage et al., 1971; Magbagbeola and Adadevoh, 1974; Brandt et al., 1976a).

The mechanism of the hyperglycemic response has received a great deal of attention, for there are many underlying factors that are complex and difficult to measure. The high blood sugar could result from one or more of the following factors:

A. Increased release of glucose from glycogen stores (gluconeogenesis)
   1. Neural via splanchnic nerves
   2. Humoral via circulating hormones, such as epinephrine or glucagon
B. Inhibition of glucose metabolism
   1. Neural or humoral inhibition of insulin excretion
   2. Neural or humoral stimulation of glucagon secretion

All these factors have been investigated, and the general pattern of response is now becoming clearer. Central or direct stimulation of the splanchnic nerves causes a rapid increase in the activities of glycogen phosphorylase and glucose-6-phosphatase in the liver, followed by an increase in the concentration of glucose in the blood (Shimazu and Fukuda, 1965; Shimazu et al., 1966). Epinephrine produces the same effect. The pancreas is also under neural control, and it secretes insulin, which lowers the blood sugar, from the B-cells of the islets of Langerhans, and glucagon, which raises the blood sugar, from the A-cells of the same islets. The autonomic nervous system exerts a significant regulatory action over the secretion of these two reciprocal hormones (Woods and Porte, 1974). Sympathetic stimulation suppresses insulin secretion and releases glucagon (Porte et al., 1973). Unfortunately, it is very difficult to assess the influence of neural blockade on the pancreatic endocrine response to surgery, because glucagon, one of the two hormones involved, is rapidly bound in the liver, and samples of blood taken from systemic veins do not reflect concentrations that are found in the pancreaticoduodenal vein and the portal blood.

Johnson (1949) showed that spinal blockade to T_4 inhibited the hyperglycemic response to surgical stress in animals, whereas blockade to levels below T_6 that did not include the whole splanchnic outflow had no effect on the blood sugar. This has been confirmed in man (Annamunthodo et al., 1958; Keating, 1958; Cullingford, 1966). Bromage et al. (1971) and Brandt et al. (1976a) have shown that prolonged epidural blockade continued for 19 to 26 hours can completely eliminate both the operative and the postoperative phases of the hyperglycemic response and maintain the blood sugar at fasting levels as long as the block lasts, as shown in Figure 10–26.

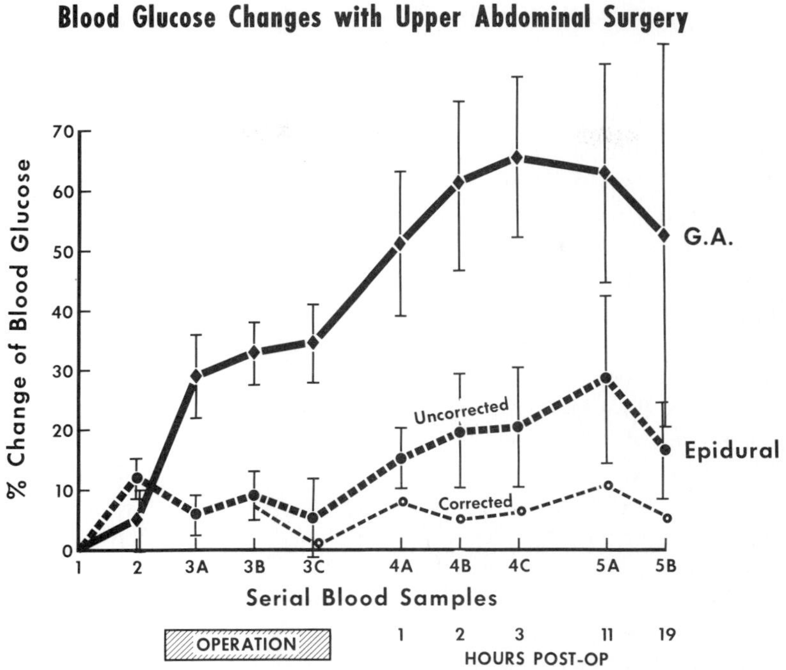

Figure 10–26. Control of hyperglycemic response to major surgery. Means ± SEM of blood glucose changes associated with upper abdominal or intrathoracic operations in 44 patients.
◆——◆ General anesthesia with curare (22 patients)
●------● General anesthesia and high spinal epidural blockade (22 patients)
○------○ Corrected epidural series after three patients were excluded in whom technical difficulties were encountered in maintaining the upper level of blockade after operation
(From Bromage et al.: Surg. Gynecol. Obstet., 1971.)

In spite of its being able to prevent the hyperglycemic response to surgery, the precise mechanism of prolonged epidural blockade is unclear, and the question remains, how much of the splanchnic control of postoperative hyperglycemia is due to neural and humoral effects on the liver, and how much is mediated through autonomic control of the reciprocal pancreatic hormones insulin and glucagon? Attempts to demonstrate changes of plasma insulin concentrations have been largely negative. Although Allison and his colleagues (1969) found a decline of plasma insulin during surgery, other investigators have failed to confirm this finding, and there is general agreement that plasma insulin does not change (Clarke et al., 1970; Magbagbeola and Adadevoh, 1974; Brandt et al., 1976a). Brandt and his colleagues (1976a) have also shown that systemic glucagon levels are unchanged and the same both in hyperglycemic patients operated under general anesthesia alone and in patients under continuous epidural blockade with low levels of blood sugar.

On the available evidence, it seems that neural blockade of the pancreas is probably not a major factor in the inhibitory effects of epidural analgesia on the hyperglycemic response to surgery. It seems more likely that other glycoregulatory pathways are concerned, probably those acting through splanchnic control of the adrenal medulla and the hepatic glycogenolytic system.

The clinical aspects of controlled hypoglycemia are both immediate and speculative. The response of diabetic patients to insulin is augmented by splanchnic blockade (Griffiths, 1953), and hyperosmolar levels of blood sugar can be restored to normal very quickly in the presence of high epidural blockade. By the same token, the blood sugar can fall to dangerously low levels if insufficient glucose is available. The anesthesiologist must be aware of the possibility that hypoglycemia may develop in rare circumstances, and he should be prepared to correct it quickly by intravenous injection of hypertonic glucose. Unexplained tachycardia or slight ST changes in lead V_5 are the warning signs to look for, and a precordial (axillary) EKG lead should be in place (Griffiths, 1953; Kaplan and King, 1976).

On the speculative side, manipulation of the blood sugar may have applications for controlling susceptibility to both microbial and neoplastic invaders. There is some evidence that gram-negative organisms are inhibited by high concentrations of blood glucose, whereas gram-positive organisms are inhibited by hypoglycemia (Robson and Heggers, 1969; Robson, 1970). It has also been suggested that successful nidation of neoplastic cells may be partially glucose-dependent, and therefore secondary deposits may be less likely to occur in a low-sugar environment than in a high one. However, these are remote possibilities that require confirmation by further work.

Temperature Control

Paralysis of the sympathetic outflow interferes with heat-regulating mechanisms in three ways. Epinephrine secretion falls, so metabolism and heat production also fall, while at the same time peripheral vasodilatation occurs and sweating stops in the area of the block. Thus, surface heat exchange is facilitated, but evaporative heat losses are reduced. It follows that body temperature may fall rapidly in cold surroundings, owing to increased blood flow through dilated skin vessels, while in hot environments there is the possibility of hyperpyrexia occurring from suppression of sweating. The peripheral vasodilatation that follows extensive segmental blockade may be used to accelerate induced hypothermia in cases in which a low body temperature is considered advantageous (Bromage, 1954; Stolar and Wynands, 1963).

The spinal canal appears to be an important temperature-sensitive zone involved in control of body heat exchange, and the temperature of fluids injected into the epidural space exerts profound effects on temperature regulation. Thauer and his colleagues at the Max-Planck Institute used implanted epidural thermodes in birds and mammals to induce reflex thermal responses. Warming the epidural space by circulating warm water through the thermodes stimulated heat-dissipating mechanisms—panting in dogs (Jessen, 1967; Jessen et al., 1967) and increased sweating in oxen (Hales and Jessen, 1969)—while cooling of the epidural space stimulated heat-generating responses—shivering and increased oxygen consumption in rabbits and dogs (Kosaka et al., 1966) and "feather fluffing" in pigeons (Rautenberg, 1969, 1971; Thauer and Simon, 1972). In dogs, the spinal canal and hypothalamus appear to be functionally equivalent temperature sensors with approximately the same degree of sensitivity to local temperature changes (Thauer and Simon, 1972). Effector mechanisms of facilitation and inhibition to whole-body or spinal canal cooling appear to be situated at different levels of the brain stem, with facilitation residing in suprapontine structures and inhibition of shivering lying within the pons (Chambers et al., 1974).

These investigations led to the assumption that the temperature sensors involved are situated in the spinal cord (Thauer and Simon, 1972). However, clinical observations in man do not support this; on the contrary, what evidence there is suggests that while the spinal epidural space is responsive to temperature changes, the subarachnoid space and spinal cord are not. Ample opportunity to observe this difference has been provided by the therapeutic use of ice-cold intrathecal saline for attempted relief of intractable pain (Hitchcock, 1967). Quite large amounts of cold saline, in the range of 15 to 90 ml, injected directly into the lumbar subarachnoid space do not induce shivering (Savitz and Mills, 1973), whereas cold solutions injected into the extradural space may do so. In two studies of epidural analgesia with bupivacaine at ambient temperature, some degree of shivering occurred in 20 per cent of cases in one series (Downing, 1969) and in 50 per cent in the other (Waters et al., 1970).

The precise reason for occasional shivering during epidural blockade is still obscure, and it is premature to attribute the cause to thermal sensors lying in the spinal canal or in the spinal cord. The simplest explanation for shivering phenomena during epidural blockade may lie in the heightened tendency to body cooling from heat losses due to cutaneous vasodilatation, as mentioned earlier. This explanation is too facile, however, and does not match the time course of events. If shivering does occur, it comes on quite rapidly within a matter of minutes after epidural injection, before enough time has elapsed for a significant amount of heat to be lost.

An alternative mechanism may lie in the anatomical arrangement of blood vessels within the epidural space, for the large extradural veins connect with the basal sinuses and represent a potentially effective heat exchange mechanism. Rapid flow through these veins is likely to carry any local thermal gradients to distal points along the azygos stream.

Perhaps the most likely cause of shivering associated with epidural blockade is to be found in the action of the local anesthetic on sensory nerves modifying thermal cues from the exterior, with resultant inappropriate thermal responses to false information that has been received. In quadriplegic patients in whom denervation is homogeneous, sensory deprivation from the greater part of the body makes them relatively insensitive to changes of external temperature, and a shivering response is triggered only by internal temperature cues, not by both internal and external temperature sensation as in normal subjects (Downey et al., 1969). However, during the onset of anesthetic spinal blockade, the character of denervation is heterogeneous until blockade of all neural modalities mimics the picture of chronic spinal man. A temporary alteration of the thermal body image of this sort is analogous to the changing proprioceptive body image that sometimes arises while sensory blockade is developing, before external sensation is completely interrupted. During the developing phase of blockade, position sense is plastic and changing. Once blockade is complete the sensory field is abandoned to internal sensory patterns that maintain the phantom body image in its stereotyped position of orthopedic rest (Bromage and Melzack, 1974). An explanation of this sort, in terms of changing afferent input, has become more attractive since the work of Fruhstorfer et al. (1974) has shown that a dissociated loss of warm and cold sensation occurs during peripheral nerve block. Blockade of cold sensation takes 27 per cent longer to develop than blockade of warm sensation, although Nathan (1976) has found that this is not an invariable order of blockade in differential subarachnoid block. Thus, in many patients there is probably a brief period during the onset of anesthesia when warm sensation is cut off but cold sensation persists, so that thermal information reaching the central nervous system is biased in favor of cold input. It would be surprising if this false picture of external cold did not trigger a programmed thermal response to raise the body temperature in its accustomed fashion. The rather high incidence of shivering reported with bupivacaine tends to support this idea, for bupivacaine is an agent with a relatively slow latency, and the prolonged onset of anesthesia might be expected to extend the interval between the onset of warm and cold blockade.

From a clinical point of view, shivering is a wasteful form of energy expenditure that places increased demands on cardiac output and oxygen consumption. Its causes should be avoided by the following measures:

1. Epidural analgesic solutions should be stored in a comfortably warm ambient temperature.

2. Cutaneous heat losses should be avoided by using adequate body coverings.

3. If shivering does occur, its cause should be sought and treated. Active hot air warming should be instituted if the body temperature is subnormal. Persistent shivering may be suppressed centrally by administering an appropriate phenothiazine drug.

Malignant Hyperthermia (MH) and Epidural Blockade

Malignant hyperthermia is a rare syndrome inherited as a mendelian dominant (Thompson, 1973; Isaacs, 1973), with an incidence of between 1:14,000 and 1:75,000 anesthetics (Kalow and Britt, 1973; Relton et al., 1973) and a mortality of 60 to 70 per cent. The syndrome consists of a rapidly rising body temperature, intense peripheral vasoconstriction (Williams et al., 1975, 1976), biochemical changes indicative of explosively accelerated metabolic processes, usually (but not invariably) muscle rigidity and myoglobinuria in survivors. Susceptible subjects usually have elevated levels of muscle enzymes in the blood, especially creatine phosphokinase (CPK), and abnormal isoenzyme patterns (Zsigmond et al., 1972). However, the correlation between high CPK levels and susceptibility to MH is poor (Ellis et al., 1972; Relton et al., 1973), which is not surprising since high levels of muscle enzymes are found in a variety of other conditions, especially acute psychosis. Meltzer and his colleagues (1969, 1970a, 1970b, 1976) made extensive enzymatic and histological studies of muscle abnormalities in acute psychosis and found significantly elevated CPK levels in about 60 per cent of acutely psychotic patients, as well as in 25 per cent of the immediate relatives of these patients. Similar findings have been reported in manic-depressive patients during the prodromal and acute phases of mania by Gosling et al. (1972a, 1972b). These findings may hint, very tentatively, at a common neural or metabolic thread running between the apparently unrelated conditions of mental disorder and MH.

The agents succinylcholine and halothane, either separately or together, have been most commonly implicated in triggering the syndrome of malignant hyperpyrexia, but other drugs, including trimeprazine, have also been involved (Moyes, 1973).

The etiology of MH is uncertain, and until recently, pathogenesis was thought to be entirely peripheral from some defect of muscle and mitochondrial membranes, but there is mounting evidence of central nervous control of the sarcoplasmic reticulum and of a neural component that can be suppressed by nerve blockade. Cross-innervation experiments between slow ("red") muscles and fast ("white") muscles have shown that the biochemical and enzymatic properties of the muscles and the sarcoplasmic reticulum are heavily dependent on the type of neural input they receive (Buller et al., 1960a and b: Buller et al., 1969; Guth and Watson, 1967; Prewitt and Salajsky, 1967; Margreth et al., 1973). For a review of cross-innervation experiments and the determination of biochemical profiles by neural input, the reader is referred to *Machina Carnis*, a definitive work on muscle by Dorothy Needham (1971). La Cour and his associates (1971) were the first to suggest a neural mechanism. In their studies of susceptible subjects they found that muscle fibers were hyperexcitable on electromyography, and on microscopy they observed an increased number of motor end plates with pronounced sprouting and abnormal forms. Using Foldes' tourniquet test for myasthenia gravis (Foldes et al., 1968), they also found that a minute dose of succinylcholine (0.1 mg/kg) gave predominantly central rather than peripheral effects in a susceptible subject.

The sympathetic autonomic nervous system seems to be heavily implicated in the hyperthermic response. Lister and his colleagues (1974) reported that MH in susceptible pigs is preceded by a massive outpouring of catecholamines and that both the hyperthermic response and the catecholamine discharge can be prevented by prior depletion of catecholamines using reserpine or by pretreatment with an alpha blocker, such as phentolamine. However, alpha blockade is useless once the hyperthermic response has started (Lister et al., 1975). Williams and his associates (1975, 1976) have confirmed that the MH syndrome is accompanied by intense peripheral vasoconstriction, leading to cessation of radiant heat losses and a fall in cardiac output.

The theme of a neural component to malignant hyperpyrexia has been developed a step further by tracing the nerve pathways back to the level of the spinal cord. One of the most intriguing discoveries in the field of thermal regulation has been the observation by Kerr et al. (1975) that porcine MH is prevented by epidural blockade. These investigators found that susceptible pigs developed characteristic muscle rigidity in all four limbs within 2 minutes of halothane inhalation. Under epidural analgesia with 2 per cent lidocaine, the same pigs continued to exhibit rigidity of unblocked forelimbs, but their blocked hind limbs remained flaccid, and the body temperature did not rise (Fig. 10–27).

These remarkable observations expand the vista of enquiry from a

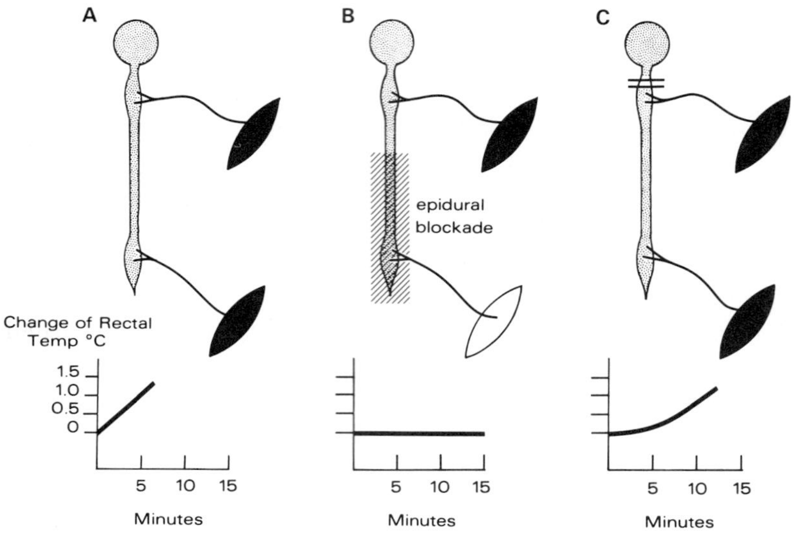

Figure 10–27. *Malignant hyperthermia in susceptible pigs.*

A, Controls. Halothane challenge causes muscle rigidity in all four limbs, and the temperature rises within 2 minutes.

B, Epidural blockade of lower body. Halothane challenge causes muscle rigidity in unblocked forelimbs. Blocked hind limbs remain flaccid. Body temperature does not rise.

C, Spinal cord transection. Section of the spinal cord delays, but does not prevent, the onset of rigidity and hyperpyrexia in response to halothane. (After Kerr et al., 1975.)

limited field in the target muscles to an entirely new philosophical view of the whole process of the malignant hyperpyrexia stress syndrome. The picture of MH is developing to include the concept of an unstable autonomic nervous system and a sort of suicidal psychosis at the level of the spinal cord. Although the disordered neural process may extend far up the neuraxis, it is relatively independent of commands from above, for high transection of the spinal cord only delays the hyperthermic response and does not prevent it. Since segmental epidural blockade seems to modify the attack and to restrict rigor to unblocked limbs, there is a strong suggestion that the major triggering process may lie somewhere in the sympathetic pathways of the cord.

It has been suggested that lidocaine is contraindicated in MH because of its effect on calcium release and uptake at a sarcoplasmic level (Relton et al., 1973). Successful clinical suppression of MH with lidocaine epidural blockade, however, shows that the neural component to the muscular response is of paramount importance, perhaps because initial calcium movements are relatively undisturbed in the presence of autonomic blockade.

The practical implications of this important work seem clear, if they can be transferred to man, and they reinforce what was already known empirically: that epidural blockade is a preferred method of analgesia in subjects who are susceptible to MH. The time course of the syndrome is too rapid to suggest the use of epidural analgesia as a form of treatment once hyperthermia has been triggered, and at present there is no evidence that neural or catecholamine blockade will halt the process once it has started (Lister et al.,

1975). However, effective interruption of neuraxial activity does appear to prevent the syndrome, so epidural blockade may be considered as a prophylactic measure for appropriate operations in subjects who are susceptible to malignant hyperpyrexia.

The technical applications of these principles are fairly obvious, but they should be stated firmly so that reported failures from technical inadequacies are not allowed to cloud fundamental issues (Katz and Krich, 1976). First, the disease and not the site of operation determines the extent of spinal blockade. Segmental blockade should extend to T_1 in order to involve *all* the spinal sympathetic outflow, for the central neuraxial fuse must be stamped out before it can trigger an explosive catecholamine discharge at the peripheral nerve endings. Second, continuous blockade should be prolonged for a few hours after operation in order to afford protection from sympathetic discharge during the period of greatest metabolic stress. Failure to observe these precautions will not provide the degree of protection that experimental data suggest is necessary.

The following summary of a case report from Poland illustrates the human counterpart of the porcine response to epidural blockade illustrated in Figure 10–27, and it emphasizes the incomplete degree of protection afforded by partial blockade of the sympathetic outflow (Klimanek et al., 1976).

> *A woman of 25 years was scheduled for hemorrhoidectomy under epidural blockade. Doses of 300 mg lidocaine and 50 mg bupivacaine with 60 μg epinephrine 1/200,000 were injected at the second lumbar interspace. Analgesia spread to an upper segmental level of about T_{10}. Thirty minutes after injection cyanosis developed in the whole body* except in the area of analgesia below the umbilicus. *The muscles of the face and upper body became rigid,* but the legs remained flaccid. *The temperature rose to 41.5° C, and the patient became comatose. Resuscitation along standard lines was successful, except for some persistent ECG evidence of myocardial damage in the posterior ventricular wall. During the attack of rigor the lower limbs were hotter than the rest of the body, indicating that heat was dissipated faster in the area of sympathetic block and vasodilatation (Klimanek, 1977).*

The hyperthermic response in this case may have been triggered by epidural epinephrine or by anxiety. Whatever the cause, the clinical picture bore a striking resemblance to the epiduralized pigs described by Kerr and his colleagues, shown diagrammatically in Figure 10–27. In both the animal and the human situations, a florid hyperthermic response stopped short at the upper segmental level of blockade, while the lower limbs escaped the general rigor, and survival followed. It is reasonable to suppose that a more extensive epidural block involving all of the sympathetic outflow might have prevented the attack entirely in this case.

RESPIRATION

Anesthesia is an exercise in reflex suppression. Modern anesthetic technique is heavily dominated by emphasis on interrupting the efferent side of the reflex arc. Attention has drifted away from attempts to control sensory input while preserving motor function, since muscle relaxants and artificial ventilation have come to be almost universally accepted as the mainstay of general anesthesia for most types of surgery. This section will consider the influence of afferent input on ventilation and the effects of deafferentation, as well as some of the functional changes that occur when spontaneous breathing is supplanted by artificial ventilation.

Neural Input and Control of Respiration

It used to be thought that respiratory motor neurons in the "respiratory center" of the medulla preserved intrinsic motor tone and that they fired continuously unless inhibited rhythmically by other neurons. Intracellular recordings by Salmoiraghi and Burns showed that this is not so (Salmoiraghi and Burns, 1960a, 1960b; Burns and Salmoiraghi, 1960; Salmoiraghi, 1963). These authors demonstrated that respiratory motor neurons, in common with all other motor cells, require afferent input before they can respond and perform their normal functions. In the absence of afferent input, respiratory motor neurons in the medulla fall silent. A similar dependence upon afferent input has been shown clinically for the phrenic reflex (Bromage, 1958a).

The respiratory reflex apparatus becomes remarkably tractable when afferent input is reduced by high epidural blockade to T_1 or T_2. Normally, under light general anesthesia there is an increase in active expiratory muscle tone (Freund et al., 1964), and noxious stimuli produce a grunting type of respiration, with increased expiratory effort that is readily detected by spirometry or by placing a hand on the abdomen (McCann, 1946; Morton, 1950; Kaul et al., 1973). However, under a combination of light general anesthesia and high spinal blockade, expiratory tone is not exaggerated (Kinnell, 1962), and spontaneous respiration is easily suppressed following five to ten moderately large artificial breaths imposed by squeezing the rebreathing bag. Spontaneous respiration resumes almost immediately and compliance falls if afferent input is increased by applying a noxious stimulus to an unanesthetized area above the segmental level of blockade (Bromage, 1958b).

The phrenic reflex arc (C_3, C_4 and C_5) shows a similar dependence upon an adequate traffic of afferent input that is easily demonstrated on the operating table. During thoracotomy under light general anesthesia, the diaphragm is extremely sensitive to direct stimulation, and pinching the central portion elicits vigorous diaphragmatic responses that are impossible to control without inducing neuromuscular blockade or deepening anesthesia. However, if epidural analgesia is induced and the upper level is carried to the first thoracic segment, the reflex responses alter dramatically. Now, pinching the central portion of the diaphragm results in a markedly attenuated response. Instead of a full coordinated contraction, there is only a localized wormlike fasciculation, and artificial ventilation is virtually undisturbed (Bromage, 1958a). Note that under these circumstances the phrenic reflex arc is still intact; blockade has fallen short of the phrenic roots by several segments, and yet there is no coordinated response to phrenic sensory input. Presumably, the normal phrenic reflex is dependent upon the summation of a number of different ascending as well as descending facilitatory stimuli, and depletion of a major part of the total afferent neuronal "pool" leads to quiescence of the phrenic nucleus and failure of a

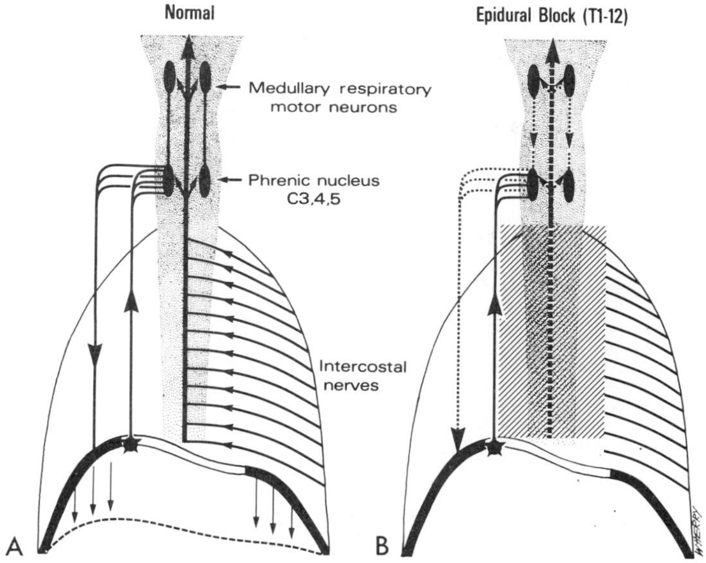

Figure 10–28. Attenuation of respiratory reflexes by reduction of collateral sensory input. *A,* Normal motor response of diaphragm to stimulation of the central portion, under light general anesthesia. Phrenic and medullary respiratory motor neurons are facilitated by sensory input from caudad sources in the chest wall and elsewhere. *B,* Abolition of facilitatory afferent input by epidural blockade to T_1. Failure of diaphragmatic response to stimulation. (After Bromage, 1958.)

normal efferent response. The neural pathways concerned in this process of partial deafferentation are shown diagrammatically in Figure 10–28. Afferent impulses traveling up the cord and through the brain stem in the reticular activating system send facilitatory stimuli to motor nuclei along the way. Reduction of this normal traffic by high spinal blockade reduces the reactivity of respiratory motor nuclei. This situation is carried a step further in cases of accidental total spinal blockade from epidural or subarachnoid overdose. Then, the cervical and cranial nerves are affected also, and deafferentation is complete. The patient is cut off from the outer world and consciousness is lost. Consciousness returns when afferent input returns along the upper cranial nerves (Gordon-Jones, 1953). An analogous dependence on external input is seen in "encéphale isolé" cats, in which bilateral destruction of the fifth nerve ganglion changes the electroencephalographic pattern from wakefulness to one of sleep (Roger et al., 1956).

In the clinical situation, deafferentation by induction of high epidural blockade ensures a gentle, easy type of spontaneous respiration, free of the expiratory effort that usually accompanies light anesthesia or surgical stimulation. Controlled ventilation is easily superimposed without the need for muscle relaxants. If an endotracheal tube is required, the trachea and larynx must also be deafferented by effective topical anesthesia, or the stimulus of intubation may be sufficient to arouse normal respiratory drive and resistance to imposed ventilation.

Neural Influences on the Thorax and Lung

The effects of neural stimulation on the thorax and underlying lung are extremely complex and only partially understood. This section will attempt no more than a brief selection of some of the relevant information available from the enormous amount of work that has been done on the subject, in order to provide a background for appreciating the effects of epidural blockade on the mechanics of respiratory exchange.

Afferent input

Sensory information from the chest wall is carried by all 12 thoracic dorsal roots. Sensation from the outer two thirds of the diaphragm passes to the lower six thoracic segments, while the central portion of the diaphragm sends its input through the phrenic nerve to the third, fourth and fifth cervical segments.

Afferent input from the lungs and airways travels along both the vagus and sympathetic nerves to the upper four thoracic segments (Widdicombe, 1963). Although anatomical studies in human fetuses had suggested that in man most of the afferent fibers are carried in the vagus (Spencer and Leof, 1964), more recent studies by Kampine's group have shown that pulmonary afferents run in the upper thoracic white rami communicantes. These pulmonary afferents are sensitive to a wide variety of stimuli and have conduction velocities of 7 to 12 m/sec, compatible with axon diameters in the A-delta range (Kostreva et al., 1975).

Efferent nerve supply

Motor supply to the bronchial tree is a mixture of parasympathetic (bronchoconstrictor) and sympathetic (bronchodilator). Normally, a balance of power is maintained between the two, but in most species the vagus has a potentially dominant role, while the sympathetic appears to function as an inhibitor of the vagus rather than as an active bronchodilator (Cabezas et al., 1971).

The autonomic supply to the lungs also plays a significant vasomotor role, with the sympathetic nerves increasing pulmonary vascular resistance (Daly and Hebb, 1952; Daly, 1958, 1961). Maximum stimulation of the stellate ganglion produces a 25 per cent increase of pulmonary vascular resistance (Kadowitz and Hyman, 1973). In addition, sympathetic stimulation increases the surface tension of lung surfactant in cats and monkeys and reduces lung compliance by about 40 per cent (Beckman et al., 1971; Droste and Beckman, 1974). In asthmatic subjects, parasympathomimetic drugs increase the pulmonary blood volume by about 60 per cent (Pierson and Grieco, 1972), and this may be related to the marked submucosal turgor and swelling that can be seen in status asthmaticus (Rodbard, 1953).

Under light general anesthesia stimulation of the lower airway by mechanical or chemical means induces vigorous coughing. Total respiratory compliance falls and then gradually returns to normal. Don and Robson (1966)

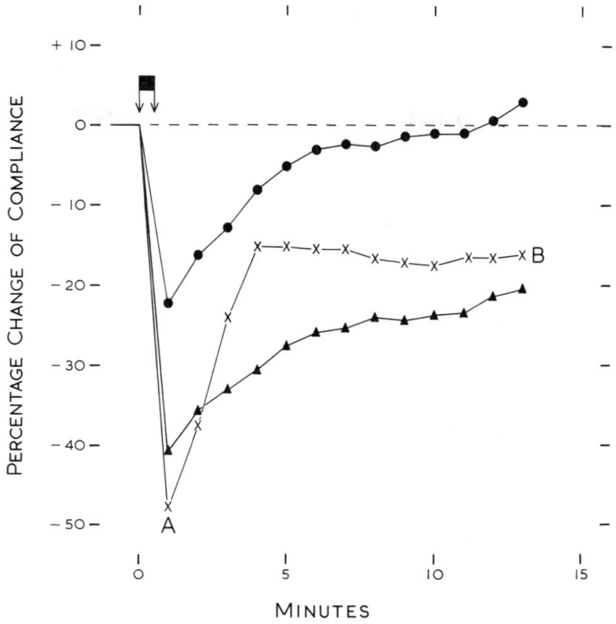

Figure 10–29. Percentage change of total respiratory compliance under light general anesthesia after chemical stimulation of the lower airways by inflation of the lungs with 40 per cent ether vapor (between arrows).
▲——▲ = Controls lightly anesthetized with thiopental and nitrous oxide–oxygen
×——× = Similar to controls, with addition of neuromuscular blockade by rapid infusion of 450 mg succinylcholine between A and B
●——● = Similar to controls, with prior induction of epidural blockade to above T_2, using 1.5 per cent plain lidocaine
(After Bromage, 1958b.)

found that average compliance returned to within 4 per cent of normal after mechanical stimulation of the bronchi in a series of six patients, although one subject had a persistent reduction of 11 per cent. Using brief inflation of the lungs with 40 per cent ether vapor as the noxious stimulus, Bromage (1958b) found a 20 to 40 per cent reduction of total compliance immediately after the induced cough reaction, and 13 minutes later there was still a 16 per cent deficit, even after full neuromuscular blockade with succinylcholine. On the other hand, in the presence of high epidural blockade to a segmental level above T_2, compliance returned to control values within 5 to 11 minutes in 17 out of 18 subjects (Fig. 10–29). Bromage's measurements were made with a simple and crude apparatus, and it would be interesting to see if the rather large difference observed between the relaxant and epidural groups could be validated using more sophisticated recording equipment.

The lung is affected not only by its own neural events but also by indirect effects from autonomic vascular events occurring at a distance in the systemic circulation. For example, a failing left ventricle and congestive heart failure are well-recognized causes of stiffened lungs and an impaired vital capacity (Christie and Meakins, 1934; Levine, 1949; Saxton et al., 1956). Excessive peripheral vasoconstriction also leads to pulmonary edema (Chen and Chai, 1974). The Framingham Heart Disease Epidemiological Study has recently reawakened interest in the vital capacity as a sensitive early warning sign of impending congestive failure before any other overt signs have become apparent, and this well-tried test has some appeal as a simple, noninvasive indicator of myocardial stress (Kannel et al., 1974). Acute reduction of peripheral vasomotor tone by subarachnoid or epidural block, or by ganglionic blockade, in congestive failure has been shown to increase vital capacity by 15 to 35 per cent, depending on the severity of symptoms (Bromage, 1956). During general anesthesia in patients with emphysema and cor pulmonale, preexisting bronchospasm tends to disappear and tidal volume increases when epidural blockade is induced (Bromage, 1954).

Denervation of the thorax by high epidural blockade does not seem to affect the posture of the rib cage, as reflected by the underlying lung volume in conscious volunteers. Measurements of functional residual capacity (FRC) before and after epidural blockade have been made by two independent groups in subjects with normal lungs, under resting conditions prior to elective surgery, and no change of FRC was found by either group (Wahba et al., 1972; McCarthy, 1976). In one series epidural puncture was performed in the lumbar region, and segmental blockade extended to T_4 (Wahba et al., 1972). In the other series epidural puncture was made in the mid-thoracic region, and segmental blockade extended between the second and third thoracic segments and the upper lumbar segments (McCarthy, 1976). These measurements were made by experienced investigators under tranquil and technically impeccable conditions, and the results can therefore be regarded as valid, in contrast to the more doubtful reliability of similar measurements attempted under postoperative conditions, when pain and fatigue impair the accuracy of FRC estimations (Wahba et al., 1975).

In summary, the tranquil breathing that follows epidural blockade is due to two major factors. First, deafferentation of the abdomen and chest wall leads to a reduction of sensory input to the respiratory motor nuclei and consequently to a subdued but adequate motor output. Second, lowered arterial and venous tone from sympathetic blockade lessens the work of the left and right sides of the heart and tends to relieve any preexisting pulmonary congestion. Clearly, if the process of vasodilatation and peripheral venous pooling is carried to excess, venous return will fall to a level where cardiac filling becomes inadequate and output will also fall. Pulmonary perfusion will then lag behind ventilation, and hypoperfusion of lung capillaries will lead to an increased alveolar-arterial oxygen gradient. Good clinical management lies in maintaining the balance between vasomotor tone and vascular volume at a point where venous and arterial pressures are adequate but never excessive.

Spontaneous versus Controlled Respiration

Muscle relaxant techniques abolish respiratory motor activity, so they cannot be used without controlled respiration. On the other hand, epidural blockade carries the option that spontaneous respiration may be adequate for surgical operations that do not intrude upon the thoracic cavity.

The question arises, is it practical to allow a patient to breathe under his own control during long operations or when the surgical procedure involves the upper abdomen, particularly if epidural blockade is combined with light general anesthesia? It may be argued that controlled ventilation is so easy to impose upon the patient that the risk of impaired respiratory exchange under spontaneous respiration is not worth taking.

Sometimes the choice is difficult, for in the presence of a low arterial and central venous pressure, imposition of controlled ventilation will raise the mean intrathoracic pressure and a further fall of cardiac output and blood pressure will occur, unless compensatory venous filling is provided by augmentation of blood volume and peripheral vasomotor tone. Common sense will usually dictate the right course, for it is certainly not worth risking impaired respiratory exchange if there is any question that the patient may not be able to maintain normal arterial oxygenation and pH. Simple measurement of tidal and minute volumes with a Wright spirometer will give a fair indication of respiratory competence. More precise information from arterial blood gas estimations should be available if there is any doubt at all about the efficacy of gas exchange.

Spontaneous respiration under high epidural blockade and light general anesthesia usually maintains satisfactory respiratory exchange surprisingly well for long periods of time, even during the course of upper abdominal surgery. Figure 11–2 (see Chapter 11) shows the acid-base situation of 41 patients breathing spontaneously under high epidural blockade combined with light thiopental and endotracheal nitrous oxide–oxygen anesthesia. It can be seen that in most instances the arterial blood gases remained within the acceptable range of normal physiological sleep.

Consideration of the geometry of the diaphragm provides an important clue to the surprisingly effective gas exchange observed with epidural blockade and spontaneous respiration during abdominal surgery. Early observations with bronchospirometry and double lumen tubes showed that in the lateral position the lower lung is better ventilated and takes up more oxygen than the upper lung (Rothstein et al., 1950). The work of Milic-Emili's group has established that in normal spontaneously breathing subjects, the dependent parts of the lung are better perfused and better ventilated than the upper parts (Kaneko et al., 1966; Milic-Emili et al., 1966). This relationship is maintained under general anesthesia, *provided the patient is breathing spontaneously.* In 1959, Potgieter found that the compliance and ventilation of the lower lung fell by about 25 to 40 per cent in curarized patients placed in the lateral jackknife position, while the upper lung remained relatively well ventilated. This reversal of the normal pattern of ventilation was attributed to the cramped position of the lower chest wall and abdomen in the lateral nephrectomy position. Nunn (1961), Rehder et al. (1964) and Wulff and Aulin (1972) confirmed Potgieter's findings that the normal pattern of ventilation is reversed in curarized subjects and the upper lung becomes better ventilated when spontaneous respiration is replaced by intermittent positive pressure ventilation (IPPV).

More recently, Froese and Bryan (1974) reexamined the effect of general anesthesia, curarization and artificial ventilation on the geometry of the diaphragm. The radiological contour of the diaphragm was recorded in supine volunteers breathing through cuffed endotracheal tubes under four conditions:

1. Awake, breathing spontaneously
2. Under light general anesthesia, breathing spontaneously
3. Awake, curarized and positive pressure ventilation
4. Under light general anesthesia, curarized and positive pressure ventilation.

The results proved to be a very beautiful and practical illustration of the law of Laplace, and they are illustrated successively in Figures 10–30, 10–31 and 10–32, redrawn from the data of Froese and Bryan. In the supine position

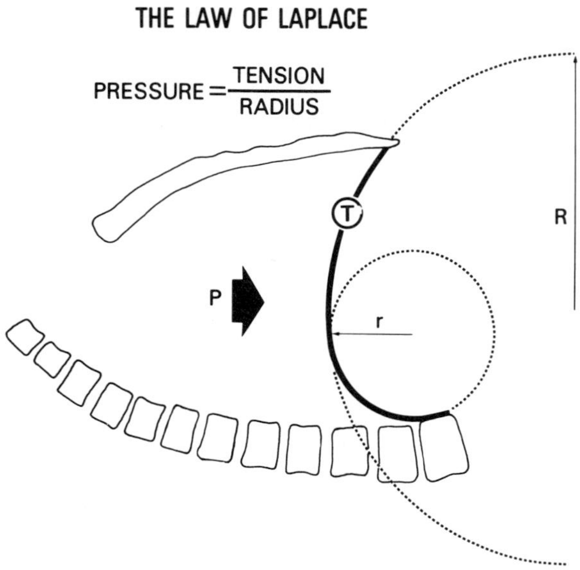

Figure 10–30. The Law of Laplace and the geometry of the diaphragm. The posterior part of the diaphragmatic dome describes an arc of small radius, and it is capable of developing a high downward pressure, since P = T/r. The anterior part of the dome describes an arc of large radius, and the pressure is small, since P = T/R. (After Froese and Bryan, 1974.)

the contour of the diaphragm may be considered as part of the circumference of two circles of different radii, with a small radius posteriorly and a large radius anteriorly (Fig. 10–30). The law of Laplace states that the pressure generated in an elastic sphere will be proportional to the tension in the wall divided by the radius. At any given tension the pressure is large when the radius is small, and the pressure falls as the radius increases. In the supine position the pressure developed along the contour of the diaphragm is evenly balanced against the vertical pressure gradient of the abdominal contents pressing against it. When the diaphragm contracts, the greatest downward pressure is exerted by the posterior portion where the radius is small, and the least pressure is exerted by the anterior portion where the radius is greatest, so during active inspiration the abdominal contents are swept before it in an even fashion, as shown in Figure 10–31.

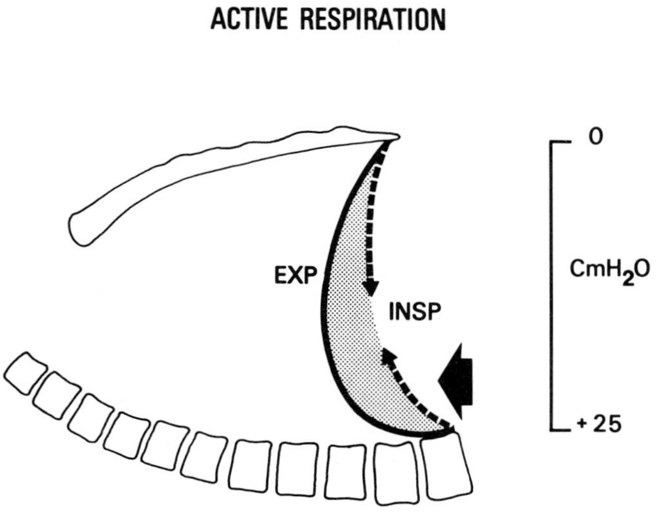

Figure 10–31. Coordinated movements of the diaphragm during spontaneous respiration. In the dorsal position the weight of the abdominal contents pressing against the underside of the diaphragm varies from zero anteriorly to about 25 cmH_2O posteriorly. (After Froese and Bryan, 1974.)

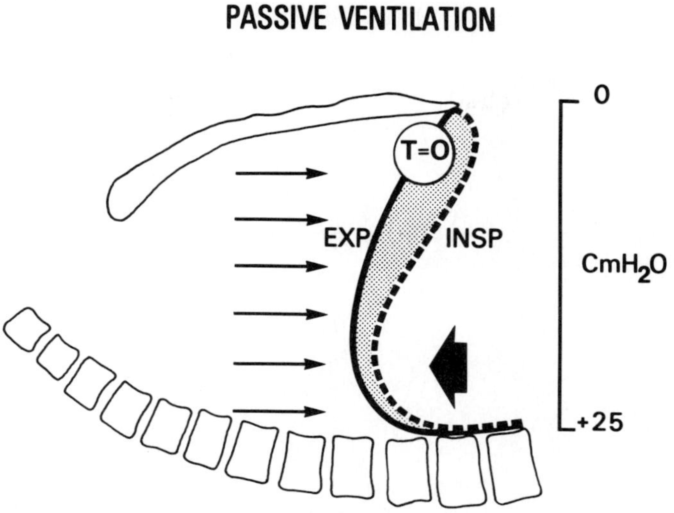

Figure 10–32. Movement of the diaphragm after curarization and during passive ventilation in the dorsal position. Tone (T) in the diaphragm is abolished (T = 0). Inspiratory pressure exerts a uniform pressure against the upper surface of the relaxed diaphragm, while the underside is exposed to the anteroposterior pressure gradient of the abdominal contents. The pattern of diaphragmatic movement is now uneven and determined by the balance of unequal forces acting upon it. (After Froese and Bryan, 1974.)

After curarization, tension is reduced toward zero, the diaphragm becomes a toneless curtain flapping passively between the abdominal and thoracic contents and the contour is determined by the balance of pressures acting upon it. The dorsal portion, being subjected to the greatest abdominal pressure, bulges upward under the weight of the abdominal viscera. Intermittent positive pressure ventilation imposes a uniform downward force during the inspiratory phase, and the abdominal contents, with the diaphragm enclosing them, are shifted most where the opposing pressure is least; the dorsal portion of the diaphragm remains elevated while the anterior part moves downward, as shown in Figure 10–32. Under these circumstances the most dependent parts of the lung move least, and ventilation and compliance may be expected to fall in them, as Potgieter found 15 years earlier.

This pattern of geometric change will occur whenever the diaphragm loses its intrinsic tone and moves passively instead of actively. Curarization is not necessary to bring it about, and the same phenomenon is seen when spontaneous respiration is suppressed and replaced by passive hyperventilation in the presence of light general anesthesia and reduced afferent input. Once tone returns to the diaphragm and spontaneous respiration begins, however, the normal geometry is restored and ventilation returns to the dependent basal portions of the lung.

These same radiological studies also showed that induction of light general anesthesia caused a slight loss of diaphragmatic tone, with a cephalad shift of the end-expiratory position of the diaphragm that was greatest in dependent parts. That is, the resting expiratory position of the diaphragm under general anesthesia is very similar to the curarized position, but in spite of

VENTILATION AND THE LUNG

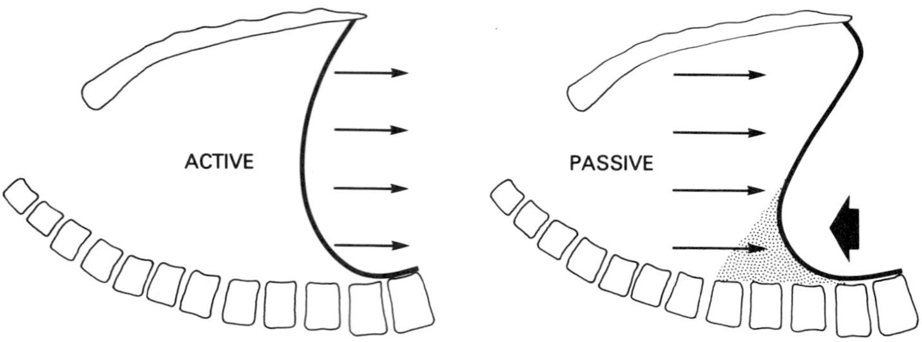

Figure 10–33. The geometry of the diaphragm during spontaneous and passive ventilation in the supine position. Stippled area denotes portions of the lung that receive little ventilation during IPPV. (After Froese and Bryan, 1974.)

this shift of the FRC position, diaphragmatic movements remain greatest in dependent parts, provided the patient breathes spontaneously. Therefore, spontaneous respiration appears to play a significant role in maintaining normal ventilation-perfusion relationships, and it is not something that should be lightly suppressed as a routine maneuver, without some thought being given to the altered respiratory geometry and efficiency that will follow (Fig. 10–33).

However, it must be pointed out that in spite of Froese and Bryan's elegant study, measurements of lung volume and compliance have not been able to distinguish very marked differences between lung mechanics in subjects who are breathing actively and in those who are paralyzed and intubated, *once general anesthesia has been induced.* Several investigations have shown that a sudden but nonprogressive fall of FRC, of between 10 and 25 per cent, occurs almost immediately after induction of light general anesthesia in the supine position (Laws, 1968; Don et al., 1970; Rehder et al., 1971; Westbrook et al., 1973; Hewlett et al., 1974), and this is associated with a fall of compliance of about the same order of magnitude (Howell and Peckett, 1957). This sudden deterioration of lung mechanics associated with induction of light general anesthesia is probably due to the upward shift of position of the diaphragm that occurs as soon as the subjects become anesthetized. As might be expected, the FRC does not fall when anesthesia and paralysis are induced in the sitting position, for then gravity keeps the viscera in their proper place and prevents them from riding upward into the thorax (Rehder et al., 1972).

From a practical point of view, the available laboratory guidance to clinical management of respiration during epidural blockade may be summarized as follows:

1. Normally, respiratory performance is at its best in awake, spontaneously breathing subjects. Diaphragmatic tone is preserved and the FRC remains unchanged, especially if the patient takes an occasional deep breath. There is no fall of compliance, and the work of breathing is not increased. From a respiratory standpoint, it is clearly advantageous to have the patient awake and

cooperative throughout his operation, if it is feasible to do so. However, it is equally plain that there will be many instances in which this ideal must take second place to other interests of the patient and to operative requirements, such as comfort and freedom from anxiety and total control of the anesthetic situation in long, difficult cases; then it is wise to superimpose light general anesthesia.

2. Induction of light general anesthesia will be followed by some loss of resting diaphragmatic tone, the FRC will fall and there will be some accompanying loss of lung compliance, with a resulting increase in respiratory work. However, the dependent parts of the lung will still be well ventilated, since inspiratory diaphragmatic tone is not appreciably affected.

These altered respiratory conditions are tolerable for operations lasting one to three hours, and normal blood gases can usually be maintained during that time, provided the FIO_2 is kept above 0.3 (i.e., an inspired oxygen concentration of 30 per cent or more). In longer operations it is probably wiser to remove the burden of the increased work of breathing and to replace spontaneous respiration with artificial ventilation.

3. Once artificial ventilation has been instituted, the diaphragm behaves as if it had been curarized, and all of its tone disappears. Respiratory mechanics and ventilation-perfusion relationships now follow exactly the same pattern as in a fully curarized patient. Dependent portions of the lung receive less ventilation than before, and in the lateral decubitus the underlying lung receives the lesser instead of the greater share of ventilation. Ventilation-perfusion imbalance occurs from underventilation of overperfused portions of dependent lung, and the alveolar-arterial oxygen gradient increases. For this reason, the inspired oxygen concentration of the ventilating gas mixture should not be allowed to fall below 30 per cent.

These are the ordinary consequences of curarization and IPPV, and the price is acceptable for the sake of sparing the patient the work of breathing. However, unlike the curarized patient, almost full respiratory function is available as soon as consciousness returns, and then coughing and deep breathing exercises can be started at once. Artificial ventilation should be imposed whenever there is any doubt about the patient's ability to maintain satisfactory gas exchange by his own efforts, or when the magnitude of the operation calls for complete control of all functions at all times.

Pain and Breathing

One of the most effective applications of epidural analgesia is the relief of abdominal and thoracic pain arising from a wide variety of causes. It is therefore important to know how pain alters respiratory mechanics and performance, and how these alterations may be modified by interruption of the relevant pain pathways by epidural blockade.

The normal respiratory response to abdominal and thoracic pain is an inhibited grunting pattern of breathing, with tightened accessory muscles of respiration, as if the body were making a cuirass of the trunk muscles to shield the vulnerable viscera from the threatening and painful situation. All the normal parameters of breathing are impaired by this cramped posture of pain. Vital capacity and peak expiratory flow rate are dramatically reduced. Functional residual capacity (FRC) falls by about 20 per cent and lung compliance by the same amount. The intrathoracic end-expiratory pressure rises within the squeezed chest, and central venous pressure also rises. The lungs are ventilated below the normal FRC, so varying degrees of airway closure follow, and coughing is weak and ineffective. Peripheral venous return is impaired for prolonged periods by the Valsalva-like effects of grunting breathing. With very severe pain, cyanosis may be visible, as in acute pancreatitis, from shunting of venous blood through collapsed and underventilated parts of the lung. In some severe cases of acute pancreatitis, the increased shunt ($\dot{Q}s/\dot{Q}t$) has been found to exceed 40 per cent of the cardiac output (Hayes et al., 1974). In the presence of chronic bronchitis or bronchiectasis, impaired coughing may allow retained secretions to collect until the patient literally drowns in his own phlegm (Bromage, 1967b).

The present state of our knowledge about the effects of pain on respiratory function has been built up gradually by laborious measurement over many years. Churchill and McNeil, in 1927, were the first to demonstrate the remarkable inhibition of respiration that follows abdominal operation. They found that vital capacity was reduced by 75 per cent after upper laparotomies and by 40 to 50 per cent after lower laparotomies. Impairment of a similar order has since been confirmed by many others (Head, 1927; Powers, 1928; Overholt, 1930; Beecher, 1933; Lassen, 1938; Pooler, 1949; Brattström, 1954; Bromage, 1955; Simpson et al., 1961; Okinaka, 1965; Diament and Palmer, 1966).

Beecher (1933) suggested that the inhibited respiration associated with abdominal pain might lead to some degree of alveolar closure, and he showed that the FRC fell by 16 per cent on the first postoperative day. Others have also found that the FRC is reduced after abdominal operations (Anscombe, 1957; Brattström, 1954), although some workers have not been able to demonstrate any change of FRC (Colgan and Malloney, 1969). In my own department we also found that FRC tended to be reduced after abdominal surgery. However, it must be pointed out that FRC measurements on postoperative patients are a singularly frustrating and unrewarding exercise, and it is extremely difficult to obtain reliable results using the helium dilution method. The patients are tired and distressed, and it is difficult to coax them into the degree of cooperation that is necessary to obtain regular, even ventilation, and to make sure that airways are close-fitting and free of leaks throughout the time necessary to carry out the test. For this reason, I believe that very little credence should be given to FRC measurements in the postoperative period, and other techniques must be used to provide evidence that pain and restricted movement of the thorax do indeed cause underlying changes in the lung. Two indirect tests that reflect collapse of lung tissue quite faithfully in the postoperative period are:

1. Measurement of lung compliance and respiratory work
2. Estimations of venous admixture by application of the shunt equation to obtain a measure of $\dot{Q}s/\dot{Q}t$

Measurement of (A-a) DO_2 will give a fairly reliable index of intrapulmonary shunting in the presence of a normal and reasonably stable cardiac output.

Both of these indirect methods have provided evidence that some degree of pulmonary collapse is an unavoidable sequel to upper abdominal surgery. Lewis and Welch (1965) found a 30 per cent fall of compliance during the first six hours after upper abdominal surgery. At the same time the proportion of cardiac output shunted through unaerated lungs rises about 12 per cent (Diament and Palmer, 1967; Sjögren and Wright, 1972).

Analgesia and Breathing

> The completeness of the pain relief produced by *successful* extradural block must be seen to be believed. The patient becomes completely unaware of the existence of an upper abdominal wound; his face loses its expression of anxiety and strain, and it is an exciting experience to see a patient, a few hours after gastrectomy, taking deep breaths, coughing vigorously and reaching enthusiastically for his dressing gown.
>
> Simpson et al. (1961)

This is not hyperbole. It is an accurate description of the remarkable change that liberates the patient from his pain, and of the sense of wonder that strikes the watchers at the bedside. The italics are mine, for the trick does not work if segmental blockade is incomplete. Bedside observations such as these are dramatic, and they can be documented visually by still photography, cinematography or videotape, and some of the films listed in Chapter 15 do this with great beauty and persuasion. These are qualitative records, however, and they tell us little of what is happening to the underlying physiological processes. Are the appearances just an illusion, or are there some deeper changes that can be measured and numbered in quantitative terms to support the outward impression of well-being?

The questions to be answered are:

1. Are lung volumes improved by epidural analgesia? Is there a significant restoration of VC and FRC to preoperative levels, and is this restoration larger than with orthodox systemic analgesics?

2. Can the patient really cough better? Is there a measurable increase in tussive force and peak expiratory flow rate?

3. If FRC has been diminished by pain and restored by epidural analgesia, can the improvement be demonstrated by: (a) Improved lung compliance? (b) A greater intrapleural negative pressure at the end-expiratory position? (c) Improved aeration of the lung bases and other possible areas of atelectasis by a diminished venous-arterial shunt ($\dot{Q}s/\dot{Q}t$) and by a smaller oxygen gradient between the alveoli and the arterial blood (i.e., a smaller (A-a) DO_2)?

Although a number of investigators have spent a great deal of time and effort trying to answer these questions, the responses have been depressingly meager. Unfortunately, the nature of the experimental material makes collection of solid repeatable data extremely difficult, particularly when those data call for sophisticated equipment and the sort of steady state that any laboratory worker would take for granted as a fundamental condition for respectable results. There is no steady state in the true sense of the word (Finer, 1970). Patients tire easily and progressively after major abdominal surgery, and they crave to be left alone. However willing and cooperative they may be, they cannot do all the things that are asked of them consistently, over a prolonged period of time, and the investigator must pay unusually obsessive attention to every detail to make sure that errors of measurement are avoided. Mouthpieces for spirometers and helium circuits are not held tightly by tired patients, and face masks tend to leak in the presence of nasal tubes from gastric or esophageal balloons left in place for measurements of abdominal and intrapleural pressure.

In order to avoid the complicating element of progressive fatigue, comparative measurements during periods of pain and analgesia must be simple and undemanding, and they should not cause unnecessary discomfort and arouse resentment in patients. In addition, they should be completed as quickly as possible, within the first four to six postoperative hours, before the patient becomes overtired and resentful. Simple isolated measurements, such as vital capacity or peak expiratory flow rate, may continue to yield satisfactory results at later stages if they are not overdone. However, the more difficult and demanding measurements of compliance, FRC and oxygen uptake are less likely to give satisfaction to the investigator, for even when done with the greatest gentleness and consideration, they are prone to antagonize the patient. Lastly, assessment of the effects of epidural analgesia demands that the investigator have rigorous objective evidence that segmental analgesia has been satisfactory throughout the run of his respiratory tests. This means that each recording run must be preceded and followed by measurement of the segmental area of cutaneous analgesia, and any patient with "missed segments," that is, a patch of ineffective cutaneous analgesia, should be excluded from the series.

Bearing in mind these constraints, it can be appreciated that a good deal of forethought must be given to designing a protocol that will give valid data. Whenever possible, comparative measurements of objective analgesic performance in the postoperative period should be planned in the following way:

1. Measurements should begin as soon as is feasible after recovery from general anesthesia and before the patient becomes exhausted and irritated by repeated testing. Gas dilution and washout techniques for estimating FRC must be postponed until elimination of inhaled gases, such as nitrous oxide, has reached insignificant proportions. In practice, this means waiting about 45 to 60 minutes before commencing this type of investigation. Most subjects will have reached the end of their patience after four to six hours of intensive study, and it is neither humane nor useful to push data collection beyond that point.

2. Because of the great variability between individuals, each patient should function as his own control, and paired comparisons should be made between analgesic methods. Pooled data require large numbers, and subtleties of individual changes are hidden in the mass, as will be seen a little further on when our compliance data are presented in a pooled and in an individual manner.

3. The protocol should not attempt to extract too much data from any one subject. It is unreasonable to attempt to measure lung volumes, lung dynamics, (A-a) DO_2, and cardiac output and venous-arterial shunts all in the same subject. For example, serial compliance measurements by themselves are enough for any one patient to tolerate cheerfully. The addition of a second test, such as serial FRC measurements, will quickly overtire the patient and spoil the quality of cooperation, to the detriment of the resultant data from both tests.

A review of the literature will show that these rather obvious constraints may explain some of the apparently divergent reports that have appeared on the subject (Holmdahl et al., 1972). In some instances, measurements have not been started until 17 hours after operation, and by that time wound edema and patchy atelectasis may have become established, adding their own fixed handicaps to hinder any functional restoration that may be attempted.

Objective Assessment of Epidural Analgesia and Breathing

Lung volume measurement

Vital Capacity (VC). A spirometer and kymograph are still among the simplest and most useful pieces of apparatus for assessing postoperative analgesia in an objective fashion after abdominal or thoracic surgery. They test both the ability and the willingness of the patient to fill and empty his lungs; timed forced expiratory volumes can be obtained by using a fast drum speed.

If the preoperative VC is regarded as the optimal standard for each patient, serial postoperative VC readings can be used to assess the effects of pain and analgesia. The results may be expressed in the form of the respiratory restoration factor (RRF). This factor gives the improvement of VC with the analgesic, as a percentage of the improvement that would occur if the VC were to return to its ideal preoperative value (Bromage, 1955), as shown in Figure 10–34. A perfect analgesic would restore the VC to its normal preoperative level, so it would have an RRF of 100 per cent, whereas an ineffectual drug would make no difference and would have an RRF of 0 per cent. Epidural blockade rates highest among postoperative analgesic procedures by this rating, as shown in Table 10–5. In this table, Bromage's figure for an 80 per cent RRF with epidural

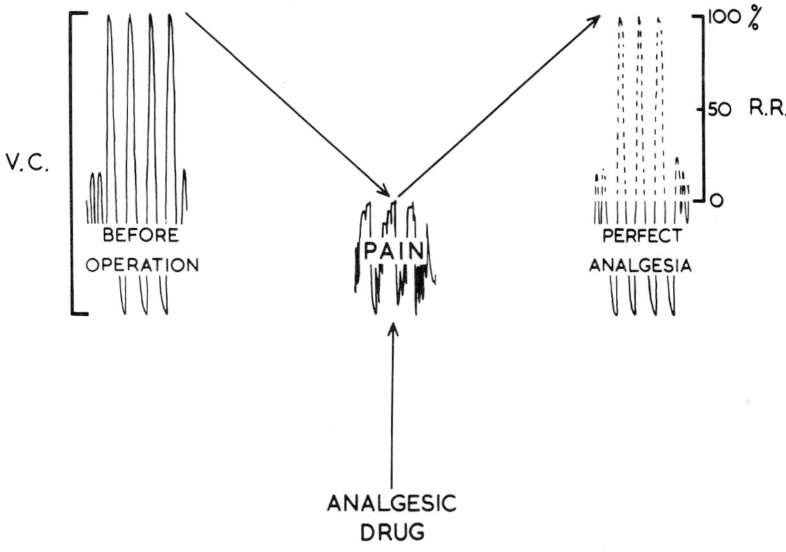

Figure 10–34. The respiratory restoration factor. The RRF is calculated thus:

$$\text{RRF} = \frac{\text{Analgesic VC} - \text{Pain VC}}{\text{Preoperative VC} - \text{Pain VC}} \times 100$$

TABLE 10–5 Comparison of Respiratory Restoration Factors

Procedure	*RRF (%)*	*Author*
Epidural	80 (corrected value 74 – see text)	Bromage (1955)
Epidural	54.5	Simpson et al. (1961)
Methadone	35.4	Bromage (1955)
Methadone	16	Parbrook (1966)
25% Nitrous oxide	23.5	Parbrook and Kennedy (1964)
Demerol	13.5	Bromage (1955)
IV lidocaine	22.8	Bromage (1955)

analgesia is artificially high, as 4 out of the 18 subjects studied had some degree of left heart strain and pulmonary congestion in the preoperative period, and their improved vital capacity may have been due, in part, to a degree of hypotension induced by the epidural blockade (Bromage, 1956). Correction of Bromage's original series, by exclusion of the cases with pulmonary congestion, reduces the average RRF due to epidural blockade to 74 per cent. Restoration of vital capacity by effective epidural analgesia is most marked during the early postoperative period. Measurements made on the day after surgery show much less effect. Holmdahl's group found an epidural RRF of only 23 per cent 24 hours after upper abdominal surgery (Holmdahl et al., 1972; Sjögren and Wright, 1972).

Peak Expiratory Flow Rate (PEFR). This measures the patient's ability and willingness to make a sharp, tussive blast. It is a simple and rapid test, but it places greater demands on the abdominal muscles and so tests the quality of analgesia more rigorously than a series of vital capacity readings. In average subjects, the peak expiratory flow rate is reduced from a preoperative level of about 300 l/min to about 90 l/min after upper abdominal surgery, and it is usually restored to about 150 to 200 l/min by effective epidural blockade. Systemic analgesics cause an appreciably smaller improvement.

Functional Residual Capacity (FRC). In theory, serial measurements of FRC should give a good estimate of changes in underlying lung volume secondary to breathing below the normal end-expiratory position. Effective analgesia followed by deep breathing should reexpand any collapsed and underventilated areas of lung, and this should be reflected in an increased FRC. Unfortunately, serial FRC measurements are difficult to perform with any degree of accuracy after major surgery. As mentioned earlier, patients are tired and find it difficult to cooperate in maintaining regular breathing and in keeping a gas-tight fit around the mouthpiece of rebreathing circuits for long enough to complete a test. Consequently, technical errors are large in relation to the small change of FRC that may be anticipated, and in our hands the method has not proved to be a practical or reliable form of measurement in the early postoperative period.

Alexander and his colleagues (1971) have used the closed-circuit nitrogen dilution technique to investigate changes of FRC after upper abdominal surgery, and they report a mean reduction of 28 per cent. This is somewhat on the high side of the figure that might be expected if the technique were entirely dependable, but these results must also be regarded with some reserve because of the difficult conditions of measurement. The same group approached this problem from a slightly different angle, using the end tidal position and an estimate of closing volume by xenon dilution, without any real success in arriving at a precise figure for postoperative loss of lung volume (Alexander et al., 1972). Wahba et al. (1975) have reported a mean FRC reduction of 21.7 per cent during pain after upper abdominal surgery, but a fall of only 16 per cent when pain was relieved by epidural analgesia.

When these data are considered, it must be reemphasized that while falls of FRC can be demonstrated with considerable accuracy under general anesthesia during which airways are reliably gas-tight and breathing is regular and well controlled (Don et al., 1970), it is quite apparent that comparable accuracy is unattainable in the conscious postoperative state using current techniques of measurement.

Blood gas measurement

Shunting through collapsed areas of lung and increased venous admixture should be reflected by arterial hypoxemia and by an alveolar-arterial oxygen gradient—(A-a) DO_2—that is increased in proportion to the degree of shunt. Again, measurements based on this assumption have been disappointing and have failed to reveal a clear correlation with different methods of postoperative analgesia. All that can be said is that most authors have reported better arterial oxygenation after epidural analgesia than after narcotic pain relief. Muneyuki et al. (1968) found an increase of PaO_2 after epidural analgesia and a fall after narcotic administration, but the difference was not very great, perhaps because they were comparing the effects of narcotics in a young group (mean age 29.2 years) with those of epidurals in a significantly older population (mean age 46.7 years). However, Spence and Smith (1971) reported that arterial oxygenation and (A-a) DO_2 were markedly better after epidural blockade than after morphine analgesia. Hollmén and Saukkonen (1972) also found appreciably improved oxygen tensions associated with less evidence of shunting after effective epidural blockade in the early postoperative period.

On the day after operation Sjögren and Wright (1972) found that shunting ($\dot{Q}s/\dot{Q}t$) and the (A-a) DO_2 were appreciably worse than in the immediate postoperative period, and after 20 hours epidural analgesia did not lessen the degree of shunting to any significant degree. Pflug et al. (1974) had similar findings.

These blood gas data suggest that the beneficial effects of epidural analgesia are more likely to be evident in the early postoperative phase than on the following day. The clinical implication is that epidural analgesia should be used fairly soon after surgery in order to obtain its best respiratory effects.

Compliance studies

So far, the idea that areas of the lungs collapse in the presence of postoperative pain and reexpand again with effective analgesia has found no experimental support in this review. Under the uniquely difficult conditions imposed on clinical measurement, technical inaccuracies have introduced a will-o'-the-wisp factor into the experimental search. FRC measurements have proved almost useless, and blood gas changes, being dependent on both cardiac and pulmonary variables, give information that is only remotely inferential.

A third approach, the study of lung dynamics, has yielded some quite suggestive results, but again these measurements give only indirect evidence of underlying changes of lung volume, and the results should not be overinterpreted.

Lewis and Welch (1965), using an esophageal balloon to indicate intrathoracic pressure and a wedge spirometer to measure volume and flow, examined the pressure-flow and pressure-volume relationships after upper abdominal and thoracic surgery in 33 patients. They found that compliance ($\Delta Vt/\Delta P$) fell by about 35 per cent within the first six hours after operation, and the work of breathing was also increased, although not significantly. The study did not attempt to obtain corroborative evidence of FRC changes by measuring end-expiratory intrathoracic pressure to indicate possible changes of end tidal position.

We studied compliance and airway resistance in 39 patients after upper abdominal surgery, an esophageal balloon being used to provide an index of intrapleural pressure and a pneumotachygraph to measure air flow at the mouth (Crowell, Pettigrew and Bromage, unpublished observations, 1961–1963). Gas leaks were avoided as far as possible by padding the nostrils under a nose clip, and by an assistant holding the facial tissues in close apposition to the mouthpiece while all measurements were made. The pneumotachograph was calibrated directly from a large rotameter reading between 0 and 500 l/min. Tidal volumes were computed from flow tracings, and pressure-volume loops were constructed by hand, taking points of no-flow as the end-inspiratory and end-expiratory positions in the conventional manner. In some cases pressure-flow loops were recorded photographically on the x and y axes of a Tektronix oscilloscope, but this system did not yield the degree of accuracy obtained by the more laborious method of loop construction by hand.

Postoperative measurements were made in the following sequence starting about one hour after full recovery from light general anesthesia:

1. During pain
2. After effective epidural blockade to T_2–T_3 to include all painful segments, using 0.9 to 1.0 per cent lidocaine plus 1/220, 000 to 1/200,000 epinephrine
3. During pain after the block had again regressed
4. After a generous dose of intravenous Demerol (0.7 mg per kilogram body weight, given slowly)
5. In a few cases, after reinstitution of epidural blockade while the Demerol was still active, in order to estimate the effect of the centrally acting narcotic combined with segmental blockade

Satisfactory measurements were obtained in 24 of the 39 patients. Typical pressure volume loops obtained during quiet and deep breathing from one patient are shown in Figure 10–35.

The most obvious feature of these comparative loops is a markedly increased inspiratory volume with epidural blockade. However, note also the shift toward greater intrapleural (esophageal) negativity during epidural

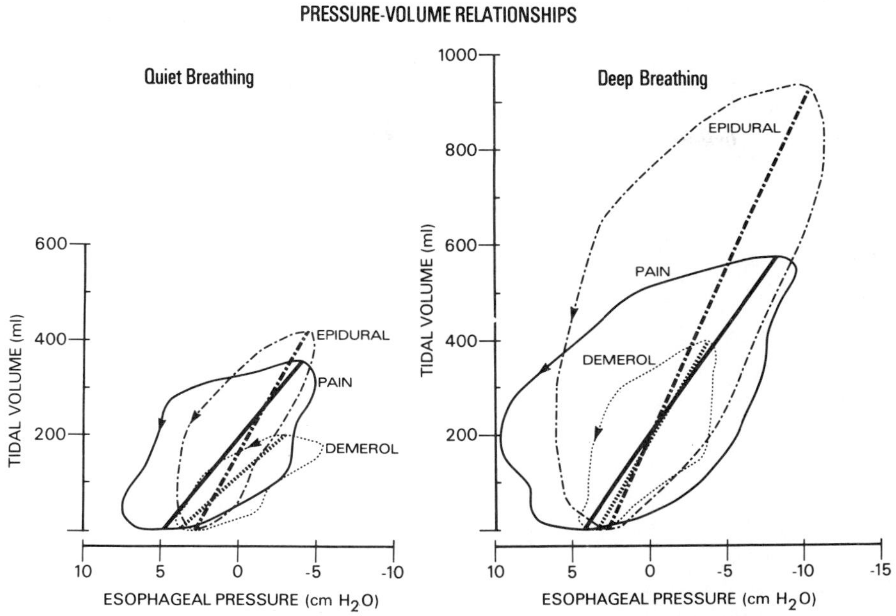

Figure 10–35. Thoracic pressure volume loops two to six hours after cholecystectomy, during pain and during analgesia produced by epidural blockade to T_2–T_3 and by demerol (IV 0.7 mg/kg). Compliance lines are drawn to connect moments of no-flow at the end-inspiratory and end-expiratory points.
——— = Pain
-·-·-·-·· = Epidural
--------- = Demerol (meperidine)

analgesia and the steeper slope in the compliance line, showing an improved pulmonary compliance. During periods of pain, the inspiratory volume is reduced and the pressure-volume loop changes to the squat type of pattern seen typically in obstructive lung disease. The dose of Demerol was clearly excessive in this particular patient, and tidal volume was markedly depressed at the time the post-Demerol recordings were made.

Table 10–6 shows the average results from 24 patients in whom satisfactory pressure-volume readings were obtained during postoperative abdominal pain and then after analgesia provided by epidural blockade or Demerol. These results are summarized graphically in Figure 10–36. End-expiratory pressure gives an indirect index of the resting position of the chest wall, assuming that the glottis is open, and this is an assumption that can be verified by the shape of the pressure-volume loops. A statistical comparison of end-expiratory pressures outlined below Table 10–6 shows the results of paired t-tests in those patients who received both types of analgesia. During quiet breathing, Demerol appears to perform almost as well as epidural analgesia in restoring intrathoracic negativity toward the normal resting position. The difference becomes much more apparent during deep breathing, when epidural analgesia stands out in a class by itself.

Consistently satisfactory measurements of nonelastic resistance were difficult to obtain because of oscillations of esophageal pressure produced by

TABLE 10-6 Respiratory Pressure-Volume Relationships in Postoperative Abdominal Pain, and after Analgesia with Epidural Blockade or Meperidine in 24 Patients*

	n	*Mean End-Expiratory Pressure (cmH_2O)*	*Mean End-Inspiratory Pressure (cmH_2O)*	*Tidal Volume (ml)*	*Compliance (ml/cmH_2O)*	*% Change of Compliance from Pain*
Quiet breathing						
Pain	24	−0.7	−7.57	489	71.2	–
Epidural	16	−2.54	−9.38	623	93.8	+31.8
Meperidine	15	−2.01	−9.54	520	69	−3.1
Deep breathing						
Pain	8	−2.06	−12.07	822	82.1	–
Epidural	8	−4.31	−17.81	1,364	101	+23
Meperidine	8	−2.35	−12.87	836	79.4	−3.3

Significance of change of end-expiratory pressure (paired t-test):

Quiet breathing
- Pain-epidural: $0.025 > p > 0.01$
- Pain-meperidine: $0.05 > p > 0.025$
- Epidural-meperidine: N.S.

Deep breathing
- Pain-epidural: $p < 0.005$
- Pain-meperidine: N.S.
- Epidural-meperidine: $p < 0.001$

*Unpublished data by Crowell, Pettigrew and Bromage (1961–1963).

transmitted cardiac action in the semisupine position. There was a general tendency for respiratory resistance to be higher in the presence of pain than after epidural blockade. This rise of airway resistance during periods of pain was probably due to glottic action and the grunting type of breathing associated with severe upper abdominal pain. However, in some cases, large airway resistances were also observed under epidural blockade at times of rapid flow during maximum deep breathing. Simpson and his colleagues remarked on a similar observation of increased airway resistance in their paper of 1961. I have interpreted this finding as arising from length-tension inappropriateness (Campbell, 1966) during partial deafferentation of the chest wall. In the absence of complete proprioceptive information, the chest wall is likely to act in the manner of a tabetic limb, exerting force that is excessive for the immediate task in hand (Davis, 1965), and this tabes-like state is likely to be expressed as a bulging type of pressure-flow loop when the patient exerts himself fully to perform maximum deep breathing. We have examined this aspect of chest wall deafferentation in cats by adding elastic loads during epidural blockade (Lynne-Davis et al., 1971), but the conditions of these experiments are too far removed from clinical conditions in the postoperative period to be able to draw any useful comparisons.

In our clinical studies, esophageal balloon pressure was taken relative to atmospheric and not airway pressure, so the measurements merely provided an index of *relative* changes of compliance rather than absolute values of lung

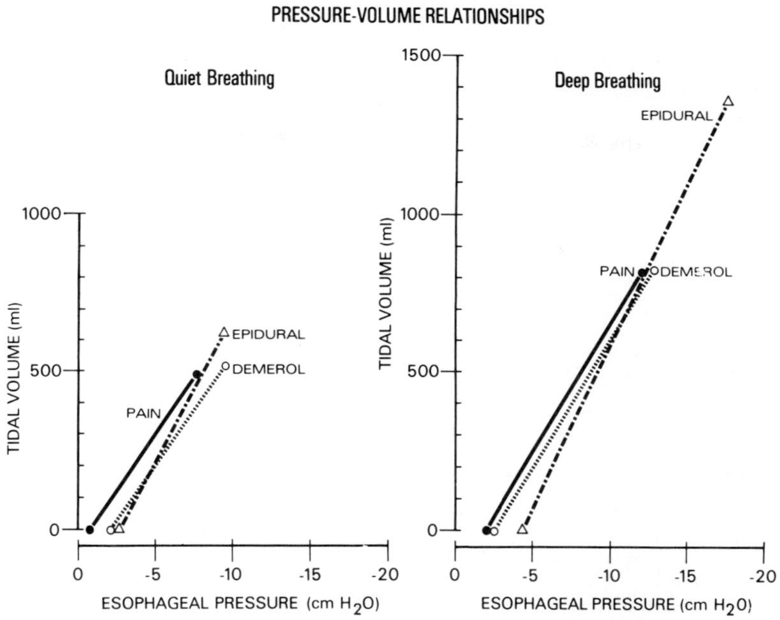

Figure 10–36. Compliance lines drawn between average points of inspiratory and expiratory no-flow in 24 patients during postoperative abdominal pain and after epidural blockade or systemic analgesia provided by intravenous Demerol. Note that the average end-expiratory position is less negative with pain and after Demerol than after effective epidural blockade.

●——● = Pain
△-·-·-△ = Epidural
○------○ = Demerol (meperidine)

compliance. Nevertheless, they do show three things in support of the idea that epidural analgesia allows reexpansion of the lung that has remained collapsed by the reflex defensive reaction to pain. First, they confirm that tidal volumes during quiet and deep breathing are larger than in the presence of pain or of analgesia supplied by a centrally acting narcotic. Second, they show that total compliance is improved during quiet and deep breathing. Thirdly, they demonstrate a significant shift of the end-expiratory pressure toward increased intrathoracic negativity in quiet and deep breathing under epidural analgesia. Demerol improves end-expiratory and end-inspiratory negativity during quiet breathing, but it does not appear to have any appreciable effect on intrathoracic negativity, or on compliance, during efforts at deep breathing.

These figures do not furnish direct proof that epidural analgesia restores the FRC after upper abdominal surgery. However, they offer quite strong circumstantial support to the claim that epidural analgesia probably does permit the chest wall to move outward to a more normal resting position than when pain is felt, and during deep breathing it appears to do this significantly better than a centrally acting narcotic.

Taking all the evidence together, the picture of improved lung expansion after effective epidural analgesia appears unequivocal, but at the present time definitive proof still eludes search, and in the end one is forced back to the beginning and to the simple tests that can be made at the bedside, with some assurance of accurate and compelling, though inconclusive, measurement.

EFFECTS ON THE PARTURIENT UTERUS AND THE FETUS

Anesthesia, whether regional or general, may affect the progress of labor and the circulation of the uterus w th its passenger inside. This section will outline a few of the relevant physiological factors; the practical applications will be dealt with in Chapter 12.

Uterine blood vessels respond to adrenergic stimuli in the same way as vascular beds in most other parts of the body. Alpha adrenergic agents cause vasoconstriction, and norepinephrine appears to be the most powerful vasoconstrictor, while some degree of vasodilatation may be caused by beta adrenergic agents, such as metaproterenol (Wallenburg et al., 1973). However, the gravid uterine vascular bed appears to be fully dilated under normal circumstances, and active vasodilatation can only occur under conditions of vasoconstriction, as in preeclampsia, when alpha adrenergic blockers, or beta adrenergic stimulators, may be expected to exert a beneficial effect by increasing uteroplacental flow.

The literature on uterine blood flow and placental perfusion contains some contradictory views stemming from differences of methodology. Until quite recently, it was customary to measure uterine activity and fetal performance with the mother lying on her back. While the supine position simplifies the observer's task when making adjustments of his monitoring equipment, unfortunately it is also the worst possible position from the point of view of uterine blood flow and fetal gas exchange, for the heavy uterus falls backward and causes varying degrees of aortocaval compression. This is the main reason why so much of the published work on uterine blood flow, uterine action and resultant fetal acid-base balance appears confusing and contradictory. The reader is cautioned to screen original papers with an eye to the crucial question of maternal posture and to discard, or at least consign to an intellectual limbo, any work that fails to state clearly whether the mother was lying on her back or on her side when the measurements were made.

Caldeyro-Barcia and his colleagues at Montevideo were the first to point out the adverse effects of the dorsal position on uterine action during labor, when they noted that basal tonus rose when the mother was on her back, while tonus fell and contractility improved when she was turned on her side (Noriega et al., 1959; Caldeyro-Barcia, 1960). Since then, data have slowly accumulated, and now the evidence is incontrovertible that of all possible positions for labor and delivery, the dorsal posture has the worst effects on both maternal and fetal circulations. The effects of the dorsal posture at term are discussed in Chapters 2 and 12; here it is only necessary to emphasize that the effects of gravity in the dorsal position may overshadow all other variables affecting uterine blood flow and fetal well-being. The most sophisticated measurements of uterine flow and fetal performance may be rendered utterly meaningless if this fundamental question of posture is overlooked.

In the simplest terms, uterine blood flow is directly proportional to the perfusion pressure (that is, arterial minus venous pressure) and inversely proportional to resistance to the perfusion pressure. Resistance is made up of several components operating in response to different stimuli, under the general headings (a) intrinsic resistance—that is, vascular resistance of myometrial and placental blood vessels, and (b) extrinsic resistance—that is, compressive resistance caused by the resting tonus in the myometrium and by the periodic contractions superimposed on the basal tonus. Each of these factors will be considered separately.

Uterine Perfusion Pressure

At term, uterine blood flow has increased 30- or 40-fold (Metcalfe et al., 1959), and uterine responses to vasoconstrictor agents are decreased (Ladner et al., 1970; Ferris et al., 1972). The enormous increase in uterine flow at term accounts for about 10 to 15 per cent of the cardiac output and appears to be due, at least partially, to local production of prostaglandins (Terragno et al., 1974).

Perfusion pressure (arterial minus venous pressure) is reduced if uterine venous pressure increases as a result of outflow obstruction arising from compression of the inferior vena cava by the gravid uterus. Normally, there is a linear relationship between arterial pressure and uterine blood flow, and this is determined by the pressure in the uterine arteries (Greiss, 1966). However, it is important to appreciate that arterial pressure measured at the arm may not necessarily be a true index of uterine arterial pressure if the aorta is partially occluded by the gravid uterus during contraction in the supine position (Bieniarz et al., 1968).

Uterine Vasoconstriction

Throughout pregnancy, the ectodermal neural elements of the uterus hold themselves aloof from the rapid process of expansion going on in the mesenchymal tissues round about them, and the static population of the adrenergic nerve endings becomes sparsely scattered throughout the burgeoning mass of muscle and blood vessels (Ryan et al., 1974). For some reason that is not entirely clear, uterine blood flow remains more responsive to neural and blood-borne adrenergic constrictor influences than might be expected, in view of the very large dilutional effects of spatial expansion and increased blood flow in the gravid uterus at term. Although the responses to vasoconstrictor influences are less than normal (Ladner et al., 1970; Ferris et al., 1972), the vasoconstrictive response to sympathetic neural stimulation is still about one half that of the nonpregnant uterus, while the responsiveness to circulating vasoconstrictor agents is only reduced by about one quarter (Ryan et al., 1974).

Vasoconstrictors are often added to local anesthetic agents to slow absorption in the epidural space, but this practice raises the possibility that they may also cause undesirable degrees of uterine vasoconstriction. Adamson et al. (1971) found that infusion of catecholamines in pregnant monkeys caused acidosis in the fetus, but the critical dose rate was above 0.5 μg/kg/min, a rate that is well in excess of the maximum that could be achieved by generally accepted epidural dosage in clinical use today. For example, a single-shot epidural dose of 16 ml of 1 per cent lidocaine with 1/200,000 epinephrine contains $16 \times 5 = 80$ μg epinephrine; this amount of epinephrine is gradually absorbed over a period of at least 10 to 15 minutes, so the peak rate of absorption is never likely to exceed 0.088 to 0.15 μg/kg/min over a relatively short period of time.

Nevertheless, the uterine responsiveness to vasoconstrictor influences is still very much in evidence, for under stress the reproductive tissues at term behave somewhat like the kidney in that placental blood flow is sacrificed to the survival of the total organism. And so catecholamines remain a power to be reckoned with when their effects on uterine vasoconstriction, uterine blood flow and fetal gas exchange are considered. Electrical stimulation of the sympathetic nerves to the uterus in sheep increases vascular resistance by about 65 per cent, while fear and stress reduce uterine blood flow by about 25 to 33 per cent (Greiss and Gobble, 1967). Angiographic studies in rabbits have shown that close arterial injection of minute amounts of catecholamines has profound effects on uteroplacental blood flow (Carter and Olin, 1972). Norepinephrine, with its predominantly alpha adrenergic effects, appears to be more potent than epinephrine in this respect, and Carter and Olin found that quantities as small as 0.01 ng of norepinephrine shut down uteroplacental flow to about the same degree as 5 ng of epinephrine. This effect is prevented by prior administration of the alpha-blocker phenoxybenzamine. Studies of uterine artery blood flow, using chronically implanted flow probes, have yielded similar results in sheep. Barton and his colleagues (1974) found that a 50 per cent reduction of uterine flow was caused by close arterial injection of norepinephrine in the dose range of 2 to 10 ng/ml or of epinephrine at a concentration of 3 to 13 ng/ml. Concentrations of norepinephrine as low as 1.5 to 2.5 ng/ml reduced uterine blood flow by about 30 per cent. These are concentrations of catecholamines that lie within the clinical range encountered during anxiety or surgery (Barton et al., 1974). The same group of investigators found that intravenous epinephrine infused at a rate of 0.1 μg/kg/min had very little effect on uterine blood flow, and doses of three times this amount were required to reduce uterine blood flow by 38 per cent (Rosenfeld et al., 1976). Closer to the fetus, within the uteroplacental unit as a whole, blood is again redistributed in favor of the mother under conditions of stress, and the placental fraction of uteroplacental flow is reduced by one third while myometrial flow is preserved (Duncan and Lewis, 1969; Duncan, 1969).

Shnider and his colleagues have also investigated the effects of small doses of epinephrine (in the range of 60 to 80 μg) added to epidural anesthetic solutions in pregnant ewes. The study was designed to see whether any redistribution of placental blood flow occurs under conditions which mimic clinical epidural analgesia very closely, and if so whether there are any ill effects on the fetus (Wallis et al., 1976). The results of this investigation were generally reassuring and in summary were as shown in Table 10–7.

TABLE 10–7 Changes of Uteroplacental Blood Flow and Fetal Status, Associated with Epidural Analgesia to T_8 with 1.5 Per Cent Chloroprocaine in Pregnant Sheep*

Uterine Blood Flow (UBF)

Total UBF remained unchanged in ewes receiving plain chloroprocaine. Added epinephrine (60 to 80 μg) caused a transient fall of UBF of 14 per cent lasting for about 15 minutes.

Uteroplacental Distribution of Blood Flow

Unchanged from control values of 84 per cent to placenta and 14 per cent to uterine tissue with both plain and epinephrine-added chloroprocaine.

Fetal Cardiovascular Changes

Fetal blood pressure and pulse rate fell slightly (5 to 10 per cent) when epinephrine was omitted but remained stable at control levels when epinephrine was added to the epidural anesthetic.

Fetal Acid-Base Status

No change, with or without added epinephrine in the epidural anesthetic solution.

*Data from Wallis et al., 1976.

Thus, epinephrine added to the epidural anesthetic in these doses of 60 to 80 μg does not appear to elicit a stress response in the mother. Blood is not shunted away from the placental circulation, and there are no demonstrably harmful effects to either placental flow or fetal well-being.

From these data it may be inferred that alpha sympathetic overactivity from any cause will reduce uterine blood flow in a manner similar to that operating in other organs, such as the liver and kidney. Conversely, blockade of alpha sympathetic activity will protect uterine blood flow from episodic vasoconstriction. This inference is true as far as it goes, but sympathetic blockade has other effects that may outweigh the benefits of uterine vasodilatation, and net uterine flow will depend upon the balance that is struck between the opposing forces. These will now be considered.

Gravity and Inferior Vena Caval Compression

Sympathetic blockade to the uterus, with accompanying loss of sympathetic tone in the pelvis and legs, has one other profoundly important and potentially dangerous effect already mentioned earlier in this chapter. The parturient uterus is unique in its capacity to either nourish or destroy its fruit under the simple influence of gravity. The supine hypotensive syndrome may arise when a parturient woman lies on her back, the weight of the gravid uterus compressing the great vessels as they traverse the lumbar region and the pelvic brim, and hypotension is likely to be more profound when sympathetic tone is suppressed in the legs and pelvis. When sympathetic tone is active in the lower limbs, venous blood returns under sufficient pressure to force a passage to the heart through the vertebral and azygos systems, even if the vena cava is occluded by the full weight of the uterus pressing on it in the dorsal position. When sympathetic tone to the legs is removed by spinal blockade or any other cause, however, the vital vis a tergo directing blood into the azygos pathway may be insufficient to ensure an adequate venous return. Then cardiac output falls, uterine perfusion also falls linearly with the declining blood pressure and fetal gas exchange deteriorates. At best, the fetus becomes acidotic, but if the process is carried far enough fetal death may ensue. It is interesting to note that recent work from Wood's group in Melbourne has shown evidence of increased fetal acidosis from caval compression during vaginal delivery in the orthodox lithotomy position, even in the absence of total sympathetic blockade (Humphrey et al., 1973, 1974). Thus, every effort must be made to avoid caval compression due to gravity, and women at term should never be allowed to lie flat on their backs. Some degree of lateral tilt must always be provided. They should be nursed on their sides, and if the lithotomy position is adopted for delivery, then a sandbag or wedge should be placed under one hip to tilt the pelvis about 15 degrees laterally, in order to displace the uterus away from the inferior vena cava.

Myometrial Tone and Oxytocin Infusion

Myometrial tone is a powerful determinant of placental perfusion by its contribution of the factor of *extrinsic vascular resistance.* Caldeyro-Barcia and Poseiro (1960) showed that placental perfusion is maximum during uterine diastole. Flow falls during a uterine contraction and then rises again as the contraction recedes. Conditions that cause an increase in diastolic or "basal tonus" of the uterus reduce perfusion to the placenta during periods between contractions. This mechanism of reduced placental perfusion is one of the principal hazards of oxytocin-induced labor.

Figure 10–37, taken from Caldeyro-Barcia and Poseiro's work (1960), shows the steady rise in basal tonus that occurs with an increasing infusion rate of oxytocin. Caldeyro-Barcia warned that an infusion rate of 16 mU oxytocin per minute was about the maximum safe upper limit, beyond which heightened diastolic tonus would rise above 12 mmHg and jeopardize fetal gas exchange. It must be appreciated that in Caldeyro-Barcia's series, as in all similar investigations at that time, measurements of maternal and fetal parameters were made with the mother lying in the dorsal position, inevitably with some degree of

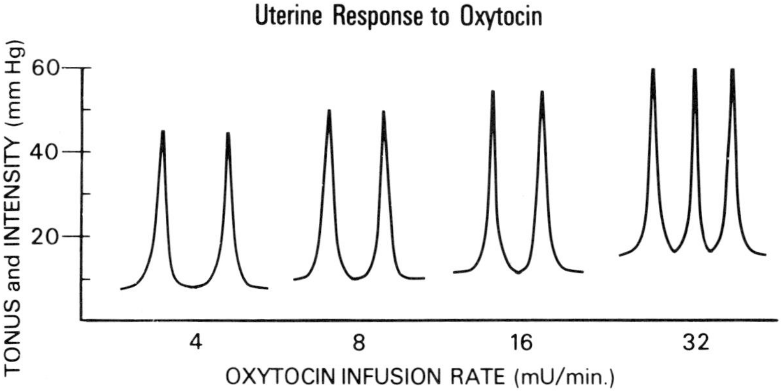

Figure 10–37. Increasing tonus, contractility and tachysystolia with increasing infusion rates of oxytocin during labor. *N.B.:* Recordings made in dorsal position. (After Caldeyro-Barcia and Poseiro, 1960.)

caval compression complicating the clinical situation. More recently, investigations of fetal acid-base balance with the mother in the lateral position have failed to show any adverse effects from oxytocin infusion raising the basal tonus to 20 mmHg, *provided the dorsal position was avoided at all times* (Weaver et al., 1974).

Debate still continues over the possible dangers, or safety, of oxytocin-driven labor and the practice of "nine-to-five o'clock obstetrics," and undoubtedly the last word in this argument has not yet been heard. Greiss (1973), with his great weight of practical and laboratory experience in the field of uterine blood flow, has sounded a warning that brings a note of wise reserve to the debate: " . . . the reason for a desultory state of labor in some patients, without obvious cause, makes for interesting speculation. Some unrecognized feedback mechanism could be at work protecting a threatened fetus. It would be wise to monitor the fetus carefully if such labors are stimulated with oxytocin." Recently, Caldeyro-Barcia's group have noted an increased incidence of Type I dips during elective induction with oxytocin infusion rates of less than 16 mU per minute, and they conclude "that an elective induction of labor at term pregnancy and without known pathology should be indicated only when important indirect medical reasons prevent more serious complications than those of the induction itself" (Schwarcz et al., 1974).

Selective β_2-receptor stimulators, such as salbutamol and terbutaline, relax uterine muscle, and these agents may be used to correct fetal distress arising from excessive uterine contractility (Andersson et al., 1975).

Neonatal Hyperbilirubinemia

High levels of unconjugated bilirubin in excess of 10 mg per 100 ml have been observed during the first week of life after the use of oxytocin during labor (Ghosh and Hudson, 1972). In other studies a large proportion of jaundiced infants were born of mothers who had received epidural analgesia as part of their induction regime (Davies et al., 1973).

Suspicion fell upon each of three factors associated with induced labor:

1. Rapid oxytocin infusion causing excessive uterine tonus, with fetal hypoxia and subsequent hepatic dysfunction
2. Epidural analgesia, absorption of local anesthetic and diminished placental flow causing hepatic dysfunction
3. Artificial and premature interruption of pregnancy before the normal surge of fetal cortisol production accompanying spontaneous labor (Murphy, 1973; Davies et al., 1973)

In a prospective study of 120 infants, Calder et al. (1974) could find no evidence that bilirubin levels were increased by epidural analgesia. Rather, the evidence seems to favor the idea that artificial interruption of pregnancy deprives the fetus, to some extent, of the normal rise of cortisol production which in turn induces a number of hepatic enzyme systems.

At the present time there is no evidence that epidural analgesia per se is responsible for neonatal hyperbilirubinemia. However, as party to an unnaturally premature form of birth, it *may* be an accessory after the fact in a situation that may handicap the liver during the early period of inducing its own enzyme systems.

Maternal Inspired Oxygen Concentration

Change of maternal inspired oxygen concentration is an added variable that may affect uterine blood flow and fetal well-being. Since supplemental oxygen may be administered for fetal distress during labor and epidural blockade, the resulting changes of oxygen delivery to the fetus are of great interest.

The effects of hypoxia are relatively well documented in animals and are seriously detrimental, placental flow being reduced between 36 per cent and 70 per cent in acute experiments (Duncan and Lewis, 1969; Karlsson, 1974). The effects of maternal hyperoxia on uterine vascular tone and placental perfusion are less well defined and have been hotly debated since Nyberg and Westin (1957) observed that high oxygen concentrations caused a 20 per cent constriction of placental vascular strips. Other in vitro experiments by Panigel (1959, 1962) showed that placental vascular resistance increased in the presence of high oxygen tension. However, more recent in vivo studies suggest that uterine blood flow is not seriously depressed when maternal arterial oxygen tensions are raised by giving the mother 100 per cent oxygen to breathe. Although acute experiments with radioactive microspheres in anesthetized rabbits have shown a 24 per cent reduction in placental flow (Karlsson and Kjellmer, 1974), chronic preparations in conscious sheep have maintained a normal uterine flow in the presence of hyperoxia (Makowski et al., 1973; Greiss et al., 1974). Fairly wide species differences are found in the net oxygen transfer to the fetus during maternal hyperoxia. In pigs, no change of uterine flow or fetal oxygenation is apparent (Hanka et al., 1975). However, in the ewe, fetal oxygenation increases in proportion to the maternal FIO_2, and in the mare the increase of fetal oxygenation is even greater (Comline and Silver, 1968). In humans, Hon's group found that fetal scalp pO_2 increases rapidly to 20 per cent above control and reaches a peak level 30 per cent above control after 45 minutes of maternal hyperoxia, then declines back to about 20 per cent above control after 60 minutes of oxygen breathing (Khazin et al., 1971). This finding suggests that in the human some degree of compensatory vasoconstriction does occur with time somewhere in the uteroplacental unit but the degree of compensation is not enough to prevent an appreciable improvement in fetal oxygenation.

The mature fetal ductus arteriosus and preductal aortic wall are exquisitely sensitive to hyperoxia (Gillman and Burton, 1966), and the possibility that hyperoxia might lead to premature closure of the ductus has been considered (Heymann and Rudolph, 1975). However, the isolated ductus does not respond to oxygen tensions in the range of 20 to 90 mmHg, so premature contraction is only likely to occur either in the presence of hypoxia or at fetal oxygen tensions above 100 mmHg, high levels that cannot be reached under clinical conditions (McMurphy et al., 1972).

In summary, uterine blood flow may be considerably reduced by alpha sympathetic stimulation or by increased concentrations of circulating catecholamines or other adrenergic substances, and these factors are lessened or eliminated by effective epidural blockade. In the absence of sympathetic uterine vasoconstriction, blood flow is linearly related to arterial pressure. Maternal hyperoxia with 100 per cent O_2 may lead to a gradual fall in placental perfusion over a period of 45 to 60 minutes, but even then the net transfer of oxygen to the fetus is still better than when the mother is breathing room air.

Impairment of uterine flow may be caused by increases of extrinsic resistance from excessive myometrial tone compressing the uterine vessels as they traverse the uterine wall. The most sinister and dangerous cause of depressed uterine blood flow arises from inferior vena caval compression in the dorsal position, especially when combined with vasodilatation in the lower limbs and pelvis. Then, inflow pressure to the placenta is reduced and outflow pressure is raised, causing a Starling resistor effect and a reduced fetal placental flow (Power and Longo, 1973). By the same token, physiological experiments on the effects of drugs or neural blockade on uterine blood flow and uterine action, carried out in the dorsal position, are likely to provide erroneous data because of the side effects arising from uncontrolled aortocaval compression.

ELECTROMYOGRAPHY

The effects of nerve blockade on axoplasmic flow have been discussed in Chapter 3. It was seen that although clinical concentrations of commonly used local anesthetics may interrupt fast axoplasmic transport for short periods of time, the process is reversible, and permanent electrical changes are not produced in the nerves or in the muscles supplied by them. However, toxic, ischemic or surgical damage to a nerve does interrupt axoplasmic flow completely, and the failure of metabolic supply leads to gradual loss of function in the distal part of the nerve and to characteristic electrical changes in the muscles supplied by it.

When a motor nerve is cut, the muscles supplied by it lose central direction and trophic sustenance, and the muscle membrane undergoes changes that are manifested by an increased sensitivity to acetylcholine at regions away from the end plate (Miledi, 1960) and by increased resistance to the blocking action of tetrodotoxin (Redfern and Thesleff, 1971). These events are thought to be due to alterations in the character of sodium channels in the membrane (Colquhoun et al., 1974). The electrical activity of a denervated fiber is characterized by a low-voltage, uncoordinated fibrillation pattern on the electromyograph (EMG) and by a prolonged response to impaling by the EMG electrode. These changes on an electromyograph can be used as an important diagnostic tool in seeking the cause of neurological lesions occurring after anesthesia, and they may help to decide whether the lesion is due to the anesthetic or whether it is attributable to other causes.

It takes time for a muscle membrane to undergo fibrillary changes. The lapse of time between nerve section and onset of fibrillation depends on the store of trophic substances remaining in the distal stump of the cut nerve, and this in turn depends upon the length of the distal stump. Thus, with short nerves the lapse of time will be comparatively short, perhaps one to two weeks, whereas with long nerves, such as the sciatic, it may take three weeks to one

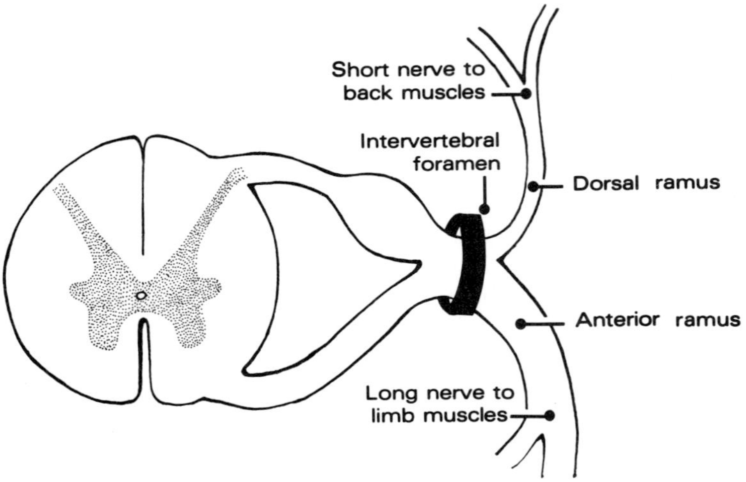

Figure 10–38. Diagram of spinal nerve to show the short posterior primary ramus going to the paraspinal muscles, and the long anterior primary ramus distributed to the more distant limb muscles.

month before a denervation pattern appears in the distant muscles (Goodgold and Eberstein, 1972).

In the event of a neurological complication, careful recordings should be made from affected limb muscles and from the corresponding paraspinal muscles in the same metameric segments as soon as symptoms become apparent. Recordings should be repeated at one- or two-week intervals for the next month, to map out the developing zone of fibrillation in muscles supplied by the short posterior primary rami and the long anterior primary rami (Fig. 10–38).

The resulting information will tell which metameres are affected and whether the lesion affects both anterior and posterior primary rami or is distal to the intervertebral foramen, occurring in a more peripheral trunk or nerve. Also, the timing of onset of the fibrillary patterns will indicate whether the lesion was likely to have occurred at the time of surgery or whether it began before operation from some preexisting disease.

Applications of these principles will be discussed in Chapter 14.

REFERENCES

Abajian, J.: Peridural segmental anesthesia with intracaine. Anesthesiology *4*:372, 1943.

Abboud, F. M.: Control of the various components of the peripheral vasculature. Fed. Proc. *31*:1226, 1972.

Abraham, J., Margolis, G., O'Loughlin, J. C., and MacCarty, W. C.: Differential reactivity of neural and extraneural vasculature. I. Role in the pathogenesis of spinal cord damage from contrast media in experimental aortography. J. Neurosurg. *25*:257, 1966.

Adamson, K., Mueller-Heubach, E., and Myers, R. E.: Production of fetal asphyxia in the rhesus monkey by administration of catecholamines to the mother. Amer. J. Obstet. Gynecol. *109*:248, 1971.

Ahlquist, R. A.: A study of adrenotropic receptors. Amer. J. Physiol. *153*:586, 1948.

Akamatsu, T. J., Ward, R. J., Bonica, J. J., Kennedy, W. F., Freund, F. G., and Takamura, J. H.: Cardiovascular response to increased epidural pressure in the elderly surgical patient. Pacific Med. Surg. *75*:161, 1967.

Alexander, J. I., Horton, P. W., Millar, W. T., and Spence, A. A.: Lung volume changes in relation to airway closure in the postoperative period: A possible mechanism of postoperative hypoxaemia. Brit. J. Anaesth. *43*:1196, 1971.

Alexander, J. I., Horton, P. W., Millar, W. T., Parikh, R. K., and Spence, A. A.: The effect of upper abdominal surgery on the relationship of airway closing point to end tidal position. Clin. Sci. *43*:137, 1972.

Allison, S. P., Tomlin, P. J., and Chamberlain, M. J.: Some effects of anaesthesia and surgery on carbohydrate and fat metabolism. Brit. J. Anaesth. *41*:588, 1969.

Andersson, K. E., Gennser, G., and Nilsson, E.: Influence of mepivacaine on isolated human foetal hearts at normal and low pH. Acta Physiol. Scand. Suppl. 353, *80*:34, 1970.

Andersson, K. E., Bengtsson, L. P., Gustafson, I., and Ingemarsson, I.: The relaxing effect of terbutaline on the human uterus during term labor. Amer. J. Obstet. Gynecol. *121*:602, 1975.

Annamunthodo, H., Keating, V. J., and Patrick, S. J.: Liver glycogen alterations in anaesthesia and surgery. Anaesthesia *13*:429, 1958.

Anscombe, A. R.: Pulmonary Complications in Abdominal Surgery. Chicago, Year Book Medical Publishers, 1957.

Avery, M. E.: Pharmacological approaches to the acceleration of fetal lung maturation. Brit. Med. Bull. *31*:13, 1975.

Barnard, J. R., MacAlpin, R., Kattus, A. A., and Buckberg, G. D.: Ischemic response to sudden strenuous exercise in healthy men. Circulation *48*:936, 1973.

Barton, M. D., Killam, A. P., and Meschia, G.: Response of ovine uterine blood flow to epinephrine and norepinephrine. Proc. Soc. Exp. Biol. Med. *145*:996, 1974.

Bauer, R. W.: Liver circulation and function. Physiol. Rev. *43*:115, 1963.

Beckman, D. L., Bean, J. W., and Baslock, D. R.: Sympathetic influence on lung compliance and surface forces in head injury. J. Appl. Physiol. *30*:394, 1971.

Beecher, H. K.: The measured effect of laparotomy on the respiration. J. Clin. Invest. *12*:639, 1933.

Bellis, C. J., and Wangensteen, O. H.: Venous circulatory changes in the abdomen and lower extremities attending intestinal distention. Proc. Soc. Exp. Biol. N.Y. *41*:490, 1939.

Bendixen, H. H., Osgood, P. F., Hall, K. V., and Laver, M. B.: Dose-dependent differences in catecholamine action on heart and periphery. J. Pharmacol. Exp. Ther. *145*:299, 1964.

Berne, R. M.: Regulation of coronary blood flow. Physiol. Rev. *44*:1, 1964.

Betz, E.: Cervical blood flow: Its measurement and regulation. Physiol. Rev. *52*:595, 1972.

Bevan, D. R.: Modification of the metabolic response to trauma under extradural analgesia. Anaesthesia *26*:188, 1971.

Bevan, D. R.: The sodium story: Effects of anaesthesia and surgery on intrarenal mechanisms concerned with sodium homeostasis. Proc. Roy. Soc. Med. *66*:1215, 1973.

Bieniarz, J., Crottogini, J. J., Curuchet, E., Romero-Salina, G., Yoshida, T., Poseiro, J. J., and Caldeyro-Barcia, R.: Aortocaval compression by the uterus in late human pregnancy. II. An arteriographic study. Amer. J. Obstet. Gynecol. *100*:203, 1968.

Bieniarz, J., Yoshida, T., Romero-Salinas, G., Curuchet, E., Caldeyro-Barcia, R., and Crottogini, J. J.: Aortocaval compression by the uterus in late human pregnancy. IV. Circulatory homeostasis by preferential perfusion of the placenta. Amer. J. Obstet. Gynecol. *103*:19, 1969.

Blake, W. D., and Jurf, A. N.: Renal sodium reabsorption after acute renal denervation in the rabbit. J. Physiol. (Lond.) *196*:65, 1968.

Bonica, J. J., Kennedy, W. F., Ward, R. J., and Tolas, A. G.: A comparison of the effects of high subarachnoid and epidural anesthesia. Acta Anaesth. Scand. *23*:429, 1966.

Bonica, J. J., Berges, P. U., and Morikawa, K.: Circulatory effects of peridural block. I. Effects of levels of analgesia and dose of lidocaine. Anesthesiology *33*:619, 1970.

Bonica, J. J., Akamatsu, T. J., Berges, P. U., Morikawa, K., and Kennedy, W. F.: Circulatory effects of peridural block. II. Effects of epinephrine. Anesthesiology *34*:514, 1971.

Bonica, J. J., Kennedy, W. F., Akamatsu, T. J., and Gerbershagen, H. U.: Circulatory effects of peridural block. III. Effects of acute blood loss. Anesthesiology *36*:219, 1972.

Bonjour, J. P., Churchill, P. C., and Malvin, R. L.: Change of tubular reabsorption of sodium and water after renal denervation in the dog. J. Physiol. (Lond.) *204*:571, 1969.

Brandt, M. R., Kehlet, H., Binder, C., Hagen, C., and McNeilly, A. S.: Effect of epidural analgesia on the glycoregulatory endocrine response to surgery. Clin. Endocr. *5*:107, 1976a.

Brandt, M. R., Kehlet, H., Skovsted, L., and Hansen, J. M.: Rapid decrease in plasma-triiodothyronine during surgery and epidural analgesia independent of afferent neurogenic stimuli and of cortisol. Lancet *2*:1333, 1976b.

Brattström, S.: Postoperative pulmonary ventilation with reference to postoperative pulmonary complications. Acta Chir. Scand. *195*:1, 1954.

Bricker, N. S., Straffon, R. A., Mahoney, E. P., and Merrill, J. P.: The functional capacity of the kidney denervated by autotransplantation in the dog. J. Clin. Invest. *37*:185, 1958.

Brigden, W., Howarth, S., and Sharpey-Schafer, E. P.: Postural changes in the peripheral blood flow of normal subjects with observations on vaso-vagal fainting reactions as a result of tilting, the lordotic posture, pregnancy and spinal anaesthesia. Clin. Sci. *9*:79, 1950.

Britt, B. A., and Gordon, R. A.: Peripheral nerve injuries associated with anaesthesia. Canad. Anaesth. Soc. J. *11*:514, 1964.

Brody, T. M., Calvert, D. N., and Schneider, A. F.: Alteration of carbon tetrachloride induced pathologic changes in the rat by spinal transection, adrenalectomy and adrenergic blocking agents. J. Pharmacol. Exp. Ther. *131*:341, 1961.

Bromage, P. R.: Vascular hypotension in 105 cases of epidural analgesia. Anaesthesia *6*:26, 1951.

Bromage, P. R.: Effect of induced vascular hypotension on the liver: Alterations in appearance and consistence. Lancet *2*:10, 1952.

Bromage, P. R.: Spinal Epidural Analgesia. Edinburgh, E. & S. Livingstone, Ltd. 1954, pp. 21, 27, 28, 30

Bromage, P. R.: Spirometry in assessment of analgesia after abdominal surgery (a method of comparing analgesic drugs). Brit. Med. J. *2*:589, 1955.

Bromage, P. R.: Hypotension and vital capacity. Anaesthesia *11*:139, 1956.

Bromage, P. R.: The phrenic reflex in epidural analgesia. Canad, Anaesth. Soc. J. *5*:29, 1958a.

Bromage, P. R.: Total respiratory compliance in anaesthetized subjects and modifications produced by noxious stimuli. Clin. Sci. *17*:217, 1958b.

Bromage, P. R.: Vasopressors. Canad. Anaesth. Soc. J. 7:310, 1960.

Bromage, P. R.: Continuous lumbar epidural analgesia for obstetrics. Canad. Med. Assoc. J. *85*:1136, 1961.

Bromage, P. R.: Physiology and pharmacology of epidural analgesia (a review). Anesthesiology *28*:592, 1967a.

Bromage, P. R.: Extradural analgesia for pain relief. Brit. J. Anaesth. *39*:721, 1967b.

Bromage, P. R.: Spinal thrombophlebitis after hypotensive anaesthesia. New Zealand Med. J. *80*:519, 1974.

Bromage, P. R., and Melzack, R.: Phantom limbs and the body schema. Canad. Anaesth. Soc. J. *21*:267, 1974.

Bromage, P. R., and Robson, J. G.: Concentrations of lignocaine in the blood after intravenous, intramuscular, epidural and endotracheal administration. Anaesthesia *16*:461, 1961.

Bromage, P. R., Shibata, H. R., and Willoughby, H. W.: Influence of prolonged epidural blockade on blood sugar and cortisol responses to operations upon the upper part of abdomen and the thorax. Surg. Gynecol. Obstet. *132*:1051, 1971.

Buchan, P. C., Milne, M. K., and Browning, M. C. K.: The effect of continuous epidural blockade on plasma 11-hydroxycorticosteroid concentrations in labour. J. Obstet. Gynecol. Brit. Cwlth. *80*:974, 1973.

Buckberg, G. D., Fixler, D. E., Archie, J. P., and Hoffman, J. I. E.: Experimental subendocardial ischemia in dogs with normal coronary arteries. Circ. Res. *30*:67, 1972.

Bull, G. M.: Postural proteinuria. Clin. Sci. 7:77, 1949.

Buller, A. J., Eccles, J. C., and Eccles, R. M.: Differentiation of fast and slow muscles in the cat hind limb. J. Physiol. (Lond.) *150*:399, 1960a.

Buller, A. J., Eccles, J. C., and Eccles, R. M.: Interactions between motoneurones and muscle in respect of the characteristic speeds of their response. J. Physiol. (Lond.) *150*:417, 1960b.

Buller, A. J., Mommaerts, W. F. H. M., and Seraydarian, K.: Enzymic properties of myosin in fast and slow twitch muscles of the cat following cross-innervation. J. Physiol. (Lond.) *205*:581, 1969.

Burfoot, M. F., and Bromage, P. R.: The effects of epinephrine on mepivacaine absorption from the spinal epidural space. Anesthesiology *35*:488, 1971.

Burn, J. H., and Rand, M. J.: Sympathetic postganglionic mechanism. Nature *184*:163, 1959.

Burns, B. D., and Salmoiraghi, G. C.: Repetitive firing of respiratory neurones during their burst activity. J. Neurophysiol. *23*:27, 1960.

Burwell, C. S., Strayhorn, W. D., Flickinger, D., Corlette, M. B., Bowerman, E. P., and Kennedy, J. A.: Circulation during pregnancy. Arch. Int. Med. *62*:979, 1938.

Cabezas, G. A., Graf, P. D., and Nadel, J. A.: Sympathetic versus parasympathetic nervous regulation of airways in dogs. J. Appl. Physiol. *31*:651, 1971.

Calder, A. A., Moar, V. A., Ounsted, M. K., and Turnbull, A. C.: Increased bilirubin levels in neonates after induction of labour by intravenous prostaglandin F_2 or oxytocin. Lancet *2*:1339, 1974.

Caldeyro-Barcia, R.: Effects of position changes on the intensity and frequency of uterine contractions during labor. Amer. J. Obstet. Gynecol. *80*:284, 1960.

Caldeyro-Barcia, R., and Poseiro, J. J.: Physiology of the uterine contraction. Clin. Obstet. Gynecol. *3*:386, 1960.

Campbell, E. J. M.: The relationship of the sensation of breathlessness to the act of breathing. *In*

Howell, J. B. L., and Campbell, E. J. M. (eds.): Breathlessness. Oxford, Blackwell Scientific Publications, 1966, pp. 55–64.
Carter, A. M., and Olin, T.: Effect of adrenergic stimulation and blockade on the uteroplacental circulation and uterine activity in the rabbit. J. Reprod. Fert. *29*:251, 1972.
Catterberg, J., and Insausti, T.: Paraplejias consecutivas a anestesia peridural (estudio clinico y experimental). Rev. Asoc. Med. Argent. *78*:1, 1964.
Celander, O.: The range of control exercised by the sympathico-adrenal system. A quantitative study on blood vessels and other smooth muscle effectors in the cat. Acta Physiol. Scand. Suppl. 116, *32*:1, 1954.
Chambers, W. W., Seigel, M. S., Liu, J. C., and Liu, C. N.: Thermoregulatory responses of decerebrate and spinal cats. Exp. Neurol. *42*:282, 1974.
Chen, H. I., and Chai, C. Y.: Pulmonary edema and hemorrhage as a consequence of systemic vasoconstriction. Amer. J. Physiol. *227*:144, 1974.
Christie, R. V., and Meakins, J. C.: The intrapleural pressure in congestive heart failure and its clinical significance. J. Clin. Invest. *13*:323, 1934.
Churchill, E. D., and McNeil, D.: The reduction of vital capacity following operations. Surg. Gynecol. Obstet. *44*:483, 1927.
Clarke, R. S. J.: The hyperglycaemic response to different types of surgery and anaesthesia. Brit. J. Anaesth. *42*:45, 1970.
Clarke, R. S. J., Johnston, H., and Sheridan, B.: The influence of anaesthesia and surgery on plasma cortisol, insulin and free fatty acids. Brit. J. Anaesth. *42*:295, 1970.
Cohen, G., Holland, B., Sha, J., and Goldenberg, M.: Plasma concentrations of epinephrine and norepinephrine during intravenous infusions in man. J. Clin. Invest. *38*:1935, 1959.
Colgan, F. J., and Mahoney, P. D.: The effects of major surgery on cardiac output and shunting. Anesthesiology *31*:213, 1969.
Colquhoun, D., Tang, H. P., and Ritchie, J. M.: The binding of tetrodotoxin and alpha-bungarotoxin to normal and denervated mammalian muscle. J. Physiol. (Lond.) *240*:199, 1974.
Comline, R. S., and Silver, M.: pO_2 levels in the placental circulation of mare and ewe. Nature *217*:76, 1968.
Cooperman, L., Warden, J. C., and Price, H. L.: Splanchnic circulation during nitrous oxide anesthesia and hypocarbia in normal man. Anesthesiology *29*:254, 1968.
Corbett, J. L., Frankel, H. L., and Harris, P. J.: Cardiovascular reflex responses to cutaneous and visceral stimuli in spinal man. J. Physiol. (Lond.) *215*:395, 1971a.
Corbett, J. L., Frankel, H. L., and Harris, P. J.: Cardiovascular response to tilting in tetraplegic man. J. Physiol. (Lond.) *215*:411, 1971b.
Corbett, J. L., Frankel, H. L., and Harris, P. J.: Cardiovascular reflexes in tetraplegia. Paraplegia *9*:113, 1971c.
Cort, J. H.: Relief of post-traumatic anuria. Amer. J. Physiol. *164*:686, 1951.
Cort, J. H.: Effect of nervous stimulation on the arteriovenous oxygen and carbon dioxide differences across the kidney. Nature *171*:784, 1953.
Cosgrove, D. O., and Jenkins, J. S.: The effects of epidural anaesthesia on the pituitary-adrenal response to surgery. Clin. Sci. Molec. Med. *46*:403, 1974.
Courington, F. W., and Little, D. M.: The role of posture in anaesthesia. Clin. Anaesth. *3*:23, 1968.
Cousins, M. J., and Wright, C. J.: Graft, muscle, skin blood flow after epidural block in vascular surgical procedures. Surg. Gynecol. Obstet. *133*:59, 1971.
Coyle, J. T., and Henry, D.: Catecholamines in fetal and newborn rat brain. J. Neurochem. *21*:61, 1973.
Crawford, J. S., Burton, M., and Davies, P.: Time and lateral tilt at Caesarean section. Brit. J. Anaesth. *44*:477, 1972.
Cullingford, D. W. J.: The blood sugar response to anaesthesia and surgery in Southern Indians. Brit. J. Anaesth. *38*:463, 1966.
Dahlström, A. D., and Zetterstrom, B. E. M.: Noradrenaline stores in nerve terminals of the spleen: Changes during hemorrhagic shock. Science *147*:1583, 1965.
Daly, I. D.: Intrinsic mechanisms of the lung. Quart. J. Exp. Physiol. *43*:2, 1958.
Daly, I. D.: An analysis of active and passive effects on the pulmonary vascular bed in response to pulmonary nerve stimulation. Quart. J. Exp. Physiol. *46*:257, 1961.
Daly, I. D., and Hebb, C.: Pulmonary vasomotor fibers in the cervical vagosympathetic nerve of the dog. Quart. J. Exp. Physiol. *37*:19, 1952.
Davies, D. P., Gomersall, R., Robertson, R., Gray, O. P., and Turnbull, A. C.: Neonatal jaundice and maternal oxytocin infusion. Brit. Med. J. *3*:476, 1973.
Davies, L. G., Goodwin, J. F., and Van Leuven, B. D.: Nature of pulmonary hypertension in mitral stenosis. Brit. Heart J. *16*:440, 1954.
Davis, J. M.: The effect of upper spinal cord lesions on the detection of increased airway resistance in man. J. Physiol. (Lond.) *179*:25P, 1965.

Dawkins, C. J. M.: Discussion on extradural spinal block. Proc. Roy. Soc. Med. *35*:547, 1945.
Defalque, R. J.: Compared effects of spinal and extradural anesthesia upon the blood pressure. Anesthesiology *23*:627, 1962.
Denecke, K.: Die Periduralanästhesie in der Chirurgie. Zbl. Chir. *64*:130, 1937.
Diament, M. L., and Palmer, K. N. V.: Postoperative changes in gas tensions of arterial blood and in ventilatory function. Lancet *2*:180, 1966.
Diament, M. L., and Palmer, K. N. V.: Venous/arterial pulmonary shunting as the principal cause of postoperative hypoxaemia. Lancet *1*:15, 1967.
Dogliotti, A. M.: Anesthesia. Chicago, S. B. Debour, 1939.
Don, H. F., and Robson, J. G.: Effect of mechanical stimulation of the lower airway on respiratory mechanics in apneic anesthetized man. Anesthesiology *27*:284, 1966.
Don, H. F., Wahba, M., Cuadrado, L., and Kelkar, K.: The effect of anesthesia and 100 per cent oxygen on the functional residual capacity of the lungs. Anesthesiology *32*:521, 1970.
Doppman, J., Rubinson, R. M., Rockoff, S. D., Vasko, J. S., Shapiro, R., and Morrow, A. G.: Mechanism of obstruction of the infradiaphragmatic portion of the inferior vena cava in the presence of increased intra-abdominal pressure. Invest. Radiol. *1*:37, 1966.
Downey, J. A., Miller, J. M., and Darling, R. C.: Thermoregulatory responses to deep and superficial cooling in spinal man. J. Appl. Phys. *27*:209, 1969.
Downing, J. W.: Bupivacaine: A clinical assessment in lumbar extradural block. Brit. J. Anaesth. *41*:427, 1969.
Dreyer, C., Bischoff, D., and Göthert, M.: Effects of methoxyflurane anesthesia on adrenal medullary catecholamine secretion: Inhibition of spontaneous secretion and secretion evoked by splanchnic-nerve stimulation. Anesthesiology *41*:18, 1974.
Droste, P. L., and Beckman, D. L.: Pulmonary effects of prolonged sympathetic stimulation. Proc. Soc. Exp. Biol. Med. *146*:352, 1974.
Duncan, S. B.: The partition of uterine blood flow in the pregnant rabbit. J. Physiol. (Lond.) *204*:421, 1969.
Duncan, S. B., and Lewis, B. V.: Maternal placental and myometrial blood flow in the pregnant rabbit. J. Physiol. (Lond.) *202*:471, 1969.
Düttmann, G.: Die peridurale segmentare Anästhesie. Zbl. Chir. *68*:530, 1941.
Ellis, F. R., Keaney, N. P., Harriman, D. G. F., Sumner, D. W., Kyei-Mensah, K., Tyrrell, J. H., Hargreaves, J. B., Parikh, R. K., and Mulrooney, P. L.: Screening for malignant hyperpyrexia. Brit. Med. J. *3*:559, 1972.
Epstein, R. M., Deutsch, S., Cooperman, L. H., Clement, A. J., and Price, H. L.: Splanchnic circulation during halothane anesthesia and hypercapnia in normal man. Anesthesiology *27*:654, 1966.
Estabrooks, R. A., Marks, L. J., Lonergan, J. C., Murtaugh, J. F., and Strobl, V. E.: The effect of surgical operation on the adrenocortical response to ACTH. Ann. Surg. *150*:941, 1959.
Euler, U. S. v., and Floding, I.: Fluorimetric micromethod for differential estimation of adrenaline and noradrenaline. Acta Physiol. Scand. (Suppl. 118) *33*:46, 1955.
Ferris, T. F., Stein, J. H., and Kauffman, J.: Uterine blood flow and uterine renin secretion. J. Clin. Invest. *51*:2827, 1972.
Figueiredo, R. R.: Nossa experiencia com 1,201 casos de anestesia extradural. Rev. Bras. de Cir. *17*:31, 1948.
Finer, B.: Studies of the variability in expiratory efforts before and after cholecystectomy. Acta Anaesth. Scand. (Suppl.) *38*:7, 1970.
Finnerty, F. A., Witkin, L., and Fazekas, J. F.: Cerebral hemodynamics during cerebral ischemia induced by acute hypotension. J. Clin. Invest. *33*:1227, 1954.
Foldes, F. F., Klonymus, D. H., Maisel, W., and Osserman, K. E.: A new curare test for the diagnosis of myasthenia gravis. J.A.M.A. *203*:649, 1968.
Folkow, B., and Langston, J.: The interrelationship of some factors influencing renal blood flow autoregulation. Acta Physiol. Scand. *61*:165, 1964.
Freund, F., Roos, A., and Dodd, R. B.: Expiratory activity of the abdominal muscles in man during general anesthesia. J. Appl. Physiol. *19*:693, 1964.
Froese, A. B., and Bryan, A. C.: Effects of anesthesia and paralysis on diaphragmatic mechanics in man. Anesthesiology *41*:242, 1974.
Fruhstorfer, H., Zenz, M., Nolte, H., and Hensel, H.: Dissociated loss of cold and warm sensibility during regional anaesthesia. Pflügers Arch. *349*:73, 1974.
Galbert, M. W., and Marx, G. F.: Extradural pressures in the parturient patient. Anesthesiology *40*:499, 1974.
Galindo, A.: Hepatic circulation and hepatic function during anaesthesia and surgery. Canad. Anaesth. Soc. J. *12*:262, 1965a.
Galindo, A.: Hepatic circulation and hepatic function during anaesthesia and surgery. Canad. Anaesth. Soc. J. *12*:337, 1965b.

Galindo, A., and Sprouse, J. H.: The influence of epidural anaesthesia on cardiac excitability in profound hypothermia. Canad. Anaesth. Soc. J. *11*:614, 1964.

Ghosh, A., and Hudson, F. P.: Oxytocin agents and neonatal hyperbilirubinaemia. Lancet *2*:823, 1972.

Gillespie, J. S., and Kirpekar, S. M.: The uptake and release of radioactive noradrenaline by the splenic nerves of cats. J. Physiol. (Lond.) *187*:51, 1966.

Gillman, R. A., and Burton, A. C.: Constriction of the neonatal aorta by raised oxygen tension. Circ. Res. *19*:755, 1966.

Glick, G., and Braunwald, E.: Relative roles of the sympathetic and parasympathetic nervous systems in the reflex control of the heart rate. Circ. Res. *16*:363, 1965.

Goepel, H.: Die Periduralanästhesie in der Chirurgie. Chirurg. *15*:136, 1943.

Goffen, B. J., Fitzpatrick, L. J., and Wood, P. M.: Control of bleeding during fenestration and similar operations by sympathetic block. Anesth. Analg. *29*:340, 1950.

Goldberg, L.: Studies on local anaesthetics. Pharmacological properties of homologues and isomers of xylocain (alkyl aminoacyl derivatives). Acta Physiol. Scand. *18*:8, 1949.

Goldenberg, I. S., Hayes, M. A., and Greene, N. M.: Endocrine responses during operative procedures. Ann. Surg. *150*:196, 1959.

Goodgold, J., and Eberstein, A.: Electrodiagnosis of Neuromuscular Diseases. Baltimore, Williams & Wilkins Co., 1972, pp. 76, 164, 165, 169.

Gordon, N. H., Scott, D. B., and Robb, I. W. P.: Modifications of plasma corticosteroid concentrations during and after surgery by epidural blockade. Brit. Med. J. *1*:581, 1973.

Gordon-Jones, R. G.: A complication of epidural technique. Anaesthesia *8*:242, 1953.

Gosling, R., Kerry, R. J., Orme, J. E., and Owen, G.: Creatine phosphokinase activity in newly admitted psychiatric patients. Brit. J. Psychiat. *121*:351, 1972a.

Gosling, R., Kerry, R. J., and Owen, G.: Creatine phosphokinase activity during lithium treatment. Brit. Med. J. *3*:327, 1972b.

Granger, H. J., and Guyton, A. C.: Autoregulation of the total systemic circulation following destruction of the central nervous system in the dog. Circ. Res. *25*:379, 1969.

Green, H. D., Hall, L. S., and Sexton, J.: Autonomic responses in the canine hepatic arterial and venous beds. Amer. J. Physiol. *196*:196, 1959.

Greiss, F. C., Jr.: Pressure-flow relationship in the gravid uterine vascular bed. Amer. J. Obstet. Gynecol. *96*:41, 1966.

Greiss, F. C., Jr.: Concepts of Uterine Blood Flow. *In* Wynn, R. M. (ed.): Obstetrics and Gynecology Annual. Vol. 2. New York, Appleton-Century-Crofts, 1973, pp. 55–83.

Greiss, F. C., and Gobble, F. L.: Effect of sympathetic nerve stimulation on the uterine vascular bed. Amer. J. Obstet Gynecol. *97*:962, 1967.

Greiss, F. C., Anderson, S. G., and King, L. C.: Uterine vascular bed: Effects of acute hyperoxia. Amer. J. Obstet. Gynecol. *118*:542, 1974.

Griffiths, I. R.: Spinal cord blood flow in dogs. I. The "normal" flow. J. Neurol. Neurosurg. Psychiat. *36*:34, 1973a.

Griffiths, I. R.: Spinal cord blood flow in dogs. 2. The effect of the blood gases. J. Neurol. Neurosurg. Psychiat. *36*:42, 1973b.

Griffiths, I. R.: Spinal cord blood flow in dogs: The effect of blood pressure. J. Neurol. Neurosurg. Psychiat. *36*:914, 1973c.

Griffiths, I. R., Rowan, J. O., and Crawford, R. A.: Spinal cord blood flow measured by a hydrogen clearance technique. J. Neurol. Sci. *26*:529, 1975.

Griffiths, J. A.: The effects of general anaesthesia, and hexamethonium on the blood-sugar in non-diabetic and diabetic surgical patients. Quart. J. Med. *22*:405, 1953.

Guth, L., and Watson, P. K.: The influence of innervation on the soluble proteins of fast and slow muscles of the rat. Exp. Neurol. *17*:107, 1969.

Gutierrez, A.: Anestesia extradural. Buenos Aires, Rev. Cirug. 1939, p. 61.

Guyton, A. C.: Circulatory Physiology: Cardiac Output and Its Regulation. Philadelphia, W. B. Saunders Co., 1963, pp. 223–234.

Guyton, A. C., Abernathy, J. B., Langston, J. B., and Fairchild, H. M.: Relative importance of venous and arterial resistances in controlling venous return and cardiac output. Amer. J. Physiol. *196*:1008, 1959.

Häggendal, J.: An improved method for fluorimetric determination of small amounts of adrenaline and noradrenaline in plasma and tissues. Acta Physiol. Scand. *59*:242, 1963.

Hales, J. R. S., and Jessen, C.: Increase of cutaneous moisture loss by local heating of the spinal cord in the ox. J. Physiol. (Lond.) *204*:40P, 1969.

Hammond, W. G., Vandam, L. D., Davis, J. M., Certer, R. D., Ball, M. R., and Moore, F. D.: Studies in surgical endocrinology. IV. Anesthetic agents as stimuli to change in corticosteroids and metabolism. Ann. Surg. *148*:199, 1958.

Hanka, R., Lawn, L., Mills, I. H., Prior, D. C., and Tweeddale, P. M.: The effects of maternal hypercapnia on foetal oxygenation and uterine blood flow in the pig. J. Physiol. (Lond.) *247*:447, 1975.

Hansen, R.: Ohnmacht und Schwangerschaft. Klin. Wschr. *21*:241, 1942.

Harp, J. R., and Wollman, H.: Cerebral effects of hyperventilation and deliberate hypotension. Brit. J. Anaesth. *45*:256, 1973.

Havers, L.: Controlled hypotension by extradural spinal block under chlorpromazine cover. Brit. J. Anaesth. *28*:83, 1956.

Hayes, M. F., Rosenbaum, R. W., Zibelman, M., and Matsumoto, T.: Adult respiratory distress syndrome in association with acute pancreatitis. Evaluation of positive end expiratory pressure ventilation and pharmacologic doses of steroids. Amer. J. Surg. *127*:314, 1974.

Head, J. R.: The effect of operation upon the vital capacity. Boston Med. Surg. *197*:83, 1927.

Hewlett, A. M., Hulands, G. H., Nunn, J. F., and Heath, J. R.: Functional residual capacity during anaesthesia. II. Spontaneous respiration. Brit. J. Anaesth. *46*:486, 1974.

Heymann, M. A., and Rudolph, A. M.: Control of the ductus arteriosus. Physiol. Rev. *55*:62, 1975.

Hipona, F. A., Yules, R., and Hehre, F. W.: Venous encroachment on the spinal peridural space due to experimental IVC occlusion: Possible clinical implications in late pregnancy. Invest. Radiol. *1*:157, 1966.

Hitchcock, E.: Hypothermic subarachnoid irrigation for intractable pain. Lancet *1*:1133, 1967.

Hix, E. L.: Uretero-renal reflux facilitating renal vasoconstrictor responses to emotional stress. Amer. J. Physiol. *192*:191, 1958.

Hoar, P. F., Hickey, R. F., and Ullyot, D. J.: Systemic hypertension following myocardial revascularization: A method of treatment using epidural anesthesia. J. Thorac. Cardiovasc. Surg. *71*:859, 1976.

Hoffman, J. I. E., and Buckberg, G. D.: Transmural variations in myocardial perfusion. *In* Yu, P., and Goodwin, J. (eds.): Progress in Cardiology. Vol. V. Philadelphia, Lea & Febiger, 1976, pp. 37–89.

Holland, W. C., and Schümann, H. J.: Formation of catechol amines during splanchnic stimulation of the adrenal of the cat. Brit. J. Pharmacol. *11*:449, 1956.

Hollenberg, N. K., Epstein, M., Guttmann, R. D., Conroy, M., Basch, R. I., and Merrill, J. P.: Effect of sodium balance on intrarenal distribution of blood flow in normal man. J. Appl. Physiol. *28*:312, 1970.

Hollenberg, N. K., Adams, D. F., Solomon, H. S., Abrams, H. L., and Merrill, J. P.: What mediates the renal vascular response to a salt load in normal man? J. Appl. Physiol. *33*:491, 1972.

Hollmén, A., and Saukkonen, J.: The effects of postoperative epidural analgesia versus centrally acting opiate on physiological shunt after upper abdominal operation. Acta Anaesth. Scand. *16*:147, 1972.

Holmdahl, M. H., Sjögren, S., Ström, G., and Wright, B.: Clinical aspects of continuous epidural blockade for postoperative pain relief. Uppsala J. Med. Sci. *77*:47, 1972.

Holmes, J.: Spinal analgesia and Caesarean section. Maternal mortality. J. Obstet. Gynaecol. Brit. Emp. *64*:229, 1957.

Howell, J. B. L., and Peckett, B. W.: Studies of the elastic properties of the thorax of supine anaesthetized paralysed human subjects. J. Physiol. (Lond.) *136*:1, 1957.

Hume, D. M., and Egdahl, R. H.: The importance of the brain in the endocrine response to surgery. Ann. Surg. *150*:697, 1959.

Hume, D. M., Bell, C. C., and Bartter, F. M. Direct measurement of adrenal secretion during operative trauma and convalescence. Surgery *52*:174, 1962.

Humphrey, M. D., Hounslow, D., Morgan, S., and Wood, C.: The influence of maternal posture at birth on the fetus. J. Obstet. Gynaecol. Brit. Cwlth. *80*:1075, 1973.

Humphrey, M. D., Chang, A., Wood, E. C., Morgan, S., and Hounslow, D.: A decrease in fetal pH during the second stage of labour, when conducted in the dorsal position. J. Obstet. Gynaecol. Brit. Cwlth. *81*:600, 1974.

Isaacs, H.: High serum creatine phosphokinase levels in asymptomatic members of the families of patients developing malignant hyperpyrexia—a genetic study. *In* Gordon, R. A., Britt, B. A., and Kalow, W. (eds.): International Symposium on Malignant Hyperthermia. Springfield, Ill., Charles C Thomas, Publisher, 1973, pp. 331–338.

Iversen, L. L., and Jarrott, B.: Modification of an enzyme radiochemical assay procedure for noradrenaline. Biochem. Pharmacol. *19*:1841, 1970.

Jarisch, A.: Vagovasale Syncope. Z. Kreisl. Forsch. *23*:267, 1941.

Jarisch, A., and Zotterman, Y.: Depressor reflexes from the heart. Acta Physiol. Scand. *16*:31, 1948.

Jessen, C.: Auslösung von Hecheln durch isolierte Wärmung des Rüchenmarks am wachen Hund. Pflügers Arch. *297*:53, 1967.

Jessen, C., Meurer, K. A., and Simon, E.: Steigerung der Hautdurchblutung durch isolierte Wärmung des Rüchenmarks am wachen Hund. Pflügers Arch. *297*:35, 1967.

Johansson, B., and Langston, J. B.: Reflex influence of mesenteric afferents on renal, intestinal and muscle blood flow and on intestinal motility. Acta Physiol. Scand. *61*:400, 1964.

Johnson, S. R.: The mechanism of hyperglycemia during anesthesia: An experimental study. Anesthesiology *10*:379, 1949.

Jordfelt, L., Löfstrom, B., Pernow, B., Persson, P., Wahren, J., and Widman, B.: The effect of local anesthetics on the central circulation and respiration in man and dog. Acta Anaesth. Scand. *12*:153, 1968.

Kadowitz, P. J., and Hyman, A. L.: Effect of sympathetic nerve stimulation on pulmonary vascular resistance in the dog. Circ. Res. *32*:221, 1973.

Kalow, W., and Britt, B. A.: Inheritance of malignant hyperthermia. *In* Gordon, R. A., Britt, B. A., and Kalow, W. (eds.): International Symposium on Malignant Hyperthermia. Springfield, Ill., Charles C Thomas, Publisher, 1973, pp. 67–76.

Kamm, D. E., and Levinsky, N. G.: The mechanism of denervation natriuresis. J. Clin. Invest. *44*:93, 1965.

Kaneko, K., Milic-Emili, J., Dolovich, M. B., Dawson, A., and Bates, D. V.: Regional distribution of ventilation and perfusion as a function of body position. J. Appl. Physiol. *21*:767, 1966.

Kannel, W. B., Seidman, J. M., Fercho, W., and Castelli, W. P.: Vital capacity and congestive heart failure. The Framingham Study. Circulation *49*:1160, 1974.

Kaplan, J. A., and King, S. B.: The precordial electrocardiographic lead (V_5) in patients who have coronary-artery disease. Anesthesiology *45*:570, 1976.

Karlsson, K.: The influence of hypoxia on uterine and maternal placental blood flow, and the effect of α-adrenergic blockade. J. Perinat. Med. *2*:176, 1974.

Karlsson, K., and Kjellmer, I.: The uterine and maternal placental blood flow during hyperoxia. J. Perinat. Med. *2*:170, 1974.

Katz, J. D., and Krich, L. B.: Acute febrile reaction complicating spinal anaesthesia in a survivor of malignant hyperthermia. Canad. Anaesth. Soc. J. *23*:285, 1976.

Kaul, S. U., Heath, J. R., and Nunn, J. F.: Factors influencing the development of expiratory muscle activity during anaesthesia. Brit. J. Anaesth. *45*:1013, 1973.

Keating, V.: Carbohydrate metabolism. The effects of surgery in a tropical population. Anaesthesia *13*:434, 1958.

Kennedy, W. F., Everett, G. B., Cobb, L. A., and Allen, G. D.: Simultaneous systemic and hepatic hemodynamic measurements during high spinal anesthesia in normal man. Anesth. Analg. *49*:1016, 1970.

Kennedy, W. F., Everett, G. B., Cobb, L. A., and Allen, G. D.: Simultaneous systemic and hepatic hemodynamic measurements during high peridural anesthesia in normal man. Anesth. Analg. *50*:1069, 1971.

Kerr, D. D., Wingard, D. W., and Gatz, E. E.: Prevention of porcine malignant hyperthermia by epidural block. Anesthesiology *42*:307, 1975.

Kerr, M. G., Scott, D. B., and Samuel, E.: Studies of the inferior vena cava in late pregnancy. Brit. Med. J. *1*:532, 1964.

Kety, S. S., King, B. D., Horvath, S. M., Jeffers, W. A., and Hafkenschiel, J. H.: The effects of an acute reduction in blood pressure by means of differential spinal sympathetic block on the cerebral circulation of hypertensive patients. J. Clin. Invest. *29*:402, 1950.

Khazin, A. F., Hon, E. H., and Hehre, F. W.: Effects of maternal hyperoxia on the fetus. I. Oxygen tension. Amer. J. Obstet. Gynecol. *109*:628, 1971.

Kinnell, J. D.: The influence of afferent block on hyperventilation anaesthesia. Anaesthesia *17*:58, 1962.

Klimanek, J.: Personal communication, 1977.

Klimanek, J., Majewski, W., and Walencik, K.: A case of malignant hyperthermia during epidural analgesia. Anaesth. Resusc. Inten. Ther. *4*:143, 1976.

Kobrine, A. I., Doyle, T. F., and Martins, A. N.: Spinal cord blood flow in the Rhesus monkey by the hydrogen clearance method. Surg. Neurol. *2*:197, 1974.

Kobrine, A. I., Doyle, T. F., and Rizzoli, H. V.: Spinal cord blood flow as affected by changes in systemic arterial blood pressure. J. Neurosurg. *44*:12, 1976.

Kosaka, M., Simon, E., and Thauer, R.: Shivering in intact and spinal rabbits during spinal cord cooling. Experientia *23*:385, 1966.

Kostreva, D. R., Zuperku, E. J., Hess, G. L., Coon, R. L., and Kampine, J. P.: Pulmonary afferent activity recorded from sympathetic nerves. J. Appl. Physiol. *39*:37, 1975.

La Cour, D., Juul-Jensen, P., and Reske-Nielsen, E.: Malignant hyperthermia during anaesthesia. A neurophysiological and neuropathological follow-up study of a patient and his family. Acta Anaesth. Scand. *15*:299, 1971.

Ladner, C., Brinkman, C. R., Weston, P., and Assali, N. S.: Dynamics of uterine circulation in pregnant and nonpregnant sheep. Amer. J. Physiol. *218*:257, 1970.

Lassen, H. K.: The influence of various operations and of postoperative complications on vital capacity. Acta Chir. Scand. *81*:361, 1938.
Lassen, N. A.: Cerebral blood flow and oxygen consumption in man. Physiol. Rev. *39*:183, 1959.
Laws, A. K.: Effects of induction of anaesthesia and muscle paralysis on functional residual capacity of the lungs. Canad. Anaesth. Soc. J. *15*:325, 1968.
Lees, M. M., Scott, D. B., and Kerr, M. G.: Haemodynamic changes associated with labour. J. Obstet. Gynaecol. Brit. Cwlth. *77*:29, 1970.
LeFemine, A. A., Marks, L. J., Teter, J. G., Leftin, J. H., Leonard, M. P., and Baker, D. V.: The adrenocortical response in surgical patients. Ann. Surg. *146*:26, 1957.
Levine, S. A.: The value of determination of the vital capacity of the lungs in the care of patients with heart disease. Arq. Bras. Cardiol. *2*:253, 1949.
Levy, M. N.: Sympathetic-parasympathetic interactions in the heart. Circ. Res. *29*:437, 1971.
Lewis, J., and Welch, J. A.: Respiratory mechanics in postoperative patients. Surg. Gynecol. Obstet. *120*:305, 1965.
Libonati, M., Malsch, E., Price, H., Cooperman, L. H., Baum, S., and Harp, J. R.: Splanchnic circulation in man during methoxyflurane anesthesia. Anesthesiology *38*:466, 1973.
Lines, J. G., Loder, R. E., and Millar, R. A.: Plasma cortisol responses during neurosurgical and abdominal operations. Brit. J. Anaesth. *43*:1136, 1971.
Lister, D., Hall, G. M., and Lucke, J. N.: Catecholamines in suxamethonium-induced hyperthermia in Pietrain pigs. Brit. J. Anaesth. *46*:803, 1974.
Lister, D., Hall, G. M., and Lucke, J. N.: Malignant hyperthermia: A human and porcine stress syndrome. Lancet *1*:519, 1975.
Lumley, J., Walker, A., Marum, J., and Wood, C.: Time an important variable at Caesarean section. J. Obstet. Gynaecol. Brit. Cwlth. 77:10, 1970.
Lund, A.: Fluorimetric determination of adrenaline in blood. III. A new sensitive and specific method. Acta Pharmacol. Toxicol. (Kbh.) *5*:231, 1949.
Lush, D., Thorpe, J. N., Richardson, D. J., and Bowen, D. J.: The effect of epidural analgesia on the adrenocortical response to surgery. Brit. J. Anaesth. *44*:1169, 1972.
Lynne-Davies, P., Couture, J., Pengelly, L. D., West, D., Bromage, P. R., and Milic-Emili, J.: Partitioning of immediate ventilatory stability to added elastic loads in cats. J. Appl. Physiol. *30*:814, 1971.
McCall, M. L.: Cerebral circulation and metabolism in toxemia and pregnancy. Observations on the effects of veratrum viride and apresoline (1-hydrazinophthalazine). Amer. J. Obstet. Gynecol. *66*:1015, 1953.
McCann, J. C.: Physiology of traumatic reflexes and respiration during surgical anesthesia. Calif. Med. J. *65*:212, 1946.
McCarthy, G. S.: The effect of thoracic epidural analgesia on pulmonary gas distribution, functional residual capacity and airway closure. Brit. J. Anaesth. *48*:243, 1976.
McDonald, L., Baker, C., Bray, C., McDonald, A., and Restieaux, A.: Plasma-catecholamines after myocardial infarction. Lancet *2*:1021, 1969.
McDowall, D. G., Keaney, N. P., Turner, J. M., Lane, J. R., and Okuda, Y.: The toxicity of sodium nitroprusside. Brit. J. Anaesth. *46*:327, 1974.
Mackay, R. L.: Observation on the blood sugar changes in general anaesthesia. Brit. J. Anaesth. *6*:15, 1928.
Mackay, R. L., and Dyke, S. C.: On certain changes in the blood during surgical anaesthesia. Brit. J. Anaesth. *6*:61, 1928.
McLean, A. P. H., Mulligan, G. W., Otton, P., and MacLean, L. D.: Hemodynamic alterations associated with epidural anesthesia. Surgery *62*:79, 1967.
McLennan, C. E.: Antecubital and femoral venous pressure in normal and toxemic pregnancy. Amer. J. Obstet. Gynecol. *45*:568, 1943.
McMurphy, D. M., Heymann, M. A., Rudolph, A. M., and Melmon, K. L.: Developmental changes in constriction of the ductus arteriosus: Responses to oxygen and vasoactive substances in the isolated ductus arteriosus of the fetal lamb. Pediat. Res. *6*:231, 1972.
Magbagbeola, J. A. O., and Adadevoh, B. K.: Metabolic response to anaesthesia and upper abdominal surgery in Nigerians: Changes in plasma cortisol, insulin and blood sugar. Brit. J. Anaesth. *46*:942, 1974.
Makowski, E. L., Hertz, R. H., and Meschia, G.: Effects of acute maternal hypoxia and hyperoxia on the blood flow to the pregnant uterus. Amer. J. Obstet. Gynecol. *115*:624, 1973.
Malatinsky, J., and Kadlic, T.: Inferior vena caval occlusion in the left lateral position. Brit. J. Anaesth. *46*:165, 1974.
Malliani, A., Peterson, D. F., Bishop, V. S., and Brown, A. M.: Spinal sympathetic cardiocardiac reflexes. Circ. Res. *30*:158, 1972.
Malliani, A., Parks, M., Tuckett, R. P., and Brown, A. M.: Reflex increases in heart rate elicited by stimulation of afferent cardiac sympathetic nerve fibers in the cat. Circ. Res. *32*:9, 1973.

Marcus, M. L., Heistad, D. D., Ehrhardt, J. C., and Abboud, F. M.: Regulation of total and regional spinal cord blood flow. Circ. Res. *41*:128, 1977.

Margolis, G., Griffin, A. T., Kenan, P. D., Tindall, E., Laughlin, H., and Phillips, R. L.: Circulatory dynamics of the canine spinal cord. J. Neurosurg. *14*:506, 1957.

Margreth, A., Salviati, G., and Carraro, U.: Neural control on the activity of the calcium-transport system in sarcoplasmic reticulum of rat skeletal muscle. Nature *241*:285, 1973.

Marley, E., and Paton, W. D. M.: The output of sympathetic amines from the cat's adrenal gland in response to splanchnic nerve activity. J. Physiol. (Lond.) *155*:1, 1961.

Mellander, S.: Comparative studies on the adrenergic neurohumoral control of resistance and capacitance blood vessels in the cat. Acta Physiol. Scand. *50*:176, 1960.

Mellander, S., and Johansson, B.: Control of resistance, exchange, and capacitance functions in the peripheral circulation. Pharmacol. Rev. *20*:117, 1968.

Meltzer, H. Y.: Serum creatine phosphokinase in schizophrenia. Amer. J. Psychiat. *133*:2, 192, 1976.

Meltzer, H. Y., and Engel, W. K.: Histochemical abnormalities of skeletal muscle in acutely psychotic patient. Arch. Gen. Psychiat. *23*:492, 1970b.

Meltzer, H. Y., and Moline, R.: Muscle abnormalities in acute psychoses. Arch. Gen. Psychiat. *23*:481, 1970a.

Meltzer, H. Y., Elkun, L., and Moline, R. A.: Serum-enzyme changes in newly admitted psychiatric patients. Arch. Gen. Psychiat. *21*:731, 1969.

Metcalfe, J., Romney, S. L., Swartwout, J. R., Pitcairn, D. M., Lethin, A. N., and Barron, D. H.: Uterine blood flow and oxygen consumption in pregnant sheep and goats. Amer. J. Physiol. *197*:929, 1959.

Miledi, R.: The acetylcholine sensitivity of frog muscle fibres after complete or partial denervation. J. Physiol. (Lond.) *151*:1, 1960.

Milic-Emili, J., Henderson, J. A. M., Dolovich, M. B., et al: Regional distribution of inspired gas in the lung. J. Appl. Physiol. *21*:749, 1966.

Millar, R. A., and Morris, M. E.: Sympatho-adrenal responses during general anaesthesia in the dog and man. Canad. Anaesth. Soc. J. *8*:356, 1961.

Miller, R. R., Vismara, L. A., Zelis, R., Amsterdam, E. A., and Mason, D. T.: Clinical use of sodium nitroprusside in chronic ischemic heart disease. Effects on peripheral vascular resistance and venous tone and on ventricular volume, pump and mechanical performance. Circulation *51*:328, 1975.

Miller, R. R., Vismara, L. A., Williams, D. O., Amsterdam, E. A., and Mason, D. T.: Pharmacological mechanisms for left ventricular unloading in clinical congestive heart failure. Differential effects of nitroprusside, phentolamine, and nitroglycerin on cardiac function and peripheral circulation. Circ. Res. *39*:127, 1976.

Moore, F. D.: Metabolic Care of the Surgical Patient. Philadelphia, W. B. Saunders Co., 1959.

Morales-Anguilerá, A., and Vaughan Williams, E. M.: The effects on cardiac muscle of betareceptor antagonists in relation to their activity as local anaesthetics. Brit. J. Pharmacol. *24*:332, 1965.

Morikawa, K. I., Bonica, J. J., Tucker, G. T., and Murphy, T. M.: Effect of acute hypovolaemia on lignocaine absorption and cardiovascular response following epidural block in dogs. Brit. J. Anaesth. *46*:631, 1974.

Morris, D. D., and Candy, J.: Anaesthesia for prostatectomy. Brit. J. Anaesth. *29*:376, 1957.

Morton, H. J. V.: Respiratory patterns during surgical anaesthesia. Anaesthesia *5*:112, 1950.

Moyes, D. G.: Malignant hyperpyrexia caused by trimeprazine: Case report. Brit. J. Anaesth. *45*:1163, 1973.

Mudge, G. H., Grossman, W., Mills, R. M., Lesch, M., and Braunwald, E.: Reflex increase in coronary vascular resistance in patients with ischemic heart disease. New Eng. J. Med. *295*:1333, 1976.

Mukherjee, S. R.: Effect of bladder distension on arterial blood pressure and renal circulation: Role of splanchnic and buffer nerves. J. Physiol. (Lond.) *138*:307, 1957.

Muneyuki, M., Ueda, Y., Urabe, N., Takeshita, H., and Inamoto, A.: Postoperative pain relief and respiratory function in man: Comparison between intermittent intravenous injections of meperidine and continuous lumbar epidural analgesia. Anesthesiology *29*:304, 1968.

Murphy, B. E. P.: Does the human fetal adrenal play a role in parturition? Am. J. Obstet. Gynecol. *115*:521, 1973.

Nathan, P. W.: Observations on sensory and sympathetic function during intrathecal analgesia. J. Neurol. Neurosurg. Psychiat. *39*:114, 1976.

Needham, D. M.: Machina Carnis: The Biochemistry of Muscular Contraction in Its Historical Development. Cambridge, Cambridge University Press, 1971, pp. 484–498.

Ngai, S. H.: Plasma catecholamines—Their significance in anesthesia. Anesthesiology *41*:429, 1974.

Nikki, P., Takki, S., Tammisto, T., and Jäättelä, A.: Effect of operative stress on plasma catecholamine levels. Ann. Clin. Res. *4*:146, 1972.

Nomura, G., Kurosaki, M., Takabatake, T., Kibe, Y., and Takeuchi, J.: Reinnervation and renin release after unilateral renal denervation in the dog. J. Appl. Physiol. *33*:649, 1972.

Nomura, G., Kibe, Y., Arai, S., Uno, D., and Takeuchi, J.: Distribution of intrarenal blood flow after renal denervation in the dog. Nephron *16*:126, 1976.

Noriega, L., Cibils, L. A., Alvarez, H., Poseiro, J. J., Posé, S. V., Sica-Blanco, Y., Mendez-Bauer, C., Fielitz, C., Gonzalez-Panizza, V. H., and Caldeyro-Barcia, R.: Efecto de los cambios de posicion de la parturienta sobre la intensidad y la frecuencia de las contracciones uterinas. Anales de la Facultad de Medicina. Montevideo *44*:383, 1959.

Norris, J. E., Foreman, R. D., and Wurster, R. D.: Responses of the canine heart to stimulation of the first five ventral thoracic roots. Amer. J. Physiol. *227*:9, 1974.

Nunn, J. F.: The distribution of inspired gas during thoracic surgery. Ann. Roy. Coll. Surg. Eng. *28*:223, 1961.

Nyberg, R., and Westin, B.: The influence of oxygen tension and some drugs on human placental vessels. Acta Physiol. Scand. *39*:216, 1957.

Öberg, B., and Thorén, P.: Studies on left ventricular receptors signalling in non-medullated vagal afferents. Acta Physiol. Scand. *85*:145, 1972a.

Öberg, B., and Thorén, P.: Increased activity in left ventricular receptors during hemorrhage or occlusion of caval veins in the cat. A possible cause of vaso-vagal reaction. Acta Physiol. Scand. *85*:164, 1972b.

Odom, C. B.: Epidural anesthesia. Amer. J. Surg. *34*:547, 1936.

Okinaka, A. J.: Closure of pulmonary air spaces following abdominal surgery. Surg. Gynecol. Obstet. *121*:1282, 1965.

Otton, P. E., and Wilson, E. J.: The cardiocirculatory effects of upper thoracic epidural analgesia. Canad. Anaesth. Soc. J. *13*:541, 1966.

Overholt, R. H.: Postoperative pulmonary hypoventilation. J.A.M.A. *95*:1484, 1930.

Oyama, T., Takiguchi, M., Aoki, N., and Kudo, T.: Adrenocortical function related to thiopental-nitrous oxide-oxygen anesthesia and surgery in man. Anesth. Analg. *50*:727, 1971.

Page, I. H., Corcoran, A. C., Dustan, H. P., and Koppanyi, T.: Cardiovascular actions of sodium nitroprusside in animals and hypertensive patients. Circulation *11*:188, 1955.

Pagés, F.: Anestesia metamerica. Rev. Sanid. Mil. Madr. *11*:351, 1921.

Palmeiro, C., Zetterstrom, B., Shamnash, J., Euchbaum, E., Frank, E., and Fine, J.: Denervation of the abdominal viscera for the treatment of shock. New Eng. J. Med. *269*:709, 1963.

Panigel, M.: Contribution à la physiologie de la circulation foeto-placentaire I. Etude de la vaso-motricité des artères du cordon ombilical humain. J. Physiol. (Paris) *51*:941, 1959.

Panigel, M.: Placental perfusion experiments. Amer. J. Obstet. Gynecol. *84*:1664, 1962.

Papper, E. M., Habif, D. V., and Bradley, S. E.: Studies on renal and hepatic function in normal man during thiopental, cyclopropane and high spinal anesthesia. J. Clin. Invest. *29*:838, 1950.

Parbrook, G. D.: Post-operative pain relief: Comparison of methadone and morphine when used concurrently with nitrous-oxide analgesia. Brit. Med. J. *2*:616, 1966.

Parbrook, G. D., and Kennedy, B. R.: Value of premixed nitrous-oxide-and-oxygen mixtures in the relief of post-operative pain. Double blind trial of 25% nitrous oxide in oxygen, 15% nitrous oxide in oxygen, and oxygen. Brit. Med. J. *2*:1303, 1964.

Payling Wright, H., Osborn, S. B., and Edmonds, D. G.: Changes in the rate of flow of venous blood in the leg during pregnancy measured with radioactive sodium. Surg. Gynecol. Obstet. *90*:481, 1950.

Perry, L. B., Van Dyke, R. A., and Theye, R. A.: Sympathoadrenal and hemodynamic effects of insoflurane, halothane and cycloproprane in dogs. Anesthesiology *40*:465, 1974.

Pflug, A. E., Murphy, T. M., Butler, S. H., and Tucker, G. T.: The effects of postoperative peridural analgesia on pulmonary therapy and pulmonary complications. Anesthesiology *41*:8, 1974.

Pierson, R. N., and Grieco, M. H.: Pulmonary blood volume in asthma. J. Appl. Physiol. *32*:391, 1972.

Pomeranz, B. H., Birtch, A. G., and Barger, A. C.: Neural control of intrarenal blood flow. Amer. J. Physiol. *215*:1067, 1968.

Pooler, H. E.: Relief of postoperative pain and its influence on the vital capacity. Brit. Med. J. *2*:1201, 1949.

Porte, D., Girardier, L., Seydoux, J., Kanazawa, Y., and Posternak, J.: Neural regulation of insulin secretion in the dog. J. Clin. Invest. *52*:210, 1973.

Potgieter, S. V.: Atelectasis: Its evolution during upper urinary tract surgery. Brit. J. Anaesth. *31*:472, 1959.

Power, G. G., and Longo, L. D.: Sluice flow in placenta: Maternal vascular pressure effects on fetal circulation. Am. J. Physiol. *225*:1490, 1973.

Powers, J. H.: Vital capacity: Its significance in relation to postoperative pulmonary complications. Arch. Surg. *304*:17, 1928.

Prewitt, M. A., and Salafsky, B.: Effect of cross innervation on biochemical characteristics of skeletal muscles. Amer. J. Physiol. *213*:295, 1967.

Price, H. L., Deutsch, S., Cooperman, L. H., Clement, A. J., and Epstein, R. M.: Splanchnic circulation during cyclopropane anesthesia in normal man. Anesthesiology *26*:312, 1965.

Price, H. L., Deutsch, S., Davidson, I. A., Clement, A. J., Behar, M. G., and Epstein, R. M.: Can general anesthetics produce splanchnic visceral hypoxia by reducing regional blood flow? Anesthesiology *27*:24, 1966.

Pugh, L. G. C., and Wyndham, C. L.: The circulatory effects of high spinal anaesthesia in hypertensive and control subjects. Clin. Sci. *9*:189, 1950.

Randall, W. C., and Armour, J. A.: Regional vagosympathetic control of the heart. Amer. J. Physiol. *227*:444, 1974.

Randall, W. C., and McNally, N.: Augmentor action of the sympathetic cardiac nerves in man. J. Appl. Physiol. *15*:629, 1960.

Ranniger, K., and Switz, D. M.: Local obstruction of the inferior vena cava by massive ascites. Amer. J. Roentgen. *93*:935, 1965.

Rautenberg, W.: Die Bedeutung der zentralnervösen Thermosensitivität für die Temperatur-regulation der Taub. Z. Vergl. Physiol. *62*:235, 1969.

Rautenberg, W.: The influence of the skin temperature on the thermoregulatory system of pigeons. J. Physiol. (Paris) *63*:396, 1971.

Redfern, P., and Thesleff, S.: Action potential generation in denervated rat skeletal muscle. II. The action of tetrodotoxin. Acta Physiol. Scand. *82*:70, 1971.

Rehder, K., Theye, R. A., and Fowler, W. S.: Function of each lung of dogs during intermittent positive-pressure breathing. Amer. J. Physiol. *206*:1031, 1964.

Rehder, K., Hatch, D. J., Sessler, A. D., Marsh, H. M., and Fowler, W. S.: Effects of general anesthesia, muscle paralysis, and mechanical ventilation on pulmonary nitrogen clearance. Anesthesiology *35*:591, 1971.

Rehder, K., Sittipong, R., and Sessler, A.: The effects of thiopental-meperidine anesthesia with succinylcholine paralysis on functional residual capacity and dynamic lung compliance in normal sitting man. Anesthesiology *37*:395, 1972.

Reivich, M.: Arterial pCO_2 and cerebral hemodynamics. Amer. J. Physiol. *206*:25, 1964.

Relton, J. E. S., Britt, B. A., and Steward, D. J.: Malignant hyperpyrexia. Brit. J. Anaesth. *45*:269, 1973.

Robson, M. C.: A new look at diabetes mellitus and infection. Amer. J. Surg. *210*:681, 1970.

Robson, M. C., and Heggers, J. P.: Effect of hyperglycemia on survival of bacteria. Surg. Forum *20*:56, 1969.

Rodbard, S.: Bronchomotor tone. A neglected factor in the regulation of the pulmonary circulation. Amer. J. Med. *15*:356, 1953.

Roger, A., Rossi, G. F., and Zirondolli, A.: Le rôle des afférences des nerfs crâniens dans le maintien de l'état vigile de la préparation "encéphale isolé." Electroenceph. Clin. Neurophysiol. *8*:1, 1956.

Roizen, M. F., Moss, J., Henry, D. P., and Kopin, I. J.: Effects of halothane on plasma catecholamines. Anesthesiology *41*:432, 1974.

Rosenfeld, C. R., Barton, M. D., and Meschia, G.: Effects of epinephrine on distribution of blood flow in the pregnant ewe. Amer. J. Obstet. Gynecol. *214*:156, 1976.

Rothstein, E., Landis, F. B., and Narodick, B. G.: Bronchospirometry in the lateral decubitus position. J. Thorac. Surg. *19*:821, 1950.

Rubinson, R. M., Vasko, J. S., Doppman, J. L., and Morrow, A. G.: Inferior vena caval obstruction from increased intra-abdominal pressure. Arch. Surg. *94*:766, 1967.

Runge, H.: Über den Venendruck in Schwangerschaft, Geburt und Wochenbett. Archiv. f. Gynaek. *122*:142, 1924.

Ryan, M. J., Clark, K. E., and Brody, M. J.: Neurogenic and mechanical control of canine uterine vascular resistance. Amer. J. Physiol. *227*:547, 1974.

Salmoiraghi, G. C.: Functional organization of brain stem respiratory neurones. Ann. N.Y. Acad. Sci. *109*:571, 1963.

Salmoiraghi, G. C., and Burns, B. D.: Localization and patterns of discharge of respiratory neurones in brain-stem of cat. J. Neurophysiol. *23*:2, 1960a.

Salmoiraghi, G. C., and Burns, B. D.: Notes on mechanism of rhythmic respiration. J. Neurophysiol. *23*:14, 1960b.

Sarnoff, S. J., and Berglund, E.: Neurohemodynamics of pulmonary edema. IV. Effect of systemic vasoconstriction and subsequent vasodilatation on the flow and pressures in systemic and pulmonary vascular beds. Amer. J. Physiol. *170*:588, 1952.

Sarnoff, S. J., and Farr, H. W.: Spinal anesthesia in therapy of pulmonary edema: A preliminary report. Anesthesiology *5*:69, 1944.

Sartorius, O. W., and Burlington, H.: Acute effects of denervation on kidney function in the dog. Amer. J. Physiol. *185*:407, 1956.

Savitz, M. H., and Mills, L. I.: Intractable pain treated with intrathecal isotonic iced saline. J. Neurol. Neurosurg. Psychiat. *36*:417, 1973.

Saxon, A., and Kattlove, H. E.: Platelet inhibition by sodium nitroprusside, a smooth muscle inhibitor. Blood *47*:957, 1976.

Saxton, G. A., Rabinowitz, M., Dexter, L., and Haynes, F.: The relationship of pulmonary compliance to pulmonary vascular pressures in patients with heart disease. J. Clin. Invest. *35*:611, 1956.

Schumacker, H. B., Riberi, A., Boone, R. D., and Kajikuri, H.: Ventricular fibrillation in the hypothermic state. IV. The role of extrinsic cardiac innervation. Ann. Surg. *143*:223, 1956.

Schwarcz, R. L., Belizan, J. M., Cifuentes, J. R., Cuadro, J. C., Marques, M. B., and Caldeyro-Barcia, R.: Fetal and maternal monitoring in spontaneous labors and in elective inductions. Amer. J. Obstet. Gynecol. *210*:356, 1974.

Scott, D. B.: Inferior vena caval pressure. Changes occurring during anaesthesia. Anaesthesia *18*:135, 1963.

Scott, D. B.: Inferior vena caval occlusion in late pregnancy. Clin. Anesth. *10*:37, 1973.

Scott, D. B., and Kerr, M. G.: Inferior vena caval pressure in late pregnancy. J. Obstet. Gynaecol. Brit. Cwlth. *70*:1044, 1963.

Scott, D. B., Davie, I. T., and Stephen, G. W.: Cardiovascular effects of intravenous lignocaine during nitrous oxide-halothane anaesthesia. Brit. J. Anaesth. *43*:595, 1971.

Scott, D. B., Jebson, P. J. R., Braid, D. P., Örtengren, B., and Frisch, P.: Factors affecting plasma levels of lignocaine and prilocaine. Brit. J. Anaesth. *44*:1040, 1972.

Scott, D. B., Littlewood, D. G., Drummond, G. B., Buckley, B. F., and Covino, B. G.: Modification of the circulatory effects of extradural block combined with general anesthesia by the addition of adrenaline to lignocaine solutions. Brit. J. Anaesth. *49*:917, 1977.

Sharpey-Schafer, E. P.: Syncope. Brit. Med. J. *1*:506, 1956.

Shaw, E. C.: Epidural anesthesia for perineal prostatectomy. J. Urol. *15*:219, 1926.

Shimazu, T., and Fukuda, A.: Increased activities of glycogenolytic enzymes in liver after splanchnic-nerve stimulation. Science *15*:1607, 1965.

Shimazu, T., Fukuda, A., and Ban, T.: Reciprocal influences of the ventromedial and lateral hypothalamic nuclei on blood glucose level and liver glycogen content. Nature *210*:1178, 1966.

Shimosato, S., and Etsten, B. E.: The role of the venous system in cardiocirculatory dynamics during spinal and epidural anesthesia in man. Anesthesiology *30*:619, 1964.

Shoemaker, C. P.: A study of hepatic hemodynamics in the dog. Circ. Res. *15*:216, 1964.

Shorr, E., Zweifach, B. W., and Furchott, R. F.: On the occurrence, sites and modes of origin and destruction, of principles affecting the compensatory vascular mechanism in experimental shock. Science *102*:489, 1945.

Silver, J. R., and Buxton, P. H.: Spinal stroke. Brain *97*:539, 1974.

Simpson, B. R., Parkhouse, J., Marshall, R., and Lambrechts, W.: Extradural analgesia and the prevention of postoperative respiratory complications. Brit. J. Anaesth. *33*:628, 1961.

Sjögren, S., and Wright, B.: Circulation, respiration and lidocaine concentration during continuous epidural blockade. Acta Anaesth. Scand. Suppl. 46, *16*:5, 1972.

Smith, A. L., Pender, J. W., and Alexander, S. C.: Effects of PCO_2 on spinal cord blood flow. Amer. J. Physiol. *216*:1158, 1969.

Smith, O. A.: Reflex and central mechanisms involved in the control of the heart and circulation. Ann. Rev. Physiol. *36*:93, 1974.

Spence, A. A., and Smith, G.: Postoperative analgesia and lung function: A comparison of morphine with extradural block. Brit. J. Anaesth. *43*:144, 1971.

Spencer, H., and Leof, D.: The innervation of the human lung. J. Anat. (Lond.) *98*:599, 1964.

Steenberg, R. W., Lennihan, R., and Moore, F. D.: Studies in surgical endocrinology. II. The free blood 17-hydroxycorticosteroids in surgical patients: Their relation to urine steroids, metabolism and convalescence. Ann. Surg. *143*:180, 1956.

Stein, J. H., Boonjarern, S., Mauk, R. C., and Ferris, T. F.: Mechanism of the redistribution of the renal cortical blood flow during hemorrhagic hypotension in the dog. J. Clin. Invest. *52*:39, 1973.

Steinhaus, J. E.: Local anesthetic toxicity: A pharmacological re-evaluation. Anesthesiology *18*:275, 1957.

Stewart, D. M., Rogers, W. P., Mahaffey, J. E., Winterspoon, S., and Woods, E. F.: Effect of local anesthetics on the cardiovascular system of the dog. Anesthesiology *24*:620, 1963.

Stolar, S. H., and Wynands, J. E.: A technique for cancer perfusion. Canad. Anaesth. Soc. J. *10*:48, 1963.

Surtshin, A., Mueller, C. B., and White, H. L.: Effect of acute changes in glomerular filtration rate on water and electrolyte excretion: Mechanism of denervation diuresis. Amer. J. Physiol. *169*:159, 1952.

Takki, S., Nikki, P., Tammisto, T., and Jäättelä, A.: Effect of epidural blockade on the pentazocine-induced increase in plasma catecholamines and blood pressure. Brit. J. Anaesth. *45*:376, 1973.

Tammisto, T., Jäätelä, A., Nikki, P., and Takki, S.: Effect of pentazocine and pethidine on plasma catecholamine levels. Ann. Clin. Res. *3*:22, 1971.

Terragno, N. A., Terragno, D. A., Pacholcyzk, D., and McGiff, J. C.: Prostaglandins and the regulation of uterine blood flow in pregnancy. Nature *249*:57, 1974.

Thauer, R., and Simon, E.: Spinal cord and temperature regulation. *In* Ito, S., Ogata, K., and Yoshimura, H. (eds.): Advances in Climatic Physiology. Tokyo, Igaku Shoin Ltd., 1972, pp. 22–49.

Thomasson, B.: Studies on the content of 17-hydroxycorticosteroids and its diurnal rhythm in the plasma of surgical patients. Scand. J. Clin. Lab. Invest. (Suppl.)*42*:1, 1959.

Thompson, M. W.: Some principles of medical genetics. *In* Gordon, R. A., Britt, B. A., and Kalow, W. (eds.): International Symposium on Malignant Hyperthermia. Springfield, Ill., Charles C Thomas, Publisher, 1973, pp. 59–66.

Thorne, T. C., Galley, H. A., and Bromage, P. R.: Present position of spinal and epidural analgesia. Proc. Roy. Soc. Med. *47*:301, 1954.

Trueta, J., Barclay, A. E., Daniel, P. M., Franklin, K. J., and Prichard, M. M. L.: Studies of the Renal Circulation. Oxford, Blackwell Scientific Publications, 1948.

Ueland, K., and Hansen, J. M.: Maternal cardiovascular dynamics. II. Posture and uterine contractions. Amer. J. Obstet. Gynecol. *103*:1, 1969.

Ueland, K., Akamatsu, T. J., Eng, M., Bonica, J. J., and Hansen, J. M.: Maternal cardiovascular dynamics. VI. Cesarean section under epidural anesthesia without epinephrine. Amer. J. Obstet. Gynecol. *114*:775, 1972.

Urquhart-Hay, D.: Paraplegia following epidural analgesia. Anaesthesia *24*:461, 1969.

Usubiaga, J. E., Gollan, F., Yannakakis, Z., and Johnson, A.: The effect of epidural and subarachnoid epinephrine upon spinal cord blood flow, Proc. A. S. A. Meeting, San Francisco, 1969, p. 57.

Valori, C., Brunori, C. A., and Renzini, V.: Improved procedure for formation of epinephrine and norepinephrine fluophors by the trihydroxyindole reaction. Anal. Biochem. *33*:158, 1970.

Virtue, R. W., Helmriech, M. L., and Gainza, E.: The adrenal cortical response to surgery. I. The effect of anesthesia on plasma 17-hydroxycorticosteroid levels. Surgery *41*:549. 1957.

Wahba, W. M., Craig, D. B., Don, H. F., and Becklake, M. R.: The cardiorespiratory effects of thoracic epidural anaesthesia. Canad. Anaesth. Soc. J. *19*:8, 1972.

Wahba, W. M., Don, H. F., and Craig, D. B.: Post-operative epidural analgesia: Effects on lung volumes. Canad. Anaesth. Soc. J. *22*:519, 1975.

Wallenburg, H. C. S., Mazer, J., and Hutchinson, D. L.: Effects of a beta-adrenergic agent (metaproterenol) on uteroplacental circulation. An angiographic study in the pregnant rhesus monkey. Amer. J. Obstet. Gynecol. *117*:1067, 1973.

Wallis, K. L., Shnider, S. M., Hicks, J. S., and Spivey, H. T.: Epidural anesthesia in the normotensive pregnant ewe: Effects on uterine blood flow and fetal acid-base status. Anesthesiology *44*:481, 1976.

Ward, R. J., Bonica, J. J., Freund, F. G., Akamatsu, T., Danziger, F., and Engelsson, S.: Epidural and subarachnoid anesthesia: Cardiovascular and respiratory effects. J.A.M.A. *191*:275, 1965.

Waters, H. R., Rosen, N., and Perkins, D. H.: Extradural blockade with bupivacaine. A double blind trial of bupivacaine with adrenaline 1/200,000 and bupivacaine plain. Anaesthesia *25*:184, 1970.

Weaver, J. B., Pearson, J. F., and Turnbull, A. C.: The effect upon the fetus of an oxytocin infusion in the absence of uterine hypertonus. J. Obstet. Gynecol. Brit. Cwlth. *81*:297, 1974.

Werner, M. H., Hayes, D. F., Lucas, C. E., and Rosenberg, I. K.: Renal vasoconstriction in association with acute pancreatitis. Amer. J. Surg. *127*:185, 1974.

Westbrook, P. R., Stubbs, S. E., Sessler, A. D., Rehder, K., and Hyatt, R. E.: Effects of anesthesia and muscle paralysis on respiratory mechanics in normal man. J. Appl. Physiol. *34*:81, 1973.

Widdicombe, J. G.: Regulation of tracheobronchial smooth muscle. Physiol. Rev. *43*:1, 1963.

Wiederman, M. P.: Dimensions of blood vessels from distributing artery to collecting vein. Circ. Res. *12*:375, 1963.

Williams, C. H., Houchins, C., and Shanklin, M. D.: Pigs susceptible to energy metabolism in the fulminant hyperthermia stress syndrome. Brit. Med. J. *2*:411, 1975.

Williams, C. H., Stubbs, D. H., Payne, C. G., and Benedict, J. D.: Role of hypertension in fulminant hyperthermia-stress syndrome. Brit. Med. J. *1*:628, 1976.

Wisehart, J. D., Archie, J. P., Kirklin, J. W., and Tracy, W. G.: Myocardial blood flow and oxygen consumption in man early after valve replacement. Circulation *49*:933, 1974.

Woods, E. F., and Richardson, J. A.: Effects of acute anoxia on cardiac contractility. Amer. J. Physiol. *196*:203, 1959.

Woods, E. F., Richardson, J. A., Richardson, A. K., and Bozeman, R. F.: Plasma concentrations of epinephrine and arterenol following the actions of various agents on the adrenals. J. Pharmacol. Exp. Ther. *116*:351, 1956.

Woods, S. C., and Porte, D.: Neural control of the endocrine pancreas. Physiol. Rev. *54*:596, 1974.

Wulff, K. E., and Aulin, I.: The regional lung function in the lateral ducubitus position during anaesthesia and operation. Acta Anaesth. Scand. *16*:195, 1972.

Yamamoto, Y. L., Hodge, C. P., Phillips, K. M., and Feindel, W.: Microflow patterns after experimental occlusion of middle cerebral artery demonstrated by fluorescein angiography and ^{133}Xenon clearance. *In* Brock, M., Fieschi, C., Ingvar, D. H., Lassen, N. A., and Schürman, K.: Cerebral Blood Flow. New York, Springer-Verlag, 1969, pp. 123–126.

Yeates, W. K.: Disorders of bladder function. Ann. Roy. Coll. Surg. Eng. *50*:335, 1972.

Zimmerman, B.: Pituitary and adrenal function in relation to surgery. Surg. Clin. N. Amer. *45*:299, 1965.

Zimmerman, H. A.: A preliminary report on intracardiac catheterization studies during pregnancy. J. Lab. Clin. Med. *36*:1007, 1950.

Zsigmond, E. K., Starkweather, W. H., Duboff, G. S., and Flynn, K. A.: Abnormal creatine phosphokinase isoenzyme patterns in families with malignant hyperpyrexia. Anesth. Analg. *51*:827, 1972.

chapter 11
Surgical Applications

It is hard for thee to kick against the pricks

Acts 9:5

INTRODUCTION

All segments of the spinal canal from the base of the skull to the sacral hiatus are available for epidural injection, and epidural analgesia can be adapted to almost any type of surgery below the chin. Whether it is used alone or in combination with general anesthesia depends on a number of factors, which include the respiratory competence of the patient and his personal preferences.

Epidural analgesia is suitable as a sole agent for lower abdominal surgery and for operations on the lower limbs and pelvis. Operations involving the upper abdomen are more comfortably performed with combinations of epidural analgesia and light general anesthesia, while intrathoracic surgery usually, but not always, demands intubation and controlled ventilation. Surgery on the shoulder or neck can be performed on awake patients under epidural analgesia alone, but operations in these areas are more comfortable and better controlled when combined with light general anesthesia. Epidural analgesia is also suited to surgery on the spine. However, there are well-recognized neurological sequelae associated with surgery of the spine, as pointed out in Chapter 12, and it is imprudent to risk unnecessary involvement in litigation if other methods of anesthesia will serve. Nevertheless, on rare occasions epidural analgesia may be the best choice for delicate surgery on the spine, as in certain vascular anomalies of the cord. Then, added safety is gained by having the patient awake and cooperative for neurological testing during the course of operation.

The rationale of epidural analgesia in surgery is simple. The technique is used to prevent afferent impulses from reaching the central nervous system and to prevent transmission of inappropriate efferent signals to target organs such as muscles, blood vessels and viscera. In doing so, epidural blockade fulfills the central aims of anesthesia, that is, prevention of pain, overall control of the patient and his reflexes and preservation of physical well-being. The reflex responses to injury outlined in Chapter 10 are remnants of ancient protective mechanisms for survival in a violent hostile environment. Reflex spasm around an injured part, whether in a limb or in the abdomen or chest, is helpful for protection in battle, but it has no meaning and no relevance in sickbed or on an operating table. Then the whole process of care and healing demands a relaxed body, while ordinary background functions are allowed to carry on as normally as possible, as if nothing had happened.

Surgery without suppression of afferent impulses conjures up the full protective program inherited from our evolutionary past. The blood sugar climbs to persistently high levels, in some instances to hyperosmolar concentrations. Each breath becomes a partial Valsalva maneuver as the clenched chest and abdominal wall restrict breathing to a fraction of normal potential, and venous pressure rises from compression of the large veins and plexuses within the rigid trunk walls. Not only are these actions inappropriate in the therapeutic context, but also they are all harmful to a greater or lesser degree, and in some circumstances they may become lethal unless steps are taken to prevent them. The most obvious ill effects are seen in the venous circulation and in hindered respiration.

This chapter will apply to the surgical situation information set out in earlier sections, first in a general way in terms of exploitation of altered physiological responses, and later in terms of detailed practical management.

CARDIOVASCULAR STATUS

The effects of epidural analgesia on the vascular system were discussed in Chapter 10. Here we will merely emphasize those modifications that may be applied to improving surgical conditions on the operating table, as well as the state of the patient after the operation is over.

Arterial Pressure

Some reduction of arterial pressure usually occurs when epidural blockade extends into the thoracic segments unless vasopressor agents are used to prevent hypotension (Bromage, 1951). A moderate degree of arterial hypotension is helpful in preventing unnecessary blood loss. More pronounced arterial hypotension and controlled vascular stability can be induced by extending blockade to involve the whole sympathetic outflow. This may be useful to reduce operative bleeding or to provide unusually stable background conditions in the vascular bed for certain operations, such as exploration for a pheochromocytoma (Bromage and Millar, 1958; Cousins and Rubin, 1973).

Venous Pressure

During surgery under light general anesthesia the venous pressure rises as a result of increased vasomotor activity and of raised intra-abdominal pressure due to increased respiratory drive and heightened tone in the expiratory muscles (McCann, 1946; Morton, 1950; Bromage, 1958a; Freund et al., 1964; Kaul et al., 1973). As a consequence venous oozing and blood loss increase. These unfavorable changes do not occur under regional anesthesia.

In the 1950's when controlled hypotension to produce a dry surgical field was in vogue, most anesthesiologists were aware of the importance of a tranquil anesthetic in obtaining the desired operating conditions. However, emphasis was focused on the arterial side of the circulation. Controlled hypotension was referred to as "controlled *arterial* hypotension," and the venous side received secondary attention. Today, thanks to the prodigious generosity of blood banks, even less attention is paid to venous oozing, and very little attempt is made to ensure low venous pressures.

One of the most striking characteristics of effective regional analgesia is the relatively bloodless appearance of the tissues, even in the presence of a normal arterial blood pressure (Fujikawa et al., 1948). There is no general response to the knife. Breathing is easy, the trunk muscles are relaxed, with a low intrathoracic pressure, and the central venous pressure follows suit. Relatively few formal studies have been undertaken to document these phenomena in terms of accurate blood loss measurements. Because of the many variables involved, it is difficult to obtain useful comparisons of blood loss between different series and different techniques (Moir, 1968). In one hospital where I worked, an estimate of blood replacement for open hip operations in children showed a saving of approximately 50 per cent with epidural blockade, but this was a small series that needed wider confirmation. Stanton-Hicks (1971) has reported a similar reduction of blood loss in elderly patients undergoing prosthetic replacement of the hip joint, and comparable savings of blood loss have been reported in prostatic surgery (Zorgniotti et al., 1970; Fasth et al., 1972). Free unimpeded respiration seems to be an important factor in preserving a low CVP and in reducing hemorrhage: in one series of total hip replacements, blood loss was 56 per cent greater with IPPV than when the patient breathed spontaneously under epidural blockade (Modig and Malmberg, 1975).

In the postoperative period the level of central venous pressure (CVP) seems to be influenced more by the presence or absence of adequate analgesia than by the overall degree of vasomotor tone determined by the number of sympathetic segments anesthetized. Figure 11–1 illustrates this point in a patient two to three hours after partial gastrectomy.

Measurements of intraplural pressure with esophageal balloons show that the central venous pressure in the postoperative period is partly dependent on the end-expiratory pressure, which in turn is dependent on the rigidity of the chest and abdominal muscles (see Chapter 10). Clearly, the sympatholytic effects of epidural blockade on the cardiovascular system will play a major role in changes of CVP, but the "clenched chest" phenomenon will produce an additional artifactual increment through a raised intrathoracic pressure.

Table 11–1 from my own data shows the influence of pain and segmental analgesia on the CVP after upper abdominal surgery. Note that while the arterial pressure is reduced by only 10 per cent after epidural blockade, the central venous pressure is reduced by more than one-half. This large proportional change of CVP may have an important secondary effect on peripheral venous flow and on the incidence of postoperative thromboembolism. Peripheral venous flow is reduced when intrathoracic pressure is raised (Dyde and Bethel, 1968; Laaksonen et al., 1974), and it is reasonable to speculate

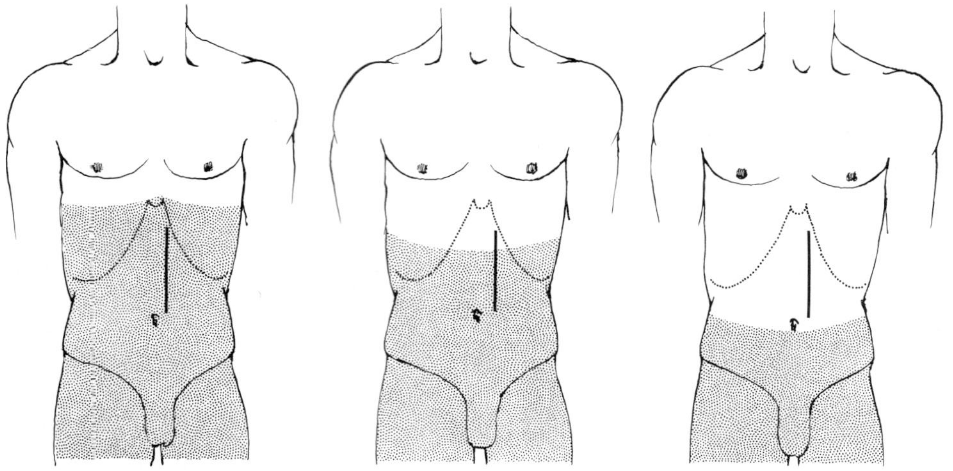

	Anaesthesia T_6	Pain T_8	Severe Pain T_{10}
VC	1600 ml	950 ml	750 ml
BP	120/80	130/90	130/80
CVP	5.0 cm H_2O	8.0 cm H_2O	12.0 cm H_2O

Figure 11–1. Segmental level of analgesia related to CVP and arterial blood pressure after subtotal gastrectomy. The CVP is low while analgesia is complete (blockade to T_6). The CVP rises as the level of analgesia falls, but the rise is greatest when wound pain is severe after analgesia has regressed to T_{10}.

that deep vein thrombosis is more likely to occur when venous return is impaired than when intrathoracic pressure and the CVP are low. Clinical data by Lahnborg and Bergström (1975), supported by ^{125}I fibrinogen scanning, suggest that thromboembolic complications are indeed less frequent after major abdominal surgery under epidural blockade and spontaneous respiration than after general anesthesia, in accordance with principles discussed in Chapter 7 on Continuous Epidural Analgesia.

TABLE 11–1 Central venous pressure after upper abdominal surgery; Influence of pain and effective epidural analgesia on CVP and arterial pressure in ten cases

Case	*CVP with Pain (cmH_2O)*	*CVP with Segmental Analgesia (cmH_2O)*	*ΔCVP with Analgesia (cmH_2O)*	*(%)*	*ΔArterial Pressure with Analgesia (%)*
1	13	8	−5	−38	−12
2	8	3	−5	−62	0
3	5.5	1	−4.5	−82	+ 7
4	9	2	−7	−78	−26
5	9	4	−5	−55	0
6	15	4	−9	−60	−21
7	14	7	−7	−50	−10
8	7.5	4.5	−3	−40	−12.5
9	12	5	−7	−58	−15
10	13	7	−6	−46	−10
Average:	10.6 ± 3.19	4.55 ± 2.27	−5.85	−56.9	−9.95

RESPIRATION

Intraoperative Respiration

Respiratory rhythm

Respiratory motor neurons are dependent upon an adequate traffic of afferent input to maintain their activity (Salmoiraghi and Burns, 1960). When this afferent traffic is reduced by high spinal blockade, the respiratory center readily surrenders its rhythm to imposed respiration (see section on Respiration in Chapter 10). Controlled respiration is easily induced in the presence of analgesia that extends into the upper thoracic segments and above the segmental level of surgical stimulation. Then a small dose of barbiturate, followed by a few inflations of the chest, is all that is required to induce controlled ventilation, and spontaneous respiration ceases. Total compliance is also increased by high blocks extending into the upper thoracic segments, and artificial ventilation can be maintained with relatively low mean intrathoracic pressures (Bromage, 1958a).

Phrenic reflex

As explained in Chapter 10, analgesia as high as T_1 obtunds the phrenic reflex by reducing the sensory input flowing past the phrenic nucleus in the mid-cervical cord. Then stimulation of the phrenic sensory territory in the central part of the diaphragm fails to elicit a characteristic coordinated diaphragmatic contraction, and diaphragmatic irritability is markedly reduced (Bromage, 1958b).

Spontaneous ventilation

General anesthesia that is deep enough to produce adequate reflex suppression and abdominal relaxation also depresses respiration to a point where carbon dioxide retention becomes dangerous. Early measurements of respiratory gases during anesthesia with spontaneous respiration revealed arterial carbon dioxide tensions in the range of 60 to 65 mmHg, and even higher when cyclopropane was used as the principal agent (Stormont et al., 1942; Dripps, 1947; Buckley et al., 1953).

Current methods of general anesthesia and neuromuscular blockade require controlled ventilation (IPPV) as an absolute necessity to maintain adequate respiratory exchange, but as we have seen in earlier sections (see Chapter 10 on Physiology), there are inherent disadvantages to IPPV, particularly in terms of pulmonary shunting and raised venous pressure in the central and peripheral circulations.

By contrast, effective regional anesthesia provides adequate relaxation without respiratory depression, and spontaneous respiration is adequate to maintain arterial blood gases within the normal range (Morgan and Norman, 1975). Several studies have shown that high epidural blockade produces insignificant changes of ventilation and acid-base balance in conscious subjects (Moir, 1963; Moir and Mone, 1964; Wahba et al., 1975; McCarthy, 1976). Even when general anesthesia is superimposed on epidural blockade for convenience or comfort's sake, the required level of central depression is so slight that respiratory performance differs little from that of normal physiological sleep. Robin and his colleagues (1958) found a range of end-tidal CO_2 in healthy sleeping volunteers between 41 and 49 mmHg, so these limits can be accepted as normal values for patients breathing spontaneously under a combination of epidural blockade and light general anesthesia.

The adequacy of spontaneous respiration was tested in a series of 41 upper abdominal operations in which lumbar or thoracic epidural blockade was used with 2 per cent lidocaine, 0.5 per cent bupivicaine or 1 per cent etidocaine. Light thiopentone, nitrous oxide and oxygen anesthesia was provided, with the patient breathing spontaneously through a cuffed endotracheal tube. Blood gas estimations were made at intervals throughout the operation. Figure 11–2 shows the results of this study plotted on standard coordinates for arterial pH, pCO_2 and bicarbonate. It can be seen that although minor degrees of respiratory acidosis were present during the second hour of spontaneous respiration, hypercapnia was relatively slight and within accepted limits for normal sleep in most of the patients.

This small series indicates that spontaneous respiration is often adequate during abdominal surgery performed under epidural analgesia and light general anesthesia. It does not imply that spontaneous breathing can be safely left to its own devices under all circumstances of physical condition, posture or length of surgery. Some degree of underventilation is bound to occur if breathing is handicapped by abnormal surgical posture, obesity or excessive motor blockade, and then the anesthesiologist must intervene and provide artificial ventilatory assistance to ensure normal gas exchange. However, in the great majority of cases spontaneous ventilation is adequate and safe if monitored by occasional checks on end-tidal CO_2 or arterial blood gases. Common sense and clinical judgment, backed by objective measurements of ventilation and blood gases, should dictate when the patient may be allowed to breathe by himself and when the anesthesiologist should step in and control respiration for

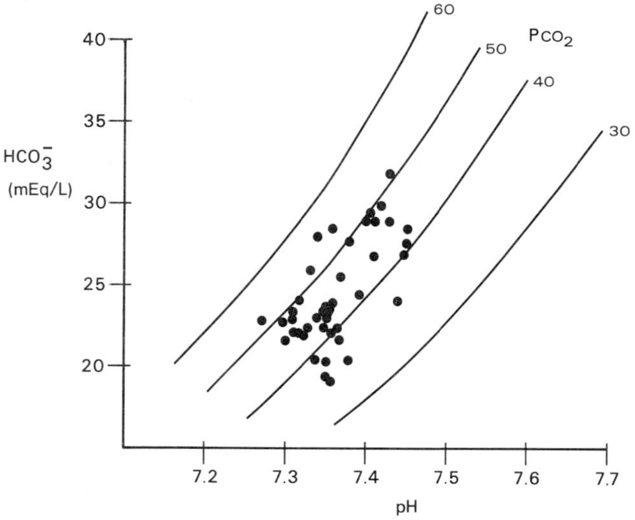

Figure 11–2. Acid-base balance in 41 patients during upper abdominal surgery under epidural blockade and light general anesthesia with spontaneous respiration. Arterial samples were drawn 60 to 120 minutes after incision.

him. As pointed out in Chapter 10, the geometry of the spontaneously moving diaphragm has a greater mechanical advantage and is more effective for gas exchange than the relaxed diaphragm passively driven under controlled respiration (Froese and Bryan, 1974).

Postoperative Respiration

It is in the postoperative phase that the respiratory handicap of abdominal and thoracic surgery is most noticeable and most susceptible to correction by segmental deafferentation. Many different methods of respiratory measurement have been used to confirm this phenomenon and to compare the effects of epidural analgesia with other methods of pain relief, as described in Chapter 10.

Centrally acting analgesics do not restore any of the impaired functions listed in Table 11–2 except vital capacity, and then only to a minor degree, whereas afferent blockade improves them all. The earliest postoperative signs of the different respiratory behavior after epidural blockade and after general anesthesia can be determined by simple measurements of total static compliance at the end of surgery, before the patient wakes up (Bromage, 1958a). Compliance falls about 15 to 25 per cent after the surgical incision under general anesthesia and remains reduced until the patient is extubated and measurements can no longer be made. Under epidural blockade and light general anesthesia, the compliance does not fall so far. Figure 11–3 shows measurements of total static compliance made after completion of surgery and immediately prior to extubation in 28 patients. Under epidural blockade, compliance fell very

TABLE 11–2 Respiratory functions affected by upper abdominal pain and modifications produced by systemic or epidural analgesia

		Restoration Toward Normal		
Function	***Change with Pain***	*SYSTEMIC ANALGESIA*	*EPIDURAL ANALGESIA*	***References***
Vital capacity	50–75% reduction	10–30%	70–100%	Churchill and McNeil, 1927; Beecher, 1933a; Bromage, 1955; Lewis and Welch, 1965; Simpson et al., 1961; Parbrook, 1966; Parbrook et al., 1964
Functional residual capacity	0–20% reduction	No change	Restoration to normal	Beecher, 1933b; Brattström, 1954; Anscombe, 1957; Lewis and Welch, 1965; Okinaka, 1965; Bromage et al., unpublished data
Peak expiratory flow rate	50–80% reduction	Less than 20% restoration	40–70% restoration	Parbrook et al., 1964; Bromage, unpublished data
Intrathoracic (esophageal) end-expiratory pressure	+1–4 cmH_2O more positive	Less than 0.5 cmH_2O more negative	3.0 cmH_2O more negative	Bromage et al., unpublished data
Total compliance	0–20% fall	?	?	Okinaka, 1965; Lewis and Welch, 1965
Central venous pressure	Raised	No change	Lowered	Bromage, unpublished data

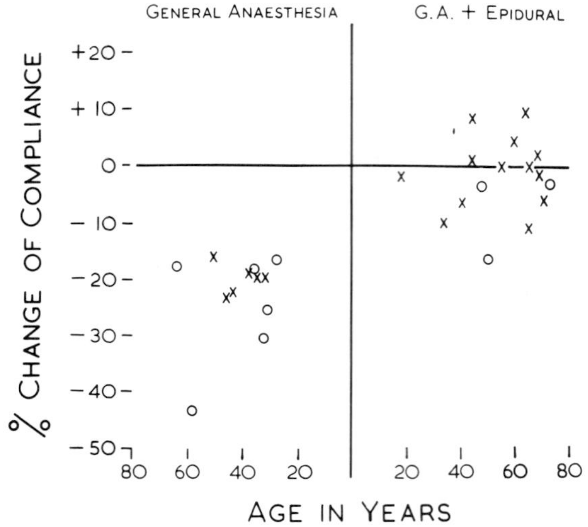

Figure 11–3. Change of total static compliance at completion of surgery in 28 patients compared with control measurements made prior to incision under resting conditions of light general anesthesia.

General anesthesia — 12 patients.

○ = Spontaneous respiration in non-abdominal surgery under general anesthesia alone

× = IPPV in abdominal surgery under general anesthesia and muscle relaxant

General anesthesia + epidural — 16 patients undergoing abdominal surgery. Segmental blockade to T_5.

○ = Spontaneous respiration

× = IPPV

(Bromage, unpublished data, 1959.)

little from preincision values. Under general anesthesia the fall was more pronounced, regardless of whether the patients breathed spontaneously or whether they were curarized and ventilated with IPPV.

Very simple bedside instruments can yield a considerable amount of useful information after the patient regains consciousness. A spirometer and variable speed kymograph provide a written record of tidal volume, vital capacity and timed vital capacity, measurements that reflect the patient's willingness and ability to breathe deeply and cough in the early postoperative period. A well-fitting face mask is better tolerated than a mouthpiece and nose clip, and under the conditions of measurement it is easier to use, while a properly gas-tight system is ensured. A few clinical examples will illustrate the magnitude of the respiratory changes that occur in response to abdominal pain and analgesia.

Figure 11–4 shows a series of VC measurements during the first 14 hours after total gastrectomy. The preoperative VC was 3850 ml. We can see that the VC increased during periods of analgesia and fell to low levels when abdominal pain returned. Restoration of VC came close to the control preoperative value during the brief period of effective epidural blockade. Demerol (pethidine) and methadone (Amidone) also improved the VC, but less effectively.

Figure 11–5 shows vital capacity tracings from a 30-year-old man before and after total gastrectomy. In this patient the VC was seriously compromised by abdominal pain. The systemic analgesics IV lidocaine and pethidine (Demerol) gave subjective relief but produced virtually no improvement in objective respiratory performance. However, epidural blockade both relieved pain and restored respiratory function very significantly.

Figure 11–6 shows the restorative effects of epidural blockade on both preoperative and postoperative pain in a man of 49 years with a perforated gastric ulcer. The first tracing of maximum deep breaths was made about one hour after an opiate injection had produced considerable subjective relief. Preoperative epidural blockade abolished his pain completely and doubled his

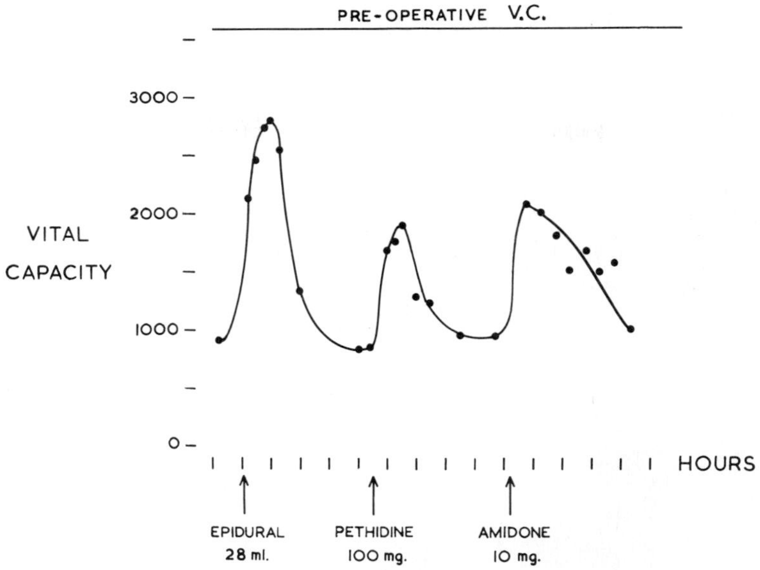

Figure 11–4. Serial vital capacity figures during the first 14 hours after total gastrectomy.
Epidural 28 ml of 0.8 per cent plain lidocaine
Pethidine (Demerol) 100 mg IV
Amidone (methadone) 10 mg IV
(From Bromage, P. R.: Spirometry in assessment of analgesia after abdominal surgery. Brit. Med. J. *2*:589, 1955.)

vital capacity. A partial gastrectomy was performed, and even within a few minutes of awakening the VC was better than before the block was instituted. Deep breathing remained effective as long as epidural analgesia was continued.

These few cases illustrate the type of permanent respiratory record that can be obtained very simply in the early postoperative period, without the use of expensive and sophisticated equipment. The differences in respiratory competence following systemic analgesia or epidural blockade are very obvious, both qualitatively in terms of the pattern of breathing and quantitatively in terms of the volume of air that the patient can move in and out of his lungs.

Table 11–3 lists comparative figures from a number of authors for the percentage restoration of vital capacity after upper abdominal surgery by the use of a variety of analgesic agents. The difficulty in obtaining comparable objective figures from this type of investigation is seen in the unusually small degree of respiratory restoration found by Sjögren and Wright (1972), compared with the much larger values obtained by Bromage (1955) and by Simpson and his colleagues (1961). The low values found by Sjögren and Wright may be partly due to the marked fatigue of their patients, who underwent more extensive and exhausting investigations than those in the other series. Parbrook and his colleagues (1966) have shown the importance of neurotic factors in determining low respiratory performance after operation, confirming that accurate comparisons can only be expected when different analgesic regimens are compared in the same patients rather than in different groups of patients (Dalrymple et al., 1973). In addition, the enthusiasm of the observer has a

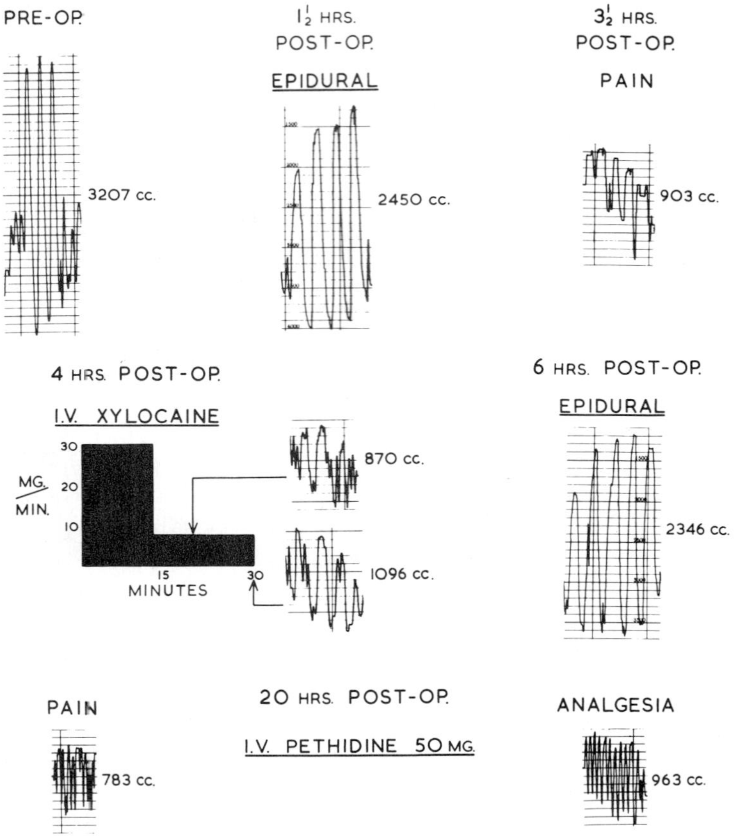

Figure 11–5. VC tracings before and after total gastrectomy in a 30-year-old man. Comparison of respiratory effects of epidural blockade, IV Xylocaine (lidocaine) and pethidine (Demerol).

Note the hesitant jagged pattern of attempted deep breathing during pain and the negligible objective improvement caused by systemic analgesics. Contrast the smooth, regular pattern of large-volume breaths under epidural blockade. (From Bromage, P. R.: Spirometry in assessment of analgesia after abdominal surgery. Brit. Med. J. *2*:589, 1955.)

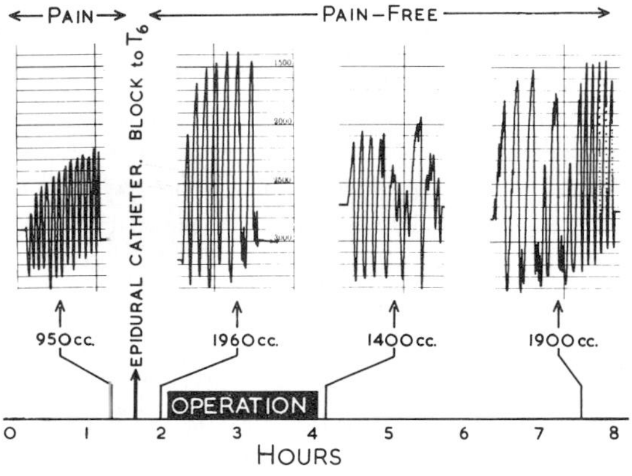

Figure 11–6. Man of 49 years with perforated gastric ulcer treated by partial gastrectomy. Vital capacity records before and after surgery. Anesthesia: continuous epidural blockade (1 per cent lidocaine with 1/200,000 epinephrine). Thiopentone 400 mg, nitrous oxide–oxygen. (From Bromage, P. R.: Spirometry in assessment of analgesia after abdominal surgery. Brit. Med. J. *2*:589, 1955.)

TABLE 11-3 Effect of different analgesic agents on percentage restoration of vital capacity (i.e., Respiratory Restoration Factor, or RRF) after upper abdominal operations

Analgesic Agent	*RRF (%)*	*Reference*
Pethidine	13.5	Bromage (1955)
IV lidocaine	22.0	Bromage (1955)
Morphine	8.3	Parbrook (1966)
25% N_2O and methadone	27.5	Parbrook (1966)
Epidural analgesia (intermittent)	70–100	Bromage (1955)
Epidural analgesia (intermittent)	54.5	Simpson et al. (1961)
Epidural analgesia (intermittent)	<10	Finer (1970)
Epidural analgesia (intermittent)	29.4	Wahba et al. (1975)
Epidural analgesia (continuous)	20	Sjögren and Wright (1972)

marked effect on the patient's respiratory performance (Finer, 1970). Valid comparisons of analgesic methods based on maximal respiratory effort demand that the same degree of supportive encouragement be given to each patient during every measurement that is made. Unless the observer applies a standardized and maximal degree of forceful motivation, the uneven stimulus will introduce a serious element of observer bias and inaccuracy into any measurements that are made.

In spite of some differences in clinical measurement between different groups of investigators, the weight of clinical observation and measurement leaves no doubt about the superiority of postoperative respiratory performance under properly managed epidural blockade, especially on the day of operation (see also data in Chapter 10). Full restoration of normal blood gases requires more than just good analgesia: the patient must also be made to breathe deeply before the full benefits of epidural blockade become apparent. In addition, ventilation and perfusion must be well matched throughout the lungs. Some degree of hypoxemia usually exists after upper abdominal surgery, and the range of fall of PaO_2 is about 10 to 25 per cent below preoperative levels (Pflug et al., 1976; Lees et al., 1976). This degree of hypoxemia usually persists after epidural blockade in spite of adequate pain relief, unless deep breathing is forcibly stimulated by command or pharmacologically by a respiratory stimulant, such as doxapram (Pflug et al., 1974, 1976). Then the combination of deafferentation and respiratory stimulation restores patency in the basal airways, and the arterial oxygen tension rises to preoperative levels. By contrast, centrally acting analgesics such as morphine in combination with doxapram do not fully restore normal PaO_2 in the early postoperative period (Aldrete, 1973; Lees et al., 1976). However, the situation is more complex than a study in ventilation alone. Normal oxygenation of the blood is dependent on a proper matching of ventilation *and* perfusion of the lung capillaries, so restoration of a normal PaO_2 requires that not only should ventilation be normal but also the quantity of blood flowing through the lungs should be normal. In other words, there must be no appreciable fall of cardiac output (James and Fisher, 1969). Hence, any significant fall in blood pressure following epidural block must be corrected by appropriate fluid replacement and vasopressor therapy. Perhaps this is another reason why a combination of epidural analgesia and doxapram is so successful in maintaining a normal PaO_2, for doxapram has an appreciable central sympathetic stimulating effect that tends to augment cardiac output.

The first few postoperative hours seem to be crucial ones from the point of view of respiratory management. Patients who can clear their chests and expand their lung bases effectively during this early period seem to do well, even if the epidural block is discontinued after four or five hours (Miller et al., 1976). However, patients with special respiratory handicaps, such as gross obesity or chronic productive cough, may require prolonged epidural support for one to three days in order to maintain adequate ventilation and normal blood gases without mechanical ventilatory support (Shuman and Peters, 1976).

VISCERA

Sympathetic blockade of the abdominal viscera occurs when anesthesia extends to include the lower six thoracic segments. Splanchnic denervation prevents the normal sympathetic response to noxious stimuli and confers a number of potential advantages on the abdominal organs.

Liver

Interruption of the splanchnic nerves protects the liver against reflex hepatic vasoconstriction and excessive glycogen depletion (Green et al., 1959; Shoemaker, 1964; Shimazu and Fukuda, 1965). In addition, it prevents depletion of norepinephrine stores in the liver and spleen (Dahlström and Zetterstrom, 1965; Gillespie and Kirpekar, 1966). Reflex vasoconstrictive ischemia is therefore prevented, and net blood flow remains even and steady, provided the systemic pressure is not allowed to fall excessively (see Chapter 10).

Blood Sugar and Osmolarity

Under normal circumstances the sympathetic response to surgery or trauma causes a glycogenolytic discharge of glucose from the liver and a rise of blood sugar that persists for 12 to 48 hours (Cullingford, 1966; Keating, 1958; Clarke, 1970). This rise is of the order of 60 to 100 mg per 100 ml in a typical North American population (Bromage et al., 1971), making an additional contribution of 3 to 5 mOsm/L to the total plasma osmolarity, that is, a rise of 1 or 2 per cent above the normal range of 285 to 295 mOsm/L. Such a small increase will have no ill effects under normal circumstances, but in diabetics the degree of hyperglycemia may be much greater and sufficient to cause severe hyperosmolarity and coma (Toker, 1974; Wulfson and Dalton, 1974).

The normal hyperglycemic response to surgery is prevented as long as splanchnic blockade is maintained (Bromage et al., 1971; Brandt et al., 1976). The blood sugar remains close to the fasting value of 80 mg per 100 ml, but it may fall below this level in the absence of exogenous glucose. Therefore, it is prudent to maintain a slow glucose drip in order to prevent inadvertent hypoglycemia during prolonged epidural blockade.

Kidney and Adrenals

Renal vasoconstriction occurs in response to trauma or pain from visceral distension, and this reflex is abolished by sympathetic denervation to T_5 (Folkow and Langston, 1964; Johansson and Langston, 1964). As in the liver, splanchnic blockade protects the renal parenchyma from local ischemia due to reflex vasoconstriction, and organ blood flow becomes dependent on the systemic perfusion pressure. Under these conditions renal blood flow is well maintained at all ranges of arterial pressure above a mean of 80 mmHg.

Neural blockade also prevents disturbances of distribution in renal blood flow. The innervated kidney reacts to trauma by shunting its reduced blood supply from outer cortical nephrons to the deeper juxtamedullary glomeruli, and sodium is retained (see Chapter 10). However, under neural blockade blood flow is distributed more evenly between cortex and medulla, and sodium loads are excreted freely (Pomeranz et al., 1968; Bevan, 1973; Davis and Freeman, 1976). Thus, patients who are subjected to heavy sodium loads through excessive saline infusion are less likely to develop tissue edema under epidural blockade than under general anesthesia.

Splanchnic nerve stimulation increases the total catecholamine output from the adrenal medulla five- to tenfold and raises the proportion of norepinephrine in the adrenal venous effluent (Holland and Schümann, 1956; Marley and Paton, 1961). This powerful vasoactive response is also prevented by splanchnic blockade, producing a very stable cardiovascular state which is particularly helpful in certain types of operation, such as exploration for pheochromocytoma (vide infra). As pointed out in Chapter 10, the adrenal medullary response to upper abdominal trauma is fully blocked by splanchnic denervation, but the adrenal cortical response is not, as one of its reflex pathways travels through the vagus and the hypothalamus.

Bladder

Bladder sensation and sphincter control is subserved by the lower thoracic and upper lumbar segments and by the second, third and fourth sacral segments, so normal voiding mechanisms are disturbed by prolonged epidural blocks. Holmdahl and his colleagues (1972) found that bladder catheterization was necessary in more than 80 per cent of cases involving prolonged lumbar blockade. However, segmental blocks confined to the thoracic and upper lumbar segments gave rise to this disadvantage much less frequently. Nevertheless, careful watch must be kept to ensure that bladder distension does not occur in the postoperative period. Regular palpation of the lower abdomen should be a normal part of the postoperative routine, and a catheter should be passed if there is any suspicion of retention. A distended bladder is a potent cause of reflex postoperative hypertension, and relatively minor degrees of distension may give rise to alarmingly high blood pressure in susceptible subjects.

Bowel

Bowel motility quickly returns after abdominal and thoracic operations under epidural blockade, and with continuous block it is often possible to hear some bowel sounds throughout the period of blockade.

Body Temperature and Induced Hypothermia

Temporary suspension of the peripheral heat-regulating mechanisms can be exploited to facilitate induction of hypothermia by surface cooling in cases in which a lowered metabolism may help to decrease tissue demands in the face of a depleted supply, for example, in oligemic shock or surgery of the liver. In an ambient temperature of 68°F (20°C), the rectal temperature commonly falls to 96 to 97°F (35.6 to 35.7°C) after a high epidural block without any active measures beyond removal of clothing from the patient's lower limbs. Greater degrees of hypothermia can be induced by active surface cooling with ice or a cooling blanket (Stolar and Wynands, 1963). Skin temperature readings are unreliable when surface cooling is being carried out, and core temperature should be measured by the esophageal route, or by the rectum if the chest is open.

POSTOPERATIVE ANALGESIA

Exercise and Locomotion

The most striking feature of deafferentation after surgery is the patient's willingness to move about freely, undisturbed by protective muscle spasm. This freedom of movement can be exploited for active physiotherapy in the immediate postoperative period. Lower limb exercises and "quadriceps drill" with straight leg raising can be started at once after arthrotomy of the knee or other operations on the leg. Caudal anesthesia for outpatient urological or rectal surgery enables the patient to travel home in comfort while the lower sacral segments are still partially anesthetized.

Early and Ultra-early Ambulation

If early postoperative ambulation is beneficial (and this assumption awaits conclusive proof), then perhaps ultra-early ambulation is better. In 1949 Cleland demonstrated that segmental epidural analgesia in the thoracic region allowed painless early ambulation after major abdominal operations. We have extended Cleland's technique to the immediate postsurgical period so that patients can get out of bed comfortably and walk about the recovery room within an hour or so of leaving the operating room (Fig. 11–7).

Ultra-early ambulation requires detailed supervision, and it is too demanding of nursing care for routine use. However, when used in selected patients it demonstrates very beautifully that postoperative immobility is

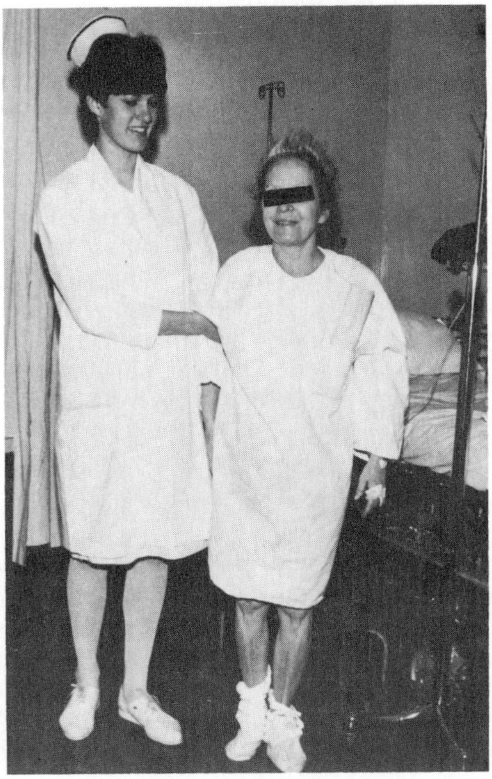

Figure 11-7. Ultra-early ambulation. Patient of 63 years walking comfortably three hours after common bile duct exploration. Mid-thoracic epidural with 4 ml of 2 per cent carbonated lidocaine. Analgesia T_4–T_{11}. (From Bromage, P. R.: Extradural analgesia for pain relief. Brit. J. Anaesth. *39*: 721, 1967.)

pain-dependent and that normal locomotion can be restored by segmental blockade of the appropriate pain pathways. Moreover, the astonishing freedom of immediate ambulation inspires the patients with great confidence and arouses their enthusiastic cooperation in early postoperative physiotherapy.

The regimen requires very close attention to technique so that a narrow segmental band of analgesia is provided only in the area of the wound, while the lower limbs are unaffected. The blood pressure must be watched carefully, and the vascular volume must be adequately filled by prior infusion with fluids and electrolytes so that hypotension does not occur on standing. A small intramuscular dose of vasopressor, such as 15 to 30 mg of ephedrine given 10 minutes before, will usually ensure a stable arterial pressure during ambulation. The lower limit of segmental blockade should be assessed before the patient leaves his bed, and leg movements and knee jerk must be tested to confirm adequate quadriceps control before ambulation is attempted. Failure to apply these obvious precautions may result in the humiliating sight of a patient crumpling to the floor from lack of effective limb control if the block has extended too far into the lumbar segments (Bromage, 1967).

CHOICE OF LOCAL ANESTHETIC AGENTS

Local anesthetic agents differ markedly in their physiochemical properties and in their clinical actions. Successful practice lies in matching drug capabilities to clinical requirements. Different degrees of blockade are needed for different operations and at different times, and the anesthesiologist must be quite clear about the precise qualities that he needs for any given situation. This is an exercise in strategy and tactics. Successful strategy requires an understanding of the aims and goals of the method, together with the strengths and weaknesses of the neural systems that must be subdued. Successful tactics lie in understanding the capabilities and limitations of the drugs available and in selecting the most appropriate agents and solutions for the required task.

This section will consider the general principles governing selection of local anesthetic solutions for surgical analgesia in terms of intensity of blockade, speed of onset and duration of action.

Quality of Blockade

As a general rule, solutions with strong sensory- and motor-blocking abilities are required during surgery, especially during abdominal operations when profound sensory block and muscular relaxation are needed. Some types of operation—for example, certain orthopedic procedures—require very little motor paralysis, and satisfactory surgical conditions are obtained with predominantly afferent blockade. Motor blockade is highly undesirable once the operation is over. At this point a differential block is required, giving effective pain relief while sparing motor activity as much as possible, so that postoperative movements and exercises can be started as soon as possible after the return to the recovery ward. Then afferent blockade should provide relaxation by interrupting the reflex arc on the afferent side of the segmental reflex arc, while motor commands from higher centers are still able to find full expression in the deafferented segments through the intact and potentially active final common motor pathway, as shown in Figure 11–8.

Agents that cause significant amounts of motor blockade in the postoperative period completely defeat one of the prime objectives of regional analgesia—that is, early restoration of function.

Although epidural analgesia never achieves such dramatic paresis as subarachnoid analgesia, the intensity of motor blockade varies over a wide range, depending on the drug and the concentration chosen. The most profound degrees of epidural blockade can come close to the motor intensity of intrathecal blockade. Figure 11–9 shows the degree of motor blockade produced by some commonly used epidural solutions. Note that the block is consistently intensified by the addition of 1/200,000 epinephrine. Three of the solutions shown in Figure 11–9 produce an outstanding degree of motor paralysis, namely 1 per cent etidocaine, 0.75 per cent bupivacaine and 1.73 per cent carbonated lidocaine, all with epinephrine added. Any one of these solutions would therefore be a suitable choice for operations requiring profound motor paralysis, as in abdominal surgery, but they would be quite unsuitable for analgesia and restoration of motor activity in the early postoperative period.

Given a sufficiently concentrated solution, most local anesthetics can produce profound sensory and motor blockade. As pointed out in Chapter 3, however, individual qualities of the various agents become more apparent with progressive dilution, and it is clear that wide differences exist between the

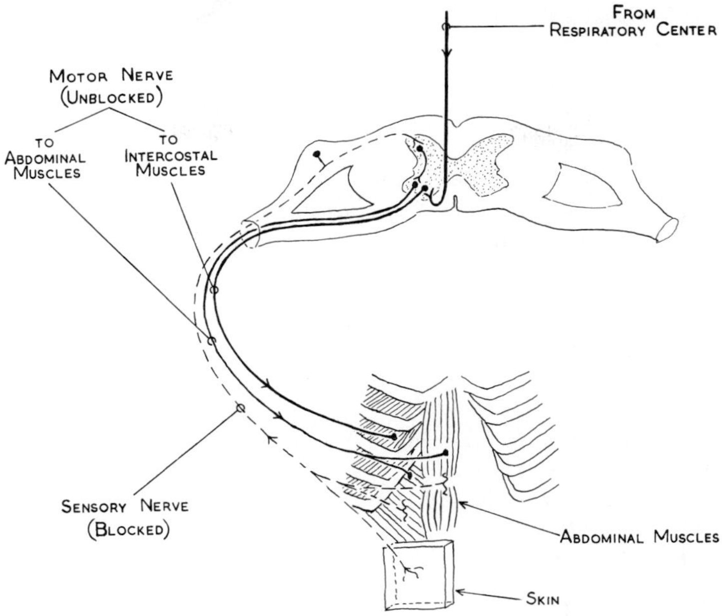

Figure 11–8. Differential neural blockade for postoperative pain relief. Correctly chosen local analgesic blocks afferent pathways but spares most of the motor nerves. Reflex flaccidity results, but the muscles can still respond to motor commands from above.

sensory and motor affinities in weak concentrations. Figure 12–21, in the next chapter, is a composite diagram compiled from data in obstetrical patients to show the general trend of motor and sensory blocking capabilities for several commonly used local anesthetic agents. The data on which this figure is based are presented more fully in Chapters 3 and 12. It seems that the various agents shown in Figure 12–21 fall on distinct isopleths that converge at increasing concentration and diverge with progressive dilution. Bupivacaine provides relatively poor motor block unless the concentration is raised to 0.75 per cent

Figure 11–9. Intensity of motor blockade of legs following epidural injection at the second lumbar interspace for 2 per cent lidocaine HCl, 1.73 per cent lidocaine–CO_2, 3 per cent chloroprocaine, 0.5 per cent and 0.75 per cent bupivacaine and 1 per cent etidocaine in plain solution or with 1/200,000 epinephrine. Means ± S.D.
■ = Plain solution
▨ = +Epinephrine
(Data from Bromage, 1969a; Bromage et al., unpublished data.)

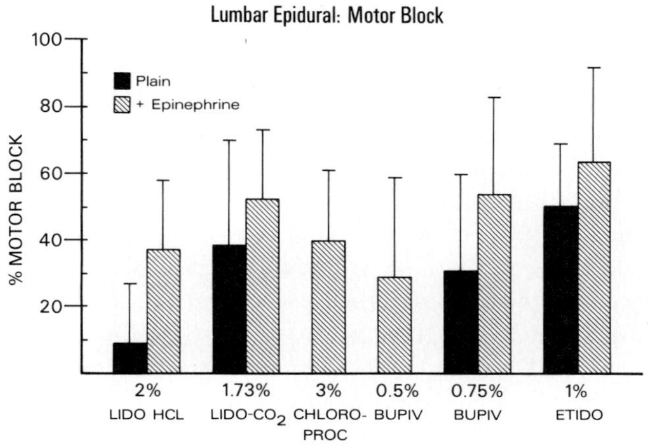

(Nolte et al., 1974). On the other hand, bupivacaine provides a relatively good quality of sensory blockade, even in low dilutions. At the other extreme, tetracaine and etidocaine cause profound motor block in high concentrations, but in more dilute solutions the quality of sensory blockade is comparatively poor despite significant motor block. On the basis of this information, bupivacaine and drugs that behave like it are clearly a suitable choice for postoperative pain relief, for which unimpaired motor activity is an important requirement.

Speed of Onset

Latency of onset is one of the most important practical attributes of any agent. The realities of busy clinical practice do not permit indefinite delays while the whole operating team waits for a sluggish analgesic agent to creep to the full extent of its segmental spread. Before the advent of the amide local anesthetics, the choice of agents was limited to such solutions as procaine 2 to 3 per cent, tetracaine 0.2 per cent and dibucaine 0.167 per cent, but the slow latency of these solutions made the technique unpopular in the hands of all but a few enthusiasts working under conditions in which patients could be prepared and effectively blocked well ahead of the scheduled operating time.

Figure 11–10 shows the segmental profiles of latency of onset and spread of analgesia for a number of contemporary solutions. Each profile is the average for a population of 25 to 35 cases. The average time required for complete spread of analgesia ranges between 10.3 minutes for 1.73 per cent carbonated lidocaine to 19 minutes for 0.5 per cent bupivacaine.

The fastest solutions in this series are 1 per cent etidocaine and 2 per cent carbonated lidocaine (i.e. 1.73 per cent carbonated base), and the two agents have very similar onset profiles. Both produce quite profound motor block, so although they are drugs of choice for induction and maintenance of surgical analgesia, the intensity of motor blockade makes them unsuitable for restoration of function in the postoperative period.

Salient of Delay (L_5 and S_1)

The fifth lumbar and first sacral segments are particularly resistant to blockade for reasons that were discussed in Chapter 2 on Anatomy. Not only is analgesia slow to appear in these two segments, as shown in Figure 11–10, but also the quality of analgesia is relatively tenuous when it does develop (Bromage, 1962; Bromage and Burfoot, 1966; Galindo et al., 1975; Stanton-Hicks et al., 1976). This salient of delay is less apparent when injection is made into the caudal canal or at the lumbosacral interspace, but even then the quality of analgesia tends to be relatively poor on the outer aspect of the ankle. For this reason epidural analgesia is sometimes judged to be a bad choice for operations involving that segmental area of the lower limbs, such as open reduction of a fractured ankle or multiple varicose vein ligations.

From inspection of the onset profiles in Figure 11–10 it is clear that 0.5 per cent bupivacaine is likely to give poor conditions for operations on the

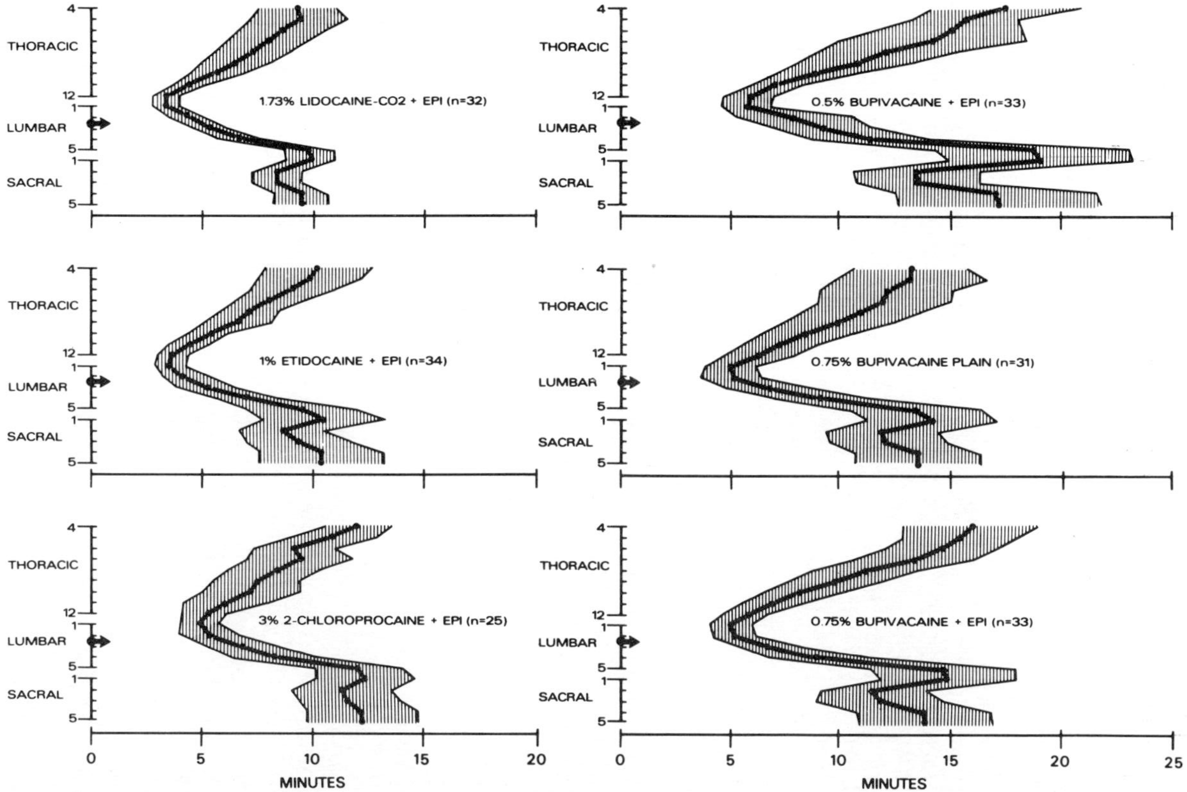

Figure 11–10. Latency of onset and spread of analgesia after epidural injection at the second lumbar interspace. Segmental profiles for 1.73 per cent lidocaine, 1 per cent etidocaine, 3 per cent chloroprocaine and 0.5 per cent bupivacaine, all with 1/200,000 epinephrine; 0.75 per cent bupivacaine with and without epinephrine. Means ± S.D. (Data from Bromage, 1969a; Bromage et al., 1967, 1974, unpublished data.)

lower leg, whereas etidocaine and carbonated lidocaine are the agents of choice, since the salient of delay in L_5 and S_1 is practically eliminated with both of these solutions, and the quality of analgesia is superior to that afforded by less penetrating agents. The following case illustrates the superiority of carbonated lidocaine under conditions in which the effects of the hydochloride and the carbonated salts of lidocaine could be compared in the same patient.

> *An anesthesiologist of 33 years required reduction of an unstable fractured ankle on three occasions, and he requested lumbar epidural blockade for each procedure.*
>
> First reduction: *epidural injection of 18 ml of 2 per cent lidocaine hydrochloride with 1/200,000 epinephrine was made at the second lumbar interspace in the sitting position. Analgesia rose to the tenth thoracic dermatome but was slow to develop in the outer ankle and was still incomplete at 20 minutes. Intravenous Demerol was required for pain relief during closed reduction.*
>
> Second reduction: *one week later the ankle was repositioned. Epidural injection of 18 ml of 2 per cent lidocaine hydrochloride with 1/200,000 epinephrine was made two spaces lower at the fourth lumbar interspace, with the patient in the sitting position. Again analgesia was slow to develop at the ankle, but this time analgesia was more satisfactory at 20 minutes.*
>
> Third reduction: *one week later open reduction of the ankle was performed, with insertion of a fibular screw. At the second lumbar interspace 18 ml of carbonated lidocaine 2 per cent (1.73 per cent base) with 1/200,000 epinephrine was injected. Analgesia rose to the eighth thoracic dermatome in 10 minutes, and analgesia at the ankles was complete in 8 minutes. No supplementation was required at any time; analgesia was intense and entirely satisfactory throughout the operation.*

This patient was a trained observer and a proponent of regional analgesia, and the unusual opportunity to test both the site of injection and the selection of an agent on three separate occasions strongly confirmed the outstanding superiority of carbonated lidocaine for surgical procedures involving L_5 and S_1 segments.

Duration of Action

Local anesthetic action does not persist for very long in the epidural space compared to blocks of peripheral nerves. If segment-minute diagrams are constructed for each case, it will be seen that the pattern of analgesia following lumbar blockade has the general shape of Figure 11–11.

Analgesia begins to wear off from above in the upper segments, and then later the lower margin creeps up from below. The last segments to regain sensation are usually the same as the first ones to become blocked, that is, the upper lumbar region after a lumbar induction, and these dermatomes contribute a long tail of analgesia to the segment-time diagram.

Thus, *total duration* is of very little practical interest, except when the operative site happens to coincide with the prolonged analgesic "tail." The point in time when the upper level of analgesia regresses significantly is of much more importance, for this determines the actual working time available during an abdominal operation. The point where analgesia has regressed downward for a distance of two dermatomes is easily measured in the conscious patient, and this has been adopted as a practical measure of duration and is termed "duration to regression of two segments." This is also the point in time to administer the first

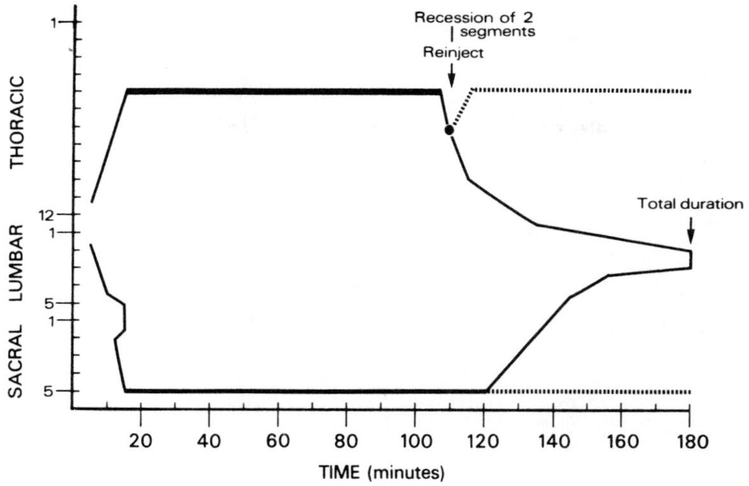

Figure 11–11. Typical segment-time diagram of onset and regression of analgesia after epidural injection at the second lumbar interspace (see text).

maintenance dose if a continuous catheter technique is being used (see Fig. 7–17).

Table 11–4 summarizes the duration to regression of two segments of seven well-known agents both in plain solution and with epinephrine 1/200,000. It can be seen that lidocaine, mepivacaine and prilocaine are relatively short-acting, and even when epinephrine is added to these solutions, full duration of more than about 1½ hours cannot be counted on. Tetracaine, bupivacaine and etidocaine have appreciably longer actions, and a duration of 2½ to 3 hours is obtainable, with bupivacaine giving the longest duration.

All these drugs have a somewhat shorter duration after injection in the thoracic region than after lumbar injection, probably because the small mass of neural and perineural tissue in the thoracic cord and roots requires about 40 per cent less local anesthetic per segment (Bromage, 1969a; Sjögren and Wright, 1972; Nakamura et al., 1972; Bromage et al., 1974).

TABLE 11–4 Duration to regression of two segments of lidocaine, mepivacaine, prilocaine, tetracaine, bupivacaine and etidocaine in plain solution and with epinephrine 1/200,000, after injection at the second lumbar interspace*

Drug	***Plain***	***+Epinephrine 1/200,000†***
Lidocaine HCl 2%	46 ± 5	97 ± 19
Lidocaine-CO_2 2%	45	108 ± 13
Mepivacaine HCl 2%		117 ± 16
Prilocaine HCl 3%	85 ± 16	99 ± 17
Tetracaine 0.5%		146 ± 22
Bupivacaine 0.5%	165	196 ± 31
Bupivacaine 0.75%	164 ± 46	201 ± 40
Etiodocaine 1%	128 ± 43	170 ± 57

*Data from Bromage, 1965, 1969a; Bromage et al., 1967, 1974.
†Epinephrine freshly added immediately prior to injection.

TABLE 11–5 Attributes required for operative and postoperative epidural blockade

Operative Blockade	*Postoperative Analgesia*
Attributes	*Attributes*
Fast onset	Good sensory analgesia
Intense sensory blockade	Weak motor blockade
Powerful motor block (usually)	Long duration
Duration according to length of operation	
Suitable solutions	*Suitable solutions*
1% Etidocaine	0.5% or 0.25% Bupivacaine
2% Lidocaine-CO_2	1% Lidocaine
2% Lidocaine HCl	1% Mepivacaine
2% Mepivacaine HCl	2% Prilocaine (restricted to a total dose of 600 mg)
3% Chloroprocaine (short procedures)	
0.75% Bupivacaine	
3% Prilocaine plain (restricted to a total dose of 600 mg)	

Catheter techniques for continuous or intermittent administration have lessened the overriding importance of long-acting agents for lengthy surgical procedures. Nevertheless, long-acting drugs are still preferable for long procedures, since the frequency of repeat injections is reduced and the onset of tachyphylaxis is correspondingly postponed.

Table 11–5 summarizes the main features that determine the choice of analgesic solution for operative and postoperative use.

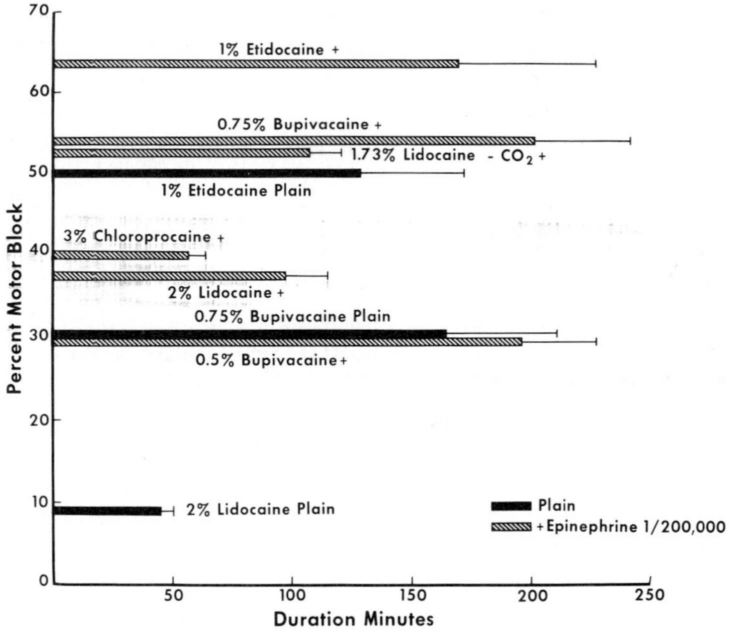

Figure 11–12. Choice of local anesthetic agents. Duration of epidural blockade to recession of two segments (mean ± S.D.), related to intensity of motor block for a number of local anesthetic solutions.
■ = Plain solution
\\\ = +1/200,000 epinephrine

The two parameters of motor blockade and duration of action are presented together in Figure 11–12 for quick reference as a visual aid to choosing the most suitable agent for any particular circumstance. Note the wide standard deviation for duration of the longer acting solutions, such as 1 per cent etidocaine and 0.75 per cent bupivacaine, indicating that it is difficult to predict the precise length of action of these solutions.

None of the solutions already discussed has all the requirements for a single-shot injection in moderately prolonged surgery. Theoretically, it could be advantageous to have an agent that would meet the three basic needs of:

1. Rapid onset
2. Profound sensory blockade
3. Sparing of motor activity in the early postoperative period.

With these aims in view, mixtures of carbonated lidocaine with bupivacaine are under trial at the time of writing.

Carbonated Lidocaine-Bupivacaine Mixtures

By restricting the concentrations of the two components of this mixture, it is possible to remain within acceptable limits of systemic toxicity. Two concentrations of bupivacaine are under investigation: (a) 1 per cent CO_2-lidocaine + 0.25 per cent bupivacaine, and (b) 1 per cent CO_2-lidocaine + 0.375 per cent bupivacaine. Preliminary results suggest that the latter mixture is preferable, as shown in Table 9–3 (Chapter 9).

The 0.375 per cent bupivacaine mixture with carbonated lidocaine gives a rapid onset with excellent sensory analgesia. The duration to two segment regression is about 2½ hours, and the degree of motor block is rather heavy at 50 per cent. This mixture, involving a single-shot technique, is admirable, therefore, for abdominal operations lasting 1½ to 2 hours, but the combination of strong motor block and moderately long duration makes it unsuitable for short outpatient procedures.

Carbonated Bupivacaine

The great improvement of carbonated lidocaine and prilocaine over their orthodox hydrochloride counterparts encouraged the view that bupivacaine would be an ideal drug for carbonation and for single-shot injection, since a shortened latency would add greatly to the existing advantages of excellent sensory block and long duration. However, initial experience with carbonated bupivacaine has been disappointing, as pointed out in Chapter 9. Schulte-Steinberg (1976) found that latency of the 0.5 per cent solution was shortened very slightly, from about 19 minutes with the hydrochloride salt to 16 minutes with carbonated bupivacaine at a pCO_2 of 200 mmHg. My own experience in a small series of cases using a higher pCO_2 found latency shortened to a mean of 14 ± 4.3 minutes. However, this shortening of onset is too variable and insufficient to offer any important practical advantage. At the same time duration was shortened by about 30 minutes, and segmental dose requirements were increased by 14 per cent.

Unfortunately, at the time of writing, available solutions of carbonated bupivacaine do not appear to have the dramatic practical advantages that were hoped for. Further work is needed for a more thorough evaluation of the agent.

MANAGEMENT OF EPIDURAL ANALGESIA FOR SURGERY

Administrative Considerations

Regional analgesia cannot be practiced satisfactorily without proper facilities and supporting personnel. An efficient operating list should run like clockwork, with not more than 5 to 10 minutes between the end of one case and the draping of the next, and regional anesthesia should not interfere with the booking schedule. While this degree of efficiency is eminently attainable and is standard practice in many institutions, it becomes an impossible goal without proper transport assistance, induction rooms and trained surveillance. Each case should be started well in advance of the scheduled time so that delays are not incurred. Transport must deliver the first patient of the day to the induction room at least half an hour before the list is due to start, so that all necessary preparations can be completed carefully and without unnecessary haste. Successive cases on an operating list should be sent for in good time and the block induced before the preceding case has finished and left the table.

Unfortunately, many North American operating suites are poorly designed for regional analgesia, or indeed for a rapid turnover of any sort, having numerous operating rooms but too few adjoining induction rooms, and sometimes none at all. In the absence of properly designed induction rooms, improved efficiency and safety may best be served by annexing an operating room for induction purposes.

A properly qualified nurse or nurse-anesthetist should be available to assist and watch over the termination of the operation while the next case is being started. In contrast to general anesthesia with relaxant techniques, in which ventilatory decisions and reversal of paralysis require intensive management at the end of operation, regional analgesia is usually uncomplicated and may be safely left to an assistant while the next case is induced without delay.

Preparation of the Patient

Psychological preparation

Patients differ widely in their preferences for remaining awake or going to sleep during surgery. Most North Americans prefer to be asleep, but a minority fear losing consciousness and ask to stay awake. Individual preference should be established at the preoperative visit and catered to whenever it is safe and practicable to do so. Fear of a "needle in the back" can be allayed by careful briefing of the patient about the subjective sensations that he will experience during induction, and afterward in the recovery room, with special emphasis on the advantages of early and painless restoration of function. Patients with underlying pulmonary disease should be given a special explanation of the respiratory benefits of postoperative epidural analgesia, and they should be admonished to take every advantage of the period of effective postoperative analgesia to carry out their early physiotherapy conscientiously.

Simple preoperative explanations given in a sympathetic but factual way are particularly important for children. Children are surprisingly cooperative candidates for regional analgesia, provided they can be made to understand exactly what is going to happen and provided the procedure is carried out carefully and gently. Effective psychological preparation and good rapport are the most valuable forms of premedication in both adults and children.

PHYSICAL ASSESSMENT

A careful review of the history and physical state of the patient should be done to decide whether any contraindications to epidural blockade exist, or whether any physical deficiencies require correction. For example, fluid and electrolyte depletion from intestinal obstruction should be corrected by infusion of appropriate quantities of electrolyte solutions before anesthesia is initiated. High segmental blocks interfere with a large proportion of the sympathetic outflow, and control of blood pressure becomes difficult if volume deficits are not replaced.

Patients receiving full doses of heparin or other agents that interfere with normal clotting mechanisms must not receive epidural blockade. However, very small doses of subcutaneous heparin may not be incompatible with epidural analgesia, provided the activated thromboplastin time is not prolonged and a very cautious watch is kept for the first signs of epidural hematoma formation.

Examination of the back and sacrum will help to decide on the most favorable level for puncture. The existence of a lumbosacral laminectomy scar may influence choice of the caudal approach for operations on the perineum and lower limbs. A tuft of hair or a local subcutaneous fat pad may give warning that an occult spina bifida lies beneath, and then puncture should be made at a more favorable spinal level.

PREMEDICATION

The choice between light and heavy premedication depends not only on the individual patient but also to a large extent on the manner of practice of the anesthesiologist and the preferred posture for epidural induction. Postural hypotension is common after heavy premedication, and then patients cannot be placed safely in the sitting position for epidural puncture. Therefore, in difficult cases, such as the grossly obese in whom the sitting position is technically helpful, it is best to withhold premedicant drugs until after the epidural catheter has been inserted.

Heavy premedication or even light general anesthesia may be required for very anxious patients, and then the lateral posture must be used for induction of blockade. After extensive experience with performing epidural puncture both under general anesthesia and in awake patients, and on the basis of my own experience as an experimental subject, I believe that excessive emphasis has been placed on the need for obtunding consciousness during induction. Properly done, induction should be painless except for the slight sting of the initial intradermal wheal, but this does not call for heavy sedation or general anesthesia. One cannot repeat too often that the best premedication is sound emotional support; heavy sedation is usually redundant, provided the anesthesiologist can win the patient's confidence by skillful and sympathetic handling.

Normal preoperative anxiety is well relieved by diazepam in a dose of 0.2 mg per kg given one hour before operation. If this is insufficient, an increment of 2.5 to 7.5 mg may be given into the intravenous drip that is set up as soon as the patient arrives in the induction room. Diazepam in this dosage has the double advantage of suppressing convulsant activity in the central nervous system and increasing tolerance to local anesthetics by about 65 per cent above control levels, thus adding a corresponding margin of safety against inadvertent overdosage of local anesthetic (De Jong and Heavner, 1974; Munson and Wagman, 1972).

Antisialagogic drugs, such as atropine and scopolamine, are seldom indicated. If the patient remains awake, these drugs become an active nuisance by inducing thirst and discomfort from an unnecessarily dry mouth. If the patient is to receive light general anesthesia, atropine may be given intravenously in small amounts on the operating table.

High segmental blocks are accompanied by extensive sympathetic paralysis, and occasionally unopposed vagal tone may cause heart rate and output to fall to undesirably low levels. Bradycardia of this nature is not prevented by the usual small dose of atropine given as a routine premedication, and larger amounts are necessary. Hypotension may occur quite suddenly from bradycardia of vagal origin in conscious patients, and then 0.3 to 0.6 mg of atropine sulfate should be given rapidly by the intravenous route to raise the pulse rate and restore cardiac output (Wetstone and Wong, 1974). Needless to say, the possibility that this type of vagal reaction may occur is a strong reason for vigilant surveillance in conscious patients and for keeping atropine ready for administration at short notice.

Choice of Puncture Site

Choice of puncture site is governed by two main factors: the anesthesiologist's skill and the segmental nerve supply of the operative site. Ideally, puncture should be as close as possible to the center of the segmental distribution of the operation area, but this aim should be subordinated to the safety of the maneuver.

As pointed out in Chapter 6, beginners should not attempt puncture above the level of the termination of the cord until they are thoroughly proficient in the lumbar region and able to demonstrate that proficiency by an acceptably low incidence of dural puncture of less than 2 per cent. Then progression to the thoracic region under supervision may be considered, but until that time, puncture should not be made above the level of the second lumbar interspace. Insistence on safety and an acceptable level of technical skill is obviously essential when one considers the serious vulnerability of the cord in unskilled hands. The lumbar route is quite versatile and suitable for most types of surgery below the diaphragm, provided enough drug is given to extend the segmental level of analgesia up to the required height, that is, to the fourth or fifth thoracic segments for upper abdominal surgery.

For reasons discussed in the chapter on Continuous Epidural Blockade, no attempt should be made to thread the epidural catheter upward from the lumbar region in an effort to bring the catheter tip to a higher vertebral level. Such attempts fail nine cases out of ten, and they introduce the possibility of complications or failure from migration of the catheter beyond the confines of the epidural space. The length of catheter inserted should not exceed 4 cm.

The rule that none but the technically elite should perform epidural puncture above the termination of the cord may seem unduly austere, but I believe it is fundamental to good practice and to maintaining the reputation of epidural analgesia as a safe technique. To compromise by inserting a needle at the thoracolumbar junction begs the question of safety and is illogical (Dawkins and Steel, 1971). The end results of trauma to the lumbar enlargement from poor technique can be just as crippling as damage to the cord at a higher level. This point is worth belaboring because the temptation to use the lower thoracic interspaces at T_{11}–T_{12} or T_{12}–L_1 is quite strong, as shown by the number of reports in which puncture is made at these levels in an effort to extend blockade into the upper thoracic region. The lower thoracic spaces are easily felt, and the interspinous ligaments are invitingly broad for use of the loss-of-resistance test in the midline. However, there must be an all-or-nothing attitude to this region, and the anesthesiologist performing the epidural puncture should be quite clear about it in his own mind. He should stay below the second lumbar vertebra in all humility and on all occasions, until his technical skill is impeccable. Then, and only then, should he be free to induce analgesia at a higher level, with full awareness of his own responsibility to the underlying cord. He should never feel that the thoracolumbar border region is a place to gain experience before graduating to higher levels of puncture.

This principle of austerity in the choice of puncture site is perhaps the most important to follow in the process of learning and teaching the art of epidural analgesia. Unfortunately, like all principles, it demands a sacrifice. Here, the price to be paid is increased dosage requirements at the lumbar level and less versatile analgesic conditions than can be obtained by exercising a free choice of puncture site at higher levels.

The difference between the small bulk of the slender thoracic roots and cord and the lumbar enlargement with its thick roots was discussed in the chapter on Anatomy. These underlying anatomical differences determine the very different dose requirements for the two regions. In the lower part of the cord the greater bulk of neural and perineural tissue demands segmental dose requirements that are 40 to 50 per cent greater than in the mid-thoracic region (Sjögren and Wright, 1972; Bromage et al., 1974). When the lumbar approach is used for upper abdominal surgery, large amounts of local anesthetic are needed, and patients in their early twenties with maximum dose requirements may need quantities that border on the toxic limit. Moreover, blockade is most intense in the lower thoracic and upper lumbar segments, but the quality of block becomes

TABLE 11-6 Lumbar versus thoracic puncture in surgery—Constraints and freedoms

Lumbar	*Thoracic*
Safe: below termination of cord	For experts only: vulnerable underlying cord
Predominant blockade in lower abdomen and legs	Predominant blockade in thorax or upper abdomen
Relatively tenuous quality of blockade at upper segmental levels	30% less dose requirements than by lumbar route
Large dose requirements	Sparing of lower limbs: ultra-early ambulation possible
Interference with micturition; high incidence of bladder catheterization in prolonged blocks	Micturition usually normal; low incidence of catheterization in prolonged segmental blocks

more tenuous toward the upper margin of analgesia. Thus, conditions are less ideal during abdominal operations after mid-lumbar puncture than after mid-thoracic puncture, and postoperatively there is more motor block in the lower limbs and a higher incidence of urinary retention (Holmdahl et al., 1972). Nevertheless, in spite of these shortcomings, lumbar blockade at the second lumbar interspace can produce acceptable conditions for all types of abdominal surgery.

A wide spectrum of options is opened once the thoracic approach has been included in the anesthesiologist's repertoire. Puncture can now be made at any level, and it can be centered effectively over the middle of the segmental area chosen for blockade. Segmental dose requirements are reduced to a minimum, and segments distal to the blocked area remain fully functional, provided agents are selected that do not penetrate too deeply into the substance of the cord (see Neural Mechanism in chapter on Mechanism of Action). These constraints and freedoms of lumbar and thoracic puncture are summarized in Table 11-6.

The ideal spinal level for induction of blockade is summarized for different types of operations in Table 11-7.

Puncture above the vertebra prominens (seventh cervical) is technically more difficult than at the easy space at C_7–T_1, and is seldom indicated.

Cervical and thoracic punctures are most easily performed with the patient sitting up and the neck well flexed. The patient sits with his legs over the side of the operating table, his feet on a stool and his arms folded across his chest. An assistant stands in front, supporting the patient's shoulders, while

TABLE 11-7 Preferred site of epidural injection related to operative site

Operative Site	*Preferred Puncture Site*
Neck, e.g., carotid endarterectomy	C_7–T_1
Arm, e.g., forequarter amputation	C_7–T_1
Breast, e.g., mammoplasty, radical excision	T_1–T_2
Thoracotomy	T_2–T_3 or T_3–T_4
Upper abdomen	T_6–T_7 or T_7–T_8
Lower abdomen	L_2–L_3
Lower limb	L_4–L_5, L_5–S_1 or Caudal
Perineum	L_4–L_5, L_5–S_1 or Caudal

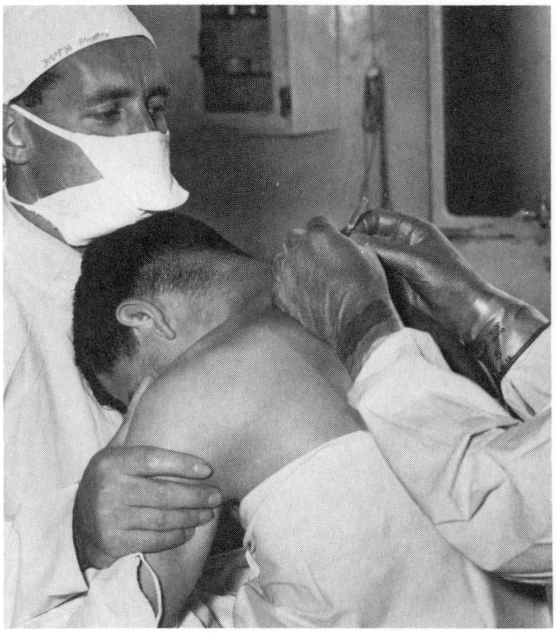

Figure 11–13. Position for cervicothoracic or upper thoracic puncture. The assistant maintains flexion of the neck to open the interspinous spaces and facilitate passage of the epidural needle. An Odom's indicator is attached to the hub of the needle (see Chapter 9 for description of Odom's indicator).

flexion of the neck is maintained by keeping the patient's head tucked under the assistant's chin, as shown in Figure 11–13 (Crawford, 1953).

Upper thoracic puncture can be done with the patient reclining in the lateral position, but in this case the head of the table should be raised to maintain a good negative intrapleural pressure (see Chapter 5), and the operative side should be underneath to obtain the benefit of gravity in aiding spread of analgesia to the downward side. In very obese patients puncture is technically much more difficult with the patient lying on his side rather than sitting up. In these patients it is not advisable to attempt puncture at any level unless the anesthesiologist has positioned the patient in the most advantageous way possible to ensure technical success, and the sitting position is usually best.

DOUBLE CATHETER TECHNIQUE

Occasionally, a double catheter technique may be helpful for special occasions when extensive segmental blockade is required, and intense analgesia is needed more in one area than another. For example, Brown and his colleagues (1974) have described a two-catheter system to provide analgesia and controlled vascular hypotension for Helmstein's hydrostatic treatment of bladder carcinoma. In this system 0.25 per cent bupivacaine is given via a thoracic catheter to provide sympathetic blockade, while 0.5 per cent bupivacaine is given through a reversed caudal catheter inserted at the fourth lumbar interspace to block the sacral segments more intensely and relieve pain arising from distension of the bladder wall.

A system similar to this was described by Cleland in 1949 for relief of pain in childbirth, and it has also been used for abdominoperineal resection of the rectum. Although it does have the merit of reducing cumulative dose requirements to a minimum, the amount saved is not very significant compared to a single catheter technique, and the refinement of technique is bought at the cost of increased complexity and risk of failure. With the local anesthetics currently available, it is possible to provide extensive blockade safely and effectively through a single catheter, and two catheters are seldom indicated (Lahiri and Boys, 1973).

Dose Requirements

The amount of drug required for epidural blockade varies with age and, to a lesser extent, height, as explained in Chapter 4. This pattern appears to be common to most of the local anesthetics in clinical use today. The average dose requirements for 2 per cent lidocaine are shown in Figure 4–12 in Chapter 4. Patients with occlusive arterial disease (OAD) behave as if they are "as old as their arteries," and their segmental dose requirements are as small as for someone 20 or 30 years older than their chronological age. Figure 11–14 summarizes the average segmental dose requirements for a number of different local anesthetic agents injected at the second lumbar interspace or in the mid-thoracic region in normal subjects. It can be seen that dose requirements for lumbar and mid-thoracic administration differ by a ratio of about 3:2, so a thoracic block will require about 30 per cent less drug than a lumbar block. Caudal blocks demand the largest amount of drug per spinal segment, and segmental dose requirements by the sacral route are approximately double the lumbar requirements (see Fig. 4–9 in Chapter 4).

This information is enough to be able to calculate the dose requirements for any particular procedure with reasonable accuracy and to allow a fairly good prediction for a single-shot injection. However, it must be remembered that in old patients the average segmental dose requirements are small in comparison to the variation about the mean, so accurate prediction of dosage

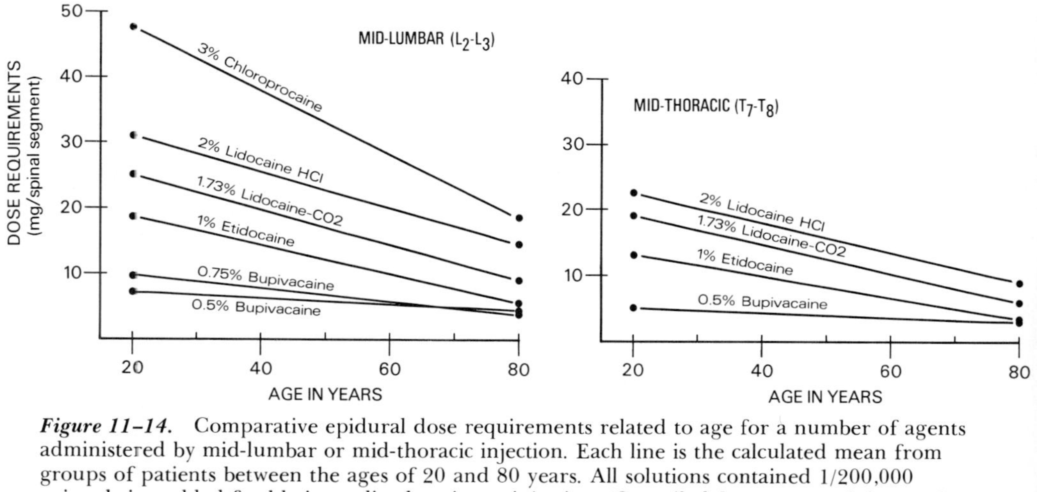

Figure 11–14. Comparative epidural dose requirements related to age for a number of agents administered by mid-lumbar or mid-thoracic injection. Each line is the calculated mean from groups of patients between the ages of 20 and 80 years. All solutions contained 1/200,000 epinephrine added freshly immediately prior to injection. (Compiled from personal data and various publications, Bromage, 1964–1974.)

and segmental levels of analgesia is more haphazard in these patients than in younger subjects. Hence, in old patients it is wise to avoid the unpredictability of single-shot injections at that age by administering the initial dose slowly in fractional amounts through an epidural catheter so that the main dose can be matched to the observed spread in each case (Bromage, 1962, 1969b).

A few actual examples will help to illustrate the general principles of calculating epidural dose requirements for surgery:

Case 1. *Man, aged 25, 6 feet tall, for appendectomy. Mean lumbar segmental dose requirements of 2 per cent lidocaine HCl at 25 years = 29 mg per seg. Number of segments to be blocked* (T_6–S_5 inclusive) = *17.* ∴ *Calculated dose* $= 29 \times 17 = 493$ *mg* = 25 ml of 2 per cent lidocaine.

Case 2. *Woman of 80 years for pinning of fractured hip. Well-preserved for her years. Mean lumbar segmental dose requirements of 2 per cent lidocaine HCl at 80 years = 15 mg per seg. Number of segments to be blocked* (T_9–S_5 *inclusive*) = *14.* ∴ *Calculated dose* $= 14 \times 15 = 210$ *mg* = 10.5 ml of 2 per cent lidocaine.

Case 3. *Man of 50 years for transthoracic repair of hiatus hernia using thoracic epidural and 0.5 per cent bupivacaine. Mean segmental dose requirements by lumbar route at 50 years = 5.5 mg per seg.* ∴ *Mean segmental dose requirements by mid-thoracic route* $= 5.5 \times \frac{2}{3} = 3.67$ *mg per seg. Number of segments to be blocked* (T_1–L_1 *inclusive*) = *13.* ∴ *Calculated dose* $= 13 \times 3.67 = 47.81$ *mg* = 9.5 ml of 0.5 per cent bupivacaine.

Case 4. *Man of 66 years with severe arteriosclerotic vascular disease and gangrene of foot, for below-knee amputation. Normal lumbar segmental dose requirements for 2 per cent lidocaine at 66 years = 18.2 mg per seg. Segmental dose requirements at physiological age of 66 + 30 (i.e., equivalent of 90 years) = 12 mg per seg. Number of segments to be blocked* (T_9–S_5 *inclusive*) = 14. ∴ *Calculated dose* $= 14 \times 12 = 168$ *mg* = 8.5 ml of 2 per cent lidocaine.

Rapid calculation of dose requirements for lidocaine

Inspection of the regression line for dose requirements of lidocaine shows that the rate of decline with age is about 1 per cent of the maximum dose per year, or 10 per cent per decade. This convenient number makes it very easy to arrive at a quick working estimate of the dose requirements of a normal patient at any given age.

For example, the dose requirements of 2 per cent lidocaine for 16 segments by lumbar injection will be roughly:

500 mg at 20 years
400 mg at 40 years
200 mg at 80 years

Maintenance doses

Simple measurements of the spread of analgesia during the induction period are informative and easy to obtain by using a disposable needle to map out the margins of cutaneous pin-prick sensation. Opinions are divided about the advisability of making this type of observation, and some authorities feel that it should be omitted since it may disturb the patients and make them anxious (Lund, 1966). However, I have not found this to be so if the measure-

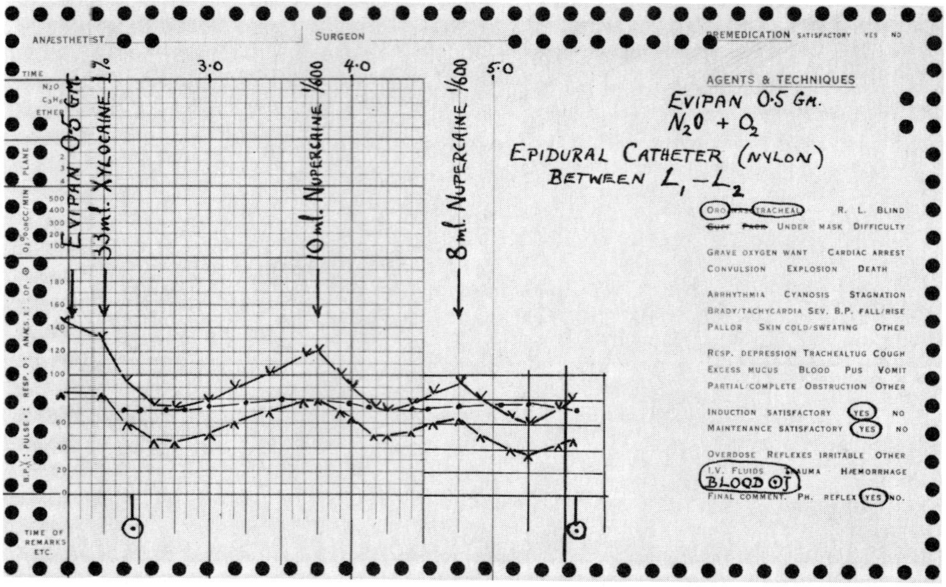

Figure 11–15. Continuous epidural analgesia combined with light general anesthesia for partial gastrectomy. A rising blood pressure indicates regression of segmental blockade and the need for a further increment of local anesthetic. (From Bromage, P. R.: Spinal Epidural Analgesia. Edinburgh, E. & S. Livingstone, Ltd., 1954.)

ments are made discreetly and gently. Valuable information is gained from this type of observation, both from the point of view of managing the individual anesthetic, and as part of a general data bank on phenomena related to epidural analgesia.

During the period of latency and analgesic spread, the anesthesiologist should check that the block is advancing symmetrically on the two sides and that the operative site will be adequately covered by the area of analgesia. Any deficiencies of spread or symmetry can then be corrected by injecting further increments of analgesic solution through the epidural catheter.

Maintenance of an adequate segmental level of blockade is easy in patients who remain conscious throughout the operation. The upper sensory level can be checked directly, and a top-up dose of local anesthetic solution can be given at the first sign that the level is falling. When patients are asleep, reliance must be placed on the calculated duration of blockade, as explained in Chapter 7. When blockade extends into the mid or upper thoracic segments, additional information may be obtained by watching the trend of blood pressure. As the block recedes, the systolic and diastolic pressures gradually climb toward resting levels. After reinjection of a maintenance dose, the blood pressure falls back to a lower level, as shown in Figure 11–15.

Sedation, Supplementary Anesthesia and Ventilation

The purist view does not favor combining regional and general anesthesia. The rhetorical question is often asked, "why give two anesthetics when one will do?" However, this question does not really appreciate that advantages may accrue when the two methods are properly used together: the object is to combine the best qualities of both. Sometimes patients are quite content to remain awake during operation, but there are also many procedures during which it is neither humane nor physically desirable for the patient to remain conscious.

Operations that interfere with respiratory mechanics through such handicaps as abnormal posture, gross obesity or an open chest demand that ventilation be supported artificially, and then it is almost essential to have the patient asleep, intubated and ventilated. The word "almost" has been used because, contrary to generally accepted teaching, it is possible, although not desirable, to conduct an open chest operation under regional anesthesia with an awake, spontaneously breathing patient (see Thoracic Surgery, page 486).

SEDATION

Diazepam (Valium) is one of the best sedative drugs available at the present time for producing amnesia and sedation during regional analgesia. It is relatively undisturbing to the respiratory and cardiovascular systems, and it confers a significant degree of protection against convulsive reactions to inadvertent overdosage of local anesthetic (Dalen et al., 1969; De Jong and Heavner, 1974). A preoperative dose of 0.2 mg per kg one hour before operation is usually sufficient to induce a calm and cooperative state in most patients. Further small increments of 2.5 to 5 mg may be given into the intravenous infusion during operation as required. Plasma concentrations of diazepam remain elevated for eight to ten hours, and the total dose administered should not exceed 0.4 mg per kg (Korttila and Linnoila, 1975).

Narcotic and Narcotic-Neuroleptic Mixtures. Narcotic and opiate drugs are best avoided in the presence of spontaneous respiration. They cause an undesirable degree of respiratory depression, and their analgesic properties are redundant if epidural blockade is effective. Droperidol, given alone or in combination with the powerful but short-acting narcotic fentanyl, produces tranquility and a degree of mental dissociation or "neuroleptanalgesia." However, fentanyl is a potent respiratory depressant, and the effects of droperidol are quite prolonged, causing some patients to complain of feeling "depressed and disconnected" in the postoperative period. Moreover, the alpha blocking effects of droperidol may lead to excessive arterial hypotension if the level of epidural analgesia extends to the mid-thoracic segments.

The anesthesiologist may be tempted to use droperidol-narcotic mixtures when regional analgesia is inadequate, but the results are often unsatisfactory and sometimes dangerous. In the event of questionable analgesia, it is better to make a firm decision to induce full anesthesia with thiopental and nitrous oxide–oxygen rather than to risk respiratory and vascular depression from opiate or neuroleptic drugs.

Ketamine. This has not proved to be a useful supplementary agent for regional analgesia in adults. Troublesome spontaneous movements are common on the operating table, and the incidence of emergence delirium is high. The agent is more satisfactory as a supplement in young children between the ages of one and ten years (Sussman, 1974), but even then the appearance of spontaneous movements may be embarrassing during the course of operation. In addition, the central sympathetic stimulating effect of ketamine raises the blood pressure and increases operative blood loss. Ketamine may be useful to produce quiescence in young children before caudal blockade is administered for operations on the lower limbs or perineum. The drug is then given intramuscularly in a dose of 10 mg per kilogram 10 to 15 minutes before the block is performed.

Barbiturates. Thiopental in intermittent intravenous doses remains the standby for inducing sleep rapidly when general anesthesia is indicated. For children under seven years of age, rectal thiopental in a dose of 25 to 30 mg per kg body weight is an excellent basal narcotic. Some anesthesiologists prefer other forms of short-acting barbiturate, such as methohexital or hexobarbital, by the intravenous route (Dawkins and Steel, 1971).

ANESTHESIA

Light thiopental–nitrous oxide–oxygen anesthesia is ideal whenever supplementary anesthesia is required. Usually, inhalational anesthesia can be given by mask, but a wider margin of safety is provided by passing a cuffed endotracheal tube to ensure a clear, watertight airway under all circumstances. Quiet operating conditions demand a tranquil airway and freedom from unexpected bouts of coughing during light anesthesia, and for this reason thorough topical anesthesia of the larynx and trachea is essential before the endotracheal tube is passed. My own preference is to avoid the use of succinylcholine, or indeed any neuromuscular blocking agent, during intubation and to rely on a combination of topical anesthesia and carefully timed intravenous anesthesia. This maintains spontaneous respiration throughout the induction period and frees the anesthesiologist from the need to impose artificial ventilation. When intubation is required, my procedure is as follows.

Transtracheal Topical Analgesia

1. The patient is told to relax his jaw and neck muscles.
2. An amnesic dose of thiopental (50 to 75 mg) or 5 to 10 mg of diazepam is given intravenously as a bolus.
3. About 45 seconds later, while the eyelash reflex is briefly obtunded, a transtracheal injection of 3.0 ml of 4 per cent lidocaine is given rapidly through a 22-gauge needle. Coughing should ensue. Laryngeal and tracheal anesthesia develops in about one minute.
4. Intravenous thiopental is given slowly until the masseter muscles are well relaxed and the jaw can be opened. About 150 to 350 mg is usually sufficient.
5. Laryngoscopy and endotracheal intubation are performed *extremely gently* and carefully. The cuff on the endotracheal tube is slowly inflated, and the tube is taped in place and connected to a source of nitrous oxide and oxygen with an FIO_2 of 0.3.

Properly done, this is not an unpleasant or traumatic procedure, and no memory of it remains on awakening. The anatomical level of transtracheal injection is not crucial; the cricothyroid membrane or any convenient ring below are equally satisfactory. However, three things are critical:

1. Careful timing is essential so that the transtracheal injection is done during a brief period of amnesia, but without having the patient too deep. Surprisingly small amounts of thiopental will suppress the cough reflex.

2. It is essential that a cough reflex be elicited by the jet of local anesthetic, so that the tussive blast will spread the anesthetic effectively over the upper trachea and vocal cords.

3. Topical lidocaine takes 50 to 60 seconds to work; therefore, one does not need to hurry the procedure. The sleep dose of thiopental is injected slowly, and a leisurely but highly controlled laryngoscopy and intubation are performed.

This method does not take any longer than a muscle relaxant intubation, and it ensures a very effective topical anesthesia of the upper airway, while at the same time maintaining spontaneous respiration. For this reason it has much to commend it when endotracheal intubation is being taught to beginners.

If plenty of time is available, the patient can be given a nebulized mist of 4 per cent lidocaine to inhale for a few minutes prior to induction of general anesthesia. This avoids the need to puncture the trachea, and it is a very gentle and effective way to anesthetize the upper airway (Abou-Madi et al., 1975).

Alternatively, the orthodox method of muscle relaxant intubation may be used, but then the anesthesiologist must take special care to spray the trachea and larynx very thoroughly with topical anesthetic before passing the endotracheal tube. In the absence of good laryngotracheal anesthesia, motor responses to the endotracheal tube may occur when the short-acting muscle relaxant wears off. These effects may range from a barely detectable expiratory effort to powerful bucking movements, but any motor response raises venous pressure and impairs the quality of the surgical field. These undesirable reactions can be avoided by effective topical anesthesia of the upper airway.

VENTILATION

As pointed out earlier in this chapter and in the chapter on Physiology, spontaneous respiration is usually adequate to maintain good gas exchange, unless mechanical conditions exist to interfere with it or fatigue sets in with the passage of time during prolonged abdominal surgery. Two hours is probably about the maximum time that a patient should be allowed to breathe spontaneously during upper abdominal surgery under epidural block with supplementary general anesthesia, and then only if the tidal volume can be monitored and an occasional check kept on the arterial blood gases.

Controlled ventilation is exceedingly easy to impose on a spontaneously breathing patient under a combination of light anesthesia and mid or high thoracic epidural blockade. The mechanism of this effect is discussed more fully in Chapter 10. Briefly, the reduced traffic of afferent input flowing past the phrenic nucleus and respiratory center reduces phrenic activity, and a slight degree of central depression and hyperventilation is all that is required to induce the respiratory apparatus to surrender its rhythm. Then five or ten good squeezes of the rebreathing bag will usually abolish spontaneous respiration, provided no noxious stimuli are allowed to reach the central nervous system from the airway or other regions above the segmental level of deafferentation (Bromage, 1958b). Mechanical ventilation can then be maintained for the remainder of the operation.

Marked hyperventilation should be avoided for two reasons. First, hypocapnia impairs tissue oxygenation by shifting the oxygen dissociation curve to the left (i.e., the Bohr effect). Second, respiratory alkalosis may delay resumption of spontaneous breathing at the end of operation. Patients who have been hyperventilated under extensive afferent blockade may be restored to consciousness and conversation, but they may fail to breathe unless commanded to do so. The ability is there, but the drive has gone.

Patients will resume spontaneous respiration very quickly once mechanical ventilation is stopped, provided respiration has been maintained within reasonable limits and the $PaCO_2$ has not been reduced below 30 mmHg. Small noxious stimuli, such as a pinch to the skin above the segmental level of blockade, will hasten return of spontaneous respiration by increasing the traffic of afferent input through the cervical cord and brain stem. This type of respiratory depression arising from a combination of deafferentation and mild hypocapnia is one of the few circumstances in which judicious use of respiratory stimulants or analeptics is justified and effective. An intravenous injection of doxapram, 1 mg per kg, will usually restart respiration and arouse the patient. Alternatively, the old-fashioned drug nikethamide (Coramine) in amounts of 1 to 2 ml (250 to 500 mg) given slowly is also effective in speeding arousal and restoring spontaneous respiration.

MANAGEMENT OF THE CARDIOVASCULAR STATUS

Sympathetic paralysis accompanying high epidural blockade dilates the vascular bed within the segmental distribution of the block. If analgesia extends into the upper thoracic segments, blockade of the cardiac sympathetic nerves also reduces inotropic and chronotropic drive to the heart. Thus, three factors may combine to cause a fall of blood pressure and cardiac output:

1. Discrepancy between the size of the vascular bed and the intravascular fluid volume.
2. Fall of inotropic drive and reduction of ejection force.
3. Bradycardia.

Each of these hypotensive factors may be treated singly, or all can be dealt with together, depending on the urgency of the situation (see Chapter 10 for a full discussion of the cardiovascular consequences of epidural blockade).

The anesthesiologist must decide whether to exploit or to correct the induced vascular hypotension, according to the nature of the case. It is impractical to make hard-and-fast rules for all types of patients, but broadly speaking three courses of action are open.

1. The blood pressure may be adjusted to normal levels throughout the operation.

2. A moderate degree of hypotension may be accepted, with a blood pressure of about 100 mmHg systolic or a fall of about 25 per cent of the resting mean arterial pressure.

3. Full hypotension may be actively sought to the lowest safe level of about 70 mmHg systolic for limited periods of time in fit patients in order to produce a dry surgical field for special purposes (Griffiths and Gillies, 1948; Bromage, 1951).

Controlled Arterial Hypotension and Surgical Blood Loss

The surge of enthusiasm for controlled arterial hypotension that swept the specialty in the 1950's has been tempered by the iatrogenic complications that arose from it, and we are now more aware of the factors that separate acceptable deviations of physiological state from unacceptable physiological trespass (Gillies, 1952). Adequate tissue blood flow is all-important, and vascular dynamics must be adjusted so that blood flow and intravascular pressure are sufficient to maintain patency of nutrient vessels in midline structures, such as heart, liver, brain and spinal cord. Ischemia of the cord from collapse of the anterior spinal artery is particularly to be feared. A free venous outflow and low venous pressure must be ensured to avoid venous infarction in the presence of low arterial pressures (see Chapter 14 on Complications). In addition, one should remember that the ill effects of physiological trespass are time-dependent. Expeditious surgery escapes many of the ill effects that arise during a slow protracted operation, so speed of surgery is a partial determinant of the level of hypotension that can be permitted. The fast surgeon may reasonably request a short period of quite profound hypotension for a particularly difficult phase of the operation; the slow worker may not. An electrocardioscope should be affixed to all patients in whom hypotension is to be allowed, so that any ischemic changes can be monitored and corrected as soon as they occur. There is no doubt that properly used controlled hypotension is a great technical boon in suitable cases, not only in simplifying the surgeon's task but also as a means of sparing the patient the danger of excessive blood loss and multiple blood transfusions.

Opinions differ over the best and safest way to provide controlled hypotension. Hypotension can be achieved by vasodilatation from ganglion blocking drugs (Enderby, 1950), by subarachnoid block (Griffiths and Gillies, 1948) or by epidural blockade (Bromage, 1951). The physiological reasons for preferring epidural analgesia have been outlined. A number of enthusiastic reports have recommended epidural analgesia as a more favorable and less bloody technique than general anesthesia (Gardner, 1958; Loudon and Scott, 1960; Moir, 1968; Fisher and James, 1968; Zorgniotti et al., 1970; Fasth et al., 1972; Thorud et al., 1975). However, careful measurements of blood loss at comparable levels of hypotension have shown that there is little real difference in the amount of blood loss under ganglionic blockade or under epidural analgesia (Donald, 1969; Urquhart-Hay et al., 1969a, 1969b). Donald (1969) experienced a 10 per cent failure rate of epidural analgesia in his comparative series and, on the basis of his findings, concluded that "epidural blockade is no more than a difficult and inconvenient method of inducing hypotension" (Donald, 1970), associated with the additional danger of paraplegia due to thrombosis of the anterior spinal artery.

The imputation of added neurological danger loses force in the light of careful comparative results published by Urquhart-Hay and his colleagues (1969a, 1969b) from two series of open prostatectomies performed under hypotensive anesthesia. One series of 103 cases was performed under epidural analgesia with an average blood loss of just over 600 ml, and a second series of 104 cases under general anesthesia and ganglionic blockade had an average blood loss of just under 500 ml. Thus, there was no appreciable difference between the two methods as far as blood loss was concerned, and the authors concluded that ganglionic blockade was preferable, as it was free of any specific neurological complications that are occasionally encountered with epidural analgesia. However, two major neurological sequelae suggestive of infarction of the lower portion of the spinal cord occurred shortly after these series were completed; one of the cases was associated with epidural blockade (Urquhart-Hay, 1969), and the other was associated with general anesthesia and ganglionic blockade (Urquhart-Hay, 1969, personal communication; Urquhart-Hay and Teague, 1974). Thus, it is erroneous to suppose that epidural analgesia adds a special and significant neurological risk in controlled hypotension. Other factors influencing cord blood flow are more important, and the syndrome of "spinal stroke" is a danger that hovers over any patient with severe arteriosclerotic disease who suffers obstruction to the arterial or venous flow in the spinal cord (Silver and Buxton, 1974). These factors will be considered in greater detail in Chapter 14.

The question of superiority of epidural blockade versus general anesthesia and ganglionic or nitroprusside blockade remains open. Both can produce excellent results if properly administered with good technique, yet both can produce equally dismal results if badly done. As with so many other technical controversies in anesthesia, the individual decision is largely a matter of personal skill and preference, combined with a sense for the overall well-being of the patient. Those of us who enjoy doing epidural analgesia and who have some measure of success with it believe it gives the best all-round results available in anatomical regions where epidural blockade is appropriate, but this is a subjective stance not yet supported by rigorous quantitative proof.

Control of the Blood Pressure

Intravascular Fluid Volume

The first line of defense against uncontrolled vascular hypotension is fluid augmentation to expand the intravascular volume and to compensate for the dilated vascular bed resulting from sympathetic paresis. This can be done adequately by saline infusion to produce a slight but deliberate reduction in the hematocrit, with a corresponding rheological improvement in flow and delivery of oxygen to the tissues (Replogle et al., 1967; Case et al., 1955). The preoperative hematocrit will be a guide to the amount of electrolyte solution to be infused.

More gradual correction of a raised hematocrit and contracted blood volume over a period of days, as in the preparation of a pheochromocytoma (vide infra), may require packed cell transfusions to maintain a satisfactory red cell mass (Crout and Brown, 1969).

Most chronically ill or bedridden patients may be expected to have a contracted blood volume, so judicious augmentation of intravascular fluid volume before induction is particularly important in these cases. Induction of total sympathetic blockade has been advocated as an objective method to assess blood volume deficits, on the basis of expanding the vascular space to its full extent and then filling up the augmented intravascular volume with appropriate replacement fluids (Henley and Kritchman, 1961, 1962). Clearly this principle needs to be applied with great caution, by an anesthesiologist who is capable of reacting swiftly to restore any cardiovascular imbalance the moment blood pressure falls below the expected level. Central venous pressure measurements may not be a very accurate guide to fluid replacement if abdominal pain is present. Intrathoracic pressures are kept artificially high by the "clenched chest" response to pain, and the CVP follows the pressure of the abdominothoracic compartments, falling back to lower levels when the trunk muscles relax, as shown in Table 11–1 on page 446.

POSTURE

The blood pressure is sensitive to posture in the presence of vasodilatation. Temporary relocation of an inadequate intravascular volume is quickly arranged by a slight head-down tilt of the table or by raising the legs. This is the first step to take as an emergency measure to fill the great veins and right heart, if it is necessary to correct an unexpected fall of pressure. Patients with high epidural blocks should be kept horizontal or very slightly head-down to ensure an adequate venous return during operation.

Patients with blocks that involve both the lumbar and thoracic outflows are more sensitive to postural changes in the postoperative period than those with analgesia confined to the thoracic segments alone. An adequate intravascular fluid volume should be maintained regardless of the site of blockade, while common sense must be used to ensure that the vascular system is not overloaded by excessive infusion therapy.

The mechanism of the supine hypotensive syndrome was discussed in Chapter 10. Pressure on the inferior vena cava for any reason, such as an abdominal tumor, ascites, surgical retractors or severe extension or lateral flexion of the spine, may obstruct venous return and cause the cardiac output and blood pressure to fall (Brigden et al., 1950; Eggers et al., 1965; Scott, 1963; Doppman et al., 1966). Acute hypotension from an obstructed venous return should be treated immediately by correcting the abnormal posture and relieving pressure on the inferior vena cava (Malatinsky and Kadlic, 1974). A combination of unrelieved caval venous obstruction and severe arterial hypotension is particularly dangerous and jeopardizes capillary flow in the spinal cord. Cord infarction and paraplegia may result if tissue flow is reduced below critical levels, as discussed in Chapters 10 and 14.

Vasopressor Drugs

Vagolytic

Cardiac output is related to heart rate, as well as to stroke volume. A sudden onset of marked bradycardia may be an important cause of abrupt arterial hypotension arising from vagal predominance in the presence of extensive sympathetic blockade. A slowing pulse in the presence of moderate arterial hypotension should warn the anesthesiologist, and a syringe of atropine should be ready for immediate injection of 0.3 to 0.6 mg if the pulse and blood pressure fall in tandem to levels that are considered inappropriate for the individual case. In these circumstances, atropine acts as a pressor drug through its chronotropic effects in terms of the simple equations:

$$\text{Blood pressure} = \text{cardiac output} \times \text{peripheral resistance}$$
$$\text{Cardiac output} = \text{stroke volume} \times \text{rate}$$

Under high epidural block, peripheral resistance is low and remains so, but cardiac output falls if the heart rate slows unduly. Thus, both output and pressure are restored by agents that increase heart rate.

Adrenergic

So far, the methods listed to maintain blood pressure in the face of sympathetic blockade have been nonadrenergic, and priority has been given to factors that influence blood volume and heart rate. If we believe that vasoconstriction does more harm than good in most circumstances under anesthesia, then vasoconstrictor drugs should be used sparingly, and if they must be used, they should be given in minimal doses to replace, or partially replace, vasomotor tone that has been suppressed by sympathetic blockade (see Chapter 10). This is not to say that vasopressor agents should be withheld in hypotensive situations when rapid restoration of pressure and flow is urgently indicated, but a general attitude of restraint should be cultivated toward their use. Routine prophylactic administration of vasopressor agents before induction of epidural analgesia is illogical and unnecessary, and the drugs should be held in reserve until indicated.

Flow is the important determinant of tissue nutrition and gas exchange. Pressure is only needed to overcome resistance to flow. Hence, there is no place for alpha stimulating drugs, such as methoxamine (Vasoxyl), that have their principal action on the peripheral vascular bed, constricting arterioles and raising the outflow resistance to the pumping action of the heart, and increasing cardiac work. The naturally occurring vasoactive substances epinephrine and norepinephrine have mixed alpha and beta stimulating effects, and tissue flow is best preserved by using agents that approximate the action of these agents on adrenergic receptors.

It is reasonable to assume that the main cardiovascular changes seen after epidural block are due to a reduced output of adrenergic amines from sympathetic stores in the segmental distribution of the block, and it may also be

TABLE 11–8 Summary of inotropic and vasoconstrictor effects of common vasopressor agents

Drug	**Receptor** *ALPHA*	*BETA*	**Inotropic**	**Arteriolar Constriction**	**Venocon-striction**
Epinephrine	+	++	++	⇅	↑
Norepinephrine	++	++	++	↑	↑
Isoproterenol	0	++	++	↓	⇅
Ephedrine	+	++	+	⇅	↑
Methamphetamine	+	++	+	⇅	↑
Metaraminol (Aramine)	++	++	+	↑	↑
Mephentermine (Wyamine)	+	++	++	⇅	↑
Methoxamine (Vasoxyl)	++	0	0	↑	↑

\+ = Reactor
++ = Strong reactor
0 = No effect
↑ = Constriction
↓ = Dilation

assumed that the level of circulating catecholamines falls during epidural blockade. Logical replacement therapy should be based on estimates of resting catecholamine production. The normal basal catecholamine output in man has been calculated to be approximately 0.05 μg per kg per minute (or 3 to 4 μg per minute in a 70-kg man), in the proportions of one-fifth epinephrine and four-fifths norepinephrine (Cohen et al., 1959), so replacement dosage of this order is required to restore vascular tone in the presence of total sympathetic blockade (Bromage, 1960). Dose rates in excess of this very small input of 3 to 4 μg per minute are beyond the physiological range and are harmful due to excessive vasoconstriction in renal and hepatic vascular beds (Bendixen et al., 1964). Provided the blood volume is adequate, rather less than this basal amount is required to restore blood pressure to resting levels, possibly because a high segmental block also interferes with the normal homeostatic depressor reflexes (Bromage, 1952). Norepinephrine in the dose range of 2 to 4 μg per minute has a marked inotropic effect on the sympathectomized heart, improving the stroke volume and ejection force, as well as having a slight constrictor effect on the capacitance vessels of the venous system, thus increasing venous return (Mellander, 1960).

Substitution therapy with synthetic vasopressor agents can be satisfactory if the chosen drug closely resembles the mixed alpha-beta receptor effects of norepinephrine, as shown in Table 11–8 (Ahlquist, 1948). Ephedrine, d-methamphetamine and mephentermine are appropriate agents, whereas methoxamine is an inappropriate choice since it is a pure alpha stimulator with overriding vasoconstrictor effects.

In summary, undesirable falls of blood pressure secondary to extensive sympathetic blockade are best controlled by augmenting the vascular volume, adjusting posture and preventing excessive bradycardia. Inotropic and vasoconstrictor drugs with mixed alpha and beta receptor effects should be used sparingly as replacement therapy and in minimal dosage.

SPECIAL APPLICATIONS

Pediatric Surgery

In spite of several enthusiastic reports in the anesthetic literature, epidural analgesia has had very little popularity for pediatric surgery (Schneider, 1951; Ruston, 1954, 1957, 1964; Spiegel, 1962; Rodriguez, 1964; Fortuna, 1967). There are a number of reasons for this lack of interest. First, very few anesthesiologists are convinced that regional analgesia has any advantages for children. Second, young children are thought to be difficult subjects from a technical point of view. They are small, and the margin of error in needle misplacement is narrower than in adults. Also, the spinal cord descends to a lower level than in the adult; therefore puncture is usually made below the third lumbar vertebra. Finally, young children tend to be reluctant subjects for regional anesthesia, and through fear they may react violently to needle punctures, so that heavy sedation or general anesthesia is often necessary before regional analgesia can be induced. In short, it may seem much simpler to put the child to sleep and to avoid the challenge of regional analgesia altogether.

However, I believe this is a mistaken view. In fact, regional analgesia in children is not technically difficult; indeed some blocks, such as caudal analgesia, are easier and more predictable than in the adult (Schulte-Steinberg and Rahlfs, 1970). Operative bleeding is less than under general anesthesia alone. Postoperative pain and distress are markedly reduced by adopting a combination of regional analgesia and light general anesthesia, and the recovery ward becomes quieter and more pleasant for all concerned.

LUMBAR ROUTE

Most children over the age of five or six years will accept epidural analgesia quite happily provided good rapport is established. The lumbar approach seems more readily accepted than the caudal route, perhaps because natural modesty or primitive fears provoke greater reluctance to bare the buttocks than the back. Dose requirements for 2 per cent lidocaine at the second lumbar interspace are shown in relation to age in Figure 11–16, with the mean

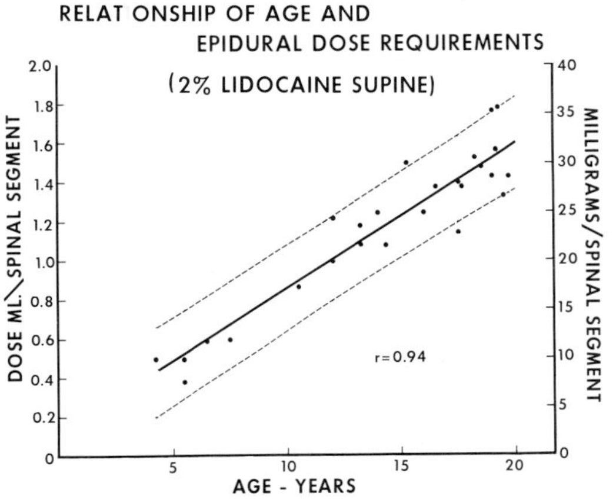

Figure 11–16. Relationship of age and segmental epidural dose requirements in children and adolescents at the second lumbar interspace for 2 per cent lidocaine HCl with 1/200,000 epinephrine (n = 26). The dotted lines show the 90 per cent confidence limits to the mean regression line. (From Bromage, P. R.: Ageing and epidural dose requirements. Brit. J. Anaesth. *41*:1016, 1969b.)

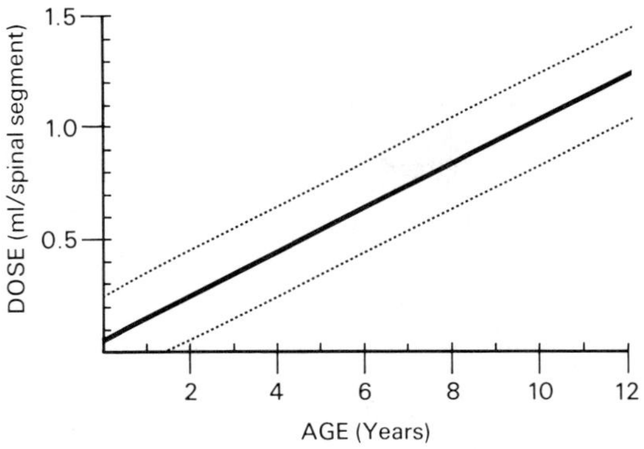

Figure 11–17. Caudal segmental dose requirements for 1 per cent lidocaine plus epinephrine, between the ages of 7 weeks and 11½ years, with 95 per cent confidence limits for the population. (Data from Schulte-Steinberg and Rahlfs, 1970.)

regression line for dose and age and the 90 per cent confidence limits to the mean.

With the approach of adulthood, dose requirements rise to a maximum level. This necessitates a large induction dose of local anesthetic for a patient in the late teens. For example, a youth of 17 years will require about 28 mg of 2 per cent lidocaine per segment, so for a laparotomy at this age, an induction dose of about 24 ml of 2 per cent lidocaine will be needed to provide analgesia of all segments up to the xiphisternum. The possible danger of a toxic reaction in these patients can be minimized by adequate premedication with diazepam, in a dose of 0.2 mg per kg given one hour before induction.

Caudal route

As mentioned in an earlier chapter, the sacral hiatus is usually very easy to identify in babies and young children. It is often the route of choice for operations on the perineum or legs, being technically easier than the lumbar approach in young subjects. However, children are often reluctant to submit to an injection at the base of the spine, and it may be necessary to induce a short period of general anesthesia with intravenous thiopental or intramuscular ketamine in order to perform the block without causing unnecessary distress.

Satisfactory caudal analgesia for children is provided by 1 per cent lidocaine with 1/200,000 epinephrine. Fortuna has proposed the following dosage schedule based on body weight:

1. For analgesia up to the twelfth thoracic segment: 10 mg per kg body weight.
2. For analgesia up to the tenth thoracic segment: 12 mg per kg body weight.
3. For anesthesia up to the xiphisternum (T_6): 15 mg per kg body weight.

A more accurate prediction can be made in terms of age. Schulte-Steinberg and Rahlfs (1970) have published a careful statistical analysis of caudal dose requirements for 1 per cent lidocaine between 7 weeks and 11½ years of age, and their results are summarized in Figure 11–17.

Postoperative pain and discomfort after circumcision in adults and children are almost entirely avoided by a small caudal epidural injection, and this has been a routine procedure at the Montreal Children's Hospital for many years. The operation may be performed under caudal block alone or in combination with light general anesthesia. Kay (1974) has described a pediatric technique using 0.5 per cent bupivacaine with 1/200,000 epinephrine in a dose of 0.5 ml per year of age. However, bupivacaine has a very slow latency, and quicker results and almost as long a duration are obtained by using a larger volume of more dilute bupivacaine mixed with carbonated lidocaine. The following dose is used: 1.0 ml per year of age of a mixture containing 1 per cent carbonated lidocaine and 0.25 per cent bupivacaine with 1/200,000 epinephrine. With this mixture, penile analgesia is established in 5 to 10 minutes and lasts for about three to four hours.

Children usually have very stable cardiovascular responses under epidural blockade, and they compensate for high segmental analgesia with a smaller fall of arterial pressure than adults. The venous pressure is lower than under general anesthesia alone, and surgical blood loss is reduced below normal expectations, probably due to diminished venous oozing.

Epidural analgesia has found very little application for postoperative pain relief in major pediatric surgery. However, there have been some enthusiastic reports in the Russian literature that continuous epidural analgesia improves respiratory performance after thoracic and upper abdominal operations in children as effectively as it does in adults (Parnes and Gordeev, 1970; Parnes et al., 1971; Isakob et al., 1971). The latter group used whole-body plethysmography to show that the work of breathing was reduced after epidural analgesia, but no data were presented to support this claim, and the reader was left wondering how the children were persuaded to cooperate effectively inside the body box so soon after major surgery (Isakob et al., 1971).

Thoracic Surgery

PERSPECTIVE

Before the mid 1950's when resection for pulmonary tuberculosis became routine, treatment of fibrotic cavitational lung disease was accomplished by collapsing the chest wall. Thoracoplasty was commonly performed in one or more stages, usually in awake patients under regional anesthesia with paravertebral blockade and local infiltration. This form of anesthesia was technically demanding, but when successfully done it provided an almost bloodless ischemic field. Satisfactory paravertebral blockade for a third-stage operation was often difficult and unsatisfactory, owing to loss of anatomical landmarks from the first two stages of rib resection, and then a high segmental epidural block provided a satisfactory but more bloody alternative form of regional analgesia (Durrans, 1947; Paletto, 1952).

In 1944, Vasconcelos of São Paulo described his technique for transthoracic total esophagectomy in awake patients under epidural analgesia, in which he used large volumes of 40 to 50 ml of a procaine-tetracaine mixture injected into one of the upper thoracic interspaces. This operation was always preceded by an adaptive pneumothorax induced some time previously, and the surgery was made tolerable by its speed, for the operation seldom lasted more than $1\frac{1}{2}$ to 2 hours (Vasconcelos, 1944). These principles were transplanted to Springfield, Missouri, by Dr. A. Neves of Rio de Janeiro, where they were adapted and successfully employed for pulmonary resections in tuberculous patients for the next ten years.

This regional anesthetic technique in conscious patients seemed to defy all the accepted canons of management of the open chest, inviting the well-known complications of paradoxical respiration, mediastinal flap and ineffective gas exchange. Nevertheless, it worked well in the right hands, and a series of articles appeared between 1948 and 1953 describing the use of thoracic epidural blockade for pulmonary resections in awake patients without intubation (Fujikawa et al., 1948; Crawford et al., 1951; Crawford, 1952, 1953).

In 1955, I had the privilege of observing Dr. Crawford and his surgical colleagues performing lobectomies under thoracic epidural blockade without general anesthesia or intubation in a number of tuberculous patients at Springfield, Missouri. There were several remarkable things about this team work which bear recall and corroboration, for this technique is now becoming a lost art, and it can help in elucidating certain other exotic anesthetic phenomena that seem puzzling to the orthodox trained anesthesiologist.

The most astonishing phenomenon of the technique was the quiet effective respiration of the patients breathing spontaneously in the lateral position throughout an open thoracotomy. There was no apparent mediastinal flap or paradoxical respiration, and breathing and speech appeared normal, even when an upper lobe bronchus was transected and held open. Five things contributed to the success of this unorthodox technique. First, analgesia was technically perfect, and the patients were comfortable. Second, the patients were well disciplined, and rapport with the anesthesiologist was excellent. Third, premedication was light and central depression was minimal, so that patients could cooperate and adjust their breathing on command. Fourth, positive pressure oxygen was given by mask as soon as the patient reported any shortness of breath, or if the mediastinum appeared to be unstable. Fifth, and very important, the surgical team was remarkably deft, gentle and expeditious. Some degree of tuberculous fibrosis may have contributed to what appeared to be an unusually stable mediastinum, but it was not obvious on direct inspection of the open chest. It seemed that the presence of consciousness with simple positive pressure support was enough to maintain adequate respiratory control in the presence of an open chest. But teamwork and patient conditioning are also important factors, for the same technique in my own hands in my own hospital was seldom so successful, and it was often necessary for me to interrupt the operation under epidural blockade to resort to the accepted methods of ventilatory support with endotracheal intubation and ventilation.

This anecdotal digression is made to dispel the belief that there is only one way to handle the open chest. There is no denying that the orthodox methods ensure the best and safest control in most hands, but given the right conditions there are other ways than the usual textbook description, and sometimes, under primitive conditions or in a disaster, it may be necessary to revert to systems that have been shown to work without sophisticated mechanical support. The success of epidural analgesia in open chest surgery may also help to explain the extraordinary cinematographic documentation of thoracotomies performed under acupuncture in the People's Republic of China. In these films it is clear that close teamwork existed, as it did in the group using epidural analgesia at Springfield, Missouri. In the Chinese films there was a similar degree of surgical gentleness and skill, and the patients showed unusual confidence and self-discipline in a milieu in which these subjective strengths could be exploited to the full.

COMBINED EPIDURAL BLOCKADE AND LIGHT GENERAL ANESTHESIA FOR THORACIC SURGERY

Current anesthetic procedure for intrathoracic operations has become standardized into a pattern which ensures full control of the airway and respiratory exchange at all times. Thanks to the work of Nosworthy and others, the reasons for this are now common knowledge, so they need not be discussed here. Prior to the introduction of curare, control of respiration under general anesthesia was obtained through central respiratory depression, usually by means of opiates and cyclopropane combined with hyperventilation. Now, apnea is induced peripherally by neuromuscular blockade, while general anesthesia is light and central depression is minimal. With this combination, the patient wakes relatively fresh and responsive, even from the longest operation, and he can attempt to cough and carry out breathing exercises from the outset, insofar as his pain will allow him. Apart from the necessity for endobronchial intubation, which the individual case may require, this technique is so easy and so safe that there may appear to be little reason to look for further improvement.

However, there are two causes for dissatisfaction with the combination of light general anesthesia and muscle relaxants. First, there is the danger of overdosage with relaxant, resulting in prolonged apnea requiring continued artificial respiration. Second, the relaxants do nothing to relieve the depressant effects of pain in the early postoperative period. The patient awakes to pain which seriously inhibits his breathing and reduces the vital capacity to a third or a quarter of the preoperative level. Effective coughing and deep breathing are impossible, and the patient may require ventilatory support specifically to overcome this inhibition. The systemic analgesics such as morphine and Amidone help a little, but the Respiratory Restoration Factor (RRF) is low, and the partial subjective pain relief which they offer is accompanied by a poor objective respiratory performance (see Fig. 11–4). All this occurs at a crucial time when bronchial secretions may be settling into peripheral parts of the lung field, sowing the seeds of postoperative pulmonary complications.

Epidural analgesia, properly used, offers a way around respiratory handicaps. The tranquillity of afferent blockade provides just as quiet a surgical field as the muscle relaxants. After operation, effective analgesia without impairment of respiration can be continued for as long as necessary, and the need for prolonged intubation and ventilation seldom arises. These two things may seem a small return for the added technical complexities of epidural analgesia, since muscle relaxants serve well enough in most cases. However, anyone who has worked extensively with both methods cannot fail to be impressed by the benefits of epidural analgesia for thoracic surgery, particularly when there is the opportunity to observe the patients for long periods of time in the recovery room. The subjective comfort and the efficient respiratory performance are striking and leave little doubt about the advantages of the method.

Thus, epidural blockade is employed both as a substitute for muscle relaxants and as a unique form of analgesia, allowing a postoperative respiratory performance that is unsurpassed by any alternative method. In other respects the anesthetic technique does not differ from currently accepted techniques for thoracic surgery. The patient is asleep with the trachea intubated, and controlled respiration is carried on throughout the operation. In the presence of afferent blockade, this type of ventilation is the genuine "controlled respiration" described by Guedel, in which spontaneous respiratory activity is kept suppressed by judicious hyperventilation and slight hypocarbia, with spontaneous breathing "just around the corner," waiting to return as soon as the arterial $PaCO_2$ is allowed to rise to normal levels (Guedel and Treweek, 1934). This is quite different from the artificial ventilation used with relaxant drugs which is often incorrectly labeled "controlled respiration"; however, it is not controlled in the true sense, since normal breathing cannot return, no matter how high the $PaCO_2$ may rise, until the effects of the relaxant have worn off.

General principles

The following conditions are necessary for good thoracic anesthesia:

1. Airway control.
2. Light anesthesia with prompt awakening.
3. Controlled respiration with quickly reversible apnea.
4. Efficient postoperative analgesia.

These factors will be considered briefly in turn before the practical details of epidural technique in thoracic surgery are dealt with.

Airway Control. As in orthodox methods of anesthesia for thoracic surgery, endotracheal intubation is essential for safety, elimination of secretions, and effective respiratory control. Bronchoscopy and endobronchial intubation may be carried out if indicated by the nature of the lesion. Thorough topical analgesia of the larynx and trachea ensures an easy intubation and a tranquil airway under light general anesthesia. This is accomplished by laryngeal spray under direct vision, or by a transtracheal injection of 2 to 4 ml of 4 per cent lidocaine.

Light General Anesthesia. Premedication is light. Anesthetic sleep is induced with 150 to 350 mg of thiopental after topical analgesia has been applied to the larynx and trachea. During induction of anesthesia, the patient is instructed to relax his face and neck muscles. This helps considerably in providing relaxation of the jaw for tracheal intubation without the aid of neuromuscular blocking agents. Anesthesia is maintained with nitrous oxide and oxygen in the proportions of 2:1, using carbon dioxide absorption or a nonrebreathing system. Traces of a volatile anesthetic agent, such as halothane, in concentrations of 0.25 to 0.5 per cent may be added if necessary to keep the patient from moving his head and arms during operation. No neuromuscular blocking agents are given except for a small dose of short-acting relaxant when the diathermy is used on the chest wall. At this point, electrical stimulation by the diathermy point causes annoying contractions of the scapular muscles, so a brief period of neuromuscular blockade is required to maintain a quiet satisfactory surgical field: 15 to 40 mg of succinylcholine is usually sufficient. An FIO_2 of at least 0.3 should be used for endotracheal anesthesia and an FIO_2 of 0.5 for endobronchial anesthesia. In certain cases of gas entrapment, as in bullous emphysema, 100 per cent oxygen should be used to avoid partial pressure expansion effects from nitrous oxide diffusion.

Apnea and Controlled Respiration. Apnea is easily induced by moderate hyperventilation under light general anesthesia, provided no noxious stimuli from the airway or operative site are allowed to reach the central nervous system and augment respiratory drive (see Chapter 10). In the presence of good topical analgesia to the larynx and trachea, five or ten inflations of the rebreathing bag are normally sufficient to suppress the patient's own respiratory rhythm. High epidural blockade prevents operative stimuli from reaching the CNS and initiating spontaneous respiration. Moderate hyperventilation is continued with a minute volume of about 8 to 12 liters per minute. This lowers the arterial $PaCO_2$ to the region of 30 to 35 mmHg and facilitates the maintenance of apnea, ensuring that spontaneous breathing does not return during intervals of tracheobronchial toilet. Artificial dead space may be added to the breathing circuit if larger minute volumes are required to maintain normal oxygenation.

At the end of the operation when the chest wall is airtight, spontaneous respiration is restored by gradually reducing the minute volume to such a point that the patient takes over his own rhythm again. If hyperventilation has been energetic and the imposed respiratory alkalosis severe, this process of weaning the respiratory center back to a normal $PaCO_2$ may take as long as 10 to 15 minutes. Sometimes, even with a normal arterial $PaCO_2$, the patient may seem to have lost the habit of automatic respiration, although he is awake and moving about and capable of breathing deeply if told to do so. In these circumstances, authoritative commands to "take a deep breath" will bring the required response, and after a few breaths the normal automatic rhythm will persist. A small intravenous dose of doxapram will hasten return of vigorous respiration.

CHOICE OF EPIDURAL SITE FOR THORACIC SURGERY

Two approaches are open. Segmental block is most easily induced by puncture in the upper thoracic spine, between C_7 and T_4, after which analgesia will spread up into the cervical region and down to the upper lumbar segments. Puncture at this level is simpler and more effective for thoracic surgery than injection in the mid-thoracic range of T_5–T_8. Alternatively, puncture may be done in the lumbar region, but then appreciably larger quantities of drug are necessary to carry analgesia up to include all the thoracic segments.

The upper thoracic approach seems the more logical of the two. The center of the block is close to the operation site, small volumes of solution are needed and it is easy to maintain postoperative analgesia even if the patient is propped up in bed. Moreover, the phrenic segments (C_3, C_4 and C_5) are often involved to some degree, so troublesome reflexes are less likely to arise from stimulation of the central portion of the diaphragm, which sends its sensory impulses through the phrenic nerve. However, thoracic punctures are relatively difficult to carry out and demand more technical skill than the lumbar approach.

The phrenic reflex must be mentioned again at this point. From evidence presented in Chapter 10 it is now apparent that in the presence of afferent blockade, light general anesthesia and hyperventilation, the phrenic reflex arc need not be blocked in order to have a quiet diaphragm, and an epidural block does not have to extend beyond T_1–T_2 in order to avoid reflex activity when the central portion of the diaphragm is stimulated (Bromage, 1958b). In other words, as far as diaphragmatic activity is concerned, similar conditions obtain at operation whether one uses a high puncture at C_7–T_4 or a lumbar approach with analgesia carried up to T_2, so the choice between the two is narrowed to consideration of (a) ease of administration, and (b) effectiveness of postoperative analgesia.

The former depends on the build of the patient and the skill and preference of the administrator. Effective analgesia is the crucial aim, and there is no question that pain after thoracic surgery is better relieved by an epidural catheter placed at an upper thoracic level than by the lumbar route. Shoulder-tip pain from diaphragmatic irritation is often troublesome, and this is not helped by injections from the lumbar area, as blockade seldom reaches the phrenic sensory roots. With high blocks, however, all the sensory inflow from the cervical and thoracic segments can be interrupted, and no pain, direct or referred, need be felt from either chest wall or diaphragm.

In summary, the best approach for thoracic work is high up between C_7 and T_4 using the hanging-drop technique, provided the anesthesiologist is competent to carry it out safely. Alternatively, the lumbar region may be chosen, using the loss-of-resistance technique, and this will serve well enough during the operation, but postoperative pain relief will not be as perfect as with a high puncture (Table 11–9).

TABLE 11–9 Comparison of thoracic and lumbar injection sites for thoracic surgery

	Thoracic Approach	*Lumbar Approach*
Posture for induction	Sitting, or tilted lateral position with operative side down	Lateral (operative side down)
Technique	Hanging-drop; caution needed in asthma or severe emphysema when intrapleural pressure is less negative than normal	Loss-of-resistance
Phrenic reflex	Obtunded	Obtunded if block extends to T_1–T_2, and if combined with light general anesthesia and hyperventilation
Analgesic solution	Dilute; requires care that motor block does not occur, or spontaneous respiration will not return at end of operation	Dilute, but no danger of diaphragmatic paralysis, since block does not extend to the phrenic outflow
Postoperative analgesia	Complete; easy to maintain upper level of analgesia, even in Fowler's position	May be difficult to maintain level high enough in sitting position; analgesia may be only partial if diaphragmatic pain is referred to cervical segments

TECHNIQUE OF EPIDURAL BLOCKADE FOR THORACIC SURGERY

Plan

1. Blockade of all thoracic segments from C_8–L_1 inclusive, with corresponding pharmacological sympathectomy. Motor blockade should be minimal at the end of operation.

2. Control of blood pressure by intravenous fluids, and replacement vasopressor therapy if required.

3. Light general anesthesia for "social sleep," with controlled endotracheal or endobronchial ventilation during operation.

4. Resumption of spontaneous respiration at the end of operation.

Materials and Drugs

1. *Vasopressor agents*
   - Atropine
   - Ephedrine, mephentermine or metaraminol
   - Norepinephrine infusion of 1 to 2 μg per ml (i.e., 1 to 2 mg of norepinephrine base in 1 liter) in reserve, in case severe hypotension occurs.
2. *Epidural tray and catheter*
3. *Epidural solutions*
   - (a) Peroperative: 1 per cent lidocaine with 1/300,000 epinephrine, or 0.5 per cent bupivacaine with epinephrine 1/300,000.
   - (b) Postoperative: 0.8 per cent lidocaine with 1/300,000 epinephrine, or 0.25 per cent plain bupivacaine. More concentrated solutions may be required if pain relief is inadequate.

Procedure

HIGH THORACIC PUNCTURE. Premedication is light so that the patient will remain cooperative during induction of the block. In the anesthetic room the blood pressure is checked, and the vasopressor drugs are prepared in readiness to correct any undesirable degree of arterial hypotension. An intravenous infusion is started and allowed to run fast to a volume of 250 to 500 ml, depending on the size and status of the patient, in order to counteract any postural hypotension which may occur while the patient is in the sitting position. The patient sits on the operating table with his feet on a stool, while an assistant steadies the shoulders and flexes the head sharply on the chest to open up the interspinous spaces (see Fig. 11–13).

The upper thoracic spines are carefully palpated, the space which is easiest from the technical point of view is chosen (this is usually somewhere between C_7 and T_4) and the skin, subcutaneous tissues and deep fascia are infiltrated with local analgesic solution. A 17- or 18-gauge thin-walled Tuohy needle is inserted in the selected interspinous space, exactly in the midline and with the orifice toward the head. The stylet is withdrawn when the needle is felt to be gripped firmly by the ligaments, and a drop of analgesic solution is placed in the hub. The needle is now advanced cautiously and intermittently, advance being made only during the inspiratory phase of respiration, so that epidural negative pressure will be greatest at the instant when the point pierces the ligamentum flavum and enters the space. The anesthesiologist must have a firm grip on the needle, so that it can be brought to an immediate halt as soon as the drop is sucked in. Once the needle enters the space the drop sign can usually be repeated several times by placing fresh drops in the hub; even more convincingly, a fine stream squirted into the hub from a 25-gauge needle will disappear up the shaft as the solution is drawn into the epidural space by the intrathoracic negative pressure (see Fig. 6–11). Fluctuations of epidural pressure, due to respiration and pulse beat, can be seen transmitted to the meniscus in the hub when the needle shaft and hub are filled with fluid. An empty 2-ml syringe is attached to the needle, and aspiration is attempted to ensure that a vein or the dura has not been pierced. Then, 15 ml of analgesic solution is injected fairly rapidly to initiate the block. The resulting temporary rise in epidural pressure may cause a fleeting ache in the arms and shoulders, so the patient is warned to remain still and is reassured that any uncomfortable feelings will quickly pass. If the patient is to remain awake, the solution chosen is usually 0.8 per cent lidocaine with 1/300,000 epinephrine, or the equivalent strength of some other local analgesic, to ensure a differential blockade with minimal motor involvement. Smaller volumes of more concentrated solutions may be used if the patient is to be asleep and ventilated under general anesthesia. A catheter is threaded in a headward direction for 3 to 4 cm, and the needle is withdrawn over the catheter. Finally, the catheter is carried up over the shoulder of the nonoperative side and taped in place with waterproof adhesive tape.

The patient is then placed on his side with the operative side downward; a 3-ml test dose is given up the catheter, and then a further 10 to 15 ml of dilute analgesic solution is injected. The patient is left in this position for a few minutes, or as long as convenient, so that the solution can gravitate to the dependent side and open up the epidural space there to establish a thoroughly effective block. Once the block has become well established in this way, it is possible to maintain effective analgesia, even when the patient is turned over and postured with the operative side uppermost. On the other hand, if this initial "soaking" is omitted and the patient is placed straightway in the operative position, the solution has to track upward against gravity from the outset, and analgesia may be uneven and incomplete. For midline operations such as thymectomy, this initial posturing is obviously unnecessary, and then the patient is placed on his back as soon as the catheter is fixed in place. The extent of the block is tested with a sharp pin before induction of general anesthesia.

Subsequent injections of local analgesic are made at appropriate intervals to maintain the level of analgesia. A volume of about half of the main dose is injected through the catheter every 60 to 70 minutes. Thus, if a total of 30 ml was given at the beginning, 15 ml of solution would be required every hour. Toward the end of the operation, the final dose should be made even more dilute in order to avoid any residual motor block, which may sometimes occur after 1.0 per cent lidocaine has been used for a long period of time. Lidocaine, 0.8 per cent, is substituted at the final injection, and this same strength is used for postoperative analgesia, either as a continuous slow drip at the rate of three to ten drops per minute, or by intermittent injection.

Mid-thoracic Punctures. Mid-thoracic punctures in the range of T_5–T_9 are not as suitable as high thoracic punctures for operations on the lung alone; however, they supply excellent conditions for thoracoabdominal procedures in which both body cavities are opened. More concentrated solutions are required, however, for satisfactory abdominal relaxation, in which case 2 per cent lidocaine or 0.5 to 0.75 per cent bupivacaine is indicated. Midline punctures are technically difficult in this region owing to the steep overhang of the thoracic spines, and the paramedian approach to the epidural space should be used, as described in Chapter 6.

THORACOLUMBAR PUNCTURES. The lumbar or lower thoracic approach has much to recommend it in thoracoabdominal procedures when the main operative site is the abdomen, as in a total gastrectomy or a portacaval anastomosis. This site is technically simple, and more concentrated analgesic solutions can be used to obtain complete motor block up to T_2 without the risk of residual phrenic paralysis remaining at the end of operation.

Epidural puncture is carried out with the patient in the lateral position and the operative side downward. A fairly high level is chosen for puncture, somewhere between T_{10} and L_2 so as to initiate blockade reasonably close to the thoracic area. The loss-of-resistance test is employed in the usual way (see Chapter 6), and a relatively large dose of analgesic solution is injected. If the operation site is entirely within the thorax, weak analgesic solutions may be used (0.8 to 1.0 per cent lidocaine with 1/200,000 epinephrine), but complete muscular flaccidity is required if the abdomen is to be opened, and then stronger solutions (e.g., 1.5 to 2.0 per cent lidocaine) are needed. Sufficient volume is injected to carry the block up to the first or second thoracic segment. As in the previous method for high puncture, the patient is kept with the operative side downward for as long as convenient in order to establish the block effectively, and the table is tilted 10 degrees head-down to encourage the solution to flow in a cephalad direction. Blockade is maintained in the usual way, and toward the end of operation the final injection is made with the same dilute analgesic solution that will be used postoperatively for pain relief (0.5 to 0.8 per cent lidocaine).

Although sensory fibers from the central portion of the diaphragm are not blocked by this technique, respiration is perfectly easy to control, even when the central part of the diaphragm is cut or stimulated. The reader is referred to Chapter 10 in which an hypothesis is outlined to account for this type of phrenic reflex suppression.

INDICATIONS FOR EPIDURAL ANALGESIA IN THORACIC SURGERY

Chest Wall

Extensive operations on the chest wall, such as radical amputation of the breast with combined internal mammary dissection, are very well tolerated under epidural block, and bleeding is minimal. Spontaneous respiration can be allowed if the chest wall is left intact, but intubation and controlled respiration must be used if the rib cage is opened.

Thoracoplasty

With changed methods of treatment, this operation for cavitational pulmonary disease is seldom performed. Blood loss, which is considerable under general anesthesia and relaxants, is minimal with good paravertebral block and local infiltration, and this remains a first choice of technique for the operation.

However, a revision thoracoplasty with new rib formation may present great technical difficulties for effective paravertebral injections, and then there is a place for epidural blockade by the high thoracic approach.

Intrathoracic

Under segmental epidural blockade, patients with simple thoracotomy wounds are capable of pain-free ambulation almost immediately after returning to the recovery room. For example, patients with open lung biopsies closed without an air leak and not requiring drainage may be allowed to walk under escort within an hour or so of operation. However, major resections are always tethered by a pleural drain, and in these cases early postoperative breathing exercises must be carried out with the patients confined to bed.

Thymectomy

Thymectomy for myasthenia gravis is managed most effectively by cervicothoracic epidural blockade. The operation is performed without muscle relaxants or powerful inhalational agents, and the patients awaken pain-free with optimal respiratory capabilities. Bedside tests of anticholinesterase requirements and ventilatory function can then be performed at intervals, to decide whether mechanically supported respiration is indicated, or whether there is sufficient muscular power to permit spontaneous respiration with safety.

Lung Resections

There are no special problems with epidural analgesia for these operations if general principles of good thoracic anesthesia are followed. The usual care in controlling tracheobronchial secretions is required, and endobronchial intubation is carried out if indicated by the presence of bronchopleural fistulas or loculated pus in diseased areas.

The tranquillity of the tracheobronchial tree produced by epidural analgesia has already been mentioned in Chapter 10. The following case of pneumonectomy illustrates how this is helpful in practice.

Powerfully built man, aged 60 years, with carcinoma of the lung; slight amount of sputum. One week before operation bronchoscopy was performed with great difficulty. Full topical analgesia of the larynx was attempted by using 4 per cent lidocaine. Krause's forceps were applied to both pyriform fossae, and two transtracheal injections of 2.5 ml each were followed by a laryngeal spray under direct vision. Thiopental, 500 mg, was given intravenously, and bronchoscopy was attempted, but persistent laryngospasm and bronchospasm prevented passage of the bronchoscope. Intermittent doses of succinylcholine were only partially effective. Finally, the patient was intubated under succinylcholine, deep ether anesthesia was induced and a direct spray of 4 per cent lidocaine was blown down the tube. After this blunderbuss assault, bronchoscopy was finally accomplished.

On the day of operation for left pneumonectomy, the same premedication was given as for previous bronchoscopy. Epidural analgesia was induced at T_{12}–L_1 and carried up to T_1, using 27 ml of 1.4 per cent plain lidocaine. Two doses of transtracheal 4 per cent lidocaine (2 ml each) were given, but the larynx was not sprayed nor were the pyriform fossae swabbed, and no muscle relaxant was used. On this occasion only 300 mg of thiopental was sufficient for an easy tranquil intubation. Subsequent tracheobronchial toilet with a suction catheter did not cause any reaction.

Thus, the tracheobronchial tree becomes much less irritable after thoracic epidural blockade, and less topical analgesia and general anesthesia are required to suppress a comparable stimulus. Part of this effect may be due to systemic absorption of local anesthetic from the epidural space, with subsequent action on involuntary muscle (Bromage and Robson, 1961; Steinhaus and Gaskin, 1963; Abou-Madi et al., 1977). However, the quantities of local anesthetic used in segmental thoracic blocks are too small to generate more than trivial blood concentrations that are below the level necessary to suppress tracheobronchial reflexes.

CARDIOVASCULAR SURGERY

Epidural analgesia for cardiac surgery has not been adequately evaluated. In the past, personal experience was limited to simple valve splitting operations for which a combination of continuous thoracic epidural block with light general anesthesia and IPPV was quite satisfactory. High epidural analgesia was also used in major vascular surgery under hypothermia, as there is evidence that total sympathetic blockade protects the myocardium against ventricular fibrillation. Induction of hypothermia itself is simplified by epidural blockade when surface cooling methods are used, since sympathetic paralysis prevents reactive vasoconstriction in the skin, and the body temperature falls rapidly (Stolar and Wynands, 1963). In operations on the thoracic aorta, epidural block was used to provide a combination of hypotension and hypothermia. The induced hypotension protected the cranium against sudden rises of pressure when the aorta was clamped, and hypothermia afforded some protection to the liver and the kidneys against ischemic anoxia when their blood supply was suddenly cut off by high aortic clamping.

Operations on the lower aorta, such as aortofemoral grafts, were commonly performed under lumbar epidural blockade because clinical impressions suggested that surgical results were more favorable after regional blockade than after general anesthesia. At McGill, Cousins and Wright (1971) confirmed these impressions by using electromagnetic flowmeters in human subjects to demonstrate the marked rise of graft blood flow that accompanies epidural blockade.

Today, epidural analgesia is precluded during major cardiovascular surgery because intraoperative heparinization is used almost routinely. Spinal bleeding and epidural hematoma formation may occur when an epidural catheter is used in the presence of full heparinization, and the advantages of epidural analgesia are outweighed by the rare but grave risk of spinal cord compression, as discussed in Chapter 14. However, epidural blockade may be used with advantage in the postoperative period, after the effects of heparinization have been reversed by protamine. Three major indications for postoperative epidural analgesia exist in cardiovascular surgery:

1. To promote blood flow in grafted vessels.
2. To relieve abdominal and thoracic pain.
3. To correct postoperative hypertension.

The first two have already been mentioned.

MANAGEMENT OF POSTOPERATIVE HYPERTENSION

Postoperative hypertension occurs very frequently after major vascular surgery and after about 50 per cent of cases of coronary revascularization (Estafanous et al., 1973; Gal and Cooperman, 1975; Hoar et al., 1976). The precise cause is unknown, and in many cases hypertension appears to be independent of common precipitating factors, such as pain, shivering, blood gas disturbances or a full bladder. Nevertheless, the clinical pattern has some features in common with the fulminating hypertension seen during bladder distension in quadriplegic patients with high cord lesions (Guttman and Whitteridge, 1947). In both situations there is some failure of depressor vascular reflexes, and the arterial pressure is set at an abnormally high level. Clearly, this derangement is undesirable. Vascular suture lines may rupture under the strain of dangerously high intraluminal pressures, and the left heart is subjected to heavy loads that may lead to subendocardial ischemia (see Chapter 10).

Since the cause of acute postoperative hypertension is unknown, treatment is symptomatic, with vasodilator therapy to reduce peripheral vascular resistance. Sodium nitroprusside is a favored agent because it is easy to administer and certain in its effects. However, sodium nitroprusside has a number of disadvantages, which are outlined in Chapter 10, and interest has returned to epidural analgesia as an alternative method for protecting the heart and major vessels from dangerously high levels of blood pressure.

Case History

Figure 11–18 illustrates the use of epidural blockade to reduce reactive hypertension in a 76-year-old man recovering from repair of a ruptured aortic graft. This patient had been moribund from hemorrhage prior to repair of his ruptured graft, and he had survived unrecordably low levels of blood pressure without apparent harm. However, reactive hypertension in the early postoperative period gave rise to anxiety that he would rerupture his graft, and hypotension was induced with sodium nitroprusside at a rate of about 250 μg per minute. The blood pressure began to rise again after 3¼ hours, so the nitroprusside infusion was stopped and a thoracic epidural block established instead, using 7 ml of 0.25 per cent bupivacaine. The patient immediately became pain-free; the blood pressure fell to 75/40 mmHg and then rose to more acceptable levels after two small doses of mephentermine (3 mg) given intravenously. The patient made a good recovery.

Hoar and his associates (1976) studied the hemodynamic effects of epidural blockade in reactive hypertension after surgery for myocardial

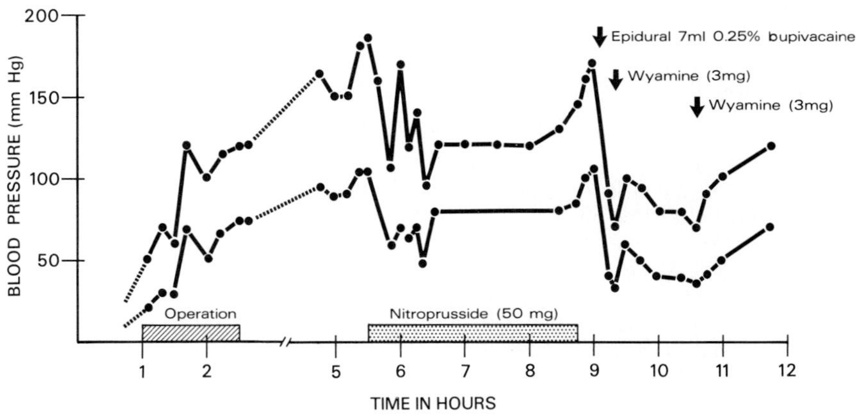

Figure 11–18. Reactive hypertension after emergency aortic surgery, controlled by vasodilator therapy. Induction of thoracic epidural blockade (T_7–T_8) following onset of tachyphylaxis to IV sodium nitroprusside (see text).

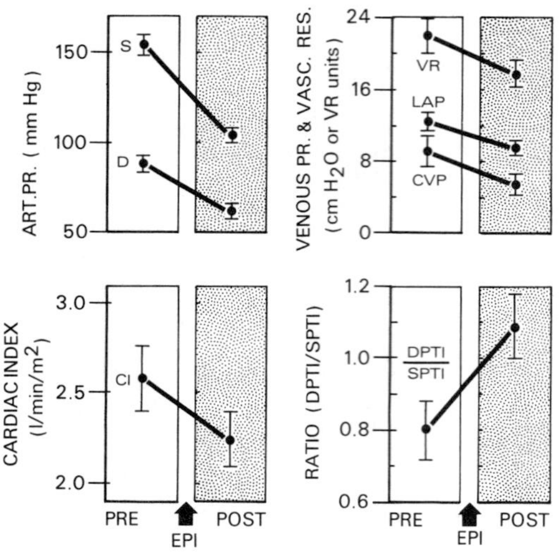

Figure 11–19. Cardiovascular responses to thoracic epidural analgesia for reactive hypertension after myocardial revascularization. Fall of systemic vascular resistance is accompanied by marked rise of ratio of diastolic to systolic pressure-time index (DPTI/SPTI)./(Data from Hoar et al., 1976.)

revascularization. They confirmed that epidural blockade not only relieved postoperative pain and controlled the systemic blood pressure but also improved indices of myocardial blood supply, as shown in Figure 11–19. It can be seen that the ratio of myocardial blood supply to myocardial demands is significantly improved in terms of the ratio of diastolic to systolic pressure-time indices, or DPTI/SPTI (see page 376, Chapter 10).

While intravenous vasodilator therapy remains a simple method for short-term management of postoperative hypertension, continuous epidural blockade is effective over longer periods, and it has the unique advantage of combining blood pressure control and outstanding control of pain without the respiratory depressant effects of systemic narcotics.

ILLUSTRATIVE CASE HISTORIES

The following case summaries give examples of the use of high epidural blockade for the operative and postoperative management of intrathoracic surgery.

Case No. TE 21

Male, aged 45 years, with bullous emphysema of the lingula, causing space-occupying effects in the left pleural space. He had undergone two previous lobar resections for bronchiectasis and removal of expanding giant bulli. Four years before, pulmonary angiograms and ^{133}*xenon studies had shown poor perfusion and ventilation in both lower lung zones, and a right lower and middle lobectomy had been performed under light general anesthesia combined with segmental epidural blockade induced at the second thoracic interspace. An elective preoperative tracheostomy had been proposed by the respiratory physicians, but this was deferred at the request of the anesthesiologist, on the grounds that ventilatory support would probably prove to be unnecessary with the anesthetic technique used. The patient awoke at the end of this first operation pain-free, with a large tidal volume and a minute volume of 11.6 liters per minute. Segmental epidural analgesia was continued for eight hours in the recovery room, and the patient was discharged to his ward without needing any artificial ventilatory support in the postoperative period.*

A second operation was necessary eight months after the first, this time for excision of the left lower lobe. The same basic technique was used, but on this occasion epidural blockade was induced in the lumbar region instead of in the upper thoracic segments. Postoperatively, analgesia did not prove to be effective in the upper thorax. Morphine was needed for control of pain, and the patient required mechanical ventilation until the fourteenth postoperative hour.

On the third occasion, four years after the first resection, remaining lung tissue comprised only the right and left upper lobes, the latter being compressed by bullous expansion of the lingula. The vital capacity was 1.93 liters instead of a predicted 4.66 liters, and the mid-expiratory flow rate was 0.18 liters per second instead of a predicted value of 1.24 liters per second. There was a mild degree of polycythemia, with a hemoglobin of 16.6 g and a hematocrit of 57 per cent. The patient begged for an upper thoracic segmental epidural as at the first operation, insisting that he did not want to undergo the operation without it.

Epidural puncture was performed between the seventh cervical and the first thoracic spines in the sitting position. The hanging-drop sign was positive but not very authoritative, probably due to loss of intrapleural negative pressure. Fifteen ml of 1.2 per cent lidocaine with 1/200,000 epinephrine was injected through the needle with the patient in the sitting position, followed by a further 5 ml through the catheter with the patient lying on his left side. Analgesia spread from C_8 to T_{10} in 10 minutes.

Intubation was performed with a transtracheal injection of 3 ml of 4 per cent lidocaine and increments of thiopental to a total of 300 mg. Anesthesia was maintained with oxygen and halothane in concentrations between 0.5 to 1.0 per cent, and respiration was controlled by hand. Succinylcholine, 40 mg, was given for muscle quiescence during electrocautery of the chest wall. Nitrous oxide was not used, in order to avoid partial pressure effects and further expansion of bulli.

The operation of lingula bronchial divorcement lasted two hours. The patient was allowed to awaken on the table before the skin incision was fully closed, in order to confirm the efficiency of spontaneous respiration. The endotracheal tube was removed after the dressing was in place, and the patient was nursed with intermittent epidural injections of 1 per cent lidocaine and 1/200,000 epinephrine in the recovery room for a period of 24 hours. Spontaneous respiration and coughing were adequate to maintain satisfactory arterial gas tensions, and no mechanical ventilatory support was required at any time in the postoperative period.

Comment: This case illustrates two points:

1. Unnecessary and invasive respiratory support can be avoided if a trial of postoperative deafferentation and spontaneous respiration seems reasonably appropriate, and if close postoperative monitoring provides a realistic basis for rapid alterations of policy should respiratory support become necessary.

2. The relative inefficiency of lumbar epidural block for relieving thoracic pain can be seen by the course of events after the second operation, when artificial ventilatory support became urgent and unavoidable in the absence of effective deafferentation. By contrast, no artificial respiratory support was needed after the third resection, although the patient's pulmonary tissue was further depleted to an extreme degree.

Case No. TE 25

Woman of 43 years with bullous emphysema of right lower and middle lobes for right lower lobectomy and middle lobe divorcement. Preoperative VC = 1.7 liters (predicted VC = 2.97 liters). Mid-expiratory flow rate = 0.22 liters per second (predicted = 3.07 liters per second).

A trial of spontaneous postoperative respiration was agreed upon, and *operation was performed under a combination of thoracic epidural block and light endotracheal anesthesia. Twenty ml of 1.2 per cent lidocaine (240 mg) with 1/200,000 epinephrine was injected at the first thoracic interspace, and this produced bilateral analgesia of 16 segments from C_7 to L_2 inclusive. At the end of operation, spontaneous respiration was allowed to return as soon as the chest wall was made gastight, and the patient was awakened and extubated before the skin incision was completely closed. Coughing and deep breathing exercises were started on the operating table. No respiratory assistance was required. However, the vital capacity fell to between 450 and 500 ml when epidural analgesia was allowed to wear off, but it returned to 1000 to 1200 ml when the block was reinstated; blockade was therefore continued intermittently for the first 24 hours after operation, and at the end of this time the block was terminated. The patient was then able to maintain adequate ventilation and vital capacity, with an arterial pO_2 of 82 mmHg breathing room air. She was discharged to her home in excellent condition on the tenth postoperative day.*

Comment: Again, this case illustrates the value of postoperative deafferentation in protecting respiratory function against reflex inhibition from pain, while sparing the patient from the dangers and discomfort of prolonged intubation and artificial ventilation.

The next three cases illustrate the use of epidural blockade as an adjuvant to both induced hypothermia and moderate arterial hypotension, as well as restoration of postoperative respiratory function.

Case No. LE 730

Man of 45 years in oligemic shock from repeated massive hematemeses, for emergency gastrectomy. Pale, sweating, pulse rate 115/minute, B.P. 78/?, rectal temperature 100.2°F (37.9°C). Blood was replaced rapidly. A lumbar epidural block was induced and its upper level carried to T_4 under light thiopental and nitrous oxide sleep. The legs were exposed. Rectal temperature fell to 96.2°F (35.6°C) during operation. The patient awoke immediately after operation but did not shiver or complain of cold. Breathing exercises were started immediately. Uneventful recovery.

Case No. LE 1562

Man of 54 years with Laennec's cirrhosis and esophageal varices. Diabetic, obese, weight 226 lbs; for Crile's operation via left thoracotomy.

Epidural block induced with 20 ml plain 1.75 per cent lidocaine at the second lumbar interspace. Analgesia rose to T_1. Transtracheal topical analgesia and light endotracheal nitrous oxide anesthesia with controlled ventilation. Surface cooling applied for 70 minutes. The rectal temperature fell to 33°C and then drifted down to 30.5°C. The blood pressure was allowed to run at a level of 95 to 100 mmHg systolic throughout the operation which lasted 3½ hours. Bleeding was minimal. Postoperative analgesia was maintained for eight hours. Recovery uneventful.

Case No. LE 1594

Man of 46 years for excision of coarctation of aorta. Slight exertional dyspnea. Cardiomegaly and marked vascular erosion of ribs. Blood pressure 160/90, weight 184 lbs.

Epidural block at eleventh thoracic interspace with 30 ml of 1 per cent plain lidocaine gave analgesia to T_1. Ventilation was maintained mechanically under light thiopental and nitrous oxide anesthesia. Surface cooling with a cooling blanket reduced the rectal temperature to 32°C, and the systolic blood pressure was allowed to run at 80 mmHg until the aorta was clamped, when the pressure rose to 140/70 mmHg. The operation was completed in five hours, with a blood loss of 2.2 liters. Epidural blockade was maintained intermittently for 12 hours to ensure optimal respiratory function, and the patient recovered uneventfully.

These last two cases illustrate the ease with which controlled hypotension and surface cooling can be applied in the presence of complete sympathetic paralysis from a high level of epidural analgesia.

Pheochromocytoma

Although pheochromocytomas are rare tumors, their management with epidural blockade illustrates the principles of imposed vascular control more vividly than many other less dramatic situations. This section will outline a technique of total epidural blockade that has proved satisfactory in eight cases of pheochromocytoma at the Royal Victoria Hospital, Montreal.

Twenty-five years ago, before alpha and beta adrenergic blocking agents were used routinely in the management of these patients, spinal anesthesia was considered dangerous because of the likelihood of hypotensive collapse arising from sympathetic blockade (Espersen and Dahl-Iversen, 1946; Apgar and Papper, 1951; Thompson and Arrowood, 1954). However, it has seemed to me that one of the most essential tasks of anesthetic management in pheochromocytoma is to ensure not only survival of the patient but also success of a demanding operation. The anesthetic should not obscure diagnostic peaks of blood pressure during the search for the primary tumor or for multiple tumors after the first one has been removed, nor should it permit irrelevant fluctuations of blood pressure arising from other causes that might mislead the surgeon during his difficult search.

The logical approach to this problem seemed to include three principal aims:

1. Retention of partial function in vascular muscle receptors so that they are capable of a modified response to challenge from vasoactive agents. This implies moderate use of adrenergic blocking agents in amounts sufficient to blunt excessive peaks of pressor and chronotropic stimulation and yet allow enough reactivity to permit a diagnostic hypertensive episode in response to handling of a vasoactive tumor.

2. Provision of a stable baseline of blood pressure under all circumstances *except* during handling of a vasoactive tumor.

3. Augmentation of intravascular volume to compensate for vasodilation caused by total sympathetic blockade.

These aims can be satisfied by careful use of high epidural blockade combined with light general anesthesia, and judicious administration of alpha blocking agents with occasional beta blocking agents when indicated. This approach was first used in 1958 for removal of a highly active 26-g tumor in an eight-year-old boy (Bromage and Millar, 1958). Since then a further seven cases have been anesthetized successfully in this way at the Royal Victoria Hospital in Montreal. Preoperative augmentation of blood and red cell mass by phenoxybenzamine treatment and packed cell transfusion has added greatly to the safety and smoothness of the technique (Crout and Brown, 1969). The technique has since been used in other centers, and it has been described by Cousins and Rubin (1973).

The following case report illustrates the general principles:

Case No. P.7

Woman of 32 years. Weight 146 lbs. Height 62 inches. Pheochromocytoma diagnosed ten years previously as the underlying cause of an "eclamptic" episode and stillbirth, but she had refused surgery. Since then she had given birth to three live children, two by vaginal delivery and one by cesarean section. Seven months before admission she had suffered a moderately large anteroseptal myocardial infarct. Blood pressure ranged between 140/80 and 180/100 mmHg. She was not in cardiac failure and she was able to do her housework.

Arteriography showed a highly vascular tumor 5 cm in diameter in the left adrenal and a similar lesion 2 cm in diameter in the right adrenal. Serum catecholamines were slightly raised, norepinephrine was 1.5 μg per L (normal range = 0 to 1.0), epinephrine 0.5 μg per L (normal range = 0 to 0.5).

The blood volume was contracted about 20 per cent below the predicted level, and the hematocrit was 44 per cent. Preoperative expansion of blood volume was accomplished by phenoxybenzamine treatment for a few days, together with a packed cell transfusion of 300 ml just prior to operation.

Epidural puncture was performed at the seventh thoracic interspace, and 12 ml of 1.73 per cent lidocaine-CO_2 *with epinephrine 1/200,000 produced blockade from* T_1–L_3. *Light thiopental and nitrous oxide anesthesia was maintained after gentle intubation with the assistance of curare and topical anesthesia to the trachea. The blood pressure chart is shown in Figure 11–20.*

A large, highly vasoactive tumor on the left side caused rapid swings of arterial pressure and pulse during surgical handling, and these were controlled with increments of phentolamine and very small amounts of propranolol. After removal of the first tumor, hypotension was corrected with a dilute norepinephrine infusion of 1 μg per ml, supplemented with 8 to 12 mg increments of methamphetamine.

The total amounts of supportive adrenergic blocking and stimulating drugs throughout the three-hour operation were phentolamine 8 mg, propranolol 0.5 mg, norepinephrine 400 μg, methamphetamine 56 mg.

The patient was awake and pain-free at the end of operation, and postoperative epidural analgesia was continued for a further six hours. Recovery was uneventful.

Comment: The very small amounts of alpha and beta blocking drugs could probably have been increased with advantage in this case.

Morbid Obesity

Grossly obese patients provide an excellent model for comparing epidural analgesia with orthodox methods of general anesthesia and muscle relaxants. All the problems associated with postoperative respiration and early movements are magnified to a point of caricature, and it is here that the advantages of epidural anesthesia become strikingly obvious.

The problems of anesthesia for fat patients have been surveyed in a number of excellent articles, and the reader is referred to these reviews for detailed discussion (Catenacci et al., 1961; Noble, 1962; Fox, 1975; Fisher et al., 1975). Here the difficulties will be presented in outline form only, and a very simple technique for management of the mordibly obese will be given in greater detail.

The problem

Obesity is considered to exist when body weight corrected for age and sex exceeds the statistically ideal weight by more than 10 per cent. This is rather a strict definition, and it includes a large proportion of the population in countries where eating is a pastime rather than a necessity. From a technical point of view, anesthesia and postoperative management present special difficulties when obesity has progressed to a more florid stage and when body

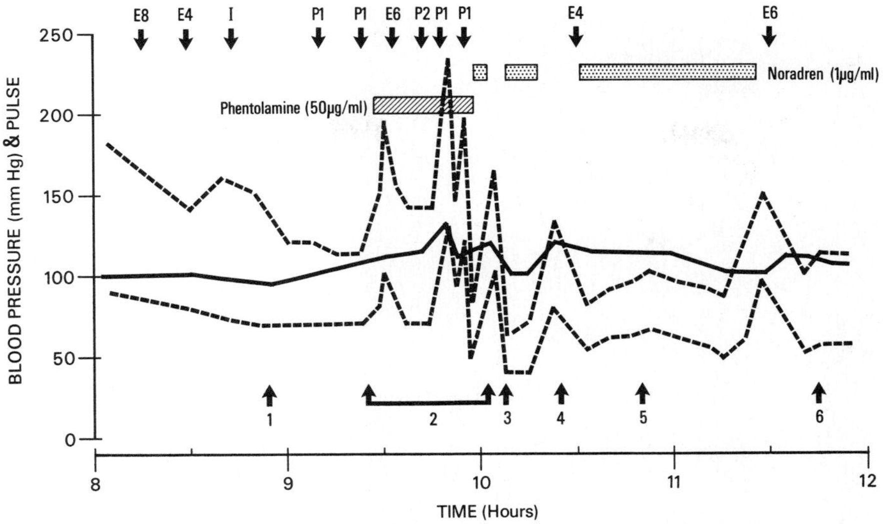

Figure 11–20. Epidural analgesia for excision of bilateral pheochromocytoma in woman of 32 years. Segmental epidural blockade from T_1–L_3 with light general anesthesia and IPPV. Preoperative preparation with phenoxybenzamine and packed red cell transfusion.

Top line: E8, E4, E4, E6 = Epidural increments in ml of 1.73 per cent lidocaine–CO_2 + 1/200,000 epinephrine at seventh thoracic interspace.

I = Induction of general anesthesia. Thiopentone 150 mg, curare 12 mg, 4 per cent topical lidocaine to larynx and trachea, nitrous oxide 4 L/min, O_2 3 L/min.

P1, P2 = Propranolol 0.1 mg or 0.2 mg IV.

Bottom line:

1 = Incision
2 = Mobilization of left tumor
3 = Excision of left tumor
4 = Exploration and mobilization of right tumor
5 = Excision of right tumor
6 = Extubation. Patient awake, talking and deep breathing.

Pulse (——); blood pressure (------).

weight exceeds the ideal by more than 50 per cent (Fig. 11–21). In referral centers where intestinal bypass operations are performed, it is commonplace to encounter patients who are more than twice their ideal weight and in the range of 130 to 210 kg. These patients present a challenge that includes the following handicaps:

Interoperative

1. Difficulties of physical bulk. Difficult veins and arteries for fluid and monitoring ports, short neck and difficult laryngoscopy.

2. Large fat reservoirs for absorption and persistence of fat-soluble depressant drugs.

3. Impaired respiratory function, with reduction of ERV and FRC (Holley et al., 1967), and FRC values below the closing volume (Craig et al., 1971). The resulting mismatch of ventilation-to-perfusion leads to lowered arterial oxygen tensions, particularly in the supine position, and large tidal volumes are required. Chest wall and total compliance are markedly reduced, and the work of breathing is increased (Naimark and Cherniack, 1960; Waltemath and Bergman, 1974).

4. Brittle fluid balance due to relatively small lean body mass in proportion to the large volume of anhydrous fat.

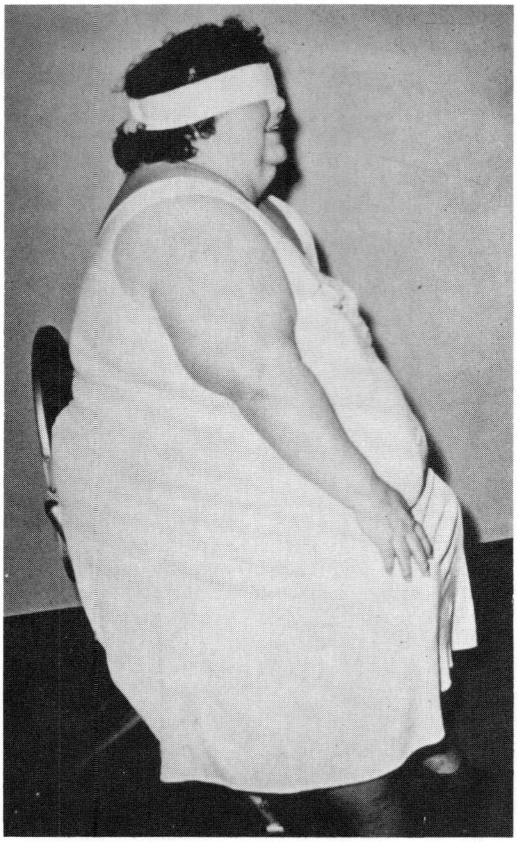

Figure 11–21. Morbid obesity and hypoventilation syndrome in woman of 53 years, weight 154.5 kilograms. Insulinoma excised under epidural analgesia and light general anesthesia. (From Noble, A. B.: The problem of obesity in anaesthesia for abdominal surgery. Canad. Anaesth. Soc. J. 9:1, 1962.)

Postoperative. Spontaneous respiration is usually out of the question after orthodox anesthetic techniques with muscle relaxants, due to the respiratory depressant effects of reduced compliance, large doses of muscle relaxants and the inhibitory effects of abdominal pain. Prolonged intubation with artificial respiration is frequently required after general anesthesia (Edelist, 1968). Paul et al. (1976) have shown that the left ventricular filling pressure rises markedly when grossly obese patients are placed in the supine position; in some cases the pressure rises to 20 cmH_2O, a level commonly associated with pulmonary congestion. Therefore it is necessary to nurse these patients in a sitting or semirecumbent posture rather than in the supine position. Obese patients are at high risk for deep vein thrombosis, and prophylactic measures should be taken to prevent thromboembolism, either in the form of minidose heparin prophylaxis (Kakkar et al., 1975) or by intermittent calf compression (Roberts and Cotton, 1974).

THE SOLUTION

The complexity and intensive care costs of using orthodox anesthetic techniques in these cases are considerable and unwarranted. The patient is subjected to the risks and discomfort of prolonged postoperative ventilation, intensive nursing care is required over several days and numerous personnel are needed to move these enormously heavy patients.

Singularly little interest has been shown in evolving techniques to circumvent these difficulties. Yet the approach can be extremely simple, turning what used to be an endurance test for all concerned into a pleasing and satisfactory experience. The secret lies in developing a philosophical approach of deafferentation instead of the traditional deefferenting technique using muscle relaxants. Once this basic attitude is cultivated, everything falls into place and the central problems are resolved. A certain amount of attention to detail is required, but no more than with any other technique under comparably difficult circumstances. We have had fairly extensive experience with the short-circuit operation for intractable obesity at the Royal Victoria Hospital, Montreal, in which a combination of continuous epidural blockade and light endotracheal anesthesia was used (Fox, 1975; Bromage and Fox, 1976).

ANESTHETIC TECHNIQUE IN THE MORBIDLY OBESE

The aim is to provide first-class operating conditions, followed by prompt awakening with immediate deep breathing and leg exercises. Postoperative respiration should be spontaneous and full, and augmented by regular deep breathing exercises.

Preoperative Visit. This is crucial to good management and to obtaining active cooperation from the patient at all stages. The basic physiological problems should be explained to the patient in simple terms, and his active help should be sought in carrying out the appropriate anesthetic strategy. A skilled interpreter should be used in the event of language difficulties. Simple respiratory measurements such as vital capacity and peak expiratory flow rate should be made and recorded as norms against which postoperative performance can be pitted. Preoperative blood gas measurements are also helpful but not essential. No premedicant sedatives or antisialagogic drugs of any sort are used; therefore, thorough psychological preparation is of paramount importance.

Anesthetic Management. An intravenous line is secured. The patient is asked to sit up, with the feet supported on a stool, and thoracic epidural blockade is induced at the sixth or seventh thoracic interspace using a paramedian approach and the hanging-drop technique. This step is usually much easier than it appears, provided the patient is comfortably placed and in the sitting position. Puncture in the lateral decubitus is technically difficult and should be avoided, as landmarks are distorted by sagging rolls of pendulous fat. Induction of blockade at lower spinal levels is acceptable but not ideal, as the subsequent analgesia will inevitably involve the lower lumbar and sacral segments, and then the patient may be incapable of performing effective leg exercises in the early postoperative period.

Epidural blockade is induced with a fast-acting and powerful agent, such as 1.73 per cent lidocaine-CO_2 with epinephrine, or 1 per cent etidocaine. Dosage is calculated on the basis of age to give a segmental block from T_4 to L_1 and is slightly less than in normal lean subjects. Volumes usually range from 4 ml in elderly subjects to 12 ml in the third decade. The patient is then placed supine with the head and shoulders slightly raised, and the segmental level of analgesia is observed by pin-prick over the next 10 minutes. Further increments of analgesic solution are given if necessary to extend blockade over the required segments. Vasopressors are not used prophylactically, but they are prepared and ready in case they are needed to maintain a systolic pressure over 90 mmHg. Mephentermine is a convenient initial vasopressor in doses of 3 to 6 mg, but a norepinephrine infusion of 1 μg per ml should also be prepared and held in readiness as a second line of defense in case it is needed.

No muscle relaxants are used for intubation or at any time throughout the operation. The nares are sprayed with 2 per cent cocaine if nasal intubation is planned. Amnesia is induced with diazepam in divided bolus doses of 5 mg to a total of 10 to 20 mg. A transtracheal injection of 3 ml of 4 per cent lidocaine provides topical anesthesia of the trachea and larynx, and this is followed by intravenous thiopental in sufficient amounts to relax the jaw (usually 200 to 350 mg). Oral or blind nasal intubation is then performed, a nasogastric tube is passed and anesthesia is continued with nitrous oxide and oxygen in equal proportions. Sufficient halothane or enflurane is added to maintain unconsciousness. Some anesthesiologists prefer nonvolatile adjuvants such as fentanyl (Lessing and de Kock, 1968), but halothane in minimal inspired concentrations of 0.25 to 0.5 per cent appears to cause no delay in awakening, provided the vaporizer is turned off as soon as the peritoneum is closed.

Moderate hyperventilation is applied manually until apnea is induced, and then the patient is ventilated mechanically with a tidal volume of 8 to 10 ml per kg, 10 to 12 times per minute. A dead space of 50 to 75 ml is added to avoid hypocapnia from the large minute volume. An arterial line is inserted for sampling blood gases and for monitoring blood pressure.

Patients are allowed to awaken as soon as the wound is closed, and if sufficiently active, they are extubated on the table before transfer to their beds. Deep breathing and leg exercises are started immediately. Patients are nursed in the semisitting position to avoid pulmonary congestion (Paul et al., 1976) and falls of FRC (Craig et al., 1971), and postoperative pain is controlled with intermittent injections of 0.5 per cent bupivacaine in sufficient volume to provide analgesia of the lower seven thoracic segments. Respiratory competence is monitored by vital capacity and peak expiratory flow rate measurements, and by arterial blood gas estimations. In the absence of complicating factors, these patients can usually be weaned from their epidural catheters and discharged from recovery room care on the second postoperative day.

With this deafferenting regimen, the patient is freed from the inhibitory effects of abdominal pain and residual depressant drugs, and he has strength enough to perform the essential tasks of deep breathing, coughing and limb exercises without special assistance. In addition, nursing duties are lightened as the patient can move himself about in bed and cooperate actively in his own care. There is one caveat: urinary retention occurs in about 30 per cent of cases, and since palpation of the bladder is impossible in these obese subjects, an indwelling catheter should be inserted while the patient is under anesthesia. Without this precaution, severe bladder distension and retention with overflow may occur.

Our series of patients had body weights that ranged from 125 to 193 kg. The following patient was not among the heaviest in this series, but he illustrates the relatively small quantities of drugs that are needed, even when the patient is unusually powerful and muscular. A summary of the anesthetic chart is shown in Figure 11–22.

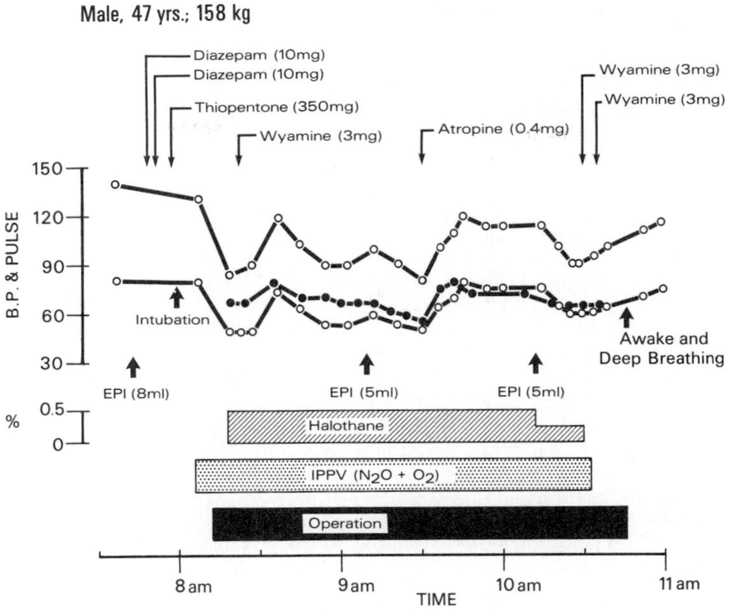

Figure 11–22. Intestinal bypass surgery for morbid obesity in male of 47 years, weight 158 kilograms (see text for explanation).

A 47-year-old bar "manager" and ex-professional wrestler presented for intestinal bypass surgery. He was 168 cm tall. His fighting weight had been steady at 80 kg until he suffered a low back injury. After several years of inactivity, his weight had risen to 158 kg, and he was short of breath and hypertensive, with a labile pressure of 140/180 to 170/95 mmHg.

The surgical and perioperative risks were fully explained to the patient. No premedicant drugs were given. Epidural puncture at the seventh thoracic interspace was very easy, and a bolus dose of 8 ml of 1.73 per cent lidocaine-CO_2 with 1/200,000 epinephrine was injected prior to inserting an epidural catheter. Analgesia extended from T_4–T_{12} inclusive in 8 minutes. In the meantime two doses of 10 mg diazepam IV produced moderate sedation. A transtracheal injection of 3 ml of 4 per cent lidocaine elicited a satisfactory cough. Thiopental, 350 mg, provided good relaxation of the jaw, and a tranquil oral intubation was performed without the aid of a muscle relaxant. Apnea was induced by moderate hyperventilation, and the patient was connected to a volume controlled ventilator with a tidal volume of 1200 ml with 50 ml of added dead space at a rate of 10 to 12 per minute. Anesthesia was maintained with equal parts of nitrous oxide and oxygen with halothane in a concentration of 0.25 to 0.5 per cent (see Fig. 11–22).

The patient awoke as the last stitches were completed and responded to commands. He was extubated on the table, and deep breathing exercises were started immediately. One hour later peak expiratory flow rate was 250 L per minute. For the next 20 hours postoperative pain was controlled by intermittent epidural injections of 0.5 per cent bupivacaine in volumes of 7 to 9 ml, and no narcotic analgesics were required during that time. He was discharged without complications on the eighth postoperative day.

REFERENCES

Abou-Madi, M., Keszler, H., and Yacoub, O.: A method for prevention of cardiovascular reactions to laryngoscopy and intubation. Canad. Anaesth. Soc. J. 22:316, 1975.

Abou-Madi, M. N., Keszler, H., and Yacoub, J. M.: Cardiovascular reactions to laryngoscopy and

tracheal intubation following small and large intravenous doses of lidocaine. Canad. Anaesth. Soc. J. *24*:12, 1977.
Ahlquist, R. A.: A study of adrenergic receptors. Amer. J. Physiol. *153*:586, 1948.
Aldrete, J. A.: Management of the postanesthetic patient. Clin. Trends Anesth. *3*:1, 1973.
Anscombe, A. R.: Pulmonary Complications in Abdominal Surgery. Chicago, Year Book Medical Publishers, 1957.
Apgar, V., and Papper, E. M.: Pheochromocytoma—Anesthetic management during surgical removal. Arch. Surg. *62*:634, 1951.
Beecher, H. K.: The measured effect of laparotomy on the respiration. J. Clin. Invest. *12*:639, 1933a.
Beecher, H. K.: Effect of laparotomy on lung volume: Demonstration of a new type of pulmonary collapse. J. Clin. Invest. *12*:651, 1933b.
Bendixen, H. H., Osgood, P. F., Hall, K. V., and Laver, M. B.: Dose-dependent differences in catecholamine action on heart and periphery. J. Pharmacol. Exp. Ther. *145*:299, 1964.
Bevan, D. R.: The sodium story: Effects of anaesthesia and surgery on intrarenal mechanisms concerned with sodium homeostasis. Proc. Roy. Soc. Med. *66*:1215, 1973.
Brandt, M., Kehlet, H., Binder, C., Hagen, C., and McNeilly, A. S.: Effect of epidural analgesia on the glycoregulatory endocrine response to surgery. Clin. Endocr. *5*:107, 1976.
Brattström, S.: Postoperative pulmonary ventilation with reference to postoperative pulmonary complications. Acta Chir. Scand. (Suppl.) *195*:69, 1954.
Brigden, W., Howarth, S., and Sharpey-Schafer, E. P.: Postural changes in the peripheral blood flow of normal subjects with observations on vaso-vagal fainting reactions as a result of tilting, the lordotic posture, pregnancy and spinal anaesthesia. Clin. Sci. *9*:79, 1950.
Bromage, P. R.: Vascular hypotension in 107 cases of epidural analgesia. Anaesthesia *6*:26, 1951.
Bromage, P. R.: Comparison of vasoactive drugs in man. Brit. Med. J. *2*:72, 1952.
Bromage, P. R.: Spirometry in assessment of analgesia after abdominal surgery. Brit. Med. J. *2*:589, 1955.
Bromage, P. R.: Total respiratory compliance in anaesthetised subjects and modifications produced by noxious stimuli. Clin. Sci. *17*:217, 1958a.
Bromage, P. R.: The phrenic reflex in epidural analgesia. Canad. Anaesth. Soc. J. *5*:29, 1958b.
Bromage, P. R.: Vasopressors. Canad. Anaesth. Soc. J. *7*:310, 1960.
Bromage, P. R.: Spread of analgesic solutions in the epidural space and their site of action: A statistical study. Brit. J. Anaesth. *34*:1961, 1962.
Bromage, P. R.: A comparison of the hydrochloride and carbon dioxide salts of lidocaine and prilocaine in epidural analgesia. Acta Anaesth. Scand. Suppl. *16*:55, 1965.
Bromage, P. R.: Extradural analgesia for pain relief. Brit. J. Anaesth. *39*:721, 1967.
Bromage, P. R.: A comparison of bupivacaine and tetracaine in epidural analgesia for surgery. Canad. Anaesth. Soc. J. *16*:37, 1969a.
Bromage, P. R.: Ageing and epidural dose requirements. Brit. J. Anaesth. *41*:1016, 1969b.
Bromage, P. R., and Burfoot, M. F.: Quality of epidural blockade. II. Influence of physicochemical factors; hyaluronidase and potassium. Brit. J. Anaesth. *38*:857, 1966.
Bromage, P. R., and Millar, R. A.: Epidural blockade and circulating catecholamine levels in a child with phaeochromocytoma. Canad. Anaesth. Soc. J. *5*:282, 1958.
Bromage, P. R., and Robson, J. G.: Concentrations of lignocaine in the blood after intravenous, intramuscular, epidural, and endotracheal administration. Anaesthesia *16*:461, 1961.
Bromage, P. R., and Fox, G. S.: Obesity: Its relation to anaesthesia. Anaesthesia *31*:557, 1976.
Bromage, P. R., Burfoot, M. F., Crowell, D. E., and Truant, A. P.: Quality of epidural blockade. III. Carbonated local anaesthetic solutions. Brit. J. Anaesth. *39*:197, 1967.
Bromage, P. R., Shibata, H. R., and Willoughby, H. W.: Influence of prolonged epidural blockade on blood sugar and cortisol responses to operations upon the upper part of abdomen and the thorax. Surg. Gynecol. Obstet. *132*:1051, 1971.
Bromage, P. R., O'Beirn, P., and Dunford, L. A.: Etidocaine: A clinical evaluation for regional analgesia in surgery. Canad. Anaesth. Soc. J. *21*:523, 1974.
Brown, P. R., Arthurs, G. J., and Glashan, R. W.: Epidural analgesia in the treatment of bladder carcinoma. Anaesthesia *29*:422, 1974.
Buckley, J. J., Van Bergen, F. H., Dobkin, A. B., Brown, E. B., and Miller, F. A.: Postanesthetic hypotension following cyclopropane; its relationship to hypercapnia. Anesthesiology *14*:226, 1953.
Case, R. B., Berglund, E., and Sarnoff, S. J.: Ventricular function. VII. Changes in coronary resistance and ventricular function resulting from acutely induced anemia and the effect thereon of coronary stenosis. Amer. J. Med. *18*:397, 1955.
Catenacci, A. J., Anderson, J. D., and Boersma, D.: Anesthetic hazards of obesity. J.A.M.A. *175*:657, 1961.
Churchill, E. D., and McNeil, D.: The reduction of vital capacity following operations. Surg. Gynecol. Obstet. *44*:483, 1927.

Clarke, R. S. J.: The hyperglycaemic response to different types of surgery and anaesthesia. Brit. J. Anaesth. *42*:45, 1970.

Cleland, J. G. P.: Continuous peridural and caudal analgesia in surgery and early ambulation. Northwest. Med. J. *48*:26, 1949.

Cohen, G., Holland, B., Sha, J., and Goldenberg, M.: Plasma concentrations of epinephrine and norepinephrine during intravenous infusions in man. J. Clin. Invest. *38*:1935, 1959.

Cousins, M. J., and Rubin, R. B.: The intraoperative management of phaeochromocytoma with total epidural sympathetic blockade. Brit. J. Anaesth. *46*:78, 1973.

Cousins, M. J., and Wright, C. J.: Graft, muscle, skin blood flow after epidural block in vascular surgical procedures. Surg. Gynecol. Obstet. *133*:59, 1971.

Craig, D. B., Wahba, W. M., Don, H. F., Couture, J. G., and Becklake, M. R.: "Closing volume" and its relationship to gas exchange in seated and supine positions. J. Appl. Physiol. *31*:717, 1971.

Crawford, O. B.: Peridural anesthesia for thoracic surgery. N. Y. State J. Med. *52*:2637, 1952.

Crawford, O. B.: The technic of continuous peridural anesthesia for thoracic surgery. Anesthesiology *14*:317, 1953.

Crawford, O. B., Ottosen, P., Buckingham, W. W., and Brasher, C. A.: Peridural anesthesia in thoracic surgery. A review of 677 cases. Anesthesiology *12*:73, 1951.

Crout, J. R., and Brown, B. R.: Anesthetic management of pheochromocytoma: The value of phenoxybenzamine and methoxyflurane. Anesthesiology *30*:29, 1969.

Cullingford, D. W. J.: The blood sugar response to anaesthesia and surgery in Southern Indians. Brit. J. Anaesth. *38*:463, 1966.

Dahlström, A. D., and Zetterstrom, B. E. M.: Noradrenaline stores in nerve terminals of the spleen: Changes during hemorrhagic shock. Science *147*:1583, 1965.

Dalen, J. E., Evans, G. L., Banas, J. S., Brooks, H. L., Paraskos, J. A., and Dexter, L.: The hemodynamic and respiratory effects of diazepam (Valium). Anesthesiology *30*:259, 1969.

Dalrymple, D. G., Parbrook, G. D., and Steel, D. F.: Factors predisposing to postoperative pain and pulmonary complications. A study of female patients undergoing elective cholecystectomy. Brit. J. Anaesth. *45*:589, 1973.

Davis, J. O., and Freeman, R. H.: Mechanisms regulating renin release. Physiol. Rev. *56*:1, 1976.

Dawkins, C. J. M., and Steel, G. C.: Thoracic extradural (epidural) block for upper abdominal surgery. Anaesthesia *26*:41, 1971.

de Jong, R. H., and Heavner, J. E.: Diazepam prevents and aborts lidocaine convulsions in monkeys. Anesthesiology *41*:226, 1974.

Donald, J. R.: The effect of anaesthesia, hypotension, and epidural analgesia on blood loss in surgery for pelvic floor repair. Brit. J. Anaesth. *41*:155, 1969.

Donald, J. R.: Conduction anaesthesia, blood pressure and haemorrhage. Brit. J. Anaesth. *42*:8, 1970.

Doppman, J., Rubinson, R. M., Rockoff, S. D., Vasko, J. S., Shapiro, R., and Morrow, A. G.: Mechanism of obstruction of the infradiaphragmatic portion of the inferior vena cava in the presence of increased intra-abdominal pressure. Invest. Radiol. *1*:37, 1966.

Dripps, R. D.: Immediate decrease in blood pressure seen at conclusion of cyclopropane anesthesia "cyclopropane shock." Anesthesiology *8*:15, 1947.

Durrans, S. F.: High extradural segmental block. Anaesthesia *2*:106, 1947.

Dyde, J. A., and Bethel, A. N.: The effect of intermittent positive-pressure respiration on the speed of blood-flow in the deep veins of the lower limb. Brit. J. Surg. *55*:917, 1968.

Edelist, G.: Extreme obesity. Anesthesiology *29*:846, 1968.

Eggers, G. W. N., de Groot, W. J., and Tanner, C. R.: Hemodynamic changes associated with various surgical positions. J.A.M.A. *185*:1, 1965.

Enderby, G. E. H.: Controlled circulation with hypotensive drugs and posture to reduce bleeding in surgery; preliminary results with pentolinium iodide. Lancet *1*:1145, 1950.

Espersen, T., and Dahl-Iversen, E.: The clinical picture and treatment of pheochromocytomas of the suprarenal. Acta. Clin. Scand. *94*:271, 1946.

Estafanous, F. G., Tarazi, R. C., Viljoen, J. F., and El Tawil, M. Y.: Systemic hypertension following myocardial revascularization. Amer. Heart J. *85*:732, 1973.

Fasth, S., Kjellgren, A., Lundström, J., and Ygge, H.: General and extradural anesthesia in connection with suprapubic prostatectomy. Scand. J. Urol. Nephrol. *6*:17, 1972.

Finer, B.: Studies of the variability in expiratory efforts before and after cholecystectomy. Acta Anaesth. Scand. (Suppl.) *38*:7, 1970.

Fisher, A., and James, M. L.: Blood loss during major vaginal surgery. Brit. J. Anaesth. *40*:710, 1968.

Fisher, A., Waterhouse, T. D., and Adams, A. P.: Obesity: Its relation to anaesthesia. Anaesthesia *30*:633, 1975.

Folkow, B., and Langston, J.: The interrelationship of some factors influencing renal blood flow autoregulation. Acta Physiol. Scand. *61*:165, 1964.

Fortuna, A.: Caudal analgesia: A simple and safe technique in paediatric surgery. Brit. J. Anaesth. *39*:165, 1967.

Fox, G. S.: Anaesthesia for intestinal short circuiting in the morbidly obese with reference to the pathophysiology of gross obesity. Canad. Anaesth. Soc. J. *22*:307, 1975.

Freund, F., Roos, A., and Dodd, R. B.: Expiratory activity of the abdominal muscles in man during general anesthesia. J. Appl. Physiol. *19*:693, 1964.

Froese, A. B., and Bryan, A. C.: Effects of anesthesia and paralysis on diaphragmatic mechanics in man. Anesthesiology *41*:242, 1974.

Fujikawa, Y. F., Neves, A., Brasher, C. A., and Buckingham, W. W.: Epidural anesthesia in thoracic surgery: A preliminary report. J. Thorac. Surg. *17*:123, 1948.

Gal, T. J., and Cooperman, L. H.: Hypertension in the immediate postoperative period. Brit. J. Anaesth. *47*:70, 1975.

Galindo, A., Hernandez, J., Benavides, O., Ortegon de Muñoz, S., and Bonica, J. J.: Quality of spinal extradural anaesthesia: The influence of spinal nerve root diameter. Brit. J. Anaesth. *47*:41, 1975.

Gardner, E. K.: Epidural analgesia for prostatectomy. Anaesthesia *13*:406, 1958.

Gillespie, J. S., and Kirpekar, S. M.: The uptake and release of radioactive noradrenaline by the splenic nerves of cats. J. Physiol. (Lond.) *187*:51, 1966.

Gillies, J.: Physiological trespass in anaesthesia. Proc. Roy. Soc. Med. *45*:1, 1952.

Green, H. D., Hall, L. S., and Sexton, J.: Autonomic responses in the canine hepatic arterial and venous beds. Amer. J. Physiol. *196*:196, 1959.

Griffiths, H. W. C., and Gillies, J.: Thoraco-lumbar splanchnicectomy and sympathectomy: Anaesthetic procedure. Anaesthesia *3*:134, 1948.

Guedel, A. E., and Treweek, D. N.: Ether apnoeas. Curr. Res. Anesth. Analg. *13*:263, 1934.

Guttman, L., and Whitteridge, D.: Effects of bladder distension on autonomic mechanisms after spinal cord injuries. Brain *70*:361, 1947.

Henley, J., and Kritchman, M. M.: A clinical method for estimation of blood volume with the use of total sympathetic blockade. Anesthesiology *22*:136, 1961.

Henley, J., and Kritchman, M. M.: Total sympathetic blockade as an adjunct to anesthesia. N. Y. Soc. J. Med. *62*:348, 1962.

Hoar, P. F., Hickey, R. F., and Ullyot, D. J.: Systemic hypertension following myocardial revascularization: A method of treatment using epidural anesthesia. J. Thorac. Cardiovasc. Surg. *71*:859, 1976.

Holland, W. C., and Schümann, H. J.: Formation of catechol amines during splanchnic stimulation of the adrenal of the cat. Brit. J. Pharmacol. *11*:449, 1956.

Holly, H. S., Milic-Emili, J., Becklake, M. R., and Bates, D. V.: Regional distribution of pulmonary ventilation and perfusion in obesity. J. Clin. Invest. *46*:475, 1967.

Holmdahl, M. H., Sjögren, S., Ström, G., and Wright, B.: Clinical aspects of continuous epidural blockade for postoperative pain relief. Uppsala J. Med. Sci. *77*:47, 1972.

Isakob, Y. F., Geraskin, B. I., and Koshevnikov, V. A.: Long-term peridural anaesthesia after operations on the organs of the chest in children. Grnd. Chirurg. *13*:104, 1971.

James, M. L., and Fisher, A.: Blood gas changes during spinal and epidural analgesia. Anaesthesia *24*:511, 1969.

Johansson, B., and Langston, J. B.: Reflex influence of mesenteric afferents on renal, intestinal and muscle blood flow and on intestinal motility. Acta Physiol. Scand. *61*:400, 1964.

Kakkar, V. V., et al.: Prevention of fatal postopertive pulmonary embolism by low doses of heparin. An international multicentre trial. Lancet *2*:45, 1975.

Kaul, S. V., Heath, J. R., and Nunn, J. F.: Factors influencing the development of expiratory muscle activity during anaesthesia. Brit. J. Anaesth. *45*:1013, 1973.

Kay, B.: Caudal block for post-operative pain relief in children. Anaesthesia *29*:610, 1974.

Keating, V.: Carbohydrate metabolism. The effects of surgery in a tropical population. Anaesthesia *13*:434, 1958.

Korttila, K., and Linnoila, M.: Recovery and skills related to driving after intravenous sedation: Dose-response relationship with diazepam. Brit. J. Anaesth. *47*:457, 1975.

Laaksonen, V. O., Arola, M. K., Kivisaari, A., and Hannelin, M.: Effect of different modes of operative anaesthesia on the clearance time of ^{125}I-fibrinogen from calf veins. Ann. Clin. Res. *6*:356, 1974.

Lahiri, S. K., and Boys, J. E.: Anaesthesia for bladder inflation therapy. Brit. J. Anaesth. *45*:1162, 1973.

Lahnborg, G., and Bergström, K.: Clinical and haemostatic parameters related to thromboembolism and low-dose heparin prophylaxis in major surgery. Ann. Chir. Scand. *141*:590, 1975.

Lees, N. W., Howie, H. B., Mellon, A., McKee, A. H., and McDiarmid, I. A.: The influence of doxapram on postoperative pulmonary function in patients undergoing upper abdominal surgery. Brit. J. Anaesth. *48*:1197, 1976.

Lessing, A. J. P., and de Kock, M. J.: Anaesthesia in a grossly obese patient. Brit. J. Anaesth. *40*:139, 1968.

Lewis, F. J., and Welch, J. A.: Respiratory mechanics in postoperative patients. Surg. Gynecol. Obstet. *120*:305, 1965.

Loudon, J. D., and Scott, D. B.: Blood loss in gynaecological operations. J. Obstet. Gynaecol. Brit. Emp. *67*:561, 1960.

Lund, P. C.: Peridural Analgesia and Anesthesia. Springfield, Ill., Charles C Thomas, Publisher, 1966, p. 268.

McCann, J. C.: Physiology of traumatic reflexes and respiration during surgical anesthesia. Calif. Med. J. *65*:212, 1946.

McCarthy, G. S.: The effect of thoracic epidural analgesia on pulmonary gas distribution, functional residual capacity and airway closure. Brit. J. Anaesth. *48*:243, 1976.

Malatinsky, J., and Kadlic, T.: Inferior vena caval occlusion in the left lateral position. Brit. J. Anaesth. *46*:165, 1974.

Marley, E., and Paton, W. D. M.: The output of sympathetic amines from the cat's adrenal gland in response to splanchnic nerve activity. J. Physiol. (Lond.) *155*:1, 1961.

Mellander, S.: Comparative studies on the adrenergic neurohumoral control of resistance and capacitance blood vessels in the cat. Acta Physiol. Scand. *50*:(Suppl.) 176, 1960.

Miller, L., Gertel, M., Fox, G. S., and MacLean, L. D.: Comparison of effect of narcotic and epidural analgesia on postoperative respiratory function. Amer. J. Surg. *131*:291, 1976.

Modig, J., and Malmberg, P.: Pulmonary and circulatory reactions during total hip replacement. Acta Anaesth. Scand. *19*:219, 1975.

Moir, D. D.: Ventilatory function during epidural analgesia. Brit. J. Anaesth. *35*:3, 1963.

Moir, D. D.: Blood loss during major vaginal surgery. Brit. J. Anaesth. *40*:233, 1968.

Moir, D. D., and Mone, J. G.: Acid-base balance during epidural analgesia. Brit. J. Anaesth. *36*:480, 1964.

Morgan, M., and Norman, J.: The effect of extradural analgesia combined with light general anaesthesia and spontaneous ventilation on arterial blood-gases and physiological deadspace. Brit. J. Anaesth. *47*:955, 1975.

Morton, H. J. V.: Respiratory patterns during surgical anaesthesia. Anaesthesia *5*:112, 1950.

Munson, E. S., and Wagman, I. H.: Diazepam treatment of local anesthetic-induced seizures. Anesthesiology *37*:523, 1972.

Naimark, A., and Cherniak, R. M.: Compliance of the respiratory system and its components in health and obesity. J. Appl. Physiol. *15*:377, 1960.

Nakamura, T., Tanaka, A., Yamamoto, T., and Sato, I.: The spread of epidural anesthesia. Hiroshima J. Anesth. *8*:197, 1972.

Noble, A. B.: The problem of obesity in anaesthesia for abdominal surgery. Canad. Anaesth. Soc. J. *9*:1, 1962.

Nolte, H., Meyer, J., Köpf, B., and Zenz, M.: Klinische und elektrophysiologische Parameter zur Differenzierung der Wirkung von Lokalanaesthetica. Anaesthesist *23*:165, 1974.

Okinaka, A. J.: Closure of pulmonary air spaces following abdominal surgery. Surg. Gynecol. Obstet. *121*:1282, 1965.

Paletto, A. E.: Peridural anesthesia in thoracoplasty. Anesth. Analg. *31*:357, 1952.

Parbrook, G. D.: Postoperative pain relief: Comparison of methadone and morphine when used concurrently with nitrous-oxide analgesia. Brit. Med. J. *2*:616, 1966.

Parbrook, G. D., Rees, G. A. D., and Robertson, G. S.: Relief of postoperative pain: Comparison of a nitrous-oxide-oxygen mixture with morphine. Brit. Med. J. *2*:480, 1964.

Parnes, D. I., and Gordeev, V. I.: Some indices of external respiration in the conduct of postoperative peridural anaesthesia in children. Lit. Vestn. Khir. *105*:66, 1970.

Parnes, D. I., Tsybulkin, E. K., Gordeev, V. I., Monashkin, E. A., Kanayeva, M. A., and Kostyuchenko, A. L.: Haemodynamic changes in the postoperative peridural blockade in children. Lit. Vestn. Khir. *106*:110, 1971.

Paul, D. R., Hoyt, J. L., and Boutros, A. R.: Cardiovascular and respiratory changes in response to change of posture in the very obese. Anesthesiology *45*:73, 1976.

Pflug, A. E., Murphy, T. M., Butler, S. H., and Tucker, G. T.: The effects of postoperative peridural analgesia on pulmonary therapy and pulmonary complications. Anesthesiology *41*:8, 1974.

Pflug, A. E., Lindop, M. J., Murphy, T. M., Aasheim, G. M., and Beck, H. A.: Early reversal of postoperative hypoxemia. Anesth. Analg. *55*:822, 1976.

Pomeranz, B. H., Birtch, A. G., and Barger, A. C.: Neural control of intrarenal blood flow. Amer. J. Physiol. *215*:1067, 1968.

Replogle, R. L., Meiselman, H. J., and Merrill, E. W.: Clinical implications of blood rheology studies. Circulation *36*:148, 1967.

Roberts, V. C., and Cotton, L. T.: Prevention of postoperative deep vein thrombosis in patients with malignant disease. Brit. Med. J. *1*:358, 1974.

Robin, E., Whaley, R. D., Crump, C. H., and Travis, D. M.: Alveolar gas tensions, pulmonary ventilation and blood pH during physiologic sleep in normal subjects. J. Clin. Invest. *37*:981, 1958.

Rodriguez, I.: A anestesia peridural no paciente pediatrico. Rev. Bras. Anest. *14*:116, 1964.
Ruston, F. G.: Epidural anaesthesia in infants and children. Canad. Anaesth. Soc. J. *1*:37, 1954.
Ruston, F. G.: Epidural anesthesia in pediatric surgery. Anesth. Analg. *36*:76, 1957.
Ruston, F. G.: Epidural anaesthesia in paediatric surgery: Present state at Hamilton General Hospital. Canad. Anaesth. Soc. J. *11*:12, 1964.
Salmoiraghi, G. C., and Burns, B. D.: Notes on mechanism of rhythmic respiration. J. Neurophysiol. *23*:14, 1960.
Schneider, H.: Peridural Anaesthesie in Kindersalter. Z. Urol. Chir. *76*:704, 1951.
Schulte-Steinberg, O.: Personal communication: Experiences with CO_2-bupivacaine, 1976.
Schulte-Steinberg, O., and Rahlfs, V. W.: Caudal anaesthesia in children and spread of 1 per cent lignocaine: A statistical study. Brit. J. Anaesth. *42*:1093, 1970.
Scott, D. B.: Inferior vena caval pressure. Changes occurring during anaesthesia. Anaesthesia *18*:135, 1963.
Shimazu, T., and Fukuda, A.: Increased activities of glycogenetic enzymes in liver after splanchnic nerve stimulation. Science *150*:1607, 1965.
Shoemaker, C. P.: A study of hepatic hemodynamics in the dog. Circ. Res. *15*:216, 1964.
Shuman, R. L., and Peters, R. M.: Epidural anesthesia following thoracotomy in patients with chronic obstructive airway disease. J. Thorac. Cardiovasc. Surg. *71*:82, 1976.
Silver, J. R., and Buxton, P. H.: Spinal stroke. Brain *97*:539, 1974.
Simpson, B. R., Parkhouse, J., Marshall, R., and Lambrechts, W.: Extradural analgesia and the prevention of postoperative respiratory complications. Brit. J. Anaesth. *33*:628, 1961.
Sjögren, S., and Wright, B.: Circulation, respiration and lidocaine concentration during continuous epidural blockade. Acta Anaesth. Scand. (Suppl.) *46*:5, 1972.
Spiegel, P.: Caudal anesthesia in pediatric surgery: A preliminary report. Anesth. Analg. *41*:218, 1962.
Stanton-Hicks, M. D'A.: A study using bupivacaine for continuous peridural analgesia in patients undergoing surgery of the hip. Acta Anaesth. Scand. *15*:65, 1971.
Stanton-Hicks, M., Murphy, T. M., Bonica, J. J., Mather, L. E., and Tucker, G. T.: Effects of extradural block: Comparison of the properties, circulatory effects and pharmacokinetics of etidocaine and bupivacaine. Brit. J. Anaesth. *48*:575, 1976.
Steinhaus, J. E., and Gaskin, L.: A study of intravenous lidocaine as suppressant of cough reflex. Anesthesiology *24*:285, 1963.
Stolar, S. H., and Wynands, J. E.: A technique of anaesthesia for cancer perfusion. Canad. Anaesth. Soc. J. *10*:48, 1963.
Stormont, R. T., Hathaway, H. R., Shideman, F. E., and Seevers, M. H.: Acid-base balance during cyclopropane anesthesia. Anesthesiology *3*:369, 1942.
Sussman, D. R.: A comparative evaluation of ketamine anesthesia in children and adults. Anesthesiology *40*:459, 1974.
Thompson, J. E., and Arrowood, J. G.: Pheochromocytoma: Surgical and anesthetic management. Anesthesiology *15*:658, 1954.
Thorud, T., Lund, I., and Holme, I.: The effect of anesthesia on intraoperative and postoperative bleeding during abdominal prostatectomies: A comparison of neurolept anesthesia, halothane anesthesia and epidural anesthesia. Acta Anaesth. Scand. (Suppl.) *57*:83, 1975.
Toker, P.: Hyperosmolar hyperglycemic nonketotic coma, a cause of delayed recovery from anesthesia. Anesthesiology *41*:284, 1974.
Urquhart-Hay, D.: Paraplegia following epidural analgesia. Anaesthesia. *24*:461, 1969.
Urquhart-Hay, D.: Personal communication, 1969.
Urquhart-Hay, D., and Teague, C. A.: Spinal thrombophlebitis after prostatectomy with hypotensive anaesthesia: Case report. New Zealand Med. J. *79*:654, 1974.
Urquhart-Hay, D., Marshall, N. G., and Marsland, J. M.: Comparison of epidural and hypotensive anaesthesia in open prostatectomy. Series 1. New Zealand Med. J. *69*:280, 1969a.
Urquhart-Hay, D., Marshall, N. G., and Marsland, J. M.: Comparison of epidural and hypotensive anaesthesia in open prostatectomy. Series 2. New Zealand Med. J. *70*:223, 1969b.
Vasconcelos, E.: Cancer of the oesophagus: Original technique for total oesophagectomy. Dis. Chest *10*:471, 1944.
Wahba, W. M., Don, H. F., and Craig, D. B.: Post-operative epidural analgesia: Effects on lung volumes. Canad. Anaesth. Soc. J. *22*:519, 1975.
Waltemath, C. L., and Bergman, N. A.: Respiratory compliance in obese patients. Anesthesiology *41*:84, 1974.
Wetstone, D. L., and Wong, K. C.: Sinus bradycardia and asystole during spinal anesthesia. Anesthesiology *41*:87, 1974.
Wulfson, H. D., and Dalton, B.: Hyperosmolar hyperglycemic nonketotic coma in a patient undergoing emergency cholecystectomy. Anesthesiology *41*:286, 1974.
Zorgniotti, A. W., Narins, D. J., and Dell'aria, S. L.: Anesthesia, hemorrhage and prostatectomy. J. Urol. *103*:774, 1970.

chapter 12
Epidural Analgesia for Obstetrics

There can be no more horrible stigma upon civilisation than the history of childbirth.

Grantly Dick Read: Revelation of Childbirth, 1946

PERSPECTIVE

Superficially, obstetrical anesthesia appears to be a simple field with a limited range of interest, but it is a deceptively demanding subspecialty. Not only are two patients involved in each anesthetic administration, but also the dynamic events of normal labor require that the muscles concerned with delivery retain their power and coordination to the full.

Traditionally, the process of labor is considered in terms of the three "P's"—the Powers, the Passages and the Passenger—and each of these three imposes its own pharmacological constraints upon any system of pain relief, for ideally, none of them should be depressed. The last of the three P's, the Passenger, is exquisitely sensitive to depressant drugs, and like a sea diver it is wholly dependent on moment to moment gas exchange through its lifeline. The mother herself presents special anesthetic risks that include the hazard of gastric regurgitation and aspiration of corrosively acid stomach contents, as well as the hemodynamic consequences of inferior vena caval obstruction by a large abdominal tumor.

These are the broad basic constraints of so-called "natural childbirth." In addition, there are other constraints superimposed by changing modes of obstetrical practice, some of which add additional complexities while others may simplify the anesthetic strategy involved.

In Europe "natural childbirth" with minimal obstetrical interference has long been the traditional mode, normal labor being handled by trained midwives and sage-femmes. The essential wisdom of the body is unquestioned in this approach, and as far as possible labor is left to its own devices. Mechanical intervention is only permitted when some physiological abnormality requires it. This approach makes for long labors, a stretched perineum and, if gynecological interventions are any guide, a high incidence of procidentia in the fifth and sixth decades.

For many years North American practice has leaned more toward a planned delivery employing what may be termed "the cult of the nulliparous perineum." That is, each vaginal delivery becomes a surgical operation, with elective episiotomy to save the perineum from unnecessary stretch, outlet forceps to ease the baby's head over the perineum and to save it from unnecessary pressure, and then a carefully tailored repair of the cut perineum. Clearly, this type of practice requires different anesthetic tactics than natural childbirth, in which forceful but controlled expulsive efforts are needed to overcome perineal resistance during expulsion of the head.

More recently, planned intervention has extended to the first stage, so that the whole process of labor is controlled from start to finish, with combined medical and surgical induction, and with the uterus driven by exogenous rather than endogenous oxytocics. In spite of being the antithesis of "natural" spontaneous labor, this practice of planned interference offers certain strategic advantages in environments in which the full panoply of consultant supervision and laboratory intensive care facilities are most easily available during office hours and in which night-time activities are covered more thinly by emergency staff (O'Driscoll et al., 1973). "Nine-to-five o'clock" obstetrics has instant appeal in many regions that had formerly seemed most conservative, since it appears to eliminate one of the harshest administrative requirements of an effective obstetrical unit, that is, full round-the-clock laboratory support and constant attendance at all levels of skilled personnel in many different disciplines (Editorial, Brit. J. Anaesth., 1974).

Again, this mode of practice modifies the demands of anesthetic technique. Indeed, it is an interesting observation that the assurance of effective safe and prolonged analgesia has been a necessary condition for the adoption of driven labor as a respectable method of practice. For without an effective and nondepressant analgesic system, the pain and discomfort of forced labor would not meet with general acceptance, and the degree of fetal depression would also be unacceptable by present standards, if pain relief were confined to systemic analgesics.

A note of caution must be sounded before the principle of daylight deliveries is embraced as a wholesale procedure. History is full of meddlesome medical fads, and the practice of induction for daylight deliveries is ground on which the narrow line between efficiency and dubious midwifery has not yet been finally drawn (Schwarcz et al., 1974). In this regard, the anesthesiologist should beware of allowing his services to become party to questionable standards. An epidural service should be able to provide its best at all times of the day and night, and this availability should be unquestioned. However, epidural services ought to be provided strictly for genuine medical indications and applied at the most advantageous time for the baby, not for purely social convenience, or the system will be in grave danger of falling into disrepute (Editorial, Lancet, 1974).

Growing concern over the dangers of general anesthesia in labor was evident in the Reports of Anaesthetic Mortality in Britain published in 1951 (Morton and Wylie, 1951) and in 1956 (Edwards et al., 1956). Dinnick estimated a death rate from aspiration of vomitus as high as 1:3,380 obstetrical anesthetics (Dinnick, 1957). A similar study in the United States by Lock and Greiss in 1955 showed a lower maternal death rate of 1:20,304 live births directly attributable to anesthesia. Of these, about one quarter were ascribed to complications of spinal anesthesia and one third to the inhalation of vomitus during general anesthesia. Pulmonary morbidity arising from Mendelson's syndrome was added to the list of hazards attributed to general anesthesia (Mendelson, 1946). The danger of vomiting and aspiration of acid gastric contents is increased by administration of narcotic analgesics such as meperidine (i.e., Demerol or pethidine), since these agents cause a marked delay in gastric emptying during labor (Nimmo, Wilson and Prescott, 1975).

In the United States a trend away from systemic analgesia and general anesthesia was stimulated by Hingson's energetic campaign to popularize caudal analgesia as a safe and effective alternative to general anesthesia or to subarachnoid blockade (Hingson and Edwards, 1943; Flowers et al., 1949; Hingson, Cull and Benzinger, 1961).

In Britain, comparatively little interest was displayed in regional analgesia for labor or delivery, and systemic methods of pain relief using combinations of meperidine and nitrous oxide remained standard practice until the late 1960's. Hypoxic mixtures of nitrous oxide and air were routinely administered for analgesia until as late as 1961, when concern for fetal hypoxia led to a change to nitrous oxide and oxygen (Tunstall, 1961). The danger of vomiting during forceps extraction under general anesthesia was countered by a hard-line policy of routine "crash" endotracheal intubation in every case, as proposed by Hamer Hodges and his colleagues in 1959.

Nevertheless, the doubtful compromise of light general anesthesia without intubation continued to be practiced in many centers on both sides of the Atlantic. To be safe, this required a very light level of unconsciousness with retention of active swallowing and cough reflexes in case of regurgitation. At the same time a tolerant attitude was needed on the part of the obstetricians, who were expected to operate on a moving target, with a perineum gyrating under light anesthesia.

With changing modes of practice based on increasing quantitative knowledge of fetal physiology, systemic analgesia and general anesthesia have almost disappeared from the obstetrical arena, leaving the field to regional analgesia as the unchallenged method of choice for relief of pain in labor. Today, general anesthesia survives only as a standby in emergency conditions, such as placenta previa, abruptio placentae and precipitate labor, and in some centers it also remains the routine method for cesarean section.

The reason for the ascendancy of lumbar epidural blockade as the paramount technique for obstetrics will become apparent when we consider the neural pathways involved in the pain of labor and the limitations of alternative methods of regional analgesia in contemporary clinical practice.

TECHNICAL EVOLUTION

In 1933 Cleland published his first account of the segmental pain pathways of the first stage of labor, showing that the pain of uterine contractions could be blocked by paravertebral injection of the eleventh and twelfth thoracic nerves, while perineal pain of the second stage required blockade of the sacral nerves (Cleland, 1933). Figure 12–1 is a diagrammatic representation of the segmental pathways involved in the pain of labor. Later, when indwelling catheter techniques became available, Cleland developed a logical

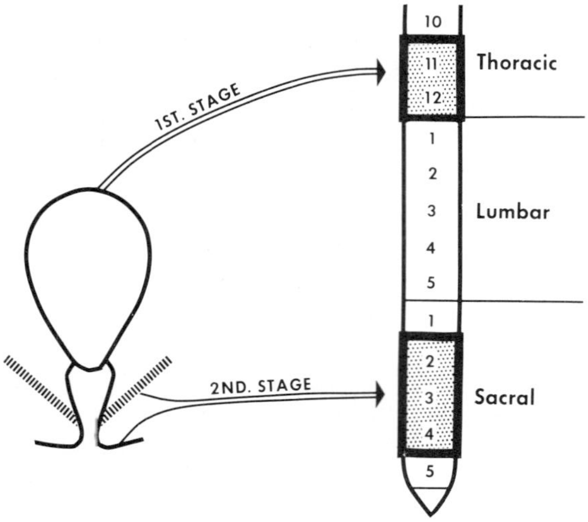

Figure 12–1. Pain pathways in labor. Pain from uterine contraction and dilatation of the cervix enters the cord through the eleventh and twelfth thoracic segments. Pain from distension of the perineum travels in the second, third and fourth sacral nerves. (After Cleland, 1949.)

method of peridural analgesia for blocking the two separate segmental levels in sequence as labor progressed. One epidural catheter was inserted in the upper lumbar or thoracolumbar region, so that small doses of local anesthetic could easily provide localized blockade of the two lowest thoracic segments during the first stage of labor. A second catheter was placed in the caudal canal via the sacral hiatus so that second-stage pain could be effectively blocked by a small caudal injection (Cleland, 1949).

This technique, somewhat complicated though it was, represented a beautiful example of sound anatomical knowledge combined with a wise clinical feeling for pharmacological parsimony. With this approach extradural dosage could be reduced to an absolute minimum, and the fetus could be spared the possible consequences of excessive local anesthetic absorption by the mother's circulation. In many ways this was ahead of the times, at a period when little thought was given to the effects of local anesthetics on the baby and when clinical and laboratory methods did not exist to quantitate them.

Cleland pointed out that in cases in which caudal puncture was technically difficult, it would still be possible to obtain satisfactory terminal sacral analgesia by injecting a supplementary dose through the lumbar catheter with the patient in the sitting position, followed by posture in a semi-Fowler's position. Alternatively, a second catheter could be placed downward into the sacral canal as a "reversed" caudal through the fourth lumbar interspace.

To many anesthesiologists a technique requiring two peridural catheters was unacceptably complicated, and the alternative of using just one catheter seemed preferable. However, reports soon appeared that perineal blockade was inadequate with a single lumbar catheter, and Flowers and his colleagues (1949) found a 45 per cent incidence of unsatisfactory perineal analgesia with a lumbar catheter alone. This led to the generally accepted view that while the lumbar approach gave good analgesia for abdominal section, caudal analgesia was much better suited for vaginal delivery (Flowers, 1954). As a result, the lumbar catheter technique fell into neglect for vaginal delivery, while continuous caudal analgesia became the method of choice for prolonged pain relief in the first and second stages of labor. Single-injection caudals or saddle block subarachnoid analgesia were used when regional analgesia was restricted to terminal pain relief at delivery.

Single-injection lumbar blockade survived as a practical technique for terminal analgesia at delivery, but very little restraint was exercised in the amounts of drug injected. Technique was oriented toward getting results in terms of a quiet, cooperative patient, without very much thought being directed to the uptake of local anesthetics and any possible depressant effects on the fetus.

As early as 1938 Graffagnino and Seyler were using 50 ml of 1 per cent procaine as a single injection at the second lumbar interspace. Similar large volumes of more toxic agents came to be recommended by other authors—for example, up to 30 ml of 2 per cent lidocaine for induction of caudal analgesia (Marmer et al., 1956), or 25 ml of 2 per cent lidocaine for a single injection in the lumbar region (Norris et al., 1960; Hellman, 1965). A rational basis for more moderate use of powerful local anesthetic agents in labor was only gradually accepted after the accumulation of clinical and laboratory data from several different disciplines over a number of years.

During the 1950's and early 1960's clinical measurement of a wide variety of physiological and pharmacological parameters was undertaken with a number of new techniques that enabled the processes of labor, delivery and medical intervention to be quantitated in a way that had not been possible before. Caldeyro-Barcia and his colleagues at Montevideo were foremost in attacking, with great energy, the problems of the physiology of labor, and their work, together with similar studies undertaken later by Hon at Yale, formed the basis for our present understanding of the mechanisms of labor. As quantitative measurement rapidly infiltrated every facet of obstetrical art, norms were set up for uterine performance (Alvarez and Caldeyro-Barcia, 1950), as well as for fetal behavior in utero and after delivery (Hon, 1959; Apgar, 1953). The limits of normality for the progression of labor in primigravida and multigravida were set by Friedman (1955, 1956). Adaptation of micro blood gas techniques meant that fetal depression could be quantitated at any time during labor in terms of fetal acid-base status (James and Adamsons, 1964; Bretscher and Saling, 1967). General and regional anesthesia became rationalized as the effects of different techniques on fetal acid-base balance were measured and assessed. Concentrations of local anesthetics in mother and baby during regional anesthesia were measured, at first somewhat coarsely by colorimetric methods (Bromage and Robson, 1961) and later by more accurate gas chromatography (Keenaghan, 1968; Tucker et al., 1970a, 1970b).

The evidence is now incontrovertible that large doses of local anesthetic given to the mother cross the placenta and depress the fetus to varying degrees (Shnider and Way, 1968a, 1968b; Shnider et al., 1968a; Andersson et al., 1970; Gennser et al., 1972). This evidence has vindicated the low-dosage regional analgesic techniques that some of us had recommended at an earlier date (Cleland, 1949; MacMillan, 1954; Bromage, 1961; Nielsen et al., 1962; Hehre et al., 1965). Today, there is no longer any place for large doses of local anesthetics in labor. The dangers are well documented, and the techniques to be considered later in the chapter must be understood in the light of these hazards. Emphasis will be placed on using the least amount of local anesthetic that is compatible with satisfactory clinical results.

ANATOMY, PHYSIOLOGY AND PHARMACOLOGY RELATED TO EPIDURAL ANALGESIA IN LABOR

The Uterus, Cardiovascular Dynamics and Posture

> During pregnancy the vascular obstruction produced by the large uterus presents a unique problem that must be constantly kept in mind when evaluating cardiovascular dynamics.
>
> Ueland and Hansen (1969)

Compression of the great vessels at the pelvic brim is one of the most important and, as Selwyn Crawford has emphasized, one of the most dangerous vascular features of the parturient woman (Crawford, 1972). Aortocaval compression at the pelvic brim is greatest when the parturient is supine, less when she is on her side, and least in the knee-elbow position. It is this vascular obstruction by the gravid uterus that gives rise to the supine hypotensive syndrome (Brigden, Howarth and Sharpey-Schafer, 1950; McRoberts, 1951; Howard et al., 1953; Holmes, 1960; Kerr et al., 1964; Hehre et al., 1965; Lees et al., 1967, 1970), to inefficient uterine contractions (Noriega et al., 1959; Caldeyro-Barcia, 1960) and to disturbances of uteroplacental perfusion with resulting fetal hypoxia and acidosis that is worst when the mother lies flat on her back. In addition, maternal capillary Po_2 falls about 13 mmHg when the mother assumes the supine position (Ang et al., 1969).

A large increase of maternal cardiac output of the order of 20 to 100 per cent occurs when caval compression is released by changing from the supine to the lateral position (Ueland et al., 1968, 1969; Ueland and Hansen, 1969; Lees et al., 1970), and there is a fall in venous pressure of 10 to 15 mmHg in the inferior vena cava below the obstruction site. These dramatic alterations in cardiac output and caval flow may not be reflected by changes of pulse and blood pressure in the arm, and ordinary bedside monitoring may arouse no suspicion of the profound disturbances of vascular dynamics that are going on in the pelvis when the mother is supine.

The pathways involved in venous return during caval compression are shown in Figure 12–2. A high venous pressure in the leg veins helps to maintain a vis a tergo to force blood through the detour of the sacral plexus and back to the heart through the superior vena cava via the veins of the spinal canal. During each uterine contraction about 300 to 500 ml of blood is forced out of the uterus to augment this flow (Hendricks, 1958), and a corresponding rise of pressure occurs in the extradural veins. Figure 12–3 shows a pressure tracing from the extradural space during first-stage labor in the supine position (Bromage, 1961). Peaks of extradural pressure rising about 8 to 10 cmH_2O above baseline accompany each uterine contraction,

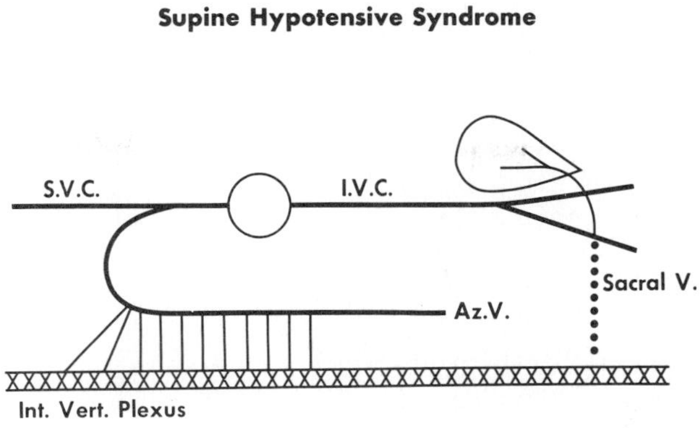

Figure 12–2. Compression of the inferior vena cava by the gravid uterus. Alternative pathway for venous return from lower limbs and pelvis via sacral veins, internal vertebral plexus (external vertebral plexus not shown) and intercostovertebral veins draining into the azygos vein (Az.V), thence back to the heart through the superior vena cava.

reflecting the distension of the extradural veins caused by augmented venous return taking the long way round back to the heart. Galbert and Marx (1974) have shown that this rise of extradural pressure is reduced, but not abolished, by displacing the uterus laterally to relieve pressure on the inferior vena cava and reopen the normal caval highway. The baseline epidural pressure upon which these peaks are superimposed increases steadily as labor progresses. This baseline pressure is also affected by caval compression, rising about 50 per cent when the patient is turned from the lateral position and allowed to lie on her back. Figure 12–4, taken from Galbert and Marx's data, shows the fall in baseline epidural pressures during labor when the patient is turned from the supine to the lateral position (Galbert and Marx, 1974). The net effect of the fluctuating venous distension is to exert a pumplike massaging force within the extradural space that spreads injected solutions more widely than under normal conditions (Bromage, 1961).

When caval compression occurs, reciprocal pressures tend to exist in the extradural veins and the right atrium, with a high extradural venous pressure and a low right atrial pressure. Figure 12–5 summarizes data from Galbert and Marx (1974) and Ueland and Hansen (1969) which emphasize the importance of using posture and uterine displacement to protect the mother and fetus from the harmful effects of the supine position and caval compression.

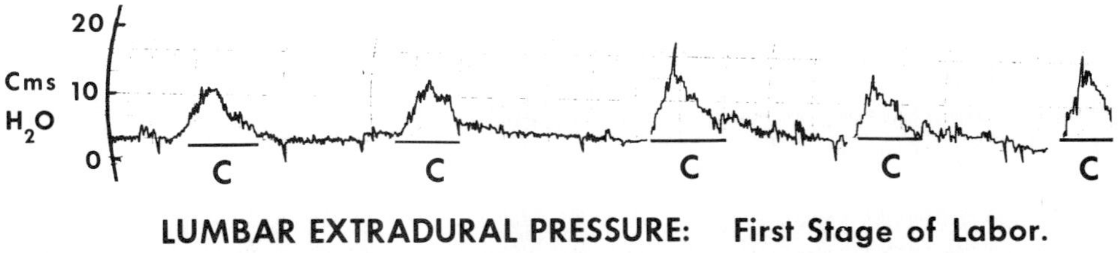

Figure 12–3. Epidural pressure tracing during labor in supine posture. Extradural catheter at L_2–L_3, and fluid-filled system attached to low-pressure strain gauge. Recordings made when patient was relaxed and pain-free, after induction of epidural analgesia, so "bearing down" artifacts were excluded. $\overline{C}$ = Duration of uterine contraction. Note marked rises of extradural pressure of 8 to 15 cmH_2O during contractions, reflecting phasic engorgement of extradural veins. (From Bromage: Canad. Med. Assoc. J., *85*:1136, 1961.)

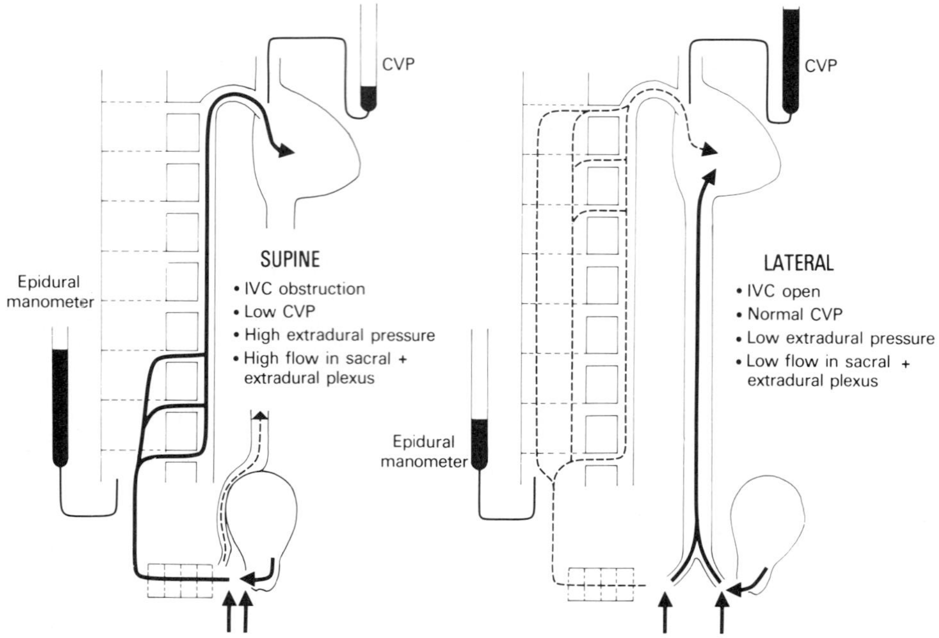

Figure 12-4. Effect of maternal posture on reciprocal pressures in extradural space and central venous compartment. *Left,* In supine position uterus compresses inferior vena cava (IVC). Venous return from legs and pelvis is shunted through the vertebral venous plexus and azygos system. Pressure and flow rise in the extradural veins. Epidural space pressure rises, and central venous pressure (CVP) falls. *Right,* In lateral position normal flow is restored in IVC. CVP rises to normal levels. Pressure and flow fall in the vertebral veins, and epidural space pressure falls. (Data from Galbert and Marx, 1974.)

Effects of Uterine Contraction on Aortocaval Compression

In the supine position, compressive phenomena are exacerbated during uterine contractions, as the uterus tenses and hardens and increases its pressure on the major arteries and veins crossing the pelvic brim, leading to

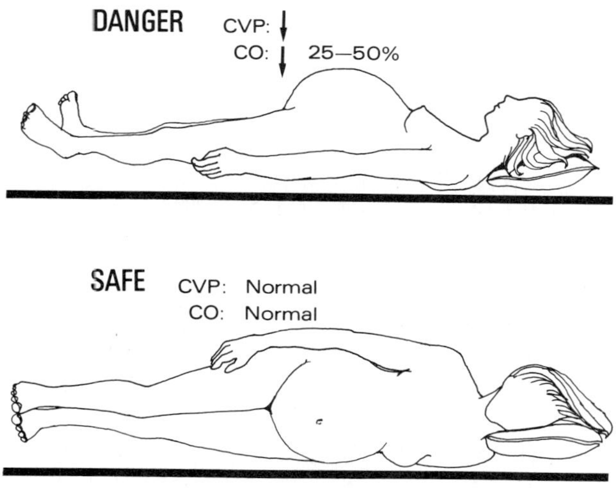

Figure 12-5. Cardiovascular hazards of supine posture in parturient patients. Supine: fall of CVP and 25 to 50 per cent fall of cardiac output. Lateral: restoration of CVP and cardiac output. (Data from Ueland and Hansen, 1969, and Galbert and Marx, 1974.)

an *apparent* improvement in the mother's circulation but to a *hidden* deterioration of the fetal environment. Thus, three things become evident:

1. Increased caval compression and obstruction intensifies the engorgement that already exists in the veins of the pelvis and uterus.

2. Almost the entire 0.3 to 0.5 liter of blood squeezed out of the uterus is forced into the extradural and azygos venous system during contraction, causing heightened peaks of extradural venous pressure. On the other hand, in the lateral position a large proportion of the increased pelvic venous return is able to take the normal pathway through the inferior vena cava without causing excessive extradural engorgement.

3. There has been some confusion about the effect of uterine contractions on aortic compression at the pelvic brim. During contraction cardiac output and blood pressure rise, so this was interpreted as an improvement of the circulation due to relief of aortic compression (Ueland and Hansen, 1969). However, the reverse is the case. Before the fetal head engages in the pelvis, each contraction tips the uterus around a fulcrum formed by the lumbosacral vertebral prominence, and aortic compression is increased, leading to a hyperdynamic circulation *above* the compression but a further deterioration below it (Bieniarz et al., 1968). Increased compression of the aorta during contraction exaggerates the coarctation effect, with a steep rise of maternal cardiac output and a hypertensive rise of blood pressure above the obstruction but a fall below it, as shown in Figure 12–6. Diminished pelvic perfusion and fall of pulse pressure in the legs accompanying uterine contraction in the supine position is known as the *Poseiro effect,* and it is present in about one third of normal spontaneous labors. Figure 12–7 shows the degree of aortic compression that can occur during uterine contraction in the supine position (Bieniarz et al., 1968).

The effects of uterine contraction and posture on the arterial system are summarized in Figure 12–8 from data by Caldeyro-Barcia's group (Bieniarz et al., 1968) and Ueland and Hansen (1969). It is clear that from the point of view of fetal environment, the supine posture is not an acceptable mode of management in late pregnancy and labor. As Selwyn Crawford has emphasized (1972), there is no excuse for allowing parturient patients to lie flat on their backs during labor. In the past, most obstetrical units have been at fault in this respect, and most of us have shared in the guilt. It is

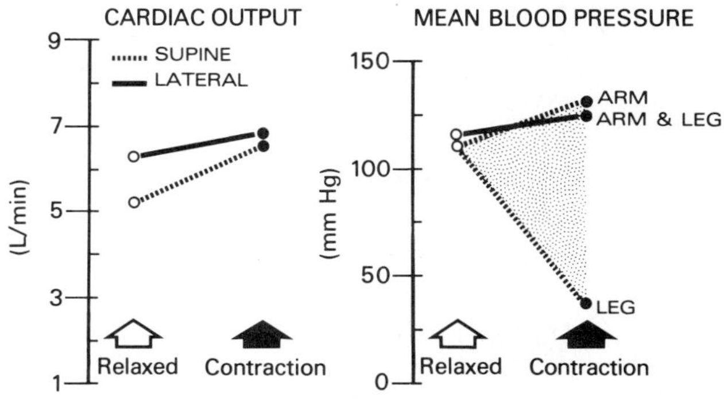

Figure 12–6. Cardiovascular effects of posture and uterine contractions. Coarctation effect of contracting gravid uterus in supine posture. Lateral position: cardiac output is augmented by increased venous return during uterine contraction, and arterial pressure rises slightly in both upper and lower limbs. Supine position: cardiac output is augmented, and pressure rises in upper limb but falls in lower limb owing to partial aortic obstruction during uterine contraction. (Data from Ueland and Hansen, 1969, and Bieniarz et al., 1968.)

Aortic Compression in Supine Posture at Term

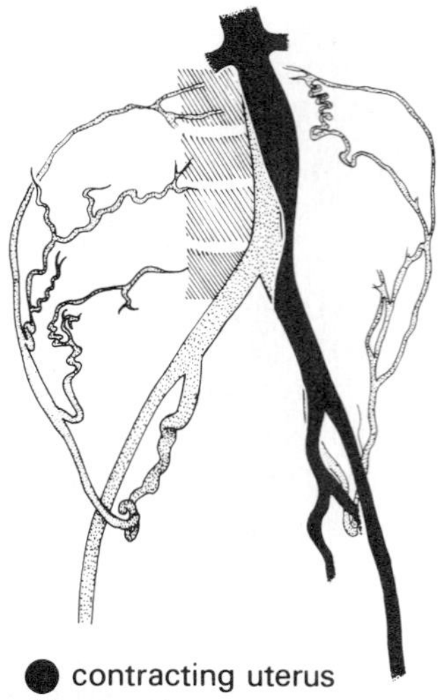

Figure 12–7. The Poseiro effect. Tracing of aortogram during uterine contraction and relaxation in supine position. Outline of aorta showing constriction of terminal aorta with complete obstruction of right common iliac artery during uterine contraction. Outline of aorta during uterine relaxation showing normal arterial filling. (After Bieniarz et al., 1968.)

temptingly convenient to nurse patients on their backs, for monitoring equipment tends to stay in place better in that position, but a constant effort must be made to insist that the mother rest on her side. If patients have to be turned supine for necessary procedures, then a wedge or a sandbag should be placed under one hip to tilt the pelvis sideways, in an effort to relieve the full weight of the uterus pressing on the vena cava and to prevent what Crawford has termed "concealed caval occlusion" (Crawford et al., 1972).

It is instructive, but disturbing, to review the slow response between published work and general clinical adoption of a massively proven idea. In this instance, the issue of maternal posture is illustrative of an unusually sluggish inertia between head and hand in everyday clinical practice. It has taken more than a decade of clear evidence for obstetricians and anesthesiologists to come to the reluctant conclusion that the supine position is harmful at term and especially harmful during labor, and even now the process of education is incomplete. The price of this inertia, in terms of unnecessary neonatal depression, can only be guessed, but from existing cardiovascular and biochemical evidence it is likely to have been high.

REDUCED EPIDURAL DOSE REQUIREMENTS IN LABOR: BASIC CONSIDERATIONS

Just as the anesthesiologist must be aware of the tendency for reduced epidural blockade to spread further than usual in diabetic and arteriosclerotic patients, so he must constantly be aware that the same tendency exists in every parturient woman.

Pregnant women at term need about one third less epidural dosage than they would in the nonpregnant state, This phenomenon was first

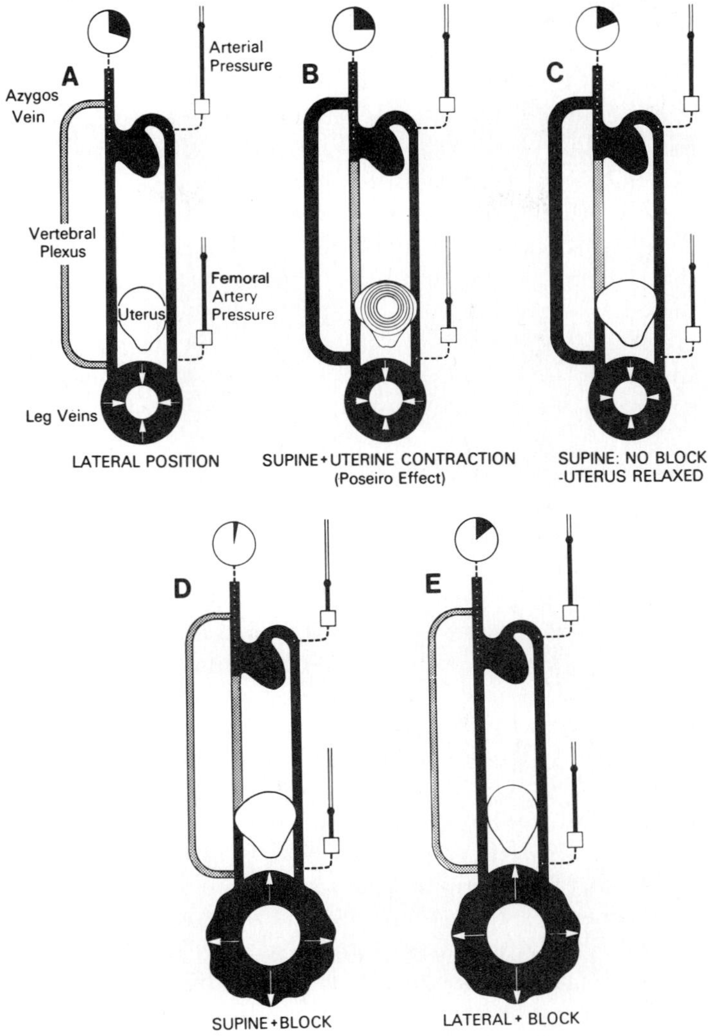

Figure 12–8. The supine hypotensive syndrome. Diagram of venous return.

A, Lateral position. No compression of aorta or inferior vena cava. Venous return through inferior vena cava is unimpeded. Cardiac output, arterial pressure and central venous pressure are all normal. Low flow through vertebral venous plexus.

B, Supine position during uterine contraction. Aorta and inferior vena cava are both compressed. Increased vascular tone in legs forces venous return through vertebral venous plexus; central venous pressure falls slightly but is maintained. Arterial pressure remains in normal range above the aortic obstruction but falls below it.

C, Supine position with relaxed uterus. Vena cava severely compressed; slight aortic compression. Increased vascular tone in legs forces venous return through vertebral venous plexus. Central venous pressure falls slightly, but arterial pressure is maintained throughout body.

D, Supine position with epidural block and loss of vasomotor tone in legs. Vena cava is compressed. The vis a tergo is lost, and venous pressure in the legs is insufficient to force an adequate venous return through the azygos system. Central venous pressure, cardiac output and arterial pressure all fall.

E, Lateral position with epidural block and loss of vasomotor tone in legs. No compression of aorta or vena cava. Venous return through the easy caval pathway is adequate to maintain a normal cardiac output. Central venous pressure and arterial pressure are slightly reduced.

described in 1949 in relation to caudal analgesia when Oral B. Crawford and R. V. Chester showed that the dermatome levels of caudal injections with a mixture of 1.5 per cent procaine and 0.15 per cent tetracaine rose as high as the eighth or ninth thoracic segment in women in labor, whereas they seldom rose above the first or second lumbar segment in nonpregnant patients. A rough calculation of caudal dose requirements from Crawford's data shows that 50 mg of procaine were required per segment in nonpregnant surgical patients, while only 35 mg per segment were needed for the parturient patient. This is a 30 per cent reduction below normal dose requirements, and Crawford and Chester attributed it to some mechanism arising out of the increased abdominal tension of pregnant patients (Crawford and Chester, 1949).

Unfortunately, this important observation escaped the attention that it should have received as an outward and highly practical manifestation of the hidden and wider phenomenon of general extradural venous engorgement. Crawford's observation appeared to have no influence on lumbar extradural technique during the next ten years, and most authors, including myself, seem to have missed this vital clue entirely.

Between 1950 and 1961 my own studies of lumbar epidural analgesia in labor showed reduced dose requirements of a similar order of magnitude to those earlier figures for caudal analgesia of Crawford and Chester. In a series published in 1961, the reduction of lumbar dose requirements was approximately one third less than normal (Bromage, 1961, 1962) as shown in Figure 12–9. Spoerel and his associates in London, Ontario (Nielsen et al., 1962; Cox and Spoerel, 1964; Kandel et al., 1966), obtained similar findings, while Hehre and his group at Yale found even greater reductions in segmental dose requirements (Hehre et al., 1965). Contrary to what Flowers et al. had reported earlier, all three groups found that relatively small doses of local anesthetics through a single lumbar catheter were sufficient to provide satisfactory analgesia for both the first and the second stages of labor.

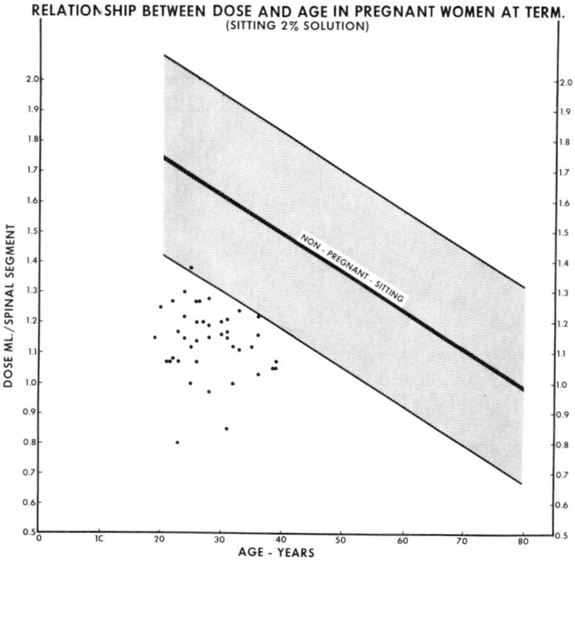

Figure 12–9. Reduced epidural dose requirements in parturient women. Dots show individual segmental dose requirements for 2 per cent lidocaine hydrochloride at term, compared to mean and 95 per cent confidence limits of normal nonpregnant population. (From Bromage: Brit. J. Anaesth., 1962.)

There is now complete agreement that epidural analgesia spreads about one third further in pregnant patients than in nonpregnant patients and that it is not only unnecessary but also potentially dangerous to administer the same size of dose to parturient patients as would be given to nonpregnant subjects. The generally accepted explanation for the difference lies in the pumplike massaging effects of the turgid epidural veins that pulse and swell with every uterine contraction (Bromage, 1961; Hipona, Yules and Hehre, 1966). However, additional mechanisms may exist in the realm of biochemical changes of membrane permeability associated with pregnancy (Bromage, 1967). The latter possibility is given some support by the interesting finding of Shnider's associates that pregnancy appears to affect the dose requirements of general anesthesia to about the same degree as it does those of epidural and spinal analgesia (Palahniuk et al., 1974). Working with sheep, these workers found that the minimal alveolar concentration (MAC) for three fluorinated hydrocarbons was reduced by 25 to 40 per cent in late pregnancy, and as an explanation they suggested that the 10- to 20-fold increase in reproductive steroids near term may have a potentiating effect on general anesthetics. If this is so, then any common link that may exist between the observed potentiation of systemic and regional anesthesia is likely to be found in a general alteration of membrane permeability and hydration affecting a wide variety of tissues. Additionally, changes of mucopolysaccharide contents of collagen and other extracellular tissue components are likely to be an important factor in altering the permeability characteristics of the meninges (McLennan, 1946; Walker and Balf, 1954; Salvatore, 1961; Bryant et al., 1968; Flint, 1972).

EFFECTS OF NEURAL BLOCKADE ON PARTURITION

The effects of spinal denervation on uterine activity are complex and depend on neural, humoral and hemodynamic factors. With epidural blockade the situation is further complicated by the possibility that a significant amount of injected local anesthetic may be absorbed into the blood stream, and this may also modify uterine action.

In the past there has been some disagreement about the role of the nervous system in controlling normal labor. This was due in some measure to confusion between *uterine contractility,* which is only one aspect of labor, and the whole process of *expulsion,* which, of course, involves much more than just intermittent contractions of the uterus. Skeletal muscle tone of all the abdominal compressors is deeply involved in the business of parturition, particularly the tone of the pelvic floor, and the contraction of the diaphragm and abdominal muscles during the act of "bearing down." The effects of neural blockade on the extrauterine forces of labor are very different from the effects on the involuntary muscle of the myometrium.

Formerly, it was thought that the motor activity of the uterus was dependent on output from its sympathetic supply through the lower seven thoracic segments and that uterine activity would be impaired by blockade of the cord up to the fifth thoracic segment (Greene, 1959). However, subsequent work showed that the uterus is remarkably independent of direct motor innervation, uterine activity being more dependent on humoral factors. Epidural or subarachnoid blockade up to the sixth and even the second thoracic segment appears to have no direct effect on uterine tone or on the frequency and intensity of contraction, provided that blood pressure and uterine blood flow are kept within normal limits (Alvarez et al., 1959; Vasicka and Kretchmer, 1961; Vasicka et al., 1964). A recent study of intrauterine pressures by Hon and his colleagues has challenged this view, suggesting that quite modest epidural doses of lidocaine of 40 to 160 mg depress uterine activity for 10 to 30 minutes. Maternal posture was not specified in this paper, however, and adoption of the supine position could have accounted for the results (Lowensohn et al., 1974).

Normal progress in the second stage of unstimulated labor is largely dependent on strong expulsive efforts by the diaphragm and abdominal muscles, combined with a nicely balanced tone in the levator ani and other pelvic muscles that form the pelvic gutter through which the descending head rotates. Premature loss of tone in these extrauterine muscles will modify or delay progress through poor expulsive efforts or failure of rotation. Motor blockade of the lower abdomen and pelvic floor is therefore to be avoided in "natural" unstimulated labor, and successful epidural technique hinges upon the difficult trick of providing sensory analgesia up to the umbilicus, without any appreciable motor paresis. For this reason local anesthetics such as tetracaine or etidocaine that cause profound motor blockade are to be avoided in this situation, whereas drugs that produce relatively little motor block, such as bupivacaine in dilute solution, allow the mother to cooperate actively in the management of her own labor.

Labor may slow down if the perineum is allowed to become anesthetized too early in labor. The exact mechanism underlying this phenomenon is still in doubt, but it is commonly known as the Ferguson reflex. The afferent components of this reflex were thought to come from receptors in the cervix or vagina and pass centrally to stimulate secretion of oxytocin from the posterior pituitary (Ferguson, 1941). Measurements of intrauterine pressure have confirmed that stimuli from cervical dilatation do increase uterine contractility (Fisch et al., 1964) and that effective epidural analgesia impairs the response to cervical dilatation (Sala et al., 1970). However, these studies did not support the idea that oxytocin was the mediator, and some other reflex mechanism is probably responsible. The degree of reflex inhibition caused by deafferentation of the perineum is not at all profound, and it is very readily overcome by small amounts of exogenous oxytocin given as an intravenous infusion (Hingson, 1961; Henry et al., 1967).

In slow incoordinate labors, progress may often be accelerated by induction of satisfactory epidural blockade. As analgesia develops, the patient relaxes and a pattern of weak irregular contractions with high basal tonus gives way to a lower baseline intra-amniotic pressure and regular, more powerful contractions (Alvarez et al., 1959; Moir and Willocks, 1967). The explanation for this change is speculative, but it may be related to the alleviation of pain, anxiety and restlessness, in turn leading to a reduced output of endogenous catecholamines (Garrett, 1954).

Freedom from pain and anxiety is also reflected in the adrenocortical response to labor and in a reduction of maternal work. During normal labor under centrally acting narcotics (e.g., meperidine), 11-hydroxycorticosteroids increase during the first stage of labor and rise to a peak during the second stage, but the response fails to appear when the mother is deafferented by epidural blockade (Buchan et al., 1973). Maternal oxygen consumption falls by about 14 per cent when pain is relieved by an effective epidural block (Sangoul et al., 1975). Using a modification of Grayson's heated thermocouple (Grayson, 1952), Brotanek and his colleagues (1973) have made the interesting observation that cervical blood flow is increased after low-dose epidural blockade in preeclamptic patients. This suggests that the conversion of incoordinate labor to regular progressive contractions by epidural blockade may have its basis in improved uterine blood flow.

In summary, then, neural blockade appears to have no direct depressant effect on uterine contractility, although it may interfere to a minor degree with the progressive reflex increase of contractile force secondary to cervical dilatation, a depression which is very easily overcome by the administration of small amounts of exogenous oxytocin by intravenous infusion. However, the indirect effects of neural blockade on cardiovascular dynamics require very careful consideration, for normal uterine activity is exquisitely dependent on adequate myometrial perfusion, and contractility fades rapidly if uterine perfusion falls off as a result of hypotension or caval compression in the dorsal position (Hon et al., 1960; Vasicka and Kretchmer, 1961; Vasicka et al., 1964; Schellenberg, 1977).

The close interrelationship between the obstructive effects of the gravid uterus, the mother's cardiovascular status and the performance of the uterus and its contents must constantly be kept in mind. It is clear that measurements of uterine activity and maternal cardiovascular status will vary according to the posture in which they are taken. Cardiac output and uterine perfusion and contractility will be optimal when measured with the patient on her side and worst when measured under conditions of caval compression with the mother lying on her back (Ueland and Hansen, 1969). The whole literature on the subject of uterine activity and fetal performance and the effects of anesthesia becomes hopelessly confused unless this key question of posture is applied to the data. Selwyn Crawford has coined the terms "revealed caval occlusion" and "concealed caval occlusion" as a reminder of the constant hidden cardiovascular hazard of the unmodified supine position. Even if caval compression is not revealed by a fall of maternal blood pressure, it is still there, reducing uteroplacental perfusion and compromising the fetus whenever the mother lies in the supine position (Crawford et al., 1972).

EFFECTS OF SYSTEMIC ABSORPTION OF EPIDURAL DRUGS ON PARTURITION

Throughout every aspect of epidural analgesia there is the recurring problem of the dual effects of neural blockade and vascular absorption and the undetermined proportional role that each plays in the final clinical picture. Twenty years ago the matter was not at all clear, since the means to measure the two components did not exist. However, it was intuitively obvious that patients would probably benefit from a philosophy of therapeutic parsimony through the cultivation of techniques that pared dosages down to a bare essential minimum. Today, methods are available to measure maternal and fetal concentrations of absorbed local anesthetics with considerable accuracy, and it is clear that these drugs are much more depressing to the baby than to the uterus and that they depress the baby a great deal more than had been supposed.

In vitro studies of the motility of gravid human uterine muscle have shown that low concentrations of local anesthetic have a net stimulating effect. McCaughey and his colleagues found an 8 per cent increase in contractility in the presence of a lidocaine concentration of 2 μg/ml, and levels of this order are very often found in maternal blood during epidural analgesia (McCaughey et al., 1962; Morishima et al., 1966; Shnider and Way, 1968a, 1968b; Fox and Houle, 1969; Lurie and Weiss, 1970; Fox et al., 1971). Much higher concentrations of about 90 μg/ml of lidocaine were needed before any appreciable uterine depression could be demonstrated in vitro. Bupivacaine in clinical concentrations also seems to have little effect on uterine contractility. Tyack and his colleagues (1973) investigated the influence of epidural analgesia with bupivacaine on uterine performance but found no correlation between plasma bupivacaine concentrations and uterine activity.

In the clinical situation moderately large epidural doses of the order of 350 mg of lidocaine may depress uterine activity for 10 to 30 minutes (Vasicka and Kretchmer, 1961; Vasicka et al., 1964), although in my experience smaller doses of 80 to 150 mg will not do this, provided the patient is lying on her side to prevent any hypotensive effects. More recently, Greiss et al. (1976) have recalled attention to McCaughey's earlier observation that modest concentrations of local anesthetics may increase uterine contractility. Greiss's observations in sheep and humans suggest that while correct epidural technique is not likely to influence uterine motility, accidental intravenous injections may well give rise to transient peak concentrations of local anesthetic that cause uterine vasoconstriction and increased uterine tonus, with consequent fetal hypoxia from depressed uteroplacental perfusion (Greiss et al., 1976).

Thus, while the pharmacological picture is complex, the clinical message is simple. Good technique with low anesthetic dosage is unlikely to influence uterine activity. However, large doses of local anesthetic, and especially large surges from accidental intravenous injection, may cause transient falls of placental perfusion with consequent fetal distress.

Epinephrine in Epidural Solutions

A considerable amount of controversy has centered around the question of whether epinephrine should or should not be added to epidural solutions in obstetrical situations. On the one hand, there is the advantage to the baby that epinephrine will reduce vascular absorption in the mother by about 20 to 30 per cent (Bromage and Robson, 1961) and spare the fetus unnecessarily high concentrations of local anesthetic; on the other hand, there is the fear that epinephrine absorption will lead to inefficient uterine action and prolonged labor.

In 1925, Rucker noticed that caudal anesthesia usually slowed labor when 330 μg of epinephrine in a concentration of 1/200,000 was added to the anesthetic solution, but labor was unaffected when the epinephrine was omitted, and he attributed this to a direct inhibiting effect of epinephrine on the uterine muscle. Rucker's conclusion was later confirmed by Kaiser and Harris (1950), who showed that a similar depressant action occurred when 200 to 500 μg of epinephrine was given by intramuscular injection or by intravenous infusion at rates of 2.5 to 5.0 μg/min.

Others have since confirmed the depressant action of epinephrine in doses of 5 to 10 μg/min. These doses are sufficient to double the resting plasma level of epinephrine, but their effects are reversible by beta receptor blockade with very small amounts of propranolol (Garrett, 1954; Zuspan et al., 1962; Barden and Stander, 1968).

However, when the concentration of epinephrine does not exceed 1/200,000 (i.e., 5 μg/ml) and epidural doses are restricted to minimal volumes of 4 to 6 ml (Bromage, 1961; Hehre, 1965), the amount of catecholamine is only about one tenth of that used by Rucker, and this is not likely to depress uterine activity to a significant degree.

It is worth noting that Rucker's original observation of the depressant effects of epinephrine on labor were made during caudal analgesia, and his results were hardly surprising, for the depressant effects are always more likely to be seen with caudal blocks than with lumbar epidurals, simply because a much larger volume of solution and mass of drug is needed by the caudal route. Gunther and Bauman (1969) also found a very significant prolongation of the first stage by the addition of 1/200,000 epinephrine to the caudal solutions, but the amounts were very large, commencing with an induction dose of 150 μg of epinephrine. In contrast, Craft and his colleagues (1972) found a very slight and transient depressant effect when the dose of epinephrine was restricted to 40 to 50 μg by the lumbar epidural route. It is not the route of injection itself that makes the difference but the size of the dose that is needed by that route.

My personal view is that epinephrine should be added to all local anesthetics that are likely to give rise to appreciable concentrations in the fetus. This includes such agents as lidocaine and mepivacaine. The position of bupivacaine is more debatable, as the protein-binding capacity of this drug is so high that very little circulating free base is left available to be transferred across the placenta to the fetus, so the need for epinephrine would appear to be less pressing than for other agents with lower protein-binding capabilities. However, published data suggest that even in the case of bupivacaine, maternal and fetal blood concentrations are lowest when epinephrine is added (Thomas et al., 1969a; Reynolds and Taylor, 1971; Hyman and Shnider, 1971; Reynolds et al., 1973), as can be seen from Figure 9–15 in Chapter 9.

LOCAL ANESTHETIC UPTAKE IN THE FETUS

The effects of local anesthetics on the fetal cardiovascular system are harmful and complex. The picture is somewhat analogous to the effects of hypercapnia on the adult cardiovascular system in that the toxic agent is directly depressant to the isolated and denervated cardiovascular system, but neurally mediated vasopressor reflexes may compensate in the intact animal, resulting in a net rise of blood pressure and an *apparent* stimulation of the cardiovascular system.

The isolated human fetal heart is measurably depressed by quite low concentrations of local anesthetic (Andersson et al., 1970a). However, higher concentrations of local anesthetic in intact animal preparations cause a brief vasostimulant effect by epileptiform stimulation of the fetal brain. At term, blood concentrations of lidocaine in excess of 7.0 μg/ml result in phasic rises of blood pressure associated with strong bursts of electrical activity in the fetal brain and convulsive respiratory movements (Teramo et al., 1974). The threshold concentration of local anesthetic necessary to produce this type of convulsive activity falls with advancing gestational age, suggesting that the phenomenon is dependent on maturation of the fetal brain and the development of reflex pathways (Teramo et al., 1976). Fetal convulsions are associated with a rapid fall of arterial pH, and this in turn leads to even greater depression of the myocardium (Andersson et al., 1970b). A vicious circle is set up in which the depressant effects of acidosis and circulating local anesthetic combine and accentuate one another, and the degree of depression is dependent on the amount of free local anesthetic circulating in the fetus.

All local anesthetics and their products pass across the placenta to a greater or lesser degree, depending on their physicochemical nature, as discussed in Chapter 3 on Pharmacology. Blood concentrations during epidural analgesia are usually found to be highest in the mother, somewhat lower in the umbilical vein and lowest in the umbilical artery, as shown in Figure 12–10. Measurements of blood concentrations of local anesthetic in the mother and baby, by gas chromatography, give an estimate of the amount of drug that crosses the placenta, but from the point of view of fetal depression, the important and much more difficult measurement is not the *total* concen-

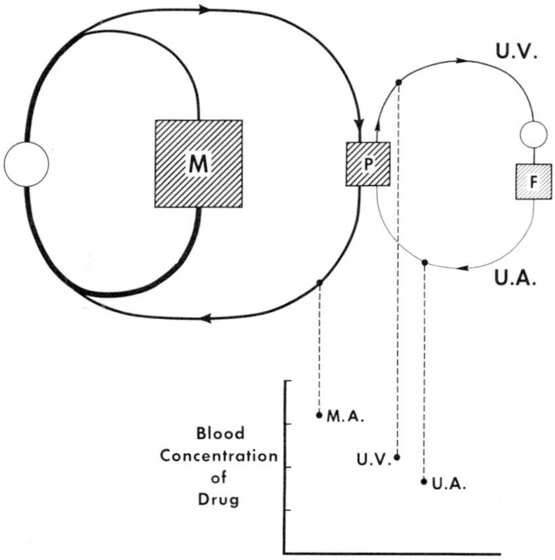

Figure 12–10. Placental transfer of local anesthetics during epidural analgesia. Diagrammatic representation of maternal (M), placental (P) and fetal (F) circulations and of relative drug concentrations found in maternal artery, umbilical vein and umbilical artery under clinical conditions.

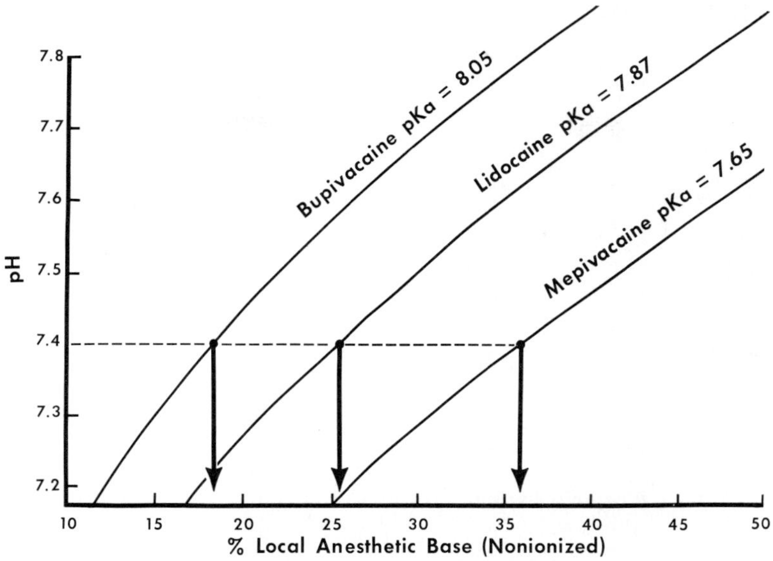

Figure 12–11. Placental transfer of local anesthetics related to pKa, ionization and pH. Comparison of bupivacaine, lidocaine and mepivacaine showing relative proportions of free base available for diffusion across the placenta at pH 7.4.

tration of drug in the baby but the concentration of free cation available in the fetal circulation (Tucker et al., 1970b). Thus, some knowledge of ionization constants, drug binding and differential binding in mother and fetus is crucial before any set of *total* concentrations presented by the gas chromatograph can be given clinical meaning by translating them into what is actually happening in terms of free active cation in the baby. A high blood concentration in the baby would be relatively inconsequential if all the circulating drug was safely bound to plasma proteins and so rendered inactive; on the other hand, a very small concentration might have disproportionate significance if none of it was bound and all the local anesthetic was free to work its depressant effects.

It will be remembered that free uncharged base is necessary to penetrate membranes, so the amount of available free base at any given pH is related to the pKa of the drug. Figure 12–11 shows the calculated percentage of free base related to pH for bupivacaine, lidocaine and mepivacaine. It can be seen that at any given pH, bupivacaine will have the least amount of base available for transfer, and mepivacaine will have the most. Thus, at pH 7.4, bupivacaine will have approximately 18 per cent base, lidocaine 26 per cent and mepivacaine 36 per cent. From this information alone, one might guess that mepivacaine would not be the best choice for regional analgesia in obstetrics, while bupivacaine would probably be a good agent.

Different degrees of protein binding in maternal and fetal blood also have profound effects, both on transfer across the placenta and on the amount of free drug available in the fetal circulation. Figure 12–12, taken from the classic paper by Tucker and his colleagues (1970b), shows the relative degrees of protein binding for local anesthetic agents in maternal and fetal blood. It can be seen that in maternal blood very little unbound

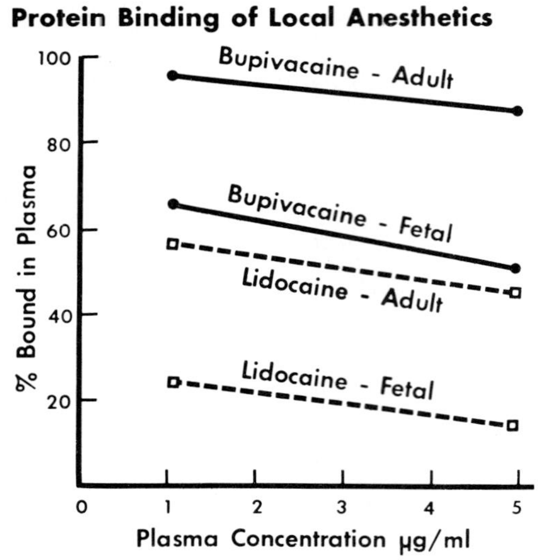

Figure 12–12. Placental transfer of local anesthetics. Relative proportions of bupivacaine and lidocaine bound to plasma proteins in adult and fetal blood at concentrations between 1 and 5 μg/ml. (After Tucker et al., 1970b.)

bupivacaine is available for placental transfer. However, once any of the local anesthetics pass the placenta, they immediately become less bound in the fetal blood and therefore relatively more toxic than in the adult circulation, as shown in Figure 12–13. There are at least two reasons for this important difference in binding capabilities on the two sides of the placenta. First, there are quantitative, and possibly qualitative, differences in the protein fractions, and

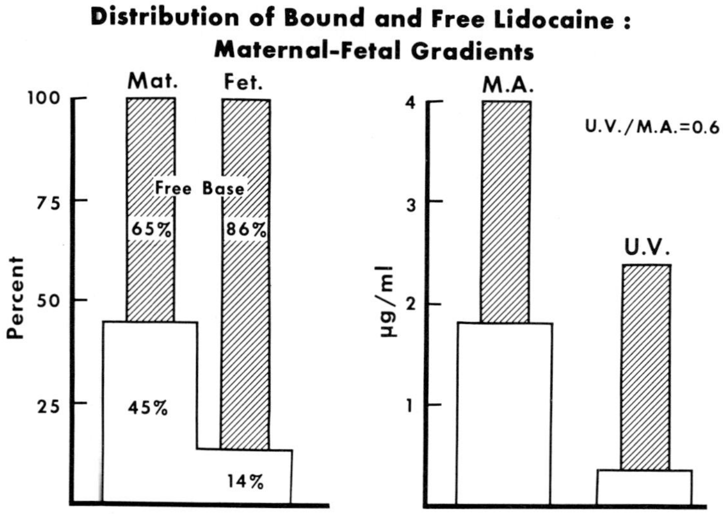

Figure 12–13. Relative toxicity of local anesthetics in maternal and fetal blood. Approximate distribution of bound and free lidocaine in adult and fetal plasma, assuming an umbilical vein/maternal artery ratio of 0.6.

□ Bound base
▨ Free base

Although the *total* concentration of lidocaine is less in the umbilical vein than in the maternal artery, the smaller degree of protein binding in fetal plasma leaves relatively more *free* unbound and pharmacologically active base available in the baby, and the real toxicity is equivalent in mother and fetus. (Data from Tucker et al., 1970b.)

TABLE 12–1 Peak Concentrations of Lidocaine in Maternal and Fetal Guinea Pig Blood and Tissues after Administration of Lidocaine, 10 mg/kg IV, to the Mother*

	Mother		*Fetus*	
Organ	*CONCⁿ OF LIDOCAINE (μg/g)*	*RATIO TISSUE CONCⁿ / BLOOD CONCⁿ*	*CONCⁿ OF LIDOCAINE (μg/g)*	*RATIO TISSUE CONCⁿ / BLOOD CONCⁿ*
Blood	7.6	–	3.6	–
Heart	17.2	2.26	8.9	2.5
Liver	7.8	1.03	22.9	6.36
Brain	31.9	4.2	9.7	2.7

*Data from Finster et al. (1972).

there are greater amounts of globulin, especially alpha-2 globulin, in the maternal blood (Mather et al., 1971). Second, the number of binding sites in fetal plasma is reduced by competition from bilirubin, which exists in higher concentrations in the fetus than in the adult (Chignell et al., 1971).

Ultimately, the toxic effects of a drug are due to its concentration and action at the tissue level rather than in the blood stream. Tissue concentration depends on the partition coefficient of the drug between blood and tissue and on the rate of tissue perfusion, the uptake being greatest in highly perfused organs. Finster and his colleagues (1972) showed that surprisingly high tissue concentrations of local anesthetic could be demonstrated in the fetal guinea pig after intravenous administration to the mother, with the greatest amounts in the fetal liver, an organ with exceptionally high perfusion rates. Some of Finster's results are summarized in Table 12–1. It can be seen that measurements of blood concentration give little indication of the tissue concentrations, some of which are three to four times higher than the blood level. For reasons discussed in Chapter 3, it will be apparent that fetal tissue uptake of local anesthetic will rise with increasing degrees of fetal acidosis, and this is a strong reason for enquiring into the effects of epidural analgesia on acid-base balance, as we will do later in this chapter.

Agents with ester linkages in their molecule, such as procaine and 2-chloroprocaine, are broken down by esterases in the blood stream, and they do not cross the placenta in appreciable amounts unless very large doses are given (Usubiaga et al., 1968). Although 2-chloroprocaine is short-acting, its rapid breakdown makes it appear to be a very safe agent from the point of view of avoiding fetal depression (Foldes and Rhodes, 1953).

Maternal Uptake and Maternal/Fetal Blood Concentration Ratios

Since 1966 a large number of papers have been published on the epidural uptake and placental transfer of regional anesthetics, both in normal labor and at cesarean section, and correlations have been made between blood levels of local anesthetic and fetal performance in terms of Apgar scores and the time lapse between birth and the onset of regular sustained respiration. In addition, material from abortion programs in Scandinavia has made it possible to study the direct action of local anesthetics on the human heart (Andersson et al., 1970a, 1970b; Gennser et al., 1972).

Lidocaine, mepivacaine and bupivacaine have been the most intensely investigated agents. Morishima and her colleagues presented an early series in 1966 in which mepivacaine was used in quite large doses up to 600 mg for caudal analgesia. Moore and his associates also measured blood concentrations in caudal analgesia and found that with repeated injections a steadily increasing accumulation of drug occurred in mother and fetus; it should be noted that large total doses of 900 to 1480 mg were also used in this caudal series (Moore et al., 1968). Later, the same group studied bupivacaine in continuous caudals and again found a cumulative rise in the mother, but with this agent fetal blood concentrations were extremely low (Moore et al., 1970). Most authors are agreed that bupivacaine gives rise to low fetal blood levels with relatively little cumulative effect (Thomas, Climie and Mather, 1969a; Reynolds and Taylor, 1970; Hyman and Shnider, 1971; Geerinckx et al., 1974; Belfrage et al., 1975; Magno et al., 1976).

Thomas and his colleagues (1969b) showed that lidocaine uptake was appreciably reduced in parturient women by adding epinephrine 1/250,000 to the epidural solution, as shown in Table 12–2. With an epidural dose of 400 mg of lidocaine, epinephrine reduced peak maternal venous concentrations by 23.6 per cent and peak umbilical vein concentrations by about 15 per cent. Shnider made an extensive study of the pharmacokinetics of lidocaine in labor in a series of papers in 1968, and he found that umbilical vein concentrations seldom rose above 3.0 μg/ml, even with total maternal doses as high as 8.5 mg/kg. Fetal performance was unimpaired in all cases in which the umbilical vein concentration of lidocaine was below 2.5 μg/ml, but low Apgar scores were found in four infants with umbilical vein levels between 2.6 and 4.0 μg/ml (Shnider and Way, 1968b). Fox and Houle at the Royal Victoria Hospital, Montreal, showed that when careful dose regimens were used, both lidocaine hydrochloride and carbonated lidocaine gave acceptably low fetal blood levels in single-shot injections for cesarean section and in continuous administration for vaginal delivery (Fox and Houle, 1969; Fox et al., 1971).

Prilocaine has had a fairly extensive trial for epidural analgesia in labor (Poppers et al., 1966; Poppers and Finster, 1968; Climie et al., 1967). However, prilocaine tends to cause methemoglobinemia in the baby, so it is probably unsuitable for obstetrical practice.

Etidocaine appears to behave similarly to bupivacaine, and it gives rise to very low concentrations in the baby. In a small series of my own in

TABLE 12–2 Influence of Epinephrine 1/250,000 on Epidural Uptake of Lidocaine in Parturient Women after Lumbar Injection of 400 mg Lidocaine*

	Lidocaine Plain	*Lidocaine + Epinephrine (μg/ml)*	*Δ Percentage with Epinephrine*
Peak maternal venous concentration	3.43	2.62	−23.6
Peak umbilical vein concentration	1.56	1.33	−14.74

*Data from Thomas et al. (1969b).

which single-shot doses of 140 to 225 mg were used for cesarean section, the average maternal venous concentration of etidocaine was 0.45 μg/ml, and the umbilical vein concentration was only 0.16 μg/ml: an umbilical vein/maternal (UV/M) ratio of 0.35 (Bromage et al., 1974).

The foregoing mass of data is somewhat heterogeneous since the clinical protocols of the numerous investigations were often varied both between drugs and within groups. All one can usefully do to synthesize these findings is to summarize a number of them in a very loose way, as has been done in Table 12–3, so that the reader can pick out a few salient points for himself. The information compiled in Table 12–3 has been presented in a very condensed form, without including the period of time over which the anesthesia was administered, as this important variable was often missing from the original data. Nevertheless, a number of points emerge:

1. Maternal and fetal blood levels are a function of the total dose administered to the mother; the larger the cumulative dose, the higher the blood levels in mother and baby.

2. From the data by Thomas et al. (1968) and Epstein et al. (1968), it can be seen that epinephrine reduces uptake by the mother even when bupivacaine is used (Hyman and Shnider, 1971); with plain lidocaine maternal blood levels are about 30 per cent higher and fetal concentrations 12 to 17 per cent higher than when epinephrine is added.

3. Caudal block requires large amounts of local anesthetic, and blood concentrations in mother and child are likely to be higher than after lumbar epidural analgesia.

4. The ratio of fetal to maternal concentration is different with different agents. With lidocaine and mepivacaine, the ratio of umbilical vein to maternal vein concentration (UV/M) is about 0.6. With prilocaine, more drug passes into the fetus and the ratio rises to about 1.0 to 1.2. On the other hand, bupivacaine has a very low UV/M ratio of about 0.2 to 0.4. This reflects the stronger degree of protein binding that inhibits the placental transfer of bupivacaine. A comparable gradient between fetal blood and fetal tissues is seen, once the drugs pass the placenta, and Hollmén (1973) has shown that the fetal tissue/blood ratio for bupivacaine is about one half that for lidocaine. Thus, in terms of minimal uptake by fetal tissues, bupivacaine appears to be a remarkably safe agent.

5. The data from Fox and Houle's four studies on analgesia in labor, as practiced at the Royal Victoria Hospital, Montreal, show that a low-dose regimen gives rise to very low maternal and fetal concentrations. Under these conditions, with average umbilical vein concentrations of lidocaine of less than 1.0 μg/ml, it is extremely unlikely that any degree of fetal depression can be attributed to the local anesthetic (Fig. 12–14) (Houle et al., 1971).

Thus, the published evidence bears out what has been said earlier: doses should be kept as small as possible, and the use of epinephrine and the avoidance of caudal blocks will contribute to this goal. Figure 12–15 shows the relationship between maternal venous and umbilical venous blood concentrations with four anesthetic techniques. The data points from each series are enclosed in a separate ellipse. The smallest ellipse is from a series of vaginal deliveries with lidocaine hydrochloride (Houle et al., 1971). The next ellipse, with a

TABLE 12-3 Placental Transfer of Local Anesthetics in Lumbar Epidural and Caudal Blockade During Labor

Authors	Anesthetic Agents	Dose (mg)	Maternal Plasma Conc[n] at Delivery ($\mu g/ml$)		Umbilical Vein (or Cord) Concentration ($\mu g/ml$)		UV/MA
			RANGE	MEAN	RANGE	MEAN	
Lumbar epidurals							
1. Schnider and Way (1968b)	Lidocaine + epinephrine	8.15 mg/kg	0.2–5.5	2.7	0.4–3.4	1.3	0.5
2. Thomas, Climie and Mather (1968)	Lidocaine plain	540 (100–900)	1.48–4.52	2.53	0.6–2.02	2.7	0.5
	Lidocaine + epinephrine	490 (300–1070)	1.10–4.68	2.75	1.0–4.28	1.72	0.6
3. Thomas et al. (1969b)	Lidocaine plain	400	1.85–5.95	3.43	1.10–2.85	1.56	0.45
	Lidocaine + epinephrine	400	1.45–3.9	2.62	0.65–2.48	1.33	0.5
4. Epstein et al. (1968)	Lidocaine plain	502 ± 218	0–6.7	2.6	0–3.6	1.8	0.7
	Lidocaine + epinephrine	424 ± 169	0–3.7	1.7	0–3.5	1.6	0.9
	Prilocaine plain 1.5%	447 ± 188	0–3.6	1.4	0–6.2	1.7	1.2
5. Hehre et al. (1969)	Prilocaine plain 2%	564 ± 250	0–5.0	1.5	0–3.4	1.5	1.0
	Lidocaine 2% + epinephrine	129 mg/hour	–	1.23 ± 0.09	–	0.80 ± 0.06	0.65
	Prilocaine 2% + epinephrine	129 mg/hour	–	1.03 ± 0.07	–	1.07 ± 0.14	1.04
6. Lurie and Weiss (1970)	Mepivacaine plain	396 (165–1025)	1.2–3.6	2.2	0.9–2.9	1.6	0.7
	Lidocaine plain	367 (135–930)	0.95–3.4	2.2	0.7–2.6	1.55	0.7
7. Fox and Houle (1969)	Lidocaine + epinephrine	315 ± 36	0.5–2.4	1.39	0.4–1.4	0.83	0.6
8. Houle et al. (1971)	Lidocaine-CO_2 + epinephrine	297 ± 31	1.0–2.6	1.93	0–2.0	0.91	0.4

9. Houle et al. (1971)	Lidocaine HCl + epinephrine	326 ± 141	–	1.3 ± 0.5	–	0.73 ± 0.4	0.5
	Lidocaine-CO_2 + epinephrine	251 ± 97	–	1.1 ± 0.5	–	0.64 ± 0.4	0.6
10. Fox et al. (1971)	Lidocaine + epinephrine	319 ± 132	–	–	–	0.84 ± 0.35	
11. Scanlon et al. (1974)	Mepivacaine	–	–	–	0.29–5.8	1.68	
12. Thomas et al. (1969a)	Bupivacaine + epinephrine	50–150	0.12–0.41	0.25	0.04–0.25	0.11	0.45
13. Reynolds and Taylor (1970)	Bupivacaine + epinephrine	120.9 (50–645)	0.10–0.76	0.26	0.02–0.25	0.077	0.3
	Lidocaine + epinephrine	860.8 (120–1875)	0.25–2.13	1.81	0.16–1.86	1.00	0.5
14. Bromage, Datta and Dunford (1974)	Etidocaine + epinephrine	185		0.45		0.16	0.35
Caudal Block							
15. Morishima et al. (1966)	1.5% Mepivacaine plain (single injection)	3.5–7.2 mg/kg	2.0–5.0	2.91	0.5–3.6	1.90	0.7
	1.5% Mepivacaine plain (continuous)	4.4–9.4 mg/kg	1.0–8.6	3.90	0.8–4.5	2.68	0.7
16. Moore et al. (1968)	1.5% Mepivacaine plain (continuous)	900–1480	3.9–8.6	6.94	2.5–7.9	4.9	0.7
17. Poppers and Finster (1968)	Prilocaine plain	195–1650	0.4–2.7	1.2	0.5–2.3	1.3	1.1
18. Moore et al. (1970, 1971)	Bupivacaine plain	125–260	0.22–0.80	–	0.06–0.24	–	–
19. Hyman and Shnider (1971)	Bupivacaine plain	82.9 (50–105)	0.04–0.72	0.39	0.02–0.17	0.098	0.26
	Bupivacaine + epinephrine	96.4 (48–160)	0.05–0.44	0.24	0.01–0.25	0.082	0.38

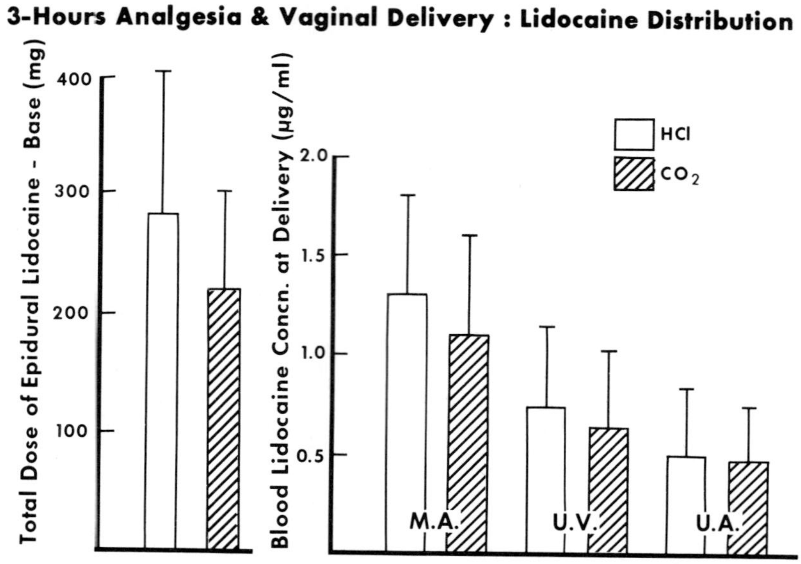

Figure 12–14. Blood concentrations of local anesthetic with low-dose regimen for epidural analgesia in labor. Maternal and fetal concentrations of lidocaine base at delivery after three hours of analgesia (means ± S.D.) With hydrochloride (❑) or carbonated (▨) salts of lidocaine. (After Houle et al., 1972.)

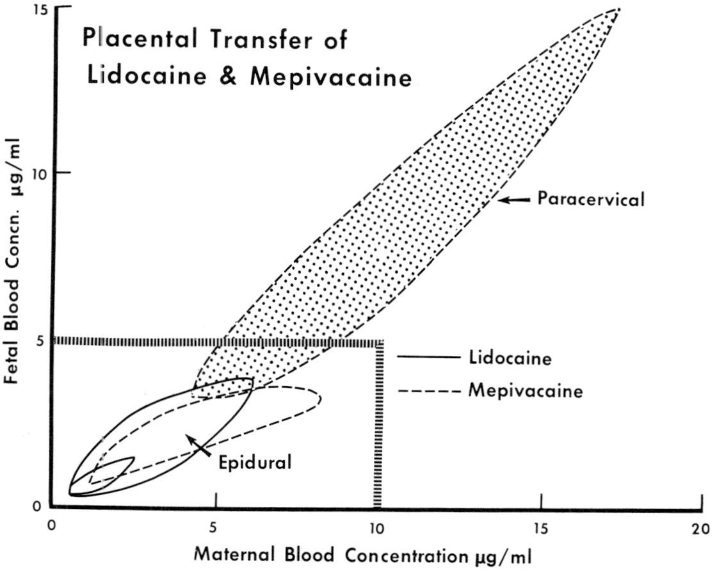

Figure 12–15. Maternal and fetal blood concentrations of local anesthetic after epidural or paracervical block. Ellipses enclose data from three epidural and one paracervical series.

——— = Lidocaine

– – – – = Mepivacaine

Barred rectangle outlines toxic limits. Smallest ellipse (lidocaine) from Houle et al. (1971). Larger ellipse (lidocaine) from unpublished data in long labors by Bromage and Crowell (1961–1965). Dotted epidural ellipse (mepivacaine) from caudal analgesia (Morishima et al., 1966.) Largest ellipse (mepivacaine) from paracervical blocks (Gordon, 1968).

solid outline, is an earlier unpublished series of long labors collected between 1961 and 1965 which were studied by using the colorimetric methyl orange method of assay (Bromage and Crowell, unpublished data). The next and dotted ellipse encloses data by Morishima et al. (1966) from caudals with mepivacaine. The largest ellipse is shown for interest and comparison, and it is drawn around data from paracervical blocks (Gordon, 1968). A barred line encloses the toxic limits for adults and newborns, based on data from my own series, which showed tolerances somewhat higher than those found by Shnider and Way (1968b) in their newborns. It can be seen that small-dose lumbar epidurals stay well within the prescribed boundaries, as illustrated by the smallest ellipse from the series by Houle et al. (1971).

This figure should not be taken to imply an outright condemnation of paracervical block, but only to show that it *may* give rise to very high fetal blood levels. Paracervical block requires scrupulous technique and minimal dosage of 40 to 50 mg of lidocaine on each side, to avoid the risk of high fetal concentrations (Gomez, 1969), and it is not a good choice in the presence of existing fetal distress (Shnider and Gildea, 1973).

In summary, undoubtedly the last word has not yet been heard on the subject of local anesthetic depression of the fetus. There is good evidence that local anesthetics, like all other depressant drugs, may impair fetal cardiovascular performance. In vitro, human hearts taken from 14- to 28-week aborted fetuses (21 to 28 cm crown-to-heel length) are significantly depressed by concentrations of local anesthetic that are commonly achieved under clinical conditions (Andersson et al., 1970a). Gennser and his colleagues (1972) measured the contractile force of human papillary muscle from fetuses of 21 to 28 cm heel-to-crown length and found a 20 per cent reduction with mepivacaine concentrations as low as 0.625 μg/ml at contraction frequencies of 120 per minute. Increasing the concentration of mepivacaine to 2.5 μg/ml did not cause any appreciable difference, as shown in Figure 12–16, but a further increase of concentration to 10 μg/ml produced a marked reduction of papillary muscle force.

Measurements of blood concentrations of local anesthetic and existing data from Apgar scores and the interval from birth to the time of sustained respiration (TSR) give no reason to suppose that contemporary low-dosage epidural techniques, properly managed, cause any detectable impairment of fetal performance. However, more refined neurobehavioral measurements, such as Brazelton's behavior assessment scale (Brazelton, 1973), may reveal changes of considerable interest that are not evident from simpler but less sensitive tests. Brackbill et al. (1974) and Scanlon et al. (1974) have applied the Brazelton scale to newborns after epidural births in two independent studies, and Scanlon has suggested the syndrome of the "floppy but alert" child born after epidural block, as opposed to the "floppy and disorientated" child born after centrally acting narcotics are given to the mother. In Scanlon's paper it should be noted that two of the babies included in their "floppy but alert" series had relatively high blood concentrations of mepivacaine, with umbilical artery levels of 3 μg/ml and 5.8 μg/ml, respectively. In the case of the second child, quite a large dose of mepivacaine (605 mg) had been given to the mother in the presence of significant maternal acidosis (pH 7.30), and the maternal venous concentration of mepivacaine at birth was 5.17

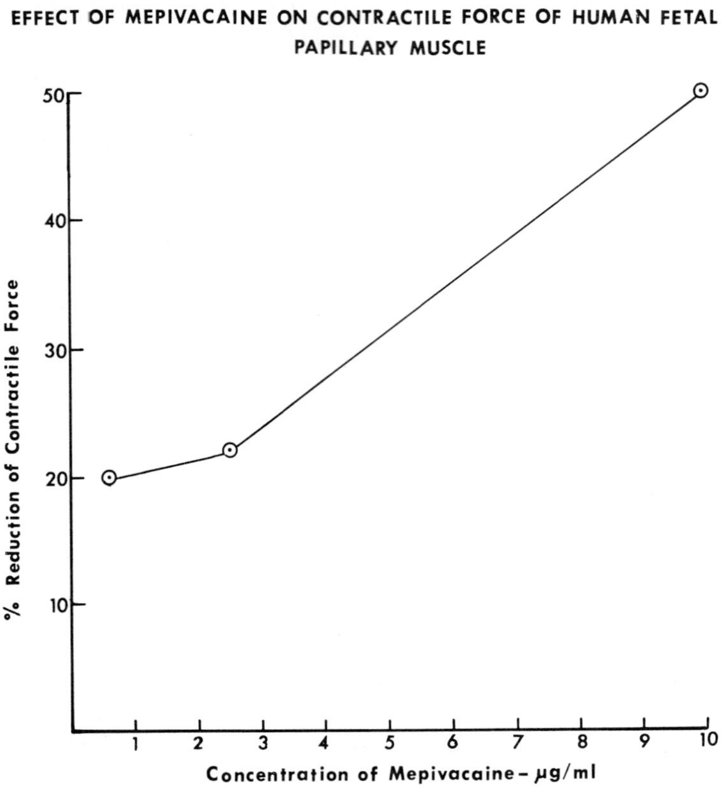

Figure 12–16. Effect of increasing concentrations of mepivacaine on contractile force of human fetal papillary muscle (age 14 to 28 weeks) at constant pH in range 7.32 to 7.41. Frequency of contractions: 120/min. (After Gennser et al., 1972.)

μg/ml, indicating considerable maternal uptake (Scanlon, 1974). In the light of Shnider and Way's data mentioned earlier, these are higher levels than one would normally wish to see, and they may have contributed to the overall picture of "floppy but alert" babies.

Neurobehavioral examinations are likely to prove a useful new tool for assessing the outcome of obstetrical and anesthetic practice, carrying on where the Apgar score leaves off. However, a sense of proportion must be preserved in their use, and results should not be overinterpreted without careful control of the major determinants of fetal well-being. For example, one statistical study using the Brazelton scale concluded that infants born by local-regional analgesia were less well coordinated than those born without analgesia, but the conclusions were reached without any supporting data involving other major factors, such as ease of labor, maternal posture and hydration, and fetal blood gases (Standley et al., 1974).

The suspicion that certain amide-type local anesthetics may possibly cause occult degrees of neonatal depression reopens the question of a return to short-lived ester-type agents, such as 2-chloroprocaine, in spite of the practical disadvantages inherent in short-acting local anesthetics. However, more extensive research into neurobehavioral patterns is needed before any definite policy along these lines can be given rational support.

PROGRESS OF LABOR AND TIMING OF EPIDURAL ANALGESIA

The effects of epidural analgesia on labor can only be assessed relatively by measuring the progress of labor against some standard. Since 1955, Friedman's cervimetric curves using cervical dilatation plotted against time as the measure of progress have been the generally accepted yardstick (Friedman, 1955, 1956). Friedman described four phases of dilatation during the first stage of labor: a latent phase up to about 2 cm dilatation, followed by a short, steeply rising acceleration phase, which then tapers off into a phase of "maximum slope," and then a deceleration phase between 8 and 10 cm dilatation. Friedman curves are shown for normal primigravidas and multigravidas in Figure 12–17. His analysis gave the following norms for the duration of normal unstimulated labor:

	First Stage	***Second Stage***	***Total Duration* (hours)**
Primigravida	13.3	0.95	14.25
Multigravida	7.73	0.29	8.0

These curves have been criticized by Hendricks and his colleagues as being unduly formalized, since very few women have zero dilatation during the last few days preceding labor (Hendricks et al., 1970). Nevertheless, Friedman's curves have played a most helpful role as a basis for measurement until stimulated labor became regular practice, and they were a useful guide for deciding the proper time for induction of epidural analgesia in unstimulated labor. Since the latent phase is often painless and progress sometimes doubtful, there has been a tendency in the past to delay induction of epidural analgesia until contractions became strong and painful in the phase of acceleration at about 4 cm dilatation. By this time, spontaneous labor is confidently established and it is reasonable to maintain blockade by intermittent epidural injection until full dilatation and delivery.

Before oxytocin infusion became generally accepted, the more conservative obstetricians would tend to blame all delays upon the epidural anesthetic and a suppressed Ferguson reflex, or worse, there would be a

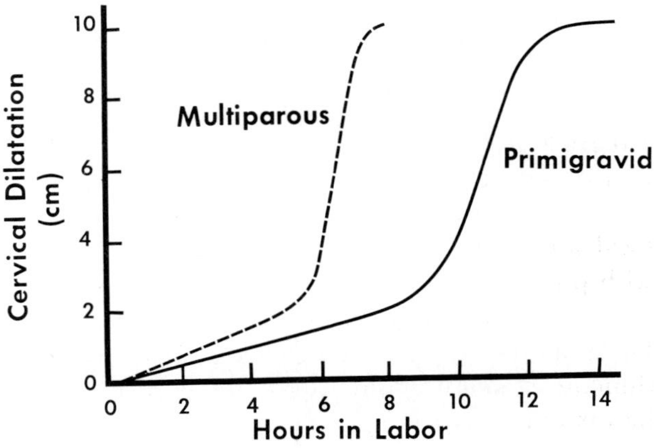

Figure 12–17. Friedman's partographs for the normal progress of labor in primigravid and multiparous births. (After Friedman, 1955, 1956.)

reluctance to embark on the combination of oxytocin infusion and epidural blockade which had been shown to be effective and safe in our department (Henry et al., 1967). This would sometimes lead to an untidy difference of opinion between obstetrician and anesthesiologist, requests being made to allow the block to wear off so that full contractions could return—a shaky course that inevitably causes unnecessarily painful and esthetically displeasing labors. Today, with general acceptance of oxytocin assistance, a better understanding of the active management of labor has come about, and the causes of delay are handled more rationally, with epidural blockade and oxytocin infusions complementing one another rather than being regarded as mutually exclusive (Steel, 1972; Boyd, 1974).

A steadily growing confidence in handling driven labor has enabled elective epidurals to be accepted more readily. Now, instead of always waiting until spontaneous labor becomes established and painful at Friedman's phase of rapid acceleration, it is commonplace to insert a catheter under calm conditions just before the surgical-medical induction of labor. Then, as contractions become painful and the need arises, local anesthetic can be injected and blockade induced without the added technical hazard of a moaning, writhing patient presenting a moving target. Various modifications of Friedman's curves are now in current use as being more applicable to driven labor, and these usually start with a basic cervical dilatation of 2 cm instead of zero.

TECHNIQUE OF EPIDURAL ANALGESIA FOR VAGINAL DELIVERY

Let us review briefly what is required of a good technique:

1. Safety
2. Effective analgesia throughout the painful period of labor; it is illogical and unnecessarily depressing to the fetus to use systemic narcotics and tranquilizers during the first stage and to reserve regional analgesia for the process of delivery
3. No depressant effects on the maternal cardiovascular system
4. No depressant effects on the progress of labor
5. No depressant effects on the baby
6. No after-effects
7. High technical success rate

Of the regional anesthetic options available, lumbar epidural blockade is the only one that comes close to fulfilling all these requirements. Subarachnoid analgesia is only appropriate for delivery at the end of labor, and it cannot be extended safely throughout the first stage.

Paracervical block has a high incidence of fetal bradycardia from local anesthetic absorption (Shnider et al., 1970), and it must be combined with pudendal block or low spinal anesthesia for episiotomy and delivery.

Continuous caudal anesthesia can be made to work, but excessively large amounts of analgesic drug are needed. Moreover, it is technically difficult in many cases, there is an unacceptably high failure rate in many hands and it is carried out in a surgically dirty area subject to fecal soiling.

During active labor the baby's head is close beneath the site of puncture, and intracranial injection is a rare and lethal consequence of pushing the needle too far and at the wrong inclination (Finster et al., 1965). Finally, caudal analgesia is a back-to-front technique for analgesia in spontaneous labor. It provides optimal perineal analgesia and a flaccid perineum at an early stage of labor when both of these factors are preferably avoided, and at the same time large doses of anesthetic are needed to reach the lower abdominal segments where first-stage pain is actually felt. It is an acceptable technique for second-stage pain relief but an irrational technique for analgesia during the first stage.

Many varieties of lumbar epidural technique for obstetrical analgesia have been published, and some of these have been alluded to earlier in this chapter. Some are single-dose injections for delivery only, and many of them use what I consider to be excessively large amounts of local anesthetic. Again, I must reiterate: dosage should be as parsimonious as efficacy will allow. The technique should work to everyone's satisfaction, but the balance is a nice one, and good anesthetic conditions should not have to be bought at the expense of luxuriant and toxic overdosage.

Cleland's original technique came as close as any to rational parsimonious perfection, but for reasons already given it is technically cumbersome, and in most practitioners' hands a single-catheter method is more likely to be successful for routine purposes. Figure 12–18 illustrates the alternatives to Cleland's double-catheter technique: its modification as a "reversed caudal" and a single lumbar epidural catheter using gravity as an aid to directional spread of anesthetic solution during the first and second stages.

Figure 12–19 shows the segmental distribution of blockade achieved during the first and second stages of labor by Cleland's technique and by single-catheter caudal and lumbar blockade. The compromise of the single-catheter lumbar block is less ideal than Cleland's technique, but with proper management its success rate is higher in a large and busy department.

Gravity has a slight but statistically significant effect on epidural spread (Bromage, 1961), and it is reasonable to use appropriate postural changes as an aid to achieving a correct segmental distribution. Thus, patients should be nursed in the lateral position during the first stage with changes from side to side as necessary to ensure even symmetrical spread, and dosage should be small enough to discourage premature downward spread to the sacral segments. It is important to avoid early sacral anesthesia during spontaneous "natural" labor in order to retain an active Ferguson reflex. However, in oxytocin-driven labors premature perineal analgesia is of little consequence.

Procedure

Fetal depression must be avoided. No centrally acting analgesic drugs should be given at any time during labor. All pain relief should be achieved by afferent blockade. The aim is to achieve an effective segmental band of analgesia from T_{10} to L_2 during the first stage of labor in order to embrace the eleventh and twelfth thoracic segments with an adequate margin

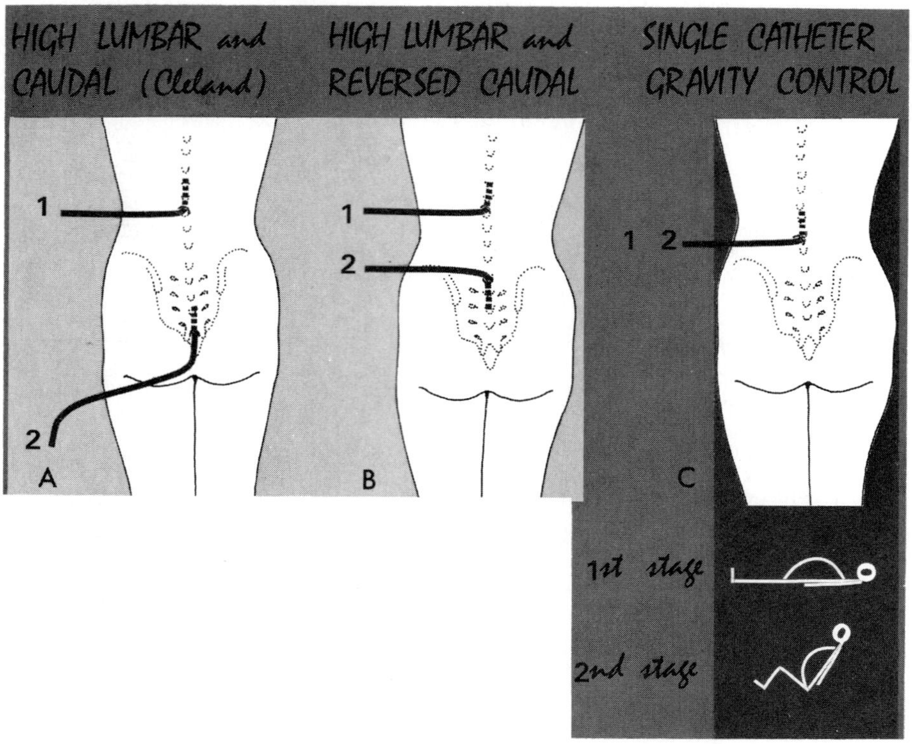

Figure 12–18. Three epidural techniques for relief of pain in labor.
A, Cleland's two-catheter technique, using upper lumbar and caudal catheters.
B, Modification of Cleland's technique, with upper lumbar and "reversed caudal" via lower lumbar catheter directed downward.
C, Single catheter technique at second lumbar interspace (L_2–L_3). Induction in lateral position for first stage pain. Tilted head-up for "perineal dose" at full dilatation.

to spare. For the second stage, analgesia must be extended caudally to include all segments from the tenth thoracic downward.

Before epidural analgesia is induced, an intravenous infusion of glucose-saline is started, and a blood pressure cuff is put in place. All necessary equipment and drugs should be readily available to carry out immediate resuscitation in case of an emergency.

The continuous technique is used almost invariably in preference to the single-injection method. In this way the mother is given the benefits of restful analgesia throughout the active and often exhausting stages of a prolonged labor. I believe that the single-shot method just before delivery is seldom warranted. In precipitous labors analgesia of the perineum can usually be achieved quite adequately by the simpler technique of pudendal nerve block or by subarachnoid saddle block anesthesia. The lumbar catheter may be inserted when labor is clearly established, or before induction if an elective epidural is to be combined with driven labor (Steel, 1972).

The patient is positioned on her side in bed or on the delivery table. The lateral position should be used whenever possible, as it tends to limit downward spread and to favor a narrow band of lower abdominal analgesia from a small induction dose, but in difficult patients with gross

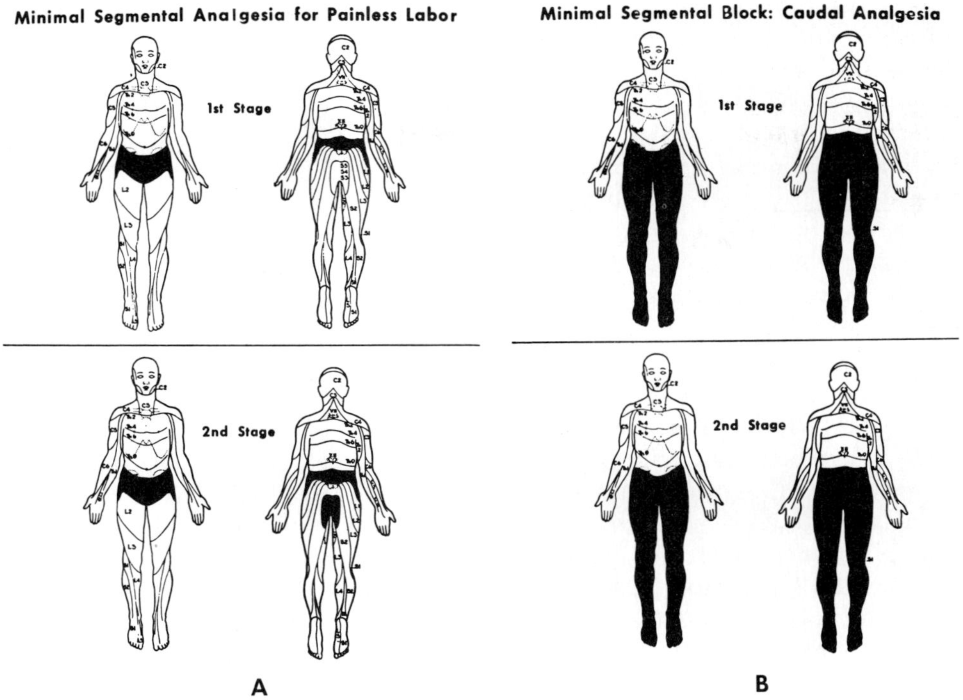

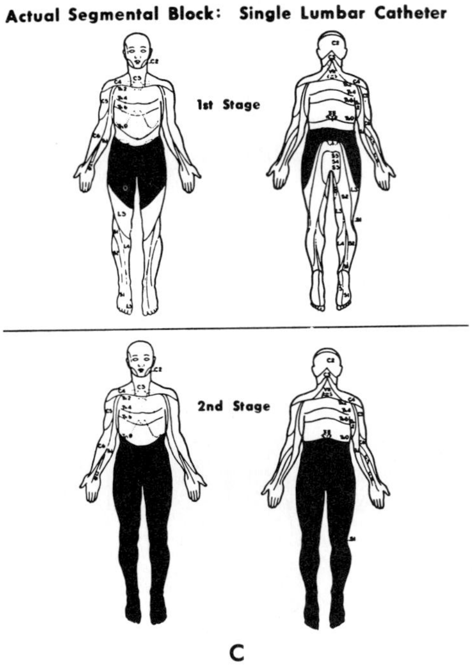

Figure 12–19. Segmental blockade for first and second stages of labor.

A, Cleland's two-catheter technique, requiring the least quantities of local anesthetic. First stage: block of T_{11}–L_1 inclusive. Second stage: T_{11}–L_1 plus S_3, S_4 and S_5. In practice, blockade should extend to include S_2 (not shown in this diagram).

B, Continuous caudal block, requiring inappropriately large quantities of local anesthetic for first-stage pain relief.

C, Single lumbar catheter technique, a satisfactory compromise for effective pain relief in first and second stages, using small doses of local anesthetic.

obesity or scoliosis it is best to abandon this advantage for the assurance of a technically successful puncture and sit the patient up instead. Excessive flexion of the spine around a gravid uterus in the lateral position may lead to just as much inferior vena cava compression as in the supine posture, so great care must be taken to see that the mother is comfortably flexed but not forcibly bent up. Scott has reported a maternal death arising from excessive flexion in the lateral position (Scott, 1972).

A 17-gauge Tuohy needle is inserted in the second or third lumbar interspace with the orifice toward the head, by use of the loss-of-resistance technique. The detailed reasons for these technical moves have already been given in Chapter 6, but they are worth repeating at this point. First, the hanging-drop technique should not be used, as anatomical conditions are least favorable for its success; the loss-of-resistance test should always be used (Galbert and Marx, 1974). Second, there may be a strong temptation to pass the epidural catheter downward in order to favor good sacral analgesia in the second stage. This temptation should be resisted or it will lead to a high incidence of transforaminal escape by the catheter; a catheter is more likely to stay correctly in the spinal canal if it is passed upward.

When the epidural space is identified, a test dose of local anesthetic is injected up the needle. The surge of extradural venous distension accompanying a contraction will tend to disperse injected solutions abnormally far in the spinal canal, with the danger of excessive segmental blockade (Webster, 1962). For this reason, *epidural injections during labor should always be made between contractions and not while a contraction is actively taking place.* One cannot make "cookbook" rules about the size of the test dose, for the volume will have to be varied inversely with the concentration. In general, it is better to employ dilute solutions in order to be able to take advantage of using a large volume. The test dose serves more than one function. First, it opens up the epidural space to facilitate passage of the catheter; second, it expedites induction by placing a priming dose in the epidural space; and third, it performs its safety function of ensuring that inadvertent subarachnoid puncture has not taken place. With 1 per cent lidocaine or 0.25 per cent bupivacaine, a volume of 4 to 5 ml serves all three functions well.

A catheter is then gently inserted for a distance of 3 to 4 cm beyond the tip of the needle, and the needle is withdrawn over the catheter. An aspiration test is made through the catheter to ensure that the tip has not entered an epidural vein or punctured the dura. A sterile dressing is placed over the puncture site, and the catheter is taped in place. A syringe full of local anesthetic is attached with or without a micropore filter, and the patient is turned onto the opposite side. Tests for skin analgesia are made in the lower lumbar segments, and the patient is asked to move her legs. If no signs of subarachnoid block have developed, it may be assumed that the original test dose was correctly placed in the epidural space. Now, a second test dose must be given through the epidural catheter to reconfirm the result of the aspiration test performed shortly before and to ensure that the catheter has not penetrated the dura and entered the subarachnoid space. The second test dose can be somewhat smaller than the first, of the order of 2 to 3 ml of 1 per cent lidocaine or 0.25 per cent bupivacaine, and this serves the secondary function of consolidating a satisfactory segmental epidural block with symmetrical analgesia on the two sides. Thus, the two test doses in fact become the epidural induction dose.

The onset of blockade is faster in pregnancy than under normal circumstances, and the pain of uterine contractions is rapidly relieved. A band of skin analgesia develops during the next 5 to 10 minutes, extending from about the tenth or eleventh thoracic segment to the second or third lumbar segment. Further increments of 3 to 4 ml may be injected if segmental analgesia has not spread far enough. Gravity should be used to assist spread if analgesia develops more on one side than on the other, and the patient should be turned with the less well-anesthetized side downward when further increments are injected.

Maintenance

Further increments of epidural solution are injected through the catheter at intervals to maintain satisfactory analgesia throughout labor. Opinions differ as to how this should be done, some preferring a continuous system using an electrically driven syringe pump, and others remaining content with intermittent injections by the clock. Personally, I prefer to avoid both of these courses and to use an "on-demand" approach with repeat injections administered when contractions become uncomfortable. In this way minimum dosage can be tailored to the mother's real needs better than by some arbitrary time scale that may not match each patient's requirements.

The anesthesiologist should remain with the patient throughout the induction period in order to observe the upper and lower limits of segmental spread and to satisfy himself that an adequate and symmetrical block has been established. He will then know the precise total induction dose that was necessary to achieve the required number of analgesic segments, and he will be in a position to base subsequent doses upon this information. Because of the small quantities of drug used, maintenance or "top-up" doses need to be almost the same amount as the initial induction dose. This is unlike the surgical situation in which a large induction dose is followed by maintenance doses of half the initial amount. Figure 12–20 shows a typical segment-time diagram after induction of segmental analgesia in labor. With repeated injections some local anesthetic agents show a tendency to creep downward to involve the lower lumbar and sacral segments, even when very small doses are used. This tendency has been most apparent with highly diffusible agents, such as carbonated lidocaine and etidocaine, and less apparent with bupivacaine (Bromage, 1967). This downward creep may be a disadvantage in spontaneous labor, since it may lead to premature loss of the Ferguson reflex, but in oxytocin-assisted labor it has the advantage that some degree of perineal analgesia is already present during the last stages of cervical dilatation, and then induction of full perineal analgesia is quicker and easier.

The question arises, who should administer the "top-up" doses? Must it be a physician, or is it reasonable to request the nursing staff to perform this function? My view is that it is entirely reasonable to ask this assistance from a nursing department; in fact, I believe an epidural service would be almost unworkable without such an arrangement. The antagonists claim that ordinary nursing staff are not permitted to administer anesthetics and therefore should not administer "top-up" doses of epidural anesthetics. The issue is partly a matter of semantics and partly of common sense. Of course, the request is not to give an anesthetic but an analgesic, and this is not

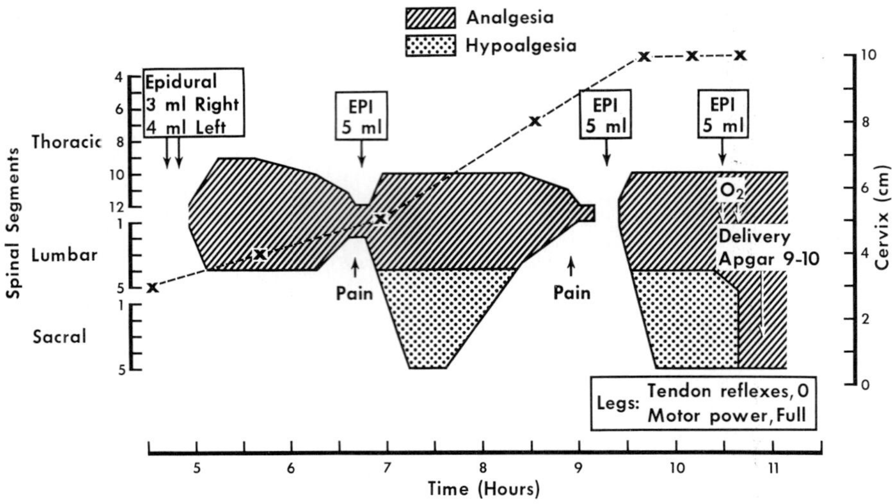

Figure 12–20. Epidural analgesia in labor with 0.25 per cent bupivacaine + 1/200,000 epinephrine. No sedative drugs used in this 24-year-old primigravida. Epidural analgesia induced when cervix 4 cm dilated. Epidural puncture at L_2–L_3 in supine position on right side. Tuohy needle used to inject 3 ml of 0.25 per cent bupivacaine + 1/200,000 epinephrine. Catheter inserted and 4 ml analgesic solution injected with patient turned on left side. Symmetrical analgesia developed. Note (1) gradual "ripening" of analgesia in sacral segments with successive injections; (2) retention of motor power in legs in spite of absent knee and ankle jerks, and analgesia extending from T_{10} to S_5 at time of delivery.
x– – – – –x Cervical dilatation (cm)

an unusual request. Common sense demands that there must be adequate safeguards against all risks involved, and this implies that close medical support must be available at all times for consultation or for treatment if unforeseen difficulties arise.

If nurses are to give "top-up" doses, then explicit orders must be written in the patient's record with details of volume and concentration of drug to be administered and the limits of frequency of injection. The order should also include instructions to check the blood pressure at 5-minute intervals for at least 15 minutes after each dose. As an additional precaution, all syringes of local anesthetic may be charged and labeled by the anesthesiologist, so that wrongful administration can be avoided. This system of interdepartmental cooperation between Nursing and Anesthesia has been in practice at the Royal Victoria Hospital, Montreal, since the introduction of an obstetrical epidural service in 1956, and it has worked well and safely in over 30,000 continuous epidurals. Such an arrangement is only feasible if close cooperation exists between departments and if anesthesia staff coverage is available in the hospital at all times.

The Perineal Dose

Perineal pain is felt when the fetal head distends the perineum, and this is the signal to block the sacral roots in preparation for a painless delivery.

The anesthesiologist returns to the scene at this point to supervise the final disposition of analgesia in readiness for delivery. The existing extent of analgesia may be checked by pinprick to establish any segmental deficiencies that remain in the caudal area and to obtain a rough estimate of the amount of analgesic solution that is likely to be needed to obtain solid sensory blockade of all segments below T_{10}. The patient is placed in the sitting or semisitting position, or if her legs are already positioned in lithotomy stirrups, the table is tilted steeply head-up while the perineal dose is injected through the catheter; the head-up position is maintained for 5 minutes. As a general practical guide, about twice the maintenance dose is usually needed. For example, if maintenance doses of 6 ml of 0.25 per cent bupivacaine have been satisfactory, then 12 ml of the same solution may be given. This volume may be reduced, or possibly omitted altogether, if prior test by pinprick has revealed that good sacral analgesia already exists. The rule should be to give as little analgesic as possible, consistent with obtaining satisfactory conditions for the mother and obstetrician.

Timing of the perineal dose is important. With most agents full perineal anesthesia, adequate for episiotomy and forceps extraction, takes about 15 to 20 minutes to develop from the time of injection, and clearly the progress of labor must be monitored accurately enough for the perineal dose to be given before it is too late. If mistiming has left an unexpectedly short interval before delivery, the anesthesiologist should change solutions to one of the rapidly acting agents, such as carbonated lidocaine, 2-chloroprocaine or etidocaine, although the latter drug will produce an undesirably intense degree of motor paralysis in the legs for the next two hours.

Choice of Analgesic Solution

A wide variety of drugs and concentrations are available, and it would be idle to insist upon any one exclusive and didactic dose schedule. It is better to keep the basic principles clearly in mind and to fit individual dose schedules to them. Essentially, the aim is to perform the anesthetic task well but at the same time as economically as possible, with the least amount of drug. There is no place in obstetrical analgesia for large volumes of concentrated solution that assure prompt effect and slick anesthetic showmanship, but at the risk of fetal depression.

In general, a given mass of drug will give satisfactory conditions for a longer time in dilute solution than in concentrated solution—that is to say, more segment-minutes per milligram can be extracted in dilute solution. However, as in surgical analgesia, the intensity of blockade is less with dilute solutions, and occasionally spotty analgesia or a "missed segment" may make it necessary to change to a stronger concentration at the cost of a higher cumulative dose.

Figure 12–21 shows the performance of solutions tested for epidural analgesia in obstetrics using a minimal dose regimen (Bromage, 1969; Bromage et al., 1974). The ordinate shows the degree of motor block in the legs measured by the simple clinical criteria outlined in Chapter 4. The sensory performance is shown on the abscissa. An individual sensory score of 100 per cent was applied when analgesia was satisfactory at all stages of labor,

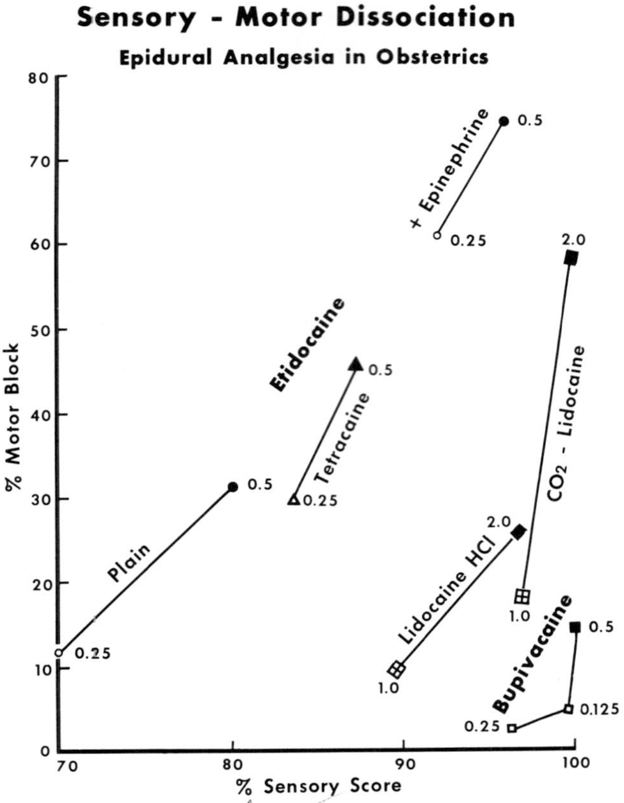

Figure 12-21. Epidural analgesia in labor. Quality of sensory and motor blockade with various analgesic solutions. Each point is the mean of 20 to 50 cases.
○ Etidocaine
△ Tetracaine
⊞ Lidocaine
□ Bupivacaine
Note the dissociation between intensity of motor and sensory blockade with the four agents tested and the most favorable ratio of sensory to motor block with bupivacaine. (After Bromage, 1969; Bromage et al., 1974.)

from induction to completion of perineal repair. A score of zero was given to any case that required supplementation by general or local anesthesia at any stage during labor or delivery. The values shown are the averages from groups of 20 to 50 patients. A simple assessment grid of this sort provides an objective guide for comparing different drugs and for planning successful analgesic tactics at various stages of labor, or under conditions of special difficulty.

In most normal labors early first-stage pain is easily relieved by small amounts of relatively dilute analgesic solutions, and power can be held in reserve. The potential failures show up at the end of the first stage when some abnormality such as a persistent occipitoposterior position gives rise to a heightened afferent input. It is at this point that the wavering battle between afferent input and neural blockade should be carried to success by throwing in the heavy reserve of analgesic power that can be made available by increasing the dose or concentration or by changing to one of the highly penetrating agents, such as carbonated lidocaine.

Another helpful way of judging local anesthetic capability in obstetrics is to plot the cumulative dosage against duration of labor. Examples of this type of data assessment are shown in Figures 12-22 and 12-23 for tetracaine, bupivacaine and etidocaine (Bromage, 1969; Bromage et al., 1974). Even without accurate statistical treatment, the eye can quickly pick out the scatter of failures and the slope of cumulative dose requirements for each

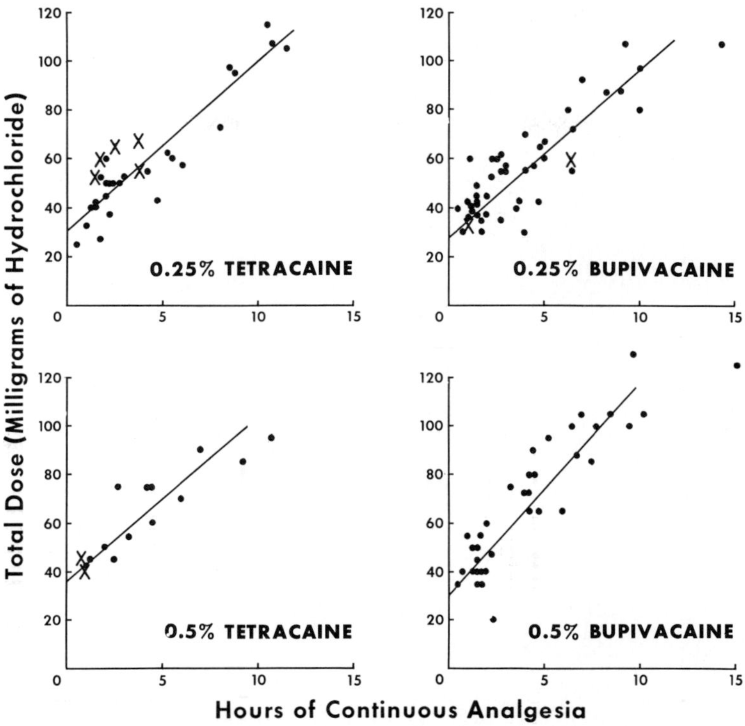

Figure 12–22. Continuous epidural analgesia in labor and delivery. Cumulative drug requirements, using low-dose regimen, for tetracaine and bupivacaine in 0.25 and 0.5 per cent solution with epinephrine 1/200,000. Calculated regression lines drawn through the data points.

● Successful analgesia for labor and delivery. No other supplementation required.

X Unsatisfactory analgesia for delivery, requiring supplementation with inhalational analgesia or anesthesia.

(From Bromage: Canad. Anaesth. Soc. J., 1969.)

solution, and it is easy to see where the pharmacological strengths and the weaknesses lie. This plot also gives a quick estimate of the total duration of analgesia to be expected from a given cumulative dose of anesthetic, as shown in Figure 12–24. It is interesting to note that in spite of the intrinsically longer duration of bupivacaine, its equitoxic cumulative dosage is very similar to that of lidocaine. However, it should be noted that in speaking of an equivalent or equitoxic dose, we are considering maternal conditions. Animal evidence of drug distribution in fetal tissues shows that the partition ratio between tissues and blood for bupivacaine is about one half that of lidocaine (Hollmén, 1973). That is to say, much less bupivacaine actually reaches fetal tissues, and this suggests that bupivacaine is an unusually safe drug from the point of view of fetal depression.

Table 12–4 lists a range of dosages that have been found to be practical in my own series under conditions of close supervision in which doses could be adjusted quickly to the needs of the patient.

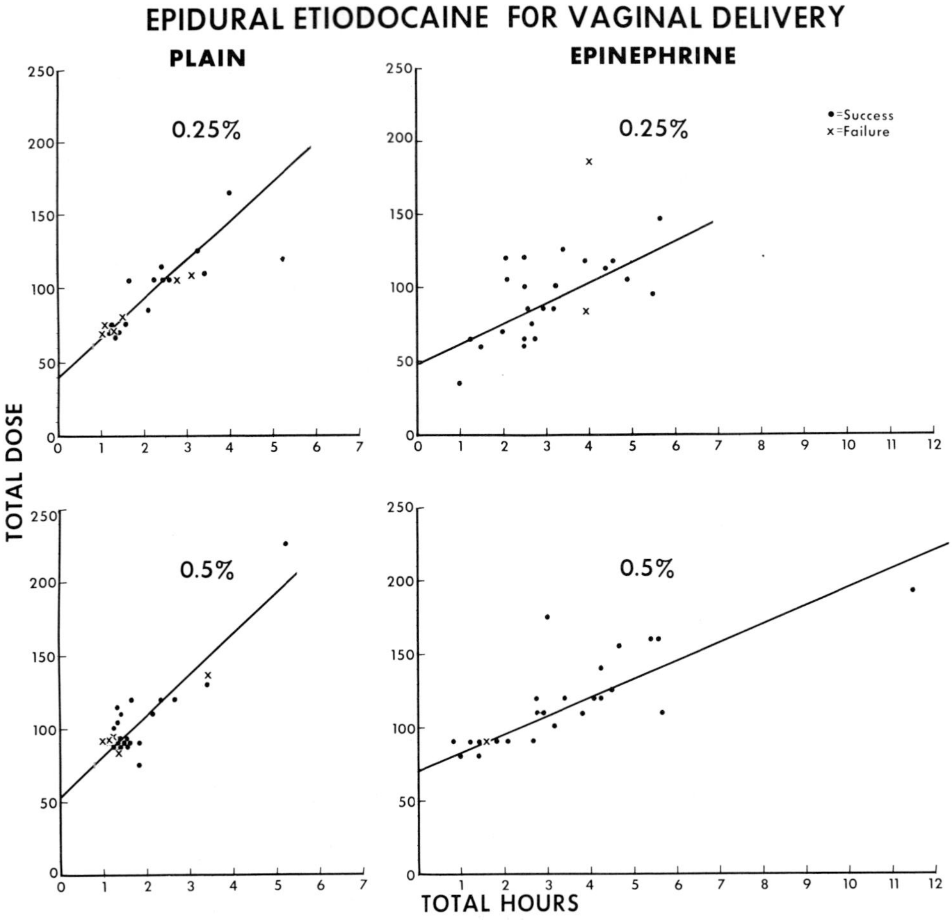

Figure 12–23. Continuous epidural analgesia in labor and delivery. Cumulative dose requirements for 0.25 and 0.5 per cent etidocaine with and without epinephrine 1/200,000. Symbols the same as in Figure 12–22. Note lower cumulative dose requirements and higher success rate when epinephrine is added. (From Bromage et al.: Canad. Anaesth. Soc. J., 1974.)

Bupivacaine 0.125% + epinephrine 1/400,000

Van Steenberge and his colleagues have shown that a dilute solution of bupivacaine in 0.125 per cent concentration with 1/400,000 epinephrine gives surprisingly effective analgesia for labor and delivery while causing very low maternal and fetal blood concentrations of bupivacaine (Vanderick et al., 1974; Geerinckx et al., 1974). These authors propose the following regimen:

Induction dose	15 ml (18.75 mg)
Maintenance doses	10 ml (12.5 mg)
Perineal dose	15 ml (18.75 mg)

They found a 93 per cent incidence of complete pain relief for labor and delivery in a series of 500 patients.

Our experience with this regimen in a small series of cases has been most gratifying and has confirmed Van Steenberge's findings. The quality of

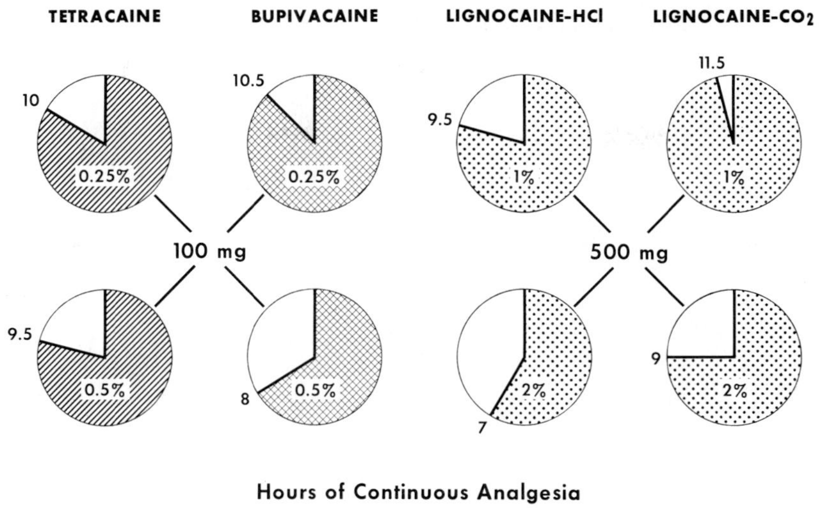

Figure 12–24. Cumulative dose requirements for continuous epidural analgesia during labor and delivery. Average hours of analgesia provided by cumulative dose of 100 mg tetracaine or bupivacaine, or 500 mg lidocaine (lignocaine) HCl or CO_2 salt in 1 or 2 per cent solution. All solutions with epinephrine 1/200,000. (After Bromage, 1967, 1969.)

analgesia was surprisingly good, and no failures were encountered in 50 patients. Moreover, the segmental spread was not excessive, and analgesia seldom rose above the ninth thoracic dermatome—a finding that confirms the impression that epidural segmental spread is determined more by the mass of local anesthetic than by the volume of solution. The cumulative dose requirements were also very low, being about 30 per cent less than for 0.5 per cent bupivacaine and about 12 per cent less than for 0.25 per cent bupivacaine, as shown in Table 12–5 and Figure 12–25.

Duration of Second Stage

Once perineal pain is abolished, the normal imperative urge to bear down is also removed, and the mother may tend to lie passively, taking no

TABLE 12–4 Lumbar Epidural Analgesia in Labor: Induction, Maintenance and Perineal Doses for Lidocaine, Bupivacaine and Etidocaine

Solution	*Epinephrine*	*Induction Dose (ml)*	*Maintenance Dose (ml)*	*Perineal Dose (ml)*
Lidocaine HCl 1%	1/200,000	4–8	4–6	6–14
Lidocaine HCl 2%	1/200,000	4–6	3–5	5–12
CO_2-Lidocaine 1%	1/200,000	4–6	3–5	6–12
CO_2-Lidocaine 2%	1/200,000	3–6	3–4	5–9
Bupivacaine 0.125%	1/400,000	15	10	15
Bupivacaine 0.25%	1/200,000	5–8	4–6	6–14
Bupivacaine 0.5%	1/200,000	4–6	3–5	5–12
Etidocaine 0.5%	1/200,000	5–7	4–6	5–10

TABLE 12–5 Bupivacaine for Continuous Epidural Analgesia in Labor: Sensory Score, Degree of Motor Block and Cumulative Dose Requirements for 0.125%, 0.25% and 0.5% Bupivacaine*

				Linear Regression of Cumulative Dose Requirements			
Concentration of Bupivacaine	*n*	*Sensory Score (%)*	*Average Motor Block at Delivery*	*INTERCEPT*	*SLOPE*	*CORRELATION COEFFICIENT*	*Cumulative Dose for 5 Hours Analgesia (mg)*
0.125	40	100	4.1 ± 12	29.01	0.8678	0.83	55
0.25	56	96.5	2.0 ± 9	33.6	0.0996	0.84	63.5
0.5	35	100	12.5 ± 20	34.3	0.1389	0.93	75.9

*Data from Bromage (1969) and Bromage and Bramwell (unpublished data).

active part in her labor (Kandel et al., 1966). The resulting prolongation of the second stage was a source of considerable criticism before the paramount importance of posture was appreciated, but with correct posture and avoidance of the supine position, lengthening of the second stage from this type of inertia is not of great importance. Provided the epidural analgesia has not caused too much motor block of the abdominal muscles, most women can substitute effective voluntary bearing-down efforts for the involuntary drive of normal painful labor. An attendant should keep a hand on the abdomen and encourage the mother to bear down actively when the uterus is felt to contract.

Much attention has been focused on the second stage and the

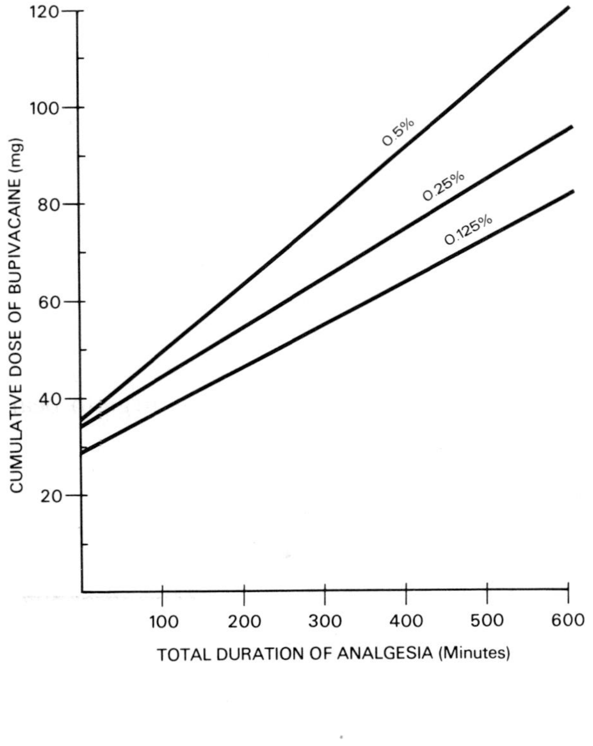

Figure 12–25. Cumulative dose requirements for continuous epidural analgesia during labor and delivery. Bupivacaine HCl, 0.5 and 0.25 per cent + 1/200,000 epinephrine, and 0.125 per cent + 1/400,000 epinephrine (regression lines calculated from original data). (After Bromage, 1969; Bromage and Bramwell, unpublished data.)

deterioration of fetal acid-base status that occurs in a prolonged second stage during natural spontaneous labor. There was a widely held belief that the second stage should not exceed one hour (Jacobson, 1970), and therefore any prolongation of the second stage by epidural analgesia would be harmful to the fetus. However, recent evidence suggests that any harm arising from a prolonged second stage is attributable to two easily identified and preventable factors unrelated to anesthesia, namely, (1) hard labor (Pearson and Davies, 1973b) and (2) enforced posture in the dorsal position that normally causes a predicted change of −0.26 pH units in fetal scalp blood when the supine position is maintained for more than 30 minutes (Wood et al., 1973a, 1973b; Humphrey et al., 1974). If both of these factors are eliminated, the acid-base status does not change and the duration of the second stage becomes inconsequential. Epidural analgesia provides a comfortable, tranquil second stage. Maternal work is reduced, oxygen consumption is lowered and maternal lactic acid does not rise as it normally would in a painful spontaneous labor (Pearson and Davies, 1973b). The second factor is dealt with by an effective pelvic tilt with a sandbag under one hip. This relieves aortocaval compression (vide infra), and the fetal pH no longer falls with elapsed time (Humphrey et al., 1974). Thus, the bogey of epidural analgesia contributing to fetal distress by prolonging the second stage is dispelled. With proper management and attention to good maternal posture, epidural analgesia becomes a positive rather than a negative factor, and it contributes in an important fashion to the maintenance of good fetal acid-base status and to the delivery of a vigorous baby.

Delivery

Having administered the perineal dose, the anesthetist should be present to ensure that analgesia develops satisfactorily, to supervise the mother's cardiovascular status and to undertake any resuscitation that may be necessary in the event of fetal distress or maternal hemorrhage after delivery. In addition, he should ensure that the mother is breathing an oxygen-enriched atmosphere, preferably 100 per cent oxygen for 5 to 20 minutes prior to delivery and until the umbilical cord is clamped.

Maternal Oxygenation and Effects on the Fetus

A great deal of controversy has centered around the question of whether or not high concentrations of oxygen should be given to the mother at vaginal delivery. The available clinical and laboratory evidence leaves little doubt that high maternal oxygen concentrations do improve fetal oxygenation and fetal performance at birth and provide an extra margin of safety for the baby, and in the light of this evidence there is no valid reason for withholding oxygen from the mother during the process of delivery.

Opponents of maternal oxygen therapy have held that hyperoxia is self-defeating because of its effect on arterioles. Large changes of oxygen tension result in small changes in the contractility of arterial muscle; high oxygen tensions tend to favor contraction, and low oxygen tensions favor relaxation (Roddie and Scott, 1965). A number of vascular beds react to hyperoxia by more marked vasoconstriction, and these include the uterine arterioles, the newborn retinal vessels and the ductus arteriosus and periductal tissue (Kovalčík, 1963; Moss et al., 1964; Gillman and Burton, 1966). Nyberg and Westin (1957) found evidence of placental vasoconstriction with 20 per cent shortening of vascular strips in high oxygen concentration. In vitro perfusion experiments by Panigel (1959, 1962) showed increased placental resistance at high oxygen tensions, and more recent studies of uterine perfusion by thermal dilution have added support to this observation (Tervila et al., 1973). Thus, there are some laboratory grounds for fearing two ill effects from high oxygen concentrations to the mother. First, premature closure of the ductus arteriosus, and second, a reduction of uteroplacental perfusion with resultant fetal acidosis and a net worsening of fetal oxygenation.

The first of these fears appears to be groundless within the range of fetal oxygenation that can be achieved by giving 100 per cent oxygen to the mother. The second objection may possibly have some basis if maternal hyperoxia is continued for long periods of time in excess of one hour (Newman et al., 1967). Shorter periods of maternal hyperoxia between 5 and 30 minutes, however, appear to have nothing but beneficial effects on uterine blood flow (Greiss et al., 1974) and on the fetus, as measured by fetal blood gases and the fetal heart rate before birth and by respiratory performance after delivery, not only in humans but also in other species (Battaglia et al., 1968; Comline and Silver, 1968; Myers et al., 1977).

Caldeyro-Barcia and his colleagues (1966) showed that maternal oxygen reduced or abolished Type 2 bouts of bradycardia in fetal distress occurring in normal labor, and maternal oxygen administration is now used routinely in this situation. Quilligan et al. (1960) found that the umbilical vein oxygen tension increased by 33 per cent when 100 per cent oxygen was breathed by the mother. Gare et al. (1969) found similar changes in fetal scalp blood, the improvement in oxygenation being inversely proportional to the initial fetal Po_2. Newman and his colleagues (1967) showed that short periods of maternal hyperoxia of 5 to 30 minutes could raise the fetal scalp Po_2 to a level of 40 mmHg but that prolonged hyperoxia for periods of more than one hour might lead to some degree of fetal acidosis, possibly from uteroplacental vasoconstriction. Rorke et al. (1968) found that the optimal effect on fetal oxygenation was obtained at a maternal Po_2 of 300 mmHg; above this level the fetal oxygenation declined slightly. Other investigators, including Baraka (1970), Künzel et al. (1970), Fox and Houle (1971) and Marx and Mateo (1971), have all found raised fetal oxygen tensions and improved clinical performance of the newborn when the mother received high inspired oxygen tensions. Hon's group at Yale found that maternal hyperoxia was fairly slow to confer its full effect on the fetus, and scalp Po_2 did not reach a maximum until after 45 minutes of oxygen administration to the mother (Khazin et al., 1971). This evidence is summarized in Table 12–6, and it can be seen that maternal hyperoxia raises the oxygen tension of the umbilical vein or fetal scalp blood by about 40 per cent in animals and in man.

Because the slope of the fetal oxygen dissociation curve is steepest at low oxygen tensions, a high maternal FIO_2 will confer greatest benefit to

TABLE 12-6 Effect of High Maternal Inspired Oxygen on Fetal Oxygenation (Fetal Scalp or Umbilical Vein)

	Fetal Umbilical Vein Po_2 *(mmHg)*		
Author	*AIR*	*OXYGEN*	*AIR-O_2* Po_2 *DIFFERENCE (mmHg)*
McClure (1958)	28.9	38.2	+9.3
Prystowsky (1959)	18.0	31.7	+13.7
Quilligan et al. (1960)			
Cesarean section	16.9	29.4	+12.5
Vaginal delivery	26.3	33.8	+7.5
Vasicka et al. (1960)	20.7	30.7	+10.0
Newman et al. (1967)	23.0 (scalp)	35.0	+12.0
Rorke et al. (1968)	29.2 (Mat FIO_2 0.33)	36.4	+6.6
Gare et al. (1969)	21.6	27.8	+6.2
Baraka (1970)	23.0	45.0	+22.0
Künzel et al. (1970)	30.6	34.3	+3.7
Khazin et al. (1971)	19.4 (scalp)	25.2	+5.8
Fox and Houle (1971)	29.0	35.0	+6.0
Marx and Mateo (1971)	28.6	41.3	+12.7
Jacobson (1970)	saturation data only		+4.0
Animals			
Battaglia et al. (1968)—Ewe	22.8	42.0	+19.2
Comline and Silver (1968)—Ewe	33.9	40.0	+6.1
Comline and Silver (1968)—Mare	57.4	80.0	+22.6
Myers et al. (1977)—Monkey	28.5*	34.0*	+5.5*

*Fetal carotid artery.

fetuses with initially low oxygen tensions. However, even a normal fetus starting higher up on the oxygen dissociation curve with an umbilical vein Po_2 of 28 mmHg may be expected to reach a tension of 40 mmHg after 15 minutes of oxygen administration to the mother. Assuming a fetal hemoglobin of 17 grams per 100 ml, this rise of Po_2 would increase the umbilical vein oxygen content from about 15.25 ml of oxygen per 100 ml to 18.25 ml per 100 ml—a 20 per cent increase in oxygen content available as extra stores in case of emergency requirements.

Thus, in balance, the fetus appears to be appreciably benefitted by a moderate period of maternal hyperoxia, and there is little solid evidence to justify denying this advantage to the newborn (Dawes, 1969). The period of delivery is perhaps one of the most important moments in the life of an individual, and it requires a cynical degree of therapeutic nihilism to withhold any possible advantage or protection that can be given at that vulnerable time. Preventable brain damage arising from inadequate supplies of substrate during labor or birth is an immensely tragic and costly legacy of ineptitude to leave to the coming generation. It is estimated that 0.5 per cent of the general population has some degree of mental retardation referable to this cause (Towbin, 1969). Towbin has pointed out that although the seeds of brain damage may have been sown in the germinal matrix early in pregnancy, a turbulent traumatic birth will seal the fate of an infant that might otherwise escape with unrecognizably slight deficiencies under gentler and more favorable conditions (Towbin, 1970, 1971). Until stronger reasons are found for not doing so, I believe it is wise for the obstetrician and anesthesiologist to ensure that every mother receives an oxygen-enriched atmosphere to breathe for at least 5 to 20 minutes before delivery and clamping of the cord. This precaution may seldom be necessary, but if unexpected complications should arise during delivery, then there is a slight extra margin of safety that may make all the difference in salvaging an unscathed central nervous system in the baby.

TECHNICAL PROBLEMS

Obstetrical analgesic technique should be deliberately parsimonious, and for the sake of the baby one must skate on thin anesthetic ice with minimal dosage. From time to time some technical deficiencies will inevitably arise from this policy, and when they do occur they must be corrected quickly by falling back on stronger analgesic solutions, such as 1 per cent or 2 per cent carbonated lidocaine, 2 per cent chloroprocaine or 1 per cent etidocaine, that have been held in reserve for this purpose. Other difficulties are related to the anatomical pecularities of the parturient epidural space, and these call for vigilance and awareness of their existence.

If basic principles are neglected, analgesia may spread excessively far into the upper thoracic region. For example, unnecessarily large doses of local anesthetics must be avoided, and repeat injections should not be made either with the mother lying on her back or during a uterine contraction, for under these circumstances the extradural veins are distended and epidural solutions spread upward for abnormally long distances within the spinal canal. Cases of upper thoracic spread with transient Horner's syndrome have been reported when one or more of these precautions have been neglected (Evans et al., 1975; Mohan and Potter, 1975).

Missed Anesthetic Segments

Epidural analgesia is "spotty" in a small proportion of cases. One or more dermatomes may escape blockade and remain sensitive in an otherwise satisfactory field of analgesia, as shown in Figure 12–26. These unblocked segments are often confined to one side, and they are more commonly seen in obstetrical patients than in a general surgical population. In regional analgesia for obstetrics there is a very narrow margin between success and failure, and "partial" successes scarcely exist. The mother either experiences complete relief or feels pain if one or more segments escape blockade. There is nothing in between. For practical purposes a "spotty" regional anesthetic is a failed anesthetic unless it can be corrected. The patient experiences pain, and if the sensory input is high enough, the quality of agony is just as acute as if no anesthesia existed in the neighboring segments.

The mechanism of unblocked or "missed" segments is still speculative, but at least two factors appear to be at work. One is failure of the local anesthetic to reach a given segment in adequate concentration, and the other

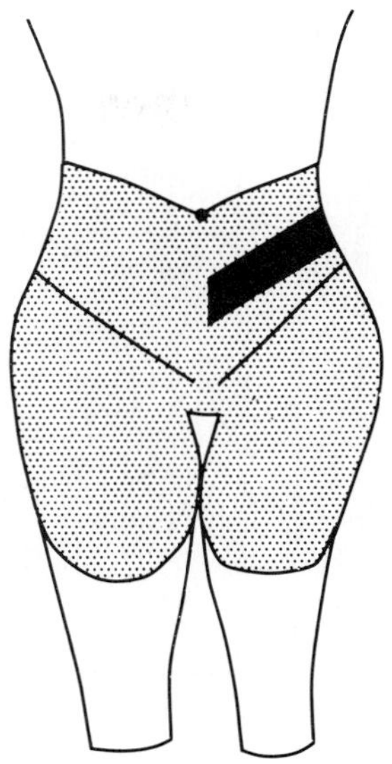

Figure 12–26. Continuous epidural analgesia for labor and delivery. Diagram of painful unblocked segment within satisfactory area of analgesia.

is a quantitative increase of afferent input through one or more segments, possibly by stretching of the round ligaments (Roberts, 1972). Bryce-Smith (1954) suggested that a missed segment could be attributed to failure of the anesthetic solution to escape from the intervertebral foramen in sufficient amount to bathe an adequate length of the paravertebral nerve. The existence of epidural membranes and adhesions has been invoked to account for the limited spread of blockade, and X-ray evidence tends to support this idea (Shanks, 1968). Usubiaga (1970) postulated that sensory block might be ineffective if the catheter tip came to lie in the anterior instead of the posterior part of the epidural space (see Chapter 7). At term, the distended epidural veins may be an additional factor limiting the spread and diffusion of local anesthetics during labor.

Missed segments from malpositioned catheter tips are often referable to insertion of an excessive length of catheter into the epidural space, and these cases can usually be corrected by withdrawing the catheter for 1 or 2 cm and trying again. Occasionally, in cases of persistently unilateral analgesia, the catheter may have to be reinserted in an adjacent space.

Ducrow (1971) found an overall incidence of spotty or unilateral anesthesia of 8.2 per cent with bupivacaine, and the condition was persistent in 2.04 per cent of cases in spite of repeated doses of bupivacaine. In my own practice the incidence of missed segments was found to vary with the local anesthetic used (Bromage, 1972). Figure 12–27 shows the incidence of unblocked segments in labor for six different anesthetic agents. For purposes of description, "persistent" unblocked segments were those that remained resistant to repeated injections of local anesthetic.

The carbonated solutions of lidocaine and prilocaine were found to have a very low incidence of painful segments compared to their hydrochloride counterparts, and carbonated lidocaine was especially potent in over-

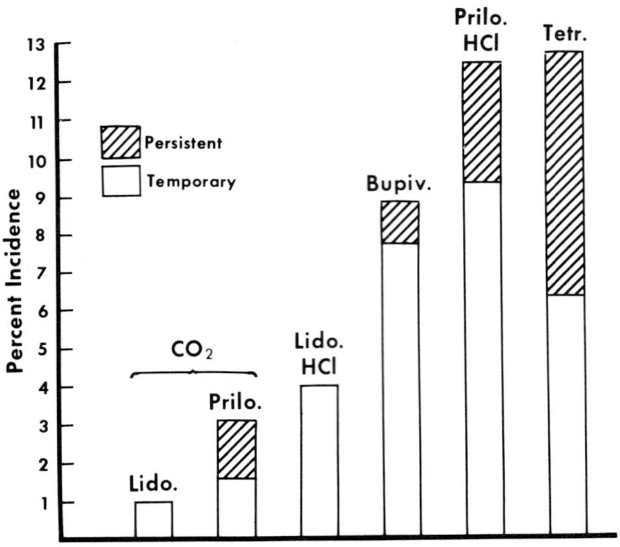

Figure 12-27. Incidence of unblocked or painful segments in analgesia for relief of pain in labor in a series of 433 patients.
▨ Persistent unblocked segments
☐ Temporary unblocked segments corrected by further increments of local anesthetic
Lido = Lidocaine
Prilo = Prilocaine
Bupiv = Bupivacaine
Tetr = Tetracaine
(From Bromage: Brit. J. Anaesth., 1972.)

coming unblocked segments that were persistently resistant to other agents. Thus, carbonated lidocaine (with epinephrine 1/200,000) is an immensely useful agent to keep in reserve in case a rapid and powerful action is needed to rescue a patchy unsatisfactory anesthetic associated with the cautious use of small doses of a less penetrating agent.

Intractable low back pain in persistent occipitoposterior positions is another example of heightened afferent input breaking through a marginally satisfactory block. Again, in these cases, a single supplementary dose of 3 to 4 ml of 2 per cent carbonated lidocaine is usually sufficient to convert an inadequate block to a complete one within a few minutes.

Epidural Vein Puncture

Inadvertent and undiagnosed venous cannulation is a potentially serious hazard of epidural analgesia in labor. The distended extradural veins are a more prominent target for accidental puncture at the end of pregnancy than at other times, so it is important to insert the epidural needle as close to the midline as possible to avoid the greater concentration of veins in the lateral parts of the spinal canal. If venous puncture occurs and blood can be aspirated through the needle, the original space should be abandoned and a fresh insertion should be made in an adjacent space. The same course should be pursued if the catheter enters a vein and blood appears in the catheter. Scrupulous care should always be taken to perform an aspiration test through the catheter after it has been inserted and before occlusive dressings and adhesive tape are put in place. Sooner or later a toxic reaction will be encountered from inadvertent intravenous injection if this simple test is forgotten (Ryan, 1973).

Accidental Dural Puncture

With care and good hand control, dural puncture should occur only very infrequently, and beginners must be impressed with the seriousness of an unnecessary dural tap. It is likely to have uncomfortable consequences for the patient, and it is a sure sign of sloppy technique on the part of the anesthesiologist if dural puncture is anything but a rarity. The steps to be taken if dural puncture does occur have already been outlined in an earlier chapter (see page 208). In the event of accidental dural puncture a second epidural insertion may be attempted in an adjacent space; if this fails, the procedure should be abandoned, or the possibility of a caudal insertion may be considered. Prophylactic hydration and epidural saline injection should be started immediately after delivery in an attempt to avoid a postpuncture headache. If severe headache does develop in spite of these precautions, then it is reasonable to proceed to perform an epidural blood patch without further delay.

The Difficult Back

Severe scoliosis or kyphoscoliosis may present technical problems due to angulation and rotation of the spinal column. However, these cases cause surprisingly little difficulty if the puncture site is chosen correctly. The point at which transition takes place from the primary to the secondary scoliotic curvature is usually between the twelfth thoracic and first lumbar vertebrae, and at this point where angulation and rotation of the vertebral bodies is minimal, epidural puncture is usually as simple as in a normal spine. In these cases puncture should be performed with the patient sitting up in order to take every possible advantage of posture and alignment of the spine. Since the catheter may have to be inserted at an unusually high level, some difficulty may be experienced in obtaining satisfactory perineal analgesia for delivery when standard solutions of lidocaine or bupivacaine are used. This is another situation in which the intensely penetating qualities of carbonated lidocaine or etidocaine may be extremely useful for supplying effective perineal analgesia with small dosage and without excessive upward segmental spread.

The presence of spinal grafts or plates will force a choice of interspace above or below the site of previous operation (Walpole, 1974). If lumbosacral or thoracolumbar insertion is technically impossible in these cases, the anesthesiologist should again consider the caudal approach as a last resort, using 25 ml of 0.25 per cent bupivacaine (i.e., 62.5 mg) as an induction dose for first-stage pain relief. Bonica recommends advancing the caudal catheter upward for a distance of 8 to 15 cm until the tip lies near the fifth lumbar vertebra. In this way less solution is required, and the usual caudal dose may be reduced by 30 to 50 per cent (Akamatsu and Bonica, 1974). It must be emphasized that since the dose of local anesthetic required for first-stage pain relief by the caudal approach is three to four times higher than that required by the lumbar route, caudal analgesia exposes the fetus to higher concentrations of local anesthetic, and it is only justified when the lumbar route is contraindicated.

Breech Delivery and Multiple Births

In the past there has been controversy over the choice of anesthesia for breech delivery and for delivery of the second twin. The conservative view has been that general anesthesia is safer than regional, since uterine relaxation can be obtained at short notice for ease of intrauterine manipulations (Crawford, 1971). It is interesting to note that with increasing experience, current views have undergone a process of conversion from categorical rejection of regional anesthesia (Little and Friedman, 1958), through a stage of cautious acknowledgment that properly handled epidural analgesia may be acceptable (Crawford, 1972; Bowen-Simpkins and Fergusson, 1974), to enthusiastic recommendation of epidural analgesia as the method of choice (Crawford, 1974a; Darby et al., 1976; James et al., 1977a).

Whatever technique is chosen, the secret is control and versatility. The anesthesiologist might be able to ensure active powers when required or a compliant relaxed uterus if intrauterine manipulations become necessary. For many years my own practice has been to employ epidural analgesia in every case of abnormal lie or multiple pregnancy, with full preparation for immediate induction of general anesthesia if required. To date, the latter has not proved necessary. Particular care has been taken to fulfil the following conditions:

1. *Active powers.* This implies (a) minimal dosage, preferably using 0.125 per cent or 0.25 per cent bupivacaine, so that extrauterine forces, and particularly the abdominal muscles, are not significantly depressed; and (b) the availability of oxytocic support by intravenous infusion in case uterine activity flags from loss of the so-called Ferguson reflex, or for any other reason.

2. *Active passenger.* One hundred per cent oxygen is delivered to the mother by a Magill circuit and a close-fitting mask throughout the period of delivery.

3. *Uterine relaxation on demand.* The anesthesiologist must be able to convert an active uterus to a passive one if fetal indications demand it. Brief uterine relaxation may be obtained with amyl nitrite by placing a capsule in a rebreathing bag of the Magill circuit and then cracking it when required, after warning the mother that she will experience a strong fruity smell and a feeling of light-headedness for a few minutes.

Intravenous infusions of selective β_2-receptor stimulators, such as salbutamol or terbutaline, may also be used to relax the uterus, but their onset of action is somewhat slower than that of amyl nitrite. Terbutaline, given at a dose rate of 10 μg/min, takes about 2 minutes to stop contractions and lower uterine tonus (Andersson et al., 1975).

If these measures do not produce adequate uterine relaxation, then general anesthesia may have to be undertaken using a "crash induction", endotracheal intubation and halothane and oxygen until the uterus is sufficiently relaxed.

Placental Hemorrhage

Active hemorrhage is wisely considered to be a contraindication to any technique that compromises the normal vasoconstrictive mechanisms which compensate for an acute loss of blood volume. One must concede that this is sound teaching from a practical point of view, especially if banked blood is not available ad libitum to replace hemorrhagic losses as they occur. Therefore, light general anesthesia with muscle relaxants will be the choice of technique in case of placenta previa or abruptio placentae.

However, I believe it is always prudent to preserve a questioning heterodox approach to even the most established ex cathedra doctrines, as occasional necessity proves. In fact, there would be no theoretical objection to using a sympathetic blocking technique, such as epidural analgesia, provided blood could be replaced as fast as it is lost, but trouble may be anticipated if losses exceed supplies. This situation may arise as a rare complication in cases of placenta accreta, in which hemorrhage may be torrential and fatal, if unsupported by immediate and adequate supplies of banked blood. Therefore, means should always be at hand to replace sympathetic constrictor tone urgently, using a dilute norepinephrine drip of 4 to 8 μg/min, in case this type of emergency should arise unexpectedly. This is one of the very rare occasions when the alpha and beta adrenergic effects of norepinephrine are needed and justified.

Toxemia and Preeclampsia

The hypertension and renal vasoconstriction of preeclamptic toxemia must be controlled by appropriate vasodilator therapy. Prolonged sympathetic blockade by epidural analgesia has been used to control preeclampsia (Ostlere, 1952; Bryce-Smith and Williams, 1955; Mylks et al., 1960), but it is a cumbersome technique when administered for many days, and it has the inherent disadvantage of being steadily overtaken by developing tachyphylaxis to the local anesthetic agents. Nevertheless, epidural blockade is a logical choice for the short-term management of labor and delivery in the preeclamptic patient (Bromage, 1954, 1961; Willocks and Moir, 1968; Moir et al., 1972; James and Davies, 1976).

Preeclamptic women, like patients with pheochromocytoma, have a reduced plasma volume, so caution must be exercised when epidural blockade is induced. It is very easy to go too far and take the patient from a state of dangerous hypertension to one of acute hypotension, as illustrated by the following case from an early series.

Case History

A secundagravida of 27 years had a normal antenatal course until slight labor pains began one week after her expected date of delivery. Severe frontal headache developed, and she was admitted with gross edema, oliguria and albuminuria, and a blood pressure of 180/100. A combination of morphine, bromide and chloral was given on admission, but three hours after admission she had a major convulsion, followed by a second one 90 minutes later.

Light general anesthesia was administered to quiet the patient, 20 ml of 1 per cent lidocaine were injected epidurally at the second lumbar interspace and a catheter was inserted. Following this, the blood pressure fell precipitously to 70/40 mmHg, but normotension was restored by posture, intravenous fluids and a small dose of methamphetamine (10 mg). Anesthesia extended to the fifth thoracic segment, and the patient awoke feeling refreshed, relaxed and free from headache. Labor progressed under continuous epidural blockade, and low-forceps delivery of an active baby was accomplished 3½ hours later. The urine was clear of albumin by 40 hours after delivery, and the patient made an excellent recovery.

Here, prehydration was omitted, and anxiety to lower the blood pressure overcame prudence in dosage. The case would have been better managed by prehydration with Ringer's lactate solution and by use of a smaller induction dose of about 80 to 100 mg of 1 per cent lidocaine, followed by further incremental doses as necessary to reduce the blood pressure in a more controlled fashion.

In preeclamptic patients epidural analgesia should be complemented by anticonvulsant therapy, with magnesium sulfate or a continuous infusion of chlormethiazole administered during the labor and for some hours after delivery (Duffus et al., 1969). The danger of convulsions does not end with delivery, and anticonvulsant precautions should be carried on in the postpartum period (Moir et al., 1972). If an epidural catheter is in place, it is wise to maintain blockade for six to eight hours after delivery in order to avoid the possibility of postpartum convulsions.

EPIDURAL ANALGESIA FOR CESAREAN SECTION

Twenty-five years ago the safety and advantages of epidural analgesia, compared to general anesthesia, were more obvious than today (Ansbro et al., 1952). But now, with improved understanding of the underlying respiratory and cardiovascular hazards, the choice between general anesthesia and epidural blockade for elective cesarian section is an open one. If done well, either method produces good results. The balance of laboratory evidence suggests that fetal conditions may be slightly better after epidural blockade, provided the mother is breathing 100 per cent oxygen (Fox and Houle, 1971). The difference is not spectacular, as will be seen in the next section on maternofetal acid-base balance, and what difference there is may be referable to the maternal FIO_2 and to posture rather than to any fundamental superiority of regional analgesia for abdominal section. Therefore, the choice between epidural analgesia and general anesthesia will revolve around other, and often minor, considerations, such as personal preference or local custom (James et al., 1977b).

In trial of labor under epidural blockade the decision is clearer. There, an epidural catheter is already in place, and it is a simple matter to extend the area and the quality of blockade to ensure maternal comfort and to include all the spinal segments below the sixth thoracic when the time comes to perform abdominal section (Bromage, 1961; Milne and Lawson, 1973).

A rapidly acting and powerful local anesthetic is required in order to provide rapid onset and comfort during intra-abdominal uterine manipulations. These patients do not receive preoperative sedation, so a high quality of analgesia is required. Unfortunately, most agents fall short of perfection, and some degree of discomfort is often felt while the lower segment is stripped, or during suture of the uterine incision after delivery. Carbonated lidocaine in 2 per cent concentration (1.73% base) with 1/200,000 epinephrine has been the most satisfactory solution in this respect that I have encountered; onset is rapid, and analgesia is profound and dependable. Bupivacaine 0.75 per cent or 1 per cent etidocaine with epinephrine also provides reliable analgesic, but at the expense of prolonged motor blockade in the postoperative period.

Technique

Premedication is omitted, but a careful psychological briefing is given. The mother is told that she must inhale oxygen by mask continuously between induction and the time of delivery of the baby. Before induction all patients should receive a 15-ml oral dose of suitable antacid medication, such as magnesium trisilicate, to raise the gastric pH in case general anesthesia becomes necessary during the course of operation (Taylor and Pryse-Davies, 1966). Also, prior to induction an intravenous cannula is inserted, and 1 liter of glucose-saline is started and allowed to run rapidly in order to ensure adequate filling of the vascular bed after sympathetic blockade and vasodilatation begin. Prophylactic vasopressor agents are not given.

Induction of blockade for elective section is most conveniently performed with the patient in the sitting position. This makes the procedure technically easier than in the lateral decubitus, and it allows the influence of gravity to encourage downward spread of the analgesic solution toward the sacral roots. Since these patients are unpremedicated, the chances of a vasovagal faint from venous pooling in the legs is much less likely than in a premedicated surgical patient. Segmental requirements are reduced by about 25 to 35 per cent below nonpregnant values, and due allowance must be made for the difference when the induction dose is calculated. Charts of dosage/age relationship may be used for guidance in making these calculations. As an example, Figure 12–28 shows the difference between segmental dose requirements in parturient and nonpregnant women receiving 2 per cent lidocaine hydrochloride or 1 per cent etidocaine for cesarean section, with injection in the sitting position. Analgesia should extend to just above the xiphisternum (i.e., the sixth thoracic segment) in order to ensure comfort during intra-abdominal manipulations, so 17 segments must be anesthetized, counting five sacral, five lumbar and seven thoracic segments. Simple calculations from Figure 12–28 show that women in their third decade require about 20 ml of either of these two agents. Other agents have slightly different volume requirements. For example, carbonated lidocaine produces more extensive segmental spread and a more solid block than the hydrochloride solution, so the volume of the 2 per cent carbonated solution must be reduced by 10 to 15 per cent, to 16 to 18 ml. Bupivacaine 0.75 per cent, being a concentrated solution, shows even more extensive spread, and 15 to 16 ml (i.e., 112.5 to 120 mg) are often adequate for cesarean section. Further increments of 4 to 6 ml of solution may be injected through the catheter if the upper limit of analgesia fails to reach the xiphisternum within 15 to 16 minutes after injection of the induction dose.

As soon as the mother is placed on the operating table, a left lateral tilt is provided by means of a foam rubber wedge or sandbag positioned under the right hip. This degree of tilt is usually sufficient to ensure that the uterus is displaced to the left, freeing the iliac vessels and minimizing aortocaval compression (Crawford, 1972). Marx and her colleagues have

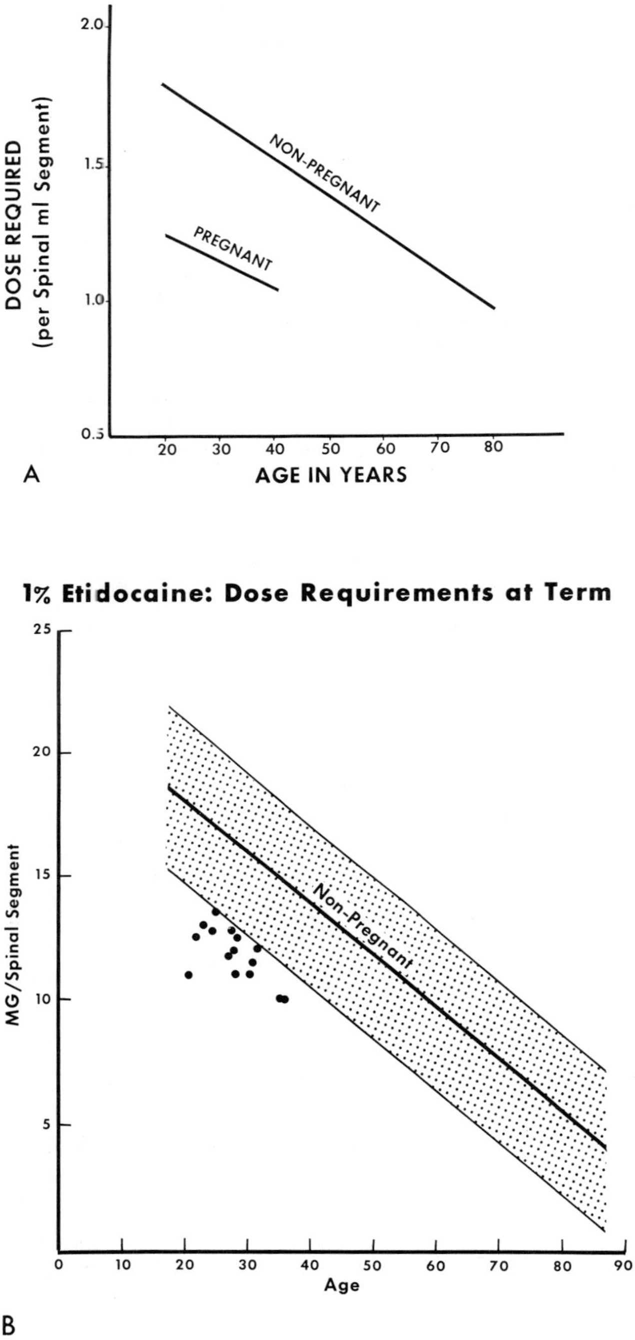

Figure 12–28. Epidural dose requirements for cesarean section, with induction in the sitting position.

A, Dose requirements in ml/segment for 2 per cent lidocaine HCl, parturient women being compared to normal population.

B, Dose requirements in milligrams per segment (10 mg = 1 ml) for 1 per cent etidocaine HCl in parturient and nonpregnant patients. Dots show data points for 15 cesarean section patients compared to the mean and 95 per cent confidence limits for a normal population. (After Bromage, 1961, Bromage et al., 1974.)

shown that a mechanical uterine displacer of the sort described by Colon-Morales (1970) may allow slightly better conditions for maternal ventilation (Jassir et al., 1973). However, the difference is not great, and a wedge under the hip is less cumbersome and is adequate for the purpose. In obese patients a wedge under the shoulder may also be necessary. The mother is given 100 per cent oxygen to breathe via a well-fitting mask until the baby is delivered and the cord is clamped.

Under these conditions, with prehydration and left uterine displacement, it is rare to find any significant degree of maternal hypotension. However, if the blood pressure should fall more than 15 to 20 per cent, other measures must be taken to raise the pressure and to ensure adequate fetal perfusion. *Ischemic fetal anoxia from low perfusion cannot be corrected by a high maternal FIO_2: the blood pressure must be restored* (Shnider et al., 1968b). The legs are raised 20 degrees to augment venous return, and a small dose of vasopressor may be given. Pure alpha-receptor stimulators, such as methoxamine, should be avoided in favor of mixed alpha and beta-receptor stimulators, such as ephedrine or methamphetamine (James et al., 1970). Ephedrine, 10 mg, given intravenously is usually an adequate dose under these circumstances.

Once the cord is clamped there is no further need for the mother to breathe an oxygen-enriched atmosphere, and the face mask may be removed. However, any deficiencies of analgesia may have to be made good by a low concentration of nitrous oxide in oxygen, so it is wise to keep the anesthetic mask close at hand. Restlessness after delivery can be managed by small intermittent doses of diazepam. Frank failure of epidural blockade due to technical difficulties is very rare, but when it does occur the anesthesiologist must be fully prepared for a rapid change of tactics to general anesthesia. This implies taking all necessary precautions for a safe, dry airway using preoperative antacids, preoxygenation, a "crash induction" and rapid intubation with Sellick's maneuver of cricoid pressure.

When trial of labor has been undertaken with first-stage epidural analgesia, it is a simple matter to extend the area of segmental blockade by injecting increments of 5 to 7 ml of a powerful agent, such as 2 per cent carbonated lidocaine, 3 per cent chloroprocaine, 0.75 per cent bupivacaine or 1 per cent etidocaine, through the epidural catheter until analgesia extends up to the sixth thoracic dermatome.

EFFECTS OF EPIDURAL ANALGESIA ON MATERNAL AND FETAL ACID-BASE BALANCE

Over the past 20 years an enormous amount of effort has been directed toward the study of the precise physicochemical changes that occur in mother and fetus during the course of labor and delivery. Distinguished work from groups at Montevideo, Oxford, Yale, Harvard, Columbia Presbyterian, Gainesville, Berlin, various Scandinavian centers and elsewhere has given us a clear understanding of the forces and chemistry of labor. The modifying effects of anesthesia have also been studied extensively, but much of the literature on the subject is confusing. Unfortunately, very little of the work has been standardized, and control values from one department do not necessarily match those from another, where important but unrecognized variables may differ significantly.

Within the past few years gradual recognition has been accorded to three fundamental nonanesthetic variables that previously had been largely ignored in assessing the effects of anesthesia on the acid-base status and performance of the fetus. These three nonanesthetic factors are:

1. The effects of hard labor
2. The effects of the supine posture on maternal and fetal cardiovascular dynamics
3. Oxytocin overdose and uterine hypertonus

Hard Labor

The first, the severity of labor, is partly a geographical variable depending on the obstetrical mores of a country, an ethnic group or a social class. Rooth has shown this very clearly in a simple comparison of acid-base data from normal deliveries in two centers in which he had worked (Rooth et al., 1973). At Lund in Sweden, normal labor was hard and unalleviated (Jacobson, 1970), while in Edmonton, Alberta, labor was eased by a combination of sedatives and regional analgesia. The values for maternal and fetal pH at delivery in the two places are shown in Table 12–7.

It can be seen that hard labor is associated with a lower maternal pH and an even lower fetal pH than the quieter, less turbulent labors at centers where pain relief is practiced routinely. The important parameter is the maternal-fetal pH difference (Δ Mat-Fet pH) that reflects worsening fetal status as Δ pH increases, and this measurement is appreciably larger after hard labors than after tranquil ones. The manner in which hard labor affects acid-base balance will be discussed at greater length, but for the moment it serves as an illustration of how easily geography can influence data in ways that are not immediately apparent to those unfamiliar with local modes of obstetrical practice.

Maternal Posture

Maternal posture is the second variable that can confuse even the most elegantly presented data. All the other variables influencing fetal well-being, such as maternal blood pressure, FIO_2 and blood concentrations of anesthetic, become meaningless in the absence of information about the mother's posture and the possible degree of aortocaval compression that may have existed because of it. All else pales into insignificance if the mother is

TABLE 12–7 Geographical Differences in Maternal-Fetal pH at Delivery Referable to Turbulence of Labor*

	Lund (No Analgesia)	*Edmonton (Analgesia)*	*Δ Edmonton-Lund*
Maternal pH	7.36	7.45	0.09
Fetal pH	7.26	7.39	0.13
Δ Mat-Fet pH	0.10	0.06	−0.04

*Data from Rooth et al. (1973).

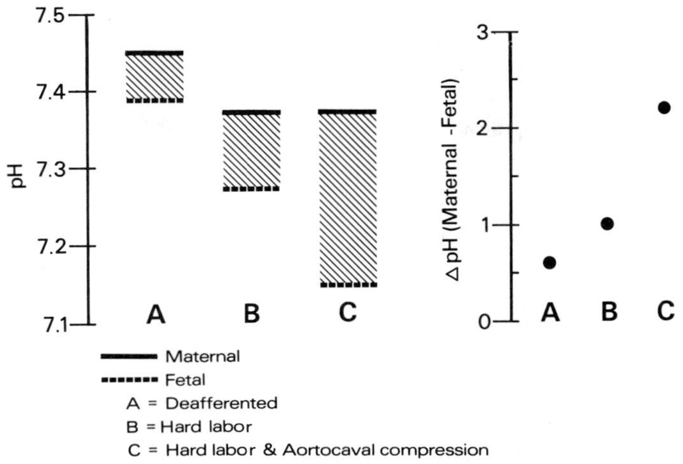

Figure 12–29. Effects of muscular effort and supine posture on maternal and fetal acidosis.

———— Maternal pH
– – – – – – – Fetal pH

A, Deafferented labor in lateral posture under epidural blockade. Labor is tranquil, and pH is not depressed in either mother or baby.

B, Hard labor depresses maternal pH, and fetal pH falls as a secondary event.

C, Hard labor and supine posture with partial aortocaval compression. Fetal and maternal pH fall in a time-dependent manner.

lying flat on her back, with a low cardiac output and a placental circulation strangled by a heavy uterus lying athwart its lifeline. And yet, a great deal of past research on anesthesia and fetal acid-base balance has been presented without this basic information, and it is often impossible for the reader to tell whether unfavorable fetal conditions in any given series were due to the noxious effects of anesthetic drugs or to the harmful results of bad obstetrical posture. The general effect of these two nonanesthetic variables on maternal and fetal pH is shown diagrammatically in Figure 12–29.

Either factor will lead to a greater accumulation of hydrogen ions and to a depression of maternal and fetal pH, and the effects on the fetus will be most harmful if both hard labor and the supine posture are operative together throughout labor and delivery. Aortocaval compression resulting from the supine posture is particularly harmful, and it gives rise to a widening of the maternal-fetal pH and base deficit differences and to associated fetal hypoxia. Table 12–8 shows the normal and abnormal range of Δ Mat-Fet pH.

Oxytocin Infusion and Uterine Hypertonus

Uterine hypertonus from excessive oxytocin administration is a third nonanesthetic variable that may affect the fetus adversely. Caldeyro-Barcia and Poseiro (1960) pointed out that rates of oxytocin infusion in excess of 16 mU/min are likely to cause a pathological degree of uterine hypertonus

TABLE 12–8 Normal and Abnormal Ranges of Maternal-Fetal pH Differences During Labor

Δ pH	*Status*
0.01–0.15	Normal
0.15–0.20	Impaired fetal gas exchange
0.20	Definitely abnormal fetal gas exchange requiring urgent correction

and fetal asphyxia, and it seems that excessive oxytocin administration at rates far above the physiological limit is a common iatrogenic cause of fetal distress (Schifrin, 1973).

Schifrin has examined the influence of oxytocin combined with general analgesia or with epidural analgesia in the supine position in a series of 360 cases. A second series of cases has since been investigated with the patients in the lateral position (Schifrin, personal communication), and the comparative results are shown in Table 12–9. Two points should be noted in evaluating the results of the supine series. First, oxytocin was administered from a manually controlled intravenous drip containing 10 mU/ml, with rates of up to 20 mU/min. With this type of simple infusion arrangement, gross inaccuracies are common, and it is reasonable to suppose that even higher rates of administration might have occurred in some instances. Second, the epidural patients were lying supine and were only turned on their sides if trouble became evident, and then the fetal heart rate tended to resume a normal pattern. In the second series the mothers were prehydrated with Ringer's lactate and were nursed on their sides, and oxytocin was given in exact amounts by a constant infusion pump. These studies emphasize three lessons of vital importance:

1. Oxytocin infusion constitutes a significant fetal hazard if given in excessive dosage or by inaccurate infusion equipment.

2. The supine posture is contraindicated during labor and delivery, especially in the presence of epidural blockade.

3. It is impossible to evaluate the effects of epidural analgesia on

TABLE 12–9 Incidence of Pathological Fetal Heart Rate Patterns Related to Oxytocin Infusion and Epidural Analgesia During Labor in Supine and Lateral Positions*

	Incidence of Fetal Heart Rate Abnormalities (%)	
Analgesia	*SUPINE (OXYTOCIN DRIP INFUSION APPROX. 8–20 mU/min)*	*LATERAL (OXYTOCIN BY CONSTANT INFUSION PUMP)*
No oxytocin; no analgesia	16.8	
Oxytocin + systemic analgesia	26.8	
Oxytocin + epidural analgesia	40	<5
No oxytocin; epidural analgesia	24.4	<2

*Data reproduced courtesy of Dr. B. Schifrin (1972; personal communication, 1974).

the fetus if other important variables, such as uterine hypertonus or adverse posture, are operating at the same time.

Having briefly discussed the three principal nonanesthetic variables that influence acid-base balance during labor, we can now turn to examine the effects of regional anesthesia itself in a more relevant perspective.

INFLUENCE OF EPIDURAL ANALGESIA ON THE METABOLIC CONSEQUENCES OF LABOR

Normal labor is accompanied by progressive metabolic acidosis in the mother (Hendricks, 1957; Derom, 1968). The very term labor is descriptive of the intense effort of uterine and extrauterine muscles necessary to expel the baby through the birth canal. The process of natural spontaneous labor is accompanied by intermittent pain, hyperventilation and restless skeletal movements during the first stage and by violent contractions of the extrauterine muscles during the second stage. The metabolic cost involved is dependent on the intensity and duration of the activity. During the first stage of labor the metabolic changes are mostly due to hyperventilation. Oxygen consumption rises by about 14 per cent (Sangoul et al., 1975), and arterial P_{CO_2} falls to about 25 mmHg. A compensatory metabolic acidosis occurs as the P_{CO_2} drops, with retention of lactate (Gemzell et al., 1957; Huckabee, 1958; Eichenholz et al., 1962; Pearson and Davies, 1973a, 1973b; Thalme et al., 1974a, 1974b).

During the second stage of natural childbirth, strong contractions of extrauterine muscles add to the heavy physical work the mother has to perform in forcing the baby through the birth canal, and metabolic demands become more compelling (Marx and Greene, 1964; Kubli, 1968). Lactate accumulates rapidly and base deficit increases in a linear time-dependent manner (Pearson and Davies, 1973b), and maternal pH falls about 0.05 units (Derom, 1968; Wood et al., 1973a, 1973b; Gårdmark, 1974). The fall of pH is greatest if the mother is forced to lie in the dorsal position, and then the pH declines at the rate of about −0.26 units per 30 minutes (Humphrey et al., 1974).

This train of response to labor pain is only slightly modified by centrally acting narcotics, such as meperidine (Demerol), but it is almost completely abolished by deafferentation at a peripheral or spinal level. Figure 12–30, redrawn from data by Pearson and Davies (1973a, 1973b), shows the effects of epidural blockade on lactate accumulation in the mother. In "natural" childbirth or with centrally acting narcotics, the duration of the second stage has great metabolic significance, but with epidural analgesia there is little or no increase in lactate so long as the mother is resting quietly, and the length of the second stage becomes metabolically unimportant provided the pelvis is tilted to one side to alleviate aortocaval compression. The difference seems to be related to the mother's response to pain. Painful *involuntary* bearing-down efforts cause the venous lactate to rise steeply at the rate of 2 mM per liter per hour. On the other hand, *voluntary* expulsive efforts under epidural analgesia lead to a negligible degree of metabolic acidosis.

Once again we see epidural analgesia acting in its role as a protec-

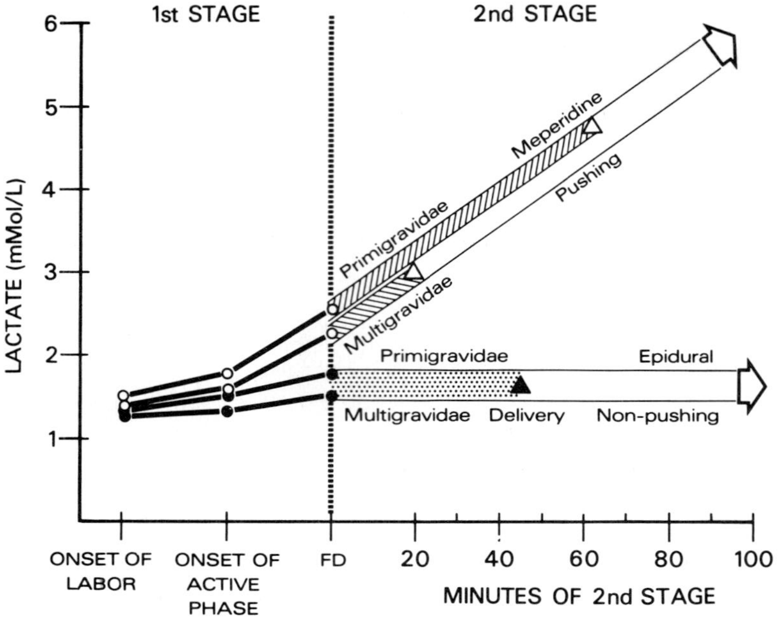

Figure 12–30. Metabolic acidosis and lactate accumulation during labor.
○ Patients receiving meperidine 100 to 150 mg and no other analgesia during "normal" active labor.
● Patients receiving continuous epidural analgesia and delivered by low forceps. No voluntary expulsive efforts during second stage.
△ Time of spontaneous delivery in patients receiving meperidine only.
▲ Average time of low forceps delivery in patients receiving epidural analgesia. (After Pearson and Davies, 1973a, 1973b.)

tor against the body's reflex response to pain. In the postsurgical situation, normal breathing and movements are inhibited by wound pain, but in labor the reverse occurs, and respiration and purposeless movements are driven by the overwhelming compulsion of pain and uterine contractions. In the postsurgical situation, respiratory function is restored toward normal by freeing inhibited movement. Here, in the obstetrical situation, metabolic function is indirectly restored to normal by quenching excessive respiratory and motor hyperactivity.

Ideally, regional analgesia should be started early before the metabolic consequences of labor have been set in train. Once severe hyperventilation has developed in response to pain, maternal pH is held down by increasing metabolic acidosis. Abrupt disturbance of this balance by sudden pain relief from any form of regional analgesia may cause an equally sudden return of respiration toward normal ventilatory levels, with maternal P_{CO_2} increasing by about 5 to 10 mmHg (Gårdmark, 1974). Sudden alleviation of respiratory alkalosis gives rise to a transient fall of maternal and fetal pH of about 0.08 units, lasting for 30 minutes or so, as carbon dioxide accumulates and before the metabolic acidosis has had time to adjust by elimination of lactate. Gårdmark (1974) has suggested that this abrupt but transient fall of pH may be partly responsible for the high incidence of fetal bradycardia seen after paracervical block with small amounts of local anesthetic.

A number of factors, including central sedation, may interfere with the hyperventilatory response to labor pain, and this is why it is so difficult to obtain true control acid-base values. Demerol, given early in labor, will attenuate hyperventilation somewhat and so modify the degree of compensatory acidosis that results. Differences in narcotic regimen are responsible for the quite wide differences in control values published by various centers, as pointed out earlier. For example, public demand in Sweden in 1972 led to a more liberal use of analgesics than formerly, so that Swedish "control" values for acid-base balance before and after 1972 are likely to differ appreciably (Gårdmark, 1974). It should be noted that the control regression line for lactate accumulation for Pearson's data in Figure 12–30 is taken from patients who had received generous amounts of meperidine in doses of 100 to 150 mg, sometimes with the addition of 25 to 50 mg promazine. Clearly, these "control" values are likely to be appreciably different from a true control situation in which the mother is allowed to labor hard, unrelieved by medication of any sort.

Fetal acid-base balance is partly determined by gradients across the placenta and partly by the competence of uterofetal communication through the placental bed and cord. Maternal acidosis per se does not cause fetal hypoxia, but as we have seen, uteroplacental perfusion may be impaired by aortocaval compression or by falls of blood pressure secondary to extensive segmental blockade and excessive vasodilatation. Fetal acidosis, secondary to placental insufficiency from any cause, is asphyxial in nature, and acidosis in these cases is associated with increasing hypoxia. Rooth and his colleagues (1973) have shown that under these circumstances there is a highly significant negative correlation between maternal-fetal pH difference and fetal oxygen tension, as shown in Figure 12–31; that is, the worse the fetal acidosis, the more the hypoxia. Apart from accidental falls of perfusion arising from poor posture and poor technique, placental perfusion is not appreciably affected by epidural analgesia, except when some improvement occurs through correction of incoordinate labor and high basal uterine tonus (Moir and Willocks, 1967).

Acidosis and lactate accumulation in the mother are passed on to the fetus, which has a pH about 0.10 unit below that of the mother (Kubli, 1968; Thalme et al., 1974a). There is little difference between the Δ Mat-Fet pH of epidural and sedated mothers while the baby is still in utero, but the

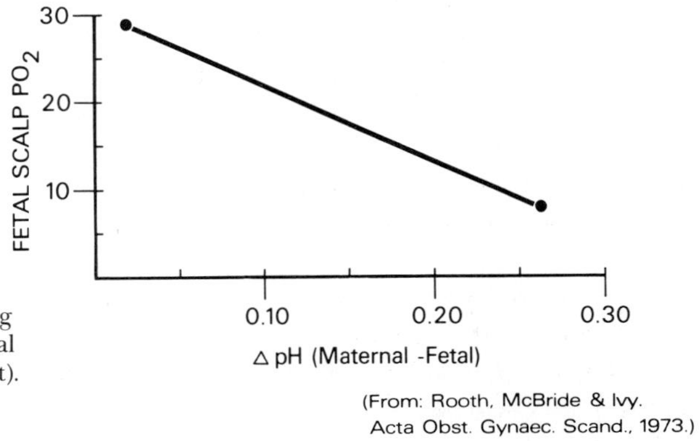

Figure 12–31. Association of fetal hypoxia with fetal acidosis (increasing maternal-fetal Δ pH) during placental insufficiency from any cause (see text). (From Rooth et al.: Acta Obst. Gynaecol. Scand., 1973.)

metabolic component, as shown by lactate levels, is less during epidural analgesia, so after delivery epidural babies recover a normal pH faster, and the incidence of neonatal depression is significantly less after epidural births (Noble et al., 1971).

It must be pointed out that clinical opinion is not unanimous about the safety of epidural analgesia for the baby. Two series have reported adverse effects on the maternal circulation during labor, with a high rate of maternal hypotension. One study showed a 77 per cent incidence of pathological changes in fetal heart rate related to maternal hypotension within 20 minutes of epidural injection (Zilianti et al., 1970). The other reported a 39 per cent incidence of maternal hypotension associated with a 55 per cent incidence of abnormal fetal heart rate during labor (Wingate et al., 1974). No prehydration regimen was undertaken. The posture of the former group was not described, but in the second group patients were in the supine position and were only turned into the lateral position to correct any hypotension when it occurred (Wingate, personal communication, 1974). In both of these series, the dose of lidocaine administered was generous, varying between 120 and 360 mg, and no epinephrine was added, so one may assume that a significant amount of drug was absorbed and in some cases passed on to the fetus.

It may be concluded that these unfavorable reports record the effects of the supine hypotensive syndrome revealed by epidural analgesia rather than a primarily deleterious effect of epidural blockade itself. Again, emphasis must be placed on the importance of the lateral position. The supine position in the presence of vasodilatation of the legs is a sure recipe for maternal hypotension in a significant number of cases (Grennell and Vandewater, 1961).

Summary

The influence of posture, labor and analgesic technique on acid-base balance are summarized in Figures 12–32 and 12–33. It can be seen that many factors affect the acid-base balance of the mother and fetus during labor, and the normal trend is toward a markedly acidotic state in both mother and child. Epidural analgesia and correct posture can influence the balance profoundly. If bad management allows maternal hypotension to develop and persist, then acidosis and fetal asphyxia may reach dangerous proportions, leading to severe fetal depression. On the other hand, with proper technique the burden of labor is lifted, and the mother rests quietly throughout the whole active period of the first and second stages. As a result, maternal acidosis does not develop, and the fetus is born with a significantly lower blood lactate and a higher postdelivery pH than in a "normal" spontaneous labor.

The question naturally arises, is this a good thing? Is it better to be born gently and with a higher pH than our forebears who entered the world roughly from an acid womb? This is a hard question to answer in terms of natural selection and survival of the species, but from the point of view of the individual, the evidence is in favor of an easy transit. However, teleological

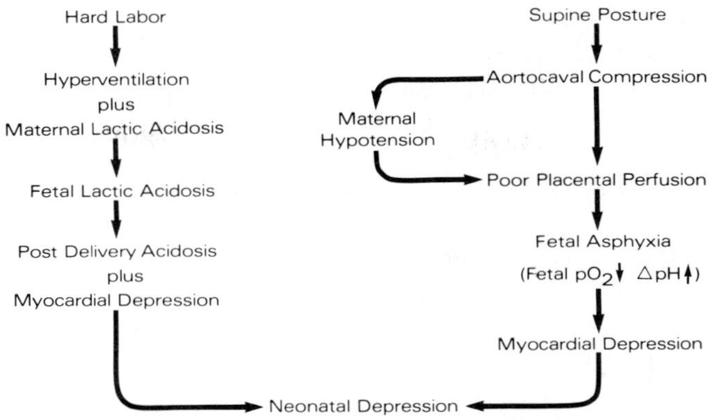

Figure 12–32. Summary of nonanalgesic fetal depressants in labor.

suspicion still lingers that nature is unlikely to have designed an acidotic entrance into the world to no purpose and that perhaps we have missed some important clue to the puzzle of acidosis in natural spontaneous labor.

Bing and his colleagues (1973) have given us a possible clue. They

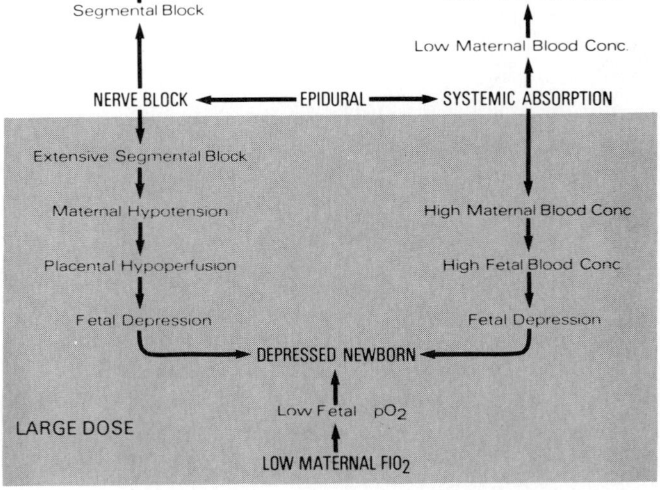

Figure 12–33. Summary of influence of epidural technique and oxygen therapy on newborn.

have shown that rat fetal heart muscle performs better under transient hypoxia if it is relatively alkalotic. This is in agreement with the previous work of others that showed deteriorating myocardial contractility with increasing acidosis (Downing et al., 1966; Gelet et al., 1969; Andersson et al., 1970). However, after extreme and almost lethal hypoxia, papillary muscle function recovered about twice as fast from a pH of 7.1 than from a pH of 7.4. Thus, in profound degrees of hypoxia, acidosis may have a function in protecting the myocardium from contracture and death. Nevertheless, this work must be seen in proportion, for in a clinical situation brain death is likely to precede myocardial death, and there would be little point in choosing an acidotic situation merely to favor the survival of a heart-lung preparation in the event of extreme hypoxia.

At the present time, the balance of evidence supports the view that the newborn is favored and assisted in his difficult adaptation to independent life by a tranquil, planned labor, freed from the acidosis of a normal delivery. Of all the analgesic regimens available to bring this about, *properly managed* lumbar epidural analgesia appears to be the safest and most effective way to protect the baby from the hazards of natural childbirth.

ACID-BASE BALANCE DURING CESAREAN SECTION

At elective abdominal section the fetus is spared the metabolic consequences of labor. However, there are some disadvantages, particularly those of the mother's supine posture on the operating table and birth by a route that fails to compress the fetal thorax and wring out the air passages. In addition, the fetus is exposed to any depressant anesthetic drugs that may reach it from the maternal circulation.

Maternal hypotension is a common accompaniment of cesarean section under epidural analgesia in the supine position. The incidence has been quoted as between 16 and 50 per cent, depending on criteria and technique (Fox and Houle, 1969; Milne and Lawson, 1973). Uncorrected maternal hypotension is a potent cause of deterioration in fetal acid-base status, so the special circumstances surrounding low blood pressure at cesarean section will be considered in some detail.

Posture

As we have seen, the supine posture is one of the most powerful, and at the same time unnecessary, forces contributing to maternal hypotension and to fetal asphyxia from aortocaval compression. This factor becomes more important in the presence of lower limb vasodilatation from either general anesthesia or from conduction blockade when regional vascular tone is reduced and insufficient to force venous return into the unobstructed azygos system. The incidence of the Poseiro effect and of maternal hypotension is greater under spinal and epidural block than under general anesthesia, unless effective steps are taken to relieve aortocaval compression (Ansari et al., 1970; Goodlin, 1971; Clemetson et al., 1973; Humphrey et al., 1973). However, the supine hypotensive syndrome can occur under general anesthesia, and the degree of collapse may be just as severe as under subarachnoid or epidural block. For example, three cases of severe supine hypotensive syndrome were reported from one center in 1970, all of them under light nitrous oxide–oxygen and relaxant anesthesia, and one of them ended fatally (Courtney, 1970). Various measures have been recommended to displace the uterus away from the great vessels, including lateral tilt of the table (Ansari et al., 1970), a self-supporting device for pushing the uterus sideways (Colon-Morales, 1970), and a simple sandbag or foam wedge under one or other hip (Crawford, 1972). None of these maneuvers does a completely effective job, and the logical step of operating in the lateral position has been taken by Waldron and Wood at Melbourne (1971). The lateral position offers two great safety advantages that may outweigh its disadvantages. Aspiration of vomitus is almost completely avoided if general anesthesia becomes necessary, and the effects of aortocaval compression on the mother and fetus are eliminated. Little is sacrificed except custom, and the surgeon becomes less fatigued because he is able to sit down throughout the performance of his task. At the present time, comparative acid-base studies have not been done to assess the degree of improvement obtained in the fetus by changing from a lateral tilt to the full lateral position.

Hydration

In the presence of aortocaval compression, the maternal circulation is highly sensitive to changes of vascular capacitance, and it is most important to ensure an adequate or augmented blood volume during spinal blockade. Marx and her colleagues have shown that maternal blood pressure is more stable and the baby is in better condition if the mother is prehydrated with 1000 ml of glucose or glucose-saline immediately before induction of spinal blockade (Wollman and Marx, 1968; Marx et al., 1969).

In cardiac failure a narrow margin exists between adequate hydration and circulatory overload, and these patients must be handled with extreme care to keep the middle path between hypotension and congestive failure. However, with a slow incremental induction, epidural blockade can be instituted safely and satisfactorily.

Oxygen

The fetus also has a narrow margin between adequate oxygenation and a state of hypoxia that draws upon its carbohydrate stores for caloric requirements by anaerobic breakdown of glycogen to glucose and lactic acid, with a resulting fall of pH and increase of lactate/pyruvate ratio. Analysis of available oxygen and carbohydrate stores shows that a 10 per cent oxygen deficit will exhaust fetal oxygen stores in about 20 to 25 minutes, and beyond this point fetal pH will fall and Δ Mat-Fet pH will increase rapidly (Rooth, 1973).

Provided some degree of placental exchange exists, maternal hy-

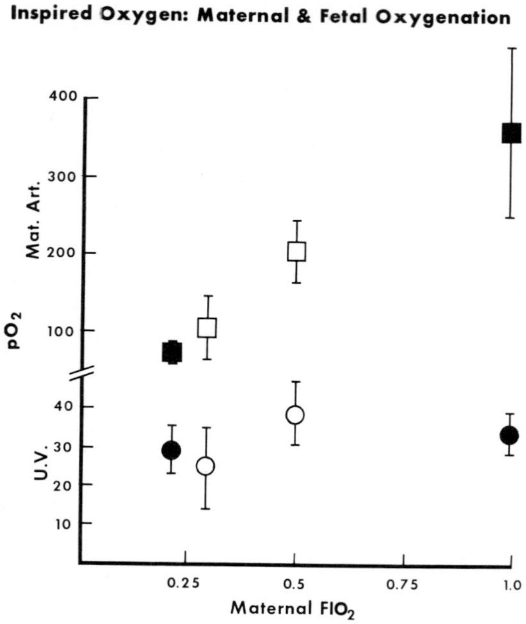

Figure 12–34. Influence of maternal inspired oxygen ratio (FIO_2) on maternal and fetal oxygenation at birth by cesarean section.
● ■ Epidural analgesia
○ □ Light general anesthesia + relaxant
(After Fox and Houle, 1971; Houle et al. 1969.)

peroxia will improve fetal oxygenation, so any situation that may conceivably jeopardize fetal oxygen supplies should be treated prophylactically by giving 100 per cent oxygen to the mother. Oxygen used in this way is analogous to a safety belt in an automobile: most of the time it seems unnecessary, but in an accident it may mean all the difference between life and death. Even in uncomplicated cesarean sections, fetal oxygenation, acid-base status and performance are at their best when the maternal FIO_2 approaches 1.0, as shown in Figures 12–34, 12–35 and 12–36 (Fox and Houle, 1971; Houle et al., 1969).

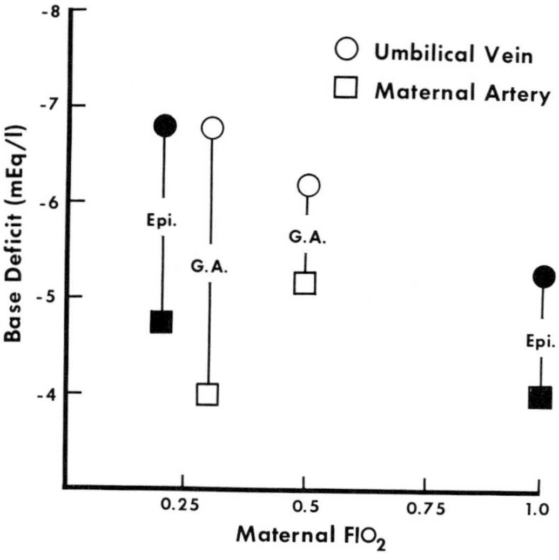

Figure 12–35. Influence of maternal FIO_2 on base deficit at birth by cesarean section (symbols as in Fig. 12–34). (After Fox and Houle, 1971; Houle et al., 1969.)

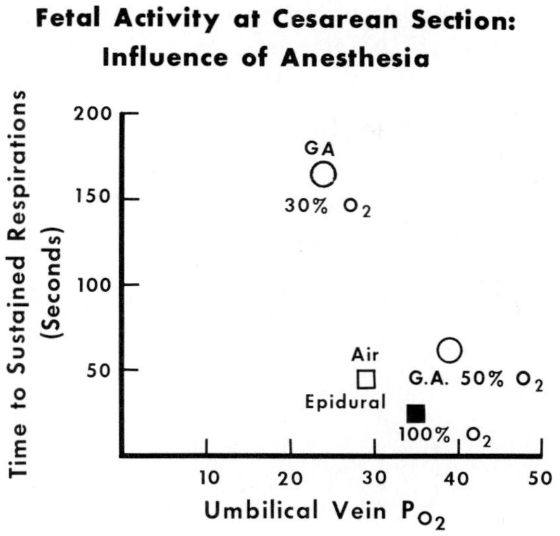

Figure 12–36. Influence of maternal FIO_2 and anesthetic technique on fetal oxygenation and performance (time to sustained respiration) at cesarean section birth (symbols as in Fig. 12–34). (After Fox and Houle, 1971; Houle et al., 1969.)

Absorption of Epidural Drugs

Excessive amounts of local anesthetic not only produce unnecessarily extensive epidural blockade but also give rise to high blood concentrations in the fetus. Although no correlations have been made between fetal blood concentrations and acid-base status, overall performance appears to suffer in the presence of high local anesthetic concentrations (Shnider and Way, 1968b).

The influence of epinephrine in the epidural solution is more subtle and controversial. Again, no direct correlations have been made between fetal acid-base status and the presence or absence of epinephrine in epidural solutions, but there is evidence that maternal cardiovascular stability is markedly affected, and therefore fetal acid-base balance is influenced indirectly.

Ueland and his associates (1972) have shown that remarkably small changes of blood pressure and cardiac output occur when blockade is performed without epinephrine added to the epidural solution, in contrast to much more serious hypotension that follows injections made with epinephrine-containing solutions (Stenger et al., 1965). This difference has been attributed to the beta-stimulating effects of absorbed epinephrine, which cause more profound peripheral vasodilatation than plain epidural solutions (Ward et al., 1965; Bonica et al., 1971). However, as mentioned in an earlier chapter, an alternative explanation lies in the more intense quality of blockade and sympathetic denervation produced by epinephrine-containing analgesic solutions. Quality of sensory, motor and sympathetic blockades tends to be interrelated, and escape from the consequences of sympathetic blockade is bought at the expense of relatively poor sensory anesthesia when local anesthetics are used in plain solution (Bromage et al., 1964; Bromage, 1965, 1975).

Vasopressors

Prophylactic vasopressor therapy before cesarean section is unnecessary and deleterious to uterine blood flow (James et al., 1970). With increased appreciation of the prime causes of hypotension, appropriate use of posture and adequate prehydration usually ensure that the maternal blood pressure remains within acceptable limits. However, vasopressors may be needed in a small proportion of cases in which segmental blockade is too extensive or lateral tilt is insufficient to relieve vascular compression at the pelvic brim.

The choice of vasopressors and technique of administration are important to obtain maximum restoration of blood pressure and cardiac output without vasoconstrictor effect on the uteroplacental circulation. Alpha-adrenergic drugs should be avoided, as they have predominant effects on the peripheral circulation, increasing vascular resistance and reducing uterine blood flow, while beta-adrenergic agents in small doses increase cardiac output and peripheral flow. Methoxamine appears to be particularly undesirable (Vasicka et al., 1964). Greiss and Crandell (1965) found that norepinephrine and phenylephrine restored central blood pressure effectively, but this was negated by a proportional reduction of uterine blood flow due to peripheral vasoconstriction. In a later paper, James, Greiss and Kemp (1970) showed that the most favorable results on uterine blood flow were obtained with small doses of pressor agents that have mixed alpha and beta activity, but with mainly beta effects. The balance between increased maternal blood pressure and improved uterine blood flow is best achieved with ephedrine and mephentermine. Effective dosage of these pressor agents could be reduced by about one half if they were given with atropine to prevent bradycardia. However, even ephedrine and mephentermine failed to return uterine blood flow completely to normal, and there was a persistent 10 to 15 per cent deficit. A very elegant study by Shnider's group, using a chronic preparation in sheep, has shown that ephedrine in clinical doses has little or no effect on resting uterine blood flow, while mephentermine causes a considerably greater reduction of uterine blood flow than was previously supposed. This same study confirmed the adverse effects of metaraminol and methoxamine, as shown in Figure 12–37 (Ralston, Shnider and deLorimier, 1974). Thus, vasopressor therapy is not ideal from the point of view of uterine blood flow and fetal acid-base balance. It should be reserved for cases in which maternal

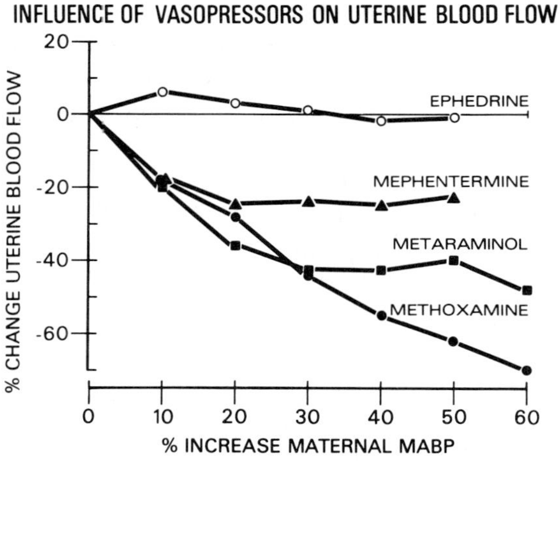

Figure 12–37. Influence of vasopressors on uterine blood flow and mean arterial blood pressure (MABP) in pregnant sheep. (After Ralston, Shnider and deLorimier, 1974.)

TABLE 12–10 Vasopressors and Uterine Blood Flow in Maternal Hypotension

Alpha and Beta Adrenergic Action	*Drug*	*Depression of Uterine Blood Flow (%)*	*Dosage*	*Indication*
Very strong alpha adrenergic effects with serious reduction of uterine blood flow	Norepinephrine Phenylephrine Methoxamine (Vasoxyl)	50–65	Contraindicated in obstetrics	
Moderately strong alpha adrenergic effects, some uterine vasoconstriction	Metaraminol (Aramine)	40–45	0.2–1 mg IV	Not ideal
	Mephentermine (Wyamine)	20–25	3–6 mg IV	
Weak alpha adrenergic effect, marked beta adrenergic effect	Ephedrine	0–5	10–20 mg IV	Almost ideal
	Methamphetamine		5–15 mg	

blood pressure cannot be kept at normal levels by other means, and then ephedrine is the drug of choice.

Table 12–10 summarizes the suitability of various vasopressors for restoring maternal blood pressure and maintaining uterine blood flow.

Comparison of Maternal and Fetal Acid-Base Status at Cesarean Section: General Anesthesia versus Epidural Analgesia

It is doubtful whether any useful comparison can be made between the published results of acid-base status at cesarean section under general anesthesia and under epidural analgesia, since so many uncontrolled variables are involved. However, it may be helpful to consider some figures from reasonably comparable series just to obtain a rough idea of the similarities and differences that have been found. Table 12–11 summarizes the maternal and fetal pH and base deficit values at elective cesarean section in four separate institutions. There is very little difference in acid-base outcome between these small samples, but what difference there is can be seen to favor epidural analgesia combined with a high maternal inspired oxygen concentration. Also, it is interesting to note the different interpretations that can be put upon the same data. For example, Hollmén and Jagerhorn (1968) concluded from their umbilical artery values that epidural analgesia caused more fetal acidosis than general anesthesia, yet the Δ M-UV results show the opposite conclusion. Two factors not shown in Table 12–11 but possibly contributing to an accumulation of hydrogen ions in Hollmén's epidural babies were a relative maternal respiratory alkalosis and the use of metaraminol (a mild uterine vasoconstrictor) in four of their ten patients.

Thus, it can be seen that there are considerable difficulties in arriving at a valid comparison between different series, even when they come from the same institution, and as far as acid-base status is concerned, the choice between epidural and general anesthesia remains open and undecided (James et al., 1977b).

In summary, fetal acid-base balance during cesarean section is at its best when satisfactory epidural analgesia is combined with a high maternal

TABLE 12–11 Comparison of Maternal and Fetal Acid-Base Status at Cesarean Section: General Anesthesia versus Lumbar Epidural Analgesia

			pH at Delivery				*Base Deficit at Delivery (mEq/L)*			
	n	*MATERNAL FIO_2*	*MATERNAL*	*UMBILICAL VEIN*	*UMBILICAL ARTERY*	*M-UV pH*	*MATERNAL*	*UMBILICAL VEIN*	*UMBILICAL ARTERY*	*M-UV*
General Anesthesia										
Hollmén et al. (1967)	12	0.37	7.35	7.23	7.21	0.12	5.7	9.7	9.9	−4.0
Rorke et al. (1968)	11	1.0	7.38	7.27	7.21	0.11	6.4	7.6	9.1	−1.2
	11	0.66	7.41	7.28	7.23	0.13	5.2	6.6	7.1	−1.4
Fox and Houle (1971)	13	0.28	7.38	7.27	7.22	0.11	4.9	6.8	8.1	−1.9
James et al. (1977b)	20	0.66	7.474	7.380	7.323	0.094	3.0	1.9	1.8	1.1
Epidural Analgesia										
Hollmén and Jägerhorn (1968)	10	0.21	7.38	7.28	7.23	0.10	6.6	8.4	12.0	−1.8
Fox and Houle (1971)	13	1.0	7.42	7.33	7.28	0.09	4.1	5.3	6.7	−1.2
James et al. (1977b)	15	1.0	7.444	7.59	7.297	0.085	3.0	1.6	1.3	1.4

FIO_2. Provided maternal hypotension is avoided, this combination produces a better fetal acid-base status and fetal performance than light general anesthesia and muscle relaxant. However, the vasodilation that accompanies effective epidural blockade increases the chances that maternal hypotension may occur in the supine position, and then uterine blood flow becomes more at risk than under light general anesthesia and relaxant.

The ideal combination probably lies in the following:

1. Epidural blockade using appropriate dosage and a local anesthetic with high protein-binding capabilities and with epinephrine added to the solution, in order to reduce maternal and fetal uptake
2. Adequate prehydration of the mother
3. The mother breathing 100 per cent oxygen
4. Operation in the full lateral position, recommended by Waldron and Wood (1971), or, failing this, adequate pelvic tilt to prevent aortocaval compression.

MASKED PATHOLOGICAL PAIN

Accidental hemorrhage (abruptio placentae) and rupture of the uterus are two obstetrical disasters that may give rise to intense boring pain in the lower abdomen and back. It is often feared that analgesia provided by epidural blockade will increase the dangers by masking early warning signs and allowing catastrophe to progress silently and unnoticed until profound oligemic shock and fetal asphyxia have developed. In fact, epidural analgesia is not a major factor clouding the diagnosis in either type of catastrophe, providing the obstetrical team is aware that the sign of pain is only one of several variables and that particular attention should be paid to the presence of *persistent* pain arising in the presence of a technically satisfactory epidural block (Eckstein et al., 1973).

Abruptio Placentae

Varying degrees of placental abruption occur with an incidence of between 1:78 deliveries and 1:200, depending on the source of material. In four out of five cases the diagnosis is apparent from "revealed" vaginal hemorrhage (Blair, 1973; Lunan, 1973). The condition is characterized by severe lower abdominal pain, a tense, spastic, "ligneous" uterus, and signs of blood loss and shock. Hemorrhage is confined within the uterine cavity and "concealed" in about one fifth of the cases, and it is only then that diagnosis may be difficult. When dilute solutions of local anesthetic are used (e.g., bupivacaine 0.125 to 0.25 per cent), the quality of analgesia is sufficient to provide relief from the intermittent pain of normal uterine contractions, but it is not enough to suppress the continuous afferent bombardment from a tetanically contracted uterus. Thus, persistent pain becomes a matter for concern, and diagnosis should be sought from among the possible causes outlined in Table 12–12.

Epidural Analgesia and Uterine Rupture

Uterine rupture during labor occurs with an incidence between 1:93 confinements and 1:8,741, depending on the source of material, and fetal mortality is said to be over 50 per cent (Oxorn and Foote, 1968). Some authors have suggested that epidural analgesia for relief of pain in labor delays the diagnosis of uterine rupture, thereby increasing the risk to mother and child (Brudenell and Chakravarti, 1975; O'Driscoll, 1975). The argument is this: effective epidural blockade relieves the pain of normal uterine contractions, but it also masks the early warning pain of uterine rupture, so that tears may extend to dangerous proportions before emergency cesarean section is undertaken. Superficially, this argument seems appealing, but in practice the situation is not so simple. First, a fair proportion of uterine tears are a silent incomplete dehiscence and are not accompanied by inordinate and diagnostic pain (Crawford, 1974b). Second, the degree of epidural analgesia that is adequate to relieve normal uterine contractions is quite tenuous and insufficient to block the more intense pain of severe rupture (Eckstein et al., 1973). Third, a sense of

TABLE 12–12 Differential Diagnosis of Persistent Pain During Labor Under Epidural Analgesia with Dilute Analgesic Solutions

Persistent occipitoposterior position:		Low back and sacral pain that may be mild or even absent in presence of technically successful epidural block
Abruptio placentae		
Rupture of uterus		
Burst uterine varix		
Torsion of uterus		
Nonuterine:	(a) Perforated or ruptured viscus	
	(b) Gallstone colic	
	(c) Strangulated diaphragmatic hernia*	

*The few cases seen by the author have given rise to pain *after* delivery and not during labor.

TABLE 12–13 Incidence of Uterine Rupture Related to Obstetrical Policy in Two Major Teaching Hospitals

Hospital	*Incidence of Uterine Rupture*	*Management of Post–Cesarean Section Labor*
Kings College Hospital, London, England	1:1,166 (Brudenell and Chakravarti, 1975)	Permissive vaginal delivery
Royal Victoria Hospital, Montreal, Canada	1:5,528 (Period 1961–1976)	Mandatory repeat section

proportion should be preserved in adapting anesthetic practice to standards of obstetrical practice. In areas where the incidence of uterine rupture is high, prudence demands that epidural analgesia be monitored extremely carefully and in doubtful circumstances sometimes avoided altogether. On the other hand, epidural analgesia can be used with greater freedom and confidence where obstetrical practice favors a very low incidence of rupture.

Key factors determining the incidence of uterine rupture are (a) obstetrical policy towards the scarred uterus; (b) standards of administration of oxytocic drugs; and (c) standards of management of labor and analgesia. Since approximately 50 per cent of uterine ruptures are associated with a scarred uterus, incidence of uterine tears will be relatively high in units where vaginal delivery is permitted after a previous cesarean section, myomectomy or tubal reimplantation, but it will be relatively low where a rigid policy of sectioning the scarred uterus is always observed. The policy of "once a cesarean section, always a cesarean section" appears to be the most important single factor in avoiding unnecessary uterine rupture and in providing an obstetrical environment in which epidural analgesia can be used with confidence that pain relief will not compound the difficulties of management. Table 12–13 illustrates this point with figures from two major teaching units.

The diagnosis and successful outcome of a uterine tear is primarily dependent on obstetrical management, and it is unlikely that epidural analgesia will delay diagnosis of uterine rupture when the appropriate policies are adopted. Experience with uterine rupture at the Royal Victoria Hospital, Montreal, over a 15½-year period has shown a lack of association between epidural analgesia and diagnostic delay. During this time 44,230 deliveries took place, and there were eight cases of partial or complete uterine rupture, an incidence of 1:5,528. Two stillbirths but no maternal deaths occurred in these cases. Epidural analgesia was used in over 30,000 deliveries, but only one case of dehiscence occurred in the presence of epidural analgesia, and even then the diagnosis was made promptly. There was not one single instance in which the diagnosis of uterine tear was delayed by the presence of epidural analgesia in this series of 44,230 deliveries and 30,500 epidurals. On the basis of our experience, we maintain that epidural analgesia does not increase the danger from a ruptured uterus, except when labor is deliberately cultivated in a scarred uterus and in the presence of profound analgesia or when labor is inadequately monitored and managed.

In conclusion, trial of labor in a scarred uterus entails a degree of risk, regardless of the mode of analgesia. However, if trial of labor is undertaken in the presence of a uterine scar, the following precautions should be observed:

1. Minimal analgesia should be provided. If epidural analgesia is chosen, only dilute solutions of local anesthetic (e.g., 0.125 per cent bupivacaine) should be used (Vanderick et al., 1974). Blockade should be intermittent and not continuous, in order to assess the site and degree of pain for brief periods during the course of labor.

2. Stringent internal and external maternal and fetal monitoring should be carried out during the whole course of labor, and frequent abdominal examinations should be made. Any one of the cardinal signs of rupture should be an indication for urgent cesarean section.

3. Oxytocin is best avoided, but if given it should be administered extremely cautiously, and then only in the presence of adequate internal monitoring.

4. The obstetrician and the anesthesiologist should be in agreement that if uterine tonus rises or uterine contractions become intense, epidural analgesia should be discontinued until uterine activity is restored to normal and dangerous stresses on the scar are reduced.

Headache, Backache and Bladder Dysfunction

The incidence of headache, backache and disturbance of micturition after delivery is higher than generally appreciated, and when these complications do occur, it is natural to blame them on some obvious and external cause. However, in the majority of cases they are coincidental and arise from causes inherent in labor and delivery rather than from the block itself. Two authorities with very extensive experience cite an appreciable incidence of headache and backache after delivery under general anesthesia. Moore (1955) estimates the occurrence rate to be about 10 per cent, and Bonica (1967) places the incidence between 10 and 15 per cent. This is in agreement with other series which recorded a 10 per cent incidence of headache after delivery under general anesthesia or pudendal block (White et al., 1962; Winkler et al., 1963).

Two independent studies carried out in England have shown that the incidence of these complications is somewhat higher and approximately the same whether epidural analgesia is used or not. Table 12–14 summarizes these results (Crawford, 1972; Grove, 1973; Moir and Davidson, 1972).

TABLE 12–14 Incidence (%) of Postpartum Headache, Backache and Bladder Dysfunction Related to Labor and Delivery, With and Without Epidural Analgesia

	Grove (1973)	*Crawford (1972)*	*Moir and Davidson (1972)*	
	***Nonepidural* n = 187**	***Epidural* n = 923**	*NONEPIDURAL* n = 50	*EPIDURAL* n = 50
Headache	23	19.4	10	18 (no dural punctures)
Backache	37.5	45	32	22
Bladder Dysfunction				
Spontaneous delivery	14.2	8.9	–	–
Forceps	37.5	25.8	20	34
Perineal pain	Not reported	Not reported	100	100

NEUROLOGICAL SEQUELAE

Neurological sequelae after childbirth may arise from a number of "natural" or obstetrical causes, some of which are listed below:

Causes of Postpartum Neural Deficits

Prevalence	*Cause*
Common 1:4,000 (approximately)	Compression and injury of peripheral nerves crossing the pelvic brim (e.g., lumbosacral trunk, femoral nerves, lateral femoral cutaneous nerve)
Moderately common 1:6,000 (approximately)	Spinal root compression from prolapsed intervertebral disc
Rare 1:15,000	Hemangioma of spinal cord; spontaneous epidural hematoma

Underlying neuropathies may predispose to neurological damage, and the prevalence of these conditions vary geographically. Diabetes is the commonest cause of mononeuropathy in North America, and investigation of a neural deficit should always include routine tests for diabetes. The overall incidence of postpartum neurological sequelae *in the absence of regional anesthesia* is in the range of 1:2,100 to 1:3,000 confinements, depending on the source of information (Tillman, 1935; Hill, 1962; Murray, 1964). Neurological problems arising after epidural analgesia for childbirth must be viewed against this "control" incidence of neural complications inherent in the obstetrical process rather than in the anesthetic (see Chapter 14).

As an example, the following case summary illustrates the type of neural injury that may result from difficult labor due to cephalopelvic disproportion.

CASE L2–59: Unilateral Footdrop (1959)

A 29 year old white primigravida had a long and painful incoordinate labor, with a right occipitoposterior presentation. After 30 hours of labor the cervix was still only 4 cm dilated; the membranes ruptured and meconium staining appeared. Epidural analgesia was induced at the second lumbar interspace. Doses of 5 ml of 2 per cent lidocaine with 1:200,000 epinephrine produced pain relief, and uterine contractions became more effective. Labor progressed slowly over the next 24 hours, and a difficult midcavity forceps rotation produced a 9-lb female infant in good condition (Apgar score not recorded). A total of 16 epidural doses were given over a 24-hour period (i.e., cumulative dose of 1600 mg lidocaine).

After delivery the patient complained of weakness of the left leg, and there was footdrop with hypoalgesia over the outer side of the left calf. Recovery was complete in four months. There was no evidence of underlying diabetes.

In this case the nature of the neurological lesion seemed quite clear, and epidural analgesia was not considered to be a direct or a contributory cause. It was assumed that pressure by the fetal head or by the forceps had caused damage to the lumbosacral trunk. This case occurred in 1959; today labor would probably be managed differently, and abdominal section for cephalopelvic disproportion would spare the lumbosacral trunk.

In addition to "natural" or unavoidable sequelae of childbirth, epidural analgesia may present its own neurological problems. However, the incidence of *serious* neurological sequelae attributable to properly conducted epidural analgesia is extremely rare and far less than that of neural injuries from obstetric and other associated but unrelated causes. This fact should be clearly appreciated in order to keep a proper perspective of the whole field of neurological safety and risk-benefit ratios. During the past 20 years more than 30,000 deliveries have been conducted under epidural analgesia at the Royal Victoria Hospital, Montreal, without a single neurologic injury attributable to the anesthetic. These anesthetics were administered by a number of staff and residents, and the experience is large enough to establish a high degree of confidence in the safety of the method. Several instances of transient nerve damage attributable to obstetrical or postural causes were encountered, as in the case above, but the anesthetic was not considered to be implicated in any of these.

Neurological Complications Attributable to Epidural Analgesia in Labor

Having dismissed serious neurological sequelae as extremely rare, it must now be said that transient neurological complications may arise relatively frequently, but they are of minor importance and of a controllable and self-limiting nature. For purposes of clarification, they may be considered as immediate and delayed.

Immediate complications

Shivering. Approximately one third of women in labor shiver after epidural blockade is induced. The shivering may be brief and last a matter of seconds, or it may continue quite violently for several minutes after the epidural solution is injected. The reason is not clear, but a disturbance of thermosensation may be the underlying cause, as suggested in Chapter 10. The rapid spread of analgesic solution at term may result in an unusually sudden and widespread segmental disturbance of thermal information. Shivering usually subsides spontaneously as the epidural block takes full effect.

Accidental Epidural Intravenous Injection. This possibility has been discussed earlier, and it may result in transient convulsions if venous cannulation is unrecognized. At term the epidural veins are distended, and accidental cannulation of the enlarged veins occurs with an incidence of about 1 per cent. The toxic effects of accidental epidural intravenous injection of local anesthetic are most florid when the patient is lying on her back. Then, the inferior vena cava is compressed by the weight of the uterus, and rapid blood flow through the alternative azygos pathway increases the bolus effect of injected local anesthetic, which travels as a "slug" to the heart and thence onward to the central nervous system.

Accidental intravenous cannulation can be avoided by the following:

1. Using soft, blunt-nosed epidural catheters.
2. Injecting a priming dose of local anesthetic through the epidural

needle before passing an epidural catheter. This seems to facilitate an atraumatic passage of the catheter.

3. Always performing aspiration through the epidural catheter to exclude the presence of blood or cerebrospinal fluid before injecting a top-up dose of local anesthetic.

Very rarely, a catheter may find its way into an epidural vein after correct placement in the epidural space, even after several uncomplicated injections of local anesthetic (Ryan, 1973). This remote possibility makes precautionary aspiration a mandatory prelude to every top-up injection of local anesthetic. Top-up doses should not be given when the patient is supine, only when she is in the lateral or tilted position.

Horner's Syndrome. Horner's syndrome has recently been noticed as a benign and relatively frequent complication of epidural analgesia in labor. It was first reported in 1972, when it was found to be associated with extensive unilateral spread of cutaneous analgesia following caudal injection of 22 ml of 3 per cent chloroprocaine (Kepes et al., 1972); an increasing number of cases have been reported since then. In some instances the miosis and ptosis accompanied an unusually extensive cephalad spread of analgesia into the upper thoracic segments, and the Horner's syndrome was not unexpected. However, an increasing number of cases have shown a Horner's syndrome in the absence of cutaneous analgesia above the level of T_7 (Mohan and Potter, 1975; Collier, 1975; Carrie and Mohan, 1976).

Mohan and Potter (1975) have reported pupillary changes in 17 out of 20 women receiving caudal analgesia for labor, and a prospective study from the same unit revealed a 75 per cent incidence after lumbar block (Carrie and Mohan, 1976). Many of us have looked for similar findings and failed to see them, except in rare instances when the presence of abnormally extensive cutaneous anesthesia has affected the upper thoracic segments (Evans, Gauci and Watkins, 1975).

This intriguing observation raises a number of questions. Why has such an apparently common phenomenon not been noticed before in the hundreds of thousands of extradural blocks administered for relief of pain in labor, and why does it seem to occur more frequently in some units than in others? Why should a cutaneous block to T_7 be accompanied by paralysis of the ocular sympathetic neurons, well above the upper limits of cutaneous analgesia? And what are the mechanisms of analgesic spread underlying this neurological oddity?

No clear explanation exists at the present time, but perhaps it may be noteworthy that the observations of pupillary changes have been made at a period when driven labor with relatively high oxytocic dosage is commonplace, suggesting that a causal relationship may possibly exist and that the incidence of Horner's syndrome may be unusually high in units where heavy doses of oxytocics are used. Extensive spread to the ocular sympathetic is another reminder of the extraordinarily wide analgesic diffusion that characterizes epidural blockade at term.

DELAYED COMPLICATIONS

Several cases of delayed recovery following epidural analgesia have been reported in the recent literature. There was no obvious cause for

TABLE 12–15 Delayed Recovery After Epidural Analgesia in Labor

Author	*Drug*	*Number of Cases*	*Duration of Residual Analgesia (hours)*
Bromage (1969)	Tetracaine 0.5% + epinephrine	3	9–48
	Bupivacaine 0.5% + epinephrine	1	10
Pathy and Rosen (1975)	Bupivacaine 0.5% + epinephrine	1	48
Cuerden et al. (1977)	Bupivacaine 0.5% + epinephrine	4	23–48

prolonged anesthesia in any of these obstetrical patients, and suspicion fell upon the anesthetic itself. In every case labor was uncomplicated, a long-acting drug such as tetracaine or bupivacaine was used in relatively strong concentration, and segmental analgesia regressed incompletely to leave a residual patchy anesthesia, sometimes with weakness of one thigh or leg. Symptoms persisted for 10 to 48 hours and then disappeared, leaving the patient completely recovered (Bromage, 1969; Pathy and Rosen, 1975; Cuerden et al., 1977). Case reports are summarized in Table 12–15.

The reason for these prolonged recoveries is not clear. However, it will be recalled that pregnant women at term show evidence of a remarkably increased susceptibility to epidural anesthesia. Analgesia is more rapid, spreads further and is more intense than in nonpregnant subjects, and it is reasonable to suppose that delayed recovery merely reflects a generally enhanced attachment for local anesthetics to binding sites in neural and perineural tissues, particularly when drugs with strong protein and lipid affinities are used. Delayed recovery has not yet been reported following obstetrical anesthesia with etidocaine, but in view of the high lipid solubility of etidocaine, it would be surprising if cases do not appear in the future.

This pattern of unusually delayed regression appears to be innocuous and fully reversible. However, prolonged recovery from anesthetic blockade could also be a warning that susceptible tissues are not invulnerable to strong concentrations of powerfully binding local anesthetics. It would seem prudent to take the hint and to use weaker solutions of long-acting analgesics at term. Shorter-acting agents, such as carbonated lidocaine or 2-chloroprocaine, would seem to be a better choice when intense analgesia is required for abdominal section.

A more general discussion of neurological sequelae unrelated to pregnancy is presented in Chapter 14.

LOGISTICS AND MANAGERIAL PRACTICES IN AN OBSTETRICAL EPIDURAL SERVICE

In former years notable differences existed between obstetrical anesthetic practice in Europe and North America (Crawford, 1959, 1966, 1972). Today, some differences still exist, but the stage is set for unifying changes. Two organizations devoted to obstetrical anesthesia have sprung into existence on opposite sides of the Atlantic. The Association of Obstetric

Anaesthetists in Britain and the Society for Obstetrical Anesthesia and Perinatology in the United States are now coordinated by closely integrated secretariats, and common problems are shared effectively. Those differences of practice that do remain between the two transatlantic groups are not related to lack of scientific agreement but rather to constraints imposed by differences of obstetrical and administrative outlook. The anesthetic skills and know-how exist; the difficulties in applying them to the whole population are mainly due to administrative, managerial and fiscal problems.

It has become increasingly evident that urban obstetrics should not be practiced in units with less than 3,000 or 4,000 deliveries per year. This is about the minimum output that can sustain a 24-hour service with all the necessary support facilities so that it can still remain economically viable in a free market. Smaller case loads are not economically feasible and cannot justify the costly intensive milieu that is necessary to provide optimal care to all comers at all times. Naturally, babies will continue to be born in remote places, and as in the past they will be given the best care that is available on the spot, but the risks of that type of environment will be higher than in specialized units, and these risks must be accepted as part of the primitive outback life, if circumstances dictate that confinement shall take place there. For the majority of the population, delivery will take place in an urban environment, and there is no excuse for perpetuating small units with dangerously limited facilities and for bringing the privations of the bush into urban and suburban practice, where every known support can and should be made available to mother and child.

The medical profession has been slow to grapple with its own logistical problems and to police its commons (Hardin, 1968; Hiatt, 1975). In some countries aggressive governmental technocracy has taken up this abandoned leadership with incisive policies of regionalization and rationalization of medical resources. In the Province of Quebec, government has tackled the problem with firmness and determination. A number of small urban obstetrical facilities have been closed by edict and obstetrical services concentrated in a few large regional centers with the physical plant, expertise and administrative capabilities to provide an effective 24-hour service offering the necessary intensive care services to cope with all eventualities; these also act as referral centers for high-risk pregnancies from outlying areas ("Projet de régroupement des services d'obstétriques 5." Ministère des Affaires Sociales; Direction des Communications 74E11–21–1974).

This type of far-seeing administrative concern is a necessary prelude to providing first class, round-the-clock anesthesia services for the obstetrical public at large. Within such an organization it is possible to arrange a sensible working schedule of 8- or 12-hour shifts that ensures freedom from overwork and the errors of judgment that arise from grinding fatigue. Indeed, changing views of medicolegal responsibility are making it clear that errors of judgment arising from fatigue are at least partly the responsibility of a culpable administration that has failed to provide an adequate establishment to cover the clinical load under safe working conditions.

In my view, an effective obstetrical anesthesia service requires that both obstetric and anesthetic consultants and junior staff should be available in the hospital at all times. This type of professional coverage is essential for the safe management of any large referral unit, particularly for one relying on an epidural service. It implies the provision of an adequate system of off-duty time, with sufficient staff for an appropriate arrangement of duty relief. In addition, suitable hospital living and sleeping quarters must be provided for physicians working at night and on weekends and public holidays. None of these expensive requirements and other supporting facilities can be justified without an adequate supply of clinical material to pay for them and enough work to ensure that all personnel are gainfully employed.

Clinical service grows rusty and empirical without the continued stimulus of self-questioning that goes with teaching and research, and wherever possible these intellectual functions should be an integral part of the group's activities. Units with an annual load of over 3,000 deliveries per year are large enough to justify inclusion in teaching and regional "recycling" programs. It is the responsibility of regional planning councils to ensure that these vital stimuli are supplied and nurtured through appropriate university affiliations.

While an elitist view should be cultivated toward obstetrical anesthetic practice, this view should not be taken as rigidly exclusive, barring the single-handed anesthesiologist from providing a personal epidural service in smaller rural units. There should always be a place for the lone enthusiast. Indeed, some of the greatest advances have been made by this type of man, and if he is skilled and sensible, he will supply a limited service of high quality. However, he should beware of extending his lines too far and falling into the error of guaranteeing an ideal he cannot humanly provide by himself, that is, a safe 24-hour service for all comers.

SUMMARY

Obstetrical anesthesia is a complex and demanding subspecialty. Not only does the obstetric-anesthetic situation affect two people, that is, both mother and child, but also it plays a powerful role in determining the well-being and neurological competence of the future generation. Perfection is therefore the only practical and acceptable goal. Less than this is too costly in terms of individual suffering and the collective toll of subnormal children falling as a charge upon the state. At present, epidural analgesia appears to be the best all-round method available for pain relief in labor. Not only does it fulfill the role of painless childbirth, but also it appears to have positive protective qualities that can improve upon the biochemical conditions of natural, unaided labor and delivery.

While a number of potential complications do exist, in practice these are rare compared to the inherent neurological risks of unaided childbirth. When epidural analgesia is practiced under appropriate conditions, the risks appear to be far outweighed by the advantages.

REFERENCES

Aburel, E.: Recherches sur les douleurs de l'accouchement et sur un nouveau procédé d'analgésie obstétricale. Bull. Soc. Obstet. Gynecol. *19*:165, 1930a.

Aburel, E.: L'anesthésie du plexus lumbo-aortique en obstétrique. Bull. Soc. Obstet. Gynecol. *19*: 616, 1930b.

Akamatsu, T. J., and Bonica, J. J.: Spinal and extradural analgesia and anesthesia for parturition. Clin. Obstet. Gynecol. *17*:183, 1974.

Alvarez, H., and Caldeyro-Barcia, R.: Contractility of the human uterus recorded by new methods. Surg. Gynecol. Obstet. *91*:1, 1950.
Alvarez, H., Poseiro, J. J., Pose, S. V., and Sica-Blanco, Y.: Effects of the anesthetic blockage of the spinal cord on the contractility of the pregnant human uterus. XXI Cong. Physiol. Sci. Buenos Aires, pp. 11, 59, 1959.
Andersson, K. E., Gennser, G., and Nilsson, E.: Contractility of isolated human foetal hearts: Influence of contraction rate, acid-base parameters and a local anaesthetic. Acta Physiol. Scand. *80*(Suppl. 353):5, 1970a.
Andersson, K. E., Gennser, G., and Nilsson, E.: Influence of mepivacaine on isolated human foetal hearts at normal and low pH. Acta Physiol. Scand. (Suppl. 353) *80*:34, 1970b.
Andersson, K. E., Bengtsson, L. Ph., Gustafson, I., and Ingemarsson, I.: The relaxing effect of terbutaline on the human uterus during term labor. Amer. J. Obstet. Gynecol. *121*:602, 1975.
Ang, C. K., Tan, T. H., Walters, W. A. W., and Wood, C.: Postural influence on maternal capillary oxygen and carbon dioxide tension. Brit. Med. J. *4*:201, 1969.
Ansari, I., Wallace, G., Clemetson, C. A. B., Mallikarjuneswara, V. R., and Clemetson, C. D. M.: Tilt caesarean section. J. Obstet. Gynaecol. Brit. Cwlth. *77*:713, 1970.
Ansbro, F. P., Gordon, C. A., Bodell, B., and Latteri, F. S.: Epidural anesthesia for Cesarean section. Report of 125 cases. N.Y. State J. Med. *52*:1901, 1952.
Apgar, V.: A proposal for a new method of evaluation of the newborn infant. Anesth. Analg. *32*: 260, 1953.
Baraka, A.: Correlation between maternal and foetal PO_2 and PCO_2 during Caesarean section. Brit. J. Anaesth. *42*:434, 1970.
Barden, T. P., and Stander, R. W.: Effects of adrenergic blocking agents and catecholamines in human pregnancy. Amer. J. Obstet. Gynecol. *102*:226, 1968.
Battaglia, F. C., Meschia, G., Makowski, E., and Bowes, W.: The effect of maternal oxygen inhalation on fetal oxygenation. J. Clin. Invest. *47*:548, 1968.
Belfrage, P., Berlin, A., Raabe, N., and Thalme, B.: Lumbar epidural analgesia with bupivacaine in labor. Drug concentration in maternal and neonatal blood at birth and during the first day of life. Amer. J. Obstet. Gynecol. *123*:839, 1975.
Bieniarz, J., Crottogini, J. J., Curuchet, E., Romero-Salinas, G., Yoshida, T., Poseiro, J. J., and Caldeyro-Barcia, R.: Aortocaval compression by the uterus in late human pregnancy. II. An arteriographic study. Amer. J. Obstet. Gynecol. *100*:203, 1968.
Bing, O. H. L., Brooks, W. W., and Messer, J. V.: Heart muscle viability following hypoxia: Protective effect of acidosis. Science *180*:1297, 1973.
Blair, R. G.: Abruption of the placenta. A review of 189 cases occurring between 1965 and 1969. J. Obstet. Gynaecol. Brit. Cwlth. *80*:242, 1973.
Bonica, J. J.: Principles and Practice of Obstetric Analgesia and Anesthesia. Philadelphia, F. A. Davis Company, 1967, pp. 725, 745.
Bonica, J. J., Akamatsu, T. J., Berges, P. U., Morikawa, K., and Kennedy, W. F.: Circulatory effects of peridural block. II. Effects of epinephrine. Anesthesiology *34*:514, 1971.
Bowen-Simpkins, P., and Fergusson, I. L. C.: Lumbar epidural block and the breech presentation. Brit. J. Anaesth. *46*:420, 1974.
Boyd, I. E.: The active management of spontaneous and induced labour. Brit. J. Hosp. Med. *11*:81, 1974.
Brackbill, Y., Kane, J., Manniello, R. L., and Abramson, D.: Obstetric meperidine usage and assessment of neonatal status. Anesthesiology *40*:116, 1974.
Brazelton, T. B.: Assessment of the infant at risk. Clin. Obstet. Gynecol. *16*:361, 1973.
Bretscher, J., and Saling, E.: pH values in human fetus during labor. Amer. J. Obstet. Gynecol. *97*: 906, 1967.
Brigden, W., Howarth, S., and Sharpey-Schafer, E. P.: Postural changes in the peripheral blood flow of normal subjects with observations on vaso-vagal fainting reactions as a result of tilting, the lordotic posture, pregnancy and spinal anaesthesia. Clin. Sci. *9*:79, 1950.
Bromage, P. R.: Spinal Epidural Analgesia. Edinburgh, E. & S. Livingstone, 1954.
Bromage, P. R.: Continuous lumbar epidural analgesia for obstetrics. Canad. Med. Assoc. J. *85*:1136, 1961.
Bromage, P. R.: Spread of analgesic solutions in the epidural space and their site of action: A statistical study. Brit. J. Anaesth. *24*:161, 1962.
Bromage, P. R.: A comparison of the hydrochloride salts of lignocaine and prilocaine for epidural analgesia. Brit. J. Anaesth. *37*:753, 1965.
Bromage, P. R.: Improved conduction blockade in surgery and obstetrics: Carbonated local anesthetics. Canad. Med. Assoc. *97*:1377, 1967.
Bromage, P. R.: An evaluation of bupivacaine in epidural analgesia for obstetrics. Canad. Anaesth. Soc. J. *16*:46, 1969.
Bromage, P. R.: Unblocked segments in epidural analgesia for relief of pain in labour. Brit. J. Anaesth. *44*:676, 1972.

Bromage, P. R.: Mechanism of action of extradural analgesia. Brit. J. Anaesth. *47*:199, 1975.
Bromage, P. R., and Robson, J. G.: Concentrations of lignocaine in the blood after intravenous, intramuscular, epidural and endotracheal administration. Anaesthesia *16*:461, 1961.
Bromage, P. R., Burfoot, M. F., Crowell, D. E., and Pettigrew, R. T.: Quality of epidural blockade. I. Influence of physical factors. Brit. J. Anaesth. *36*:342, 1964.
Bromage, P. R., Datta, S., and Dunford, L. A.: Etidocaine: An evaluation in epidural analgesia for obstetrics. Canad. Anaesth. Soc. J. *21*:535, 1974.
Brotanek, V., Vasicka, A., Santiago, A., and Brotanek, J. D.: The influence of epidural anesthesia on uterine blood flow. Obstet. Gynecol. *42*:276, 1973.
Brudenell, M., and Chakravarti, S.: Uterine rupture in labour. Brit. Med. J. *2*:122, 1975.
Bryant, W. M., Greenwell, J. E., and Weeks, P. M.: Alterations in collagen organization during dilatation of the cervix uteri. Surg. Gynecol. Obstet. *126*:27, 1968.
Bryce-Smith, R.: The spread of solutions in the extradural space. Anaesthesia *9*:201, 1954.
Bryce-Smith, R., and Williams, E. O.: The treatment of eclampsia (imminent or actual) by continuous condution analgesia. Lancet *1*:1241, 1955.
Buchan, P. C., Milne, M. K., and Browning, M. C. K.: The effect of continuous epidural blockade on plasma 11-hydroxycorticosteroid concentrations in labour. J. Obstet. Gynaecol. Brit. Cwlth. *80*:974, 1973.
Caldeyro-Barcia, R.: Effect of position changes on the intensity and frequency of uterine contractions during labor. Amer. J. Obstet. Gynecol. *80*:284, 1960.
Caldeyro-Barcia, R., and Poseiro, J. J.: Physiology of the uterine contraction. Clin. Obstet. Gynecol. *3*:386, 1960.
Caldeyro-Barcia, R., Méndez-Bauer, C., Poseiro, J. J., Escarcena, L. A., Pose, S. V., Bieniarz, J., Arnt, I., Gulin, L., and Althabe, O.: Control of human fetal heart rate during labor. *In* Cassels, D. E. (ed.): The Heart and Circulation in the Newborn and Infant. New York, Grune & Stratton, Inc., 1966, pp. 7–36.
Carrie, L. E. S., and Mohan, J.: Horner's syndrome following obstetric extradural block. Brit. J. Anaesth. *48*:611, 1976.
Chignell, C. F., Vesell, E. S., Starkweather, D. K., and Berlin, C. M.: The binding of sulfaphenazole to fetal, neonatal and adult plasma albumin. Clin. Pharmacol. Ther. *12*:897, 1971.
Cleland, J. G. P.: Paravertebral anesthesia in obstetrics. Experimental and clinical basis. Surg. Gynecol. Obstet. *57*:51, 1933.
Cleland, J. G. P.: Continuous peridural and caudal analgesia in obstetrics. Anesth. Analg. *28*:61, 1949.
Clemetson, C. A. B., Hasan, R., Mallikarjuneswara, V., and Wallace, G.: Tilt-bend Cesarean section. Obstet. Gynecol. *42*:290, 1973.
Climie, C. R., McLean, S., Starmer, G. A., and Thomas J.: Methaemoglobinaemia in mother and foetus following continuous epidural analgesia with prilocaine. Brit. J. Anaesth. *39*:155, 1967.
Collier, C. B.: Horner's syndrome following obstetric extradural block analgesia. Brit. J. Anaesth. *47*:1342, 1975.
Colon-Morales, M. A.: Self-supporting device for continuous left uterine displacement during Cesarean section. Anesth. Analg. *49*:223, 1970.
Comline, R. S., and Silver, M.: pO_2 levels in the placental circulation of the mare and ewe. Nature *217*:76, 1968.
Courtney, L.: Supine hypotensive syndrome during Caesarean section. Brit. Med. J. *1*:797, 1970.
Cox, J. M. R., and Spoerel, W. E.: Continuous epidural analgesia—The use of an intermittent injection device. Canad. Anaesth. Soc. J. *11*:72, 1964.
Craft, J. B., Epstein, B. S., and Coakley, C. S.: Effect of lidocaine with epinephrine versus lidocaine (plain) on induced labor. Anesth. Analg. *51*:243, 1972.
Crawford, J. S.: Principles and Practice of Obstetric Anaesthesia. Oxford, Blackwell Scientific Publications, 1959.
Crawford, J. S.: Principles and Practice of Obstetric Anaesthesia. 2d ed. Oxford, Blackwell Scientific Publications, 1966.
Crawford, J. S.: Anaesthesia for obstetric emergencies. Brit. J. Anaesth. *43*:864, 1971.
Crawford, J. S.: Principles and Practice of Obstetric Anaesthesia. 3d ed. Oxford, Blackwell Scientific Publications, 1972, pp. 179, 217.
Crawford, J. S.: An appraisal of lumbar epidural blockade in patients with a singleton fetus presenting by the breech. J. Obstet. Gynaecol. Brit. Cwlth. *81*:867, 1974a.
Crawford, J. S.: Epidural analgesia and uterine rupture. Lancet *1*:361, 1974b.
Crawford, O. B., and Chester, R. V.: Caudal anesthesia in obstetrics: A combined procaine-Pontocaine single injection technic. Anesthesiology *10*:473, 1949.
Crawford, J. S., Burton, M., and Davies, P.: Time and lateral tilt at Caesarean section. Brit. J. Anaesth. *44*:477, 1972.
Cuerden, C., Buley, R., and Downing, J. W.: Delayed recovery after epidural block in labour. A report of four cases. Anaesthesia *32*:773, 1977.

Darby, S., Thornton, C. A., ahd Hunter, D. J.: Extradural analgesia in labour when the breech presents. Brit. J. Obstet. Gynaecol. *83*:35, 1976.

Dawes, G. S.: Foetal and Neonatal Physiology: A Comparative Study of the Changes at Birth. Chicago, Year Book Medical Publishers, 1969, pp. 122, 123.

Derom, R. M.: Maternal acid-base balance during labor. Clin. Obstet. Gynecol. *11*:110, 1968.

Dinnick, O. P.: Discussion on general anaesthesia for obstetrics. Proc. Roy. Soc. Med. *50*:547, 1957.

Downing, S. E., Talner, N. S., and Gardner, T. H.: Influences of arterial oxygen tension and pH on cardiac function in the newborn lamb. Amer. J. Physiol. *211*:203, 1966.

Ducrow, M.: The occurrence of unblocked segments during continuous lumbar epidural analgesia for relief of pain in labour. Brit. J. Anaesth. *43*:1172, 1971.

Duffus, G. M., Tunstall, M. E., Condie, R. G., and McGillivray, I.: Chlormethiazole in the prevention of eclampsia and the reduction of perinatal mortality. J. Obstet. Gynaecol. Brit. Cwlth. *76*:645, 1969.

Eckstein, K. L., Oberlander, S. G., and Marx, G. F.: Uterine rupture during extradural blockade. Canad. Anaesth. Soc. J. *20*:566, 1973.

Editorial: A painless revolution. Brit. J. Anaesth. *46*:391, 1974a.

Editorial: A time to be born. Lancet 2(*2*):1183, 1974b.

Edwards, G., Morton, H. J. V., Pask, E. A., and Wylie, W. D.: Deaths associated with anaesthesia: A report of 1000 cases. Anaesthesia *11*:194, 1956.

Eichenholz, A., Mulhansen, R. O., Anderson, W. E., and MacDonald, F. M.: Primary hypocarbia: A cause of metabolic acidosis. J. Appl. Physiol. *17*:283, 1962.

Epstein, B. S., Banerjee, S. G., and Coakley, C. S.: Passage of lidocaine and prilocaine across the placenta. Anesth. Analg. *47*:223, 1968.

Evans, J. M., Gauci, C. A., and Watkins, G.: Horner's syndrome as a complication of lumbar extradural block. Anaesthesia *30*:774, 1975.

Ferguson, J. K. W.: A study of the motility of the intact uterus at term. Surg. Gynecol. Obstet. *73*:359, 1941.

Finster, M., Poppers, P. J., Sinclair, J. C., Morishima, H. O., and Daniel, S. S.: Accidental intoxication of the fetus with local anesthetic drug during caudal anesthesia. Amer. J. Obstet. Gynecol. *92*:922, 1965.

Finster, M., Morishima, H. O., Boyes, R. N., and Covino, B. G.: The placental transfer of lidocaine and its uptake by fetal tissues. Anesthesiology *36*:159, 1972.

Fisch, L., Sala, N. K., and Schwarcz, R. L.: Effect of cervical dilatation upon uterine contractility in pregnant women and its relation to oxytocin secretion. Amer. J. Obstet. Gynecol. *90*:108, 1964.

Flint, M.: Interrelationships of mucopolysaccharide and collagen in connective tissue remodelling. J. Embryol. Exp. Morphol. *27*:481, 1972.

Flowers, C. E.: Continuous peridural analgesia in obstetrics. Anaesthesia *9*:146, 1954.

Flowers, C. E., Helman, L. M., and Hingson, R. A.: Continuous peridural anesthesia and analgesia for labor, delivery and cesarean section. Anesth. Analg. *28*:181, 1949.

Foldes, F F., and Rhodes, D. H.: Role of plasma cholinesterase in anesthesiology. Curr. Res. Anesth. Analg. *32*:305, 1953.

Fox, G. S., and Houle, G. L.: Transmission of lidocaine hydrochloride across the placenta during Caesarean section. Canad. Anaesth. Soc. J. *16*:135, 1969.

Fox, G. S., and Houle, G. L.: Acid-base studies in elective Caesarean sections during epidural and general anaesthesia. Canad. Anaesth. Soc. J. *18*:60, 1971.

Fox, G. S., Houle, G. L., Desjardins, P. D., and Mercier, G.: Intrauterine fetal lidocaine concentrations during continuous epidural anesthesia. Amer. J. Obstet. Gynecol. *110*:896, 1971.

Friedman, E. A.: Primigravid labor: A graphico-statistical analysis. Obstet. Gynecol. *6*:567, 1955.

Friedman, E. A.: Labor in multiparas: A graphico-statistical analysis. Obstet. Gynecol. *8*:691, 1956.

Galbert, M. W., and Marx, G. F.: Extradural pressures in the parturient patient. Anesthesiology *40*: 499, 1974.

Gårdmark, S.: Studies on acid-base balance, carbohydrate and lipid metabolism in human fetal and maternal blood, in clinical and experimental conditions during labour. Studentlitteratur, Lund, 1974.

Gare, D. J., Shrine, J., Paul, W. M., and Hoskins, M.: Oxygen administration during labor. Amer. J. Obstet. Gynecol. *105*:954, 1969.

Garrett, W. J.: The effects of adrenaline and noradrenaline on the intact human uterus in late pregnancy and labour. J. Obstet. Gynaecol. Brit. Emp. *61*:586, 1954.

Geerinckx, K., Vanderick, G., Van Steenberge, A. L., Bouche, R., and De Muylder, E.: Bupivacaine 0.125% in epidural block analgesia during childbirth: Maternal and foetal plasma concentrations. Brit. J. Anaesth. *46*:939, 1974.

Gelet, T. R., Altschuld, R. A., and Weissler, A. M.: Effects of acidosis on the performance and metabolism of the anoxic heart. Circulation (Suppl.) *39–40*:60, 1969.

Gemzell, C. A., Robbe, H., Stern, B., and Strom, G.: Observations on circulatory changes and muscular work in normal labour. Acta Obstet. Gynecol. Scand. *36*:75, 1957.

Gennser, G., Johannsson, M., and Nilsson, E.: The influence of contraction frequency and of a local anesthetic (Mepivacaine) on human fetal myocardium. Acta Physiol. Scand. *85*:559, 1972.

Gillman, R. G., and Burton, A. C.: Constriction of the neonatal aorta by a raised oxygen tension. Circ. Res. *19*:755, 1966.

Gomez, D.: Paracervical block in obstetrics. Lancet *1*:1163, 1969.

Goodlin, R. C.: Aortocaval compression during Cesarean section. Obstet. Gynecol. *37*:702, 1971.

Gordon, H. R.: Fetal bradycardia after paracervical block. Correlation with fetal and maternal levels of local anesthetic (mepivacaine). New Eng. J. Med. *279*:910, 1968.

Graffagnino, P., and Seyler, L. W.: Epidural anesthesia in obstetrics. Amer. J. Obstet. Gynecol. *35*:597, 1938.

Grayson, J.: Internal calorimetry in determination of thermal conductivity and blood flow. J. Physiol. *118*:54, 1952.

Greene, N. M.: Physiology of Spinal Anesthesia. Baltimore, The Williams & Wilkins Company, 1959, p. 170.

Greiss, F. C., and Crandell, D. L.: Therapy for hypotension induced by spinal anesthesia during pregnancy. J.A.M.A. *191*:793, 1965.

Greiss, F. C., Anderson, S. G., and King, L. C.: Uterine vascular bed: Effects of acute hyperoxia. Amer. J. Obstet. Gynecol. *118*:542, 1974.

Greiss, F. C., Still, J. G., and Anderson, S. G.: Effects of local anesthetic agents on the uterine vasculatures and myometrium. Amer. J. Obstet. Gynecol. *124*:889, 1976.

Grennell, H. J., and Vandewater, S. L.: The supine hypotensive syndrome during conduction anaesthesia for the near term gravid patient: Case reports. Canad. Anaesth. Soc. J. *8*:417, 1961.

Grove, L. H.: Backache, headache and bladder dysfunction after delivery. Brit. J. Anaesth. *45*:1147, 1973.

Gunther, R. E., and Bauman, J.: Obstetrical caudal anesthesia. I. A randomized study comparing 1% mepivacaine with 1% lidocaine with epinephrine. Anesthesiology *31*:5, 1969.

Hardin, G.: The tragedy of the commons. Science *162*:1243, 1968.

Hehre, F. W., Moyes, A. Z., Senfield, R. M., and Lilly, E. J.: Continuous lumbar peridural anesthesia in obstetrics. II. Use of minimal amounts of local anesthetics during labor. Anesth. Analg. *44*:89, 1965.

Hehre, F. W., Yules, R. B., and Hipona, F. A.: Continuous lumbar peridural anesthesia in obstetrics. III. Attempts to produce spread of contrast media by acute vena caval obstruction in dogs. Anesth. Analg. *45*:551, 1966.

Hehre, F. W., Hook, R., and Hon, E. H.: Continuous lumbar peridural anesthesia in obstetrics. VI. The fetal effects of transplacental passage of local anesthetic agents. Anesth. Analg. *48*:909, 1969.

Hellmann, K.: Epidural anesthesia in obstetrics: A second look at 26,127 cases. Canad. Anaesth. Soc. J. *12*:398, 1965.

Hendricks, C. H.: Studies on lactic acid metabolism in pregnancy and labor. Amer. J. Obstet. Gynecol. *73*:492, 1957.

Hendricks, C. H.: The hemodynamics of uterine contraction. Amer. J. Obstet. Gynecol. *76*:969, 1958.

Hendricks, C. H., Brenner, W. E., and Kraus, G.: Normal cervical dilatation pattern in late pregnancy and labor. Amer. J. Obstet. Gynecol. *106*:1065, 1970.

Henry, J. S., Kingston, M. B., and Maughan, G. B.: The effect of epidural anesthesia on oxytocin-induced labor. Amer. J. Obstet. Gynecol. *97*:350, 1967.

Hiatt, H. H.: Protecting the medical commons: Who is responsible? New Eng. J. Med. *293*:235, 1975.

Hill, E. C.: Maternal obstetric paralysis. Amer. J. Obstet. Gynecol. *83*:1452, 1962.

Hingson, R. A., and Edwards, W. B.: An analysis of the first ten thousand confinements managed with continuous caudal analgesia with a report of the authors' first one thousand cases. J.A.M.A. *123*:538, 1943.

Hingson, R. A., Cull, W. A., and Benzinger, M.: Continuous caudal analgesia in obstetrics. Anesth. Analg. *40*:119, 1961.

Hipona, F. A., Yules, R., and Hehre, F. W.: Venous encroachment on the spinal peridural space due to experimental IVC occlusion: Possible clinical implications in late pregnancy. Invest. Radiol. *1*:157, 1966.

Hodges, R. J. H., Burnett, J. R., Tunstall, M. E., and Knight, R. F.: General anaesthesia for operative obstetrics, with special reference to the use of thiopentone and suxamethonium. Brit. J. Anaesth. *31*:152, 1959.

Hollmén, A.: The placental transfer of bupivacaine and lidocaine and their myocardial and cerebral uptake in the rabbit. Acta Anaesth. Scand. *17*:149, 1973.

Hollmén, A., and Jägerhorn, M.: The effects of epidural anaesthesia and Caesarean section on foetal and maternal acid-base balance at birth. Acta Anaesth. Scand. *12*:115, 1968.

Hollmén, A., Jägerhorn, M., and Pystynnen, P.: Foetal and maternal acid-base balance during labour and at birth. The effects of general anaesthesia and Caesarean section on the physiological foetal acidosis of normal delivery. Acta Anaesth. Scand. *11*:341, 1967.

Holmes, F.: Incidence of the supine hypotensive syndrome in late pregnancy: A clinical study in 500 subjects. J. Obstet. Gynaecol. Brit. Emp. *67*:254, 1960.

Hon, E. H.: Fetal heart rate patterns preceding death in utero. Amer. J. Obstet. Gynecol. *78*:47, 1959.

Hon, E. H., Reid, B. L., and Hehre, F. W.: The electronic evaluation of fetal heart rate. II. Changes with maternal hypotension. Amer. J. Obstet. Gynecol. *79*:209, 1960.

Houle, G. L., Fox, G. S., and Gertel, M.: Methoxyflurane: clinical and laboratory studies during Cesarean section. Anesth. Analg. *48*:1011, 1969.

Houle, G. L., Fox, G. S., and Torkington, I. M. G.: A comparison between lignocaine hydrochloride and lignocaine carbon dioxide base for epidural analgesia during vaginal delivery. Brit. J. Anaesth. *43*:1145, 1971.

Howard, B. K., Goodson, J. H., and Mengert, W. F.: Supine hypotensive syndrome in late pregnancy. Obstet. Gynecol. *1*:371, 1953.

Huckabee, W. E.: Relationships of pyruvate and lactate during anaerobic metabolism. I. Effects of infusion of pyruvate or glucose and of hyperventilation. J. Clin. Invest. *37*:244, 1958.

Humphrey, M., Hounslow, D., Morgan, S., and Wood, C.: The influence of maternal posture at birth on the fetus. J. Obstet. Gynaecol. Brit. Cwlth. *80*:1075, 1973.

Humphrey, M. D., Chang, A., Wood, E. C., and Hounslow, D.: A decrease in fetal pH during the second stage of labour, when conducted in the dorsal position. J. Obstet. Gynaecol. Brit. Cwlth. *81*:600, 1974.

Hyman, M., and Shnider, S. M.: Maternal and neonatal blood concentrations of bupivacaine associated with obstetrical conduction anesthesia. Anesthesiology *34*:81, 1971.

Jacobson, L.: Studies on Acid-Base and Electrolyte Components of Human Foetal and Maternal Blood During Labour. Studentlitteratur, Lund, 1970, p. 92.

James, F. M., and Davies, P.: Maternal and fetal effects of lumbar epidural analgesia for labor and delivery in patients with gestational hypertension. Amer. J. Obstet. Gynecol. *126*:195, 1976.

James, F. M., Greiss, F. C., and Kemp, R. A.: An evaluation of vasopressor therapy for maternal hypotension during spinal anesthesia. Anesthesiology *33*:25, 1970.

James, F. M., Crawford, J. S., Davies, P., and Naiem, H.: Lumbar epidural analgesia for labor and delivery of twins. Amer. J. Obstet. Gynecol. *127*:176, 1977a.

James, F. M., Crawford, J. S., Hopkinson, R., Davies, P., and Naiem, H.: A comparison of general anesthesia and lumbar epidural analgesia for elective Cesarean section. Anesth. Analg. *56*:228, 1977b.

James, L. S., and Adamsons, K.: Respiratory physiology of the fetus and newborn infant. New Eng. J. Med. *271*:1352 and 1407, 1964.

Jassir, C. Yu, K. C., and Marx, G. F.: Alveolar-arterial oxygen difference in parturient women with two types of uterine displacement. Anesth. Analg. *52*:43, 1973.

Kaiser, I., and Harris, J.: The effect of adrenalin on the pregnant human uterus. Amer. J. Obstet. Gynecol. *59*:775, 1950.

Kandel, P. F., Spoerel, W. E., and Kinch, R. A.: Continuous epidural analgesia for labour and delivery: Review of 1000 cases. Canad. Med. Assoc. J. *95*:947, 1966.

Keenaghan, J. B.: The determination of lidocaine and prilocaine in whole blood by gas chromatography. Anesthesiology *29*:110, 1968.

Kepes, E. R., Martinez, L. R., Pantuck, E., and Stark, D. C. C.: Horner's syndrome following caudal anesthesia. N.Y. State J. Med. *72*:946, 1972.

Kerr, M. G., Scott, D. B., and Samuel, E.: Studies of the inferior vena cava in late pregnancy. Brit. Med. J. *1*:532, 1964.

Khazin, A. F., Hon, E. H., and Hehre, F. W.: Effects of maternal hyperoxia on the fetus. I. Oxygen tension. Amer. J. Obstet. Gynecol. *109*:628, 1971.

Kovalčík, V.: The response of the isolated ductus arteriosus to oxygen and anoxia. J. Physiol. (Lond.) *169*:185, 1963.

Kubli, F. W.: Influence of labor on fetal acid-base balance. Clin. Obstet. Gynecol. *11*:168, 1968.

Künzel, W., Wulf, H., and Busse, A.: Der Einfluss der maternen ventilation auf die aktuellen Blutzgase und den Säure-Base-Status des Feten. Zeit. Geburt. Gynäk. *172*:1, 1970.

Lees, M. M., Scott, D. B., Kerr, M. G., and Taylor, S. H.: Circulatory effects of recumbent postural change in late pregnancy. Clin. Sci. *32*:453, 1967.

Lees, M. M., Scott, D. B., and Kerr, M. G.: Haemodynamic changes associated with labour. J. Obstet. Gynaecol. Brit. Cwlth. *77*:29, 1970.

Little, W. A., and Friedman, E. A.: Anesthesia for the twin delivery. Anesthesiology *19*:515, 1958.

Lock, F. R., and Greiss, F. C.: Anesthetic hazards in obstetrics. Amer. J. Obstet. Gynecol. *70*:861, 1955.

Lowensohn, R. I.: Intrapartum epidural anesthesia: An evaluation of effects on uterine activity. Obstet. Gynecol. *44*:388, 1974.
Lunan, C. B.: The management of abruptio placentae. J. Obstet. Gynaecol. Brit. Cwlth. *80*:120, 1973.
Lurie, A. O., and Weiss, J. B.: Blood concentrations of mepivacaine and lidocaine in mother and baby after epidural anesthesia. Amer. J. Obstet. Gynecol. *106*:850, 1970.
McCaughey, H. S., Corey, E. L., Eastwood, D., and Thornton, W. N.: Effect of synthetic anesthetics on the spontaneous motility of human uterine muscle in vitro. Obstet. Gynecol. *19*:233, 1962.
McClure, J. H.: Newborn blood oxygen. A method of increasing the partial pressure of oxygen in the blood of the newborn infant. Obstet. Gynecol. *11*:696, 1958.
McLennan, C. E.: Further observations on capillary filtration rate during pregnancy. Amer. J. Obstet. Gynecol. *52*:837, 1946.
MacMillan, A.: Peridural anaesthesia for obstetrics. Canad. Anesth. Soc. J. *1*:75, 1954.
McRoberts, W. A.: Postural shock in pregnancy. Amer. J. Obstet. Gynecol. *62*:627, 1951.
Magno, R., Berlin, A., Karlsson, K., and Kjellmer, I.: Anesthesia for Cesarean section. IV. Placental transfer and neonatal elimination of bupivacaine following epidural analgesia for elective Cesarean section. Acta Anaesth. Scand. *20*:141, 1976.
Marmer, M. J., Cadranel, J. L., and Krohn, L.: Lidocaine-norepinephrine anesthesia in obstetrics; Xylocaine and Levophed combination in caudal block. Obstet. Gynecol. *7*:315, 1956.
Marx, G. F., and Greene, N. M.: Maternal lactate, pyruvate, and excess lactate production during labor and delivery. Amer. J. Obstet. Gynecol. *90*:786, 1964.
Marx, G. F., and Mateo, C. V.: Effects of different oxygen concentrations during general anaesthesia for elective Caesarean section. Canad. Anaesth. Soc. J. *18*:587, 1971.
Marx, G. F., Cosmi, E. V., and Wollman, S. B.: Biochemical status and clinical condition of mother and infant at Cesarean section. Anesth. Analg. *48*:986, 1969.
Mather, L. E., Long, G. J., and Thomas, J.: The binding of bupivacaine to maternal and foetal plasma proteins. J. Pharm. Pharmacol. *23*:359, 1971.
Mendelson, C. L.: Aspiration of stomach contents into the lungs during obstetric anesthesia. Amer. J. Obstet. Gynecol. *52*:191, 1946.
Milne, M. K., and Murray Lawson, J. I.: Epidural analgesia for Caesarean section. Brit. J. Anaesth. *45*:1206, 1973.
Mohan, J., and Potter, J. M.: Pupillary constriction and ptosis following caudal epidural analgesia. Anaesthesia *30*:769, 1975.
Moir, D. D., and Davidson, S.: Postpartum complications of forceps delivery performed under epidural and pudendal nerve block. Brit. J. Anaesth. *44*:1197, 1972.
Moir, D. D., and Willocks, J.: Management of incoordinate uterine contraction under continuous epidural analgesia. Brit. Med. J. *3*:396, 1967.
Moir, D. D., Victor-Rodriguez, L., and Willocks, J.: Epidural analgesia during labour in patients with pre-eclampsia. J. Obstet. Gynaecol. Brit. Cwlth. *79*:465, 1972.
Moore, D. C.: Complications of Regional Anesthesia: Etiology, Signs and Symptoms, Treatment. Springfield, Ill., Charles C Thomas, Publisher, 1955.
Moore, D. C., Bridenbaugh, L. D., Bagdi, P. A., and Bridenbaugh, P. O.: Accumulcation of mepivacaine hydrochloride during caudal block. Anesthesiology *29*:585, 1968.
Moore, D. C., Bridenbaugh, L. D., Bridenbaugh, P. O., and Tucker, G. T.: Bupivacaine – A review of 2,077 cases. J.A.M.A. *214*:713, 1970.
Moore, D. C., Bridenbaugh, L. D., Bridenbaugh, P. O., and Tucker, G. T.: Caudal and epidural blocks with bupivacaine for childbirth. Report of 657 parturients. Obstet. Gynecol. *37*: 667, 1971.
Morishima, H. O., Daniel, S. S., Finster, M., Poppers, P. J., and James, L. S.: Transmission of mepivacaine hydrochloride (Carbocaine) across the human placenta. Anesthesiology *27*:147, 1966.
Morton, H. J. V., and Wylie, W. D.: Anaesthetic deaths due to regurgitation or vomiting. Anaesthesia *6*:190, 1951.
Moss, A. J., Emmanouilides, G. C., Adams, F. H., and Chuang, K.: Response of ductus arteriosus and pulmonary and systemic arterial pressure to changes in oxygen environment in newborn infants. Pediatrics *33*:937, 1964.
Murray, R. R.: Maternal obstetrical paralysis. Amer. J. Obstet. Gynecol. *88*:399, 1964.
Myers, R. E., Stånge, L., Joelsson, I., Huzell, B., and Wussow, C.: Effects upon the fetus of oxygen administration to the mother. A study in the monkey. Acta Obstet. Gynecol. Scand. *56*: 195, 1977.
Mylks, G. W., Jones, K., and Douglas-Murray, G. M.: Acute fulminating eclampsia – Management in conjunction with prolonged epidural sympathetic block. Canad. Med. Assoc. J. *82*:422, 1960.
Newman, W., McKinnon, L., Phillips, L., Paterson, P., and Wood, C.: Oxygen transfer from mother to fetus during labor. Amer. J. Obstet. Gynecol. *99*:61, 1967.

Nielsen, J. S., Spoerel, W. E., Keenleyside, H. B., Slater, P. E., and Clancy, P. R.: Continuous epidural analgesia for labour and delivery. Canad. Anaesth. Soc. J. *9*:143, 1962.

Nimmo, W. S., Wilson, J., and Prescott, L. F.: Narcotic analgesics and delayed gastric emptying during labour. Lancet *1*:890, 1975.

Noble, A. D., Craft, I. L., Bootes, J. A. H., Edwards, P. A., Thomas, D. J., and Mills, K. L. M.: Continuous lumbar epidural analgesia using bupivacaine: A study of the fetus and newborn child. J. Obstet. Gynaecol. Brit. Cwlth. *78*:559, 1971.

Noriega, L., Cibils, L. A., Alvarez, H., Posiero, J. J., Pose, S. V., Sica- Blanco, Y., Mendez-Bauer, C., Fielitz, C., Gonzalez-Panizza, V. H., and Caldeyro-Barcia, R.: Efecto de los cambios de posicion de la parturienta sobre la intensidad y la frecuencia de las contracciones uterinas. Anales de la Facultad de Medicina, Montevideo *44*:383, 1959.

Nyberg, R., and Westin, B.: The influence of oxygen tension and some drugs on human placental vessels. Acta Physiol. Scand. *39*:216, 1957.

O'Driscoll, K.: An obstetrician's view of pain. Brit. J. Anaesth. *47*:1053, 1975.

O'Driscoll, K., Stronge, J. M., and Minogue, M.: Active management of labour. Brit. Med. J. *3*:135, 1973.

Ostlere, G.: Epidural analgesia in the treatment of hypertension due to toxaemia of pregnancy. Anaesthesia *7*:169, 1952.

Oxorn, H., and Foote, W. R.: Human Labor and Birth. 3d ed. New York, Appleton-Century-Crofts, 1975.

Palahniuk, R. J., Shnider, S. M., and Eger, E. I.: Pregnancy decreases the requirements for inhaled anesthetic agents. Anesthesiology *41*:82, 1974.

Panigel, M.: Contribution à la physiologie de la circulation foeto-placentaire I. Etude de la vasomotricité des artêres du cordon ombilical humain. J. Physiol. (Paris) *51*:941, 1959.

Panigel, M.: Placental perfusion experiments. Amer. J. Obstet. Gynecol. *84*:1664, 1962.

Pathy, G. V., and Rosen, M.: Prolonged block with recovery after extradural analgesia for labour. Brit. J. Anaesth. *47*:520, 1975.

Pearson, J. F., and Davies, P.: The effects of continuous lumbar epidural analgesia on the acid-base status of maternal arterial blood during the first stage of labour. J. Obstet. Gynaecol. Brit. Cwlth. *80*:218, 1973a.

Pearson, J. F., and Davies, P.: The effect of continuous lumbar epidural analgesia on maternal acid-base balance and arterial lactate concentration during the second stage of labour. J. Obstet. Gynaecol. Brit. Cwlth. *80*:225, 1973b.

Poppers, P. J., and Finster, M.: The use of prilocaine hydrochloride (Citanest) for epidural analgesia in obstetrics. Anesthesiology *29*:1134, 1968.

Poppers, P. J., Vosburgh, G. J., and Finster, M.: Methemoglobinemia following epidural analgesia during labor: A case report and literature review. Amer. J. Obstet. Gynecol. *95*:630, 1966.

Prystowsky, H.: Fetal blood studies. XI. The effect of prophylactic oxygen on the oxygen pressure gradient between the maternal and fetal blood of the human in normal and abnormal pregnancy. Amer. J. Obstet. Gynecol. *78*:483, 1959.

Quilligan, E. J., Vasicka, A., Aznar, R., Moore, T., and Bloor, B. M.: Partial pressure of oxygen in the intervillous space and the umbilical vessels. Amer. J. Obstet. Gynecol. *79*:1048, 1960.

Ralston, D. H., Shnider, S. M., and deLorimier, A. A.: Effects of equipotent ephedrine, metaraminol, mephentermine, and methoxamine on uterine blood flow in the pregnant ewe. Anesthesiology *40*:354, 1974.

Reynolds, F., and Taylor, G.: Maternal and neonatal blood concentrations of bupivacaine. Anaesthesia *25*:14, 1970.

Reynolds, F., and Taylor, G.: Plasma concentrations of bupivacaine during continuous epidural analgesia in labour: The effect of adrenaline. Brit. J. Anaesth. *43*:436, 1971.

Reynolds, F., Hargrove, R. L., and Wyman, J. B.: Maternal and foetal plasma concentrations of bupivacaine after epidural block. Brit. J. Anaesth. *45*:1049, 1973.

Roberts, R. B.: The occurrence of unblocked segments during continuous lumbar epidural analgesia for pain relief in labour. Brit. J. Anaesth. *44*:628, 1972.

Roddie, I. C., and Scott, A. C.: Some effects of oxygen tension on isolated arterial segments. J. Physiol. (Lond.) *179*:59, 1965.

Rooth, G.: The time factor in fetal distress. J. Perinat. Med. *1*:7, 1973.

Rooth, G., McBride, R., and Ivy, B. J.: Fetal and maternal pH measurements—A basis for common normal values. Acta Obstet. Gynecol. Scand. *52*:47, 1973.

Rorke, M. J., Davey, D. A., and Du Tort, H. J.: Foetal oxygenation during Caesarean section. Anaesthesia *23*:585, 1968.

Rucker, M. P.: The action of adrenalin on the pregnant uterus. South. Med. J. *18*:412, 1925.

Ryan, D. W.: Accidental intravenous injection of bupivacaine: A complication of obstetrical epidural anaesthesia. Brit. J. Anaesth. *45*:907, 1973.

Sala, N. L., Schwarcz, R. L., Althabe, O., Fisch, L., and Fuente, O.: Effect of epidural anesthesia upon uterine contractility induced by artificial cervical dilatation in human pregnancy. Amer. J. Obstet. Gynecol. *106*:26, 1970.

Salvatore, C. A.: Capillary resistance during pregnancy. Obstet. Gynecol. *18*:96, 1961.

Sangoul, F., Fox, G. S., and Houle, G. L.: Effect of regional analgesia on maternal oxygen consumption during the first stage of labour. Amer. J. Obstet. Gynecol. *121*:1080, 1975.

Scanlon, J. W., Brown, W. U., Weiss, J. B., and Alper, M. H.: Neurobehavioral responses of newborn infants after maternal epidural anesthesia. Anesthesiology *40*:121, 1974.

Schellenberg, J. C.: Uterine activity during lumbar epidural analgesia with bupivacaine. Amer. J. Obstet. Gynecol. *127*:26, 1977.

Schifrin, B. S.: Fetal heart rate patterns following epidural anaesthesia and oxytocin infusion during labour. J. Obstet. Gynaecol. Brit. Cwlth. *79*:332, 1972.

Schifrin, B. S.: Iatrogenic fetal distress. Int. Anesth. Clin. *11*(2):119, 1973.

Schwarcz, R. L., Belizan, J. M., Cifuentes, J. R., Cuadro, J. C., Marques, M. B., and Caldeyro-Barcia, R.: Fetal and maternal monitoring in spontaneous labors and in elective inductions. Amer. J. Obstet. Gynecol. *120*:356, 1974.

Scott, D. B.: Inferior vena caval occlusion during epidural block. *In* Doughty, A. (ed.): Proceedings of the Symposium on Epidural Analgesia for Obstetrics. London, H. K. Lewis & Co., Ltd., 1972, pp. 59–63.

Shanks, C. A.: Four cases of unilateral epidural analgesia. Brit. J. Anaesth. *40*:999, 1968.

Shnider, S. M., and Gildea, J.: Paracervical block anesthesia in obstetrics. III. Choice of drug: Fetal bradycardia following administration of lidocaine, mepivacaine and prilocaine. Amer. J. Obstet. Gynecol. *116*:320, 1973.

Shnider, S. M., and Way, E. L.: The kinetics of transfer of lidocaine (Xylocaine) across the human placenta. Anesthesiology *29*:944, 1968a.

Shnider, S. M., and Way, E. L.: Plasma levels of lidocaine (Xylocaine) in mother and newborn following obstetrical conduction anesthesia: Clinical applications. Anesthesiology *29*:951, 1968b.

Shnider, S. M., Asling, J. H., Margolis, A. J., Way, E. L., and Wilkinson, G. R.: High fetal blood levels of mepivacaine and fetal bradycardia. New Eng. J. Med. *279*:947, 1968a.

Shnider, S. M., deLorimier, A. A., Holl, J. W., Chapler, F. K., and Morishima, H. O.: Vasopressors in obstetrics. I. Correction of fetal acidosis with ephedrine during spinal anesthesia. Amer. J. Obstet. Gynecol. *102*:911, 1968b.

Standley, K., Soule, A. B., Copans, S. A., and Duchowny, M. S.: Local-regional anesthesia during childbirth: Effect on newborn behaviors. Science *186*:634, 1974.

Steel, G. C.: Epidural nerve block in obstetrics. Brit. J. Hosp. Med. *1*:595, 1972.

Stenger, V., Andersen, T., Eitzman, D., and Prystowsky, H.: Extradural anesthesia for Cesarean section. Physiologic and biochemical observations. Obstet. Gynecol. *25*:802, 1965.

Taylor, G., and Pryse-Davies, J.: Prophylactic use of antacids in the prevention of the acid-pulmonary-aspiration syndrome (Mendelson's syndrome). Lancet *1*:288, 1966.

Teramo, K., Benowitz, N., Heymann, M. A., Kahanpää, K., Siimes, A., and Rudolph, A. M.: Effects of lidocaine on heart rate, blood pressure, and electrocorticogram in fetal sheep. Amer. J. Obstet. Gynecol. *118*:935, 1974.

Teramo, K., Benowitz, N., Heymann, M. A., and Rudolph, A. M.: Gestational differences in lidocaine toxicity in the fetal lamb. Anesthesiology *44*:133, 1976.

Tervila, L., Vertiainen, E., Kivalo, I., Finnilä, M. J., and Väyrynen, M.: The effect of oxygen ventilation and a vasodilator on uterine perfusion, foetal oxygen and acid-base balance. I. A study in healthy gravidae. Acta Obstet. Gynecol. Scand. *52*:177, 1973.

Thalme, B., Belfrage, P., and Raabe, N.: Lumbar epidural analgesia in labour. I. Acid-base balance and clinical condition of mother, fetus and newborn child. Acta Obstet. Gynecol. Scand. *53*:27, 1974a.

Thalme, B., Raabe, N., and Belfrage, P.: Lumbar epidural analgesia in labour. II. Effects on glucose, lactate, sodium, chloride, total protein, haematocrit and haemoglobin in maternal, fetal and neonatal blood. Acta Obstet. Gynecol. Scand. *53*:113, 1974b.

Thomas, J., Climie, C. R., and Mather, L. E.: Placental transfer of lignocaine following lumbar epidural administration. Brit. J. Anaesth. *40*:965, 1968.

Thomas, J., Climie, C. R., and Mather, L. E.: The maternal plasma levels and placental transfer of bupivacaine following epidural analgesia. Brit. J. Anaesth. *41*:1035, 1969a.

Thomas, J., Climie, C. R., Long, G., and Nighjoy, L. E.: The influence of adrenaline on the maternal plasma levels and placental transfer of lignocaine following lumbar epidural administration. Brit. J. Anaesth. *41*:1029, 1969b.

Tillman, A. J. B.: Traumatic neuritis in the puerperium. Amer. J. Obstet. Gynecol. *29*:660, 1935.

Towbin, A.: Mental retardation due to germinal matrix infarction. Science *164*:156, 1969.

Towbin, A.: Central nervous system damage in the human fetus and newborn infant. Dis. Child. *119*:529, 1970.

Towbin, A.: Organic causes of minimal brain dysfunction. Perinatal origin of minimal cerebral lesions. J.A.M.A. *217*:1207, 1971.

Tucker, G. T., Boyes, R. N., Bridenbaugh, P. O., and Moore, D. C.: Binding of anilide-type local anesthetics in human plasma. I. Relationship between binding, physicochemical properties, and anesthetic activity. Anesthesiology *33*:287, 1970a.

Tucker, G. T., Boyes, R. N., Bridenbaugh, P. O., and Moore, D. C.: Binding of anilide-type local anesthetics in human plasma. II. Implications in vivo, with special reference to transplacental distribution. Anesthesiology *33*:304, 1970b.

Tunstall, M. E.: Obstetric analgesia. The use of a fixed nitrous oxide and oxygen mixture from one cylinder. Lancet *2*:964, 1961.

Tyack, A. J., Parsons, R. J., Millar, D. R., and Nicholas, A. D. G.: Uterine activity and plasma bupivacaine levels after caudal epidural analgesia. J. Obstet. Gynaecol. Brit. Cwlth. *80*:896, 1973.

Ueland, K., and Hansen, J. M.: Maternal cardiovascular dynamics. II. Posture and uterine contractions. Amer. J. Obstet. Gynecol. *103*:1, 1969.

Ueland, K., Gills, R. E., and Hansen, J. M.: Maternal cardiovascular dynamics. I. Cesarean section under subarachnoid block anesthesia. Amer. J. Obstet. Gynecol. *100*:42, 1968.

Ueland, K., Novy, M. J., Peterson, E. N., and Metcalfe, J.: Maternal cardiovascular dynamics. IV. The influence of gestational age on the maternal cardiovascular response to posture and exercise. Amer. J. Obstet. Gynecol. *104*:856, 1969.

Ueland, K., Akamatsu, T. J., Eng, M., Bonica, J. J., and Hansen, J. M.: Maternal cardiovascular dynamics. VI. Cesarean section under epidural anesthesia without epinephrine. Amer. J. Obstet. Gynecol. *114*:775, 1972.

Usubiaga, J. E., La Iuppa, M., Moya, F., Wikinski, J. A., and Velazco, R.: Passage of procaine hydrochloride and para-aminobenzoic acid across the human placenta. Amer. J. Obstet. Gynecol. *100*:918, 1968.

Usubiaga, J. E., Dos Reis, A., and Usubiaga, L. E.: Epidural misplacement of catheters and mechanisms of unilateral blockade. Anesthesiology *32*:158, 1970.

Vanderick, G., Geerinckx, K., Van Steenberge, A. L., and De Muylder, E.: Bupivacaine 0.125% in epidural block analgesia during childbirth: Clinical evaluation. Brit. J. Anaesth. *46*:838, 1974.

Vasicka, A., and Kretchmer, H. E.: Uterine dynamics. Clin. Obstet. Gynecol. *4*:17, 1961.

Vasicka, A., Quilligan, E. J., Aznar, R., Lipsitz, P. J., and Bloor, B. M.: Oxygen tension in maternal and fetal blood, amniotic fluid and cerebrospinal fluid of the mother and the baby. Amer. J. Obstet. Gynecol. *79*:1041, 1960.

Vasicka, A., Hutchinson, H. T., Eng, M., and Allen, C. R.: Spinal and epidural anesthesia, fetal and uterine response to acute hypo- and hypertension. Amer. J. Obstet. Gynecol. *90*:800, 1964.

Waldron, K. W., and Wood, C.: Cesarean section in the lateral position. Obstet. Gynecol. *37*:706, 1971.

Walker, C. H. M., and Balf, C. L.: Capillary resistance studies. II. Late pregnancy, labour and early puerperium. J. Obstet. Gynaecol. Brit. Emp. *61*:17, 1954.

Walpole, J. B.: Continuous lumbar epidural block in labour in the presence of a Neureig Williams plate from L_1–L_4. Brit. J. Anaesth. *46*:163, 1974.

Ward, R. J., Bonica, J. J., Freund, F. G., Akamatsu, T., Danziger, F., and Engelsson, S.: Epidural and subarachnoid anesthesia: Cardiovascular and respiratory effects. J.A.M.A. *191*:275, 1965.

Webster, A. C.: A hazard of epidural anaesthesia in obstetrics. Canad. Anaesth. Soc. J. *9*:433, 1962.

White, C. W., Weiss, J. B., Alver, E. C., and Heerdegen, D. K.: Anesthesia and postpartum headache. Obstet. Gynecol. *20*:734, 1962.

Willocks, J., and Moir, D. D.: Epidural analgesia in the management of hypertension in labour. J. Obstet. Gynaecol. Brit. Cwlth. *75*:225, 1968.

Wingate, M. B., Wingate, L., Iffy, L., Freundlich, J., and Gottsegen, D.: The effect of epidural analgesia upon fetal and neonatal states. Amer. J. Obstet. Gynecol. *119*:1101, 1974.

Winkler, W. P., Sherk, W. M., and Hale, R.: Postpartum spinal headache. Amer. J. Obstet. Gynecol. *85*:500, 1963.

Wollman, S. B., and Marx, G. F.: Acute hydration for prevention of hypotension of spinal anesthesia in parturients. Anesthesiology *29*:374, 1968.

Wood, C., Ng, K. H., Hounslow, D., and Benning, H.: The influence of differences of birth times upon fetal condition in normal deliveries. J. Obstet. Gynaecol. Brit. Cwlth. *80*:289, 1973a.

Wood, C. Ng, K. H., Hounslow, D., and Benning, H.: Time—An important variable in normal delivery. J. Obstet. Gynaecol. Brit. Cwlth. *80*:295, 1973b.

Zilianti, M., Salazar, R., Aller, J., and Aguero, O.: Fetal heart rate, and pH of fetal capillary blood during epidural analgesia in labor. Obstet. Gynecol. *36*:881, 1970.

Zuspan, F. P., Cibils, L. A., and Pose, S. V.: Myometrial and cardiovascular responses to alterations in plasma epinephrine and norepinephrine. Amer. J. Obstet. Gynecol. *84*:841, 1962.

chapter 13
Diagnostic and Therapeutic Applications

In the shadow of your wings I take refuge, till harm pass by.
Psalms 57:2 (Authorized Version)

INTRODUCTION

During the past 20 years epidural analgesia has become widely used in diagnosis and treatment. The ability to produce reversible somatic and autonomic blockade at any spinal level has numerous applications in the management of ischemic or painful disorders. Patients can be treated on an ambulant basis, since epidural blockade avoids puncturing the dura, and the risk of spinal headache from cerebrospinal fluid leak is not a serious consideration.

Injection techniques for the management of chronic pain have been based on the theoretical assumptions of differential neural blockade, in the belief that pain-free function can be restored by local anesthetics in concentrations selected to block small "pain" fibers while sparing larger proprioceptive and motor nerves. However, as pointed out in Chapter 2, earlier simplistic views of differential blockade have had to be modified. The idea that dilute solutions of local anesthetic will interrupt small pain-carrying nerves preferentially, without affecting large fibers, is not necessarily true under all clinical conditions. Unmyelinated C-fibers appear to be relatively resistant at very low concentrations of local anesthetic, and some of the unmyelinated population may continue to carry an appreciable traffic of afferent and efferent impulses at a time when a substantial number of larger fibers have been blocked (Franz and Perry, 1974). Differential blockade is much less precise than was generally believed, and clinical improvement in painful states probably comes about from a quantitative reduction of total afferent neural traffic, as well as from a qualitative reduction of small fiber input, as will be seen later in this section.

The anatomy of the epidural space also presents opportunities for outlining space-occupying lesions of the spinal canal with radiopaque solutions. Recent developments in the pharmacology of nonirritant water-soluble contrast media have rekindled interest in extradural myelography or "peridurography" as a practical diagnostic procedure for outpatient examination of the spinal canal and as a complementary technique to orthodox intrathecal myelography.

Patients who are treated by epidural blockade on an ambulant basis should be issued with the usual precautionary instructions that are given to all outpatients receiving anesthesia. That is to say, they should be told not to operate a vehicle or to use power tools until the effects of the block are fully dissipated and normal coordination is assured. Ambulant patients should therefore be instructed to come for treatment accompanied by a friend or relative who will escort them home afterward. The patient should also be warned not to drive himself home, since in the event of a traffic accident it might be argued (however incorrectly) that the patient was at fault due to imperfect muscular coordination at the time of the accident.

PERIDUROGRAPHY

The anatomy of the epidural space is well suited for diagnostic radiology. The space extends throughout the length of the spinal canal and outward through the intervertebral foramina. Contrast media of the right consistency can be used to display abnormalities within the confines of the space, as well as obstructions to flow through the intervertebral foramina. A number of authors have written extensively on the subject of peridurography or extradural myelography, some with wide experience and considerable enthusiasm. Peridurograms are difficult to interpret, and the technique has never been able to rival the precision, versatility and ease of interpretation of intrathecal myelography in neuroradiological diagnosis. Nevertheless, peridurography has come to be seen as complementary to intrathecal myelography, with special and rather limited indications and with definite advantages for ambulant patients.

Sicard and Forestier were the first to experiment with peridurography in 1926. They used Lipiodol in small amounts of 3 to 6 ml to define the limits of extradural lesions, such as metastatic carcinoma or tuberculous pachymeningitis from Pott's disease of the spine. Peridurograms of satisfactory quality could be obtained by injecting 20 to 30 ml of aqueous local anesthetic solution, followed by 3 to 6 ml of warmed Lipiodol. The radiopaque oil then seemed to follow the track of the aqueous solution, outlining any irregularities in the epidural space. Figure 13–1 shows a typical lateral view of a protruding intervertebral disc at the second lumbar interspace from one of my early cases using this technique. Unfortunately, Lipiodol was difficult to sterilize, and it was abandoned in favor of other agents.

Sanford and Doub (1941) used air contrast peridurography to outline protruded intervertebral discs, but accurate visualization was achieved in only 55 per cent of cases. Moreover, large volumes of air were needed in the range of 200 to 600 ml, and the risks of air embolism appear to have outweighed the benefits. The method did not find wide acceptance.

In the 1940's several German investigators began to use water-soluble contrast media with encouraging results. These early water-soluble agents were irritating and painful in the epidural space, and another 30 years passed before a nonirritating water-soluble agent was developed to a stage where routine peridurography could become a safe and satisfactory procedure for outpatients.

Junge (1949) reported 50 cases of peridurography by the lumbar or

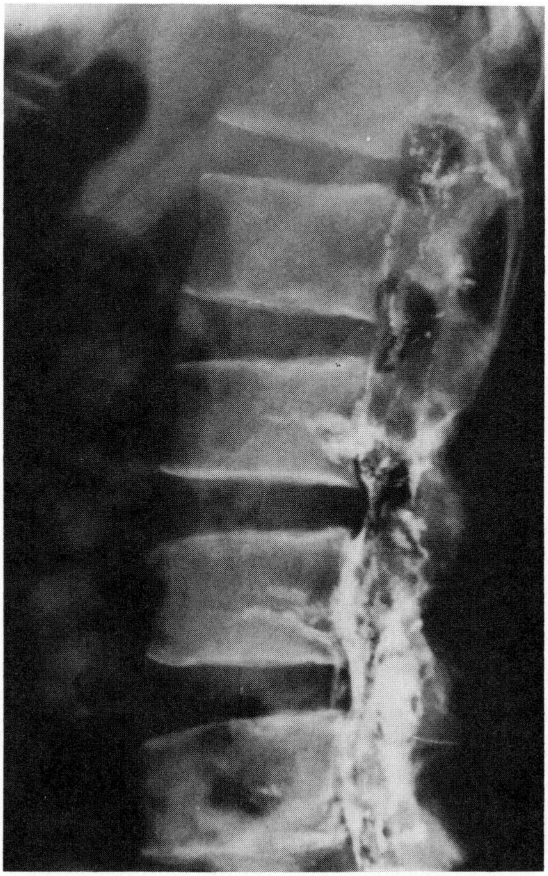

Figure 13–1. Lipiodol peridurogram. Lateral view of lumbar spine (see text).

caudal routes using the water-soluble contrast medium "Per-abrodil" mixed with polyvinylpyrrolidone (PVP) to increase viscosity and with 1 per cent procaine to make it relatively painless. In this series there were only 17 positive peridurograms out of 27 proven cases of disc prolapse, and Junge noted that lesions less than 6 mm in diameter were difficult to identify. Other German authors had even less success with the method at that stage (Frère, 1950; Tiwisina, 1951).

With the passage of time peridurography gradually gained ground as a practical diagnostic procedure. Nakamoto and his colleagues (1955), using sacral peridurography to outline the dural sac and nerve root extensions in the lumbosacral region, reported favorably on a series of 40 patients. Other encouraging reports followed. Fregnani et al. (1962) found a very high correlation between peridurographic and operative findings in patients undergoing lumbar discoidectomy for protruding intervertebral discs. Luyendijk and van Voorthuisen (1966), using 20 ml of sodium diatrizoate (Urografin) injected through the sacral hiatus, also reported very favorably on a series of 600 cases. These authors found that in their hands peridurography correlated more faithfully with the anatomical situation encountered at laminectomy than intrathecal myelography. However, they emphasized that considerable experience is required for accurate interpretation of peridurograms.

Yates (1965) and Mathews (1968) have also found peridurography to be a useful diagnostic tool in the outpatient management of low back pain from lumbar disc protrusion. These authors used 76 per cent Urografin diluted with procaine to produce a final mixture of 52 per cent Urografin and 0.3 per cent procaine, 10 to 20 ml of this mixture being injected through a catheter placed in the caudal canal (Mathews and Yates, 1969; Mathews, 1972). The procedure is easily done on an ambulant basis, and Mathews considers that peridurography outlines small disc protrusions more faithfully than standard myelography and that it is therefore preferable for studying the effects of manipulation and traction on this type of disc lesion (Mathews, 1972, personal communication 1976).

Until recently none of the water-soluble contrast media were ideally suited for peridurography. All the available agents were hyperosmolar, irritant to the tissues, and to varying degrees, all were painful unless mixed with a local anesthetic to render the epidural injection painless. Because of the irritant nature of these solutions, accidental injection into the subarachnoid space was likely to be followed by a type of massive sympathetic discharge similar to that seen after intrathecal injection of hypertonic saline. Acute arterial hypertension, cardiac arrhythmias and even death could occur unless the fulminant reflex response to intrathecal injection was attenuated by mixing local anesthetic with the irritant solution (Squire et al., 1974).

The inconvenience and potential dangers of hyperosmolar contrast solutions were overcome in 1973 with the introduction of a new series of nonionic contrast media that could provide adequate radiopacity in iso-osmolar concentration. Metrizamide, or Amipaque, was the first of the series to be used

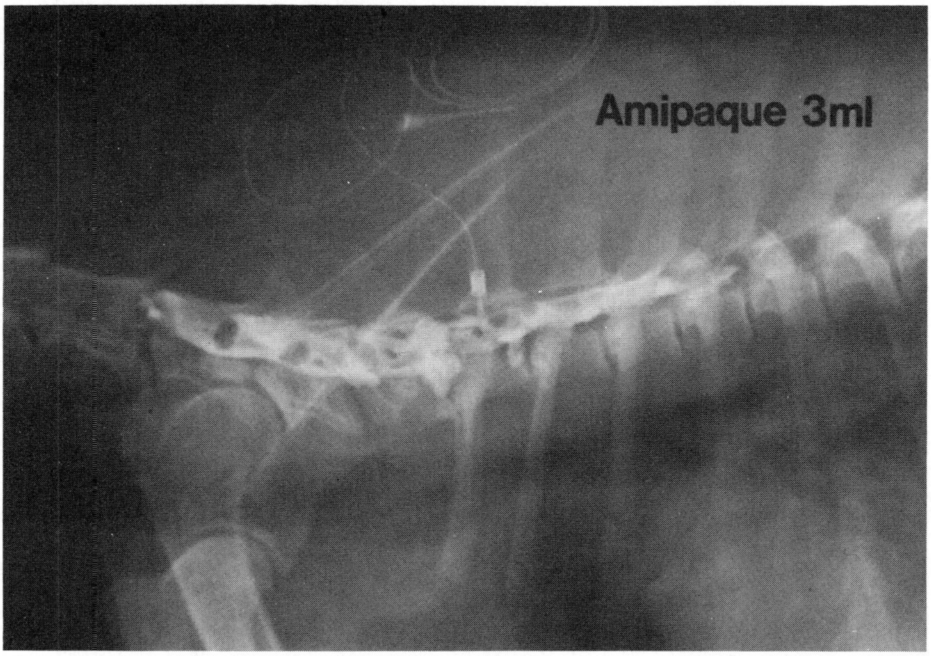

Figure 13–2. Metrizamide ("Amipaque") peridurogram in dog via catheter imbedded in lamina of first thoracic vertebra. Three ml of "Amipaque" has spread through the extradural space from C_{4-5} to T_{4-5}.

extensively for intrathecal myelography, and excellent results were reported (Gonsette, 1973a, 1973b; Hindmarsh, 1973).

Metrizamide is iso-osmolar (300 mOs/L) at an iodine content of about 170 mg I per milliliter. However, satisfactory contrast in spinal films often requires a higher iodine content of up to 300 mg I/ml at an osmolarity of 484 mOs/L. It was feared that this moderate increase of osmolarity might give rise to some discomfort when volumes as large as 12 to 20 ml were injected into the epidural space. Accordingly, trials were done in dogs with chronically implanted epidural catheters, and epidurograms were compared using 60 to 75 per cent sodium diatrizoate (Hypaque) or metrizamide (Amipaque) 300 mg I/ml (Bromage et al., 1978). All the animals showed some evidence of pain or discomfort by struggling or vocalizing when Hypaque was injected, but none of them gave any sign of discomfort or concern when metrizamide was given. Figure 13–2 shows a typical thoracocervical peridurogram in a dog, with 3 ml of metrizamide 300 mg I/ml injected through a chronically implanted catheter.

Preliminary studies in humans yielded similar encouraging results, and volumes up to 18 ml of 300 mg I/ml were tolerated in comfort, without premedication or admixture of local anesthetic. A few patients mentioned a transient feeling of soreness between the shoulder blades when large volumes were injected and when the contrast material rose to the upper thoracic region, but none complained of discomfort in the lumbar region. Radiopaque contrast was satisfactory, as shown in Figure 13–3.

In adults resistance to epidural spread was apparent at the lumbosacral junction. While lumbar injections flowed freely in a cephalad direction, sacral spread was scant and inadequate to outline all the sacral roots clearly. Similarly, caudal injections spread extensively in the sacral canal and outward through the anterior sacral foramina, but very little contrast material penetrated upward beyond the L_5–S_1 region and into the lumbar reaches of the spinal canal. The anatomical obstruction at this point is probably due to local fibrous bands within the epidural fat. As mentioned in Chapter 2, these bands seem to develop at about the age of puberty, and radiopaque solutions flow past the lumbosacral junction more freely in children than in adults (Schulte-Steinberg, 1976).

The management of intractable pain by epidural neurolytic injections will be discussed later in this chapter. In these cases a preliminary peridurogram gives some indication of the probable spread of the neurolytic solution within the epidural space, although the radiographic spread does not correlate completely with the ultimate segmental distribution of neurolysis.

In summary, new contrast materials have made peridurography independent of anesthesia. Nevertheless, any anesthesiologist interested in epidural analgesia will find peridurography a most instructive way to visualize the physical spread of solutions in the epidural space. The technique is simple to perform and can be done in outpatients. However, interpretation of the films requires considerable experience. Lateral views give relatively unambiguous information about space-occupying lesions lying in front or behind the dural tube, but the flow of contrast material is difficult to interpret in sagittal views, due to the streaked and patchy appearance imparted by the extradural venous plexus. In late pregnancy this unevenness of flow may amount to almost complete arrest of the contrast media by the grossly distended extradural veins (Burn et al., 1973). At present, peridurography is unlikely to replace intrathecal

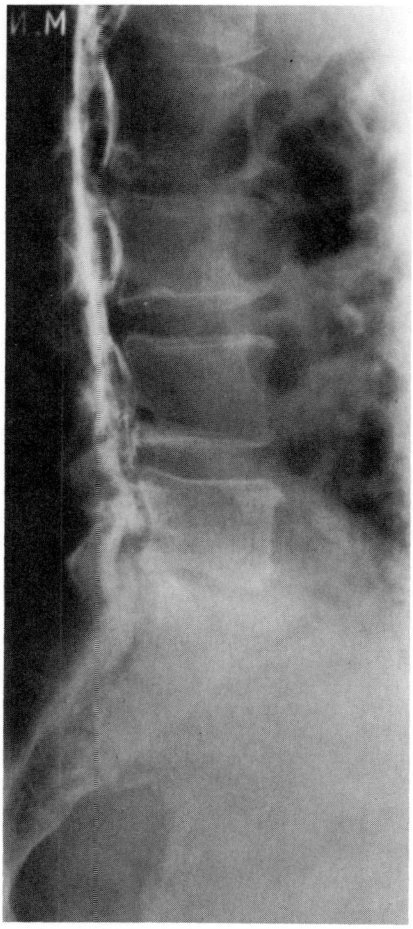

Figure 13–3. Lateral peridurogram in 52-year-old male complaining of low back pain and left sciatica; 12 ml 300 mg I/ml injected at second lumbar interspace. Lateral view shows slight retropulsion of L_3–L_4 disc, together with a moderate degree of reversed spondylolisthesis and distortion of the spinal canal at L_5–S_1. (From Bromage et al.: Peridurography with metrizamide: Animal and human studies. Radiology, 1978.)

myelography as a diagnostic procedure, and the two techniques should be considered as complementary to each other rather than mutually exclusive.

ACUTE PAIN AND TRAUMA

Epidural techniques used to block surgical pain can be adapted and extended to provide analgesia and sympathetic blockade over long periods of hours, days and occasionally weeks at a time for therapeutic indications in serious pain arising from trauma or disease. The objective is to replace centrally depressing narcotics with a sufficient degree of peripheral deafferentation to produce adequate comfort while retaining motor activity as fully as possible, as well as to induce a situation in which the patient can move about freely, breathe deeply and cough, and perform any necessary physiotherapy. In many instances the very process of deafferentation and regional analgesia will restore motor function in a part where movement was previously inhibited by pain. These objectives will be defeated if blockade is intense enough to involve motor pathways to a significant degree, for then function is impaired, and the clinical effects are little better than heavy sedation and immobility arising from large doses of orthodox narcotics.

These aims must be kept clearly in mind, for rules of management are determined by them. The following principles govern technical management.

Austerity

The block should be minimal for the task in hand. As few segments and as few axons should be blocked as is compatible with adequate analgesia. It follows that the site of injection should be as close as possible to the segmental level of pain.

Vigilance

The effects should be observed closely, so that doses can be adjusted for a parsimonious but effective blockade.

Selection of agent

Choice of local anesthetic agent should be appropriate for the task. Short-acting agents are useful for diagnostic procedures in outpatients, but long-acting drugs are more appropriate for therapeutic indications in inpatients. The agent should produce the maximum sensory block with the minimum of motor paresis. Tetracaine is a poor choice in these circumstances, as it causes too much motor blockade. By contrast, bupivacaine is a very suitable drug, as it produces very little motor block in comparison to the degree of analgesia that it provides (see Chapter 9).

Mobility of site

With the passage of time, a foreign body reaction in the epidural tissues tends to seal off an indwelling catheter, so the site of catheterization must be changed at intervals. During prolonged blockade the site of puncture should be changed every 72 hours.

Response to tachyphylaxis

Prolonged blockade with local anesthetics will inevitably provoke some degree of tachyphylaxis. Acute tolerance can be minimized by using long-acting agents with weak dilutions of epinephrine (1/200,000 to 1/300,000) and by keeping the dose of local anesthetic agent as small as possible from the outset. With the onset of tachyphylaxis, dosage must be increased to keep pace with the diminishing effect. Changing the agent and maintaining a high pH of the injected solution (see pages 104 and 233) may also help in delaying tachyphylaxis.

TECHNICAL SIMPLICITY

Be content with simple equipment and intermittent injections. A number of ingenious devices have been proposed to maintain a constant segmental level of blockade for long periods of time. These include pumps, drips and motorized syringes of various sorts. My own experience with these devices has not been encouraging, and I suspect that by the nature of things and the number of variables involved, they are likely to be unsatisfactory in most hands. Dose requirements are not constant but change with tachyphylaxis and with the degree of subjective pain. A fixed dose schedule will usually err one way or the other by falling short or by extending the analgesic segments too far. There is little to be lost by settling for intermittent injections, with close observation of the clinical results. Then the severity of pain and the size of the next dose can be assessed with greater precision than when fixed-dose systems are used.

CARDIOVASCULAR EVENTS

Be prepared for side effects or for unrelated but dangerous disease processes that may arise while their effects are masked by the blockade. Some degree of vasodilatation and peripheral pooling is inevitable when blockade involves the thoracic segments. Cardiac inotropic drive will be reduced as well if the block extends to the upper four thoracic segments. Hence, it is essential that a careful watch be kept on pulse and blood pressure, with adequate hydration and the occasional use of small doses of vasopressors, if indicated. The warning effects of sudden hemorrhage or perforation of a viscus may be masked by high epidural blockade, and these possibilities should also be borne in mind.

TRAUMA

Pain arising from peripheral trauma can usually be controlled by systemic analgesics, but when the trunk is involved the question of respiratory depression arises. In chest trauma respiration may become inadequate from one or more of three factors. The first is mechanical incompetence due to a damaged rib cage or an injured airway, and this type of difficulty requires mechanical correction. Flail chest is one of the commonest examples of mechanical injury. If a large number of ribs are broken in two places, the chest wall loses its mechanical integrity and cannot support the underlying lung. A "pendeluft" form of paradoxical respiration results, and gas exchange is impaired. When this happens there is no choice but to take full command of the patient's respiration by intubation, mechanical ventilation and aspiration of secretions. Moderate degrees of flail may be managed more conservatively, provided the underlying lungs are sound and gas exchange remains satisfactory (Lloyd et al., 1965).

A second hazard to respiratory exchange arises even when the chest wall is intact, if there is preexisting lung pathology with copious sputum and if the injury causes pain on deep breathing or coughing. Then the patient may be unable to overcome the reflex inhibition caused by pain, and accumulation of bronchial secretions may lead to asphyxial death unless appropriate measures are taken to clear the tracheobronchial tree.

A third hazard may arise from injudicious treatment with central respiratory depressants. Narcotic analgesics depress respiratory drive and hasten the need for mechanical assistance if either of the previous two factors are present to any appreciable degree.

Pain, and respiratory inhibition from pain, can be managed very effectively by continuous epidural blockade, provided the mechanical integrity of the chest wall remains adequate. Many trauma patients with chest injuries can be spared the need for intubation and respiratory therapy by the judicious use of continuous epidural analgesia (Dittmann et al., 1975). Basically the problem is very similar to that of managing postoperative abdominal pain in morbidly obese patients, as outlined in Chapter 11. In both instances there are two separate handicaps working together to hinder respiration. One is mechanical and irremovable: a massive thoracic wall in extreme obesity and a damaged one in trauma. The other factor is the patient's own inappropriate response to pain under the imperative of archaic reflexes that demand a fixed protective stance in the face of trauma instead of the coordinated mobility that is necessary for effective gas exchange.

So long as the chest wall is intact, logical management of chest injuries with complicating lung disease lies in a trial of deafferentation by limited segmental block, followed by assessment of active respiratory performance after the patient has been freed from the inhibitory effects of his protective reflexes. If performance is still inadequate, then clearly there is no recourse but to fall back on more orthodox lines of management with tracheal intubation and mechanical ventilation. However, in many instances this will prove to be unnecessary, and the patient will be spared several days of uncomfortable and expensive intensive care, with attendant invasive monitoring and all the secondary risks of tracheal damage and infection and other hazards of prolonged ventilation. The following case illustrates this point:

A man of 54 years was struck by a car and sustained fractures of the clavicle, scapula and second and third ribs on his right side (Fig. 13–4). There was no flail chest and no evidence of air or blood in the pleural cavity. However, the patient was a chronic bronchitic with a productive cough. Normal efforts to clear his lungs were impaired by pain, and within 24 hours he was gravely ill from the asphyxial effects of retained secretions. He was ashen grey and sweating, with a rapid thready pulse, a blood pressure of 85/60 mmHg and a temperature of 39.4°C (103°F). Air entry was absent over both lung bases, and loud rattling rales were heard all over the rest of the lung fields. Vital capacity was reduced to 350 ml, and he was unable to cough. He appeared to be a candidate for urgent intubation, tracheobronchial toilet and mechanical ventilation. Instead, a decision was made to treat his pain at the periphery, since this was the precipitating cause of his trouble. An epidural block was performed at the second thoracic interspace using 8 ml of 1 per cent lidocaine with 1/200,000 epinephrine. This provided analgesia that extended from the seventh cervical to the first lumbar segment. Subjective relief began 5 minutes after injection. He started coughing and in 15 minutes had produced several ounces of purulent sputum. Later the vital capacity rose from 350 ml to 1000 ml, his color improved and both lungs became fully aerated. The epidural block was continued for 12 hours, and from then on no further treatment was required.

Here, the simplicity, comfort and speed of recovery may be contrasted with the discomfort and complexity and additional hazards that would have attended the alternative regimen of intubation and IPPV. This case is a clear-cut

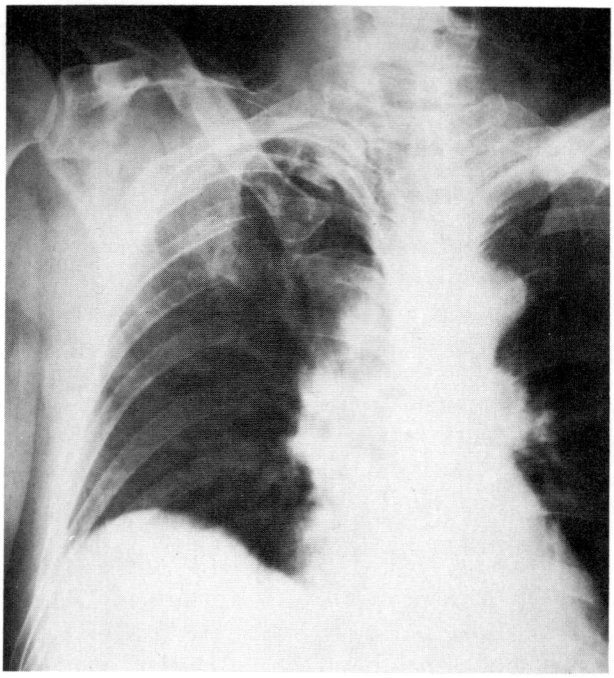

Figure 13–4. Potentially lethal pain following automobile accident. Chest X-ray of 54-year-old bronchitic, showing fractures of right scapula, clavicle and second and third ribs. Pain successfully treated by thoracic epidural blockade (see text). (From Bromage, P. R.: Extradural analgesia for pain relief. Brit. J. Anaesth. *39*:721, 1967.)

example of dramatic cure by epidural block alone. Flail was minimal or nonexistent, and it was only necessary to break the afferent side of the reflex arc inhibiting respiration. However, epidural pain relief and IPPV should not be regarded as mutually exclusive forms of therapy; rather, the two should complement each other. In a study of 121 cases of thoracic injury at Oxford, Lloyd et al. (1965) showed how epidural block, alone or in combination with IPPV and central narcotics, could be used to provide optimal conditions for each individual patient while keeping the period of respirator management as short as possible.

Gibbons and her colleagues (1973a, 1973b) have applied these principles to the management of thoracic and thoracoabdominal injuries with considerable success; only 22 per cent of their patients treated with epidural blockade deteriorated sufficiently to require additional ventilatory support with a respirator. These authors warn that epidural blockade should not be used for injuries above the fifth thoracic segment because of the danger of cardiovascular depression from interruption of the cardiac sympathetic nerves. However, in my experience this is a groundless fear, and patients with upper thoracic injuries have done extremely well with high thoracic blocks, the benefit being most dramatic when preexisting pulmonary disease was present, as illustrated by the case shown in Figure 13–4. Any vascular hypotension that may occur as a result of high epidural blockade can be treated satisfactorily by blood volume augmentation and by the judicious use of mixed alpha- and beta-adrenergic vasopressors, such as methamphetamine, ephedrine or mephentermine.

While thoracic injuries with unstable chest walls must be treated with mechanical ventilation, satisfactory control of breathing may still be difficult if there is a great deal of associated pain, and especially if an element of bronchospasm is present as well. In these cases a continuous epidural block lessens the bronchospasm, eases pain and makes it much easier for the patient to surrender himself to the imposed rhythm of the ventilator.

The new long-acting agents bupivacaine and etidocaine have made repeated intercostal blocks a feasible alternative to segmental epidural analgesia in these cases, for peripheral nerve blocks with etidocaine may last as long as 24 hours (Bromage et al., 1974). However, it must be remembered that each intercostal block carries with it the danger of accidental pneumothorax and possibly even accidental total spinal anesthesia (Benumof and Semenza, 1975). When these risks are multiplied by the several intercostal injections that must be made every time a block is repeated, it seems safer and more practical to choose the single injection required to insert a continuous epidural catheter.

Phantom Limbs and Traumatic Causalgia

Spinal and epidural analgesia have been recommended for diagnostic and therapeutic applications in phantom limb pain (Lund, 1966; Greene, 1969). While epidural analgesia will indeed produce temporary relief, in my own experience it has only very limited use for diagnosis or treatment of phantom pain arising from severed or partially severed nerves. A glance at the underlying pathology may help to show why this is so.

Phantom phenomena are poorly understood, but two aspects can be recognized and their roles differentiated. Both peripheral and central mechanisms are at work. A latent phantom image is present in all of us, related to the postural body schema or body image proposed by Head and Holmes (1912) and probably closely concerned with preconscious control of joint position, movement and coordination in three dimensions. This noumenal phantom image can be conjured up under conditions of peripheral deafferentation (Melzack and Bromage, 1973; Bromage and Melzack, 1974). Distortion of the phantom image is brought about by disturbance of neural information entering through severed or damaged peripheral nerves, or by gliosis in central lesions. It is this abnormal input in the presence of complete or partial deafferentation that seems to give rise to painful phantom phenomena and to causalgic pain.

Painful phantoms in amputees are usually associated with abnormal peripheral stimulation arising from physical conditions in or around the terminal neuromas on the peripheral nerves, and these are subject to pressure from external causes or from internal turgor, as in premenstrual edema. Thus, pain in stump or phantom is usually due to peripheral conditions such as limb-fitting problems, a stump that requires trimming and revision, tissue ischemia or just the intrinsic tissue pressure within an encapsulated neuroma. In addition, pain pathways from the periphery are not altogether clear-cut, and there is circumstantial evidence that some C-fiber limb afferents may travel for varying distances in extraspinal autonomic trunks before entering the spinal cord at a relatively high segmental level (De Jong and Cullen, 1963).

Therefore, from a diagnostic point of view it is not likely that the imprecise effects of epidural blockade, acting on spinal roots and probably on the cord as well, will tell us very much about the neural origin or pathways of pain in any individual case, except to eliminate the possibility of thalamic or other intracranial cause for the pain. We may expect that epidural blockade will relieve pain for the duration of the block, but the mechanism of the relief may be one or more of several causes. Epidural blockade is also rather disappointing as a therapeutic measure in this type of pain, for analgesia usually lasts only for the duration of the block, and during this time coordination in the limb is impaired.

More promising therapeutic results follow from local infiltration of the neuroma with long-acting agents such as etidocaine, or occasionally from blockade of the sympathetic chain.

VISCERAL DISEASE

Acute Pancreatitis

Acute pancreatitis may lead to secondary deleterious effects in major organ systems. The blood pressure rises at first as part of a generalized vasoconstrictive response and renal vasoconstriction occurs (Werner et al., 1974); renal failure may follow (Frey, 1965). Breathing is inhibited by pain, and respiration becomes rapid and shallow. A form of adult respiratory distress syndrome may develop, with respiratory alkalosis and arterial hypoxia due to tachypnea, diminished tidal volume and a marked physiological shunt (Kellum et al., 1972; Ransom et al., 1973; Hayes et al., 1974). The arterial oxygen tension falls steadily in the first 48 hours. In one series over 40 per cent of patients with acute pancreatitis developed arterial PaO_2 levels of less than 60 mmHg while breathing room air at some time during the first week of illness (Imrie et al., 1976). These changes are frequently associated with pleural effusion or atelectasis, while pulmonary arterial pressure tends to rise and pulmonary edema may occur (Rovner and Westcott, 1976).

Present trends in supportive therapy of these cardiovascular and respiratory abnormalities are mainly along orthodox lines—that is: (a) supplementary inspired oxygen; (b) tracheal intubation and volume-cycled ventilation with positive end-expiratory pressure (PEEP); (c) augmented plasma oncotic pressure by plasma or albumin infusions and by diuretics; (d) digitalization.

Segmental epidural blockade has been favored by a number of authors as a supplementary form of treatment in acute pancreatitis. This approach developed from the work of Marion and Mallet-Guy at Lyons, who reported the benefits of splanchnic blockade in the mid-1940's (Marion, 1945). Orr and Warren (1950) at the Lahey Clinic then extended the possibility of prolonged splanchnic blockade by using continuous epidural analgesia to block the spinal segments innervating the pancreas (Fig. 13–5). Other favorable reports soon followed (Berk and Krumperman, 1952; Walker and Pemberton, 1953; Bromage, 1954; Browne and Ashworth, 1969).

The logic of using epidural blockade in acute pancreatitis is analogous to the use of continuous epidural analgesia for postoperative pain relief, or to prevent the adverse effects of acute hypertension, as outlined in Chapters 10 and 11. Interruption of the spinal reflex arc in the lower six or seven thoracic

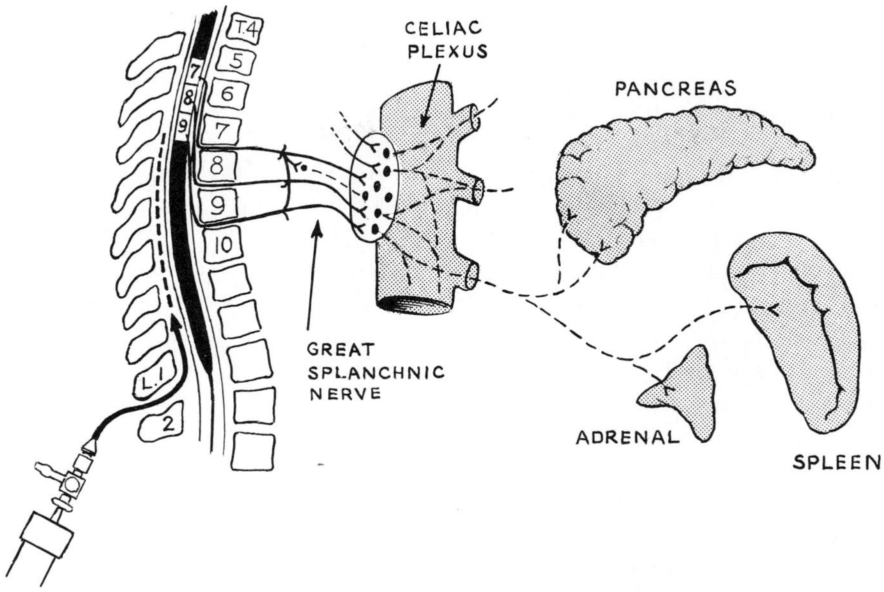

Figure 13–5. The pain of acute pancreatitis. Diagram showing the nerve pathways involved. (After Orr and Warren, 1950.)

segments relieves abdominal pain, prevents splanchnic vasoconstriction and restores respiratory function toward normal, allowing the patient to breathe slowly and deeply and to expand the atelectatic portions of the lung bases. In addition, it has been suggested that the sympathetic blockade relaxes the sphincter of Oddi and improves biliary drainage (Gage and Gillespie, 1951; White et al., 1952; Green et al., 1959). Claims have also been made that epidural blockade diminishes local vasospasm and increases pancreatic blood flow (Ochsner, 1963), but these benefits are unproven.

TECHNIQUE

Hypovolemia is often present in acute pancreatitis, so splanchnic blockade should be preceded by adequate replacement of fluids, electrolytes and glucose, in order to avoid unnecessary hypotension from vasodilatation after the block. The pain of pancreatitis travels mainly by the seventh, eighth and ninth thoracic segments, so blockade should be centered around these dermatomes (see Fig. 13–5). Puncture is best done in the mid-thoracic region with the patient on the side, small amounts of 0.5 per cent bupivacaine being used according to age, with the aim of producing segmental blockade from the fifth or sixth thoracic dermatome to the eleventh or twelfth thoracic segment in order to provide splanchnic blockade and complete relief of abdominal pain without interfering with mobility of the legs. If mid-thoracic puncture is technically difficult or if the patient is poorly responsive, it may be safer to introduce an epidural catheter lower down at the first or second lumbar interspace, a larger dose of analgesic solution being used in order to extend the block upward as far as the sixth thoracic dermatome.

The blood pressure and respiration should be checked frequently until the block is stabilized. Intravenous fluids and vasopressors should be at hand in case of vascular hypotension. Respiration becomes easier and smoother once segmental analgesia is established. The vital capacity increases, and the mucous membranes lose their cyanotic tinge. Blockade may have to be maintained for several days, so it is wise to take steps to minimize tachyphylaxis by using minimal quantities of a long-acting local anesthetic, such as bupivacaine, with 1/200,000 epinephrine added to it.

Unfortunately, the apparent benefits of epidural blockade in acute pancreatitis have only been assessed by the relatively crude criteria of vital capacity changes, arterial blood gas measurements and clinical impressions. The author is not aware of any recent studies to test the effects of epidural blockade by the same objective methods of measurement that have been applied to more orthodox modes of treatment. Such a critical study would have to include a wide range of sophisticated tests including pulmonary function and pulmonary vascular dynamics, cardiac output and shunt measurements, as well as observations on renal vascular dynamics and renal function. Superficially, epidural blockade seems to do all the right things, and patients appear to benefit by it, but so far we have neglected to corroborate these encouraging clinical results by rigorous measurement, and the method remains virtually untested by current physiological standards of critical care.

Ureteric Colic

Severe spasmodic pain is caused when small renal stones block the ureter. Impacted ureteric stones are passed spontaneously in about one quarter of all cases, and Hellstrom (1949) found a 23 per cent rate of spontaneous expulsion in a large series of 275 cases treated by conventional methods. Afferent impulses from ureteric colic are transmitted to segments T_{11} to L_2 inclusive. Blockade of these segments by epidural analgesia relieves pain and spasm dramatically and facilitates passage of the impacted stone (Bonica, 1953). Lloyd and Carrie (1965) reported successful passage of stones in more than 50 per cent of cases using this technique. Forced hydration increases the chances that the impacted stone will be passed spontaneously, and Romagnoli and Batra (1973) reported successful expulsion of impacted stones in 16 out of 22 cases (73 per cent) treated by a combination of forced fluids and continuous lumbar epidural blockade. Their success rate with epidural analgesia is three times better than the incidence of spontaneous expulsion by conventional nonsurgical methods.

VASCULAR DISORDERS

Overreaction of the sympathetic nervous system is thought to underlie many types of vascular disorders, such as Raynaud's phenomenon, acrocyanosis, Sudeck's post-traumatic dystrophy and cold injury. Leriche (1939) proposed that a form of vicious circle is set up in patients with unstable autonomic systems in whom injury elicits a segmental sympathetic response and vasoconstriction; this in turn reduces tissue perfusion and nutrition. Tissue asphyxia stimulates local afferent nerve endings which generate further sympathetic responses, and the loop of the vicious cycle is completed. Leriche reasoned that the vicious circle should be broken by interruption of the appropriate autonomic pathways in order to restore normal vascular dynamics and allow natural healing processes to take their course. This teaching has led to the adoption of sympathetic blockade as a major diagnostic and therapeutic tool in the management of vascular disorders.

Epidural blockade offers a very convenient way to provide sympathetic blockade to the upper or lower limbs. In addition, the accompanying analgesia is extremely valuable in painful vasopathies, providing a degree of comfort that is unparalleled by any other form of therapy. This section will discuss some of the factors that should be considered when epidural analgesia is used for the management of peripheral vascular disorders of the limbs.

Indications and Contraindications

Leriche's enthusiastic support of sympathectomy was based on the premise that the vicious circle underlying such reflex dystrophic conditions as Raynaud's disease and Sudeck's atrophy is reversible and that elimination of the unstable sympathetic element restores the normal balance of reparative forces. Unfortunately, this is not always the case. It is important to understand that the syndromes of peripheral vascular inadequacy are often manifestations of progressive underlying conditions that either are not susceptible to sympathetic blockade or show only a very temporary response in a remorselessly ongoing illness.

In the past, epidural analgesia has been recommended for all of the following conditions. Today, the field has narrowed somewhat as therapy has become more rationalized.

Raynaud's Phenomenon

Cold sensitivity causing peripheral vasospasm and white "dead" fingers may be due to Raynaud's disease—a benign condition—or it may be secondary to one of many other possible causes. Local treatment of the limb should always be accompanied by a diligent search for underlying disease which may or may not be curable. The following possibilities should be considered and excluded:

1. Continued local stimulus. For example, local vibration trauma may lead to persistent vasospasm and permanent arterial occlusion (Gurdjian and Walker, 1945; Laroche, 1976). Operators of vibrating tools, such as pneumatic hammers and/or chainsaws, may sustain irreversible arterial damage if they do not change their occupation.

2. Neurovascular entrapment at any level. For example, disease of the cervical spine or cervical discs, cervical rib, carpal tunnel syndrome, etc.

3. Systemic disease. For example, diabetes, scleroderma, systemic lupus erythematosus, dysproteinemias, hypothyroidism, primary pulmonary hypertension, occult carcinoma, etc. (Strandness, 1974).

4. Drug intoxication. For example, ergotamine, methysergide, lead or arsenic.

Unilateral Raynaud's disease is best treated by unilateral block of the sympathetic chain, but in severe cases of bilateral disease, treatment time may be shortened by using epidural analgesia to produce vasodilatation in both limbs simultaneously. Cervical epidural block is induced for Raynaud's disease of the hands, and lumbar block is induced if the feet are involved.

Cold Injuries of the Extremities

Frostbite, "trench foot" and "immersion foot" are disabling injuries of the greatest concern to dwellers in cold climates. Few practitioners have the opportunity to gain extensive experience with the management of frostbite, and because individual cases tend to differ so widely, opinions on pathogenesis and treatment are still less uniform than they should be. One of the largest military experiences in recent times comes from Finland where more than 8,000 soldiers suffered frostbite during the single campaign of the Winter War of 1939–1940, and where civilian experience continues to accumulate on a significant scale (Ervasti, 1962; Kyösola, 1974).

Severe cold injury of the extremities is followed by pain, local vasospasm and agglutination of intravascular cellular elements, leading to thrombosis and local gangrene. Vasospasm of neighboring tissue tends to persist into the chronic phase of frostbite (Edwards and Leeper, 1952). Therapy should aim at augmenting tissue perfusion, preventing extension of intravascular clotting and, if possible, aiding the resolution of existing thrombi. Manipulation of intravascular viscosity and coagulability by infusions of low-molecular-weight dextran and by heparinization has been clinically disappointing (Meryman, 1957; Penn and Schwartz, 1964; Kyösola, 1974). The alternative approach of enhancing local blood flow by preventing vascular spasm has proved much more promising, and cumulative laboratory and clinical evidence from the largest published series is heavily in favor of sympathectomy as a cornerstone in promoting healing and in preventing the late sequelae of frostbite (Golding et al., 1965; Martinez et al., 1966; Ervasti, 1962; Kyösola, 1974).

Bilateral lumbar sympathectomy effectively abolishes vasoconstrictor tone in the lower extremities, but it also carries operative risks, and in the male it causes infertility through loss of ejaculation. The nonsurgical alternative of temporary pharmacological sympathectomy can be accomplished by (1) depleting sympathetic nerve endings of the affected limb with intravenous regional guanethidine or reserpine (Hannington-Kiff, 1974); (2) repeated paravertebral sympathetic blocks; (3) continuous epidural blockade.

The technique of regional catecholamine depletion requires temporary exsanguination of the limb and tourniquet stasis lasting 10 to 20 minutes. While this is an effective form of treatment in some other vasospastic conditions, the method has not been extensively investigated in frostbite, and the rather long period of vascular stasis required would seem to be undesirable for tissues that are already critically ischemic. Repeated paravertebral blocks have not met with much enthusiasm or success, probably because of the large number of individual injections that are necessary and because it is difficult to guarantee a technically perfect block and complete sympathetic interruption on each occasion (Ervasti, 1962). Continuous epidural analgesia, on the other hand, is a practical and effective way to maintain sympathetic blockade for several days on end, and at the same time pain is relieved more thoroughly than by any other method (Campbell and Walker, 1961). The benefits are the same as those of operative sympathectomy. Voluntary movements of the extremity become easier as pain is relieved, limb color and perfusion improve, edema lessens and demarcation is hastened. Aseptic or infectious processes of the bone, cartilage and joints are less likely to occur and they heal more quickly, while skin grafts attach and survive more surely (Kyösola, 1974).

My own experience has been limited to relatively few civilian cases of frostbite arising from accidental exposure in Canadian winter conditions, but the effects of epidural blockade have been vivid enough to convince me of its uniquely useful place in the treatment of this condition. The following case is a typical example.

M. W., a woman of 45 years, suffered cold exposure while lingering out of doors in bitter weather after an alcoholic bout. Both hands and both feet were frostbitten, extremely painful and immobile. Two fingers of one hand and one great toe were pregangrenous on admission 24 hours after exposure. Epidural catheters were inserted at C_8–T_1 *and at* L_2–L_3, *and blockade was induced with 0.7 per cent lidocaine with 1/300,000 epinephrine. Pain was relieved immediately, color improved in all four extremities and active finger movements were begun for the first time since injury. Epidural blockade was maintained for three days and then discontinued in view of the dramatic improvement; however, intermittent stellate ganglion blocks of the worse hand were continued for the next week. Tissue loss was minimal, but the terminal phalanges of one index finger and one great toe demarcated and required amputation at a later date. There were no long-term sequelae.*

In the past, difficulties sometimes arose in choosing between anticoagulation and epidural blockade as the most effective means of therapy for frostbite. The two are not compatible, and it is unsafe to use heparinization and epidural analgesia at the same time (see Chapter 4 for detailed discussion on anticoagulation). However, the current consensus of opinion from the most authoritative sources seems clear that the dilemma is no longer a problem. Heparinization appears to have little value in these cases, whereas effective sympathetic blockade in one form or another is the best line of supportive treatment. At present, epidural blockade seems to be the most practical way to induce vasodilatation and to restore pain-free function in the damaged extremities.

Postpoliomyelitis Vasospasm

The residual paralysis from an attack of poliomyelitis is sometimes associated with cold sensitivity and a cold, blue, painful limb. The condition is thought to be due to relative sympathetic overaction, and it is improved by sympathectomy (Ogilvie, 1933; Leriche, 1949). Allison (1958) has reported that temporary improvement lasting several months is obtained by a course of two or three lumbar epidural blocks at intervals of three to four weeks, and he recommends that patients with this condition should be tided over the cold winter months by a course of epidural blocks in the late autumn. It should be noted that these are clinical impressions that are unsupported by physiological measurements, and there is a need for further study to eliminate placebo effects and to confirm the intriguing report that a short course of epidural blocks appears to have such lasting beneficial effects on limb perfusion.

Acute Arterial or Venous Occlusion

Spasm of collateral vessels accompanies acute arterial embolus or venous thrombosis in a limb, and at one time sympathetic blockade was a popular form of vasodilator treatment for thrombophlebitis or arterial embolism (Ochsner and De Bakey, 1940; Hingson et al., 1947; Halligan et al., 1953; Lund, 1966). Today, anticoagulation therapy, with or without vascular surgery, is the accepted method of management, and epidural blockade has been virtually eliminated as a redundant form of therapy in these conditions (Strandness, 1974).

Arteriosclerosis Obliterans

Chronic arterial occlusion may lead to rest pain and gangrene in the affected limbs. Severe cases with large vessel disease must be treated by arterial surgery, but patients with minor degrees of rest pain may be given a trial of lumbar sympathectomy as a form of temporization until more definitive surgical procedures become inevitable. There is little indication for epidural blockade in these cases, except as an initial screening method to assess the probable effects of sympathectomy before proceeding to lumbar sympathetic phenol blockade or surgical sympathectomy as a palliative measure.

CHRONIC NONMALIGNANT PAIN

> It is in the diagnosis and treatment of strains, both acute and chronic, that there is a tendency to surrender judgement to the fascination of a name.
>
> Sir Henry Cohen, 1948

Back Pain and Sciatica

The aphorism "diagnosis before treatment" is central to the management of chronic pain. While it is not always possible to arrive at a conclusive diagnosis, the various possibilities should always be kept in mind and a high index of suspicion cultivated so that every effort is made to exclude organic disease before palliative therapy is begun. A missed cord tumor, tuberculosis or a spinal deposit from carcinoma of the lung or genitals leads to foolish tragedy if the physician has not performed the necessary routine examinations at the outset (Shealy, 1966). Equally important are the assessment and management of the psychiatric aspects of chronic pain, and patients should be screened for primary or secondary elements of depression before palliative therapy is initiated (Pos, 1974).

Backache and sciatica are often lumped together under the umbrella diagnosis of "prolapsed intervertebral disc," but stimulation of any deep structure of the lumbosacral region may cause a nonspecific and widespread muscle spasm (Pedersen et al., 1956). Pain clinics all over the world are haunted by the wreckage of laminectomies and discoidectomies performed for inadequate or wrong reasons. For many years James Cyriax at St. Thomas's Hospital, England, pioneered for a more conservative approach to low back pain and sciatica and, based on a large experience with London policemen, proposed instead a regimen of large-volume caudal injections of dilute local anesthetic solutions, usually followed by manipulation or traction (Cyriax, 1957). In the absence of frank disc prolapse with signs of paresis or progressive sensory loss, this is a safe and effective, if empirical, technique (Mount, 1971).

From time to time during the past 70 years the epidural space has been made the repository of a widely assorted variety of therapeutic materials and, according to published reports, mostly with good effects. Among these nostrums were such unlikely substances as pitcher plant extract, air and large quantities of petrolatum. Accidental injections have included such pharmacological assaults as 2 per cent thiopental (Forestner and Raj, 1975) and 6 per cent potassium chloride (see Chapter 14) without producing any lasting damage. It is salutary to recall these past insults that have been heaped upon the epidural space, not only to appreciate its remarkable tolerance but also to view current enthusiasms and fads with a proper sense of proportion and humility.

Sicard (1901) pioneered the caudal approach to relieve back pain, and in 1913 Heile in Germany was using epidural injections of 100 to 150 ml of saline for the treatment of sciatica. Early in their radiological researches, Sicard and Forestier (1921, 1926) noted that in many cases diagnostic injection of Lipiodol into the epidural space for lumbago and sciatica was followed by immediate and lasting relief of pain. They used volumes of 8 to 10 ml of warmed iodized oil injected via the sacral hiatus, and they coined the general term "lipiodotherapy" for this type of treatment. It was assumed that the coating of iodized oil would exert a protective effect on the root funiculus as it passed through the intervertebral foramen (Sicard and Forestier, 1932). This physical explanation had contemporary appeal, and before long others were enthusiastically injecting large volumes of oily substances, including petrolatum, into the epidural space for lumbago and sciatica, much as a mechanic would in greasing the moving parts of a motorcar.

In 1925 Viner in Montreal used petrolatum in amounts up to 100 ml, and he also reported excellent results from caudal procaine injections in sciatica (Viner, 1925, 1928). Further encouraging reports of caudal procaine followed from a number of authors (Evans, 1930; Odom, 1940; Kelman, 1944; Bresgen, 1951; Cyriax, 1957; Coomes, 1961). Good results were thought to be due to a combination of local analgesia with mechanical stretching and freeing of the affected nerve roots within the spinal canal and foramina; consequently, large volumes were administered very rapidly. Some of these early therapeutic applications enjoyed remarkable luck in avoiding serious trouble when enthusiasm exceeded pharmacological prudence. For example, Evans used up to 145 ml of 1 per cent procaine given rapidly in 25-ml increments, and although many patients complained of feelings of great anxiety during the procedure, only one case of frank toxic convulsions occurred following an injection of 120 ml of 2 per cent procaine (i.e., 2400 mg) (Evans, 1930). This low incidence of toxic reactions is undoubtedly a tribute to the rapid breakdown of procaine by pseudocholinesterase in the blood. One author reported a 66 per cent success rate from injecting 30 ml of air into the caudal canal for lumbago and sciatica; a total of 186 patients were subjected to this treatment for a variety of conditions, without any evidence of air embolism (Matyas, 1953).

In 1953 Lièvre and his associates injected hydrocortisone into the epidural space via the first posterior sacral foramen for sciatica (Lièvre et al., 1953). The more convenient caudal or lumbar approaches were soon adopted, and local anesthetic and steroid mixtures quickly became a popular method for the conservative management of sciatica (Cappio, 1957; Goebert et al., 1961; Barry and Kendall, 1962; Swerdlow and Sayle-Creer, 1970).

It is generally supposed that the corticoid preparations act locally in the epidural space, resolving edema of perineural tissues and reducing pressure on irritated and compressed roots (Goebert et al., 1961; Swerdlow and Sayle-Creer, 1970; Dilke et al., 1973). Corticoids are unlikely to act on adhesions that are already formed, but the combination of local analgesia, increased range of movement and local corticoid may induce a situation in which old adhesions can be stretched and broken down painlessly, without inducing a florid regrowth of new ones. However, it is also possible that the beneficial results of the epidural corticoids may be general as much as local, due to an unknown proportion of the drug acting after vascular absorption in a manner similar to the systemic effects that have been shown to persist for 3 to 16 days after intra-articular steroid therapy (Shuster and Williams, 1961; Koehler et al., 1974). While very little systemic absorption occurs when steroids are injected into the subarachnoid space (Sehgal et al., 1963), there may be sufficient absorption from the epidural space to cause appreciable salt and water retention, and Goebert and his colleages described one case of congestive heart failure attributable to this mechanism (Goebert et al., 1961).

A note of caution must be sounded. Certain brands of steroid suspensions are dispensed containing 2.9 per cent polyethylene glycol. This concentration of polyethylene glycol has been shown to cause demyelination and neurolysis when injected perineurally in rats (Wood and Arguelles, 1977). Therefore, the ironic possibility exists that some of the subjective improvement observed after epidural steroid suspensions may be due to actual destruction of afferent nerve fibers rather than to restoration of their normal function, as discussed in Chapter 9. However, in our technique, described further on, the steroid suspension was diluted with lidocaine in a proportion of one part steroid suspension to 12 parts local anesthetic solution, thus reducing the concentration of polyethylene glycol to about 0.2 to 0.3 per cent. At the present time there is no evidence that epidural polyethylene glycol will cause neural damage in this range of dilution. Nevertheless, the apparent beneficial effects of epidural steroid suspensions should be viewed with reserve until more thorough neurohistologic assessment has shown them to be entirely free of neurolytic consequences.

TECHNIQUE

Comparison of large-volume injections using 30 to 50 ml of local anesthetic solution with smaller volumes using 5 to 10 ml of local anesthetic-steroid mixtures suggests that the latter is more efficacious (Swerdlow and Sayle-Creer, 1970), especially when injected as close as possible to the site of the lesion (Winnie et al., 1972). My own preference is to choose a middle course using moderately large volumes of dilute local anesthetic solution mixed with a suspension of methylprednisolone.

Epidural puncture is made at the segmental level of pain—caudal for low back pain and sciatica, lumbar for lumbar root involvement and upper thoracic or cervical puncture for root pain in the brachial plexus or cervical distribution. Low dilutions of local anesthetic are adequate to produce symptomatic relief, but it is more informative to use concentrations that are strong enough to provide cutaneous analgesia so that the sensory margins of the block can be mapped out and recorded. Consistently missed segments may provide a clue to underlying structural abnormalities that will require surgical correction. Lidocaine in 0.7 to 1.0 per cent concentration is sufficient, and 40 ml of this solution is prepared with 120 mg methylprednisolone added to it. Ten to 15 ml of the suspension is injected through the epidural needle, and a catheter is then passed and the needle removed. In caudal blocks a larger volume is required, and 20 to 30 ml is injected before the catheter is inserted. The patient is then observed, and the distribution of cutaneous analgesia is mapped out with a skin pencil. More solution is injected if analgesic spread is insufficient after 20 minutes. The epidural catheter is left in position, with the patient lying on the affected side, and further increments of the steroid suspension are injected at intervals of 45 minutes to one hour until the total dose of 40 ml has been given, and the catheter is then withdrawn. Appropriate physiotherapy is undertaken while the block is working. This procedure can be done on an outpatient basis, provided there are adequate facilities for observing the patient in recovery room surroundings. Extradural steroids should not be given more frequently than every ten days to two weeks, as the suspension is slow to absorb.

We have used this technique for a wide variety of musculoskeletal conditions giving rise to root pain, such as "whiplash" injuries of the neck, recurrent postlaminectomy pain, and root entrapment from cervical spondylosis. The results are less spectacular than in some series, as shown in Table 13–1; nevertheless, they are encouraging enough to retain the method on an empirical basis for the time being. However, it is well to bear in mind the cautioning words of Sir Henry Cohen quoted at the beginning of this section and to maintain a cool detachment from any method that is so shallowly understood. He continues, "Lumbago—its history teaches many lessons to the discerning; it is a graveyard in which are buried once-fashionable methods of treatment which were founded on a speculative pathology; the ghosts of these are restless, and

TABLE 13–1 Clinical Results of Extradural Steroid Injections for Lumbosciatic Pain

Author	*Good* (%)	*Fair* (%)	*No Effect* (%)
Goebert et al. (1961)	72	11	17
Swerdlow and Sayle-Creer (1970)	38	26	36
Bromage (unpublished data)	35	31	34

one must beware of their reappearance even when clothed in a different garb."

Once again I would stress the lurking presence of tragedy when chronic pain is being treated symptomatically without a clear diagnosis. The following case illustrates this point and at the same time shows how partial relief by steroid therapy may actually hinder diagnosis and delay appropriate treatment.

A man aged 53 presented with burning pain in the left chest, left arm and hand. There was a history of sudden onset of stiffness and pain in the left trunk radiating into the left armpit after a long car drive four years before. The pain gradually worsened and radiated down the inner side of the left arm into the hand and all fingers and down the outer side of the left chest to below the costal margin. The chest and arm felt on fire. In all other aspects the patient was well.

Extensive neurological examinations had been carried out at the Montreal Neurological Institute to exclude the possibility of intraspinal pathology. Myelography was done twice and a bilateral vertebral angiogram on one occasion. All tests were negative except for a slight elevation of cerebrospinal fluid protein to 50 mg per 100 ml and 88 mg per 100 ml on two occasions. The possibilities of spinal cord tumor or early syringomyelia were considered and exploratory laminectomy was discussed, but in the absence of any objective supporting evidence this was deferred. The patient was referred to the Pain Clinic for assessment and consideration of symptomatic treatment. Psychiatric evaluation showed a well-balanced personality with some depressive traits secondary to his unrelieved pain. Neurological examination showed complete absence of sensory and motor deficits, but subjective pain was severe and the patient could not bear to be touched in the area of his pain. He drew a diagram to illustrate the distribution of his symptoms (Fig. 13–6). Within

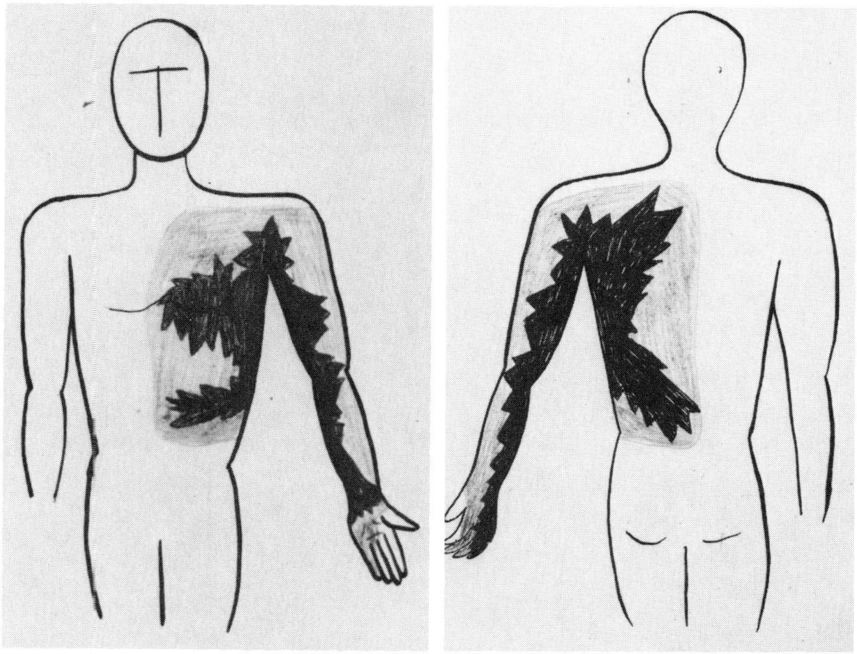

Figure 13–6. Severe causalgic pain of chest and left arm in segmental distribution of C_5 to T_{11} before treatment (see text). Patient's own sketch of distribution and quality of pain. *A*, Anterior distribution; *B*, posterior distribution.

■ Interior—burning, crampy, fish-hook, stabbing pain.
□ Exterior—hypersensitive to touch, wind, hot and cold.

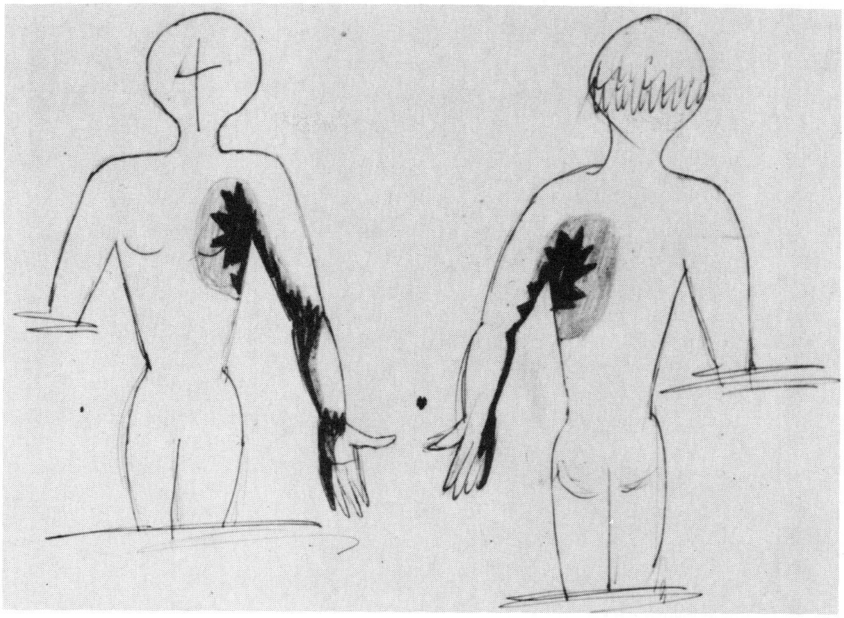

Figure 13–7. Causalgic pain of left chest and arm. Same patient as in Figure 13–6. Reduced area of pain (C_8 to T_6) after thoracic epidural injections of steroids.

this area there was marked hyperalgesia to pin-prick and light touch but no loss of temperature sensation. Use of the left hand was restricted by pain, and the fourth and fifth fingers were stiff and atrophied from disuse.

A trial epidural block was done at the second thoracic interspace using 8 ml of 2 per cent lidocaine followed by supplementary injections of 1 per cent lidocaine. Analgesia extended from C_5 to T_{11}, with complete relief of pain. While analgesia lasted, grip strength returned in his left hand, and although his fourth and fifth fingers remained stiff, he was able to move the remaining fingers freely and painlessly for the first time in many months. The block was repeated on several other occasions using a suspension of methylprednisolone acetate, 120 mg in 8 ml of 1 or 2 per cent lidocaine. Each time pain was temporarily relieved, the painful area gradually shrank in size to the distribution shown in Figure 13–7 and he regained use of his left hand. However, between blocks the pain was as intense as ever in the causalgic segments that remained, but it was now possible to touch the skin without evoking a severe response.

No further progress could be made. A neurosurgical consultation was obtained, and the possibility of operation was again considered. However, shortly afterward the patient was found dead from drug intoxication. At postmortem examination the only detectable abnormality was a small cleftlike syrinx running from the central canal of the spinal cord into the base of the left dorsal horn and extending from the eighth cervical to the eighth thoracic segments. Figure 13–8 shows a section of the spinal cord taken at the second thoracic segment.

It is interesting that epidural blockade could provide temporary but complete relief of pain arising from a deep cord lesion. The question of reduction of peripheral input, or possibly penetration of the cord, again comes to mind. Restoration of function in the affected hand was a normal accompaniment of release from painful inhibition. It is also interesting that epidural steroids improved the symptoms of this lesion over a long period of time. Possibly the partial improvement may have been due to a reduction of

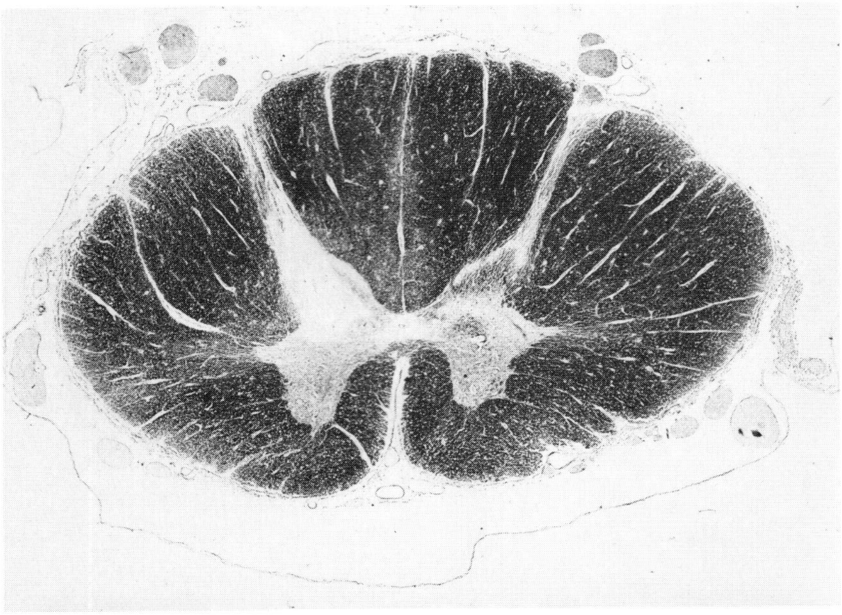

Figure 13–8. Undiagnosed atypical syringomyelia in patient shown in Figures 13–6 and 13–7. Transverse section of spinal cord at level of second thoracic segment. A cleftlike syrinx in base of left lateral horn extended from eighth cervical to eighth thoracic segment (see text).

edema within the cord, analogous to the resolution of edema and paresis seen with steroid therapy in metastatic tumors of the spinal cord (Cantu, 1968; Ushio et al., 1977a, 1977b).

Here, the basic rule of "diagnosis before treatment" was broken, but even exploration of the cord would not have revealed this tiny atypical syringomyelia. If the rule had been broken earlier, and more radically, with a spinothalamic tractotomy, as had indeed been discussed with the patient, perhaps his pain might have been relieved and the tragedy of despairing self-destruction might have been avoided.

Postherpetic Neuralgia

Herpes zoster frequently gives rise to intractable neuralgic pain in the segmental distribution of the lesions. Postherpetic neuralgia is more likely to occur in the old than in the young, and one series reported that about 50 per cent of patients over 70 still suffered pain 12 months after the acute attack had subsided (De Morages and Kierland, 1957). Pain of the acute attack is relieved and the incidence of postherpetic neuralgia markedly reduced by sympathetic blockade of the affected segments (Rosenak, 1938; Lund, 1966; Colding, 1969). Marmer (1965), using an epidural drip with 0.4 per cent lidocaine over a period of 11 days, reported relief of pain and satisfactory healing in a 70-year-old man. Relief of pain and accelerated healing is also obtained by the administration of systemic corticosteroids (Eaglstein et al., 1970). The benefits of both forms of therapy can be combined by inducing epidural blockade of the affected segments with mixtures of local anesthetic and corticosteroids. In this way the steroids are introduced close to the site of infection in the dorsal root ganglia, and systemic absorption occurs through the epidural venous and capillary plexuses.

Safety and a successful outcome depend on correct timing, and whenever possible treatment should be started after the vesicles have dried and crusted. Premature administration of steroids while the disease is still in the acute stage is potentially dangerous, for suppression of the normal immune response may allow the herpes virus to disseminate through the spinal cord, with the disastrous consequences of zoster myelitis (Juel-Jensen, 1973). On the other hand, results are poor if treatment is neglected for many months after postherpetic pain has become established. In one large series of patients with acute zoster treated with sympathetic blocks alone, Colding (1969) reported that about 80 per cent of patients over 60 years of age had complete and permanent relief without developing the postherpetic syndrome. However, patients who had already developed a postherpetic syndrome obtained very little relief. Only 40 per cent of patients with chronic disease experienced temporary improvement at the time of blockade, and less than 25 per cent found any lasting degree of benefit. My own experience has been in agreement with these findings: acute cases have generally done well with epidural steroids, but chronic cases have been disappointing. Nevertheless, the practice in our Pain Clinic has been to offer a trial course of epidural steroids to patients with long-standing postherpetic neuralgia, and a few have experienced satisfactory and lasting relief. While a placebo effect may have been responsible, I believe it is still worth offering even the slenderest hope to these stubborn cases with all the enthusiasm that can be mustered.

Management of acute cases

Epidural steroid treatment must be deferred during the acute stages of herpes zoster until viral replication has ceased, the eruption is healing and the vesicles have crusted. Aggressive early treatment with specific chemotherapy against the varicella-zoster virus may abort the attack effectively, prevent neural scarring and entirely eliminate the need for subsequent epidural injection therapy (Juel Jensen, 1973). Therefore, when cases are seen early enough, they should be referred to a virologist for antiviral treatment with one of the DNA inhibitors, such as topical idoxuridine in dimethyl sulphoxide (DMSD), or intravenous cytosine arabinoside (cytarabine). Epidural steroids should only be considered if early antiviral therapy has been omitted or has failed and if segmental pain continues.

The technical procedure of epidural steroid injection is very similar to that described for chronic postlaminectomy pain. The epidural space is punctured at the segmental level of the eruption, and a catheter is inserted. A suspension of methylprednisolone acetate is freshly prepared by adding 100 mg of methylprednisolone to 20 ml of 1 per cent lidocaine. Eight to 12 ml of this suspension is injected through the catheter, and the effects are observed. A second dose of 6 to 8 ml may be given 20 minutes later if spread of cutaneous analgesia is insufficient to cover the whole of the painful area. Epidural steroids may be repeated at intervals of two to three weeks for a maximum of four injections.

CHRONIC MALIGNANT PAIN

Epidural Chemical Neurolysis

Treatment of intractable pain due to malignancy is directed to reducing afferent input from the painful area. Since the "gate control theory" was introduced by Melzack and Wall in 1965, there has been renewed interest in applying nondestructive techniques designed to augment large-fiber afferent input, with the object of "closing the gate" at the dorsal horn (Wall and Sweet, 1967). These possibilities have been exploited with considerable sophistication and enthusiasm. In some centers electrical stimulating devices have been surgically implanted around peripheral nerves, and either epidurally or subdurally within the spinal canal (Shealy et al., 1970; Nashold and Friedman, 1972; Shealy, 1974). However, it is clear that the so-called dorsal column stimulator (DCS) is an optimistic misnomer for a device with less anatomical specificity and more pathological potential than originally supposed (Taub, 1974).

While there is no denying that analgesic techniques employing augmented afferent input by transcutaneous or implanted devices do produce effective results in selected cases, my own experience, as well as that of others, suggests that they have a limited application, and their proper use requires further evaluation.

In the meantime the older destructive methods of cordotomy and chemical posterior rhizotomy, when properly applied, still play a useful role in the management of malignant intractable pain. These techniques aim at reducing the traffic of painful afferent input by permanent destruction of sensory pathways. Cordotomy is usually reserved for patients with a life expectancy of more than six months, in which case the period of benefit is long enough to make a major operation worthwhile. Chemical rhizotomy is best used for patients with a shorter prognosis (Evans and Mackay, 1972).

Neurolysis by epidural injection has a very limited application in the management of intractable pain; nevertheless, it is a useful technique in the small number of cases in which it is indicated. This section will deal with the rationale and technique of epidural "chemical rhizotomy" and will attempt to place it in perspective along with other procedures for neurolytic "rhizotomy."

In 1931 Dogliotti suggested using intrathecal alcohol for the selective destruction of pain pathways in the dorsal roots, with the object of reducing the total amount of afferent input from painful segments. The patients were postured so that a bubble of absolute alcohol floated up through the cerebrospinal fluid and bathed the offending roots chosen as the target for chemical neurolysis. Variations of this principle were developed by Maher (1955, 1957), using hyperbaric solutions of 5 per cent to 7.5 per cent phenol in glycerine or Myodil (ethyl iodophenylundecylate). The assumption was made that the neurolytic agent would destroy small fibers while sparing the large ones (Brown, 1958).

These intrathecal techniques are accurate ways of attacking afferent input when pain is confined to two or three adjacent segments at any spinal level, but the method has limitations when pain arises from a large number of segments or from scattered sites, and it is in widespread pain that epidural neurolytic injections are most useful.

The idea of extradural chemical neurolysis was introduced in 1930, a year before Dogliotti published his paper on intrathecal alcohol, when Woodbridge reported using 80 per cent alcohol by the caudal route for relief of pain in carcinoma of the prostate. Since then a few reports have appeared from time to time, but nothing very systematic was carried out with epidural alcohol until Groenendijk published his monograph on epidural analgesia in the Dutch language in 1954. Groenendijk described his results with 17 cases of inoperable carcinoma; he had varying degrees of success, and one death was attributed to the method. It is interesting to note that he also found that epidural alcohol diffused into the subarachnoid space in appreciable quantities, giving rise to cerebrospinal fluid concentrations of between 0.2 and 0.9 per cent, 25 to 30 minutes after 10 ml of 30 per cent alcohol was injected in the epidural space (Groenendijk, 1954).

In all these reports the authors used varying dilutions of alcohol between 30 per cent and 95 per cent and gave it by a single injection (Woodbridge, 1930; Gillcreest and Mullen, 1931; DeBeule and Schotte, 1934; Odom, 1940). In 1963 Maher reported a series of 31 cases in which caudal aqueous phenol was used in concentrations of 0.5 to 5 per cent, and Lourie and Vanasupa also reported using extradural phenol in the same year (Lourie and Vanasupa, 1963). My own unpublished experience amounts to 55 cases, the earlier injections having been made with alcohol or alcohol mixtures and the more recent ones with phenol, an indwelling epidural catheter being used in all cases. Before details of technique and clinical results are discussed, it will be helpful to review the laboratory evidence that has led to a reassessment of the basic assumptions behind the original idea of chemical rhizotomy.

PATHOPHYSIOLOGY AND HISTOLOGY OF NEUROLYTIC BLOCKADE

Early postmortem studies in animals and man supported the idea that spinal roots were primarily affected by intrathecal neurolytic agents. In addition, slight degeneration of the posterior column and Lissauer's tract was described (Aird and Naffziger, 1935; Peyton et al., 1937). Peyton and French (1942) made the important observation that the rootlet lesions were patchy.

Electrical recordings of the effects of phenol on the compound spike potential of cat dorsal roots were made independently by Iggo and Walsh (1959, 1960) and by Nathan and Sears (1960). These experiments from different laboratories gave strong support to the assumption that phenol solutions cause a qualitative reduction of sensory input by irreversibly damaging C-fibers while reversibly blocking the large A-fibers. However, the results of these short-term experiments were not subjected to confirmation by histological examination.

Subsequent histological evidence by Baxter and Schacherl (1962) and Stewart and Lourie (1963) told a different story. They showed that intrathecal lesions produced by phenol in cats have the following characteristics:

1. They are patchy, as shown by Peyton and French in 1942; they have the appearance of attacking the rootlet from the periphery. That is, small lesions are crescentic around part of the surface of the fasciculus, while larger ones are completely circumferential or involve the whole fasciculus.
2. Some peripheral cells in the spinal cord may be affected.

3. Within patches of demyelination nerve axons of *all* sizes are destroyed.

4. Cell bodies of the dorsal root ganglia are not affected.

5. Regeneration of axon cylinders can be seen in the demyelinated areas after three months.

6. Patchy vascular damage to the subarachnoid arteries and arterioles and proliferative arachnoiditis occur with large doses.

These findings were later confirmed by Nathan, Sears and Smith (1965) in an elegant combination of electrophysiological and histological studies. They resolved the difference between their earlier contrary conclusions of 1960 and their later work by pointing out the dual nature of neurolytic agents. Phenol and alcohol, as well as local anesthetics in strong concentrations have both a reversible anesthetic action and an irreversible destructive action. The former reversible action shows all the laboratory characteristics of differential blockade on electrical recording, while the latter irreversible effects are nondifferential and revealed only by careful histology.

Stewart and Lourie's histological studies showed one other very interesting point. Degeneration preparations revealed that the effects of phenol on the dorsal roots could be traced into the spinal cord. Degenerating fibers could be found in the dorsal horn and beyond, throughout all parts of the gray matter, with some degenerating fibers passing to the opposite ventral horn. These axons are unlikely to have been injured in the spinal cord, and their site of injury must have been in the dorsal roots. This suggests that these sensory fibers may have followed the unorthodox anatomical course proposed in Chapter 2, with their distal axons doubling back in the dorsal root to travel through the gray matter and out through the ventral roots.

Thus, we are left with the impression that epidural phenol probably does not produce a qualitative reduction of small-fiber input but rather a quantitative reduction of fibers of all sizes in both anterior and posterior roots. Presumably it is this reduction in the algebraic sum of segmental input that produces clinical pain relief and not closure of a "gate" in the dorsal horn by selective suppression of small fiber activity, as might be imagined in terms of the gate control theory by Melzack and Wall. Moreover, the lesion is temporary. Regeneration of damaged fibers is likely to make repeated injections necessary at intervals of weeks or at most, two or three months, and this is in accordance with clinical experience.

Thus, the wide safety margin that would exist if qualitative neurolysis were possible is a mirage. It is not possible to say with any assurance that a specific dose or a specific concentration will destroy only C-fibers, while a larger dose or stronger concentration will begin to involve A-fibers as well. We can only envisage increasingly larger areas of destruction as dosage increases. Therapy must be planned on the assumption that a point can be reached where just the right number of fibers can be interrupted to relieve pain, without destroying so many that function will be impaired.

All neurolytic procedures walk the razor's edge. The balance between caution, with too little damage and inadequate results on the one hand, and boldness, with too much damage and paralysis on the other, is delicate and elusive, so it is no surprise that therapy is seldom in satisfactory equilibrium for long. Neurolytic strategy must be planned with these discomforting thoughts in mind in such a way that dosage can be monitored most critically. It also follows that we should avoid discouraging our patients and ourselves by false optimism, for by the nature of things our efforts are doomed to only partial success at the outset, and this situation must be clearly understood and accepted courageously before an imperfect but nevertheless worthwhile procedure is embarked upon.

Technique

Published reports of therapeutic procedures often gloss over what the patient feels. Let me start by saying that the dura mater is sensitive and that unlike subarachnoid alcohol, which is painless, extradural alcohol is agonizing. Alcohol should never be put in the extradural space unless it is diluted with local anesthetic or unless the patient is asleep under general anesthesia. Heavy premedication alone is not enough. By contrast, saturated aqueous phenol (6 per cent) has a local anesthetic effect and is completely painless. Patients receiving phenol injections can therefore be fully awake and unpremedicated, and the procedure is more controllable, safer and far less complicated than when alcohol is used. Nevertheless, my personal results with undiluted alcohol are slightly better than those with aqueous phenol, so I am hesitant to abandon it completely. Moreover, phenol is nephrotoxic, and large doses may cause renal tubular necrosis. About 15 mg per kg seems to be the maximum safe dose (Esplin, 1970), and this imposes a limit of 15 ml of 6 per cent phenol in a 60-kg patient.

Single-injection methods lack precision in the epidural space and should be avoided for neurolytic procedures. The placement of large volumes of neurolytic solutions in the extradural space is a potentially hazardous undertaking that calls for every reasonable precaution to ensure that the solutions are placed exactly where intended and under the most controllable conditions. The solutions used are either ethyl alcohol 90 to 100 per cent (Abbott Laboratories prepare a sterile ampule of dehydrated ethyl alcohol) or saturated aqueous phenol (i.e., 6 per cent in water).

The procedure is as follows:

1. Epidural puncture is performed as close as possible to the segmental origin of the pain, with the patient recumbent and the painful side downward. For lumbar injections a 17-gauge Tuohy needle is used with the loss-of-resistance test. For thoracic injections an 18-gauge thin-walled Bromage needle is used, with the hanging-drop sign to identify the epidural space.

2. A plastic catheter is then inserted for 2 to 4 cm beyond the tip of the needle. The needle is removed and the catheter taped in place. A careful aspiration test is made to ensure that the catheter does not lie in a vein or in the subarachnoid space.

3. A test dose of 5 to 14 ml of 1 per cent lidocaine is injected up the catheter. The size of the dose is judged by the age of the patient and the number of segments to be treated. The object of this test is twofold: first, to assess the subjective relief that follows, and second, to be able to measure the segmental analgesia obtained by a given volume of local anesthetic solution in order to have a close estimate of the volume of neurolytic solution to be used subsequently.

Alcohol and 6 per cent aqueous phenol both appear to spread about the same segmental distance as 1 per cent lidocaine.

4. One must wait now for a period of at least one hour to allow complete absorption of the local anesthetic, for if the neurolytic solution is injected up the catheter before that time, the water remaining in the epidural space may dilute and spread the neurolytic agent further than necessary. During this period a segmental diagram is constructed of the spread and regression of cutaneous analgesia resulting from the test dose of 1 per cent lidocaine, and the degree of subjective relief of pain is noted. These observations give a firm basis for deciding on the dose of neurolytic agent to be employed.

5. During the waiting period the correct position of the epidural catheter is verified by radiography. Whether the catheter is radiopaque or not, its image will be improved by injecting a small amount of radiopaque material through its lumen. Iophendylate or metrizamide, 0.5 ml, is sufficient to fill a 30-cm length of catheter and leave a small blob of radiodense material at its tip. The position of the catheter is then checked by an image intensifier in two planes, and a radiograph is taken for record purposes. A permanent picture is prudent medicolegal protection for the physician in the unlikely event of future legal action. A peridurogram may also be helpful if there is still any doubt about the precise position of the catheter and the flow of injectate in the epidural space. An hour is allowed to elapse if a peridurogram is decided upon, in order to ensure complete resorption of the lidocaine solution. Then 5 to 14 ml of metrizamide 300 mg I/ml is injected through the catheter and X-rays are taken in two planes. If the catheter is correctly placed one may proceed; if not, the position of the catheter must be adjusted, or it may even have to be withdrawn and reinserted.

6. The determined volume of neurolytic agent is now injected one hour after the initial test injection of lidocaine or two hours afterward if a peridurogram has been performed. It is prudent to inject the first milliliter and then wait a further 5 minutes before the remainder of the dose is given. This provides an opportunity to observe the effects of a safe test dose and to make absolutely certain that the catheter is safely in the epidural space and that is has not accidentally perforated the dura and entered the subarachnoid space or the subdural space.

If ethyl alcohol is to be used, the patient should be lightly anesthetized with short-acting barbiturate and nitrous oxide and oxygen. Under these circumstances a 1-ml test dose of alcohol is worthless, and the full dose must be injected on the basis of the previous tests. It is mainly for this reason that I have changed from ethyl alcohol to 6 per cent aqueous phenol in order to be able to watch the effects of incremental doses with the patient awake and comfortable. Mixtures of alcohol and lidocaine are painless on injection, and concentrations of alcohol in the range of 50 to 80 per cent can be used without the need for general anesthesia. However, in my hands the results with these mixtures have been less effective than with 100 per cent alcohol or with 6 per cent phenol.

7. Phenol has a temporary local anesthetic effect, as well as a destructive neurolytic action, so a second segment-time diagram of cutaneous analgesia may be made after the phenol injection. The quality of cutaneous analgesia from epidural phenol is quite tenuous and short-lived, lasting only

about half an hour, and then skin sensation returns and scarcely any objective effects remain.

The catheter may be removed after one hour if subjective analgesia is satisfactory. Movements and tendon reflexes in the lower limbs should be normal at this time. Two further increments of phenol solution may be injected cautiously at intervals of 20 minutes if the initial dose fails to produce good pain relief. In the meantime the legs are carefully observed for motor and reflex activity to ensure that blockade is not extending too far or becoming functionally excessive.

RESULTS

Table 13–2 outlines the results in 55 cases. It can be seen that the most satisfactory effects were obtained by using absolute alcohol or 6 per cent phenol for pain involving thoracic segments. The least effective results were obtained by using alcohol mixtures in cases of pain of sacral origin.

These figures are very similar to results obtained by Grunwald (1976) of Montevideo in a more recent and larger series of 221 patients with cancer pain treated by extradural aqueous phenol. Grunwald also found that about one-quarter of the patients received no benefit, while good or partial relief was obtained in about 75 per cent of the cases.

In my own series, pain relief was often short-lived for a period of only 5 to 20 days, and then the procedure had to be repeated or some other regime

TABLE 13–2 Clinical Results from 55 Epidural Neurolytic Injections for Intractable Pain of Malignancy

Neurolytic Agent	*Good**	*Partial†*	*Nil‡*	*Complications*
Alcohol 100% (under general anaesthesia)				
Thoracic	6	4	–	1 – motor weakness of arm and intercostal muscles for one week
Lumbar	2	1	–	1 – slight motor weakness of legs for one week
Sacral	1	4	3	–
70% Alcohol-lidocaine mixxure				
Thoracic	1	5	–	–
Lumbar	2	2	1	–
Sacral	1	4	4	1 – urinary retention for 10 days
Phenol 6% in water				
Thoracic	4	2	1	–
Lumbar	–	1	–	–
Sacral	1	2	3	1 – urinary retention for 4 days
Total:	18	25	12	

*Good = Complete relief for more than one week.
†Partial = Complete relief for less than one week or reduction of narcotic requirements.
‡Nil = No change.

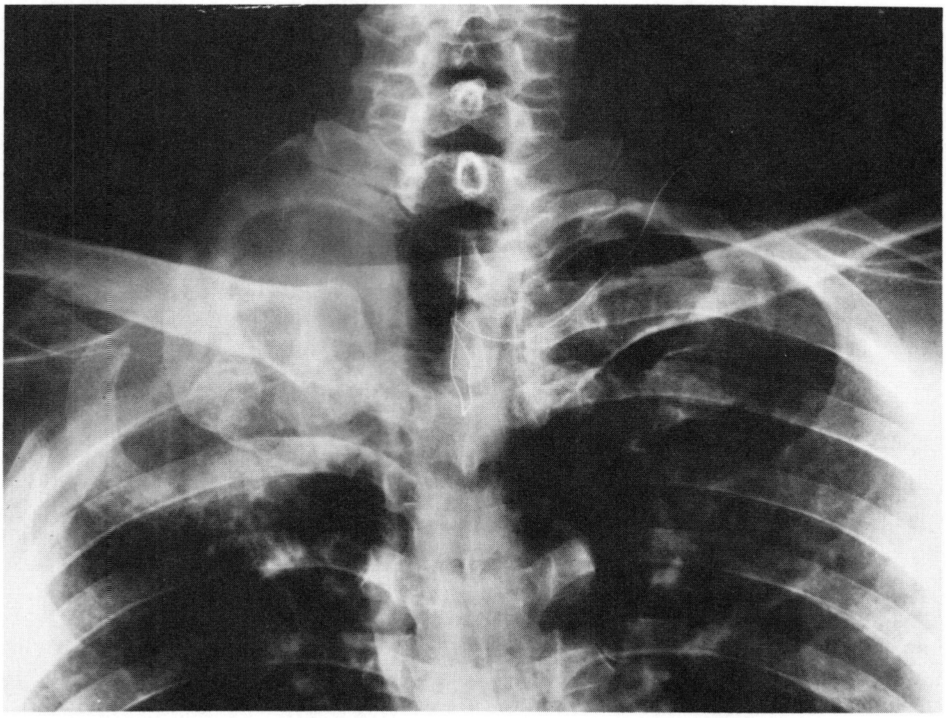

Figure 13–9. A man of 56 years with Pancoast syndrome and intractable pain of right arm, with erosion of bodies of second, third and fourth thoracic vertebrae. Successful palliative treatment with extradural alcohol (see text).

decided upon. In several instances of terminal cancer, the pain relief outlived the patient. For example:

Case 9. E. M. Man aged 56. Upper sulcus tumor of right lung. Pancoast syndrome, with erosion of the upper ribs and adjacent vertebral bodies, agonizing pain in the right arm and hand and loss of function of the right hand. An epidural catheter was inserted at T_2–T_3 *(Fig. 13–9). A preliminary injection of 5 ml of 0.8 per cent lidocaine in a water-soluble radiopaque medium relieved the pain and produced analgesia in segments* T_1–T_6. *Forty minutes later light general anesthesia was induced with the patient tilted head down on his right side, and 5 ml of absolute alcohol was injected through the epidural catheter. This produced complete pain relief and slight hypalgesia to pin-prick in segments* T_1–T_6 *on the right. Relief of pain was followed by increased range of movement in arm and fingers, and the patient was able to perform simple tasks with his right hand. The patient remained free of pain until his death six weeks later.*

Case 49. O. H. Male aged 56. Anaplastic carcinoma of the left lung, with Pancoast syndrome. Complete opacity of the left lung field (Fig. 13–10). Intense pain in left shoulder, upper chest and left upper arm. Recurrent bouts of asphyxial coughing with reflex laryngospasm. Pain poorly relieved by morphine.

An epidural catheter was inserted at T_2–T_3, *and a test dose of 11 ml of 1 per cent lidocaine gave complete relief of pain, with hypalgesia from* C_8–T_{10}. *Surprisingly, his bouts of coughing were also relieved. Eleven ml of 6 per cent phenol gave complete relief of pain and remission of reflex laryngospasm until death eight days later. No objective neurological sequelae were apparent after the block.*

Complications were few in this series, and there was no mortality. A

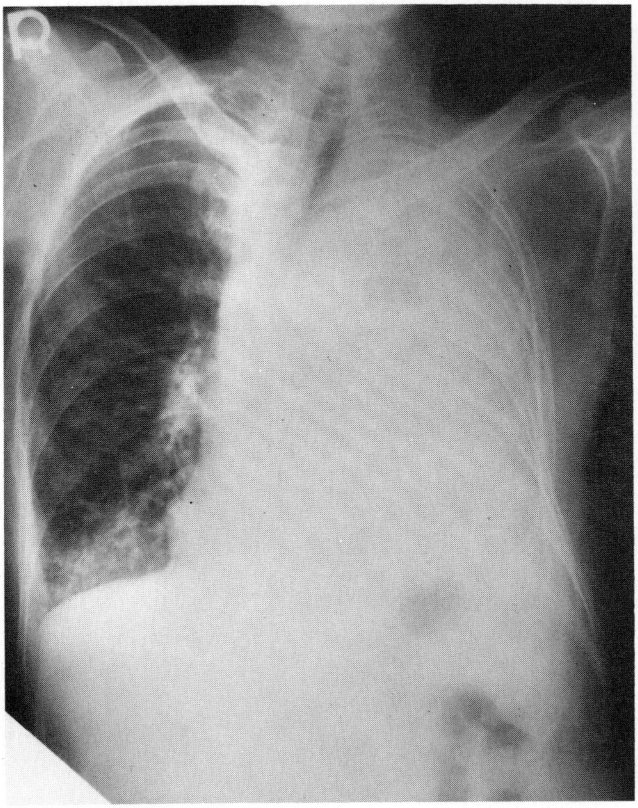

Figure 13–10. Carcinoma of left lung in man of 56 years. Intractable pain of left arm, shoulder and chest, with recurrent bouts of asphyxial coughing. Successful palliative relief after epidural injection of 11 ml of 6 per cent aqueous phenol at T_2–T_3 (see text).

few patients had insensitive bladders for a day or two, requiring catheter drainage. With the exception of one case, objective neurological signs were minimal. There was seldom complete loss of pin-prick or tactile sensations in the segments affected, although sometimes there was a barely detectable hypalgesia to pin-prick. One patient suffered a degree of motor weakness that normally would have been insignificant but in the circumstances was troublesome.

Case No. 16. Woman of 36 years suffering from severe lower chest and upper abdominal pain due to hemangiosarcoma of the liver. A right phrenic crush had been done in the belief that this might benefit her pain, and only the left hemidiaphragm moved. She was suicidal from her pain.

An epidural catheter was inserted with the tip at the vertebral level of the third thoracic body. Twelve ml of absolute alcohol was injected under general anesthesia with the patient in a semi-sitting position. Hypalgesia extended from C_8–T_8, *and there was considerable relief of pain, but the block was too high, and some residual pain was still felt in the distribution of* T_9 *and* T_{10}. *There was a serious degree of motor weakness of the right hand with wrist-drop lasting one week, and there was considerable impairment of ventilation with dyspnea on effort. Her respiratory embarrassment was presumably due to the combination of a unilateral phrenic crush with motor weakness of her upper intercostal muscles, so that the only effective respiratory muscle remaining was the left half of her diaphragm.*

This case illustrates three technical points:

1. The tip of the epidural catheter was not opposite the correct spinal

segment. It was placed too high and should have been opposite the sixth thoracic vertebra instead of at the level of the third.

2. The dose of neurolytic agent should be kept as low as possible. Here there was a spread of nine segments when only six would have been necessary with proper positioning of the catheter.

3. The permeability of the dura is not constant, and in some cases, such as this one, penetration and motor involvement may be unusually severe.

With hindsight, this case would have been better handled using small increments of 6 per cent aqueous phenol instead of alcohol, in order to be able to observe the effect with the patient awake.

INDICATIONS FOR EPIDURAL NEUROLYTIC INJECTIONS

Because of the potential hazards, neurolytic rhizotomy should be reserved for pain of malignancy. The basic aims of management of intractable malignant pain are the same as in other pain states – that is:(1) relief of pain, and (2) restoration of function. Narcotics should not be withheld if needed at night, but heavy disabling doses during the day should be staved off by using other methods in order to keep the patient comfortably at his normal occupations for as long as possible. Deafferenting procedures may be surgical, or chemical, and the appropriate choice depends on the prognosis. When life expectancy exceeds six months, chemical injections are too short-lived and require too frequent repetition to be practical; in these cases neurosurgical procedures such as cordotomy are a more appropriate choice. Evans proposed two simple criteria as useful prognostic indices of impending death in planning the management of malignant pain. These are weight loss and anemia, as shown in Table 13–3. While these signs are approximate indices that may require modification in the presence of cytotoxic therapy, they do give a practical guide for choosing between chemical neurolysis and neurosurgical intervention.

For reasons already discussed, the analgesic effects of neurolytic rhizotomy are short and in the range of days to weeks. Also, neurolytic techniques require great attention to detail, and they may be hazardous unless performed with meticulous care. The results of epidural chemical rhizotomy shown in Table 13–2 are modest and a little discouraging at first sight, but compared with other methods of pain relief in malignancy, the results are satisfactory enough to justify retaining the technique for cases with a short prognosis.

Once the decision has been made to use chemical rhizotomy, the

TABLE 13–3 Prognostic Indices in Pain of Malignant Origin

Signs	*Probability of impending death*
Time from onset of intractable pain	90% within 12 months
Weight loss of more than 20 lbs in less than 3 months, plus anemia to a Hgb concentration of less than 10 g/100 ml	100% within 3 months

Data from R. Evans, personal communication.

appropriate technique must be selected. A number of options are open (Mehta, 1973), but intrathecal procedures can be broadly classified as either proteolytic, using substances such as alcohol, phenol and chlorocresol (Maher, 1957), or hyperosmolar, using hypertonic saline (Hitchcock, 1967, 1969; Jewett and King, 1971; King et al., 1972). Each is peculiarly suited to a special set of circumstances, depending on the number and distribution of painful segments involved, and choice of technique should be based on these considerations.

Intrathecal alcohol and phenol are effective in producing a localized lesion of two or three adjacent roots, but they are not suitable for wide distribution over a large number of segments. Intrathecal hypertonic saline in a concentration of less than 10 per cent is not strikingly effective (Squire et al., 1974), but because it is also relatively innocuous at that concentration, it can be used in quite large amounts for pain that is distributed over a number of widely scattered segments. Epidural neurolytic agents fall between these two types of cases, and they are particularly useful when pain involves a number of adjacent segments either unilaterally or bilaterally, especially in the thoracic region, as in tumors involving the chest wall. These broad categories are summarized in Figure 13–11.

Dogliotti and Ciocatto (1955) reported that intermittent epidural blockade with weak local anesthetic solutions given over a period of three or four days can lead to lasting relief in cases of intractable pain from malignancy. They suggested that the effect was due to permanent damage to a proportion of the smaller nerve fibers. Other workers (Ditzler, 1966), including the author, have not been able to confirm this finding in cases of malignancy, nor does there appear to be any objective support for the claim that prolonged epidural blockade with weak anesthetic solutions will produce irreversible nerve damage. As pointed out in Chapter 3, high intraneural concentrations of local anesthetic may lead to reversible blockade of rapid axoplasmic transport, and very high levels may cause irreversible axoplasmic block and permanent loss of nerve function. However, the intraneural levels of local anesthetic required to do this are ten times greater than those needed for conduction blockade, and all the available animal data suggest that irreversible changes cannot be achieved by

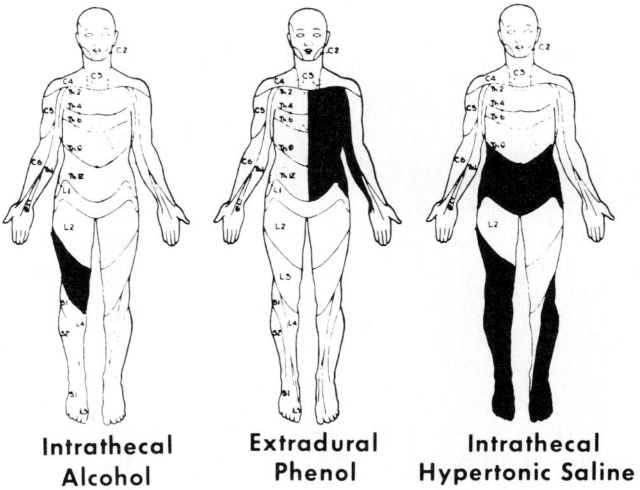

Figure 13–11. Selection of palliative neurolytic procedures for intractable malignant pain (see text): intrathecal alcohol—in discrete lesions involving a small number of segments; extradural phenol—for lesions involving a large number of contiguous segments; intrathecal hypertonic saline—for multiple sites and scattered segmental input.

ordinary clinical doses of local anesthetics. In malignant pain, relief persists for as long as the local anesthetic is working, but pain returns as soon as the anesthetic wears off (Lund, 1966).

Repeated or prolonged epidural block with local anesthetics may bring lasting relief in certain types of nonmalignant pain, but this is more likely to be due to other less easily definable factors, such as stretching of adhesions. Malignant pain is unremitting and requires direct neurolytic deafferentation.

Electrical Epidural Stimulation

Electrical means of suppressing pain are arousing widespread interest, fostered by industrial companies manufacturing the necessary hardware. The idea of controlling pain by pressing a switch has enormous appeal as being an ultimate ideal in analgesia. It is nondepressant, nontoxic and nonpharmacological, and it is sufficiently exotic to satisfy the primitive need for magic that still lingers in most of us. However, evidence to date suggests that electrical stimulation may not be entirely innocuous when carried out over long periods of time (Taub, 1974). Moreover, there are quite well-founded reasons for thinking that electrical stimulation is not strictly nonpharmacological but rather due to forced mobilization of intracellular substances from active neurons under the influence of supramaximal stimulation. One possible and quite simple mechanism would be excessive passage of intracellular potassium into extracellular spaces within the dorsal horn and subsequent depolarization of neighboring cells (Krnjevic and Morris, 1972). Another explanation could lie in the release of endogenous analgesic polypeptides or "endorphins" from central brain sites producing a generalized state of analgesia (Hughes, 1975; Pasternak et al., 1975). Although the basic analgesic mechanism of electrical stimulation of the cord remains undecided at the present time, enough empirical data have been collected by various authors to encourage further investigation and limited clinical application in special centers.

Electrical stimulation of the spinal cord has been used to produce analgesia with varying success since 1967 (Shealy et al., 1967a, 1967b; Nashold and Friedman, 1972). The amount of current required varies with the square of the distance from the cord, and the closer the stimulation, the less current is needed—hence the development of the so-called "dorsal column" stimulator electrode that is implanted as close as possible in the subdural space between the dura mater and the pia-arachnoid.

A reliable extradural stimulating device would obviously have many practical advantages in terms of simplicity of use, if a safe current density could be assured. Shimoji and his associates at Tokyo achieved reversible segmental analgesia in animals and human volunteers using a fine extradural stimulator inserted percutaneously through an ordinary Tuohy needle (Shimoji et al., 1971, 1972, 1973, 1974). In these experiments bilateral hypalgesia or analgesia was produced in six out of eight subjects using a low frequency current of 3.5 to 11.5 mA for a duration of 0.5 msec five times per second. With stimulation in the lower thoracic or lumbar region, hypalgesia spread rostrally for five to six segments, but when applied in the cervical region, it spread caudally over a much larger segmental area. Hypalgesia persisted for about 15 minutes after

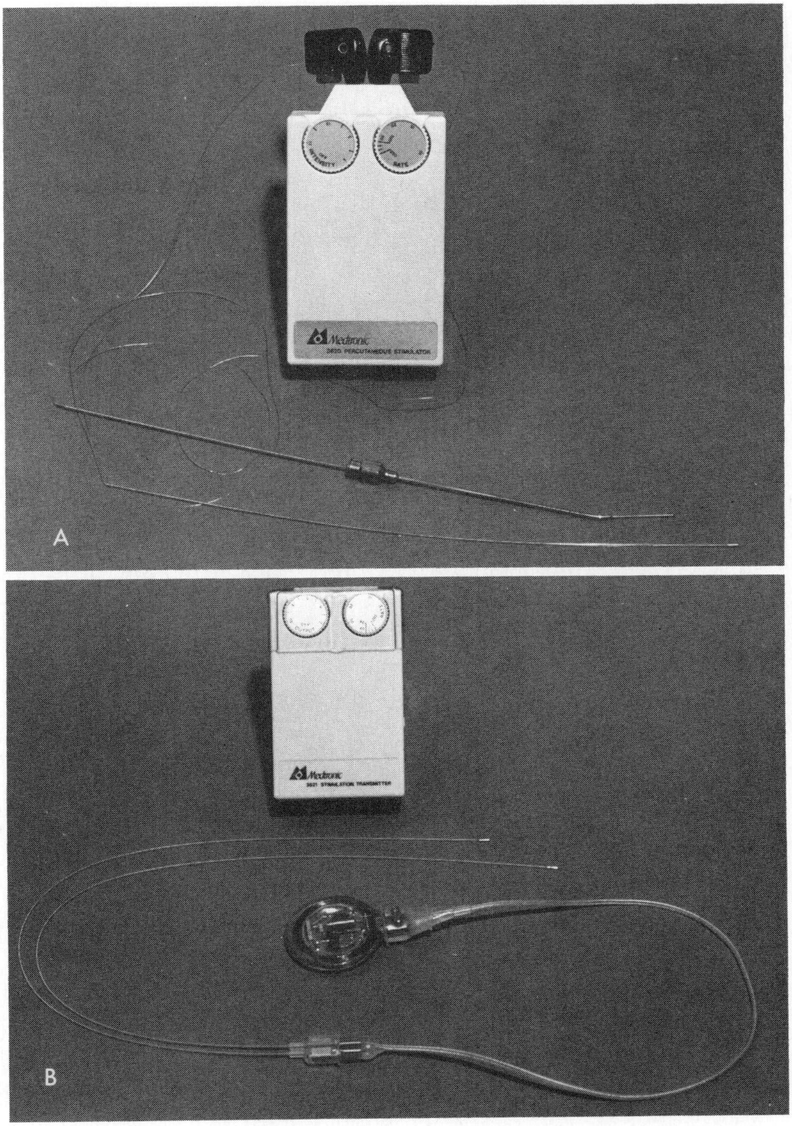

Figure 13–12. Epidural electrical stimulator for intractable pain. *A*, Temporary percutaneous electrodes, inserted via Tuohy needle. *B*, "Permanent" epidural stimulating unit for subcutaneous implantation, with external stimulator. (Courtesy of Medtronic, Inc., U.S.A.)

cessation of stimulation. Figure 13–12 shows a comparable system developed in North America for either temporary epidural stimulation or permanent implantation.

A safe stimulating device with satisfactory clinical capabilities would be attractive as a short-term analgesic system for relief of acute pain or as a screening device for decisions in long-term management of chronic pain. In addition, it would have possibilities as a recording device for evoked potentials in the spinal cord (Shimoji et al., 1972). Urban and Nashold (1978) obtained encouraging results with such a system in 20 patients suffering from intractable pain. Stimulating epidural electrodes were implanted percutaneously through

Tuohy-type needles under local anesthesia and manipulated to produce a satisfactory degree of paresthesia in the painful area. The position of the electrodes was checked by fluoroscopic control in two planes. Epidural stimulation gave satisfactory and prolonged relief in 7 out of 20 patients. The method has several desirable features:

1. It is relatively simple to perform.
2. It is less hazardous and less invasive than an open neurosurgical operation, and it is a suitable alternative to a dorsal column stimulator implant.
3. It rapidly distinguishes between patients who will be unsuitable for extended stimulation and those who are likely to benefit. However, more concrete assurance of the innocuous nature of extended epidural stimulation is needed before it can be recommended for general clinical use.

STATUS ASTHMATICUS

Attempts have been made to treat bronchial asthma by a variety of surgical procedures involving the autonomic nerves to the lungs (Szokodi-Dimitrov, 1953, 1956; Nakayama, 1961; Wood et al., 1965), but lasting relief is seldom obtained by these operations. However, transient relief has been claimed after local anesthetic infiltrations aimed at the vagus or upper sympathetic nerves. Reports of paravertebral sympathetic blockade to relieve status asthmaticus have appeared in the literature from time to time (Flothow, 1931; DuBose, 1931; Ruth, 1934; Levin, 1934), and epidural analgesia has also been recommended for the same purpose. Unfortunately, these isolated reports were published before objective measurements of pulmonary function became easily available at the bedside, and so it is difficult to assess the actual value of the procedures that were done.

This section describes four asthmatic patients whose condition was improved to varying degrees by epidural blockade. Three of these patients were indifferently documented, but one was well-documented, with serial blood gases; in this instance the transition from a moribund asphyxial state to a full recovery was sudden and complete, and induction of epidural analgesia appeared to have been life-saving. No adequate explanation has been found to explain this phenomenon, and it is presented only as an example of what may be a useful measure in rare instances, and the possible mechanisms of action are discussed.

Case Reports

Case 1. K. C. Female aged 44. *Two or three asthmatic attacks per day with moderately severe bronchospasm, but not in status. The attacks were controlled by aminophylline suppositories and phenylephrine inhalations. The frequency of the attacks appeared to depend upon a strong psychogenic element. On April 11, 1957, an epidural catheter was inserted under X-ray control with the tip at the tenth thoracic vertebra. Fifteen ml of 0.55 per cent lidocaine was injected. It was difficult to determine the sensory level accurately, but the hands became warm and dry, indicating cranial extension of blockade to at least the first thoracic segment. The injection was followed by complete relief of all asthmatic attacks for one week. Two weeks later (April 25th) very little bronchospasm was present, and the patient's condition was considerably improved. A second epidural injection was given in an attempt to assess the effect on respiratory volumes, but no further objective improvement could be demonstrated after this second block.*

Impression: The strong psychogenic element in this patient's illness made it difficult to assess therapeutic results. However, the first epidural injection did appear to produce real relief at a time when bronchospasm was moderately severe. Later, when the disease was less active, a comparable degree of improvement was not seen.

Case 2. E. S. Female aged 42. *Severe bronchospasm and underlying bronchopneumonia, cyanosed and comatose for six hours. Areflexic except for upgoing right toe. Negligible air entry at lung bases. Tidal volume 100 to 200 ml. No response to corticoids, aminophylline or epinephrine.*

An epidural injection was made at the second thoracic interspace using 11 ml of 0.5 per cent plain lidocaine. Owing to the depth of coma, it was impossible to judge the segmental extent of the resultant analgesia. Three-quarters of an hour later bronchoscopy revealed a scant amount of viscid sputum deep in the bronchial tree, and a small quantity was aspirated through the bronchoscope. Tidal volume rose slightly to 225 ml. Bronchoscopic suction was repeated 1½ hours later. Shortly after this the patient recovered consciousness and responded to instructions. Two hours later the tidal volume had risen to 250 ml and the patient was talking. An elective tracheostomy was carried out to reduce dead space and to simplify tracheobronchial toilet.

Impression: Here, a slight but definite improvement occurred during a period of one to three hours after thoracic epidural blockade. However, the clinical picture was not one of pure bronchospasm, but was complicated by the underlying bronchopneumonia.

Case 3. I. H. Male aged 52. *One-time anthracite miner. No radiological evidence of silicosis, but chronic obstructive respiratory disease labeled as "chronic bronchitis and asthma." In status asthmaticus for five days despite treatment with corticoids, aminophylline and phenylephrine inhalations. Somewhat confused but not comatose. Nonproductive cough. Vital capacity 850 ml. The arterial* pO_2 *was 40 mmHg while patient was breathing room air.*

An epidural injection was made at the second thoracic interspace using 7 ml of 1 per cent plain mepivacaine. Half an hour later the bronchospasm became less intense on auscultation, and the patient began to cough up viscid secretions. The secretions became more copious, and the patient remarked, "I can't understand where all this phlegm is suddenly coming from." One hour after the block the arterial pO_2 *had improved slightly to 54 mmHg. Two hours later the vital capacity was 1550 ml, almost double the preinjection value.*

Impression: Epidural injection produced a relaxation of bronchial spasm and an increase of vital capacity. Bronchial secretions became more available during the next three hours, and they appeared to become more watery and less viscid.

Case 4. B. H. Female aged 25. *Decompensated status asthmaticus. The patient became increasingly dyspneic, then cyanosed and somnolent at 1:45 P.M. While breathing room air, the patient's arterial blood gases were pH 7.285,* pCO_2 *69 mmHg and* pO_2 *43.8 mmHg. Hydrocortisone 300 mg and aminophylline 0.75 g were given together with epinephrine 0.5 mg subcutaneously. In spite of this treatment the patient's condition deteriorated; 3½ hours later she was comatose with arterial readings of pH 7.12,* pCO_2 *above 105 mmHg and* pO_2 *40.8 mmHg. She was curarized, an endo-*

tracheal tube was passed and ventilation was maintained automatically by an Engstrom ventilator with 40 cmH$_2$O inspiratory pressure at first, rising to 60 cmH$_2$O later.

By 7 P.M. no improvement had occurred. Curarization had been maintained, and the skeletal musculature was quite flaccid. However, total compliance was extremely low at about 15 ml per cmH$_2$O, and very little air entry could be heard. Coma was deep, and the arterial pH was still in the region of 7.12 to 7.14. A decision was made to bronchoscope the patient in the hope of removing any inspissated viscid secretions and also to try the effect of deep ether in an attempt to relax the bronchial musculature. No secretions were visible on bronchoscopy, and the bronchial mucosa was dry, red and turgid. Ventilation was carried out with 20 per cent ether vapor in oxygen for 20 minutes at 40 to 50 cmH$_2$O inspiratory pressure. This produced a slight improvement of air entry, and the arterial pH rose to 7.30, while the pCO$_2$ fell to 87 mmHg. However, the patient deteriorated again after the ether was stopped, and the pH fell to 7.25 while the pCO$_2$ rose to 98 by 8:30 P.M. There was no evidence of pneumothorax. An intravenous epinephrine infusion at the rate of 2.5 to 5.0 μg per min gave no improvement.

An epidural block was now performed at the sixth thoracic interspace using 14 ml of 1 per cent lidocaine with 1/200,000 epinephrine. Within 10 minutes the total compliance rose from 18.5 to 33 cmH$_2$O, and air entry improved all over both lung fields. Loose rales were heard for the first time, and it was possible to aspirate some bronchial secretions; the compliance improved further. The patient regained consciousness 50 minutes later, and one hour after induction of epidural block the pH had risen to 7.395 and the pCO$_2$ had fallen to 68 mmHg. At this time skin analgesia extended from the first to the tenth thoracic dermatomes inclusive. Artifical ventilation was continued for a further 70 minutes, but by this time the patient indicated vigorously that she would rather breathe by her own efforts. Two hours after the epidural block the endotracheal tube was removed, and spontaneous respiration was performed freely and easily with slight residual bronchospasm. The patient was fully conscious, talking and in good spirits. Coughing was effective and produced small quantities of tenacious sputum which gradually became less viscid as time went by. One hour later the pCO$_2$ was 45 mmHg. The patient made an uninterrupted recovery. The sequence of events and the serial blood gas estimations are summarized in Figure 13–13.

Impression: In this case the patient appeared gravely ill and likely to die. When all other methods of treatment had failed, a dramatic and unequivocal recovery followed epidural blockade of the upper ten thoracic segments.

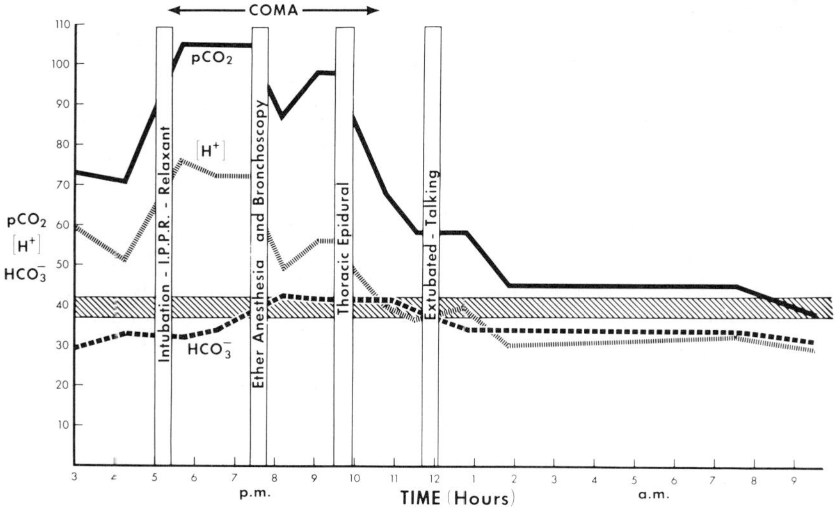

Figure 13–13. Serial blood gases in 25-year-old female moribund with status asthmaticus. Rapid recovery followed thoracic epidural blockade (see text).

Of the four asthmatics cited, two were only slightly improved by epidural block, one was considerably improved and one (Case 4) showed a dramatic and sudden response, almost as if a tap had been turned on in her chest allowing air to enter and trapped secretions to escape. In this case serial blood gas estimations confirmed the immediate change from a profound asphyxial process to a condition of relatively normal gas exchange.

A number of similar cases have been described in the literature in which a variety of injection techniques aimed at the upper thoracic sympathetic nerves, or at the vagi, have produced sudden relief of bronchospasm. However, no satisfactory theory has been proposed to explain the beneficial results of these procedures on a neurological basis (DuBose, 1931; Flothow, 1931; Odom, 1940; Levin, 1934; Descomps and Dorgeuille, 1963).

The empirical success of these local anesthetic techniques appeared to confirm the assumption that disordered autonomic neural impulses were at the root of the asthmatic process, and this emboldened surgeons to devise various denervating operations on the lung and adjacent structures (Nakayama, 1961; Szokodi-Dimitrov, 1953). The operation of glomectomy enjoyed an intense vogue in Japan, where 3,914 asthmatic patients underwent bilateral carotid sinus denervation (Nakayama, 1961). However, wider trial of these denervating operations and critical examination of their results did not give enough objective evidence to support their continued use (Wood et al., 1965; Segal, 1965; Dulfano et al., 1967).

If one assumes that the vegetative nervous system controls the asthmatic process, it would be logical to use parasympatholytic techniques while sympathetic activity is being preserved. Bronchodilator fibers are supposed to travel in the sympathetic nerves, while bronchoconstrictor nerves are carried by the vagi, so any technique which interrupts the sympathetic outflow while sparing the cranial parasympathetic would be expected to aggravate an asthmatic attack rather than abort it. For this reason epidural analgesia or paravertebral blocks of the sympathetic nerves would appear to be the worst possible form of treatment, yet there is evidence that sympathetic influences cause acute and marked changes in the character of lung surfactant (Beckman et al., 1971). Stimulation of the stellate ganglion in monkeys leads to a fourfold increase in surface tension of airways fluid and a 20 per cent fall in lung compliance (Beckman et al., 1974); in cats the fall of compliance is about double that found in monkeys (Droste and Beckman, 1974). These acute changes of lung surfactant and compliance in response to sympathetic stimulation appear to be independent of pulmonary vascular changes and are associated with an increased concentration of cholesterol in the airways fluid (Bergren and Beckman, 1975; Sexton and Beckman, 1975). Possibly changes of this nature may be involved in the process of status asthmaticus and in the occasional good results reported from sympathetic blockade. Certainly in two of the cases described above (Cases 3 and 4), the sudden change from dry bronchial "spasm" to bronchodilatation with less viscid, watery secretions was a notable and, at the time, a puzzling feature.

Local anesthetic injections of the sympathetic nerves in the paravertebral spaces, or in the extradural space, produce several effects apart from an efferent block of the sympathetic impulses, so it is necessary to examine these effects in turn to see if some mechanism other than blockade of the efferent vegetative fibers could be responsible for the beneficial results observed.

Blockade of Afferent Impulses From the Airways

Asthmatic bronchospasm is exacerbated by stimuli from the tracheobronchial tree, so it is reasonable to suppose that a reduction of afferent input from the airways might break a vicious circle and perhaps initiate bronchial relaxation.

Sensory input from the lungs and airways travels in both vagal and sympathetic pathways (Craigie, 1922; Larsell and Burgett, 1924; Cromer and Ivy, 1933; Torrance and Whitteridge, 1948; Daly et al., 1958; Banister et al., 1949; Brücke et al., 1952; Widdicombe, 1954; von Euler and Fritts, 1963), but there are considerable species differences in the proportion of afferent traffic carried by the two systems (Dawes and Comroe, 1954). For example, nonvagal pathways carry little or no afferent input in the cat and rabbit, whereas in the dog extravagal pathways exist via the stellate ganglion and the dorsal roots of the upper four thoracic ganglia (Banister et al., 1949).

The precise distribution of pulmonary afferent input between the vagal and nonvagal pathways is unknown in man. However, if a substantial proportion of the input does travel along sympathetic pathways, it is possible that interruption of this traffic might reduce intense peaks of bronchomotor activity to a point where clinical improvement could occur.

Parietal Afferent Impulses

Reciprocal facilitation between phrenic nerve roots and intercostal nerves has been demonstrated in cats, illustrating the integration of afferent input and outgoing motor activity involved in widely separated neural segments of the respiratory apparatus (Decima et al., 1967). In man, afferent stimuli from the thoracic or abdominal parietes elicit a characteristic expiratory drive that reduces total compliance (McCann, 1946; Bromage, 1958). The clinical picture of expiratory effort in the presence of noxious stimulation and that seen in severe asthma bear some resemblance to each other, and it seems possible that in both instances afferent information from the thoracic or abdominal wall may play a common role in perpetuating the disordered thoracic posture. This does not imply that the modalities of sensation are necessarily the same in each case, but only that a similar "resetting" of fusimotor tone and muscle spindle activity may be involved (Campbell, 1966; Priban and Fincham, 1965). Deafferentation of the chest wall might be sufficient to bring about a readjustment of motor output to the thoracic muscles and a more appropriate balance of respiratory forces.

Vascular Absorption

It is possible that the bronchodilator effect of epidural analgesia may be entirely independent of neural events. Rather, it may be due to the smooth muscle depressant effect of circulating local anesthetic absorbed from the site of injection. Appreciable concentrations of local anesthetic drugs appear in the peripheral venous blood after epidural or paravertebral injection, reaching a maximum concentration after an interval of 10 to 15 minutes (Bromage and Robson, 1961; Braid and Scott, 1965, 1966; Lund, 1965; Mazze and Dunbar, 1966), and there is a straight line relationship between dose and plasma concentration (Braid and Scott, 1966).

Very small quantities of local anesthetic were used in the four cases described (55 to 140 mg lidocaine or mepivacaine). Such small doses would not be expected to produce peripheral blood levels greater than 0.5 to 1.0 μg per ml, and this is probably too low to relax contracted smooth muscle. However, there is suggestive evidence that under certain circumstances the bronchial circulation may receive a disproportionately large share of local anesthetic absorbed from epidural and paravertebral sites, and this could be sufficient to depress the contractility of bronchial smooth muscles. The azygos venous system receives most of the venous drainage from the vertebral and paravertebral veins, as well as the bronchial venous drainage. The vertebral-azygos system is an important pressure equalizer for venous blood returning from the various body compartments, and within this system circulation has an ebb-and-flow quality in the ancient galenic sense, depending on the relative pressures within the thorax and abdomen respectively (Batson, 1957; Aramendia et al., 1962). Thus, under conditions of high intra-abdominal pressure, blood could be deflected from one drainage source into the other, and the forced expiratory efforts of an asthmatic attack could provide the conditions for this to occur, with blood from the vertebral system entering the bronchopulmonary system past an incompetent bronchial valve (Liebow et al., 1959).

Observations on the vascular uptake of ^{14}C-labeled local anesthetics in our laboratory have shown that after epidural injection the maximum azygos concentration of local anesthetic is about three times higher than the peak concentration in the peripheral venous blood (Burfoot and Bromage, 1971). Thus, when an epidural injection of lidocaine produces a peripheral concentration of 1 to 2 μg per ml, one may infer that the corresponding azygos level is probably in the range of 3 to 6 μg per ml. If this concentration of lidocaine were to reach the bronchial circulation, it might be expected to depress bronchial smooth muscle to a significant degree.

At present, there are insufficient data to explain the exact mode of action of epidural or paravertebral injections in aborting an asthmatic attack, but the evidence for a vascular, non-neural mechanism is almost as strong as for a neural explanation. Nevertheless, new work referred to earlier on the autonomic control of the viscous properties of bronchial and lung surfactant is suggestive enough to rekindle interest in the role of the sympathetic system in the genesis of status asthmaticus and in the possible application of sympathetic blockade as a form of adjuvant therapy.

HEMODYNAMIC THERAPY OF MYOCARDIAL INFARCTION

This section is mainly speculative, for very little human data exist on the use of epidural analgesia in the management of myocardial ischemia and the failing heart. However, circumstantial evidence exists to support the view that carefully controlled epidural blockade would be a most appropriate form of supportive therapy in acute myocardial infarction. Some of this evidence has already been discussed in Chapter 10 under "The Effects of Epidural Block on Organ Blood Flow." Here further evidence will be reviewed, together with recent animal work, which shows that epidural blockade promotes a favorable redistribution of transmural myocardial blood flow in the acutely infarcted heart.

Theoretical Considerations

More than 30 years ago Sarnoff and Farr (1944) showed that pulmonary edema could be relieved by the vasodilatation that accompanies high spinal anesthesia. Later Davies et al. (1954) demonstrated that ganglion-blocking drugs reduced pulmonary hypertension, and they suggested that the beneficial effect was due to a direct vasodilator action on the pulmonary arteries rather than to a shift of blood from the lungs to the systemic circulation. Bromage (1956) showed that vital capacity could be increased by up to 35 per cent by induced arterial hypotension with ganglion-blocking drugs or high epidural blockade in patients with varying degrees of left or right heart failure, and this enlargement of the vital capacity was interpreted as being secondary to decongestion of the pulmonary bed from reduction of peripheral vascular resistance and unloading an impedance strain on the left ventricle.

Since the advent of convenient bedside methods for measuring cardiac output and pulmonary arterial pressures, it has become clear that the failing heart is indeed helped by reducing afterload. Furthermore, it is also clear that ventricular wall tension is the principal determinant of myocardial oxygen consumption (Graham et al., 1968), and *within limits* the ischemic or the failing heart is helped by reducing sympathetic tone rather than by increasing inotropic drive, once the afterload has been reduced (Shell and Sobel, 1974; Forrester et al., 1976a, 1976b; Mudge et al., 1976). The optimal amount and distribution of sympathetic tone require very delicately balanced control, for while on the one hand myocardial work must be reduced to minimize its metabolic demands, on the other hand the heart muscle is dependent on its own efforts for its coronary blood supply, and the best compromise must be found to satisfy both requirements for rest and supply while essential organ perfusion is maintained in the rest of the body.

Vasodilator therapy is now a recognized form of management in myocardial failure (Braunwald, 1977), but clinical interest has been confined to systemic administration of vasodilator drugs, such as nitroprusside, phentolamine and nitroglycerine, that act on the vascular muscles or their receptors. Little or no attention has been paid to the alternative philosophic approach of controlling sympathetic action at other points along the autonomic reflex arc while maintaining competence of the vascular end organs and their receptors. This is a strange oversight, because it is now clear that a number of powerful reflex pathways originate and end in the heart, with their segmental stations lying in the narrow spinal region between T_1 and T_5 inclusive (Randall et al., 1971; Malliani et al., 1972, 1973; Norris et al., 1974; Hess et al., 1974; James et al., 1975; Miller et al., 1976). Tonic vasomotor control of the coronary arterial bed appears to be heavily influenced by neural traffic through the left cardiac sympathetic nerves (Schwartz and Stone, 1977). Thus, there is a great deal of sound evidence to suggest that carefully manipulated blockade of the key segments in the upper thoracic cord could be a simple and effective way to limit the baneful effects of uncontrolled reflex sympathetic action on a weakened and failing myocardium. In addition, such a segmental blockade of the upper thoracic segments would also interrupt associated pain pathways and provide a welcome degree of analgesia without central depression in cases in which cardiac pain was intense enough to require treatment. Our animal experiments tend to support this view.

Experimental Evidence

In collaboration with Dr. G. A. Klassen, we studied the effects of thoracic epidural blockade in dogs by using a multiple-labeled microsphere technique. Particular attention was paid to the possibility of manipulating the distribution of transmural myocardial blood flow in order to favor the proportion of blood going to the vulnerable subendocardial muscle (Uchida and Ueda, 1975). In these experiments the transmural distribution of myocardial blood flow was measured at different coronary flow rates in normal hearts and after acute myocardial infarction (septal branch). Epidural blockade of the thoracic segments had no effect on transmural distribution at normal rates of coronary flow, but when coronary flow was reduced, epidural block was followed by a redistribution of blood away from the epicardium toward the inner layers of the subendocardial muscle, and the ratio of endocardial to epicardial blood flow was increased, as shown in Figure 13–14 (Bramwell et al., 1976). These results suggest that epidural blockade causes an internal redistribution of coronary flow that is particularly favorable to the subendocardial layers in dangerously low flow states.

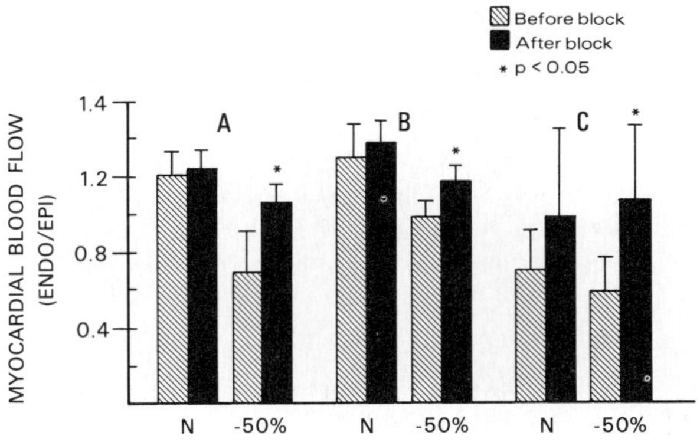

Figure 13–14. Influence of thoracic epidural blockade on transmural distribution of myocardial blood flow in dogs, showing ratio of endocardial (endo) to epicardial (epi) blood flow before and after epidural blockade under different conditions. *Group A*, Aortic pressure allowed to fall freely to about 40 per cent below resting level after epidural blockade. *Group B*, Aortic pressure sustained within 20 per cent of resting level by blood transfusion. *Group C*, Post myocardial infarction (acute occlusion of septal branch). Aortic pressure allowed to fall freely. No transfusion. *N* = Normal coronary flow rate; −50%, coronary flow rate reduced by one-half below normal flow rate.
▧ Before epidural block
■ After epidural block
* $p<0.05$
(Unpublished data from Bramwell et al., 1976.)

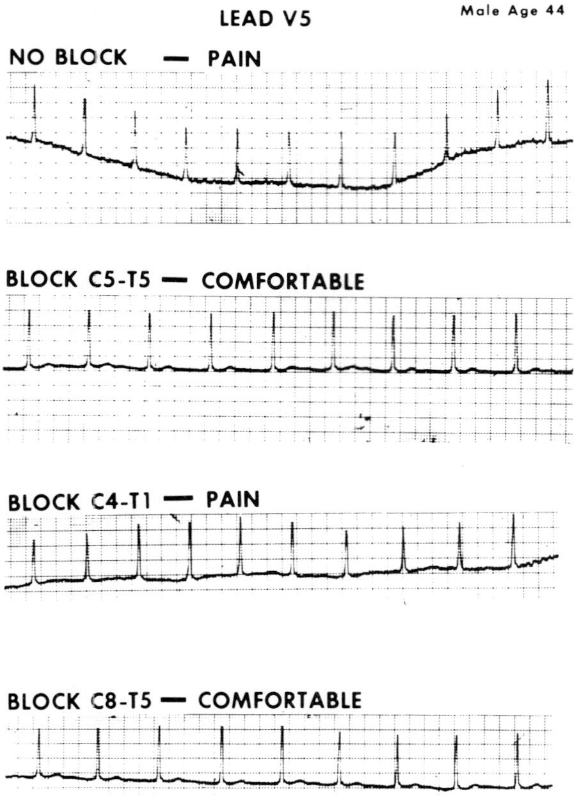

Figure 13–15. Intractable angina pectoris with alteration of T-waves in man of 44 years. Note absence of T-waves in presence of pain and restoration of T-waves when pain was abolished by block of upper five thoracic segments. (From Bromage, P. R.: Extradural analgesia for pain relief. Brit. J. Anaesth. *39*:721, 1967.)

Clinical Evidence

There has been considerable reluctance to translate the available experimental evidence into clinical practice, and at the time of writing, very little clinical data exist to confirm the view that epidural blockade would provide a useful degree of protection to a damaged myocardium on the brink of failure. Some empirical support comes from the following case, which, although atypical and anecdotal, nevertheless illustrates the beneficial effects of segmental epidural blockade on severe cardiac pain accompanied by EKG abnormalities.

A professional man of 44 years suffered from a form of migrating thrombophlebitis, with angina decubitus of uncertain origin. Attacks of intense substernal pain were accompanied by dyspnea and signs of sympathetic discharge, with drenching sweats, peripheral vasoconstriction, rapid thready pulse and flattened or inverted T-waves.

An epidural catheter was inserted at C_7–T_1, *and 8 ml of 1 per cent lidocaine produced segmental blockade from the fifth cervical to the fifth thoracic dermatome inclusive. Pain and dyspnea were relieved completely, the pulse slowed from 90 per minute to 75 per minute, and T-waves were restored (Fig. 13–15).*

There is a need to evaluate this therapeutic application of epidural blockade in myocardial disease with the same degree of physiological rigor that has been accorded the systemic vasodilators and sympatholytics, such as nitroprusside, propranolol and phentolamine. As a minimum such a trial would require continuous recording of pressures in the systemic arterial, central venous and pulmonary arterial compartments, together with serial measurements of cardiac output.

If controlled epidural blockade is shown to be helpful in selected cases of myocardial ischemia, it is likely that the technique will not prove to be an exclusive form of therapy, but rather it would offer just one more option in the difficult task of controlling inappropriate reflexes in such a way as to eliminate unnecessary cardiac work and to minimize myocardial damage. In short, epidural blockade would fit the role that it fills in its other applications—that is, to relieve pain and to restore function.

REFERENCES

Aird, R. B., and Naffziger, H. C.: Experimental injection of ethyl alcohol into the lumbar subarachnoid space: With neuropathological studies. Western J. Surg. Obstet. Gynecol. *43*:377, 1935.

Allison, R. C.: Epidural block in the treatment of circulatory disturbance after poliomyelitis. Anaesthesia *13*:157, 1958.

Aramendia, P., Martinez, J., De Letona, L., and Aviado, D. M.: Exchange of blood between pulmonary and systemic circulation via bronchopulmonary anastomosis. Circ. Res. *11*:870, 1962.

Banister, J., Fegler, G., and Hebb, C.: Initial respiratory responses to the intratracheal inhalation of phosgene or ammonia. Quart. J. Exp. Physiol. *35*:233, 1949.

Barry, P. J. C., and Kendall, P. H.: Corticosteroid infiltration of the extradural space. Ann. Phys. Med. *6*:267, 1962.

Batson, O. V.: The vertebral vein system. Amer. J. Roentgen. *128*:195, 1957.

Baxter, D. W., and Schacherl, U.: Experimental studies on the morphological changes produced by intrathecal phenol. Canad. Med. Assoc. J. *86*:1206, 1962.

Beckman, D. L., Bean, J. W., and Baslock, D. R.: Sympathetic influence on lung compliance and surface forces in head injury. J. Appl. Physiol. *30*:394, 1971.

Beckman, D. L., Bean, J. W., and Baslock, D. R.: Neurogenic influence on pulmonary compliance. J. Trauma *14*:111, 1974.

Benumof, J. L., and Semenza, J.: Total spinal anesthesia following intrathoracic intercostal nerve blocks. Anesthesiology *43*:124, 1975.

Bergren, D. R., and Beckman, D. L.: Pulmonary surface tension and head injury. J. Trauma *15*:336, 1975.

Berk, J. E., and Krumperman, L. W.: The use of fractional epidural block in the management of acute pancreatitis. Amer. J. Med. Sci. *334*:507, 1952.

Bonica, J. J.: The Management of Pain, with Special Emphasis on the Use of Analgesic Block in Diagnosis, Prognosis and Treatment. Philadelphia, Lea and Febiger, 1953, pp. 1404, 1405.

Braid, D. P., and Scott, D. B.: The systemic absorption of local anaesthetic drugs. Brit. J. Anaesth. *37*:394, 1965.

Braid, D. P., and Scott, D. B.: Dosage of lignocaine in epidural block in relation to toxicity. Brit. J. Anaesth. *38*:596, 1966.

Bramwell, R. S., Zborowski-Sluis, D. T., Bromage, P. R., and Klassen, G. A.: The effect of epidural blockade on the canine coronary circulation (unpublished data, 1976).

Braunwald, E.: Vasodilator therapy—A physiologic approach to the treatment of heart failure. New Eng. J. Med. *297*:331, 1977.

Bresgen, C.: Über Ischiassimulation—die diagnostiche Bedeutung der epiduralen Novocaininjektion. Munch. Med. Wschr. *93*:936, 1951.

Bromage, P. R.: Hypotension and vital capacity. Anaesthesia *11*:139, 1956.

Bromage, P. R.: Total respiratory compliance in anaesthetized subjects and modifications produced by noxious stimuli. Clin. Sci. *17*:217, 1958.

Bromage, P. R.: Extradural analgesia for pain relief. Brit. J. Anaesth. *39*:721, 1967.

Bromage, P. R., and Melzack, R.: Phantom limbs and the body schema. Canad. Anaesth. Soc. J. *21*:267, 1974.

Bromage, P. R., and Robson, J. G.: Concentrations of lignocaine in the blood after intravenous, intramuscular, epidural and endotracheal administration. Anaesthesia *16*:461, 1961.

Bromage, P. R., O'Beirn, P., and Dunford, L. A.: Etidocaine: A clinical evaluation for regional analgesia in surgery. Canad. Anaesth. Soc. J. *21*:523, 1974.

Bromage, P. R., Bramwell, R. S. B., Catchlove, R. F. H., Belanger, H., and Pierce, C. G. A.: Peridurography with metrizamide: Animal and human studies. Radiology, in press, 1978.

Brown, A. S.: Treatment of intractable pain by subarachnoid injection of carbolic acid. Lancet *2*:975, 1958.

Browne, R. A., and Ashworth, E. J.: The use of epidural block in acute pancreatitis: A report of eight cases. Canad. Anaesth. Soc. J. *16*:416, 1969.

Brücke, F., Kaindl, F., Maier, H., and Neumayz, A.: Über bronchokonstriktorische Reflexe von Sympathicus. Arch. Exp. Path. *215*:363, 1952.

Burfoot, M. F., and Bromage, P. R.: The effects of epinephrine on mepivacaine absorption from the spinal epidural space. Anesthesiology *35*:488, 1971.

Burn, J. M., Guyer, P. B., and Langdon, L.: The spread of solutions injected into the epidural space: A study using epidurograms in patients with the lumbosciatic syndrome. Brit. J. Anaesth. *45*:338, 1973.

Campbell E. J. M.: The relationship of the sensation of breathlessness to the act of breathing. *In* Howell, J. B. L., and Campbell, E. J. M.: Breathlessness. Oxford, Blackwell Scientific Publications, 1966, pp. 55–64.

Campbell H. H., and Walker, F. G.: Continuous epidural analgesia in the treatment of frostbite. A report of three cases. Canad. Med. Assoc. J. *84*:87, 1961.

Cantu, R. C.: Corticosteroids for spinal metastases. Lancet 2:912, 1968.

Cappio, M.: Il trattamento idrocortisonico per via epidurale sacrale delle lombosciatalgie: (osservazione su 80 casi). Reumatismo (Milano) *9*:60, 1957.

Cohen, H.: *In* Carling, E. R., and Ross, P. J. (eds.): British Surgical Practice. Vol. 2 London, Butterworth and Co. (Publishers) Ltd., 1948. pp. 1, 3.

Colding, A.: The effect of regional sympathetic blocks in the treatment of herpes zoster. A survey of 300 cases. Acta Anaesth. Scand. *13*:133, 1969.

Coomes, E. N.: A comparison between epidural anaesthesia and bed rest in sciatica. Brit. Med. J. *1*:20, 1961.

Craigie, E. H.: The reflex produced by chemical stimulation of the deeper respiratory passages. Amer. J. Physiol. *59*:346, 1922.

Cromer, S. P., and Ivy, A. C.: Respiratory death from central vagus stimulation after removal of stellate ganglia. Amer. J. Physiol. *104*:457, 1933.

Cyriax, J. H.: Textbook of Orthopaedic Medicine. 3d ed. London, Cassell, 1957, pp. 460, 469.

Daly, I. de B.: Intrinsic mechanisms of the lung. Quart. J. Exp. Physiol. *43*:2, 1958.

Davies, L. G., Goodwin, J. F., and Van Leuven, B. D.: The nature of pulmonary hypertension in mitral stenosis. Brit. Heart J. *16*:440, 1954.

Dawes, G S., and Comroe, J. H.: Chemoreflexes from heart and lungs. Physiol. Rev. *34*:167, 1954.

De Beule, F., and Schotte, A.: Nouvelles étapes dans la lutte contre la douleur. Rev. Belge Sci. Méd. *6*:357, 1934.

De Jong, R. H., and Cullen, S. C.: Theoretical aspects of pain: Bizarre pain phenomena during low spinal anesthesia. Anesthesiology *24*:628, 1963.

De Moragues, J. M., and Kierland, R. R.: The outcome of patients with herpes zoster. Arch. Derm. Syph. *75*:193, 1957.

Decima, E. E., Euler, C. von, and Thoden, U.: Spinal intercostal-phrenic reflexes. Nature *214*:312, 1967.

Descomps, H., and Dorgeuille, C.: Traitement de l'asthme par l'infiltration anesthésique rétrostylienne. Résultats sur 564 cas. J. Fr. Med. Chir. Thorac. *17*:285, 1963.

Dilke, T. F. W., Burry, H. C., and Grahame, R.: Extradural corticosteroid injection in the management of lumbar nerve root compression. Brit. Med. J. *2*:635, 1973.

Dittmann, M., Ferstl, A., and Wolff, G.: Epidural analgesia for the treatment of multiple rib fractures. Eur. J. Intensive Care Medicine *1*:71, 1975.

Ditzler, J. W.: Discussion on prolonged reversible nerve block. Anesth. Analg. *45*:662, 1966.

Dogliotti, A. M.: Traitement des syndromes douloureux de la periphérie par l'alcoolisation subarachnoïdienne des racines postérieures a leur émergence de la moelle epinière. Presse Méd. *39*:1249, 1931.

Dogliotti, A. M., and Ciocatto, E.: Method of differential block in pain relief. Anesthesiology *16*:623, 1955.

Droste, P. L., and Beckman, D. L.: Pulmonary effects of prolonged sympathetic stimulation. Proc. Soc. Exp. Biol. Med. *146*:352, 1974.

DuBose, F. G.: Therapeutic paravertebral alcohol block. Observations of its effect following its use in angina, asthma, and Raynaud's disease. Amer. J. Surg. *11*:497, 1931.

Dulfano, M. F., Schlessinger, R., Marvitt, R. C., Brogan, J. J., Sarnoff, H. S., Schwartz, M. S., and Segal, M. S.: Acute effects of bilateral glomectomy on lung mechanics at rest and during induced airway obstruction. Amer. Rev. Resp. Dis. *95*:48, 1967.

Eaglstein, W. H., Katz, R., and Brown, J. A.: The effects of early corticosteroid therapy on the skin eruption and pain of herpes zoster. J.A.M.A. *211*:1681, 1970.

Edwards, E., and Leeper, F.: Frostbite: An analysis of seventy-one cases. J.A.M.A. *149*:1199, 1952.

Ervasti, E.: Frostbites of the extremities and their sequelae. A clinical study. Acta Chir. Scand. (Suppl.) *299*:62, 1962.

Esplin, D. W.: Antiseptics and disinfectants; fungicides; ectoparasiticides. *In* Goodman, L. S., and Gillman, A. (eds.): The Pharmacological Basis of Therapeutics. London, The Macmillan Company, 1970, p. 1036.

Euler, C. von, and Fritts, H. W.: Quantitative aspects of respiratory reflexes from the lungs and chest walls of cats. Acta Physiol. Scand. *57*:284, 1963.

Evans, R. J., and Mackay, I. M.: Subarachnoid phenol nerve blocks for relief of pain in advanced malignancy. Canad. J. Surg. *15*:50, 1972.

Evans, W.: Intrasacral epidural injection in the treatment of sciatica. Lancet *2*:1225, 1930.

Flothow, P. G.: Diagnostic and therapeutic injections of the sympathetic nerves. Amer. J. Surg. *14*:591, 1931.

Forestner, J. E., and Raj, P. P.: Inadvertent epidural injection of thiopentone: A case report. Anesth. Analg. *54*:406, 1975.

Forrester, J. S., Diamond, G., Chatterjee, K., and Swan, H. J. C.: Hemodynamic therapy of myocardial infarction. New Eng. J. Med. *295*:1356, 1976a.

Forrester, J. S., Diamond, G., Chatterjee, K., and Swan, H. J. C.: Medical therapy of acute myocardial infarction by application of hemodynamic subsets. New Eng. J. Med. *295*:1404, 1976b.

Franz, D. N., and Perry, R. S.: Mechanisms for differential block among single myelinated and non-myelinated axons by procaine. J. Physiol. (Lond.) *236*:193, 1974.

Fregnani, L., De Marco, G., and Fabbri, F. L.: La peridurografia nello studio della sindrome lombosciatalgica. Arch. Putti Chir. Organi Mov. *17*:230, 1962.

Frère, R.: Bedeutung und Möglichkeiten des Periduralraumes zum Nachweis des hinteren Bandscheibenvorfalles. Zbl. Chir. *75*:586, 1950.

Frey, C. F.: Pathogenesis of nitrogen retention in pancreatitis. Amer. J. Surg. *109*:747, 1965.

Gage, M., and Gillespie, G.: Acute pancreatitis and its treatment. South. Med. J. *44*:769, 1951.

Gibbons, J., James, O., and Quail, A.: Management of 130 cases of chest injury with respiratory failure. Brit. J. Anaesth. *45*:1130, 1973a.

Gibbons, J., James, O., and Quail, A.: Relief of pain in chest injury. Brit. J. Anaesth. *45*:1136, 1973b.

Gilcreest, E. L., and Mullen, T. F.: The epidural and trans-sacral injection of alcohol for the relief of pain. Surg. Clin. N. Amer. *11*:989, 1931.

Goebert, H. W., Jallo, S. J., Gardner, W. J., and Wasmuth, C. E.: Painful radiculopathy treated with epidural injections of procaine and hydrocortisone acetate: Results in 113 patients. Anesth. Analg. *40*:130, 1961.

Golding, M. R., Martinez, A., de Jong, P., Murdosa, M., Fries, C. C., Sawyer, P. N., Henniger, G. R., and Wesolowski, S. A.: The role of sympathectomy in frostbite, with a review of 68 cases. Surgery *57*:774, 1965.

Gonsette, R. E.: Biologic tolerance of the central nervous system to metrizamide. Acta Radiol. (Suppl.) *335*:25, 1973a.

Gonsette, R. E.: Metrizamide as contrast medium for myelography and ventriculography. Preliminary clinical experiences. Acta. Radiol. (Suppl.) *335*:346, 1973b.

Graham, T. P., Jr., Covel, J. W., Sonnenblick, E. H., Ross, J., Jr., and Braunwald, E.: Control of myocardial oxygen consumption; relative influence of contractile state and tension development. J. Clin. Invest. *47*:375, 1968.

Green, H. D., Hall, L. S., and Sexton, J.: Autonomic responses in the canine hepatic arterial and venous beds. Amer. J. Physiol. *196*:196, 1959.

Greene, N. M.: Physiology of Spinal Anesthesia. Baltimore, The Williams & Wilkins Company, 1969, pp. 38–39.

Groenendijk, H. J.: De peridurale anaesthesie. Amsterdam, J. H. De Bussy, 1954, pp. 110–118.

Grunwald, I.: Neurolise com fenol: Uso da via peridural no tratamento da dor de cancer. Rev. Bras. Anest. *26*:628, 1976.

Gurdjian, E. S., and Walker, L. W.: Traumatic vasospastic disease of the hand (white fingers) with particular reference to biopsy findings. J.A.M.A. *129*:668, 1945.

Halligan, E. J., Costello, J. L., and Lewis, T. F.: Acute massive venous occlusion of the lower extremity. Ann. Surg. *137*:543, 1953.

Hannington-Kiff, J. G.: Intravenous regional sympathetic block with guanethidine. Lancet *1*:1019, 1974.

Hayes, M. F., Rosenbaum, R. W., Zibelman, M., and Matsumoto, T.: Adult respiratory distress syndrome in association with acute pancreatitis. Evaluation of positive end expiratory pressure ventilation and pharmacologic doses of steroids. Amer. J. Surg. *127*:314, 1974.

Head, H., and Holmes, G.: Sensory disturbances from cerebral lesions. Brain *34*:102, 1912.

Heile, B.: Der epidurale Raum. Arch. Klin. Chir. *101*:845, 1913.

Hellstrom, J.: Aetiological and therapeutic experiences concerning kidney and ureteric stones. Brit. J. Urol. *21*:9, 1949.

Hess, G. L., Zuperku, E. J., Coon, R. L., and Kampine, J. P.: Sympathetic afferent nerve activity of left ventricular origin. Amer. J. Physiol. *227*:543, 1974.

Hindmarsh, T.: Methiodal sodium and metrizamide in lumbar myelography. Acta Radiol. (Suppl.) *335*:359, 1973.

Hingson, R. A., Whitacre, F. E., Hughes, J. G., Turner, H. B., and Barnett, J. M.: New horizons in therapeutic nerve block in the treatment of vascular and renal emergencies with continued caudal and continuous spinal analgesia and anesthesia. South. Surg. *13*:580, 1947.

Hitchcock, E.: Hypothermic subarachnoid irrigation for intractable pain. Lancet *1*:1133, 1967.

Hitchcock, E.: Osmolytic neurolysis for intractable facial pain. Lancet *1*:434, 1969.

Hughes, J.: Isolation of an endogenous compound from the brain with pharmacological properties similar to morphine. Brain. Res. *88*:295, 1975.

Iggo, A., and Walsh, E. G.: Selective block of small fibres in the spinal roots by phenol. J. Physiol. (Lond.) *146*:6P, 1959.

Iggo, A., and Walsh, E. G.: Selective block of small fibres in the spinal roots by phenol. Brain *88*:701, 1960.

Imrie, C. W., Murphy, D., Ferguson, J. C., and Blumgart, L. H.: Arterial hypoxia in acute pancreatitis. Ann. Roy. Coll. Surg. Eng. *58*:322, 1976.

James, T. N., Isobe, J. H., and Urthaler, F.: Analysis of components in a cardiogenic hypertensive chemoreflex. Circulation *52*:179, 1975.

Jewett, D. L., and King, J. S.: Conduction block of monkey dorsal rootlets by water and hypertonic saline solutions. Exp. Neurol. *33*:225, 1971.

Juel-Jensen, B. E.: Herpes simplex and zoster. Brit. Med. J. *1*:406, 1973.

Junge, H.: Peridurographie. Dtsch. Med. Wschr. *74*:682, 1949.

Kellum, J. M., DeMeester, T. R., Elkins, R. C., and Zuidema, G. D.: Respiratory insufficiency secondary to acute pancreatitis. Ann. Surg. *175*:657, 1972.

Kelman, H.: Epidural injection therapy for sciatica pain. Amer. J. Surg. *64*:183, 1944.

King, J. S., Jewett, D. L., and Sundberg, H. R.: Differential blockade of cat dorsal root C-fibers by various chloride solutions. J. Neurosurg. *36*:569, 1972.

Koehler, B. E., Urowitz, M. W., and Killinger, D. W.: The systemic effects of intra-articular corticosteroid. J. Rheumatol. *1*:117, 1974.

Krnjevic, K., and Morris, M. E.: Extracellular K^+ activity and slow potential changes in spinal cord and medulla. Canad. J. Physiol. Pharmacol. *50*:1214, 1972.

Kyösola, K.: Clinical experiences in the management of cold injuries: A study of 110 cases. J. Trauma *14*:32, 1974.

Laroche, G. P.: Traumatic vasospastic disease in chain-saw operators. Canad. Med. Assoc. J. *115*:1217, 1976.

Larsell, O., and Burgett, G. E.: The effects of mechanical and chemical stimulation of the tracheo-bronchial mucous membrane. Amer. J. Physiol. *70*:311, 1924.

Leriche, R.: The surgery of pain. Translated by Young, A. Baltimore, The Williams & Wilkins Company, 1939, pp. 140–145.

Leriche, R.: Résultat éloigné de la ganglionectomie lombaire dans les troubles trophiques et vasomoteurs de la poliomyélite infantile. Lyon Chir. *44*:399, 1949.

Levin, G. L. L.: Treatment of bronchial asthma by dorsal perisympathetic injection of absolute alcohol. Lancet *2*:249, 1934.

Liebow, A. A., Hales, M. R., and Bloomer, W. E.: Relation of bronchial to pulmonary vascular tree. *In* Adams, W., and Veith, I.: Pulmonary Circulation. New York, Grune and Stratton, Inc., 1959, pp. 79–98.

Lièvre, J. A., Bloch-Michel, H., Pean, G., and Uro, J.: L'hydrocortisone en injection locale. Rev. du Rhum. *20*:310, 1953.

Lloyd, J. W., and Carrie, L. E. S.: A method of treating renal colic. Proc. Roy. Soc. Med. *58*:634, 1965.

Lloyd, J. W., Crampton Smith, A., and O'Connor, B. T.: Classification of chest injuries as an aid to treatment. Brit. Med. J. *1*:1518, 1965.

Lourie, H., and Vanasupa, P.: Comments on the use of intraspinal phenol-Pantopaque for relief of pain and spasticity. J. Neurosurg. *20*:60, 1963.

Lund, P. C.: A correlation of venous blood concentrations and spinal fluid concentrations of Xylocaine® and Citanest® during peridural analgesia. Acta Anaesth. Scand. (Suppl.) *16*:97, 1965.
Lund, P. C.: Peridural Analgesia and Anesthesia. Springfield, Ill., Charles C Thomas, Publisher, 1966, pp. 336, 339, 352, 356.
Luyendijk, W., and van Voorthuisen, A. E.: Contrast examination of the spinal epidural space. Acta Radiol. Diag. *5*:1051, 1966.
McCann, J. C.: Physiology of traumatic reflexes and respiration during surgical anesthesia. Calif. Med. J. *65*:212, 1946.
Maher, R. M.: Relief of pain in incurable cancer. Lancet *1*:18, 1955.
Maher, R. M.: Neurone selection in relief of pain: Further experiences with intrathecal injections. Lancet *1*:16, 1957.
Maher, R. M.: Intrathecal chlorocresol in the treatment of pain in cancer. Lancet *1*:965, 1963.
Malliani, A., Peterson, D. F., Bishop, V. S., and Brown, A. M.: Spinal sympathetic cardiocardiac reflexes. Circ. Res. *30*:158, 1972.
Malliani, A., Parks, M., Tuckett, R. P., and Brown, A. M.: Reflex increases in heart rate elicited by stimulation of afferent cardiac sympathetic nerve fibers in the cat. Circ. Res. *32*:9, 1973.
Marion, P.: Sur le traitement des pancréatites aiguës par les infiltrations splanchniques. Lyon Chir. *40*:315, 1945.
Marmer, M. J.: Acute herpes zoster: Successful treatment by continuous epidural analgesia. Calif. Med. J. *103*:277, 1965.
Martinez, A., Golding, M., Sawyer, P. N., and Wesolowski, S. A.: The specific arterial lesions in mild and severe frostbite: Effect of sympathectomy. J. Cardiovasc. Surg. *7*:495, 1966.
Mathews, J. A.: Dynamic discography: A study of lumbar traction. Ann. Phys. Med. *9*:275, 1968.
Mathews, J. A.: Epidurography. *In* Apley, A. G.: Modern Trends in Orthopaedics. London, Butterworths, 1972, pp. 148–166.
Mathews, J. A., and Yates, D. A. H.: Reduction of lumbar disc prolapse by manipulation. Brit. Med. J. *3*:696, 1969.
Matyas, M.: Treatment of backache by epidural air injection. Z. Gynäk. *75*:1096, 1953.
Mazze, R. I., and Dunbar, R. W.: Plasma lidocaine concentrations after caudal, lumbar epidural, axillary block and intravenous regional anesthesia. Anesthesiology *27*:574, 1966.
Mehta, M.: Intractable Pain. London, W. B. Saunders Company, Ltd., 1973, p. 172.
Melzack, R., and Bromage, P. R.: Experimental phantom limbs. Exp. Neurol. *39*:261, 1973.
Melzack, R., and Wall, P. D.: Pain mechanisms: A new theory. Science *150*:971, 1965.
Meryman, H. T.: Tissue freezing and local cold injury. Physiol. Rev. *37*:233, 1957.
Miller, R. R., Vismara, L. A., Williams, D. O., Amsterdam, E. A., and Mason, D. T.: Pharmacological mechanisms for left ventricular unloading in clinical congestive heart failure. Differential effects of nitroprusside, phentolamine, and nitroglycerin on cardiac function and peripheral circulation. Circ. Res. *39*:127, 1976.
Mount, H. T. R.: Hydrocortisone in the treatment of intervertebral disc protrusion. Canad. Med. Assoc. J. *105*:1279, 1971.
Mudge, G. H., Grossman, W., and Mills, R. M.: Reflex increase in coronary vascular resistance in patients with ischemic heart disease. New Eng. J. Med. *295*:1333, 1976.
Nakamoto, M. F., Unemoto, M., Yutaka, S., Wakita, S., and Katayama, N.: Extradural myelography of lumbosacral vertebrae by means of water soluble contrast media—Various positions. J. Bone Joint Surg. *37A*:1309, 1955.
Nakayama, K.: Surgical removal of the carotid body for bronchial asthma. Dis. Chest. *40*:565, 1961.
Nashold, B. S., and Friedman, H.: Dorsal column stimulation for control of pain. Preliminary report on 30 patients. J. Neurosurg. *36*:590, 1972.
Nathan, P. W., and Sears, T. A.: Effects of phenol on nervous conduction. J. Physiol. (Lond.) *150*:565, 1960.
Nathan, P. W., Sears, T. A., and Smith, M. C.: Effects of phenol solutions on the nerve roots of the cat: An electrophysiological and histological study. J. Neurol. Sci. *2*:7, 1965.
Norris, J., Foreman, R. D., Wurster, R. D.: Responses of the canine heart to stimulation of the first five ventral thoracic roots. Amer. J. Physiol. *227*:9, 1974.
Ochsner, A.: Splanchnic block in treatment of acute pancreatitis. Int. Anesth. Clin. *1*:3, 1963.
Ochsner, A., and DeBakey, M.: Therapy of phlebothrombosis and thrombophlebitis. Arch. Surg. (Chicago) *40*:208, 1940.
Odom, C. B.: Epidural anesthesia in resumé and prospect. Anesth Analg. *19*:106, 1940.
Ogilvie, W. H.: The place of operations upon the sympathetic system in the treatment of poliomyelitis. Proc. Roy. Soc. Med. *26*:429, 1933.
Orr, R. B., and Warren, K. W.: Continuous epidural analgesia in acute pancreatitis. Lahey Clin. Bull. *6*:204, 1950.

Pasternak, G. W., Goodman, R., and Snyder, S. H.: An endogenous morphine-like factor in mammalian brain. Life Sciences *16*:1765, 1975.

Pedersen, H. E., Blunck, C. F. J., and Gardner, E.: The anatomy of the lumbosacral posterior rami meningeal branches of spinal nerves (sinuvertebral nerves). J. Bone Joint Surg. *38*:377, 1956.

Penn, I., and Schwartz, S. I.: Evaluation of low molecular weight dextran in the treatment of frostbite. J. Trauma *4*:784, 1964.

Peyton, W. T., and French, L. A.: Surgical relief of intractable pain. Trans. West Surg. Assoc. *51*:140, 1942.

Peyton, W. T., Semansky, E. J., and Baker, A. B.: Subarachnoid injection of alcohol for relief of intractable pain with discussion of cord changes found at autopsy. Amer. J. Cancer *30*:709, 1937.

Pos, R.: Psychological assessment of factors affecting pain. Canad. Med. Assoc. J. *111*:1213, 1974.

Priban, I. P., and Fincham, W. F.: Self-adaptive control and the respiratory system. Nature *208*:339, 1965.

Randall, D. C., Armour, J. A., and Randall, W. C.: Dynamic responses to cardiac nerve stimulation in the baboon. Amer. J. Physiol. *220*:526, 1971.

Ranson, J. H. C., Roses, D. F., and Fink, S. D.: Early respiratory insufficiency in acute pancreatitis. Ann. Surg. *178*:75, 1973.

Romagnoli, A., and Batra, M. S.: Continuous epidural block in the treatment of impacted ureteric stones. Canad. Med. Assoc. J. *109*:968, 1973.

Rosenak S.: Procaine injection treatment of herpes zoster. Lancet *2*:1056, 1938.

Rovner, A. J., and Westcott, J. L.: Pulmonary edema and respiratory insufficiency in acute pancreatitis. Radiology *118*:513, 1976.

Ruth, H. S.: Diagnostic, prognostic and therapeutic nerve blocks. J.A.M.A. *102*:419, 1934.

Sanford, H., and Doub, H. P.: Epidurography. A method of roentgenologic visualization of protruded intervertebral discs. Radiology *36*:712, 1941.

Sarnoff, S. J., and Farr, H. W.: Spinal anesthesia in the therapy of pulmonary edema: A preliminary report. Anesthesiology *5*:69, 1944.

Schulte-Steinberg, O.: Spread of local anesthetic solutions in caudal blocks in children. Sixth World Congress of Anesthesiology Abstracts, Mexico City, 1976, Excerpta Medica, Int. Cong. Series No. 387, p. 132.

Schwartz, P. J., and Stone, H. L.: Tonic influence of the sympathetic nervous system on myocardial reactive hyperemia and on coronary blood flow distribution in dogs. Circ. Res. *41*:51, 1977.

Segal, M. S.: Glomectomy for chronic bronchial asthma: A three phase study. Ann. Allergy *23*:377, 1965.

Sehgal, A. D., Tweed, D. C., Gardner, W. J., and Foote, M. S.: Laboratory studies after intrathecal corticosteroids. Arch. Neurol. (Chicago) *9*:64, 1963.

Sexton, J. D., and Beckman, D. L.: Neurogenic influence on pulmonary surface tension and cholesterol in cats. Exp. Biol. Med. *148*:679, 1975.

Shealy, C. N.: Dangers of spinal injections without proper diagnosis. J.A.M.A. *197*:1104, 1966.

Shealy, C. N.: Six years of experience with electrical stimulation for control of pain. Adv. Neurol. *4*:775, 1974.

Shealy, C. N., Taslitz, N., Mortimer, J. T., and Becker, D. P.: Electrical inhibition of pain: Experimental evaluation. Anesth. Analg. *46*:299, 1967a.

Shealy, C. N., Mortimer, J. T., and Reswick, J. B.: Electrical inhibition of pain by stimulation of the dorsal columns: Preliminary clinical report. Anesth. Analg. *46*:489, 1967b.

Shealy, C. N., Mortimer, J. T., and Hagfors, N. R.: Dorsal column electroanalgesia. J. Neurosurg. *32*:560, 1970.

Shell, W. E., and Sobel, B. E.: Protection of jeopardized ischemic myocardium by reduction of ventricular afterload. New Eng. J. Med. *291*:481, 1974.

Shimoji, K., Higashi, H., Kano, T., et al.: Electrical management of intractable pain. Jap. J. Anesth. *20*:444, 1971.

Shimoji, K., Kano, T., Higashi, H., et al.: Evoked spinal electrograms recorded from epidural space in man. J. Appl. Physiol. *33*:468, 1972.

Shimoji, K., Kano, T., Morioka, T., and Ikezono, E.: Evoked spinal electrograms in a quadriplegic patient. Electroenceph. Clin. Neurophysiol. *35*:659, 1973.

Shimoji, K., Kitamura, H., Ikezono, E., Shimizu, H., Okamoto, K., and Iwakura, Y.: Spinal hypalgesia and analgesia by low-frequency electric stimulation in the epidural space. Anesthesiology *41*:91, 1974.

Shuster, S., and Williams, I. A.: Adrenal suppression due to intra-articular corticosteroid therapy. Lancet *2*:171, 1961.

Sicard, A.: Les injections médicamenteuses extra-durales par voie sacro-coccygienne. C. R. Soc. Biol. Paris *53*:396, 1901.

Sicard, J. A., and Forestier, J.: Méthode radiographique d'exploration de la cavité épidurale par le Lipiodol. Rev. Neurol. *28*:1264, 1921.

Sicard, J. A., and Forestier, J.: Roentgenologic exploration of the central nervous system with iodized oil (Lipiodol). Arch. Neurol. Psychiat. *16*:420, 1926.

Sicard, J. A., and Forestier, J.: The Use of Lipiodol in Diagnosis and Treatment. London, Oxford University Press, 1932, p. 178.

Squire, A. W., Calvillo, O., and Bromage, P. R.: Painless intrathecal hypertonic saline. Canad. Anaesth. Soc. J. *21*:308, 1974.

Stewart, W. A., and Lourie, H.: An experimental evaluation of the effects of subarachnoid injection of phenol-Pantopaque in cats. A histological study. J. Neurosurg. *20*:64, 1963.

Strandness, D. E.: Vascular diseases of the extremities. *In* Wintrobe, M. M., et al. (eds.): Harrison's Principles of Internal Medicine. New York, McGraw-Hill Book Company, 1974, p. 1254.

Swerdlow, M., and Sayle-Creer, W.: A study of extradural medication in the relief of the lumbosciatic syndrome. Anaesthesia *25*:341, 1970.

Szokodi-Dimitrov, J. D.: Surgical treatment of bronchial asthma by modified operative procedure. J. Internat. Chir. *13*:588, 1953.

Szokodi-Dimitrov, J. D.: Die Lungendenervation in der Therapie des Status Asthmaticus. Zbl. Chir. *81*:1771, 1956.

Taub, A.: Discussion on dorsal column stimulators. Adv. Neurol. *4*:796, 1974.

Tiwisina, T.: Kontrastdarstellung des Periduralraums mit Perabrodil zum Nachweis des hinteren Bandscheibenvorfalles (Peridurographie). Chirurg *22*:247, 1951.

Torrance, R. W., and Whitteridge, D.: Technical aids in the study of respiratory reflexes. J. Physiol. (Lond.) *107*:6P, 1948.

Uchida, Y., and Ueda, H.: Non-uniform myocardial blood flow caused by stellate ganglion stimulation. Jap. Heart. J. *16*:162, 1975.

Urban, B. J., and Nashold, B. S.: Percutaneous epidural stimulation of the spinal cord for relief of pain: Long term results. J. Neurosurg. *48*:323, 1978.

Ushio, Y., Posner, R., Posner, J. B., and Shapiro, W. R.: Experimental spinal cord compression by epidural neoplasms. Neurology *27*:422, 1977a.

Ushio, Y., Posner, R., Kim, J-H., Shapiro, W. R., and Posner, J. B.: Treatment of experimental spinal cord compression caused by extradural neoplasms. J. Neurosurg. *47*:380, 1977b.

Viner, N.: Intractable sciatica—the sacral epidural injection—an effective method of giving relief. Canad. Med. Assoc. J. *15*:630, 1925.

Viner, N.: Intractable chronic pain in the lower segments of the body: Relief by means of sacral epidural injections. Arch. Neurol. Psychiat. *20*:336, 1928.

Walker, T., and Pemberton, W. E.: Continuous epidural block in the treatment of pancreatitis. Anesthesiology *14*:33, 1953.

Wall, P. D., and Sweet, W. H.: Temporary abolition of pain in man. Science *155*:108, 1967.

Werner, M. H., Hayes, D. F., Lucas, C. E., and Rosenberg, I. K.: Renal vasoconstriction in association with acute pancreatitis. Amer. J. Surg. *127*:185, 1974.

White, J. C., Smithwick, R. H., and Simeone, F. A.: The Autonomic Nervous System. 3d ed. New York. The Macmillan Company, 1952. p. 363.

Widdicombe, J. G.: Respiratory reflexes from the trachea and bronchi of the cat. J. Physiol. (Lond.) *123*:55, 1954.

Winnie, A. P., Hartman, J. H., Meyers, H. L., Ramamurthy, S., and Baragan, V.: Pain clinic. II. Intradural and extradural corticosteroids for sciatica. Anesth. Analg. *51*:990, 1972.

Wood, K. M., and Arguelles, J. E.: A study of the effect of methylprednisolone acetate, in sterile aqueous suspension, on peripheral nerves. 1977 ASA Annual Meeting, Abstracts of Scientific Papers, p. 631.

Wood, J. B., Frankland, A. W., and Eastcott, H. H. G.: Bilateral removal of carotid bodies for asthma. Thorax *20*:570, 1965.

Woodbridge, P. D.: Therapeutic nerve block with procaine and alcohol. Amer. J. Surg. *9*:278, 1930.

Yates, D. A. H.: Epidural myelography with water-soluble contrast material (Urografin). Ann. Phys. Med. *8*:81, 1965.

chapter 14
Complications and Contraindications

From wrong to wrong the exasperated spirit proceeds, unless restored by that refining fire where you must move in measure, like a dancer.

Little Gidding
T. S. Eliot

Epidural analgesia is a technique that demands a high level of precision and accurate clinical observation for routine success. Complications may arise from many different causes, some with immediate effects and some remote, and the anesthesiologist should be familiar with the difficulties and dangers that may accompany each phase of the anesthetic. In addition, he should be aware of the unrelated conditions and complications that may be erroneously attributed to epidural analgesia, with resulting confusion of treatment, prognosis and medicolegal status.

The incidence of epidural complications varies between different series. Precise statistics on the overall incidence of epidural complications do not exist, and the figures that are available are often difficult to interpret for two principal reasons. First, a lack of adequate reporting is evident from the number of anecdotal but often very incomplete "personal communications" referred to in the more extensive reviews (Catterberg and Insausti, 1964; Usubiaga, 1975). Second, some reports, particularly of neurological complications, wrongly impute the clinical outcome to epidural anesthesia instead of to the true cause, which may be either primarily surgical or cardiovascular or coincidentally due to pre-existing disease. Examples of this type of erroneous reporting will be given later in the chapter.

IMMEDIATE TECHNICAL COMPLICATIONS

Most of the complications have been discussed in earlier sections dealing with the technique (see Chapter 6). Here, they will be summarized briefly for reference purposes and to underline the more common ones.

Inadvertent Dural Puncture

Accidental dural puncture during induction is more of a nuisance than a serious danger, but it is an important cause of headache and discomfort, and it should not be dismissed lightly. As stated before, this accident should not happen as frequently as it does. An incidence of more than 1 per cent suggests that something is wrong with the anesthesiologist's technique and it needs correcting. Either he is using the wrong type of needle and should change to a better one, or he should undergo further training or reeducation of faulty habits. The use of a training simulator model (e.g., Ansco lumbar puncture model) is very helpful for this purpose. Alternatively, time may be usefully spent practicing with a needle and syringe in the postmortem room or anatomy department. In the caudal region the dural sac extends as far down as the lower border of the second sacral vertebra and occasionally lower. Needles should not be advanced more than 3 to 4 cm within the caudal canal for fear of massive subarachnoid injection.

Dural puncture by epidural catheter is a much rarer event, but it is more subtle and dangerous as it may be easily missed, and then a *massive subarachnoid injection* of local anesthetic will occur when the next top-up dose is administered. Philip and Brown (1976) reported one case of total spinal anesthesia in which an epidural catheter appears to have penetrated into the subarachnoid space *after* a previous injection through the catheter had produced a normal epidural block. In this case only 2 cm of polyvinyl catheter was inserted beyond the needle tip. An initial induction dose of 14 ml of 0.5 per cent bupivacaine (70 mg) given through the catheter produced blockade to T_6. However, 2¾ hours later a second dose of only half the amount (i.e., 35 mg) of 0.5 per cent bupivacaine (7 ml) was followed by total spinal blockade (Case No. 17 in Table 14–1). A test dose must always be given through the catheter, once it is in place, and aspiration with a 2-ml syringe should be carried out from time to time. It would seem that a test dose of 2 ml before each top-up injection might be a worthwhile precautionary measure.

Massive Subarachnoid Injection

The most serious immediate complication is massive injection of local anesthetic into the wrong place, either subarachnoid, subdural or intravenous. This complication can occur by the needle being wrongly placed or by an epidural catheter penetrating the dura or an epidural vein. Massive subarachnoid injection is followed by *rapid* total spinal analgesia, vascular hypotension, and unconsciousness and apnea. Treatment is directed toward supporting the circulation and respiration until the effects of the block wear off. If any cause for inferior vena caval compression exists, the patient should be turned on the side to relieve caval obstruction and aid venous return. Endotracheal intubation is performed, and ventilation with air or oxygen is continued until afferent input returns and respiration recommences. Arterial pressure is maintained with a suitable vasopressor. Table 14–1 outlines 17 reported cases showing the duration of apnea and unconsciousness associated with massive subarachnoid injection of various agents and doses. It can be seen that large doses of dibucaine

TABLE 14–1 Inadvertent Subarachnoid Injection in Attempted Epidural Blockade

Patient	Volume	Epidural Dose: DOSE OF ANALGESIC AGENT	Epidural Dose: EPINEPHRINE	Duration of Apnea (min)	Duration of Unconsciousness (min)	Authors
1. Male, 41 years	40 ml	60 mg dibucaine 600 mg procaine	1/300,000	360	240	Gordon-Jones (1953)
2. Female, 65 years	40 ml	60 mg dibucaine 600 mg procaine	1/300,000	360	240	Gordon-Jones (1953)
3. Male, 54 years	41 ml	66.75 mg dibucaine	1/200,000	315	Sedated for 345 minutes until respiration normal	Bromage (1954)
4. Female, 55 years	17 ml	255 mg lidocaine	1/100,000	45	125	De Saram (1956)
5. Female, 39 years	24 ml	420 mg lidocaine	Yes	60	240	De Saram (1956)
6. Female, 50 years	24 ml	420 mg lidocaine	Yes	90	210	De Saram (1956)
7. Female, 76 years	10 ml	200 mg lidocaine	No	30	90	Bonica et al. (1957)
8. Female, 44 years	23 ml	345 mg lidocaine	1/160,000	59	118	Sykes (1958)
9. Female, 76 years	20 ml	Lidocaine (concentration not recorded)		60	65	Scott and Kyles (1961)
10. Not recorded	30 ml	300 mg mepivacaine	No	30	Not recorded	Sheffield (1964)
11. Female, 58 years	10 ml	150 mg lidocaine	1/200,000	Nil	Nil*	Gavin (1965)
12. Female	4 ml	80 mg lidocaine	No	30	90*	Moir and Hesson (1965)
13. Male, 30 years	20 ml	300 mg lidocaine	1/110,000	30	60	Mandlekar (1970)
14. Female, 43 years	20 ml	100 mg bupivacaine	1/200,000	120	185	Gillies and Morgan (1973)
15. Female, 65 years	22 ml	110 mg bupivacaine	1/200,000	95	120	Gillies and Morgan (1973)
16. Male, 57 years	30 ml	75 mg bupivacaine	1/200,000	100	60	Gillies and Morgan (1973)
17. Female, 27 years	7 ml	35 mg bupivacaine	No	75	50*	Philip and Brown (1976)

*Catheter perforation of dura.

with epinephrine produced the longest periods of paralysis and unconsciousness, whereas the duration was relatively short with less massive doses of plain lidocaine or mepivacaine. Case Nos. 11 and 12 arose after inadvertent puncture of the dura by a catheter, after a negative test dose through the needle, emphasizing again the importance of using a test dose through the catheter. Case No. 11 was the first report of an inadvertent dural puncture with a catheter. It was also the first report that used a glucose reagent strip to determine the presence of cerebrospinal fluid in the fluid effluent. This case was handled deliberately and very skillfully as a continuous spinal anesthetic without excessive spread of analgesia. Case No. 15 is interesting in that the onset of paralysis was atypically slow, and the epidural dose of 110 mg of bupivacaine was large enough to expect blockade of about 23 spinal segments (i.e., up to C_7–C_8) in a person of normal cardiovascular status. If any significant degree of diabetes or arteriosclerosis had been present, the block could be expected to continue appreciably higher and to mimic a massive subarachnoid injection, even though it had been correctly placed in the epidural space: the case would then fall under the category of massive epidural injection.

Massive Subdural Injection

A potential space exists between the dura mater and the pia-arachnoid membranes. The danger of entering this space has been mentioned in the chapters on Anatomy and on Continuous Epidural Analgesia. Rough handling of the epidural needle and unnecessary rotation of the bevel are technical factors that may cause a breach in the dura, making possible the injection of solutions into the subdural space or inadvertent passage of a catheter directly into it. It has been suggested that this mishap may be a possible explanation for rare cases of apparent massive epidural blockade. Injected solutions spread quite extensively in the subdural space, mainly along the dorsal aspect and in a cephalad direction (Taveras and Wood, 1972). It is difficult to obtain definite evidence of this type of accident, since anesthetic solutions are not usually radiopaque. However, Boys and Norman (1975) reported a case of accidental subdural catheterization, documented radiographically with X-ray contrast material injected into the subdural space after anesthetic spread had been unduly extensive from C_7 to L_2, following an injection of 40 mg of bupivacaine (0.5 per cent).

Subdural injection, in common with other forms of epidural mishap, can usually be avoided by care, by good needle control and by avoiding fussy movements of the bevel once the needle has reached the epidural space.

Massive Epidural Blockade

Overdosage from disregard of the normal relationships between dose requirements and age will lead to excessive segmental spread, simulating inadvertent subarachnoid injection. In 1954, Stringer reported four cases of excessively high segmental block, two being in patients with arteriosclerotic disease. These cases all involved doses that were large for the patient's chronological age. Later, Morrow (1959) and Mostert (1960) also reported unusually extensive spread in two arteriosclerotic patients. A curious feature of these last two cases was the extraordinarily long time taken for blockade to spread upward to involve the cervical segments, one case taking 40 minutes for this bizarre type of spread. In a subsequent series of 56 blocks in 53 severely arteriosclerotic patients, Bromage (1962) found that dose requirements in these patients were reduced on the average by 42 per cent; that is, blockade spread almost twice as far as would be expected in a normal population. Furthermore, full segmental spread took significantly longer to reach its full extent than in normal patients, sometimes taking over 30 minutes with 2 per cent lidocaine instead of the average time of about 16 minutes (see Chapter 4).

Figure 14–1 is a segment-time diagram illustrating the very extensive segmental spread that may follow quite small doses in severely arteriosclerotic patients. In this instance the upper band of analgesia rose to T_3 on one side and T_7 on the other, although the lower level only extended as far as S_3, giving an average spread for the two sides of 15 segments from a dose of 120 mg lidocaine. In a normal subject of the same age, this dose would be expected to anesthetize no more than 6 to 7 segments.

Defalque (1967) also reported a typical case of exaggerated spread in a 69-year-old man suffering from severe degenerative arterial disease, hypertension and slight hemiparesis. In this patient a lumbar epidural injection of 25 ml of 1 per cent lidocaine with 0.1 per cent tetracaine and 1/200,000 epinephrine produced analgesia up to T_4 in 10 minutes, but a few minutes later the block mounted higher and massive epidural blockade occurred with apnea lasting 3½ hours.

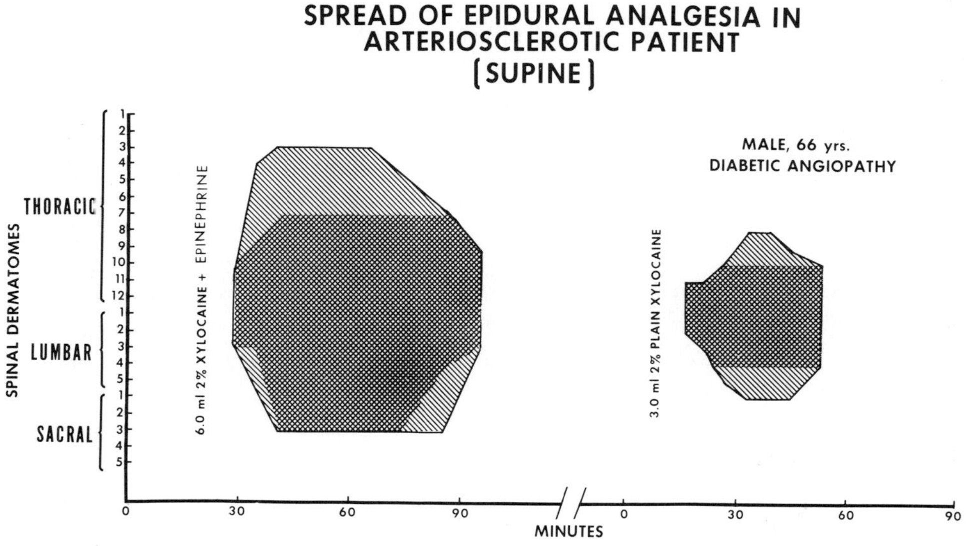

Figure 14–1. Excessive segmental spread of epidural analgesia in 66-year-old diabetic male with severe arteriosclerosis. Light hatched area: analgesia on left side. Dark hatched area: analgesia on right side. Expected segmental spread with 6 ml of 2 per cent lidocaine at 66 years = 6.6 segments. Observed segmental spread = 15 segments (average of two sides). (From Bromage, 1962.)

Diabetics are victims of microangiopathy, whether overt signs of vascular disease exist or not (Moore and Frew, 1965). In a small series of controlled diabetics without clinical evidence of vascular disease, I found there was a variable increase of segmental spread ranging from nil to 42 per cent, with an average of 25 per cent increased spread (Bromage, unpublished data).

Thus, three known conditions give rise to unusually extensive epidural spread:

Condition	***Average Increased Epidural Spread***
1. Severe arteriosclerosis	+42%
2. Controlled diabetes mellitus	+25%
3. Pregnancy at term and other conditions involving inferior vena caval obstruction and distended extradural veins	+30%

Failure to recognize the need for reduced dosage in these patients is likely to result in excessive segmental spread from *relative* overdosage, with a clinical picture that is very similar to that of massive subarachnoid injection. The distinguishing feature between the two is the speed of onset and spread of blockade, which is rapid for massive subarachnoid injection but much slower in the case of epidural overdose. Treatment is precisely the same as for massive subarachnoid injection, but since the onset is slower in relative overdose, there is more time to institute supportive measures.

Gadgetry is always at risk to go wrong, and mechanical or gravity-controlled systems for continuous or intermittent epidural administration may run out of control and cause a dangerously extensive blockade. The following case report by Edmonds-Seal (1964) is illustrative of this sort of danger:

CASE REPORT

A 63-year-old chronic bronchitic underwent left upper lobectomy for carcinoma of the lung.

An epidural catheter was inserted at the fifth thoracic interspace to provide postoperative pain relief. A closed plastic drip system was set up containing 1 per cent lidocaine, and 5 to 6 ml of this solution were allowed to drip in three times per day, with excellent relief of pain. On the evening of the second postoperative day the patient was found collapsed and twitching. His blood pressure was 60/? mm Hg, and he was analgesic in all segments up to the eighth cervical. The drip system was found to be running in spite of the fact that all four safety clips had been firmly closed on the inflow tubing. A total of 174 ml of lidocaine (i.e., 1740 mg) had been given inadvertently over the course of two hours. The patient recovered quickly.

Comment

A devil lurks in every machine. In this case the occluding clips on the lidocaine reservoir were faulty. I have encountered a similar but less florid accident after an enterprising patient had surreptitiously opened the infusion line himself. Fortunately the drip was noticed and shut off before serious harm was done.

Epidural Intravenous Injection

Puncture of an epidural vein is a relatively frequent occurrence, but bleeding usually stops within a short time. The danger of prolonged bleeding in patients with coagulation defects will be considered later under Neurological Complications.

Direct venous puncture from a needle or by inadvertent venous cannulation with a catheter occurs in about 1 per cent of cases, and then most commonly in pregnant patients at term with distended epidural veins. This technical error occurs less frequently if the needle is inserted precisely in the midline away from the lateral parts of the space where the veins are more densely clustered.

Injection of local anesthetic directly into an epidural vein is very likely to give rise to toxic effects from systemic action of the local anesthetic, with convulsions and possible cardiovascular collapse (Youngman, 1956; Hylton et al., 1964; Duncalf and Foldes, 1964). The influence of epidural venous dynamics on the outcome of an intravenous epidural bolus of local anesthetic has been discussed in Chapter 3. Treatment involves the following:

1. Diminish epidural venous flow and encourage optimal venous return through the inferior vena cava *by turning the patient into the lateral position*. This is particularly important in pregnant women at term, and it is a crucial step that is often forgotten.

2. Suppress convulsions with 5 to 15 mg of intravenous diazepam. If convulsions persist, institute neuromuscular paralysis with 50 to 80 mg of succinylcholine.

3. Administer oxygen by mask, or by cuffed endotracheal tube if apnea has ensued. Endotracheal intubation in the lateral position is not difficult, and anesthesiologists should accustom themselves to this maneuver.

4. Use a vasopressor agent if necessary to counteract arterial hypotension. Ephedrine, 15 to 30 mg intravenously, is adequate. Patients who have been receiving reserpine may have depleted norepinephrine stores, making them unresponsive to ephedrine, in which case a dilute norepinephrine infusion of 2μg/ml at the rate of 4 μg/min may be necessary for a short period of time.

Inadvertent intravenous injection should be studiously avoided by:

1. Very gentle insertion of the epidural catheter in the midline.

2. Aspiration through the catheter before it is taped in place at induction.

3. Routine use of a test dose through the catheter.

4. Aspiration through the catheter before a "top-up" dose is reinjected. Any trace of blood in the catheter or attached syringe should give warning that the catheter may have entered a vein. Very rarely a catheter may find its way into a vein although previous injections were normal (Ryan, 1973), so this remote possibility should be borne in mind.

Headache

Headaches may arise independent of dural puncture or epidural block. Headache from other unrelated causes is quite frequent, particularly in obstetrical patients. Figures from two centers in Britain showed very little difference between the incidence of headache in obstetrical patients receiving epidural analgesia and in those who did not, with a rate of about 10 to 20 per cent in both (Moir and Davidson, 1972; Crawford, 1972; Grove, 1973).

When the dura is accidentally punctured with a large needle in the size range of 18 to 16 gauge, the incidence of headache is much higher and stands at about 70 to 80 per cent (Arner, 1952; Crawford, 1972; Craft et al., 1973). Thus, accidental dural puncture is a cause of serious discomfort and possibly prolonged hospital stay, and it should not be accepted lightly as a regular minor annoyance inherent in the technique. It must be emphasized that dural puncture should not happen more than once in 100 cases. If it does, then something is wrong with the anesthesiologist's routine that needs to be changed.

The prevention and management of postdural puncture headache have been discussed fully in Chapter 6. Two approaches to treatment may be summarized as follows:

Conservative

1. Discourage cerebrospinal fluid leakage by rest and recumbency.
2. Encourage cerebrospinal fluid formation by hydration with oral or intravenous fluids or both.
3. Provide dural support by raising the extradural venous pressure with a tight abdominal binder.
4. Administer systemic analgesics.

Active

1. Administer extradural saline injections or infusions (Rice and Dabbs, 1950; Kaplan and Arrowood, 1952; Crawford, 1972; Craft et al., 1973).
2. Perform an epidural autologous blood patch (Gormley, 1960; DiGiovanni and Dunbar, 1970; DiGiovanni et al., 1972; Ostheimer et al., 1974).

In the event of accidental dural puncture, the order of procedure should be as follows: conservative prophylactic treatment first for 24 hours, combined with epidural saline by continuous infusion of 1.0 to 1.5 liters or by intermittent injections of 40 to 60 ml. If severe headache persists for more than 24 hours, an autologous blood patch may be performed and shortly afterward the patient allowed out of bed.

Backache

The incidence of backache after a successful and atraumatic epidural block is no higher than that in a normal surgical population receiving general anesthesia. Lund (1966) places the incidence at 2 per cent, although higher rates are found in some other series (Moore, 1969). In an obstetrical population the incidence is much higher, about 30 to 40 per cent in a normal control group, and again the occurrence rate is the same whether an epidural block is used or not (Moir and Davidson, 1972; Crawford, 1972; Grove, 1973).

Inadvertent injection of a large volume of solution into tissues around the epidural space may cause transient backache for a day or so that is worse on ambulation and relieved by rest. A personal experience of this nature followed an intended epidural injection of 50 ml 1/600 Nupercaine at the second lumbar interspace for experimental purposes. Injection was mistakenly made superficial to the ligamentum flavum, and aching pain accompanied the last few milliliters. I experienced low back pain and discomfort, which became worse on walking when the local anesthetic effects wore off several hours later, but symptoms disappeared after 36 hours without further sequelae.

Bladder Dysfunction

Disturbance of micturition and retention of urine are common after many operations regardless of the type of anesthesia used. The incidence of bladder dysfunction after gynecological and obstetrical procedures is high and in the region of 30 per cent (Järvinen et al., 1961), but the incidence is not appreciably affected by using epidural analgesia (Moir and Davidson, 1972; Crawford, 1972; Grove, 1973). Epidural blockade may increase the incidence of retention if it is carried on after operation to provide postoperative pain relief. Holmdahl et al. (1972) found a 90 per cent incidence of retention throughout the duration of continuous lumbar blockade, but with continuous thoracic segmental block most patients are able to micturate spontaneously.

Wrong Solution

Any patient with a catheter line opening into one of his body cavities is at risk of receiving an erroneous injection from someone misreading or failing to read an ampule or a labeled syringe. As an example of how easily this can happen, I narrowly missed becoming a statistic in this category while the subject of an experiment when a collaborator injected an intravenous bolus of 1 mg of norepinephrine from a clearly labeled syringe, thinking it was atropine; the resulting hypertension and left ventricular failure were dramatic but transient. Ampules must be carefully read; charged syringes attached to catheters must be clearly labeled, with identification of the contents and dose, and the label should be checked before the contents are injected.

The epidural space appears to be relatively tolerant of abuse, for a variety of startlingly inappropriate solutions have been erroneously injected into it without apparent harm. On the other hand, there have been tragedies. Usubiaga (1975) reported two cases of paraplegia, one arising from an erroneous injection of epidural collodion and the other from injection of hypertonic saline, but details of concentration were not given. The latter case involving hypertonic saline is surprising, as the subarachnoid space appears to tolerate appreciable amounts of 8 to 10 per cent brine without permanent effect (Squire et al., 1974). Thiopental has been erroneously injected into the epidural space without ill effects (Forestner and Raj, 1975). Potassium chloride has also been injected inadvertently, with resulting profound motor blockade and depolarizing spasms lasting for four hours, but without any untoward effects. Details of the case are as follows:

INADVERTENT EPIDURAL INJECTION OF 6.4 PER CENT POTASSIUM CHLORIDE

A fit 48-year-old man, 72 inches tall, underwent gastrectomy. Anesthesia was provided by continuous epidural analgesia and light endotracheal nitrous oxide and oxygen. An epidural catheter was inserted at T_{12}–L_1, and 23 ml of 2 per cent prilocaine with 1/200,000 epinephrine produced analgesia to T_4–T_5. The operation was uneventful, and the patient awoke immediately and commenced deep breathing exercises in comfort. The patient was nursed in the recovery ward for surveillance of postoperative analgesia and physiotherapy. The first postoperative "top-up" epidural dose consisted of 17 ml of 1.2 per cent prilocaine with 1/350,000 epinephrine; this provided complete relief of postoperative pain for about two hours, with little or no motor block of the legs.

When analgesia regressed and pain returned, the recovery room was busy and the anesthesiologist in charge was attending to several sick patients. He decided to reinstate the block with 14 ml of 1.15 per cent lidocaine using a mixture of 8 ml of 2 per cent lidocaine diluted with 6 ml saline. The patient in the next bed was about to receive a potassium supplement to his intravenous solution, consisting of 40 mEq of 15 per cent potassium chloride. In error, the anesthesiologist mistook the ampule of potassium chloride for saline and diluted the lidocaine with 15 per cent KCl. The resultant mixture consisted of 14 ml of 1.15 per cent lidocaine, 1/350,000 epinephrine and 6.43 per cent KCl; this was injected through the epidural catheter.

The resulting blockade was profound. Abdominal pain was completely relieved and skin analgesia extended to T_5. There was intense motor block below this level, with complete immobility of the legs. The patient was comfortable, but the anesthesiologist, discovering his error, was in an agony of anxiety. Intravenous corticosteroids were administered in the hope of reducing any epidural edema. One hour after injection of the potassium mixture, the patient complained of cramping pain in the legs and abdomen up to the level of T_6, accompanied by pain in the lumbar spine. Two hours after injection analgesia had receded to T_{10}, but complete motor paralysis of the legs persisted. Motor power of the legs returned four hours after injection, but residual analgesia was still present in the left buttock. By the sixth hour all sensation and movement were normal. Recovery was normal, and there were no sequelae.

Comment

This case illustrates several practical points:

1. The essential need for constant vigilance in identifying solutions for injection.

2. The unsuitability of potassium salts as adjuvants for local anesthetic solutions (this is discussed in Chapter 3). This episode involved a strong concentration of potassium chloride, and the transient symptoms of backache may have been partly due to the irritant effects of a hyperosmolar solution in the epidural space. However, the complaints of cramps and spasms were probably due to depolarizing phenomena arising from a high extracellular concentration of potassium (Bromage and Burfoot, 1966).

3. Corticosteroids may be helpful in limiting reactive edema after a chemical or osmotic insult such as this one. They should be given early, *however.*

Methemoglobinemia

Methemoglobinemia is mentioned only for the sake of completeness, for it is not strictly a complication of epidural analgesia as such, but it arises from systemic absorption of epidural drugs that may give rise to the condition. Prilocaine (Citanest) is the classic example of a local anesthetic that may cause methemoglobinemia. While in other respects prilocaine is a dependable drug with low acute toxicity, it rapidly breaks down to form orthotoluidine; this metabolic product enters the red cells, interfering with the redox mechanism and allowing hemoglobin to become oxidized to methemoglobin.

The amount of methemoglobin found is not likely to be significant if the total dose of prilocaine does not exceed 600 mg (Fujimori et al., 1964). If methemoglobinemia does occur, it is readily corrected by a single intravenous injection of 1 mg/kg methylene blue (Finch, 1948; Mangelsdorff, 1956). However, during labor quite small amounts of prilocaine cause significant degrees of methemoglobinemia in the fetus, and the UV/M ratio for prilocaine is appreciably higher than for other local anesthetics. For these reasons prilocaine is not considered a suitable drug for routine epidural use in obstetrics.

Broken Epidural Catheters

This complication was mentioned in Chapter 7. The causes of broken catheters are:

1. *Shearing at the needle tip.* Difficulty is sometimes encountered in advancing the catheter more than a centimeter or so beyond the tip of the needle. The beginner is tempted to withdraw the catheter with the needle still in place. Do not do this. If the catheter is bent at its exit from the Tuohy needle, traction on the catheter may cause the upper edge of the needle orifice to shear through the catheter, leaving the distal piece sequestered in the epidural space. If the catheter will not advance, take the needle and catheter out together as one unit and then remove the catheter from the needle before reinserting the needle.

2. *Brittle catheters.* Some types of plastic catheter tend to become hard and brittle if left in place for several days, and then they may break at or below the skin surface. Today modern catheters are more robust than formerly, and some materials such as Teflon are almost unbreakable. However, for other reasons catheters should not be left in place for more than 72 hours; tissue reaction around the tip tends to seal off the catheter in a fibrin pocket, and then further injection becomes painful and ineffective. In prolonged therapeutic block the catheter should be changed every third day, an adjacent space being used for a fresh insertion.

3. *Laminar "pincer."* In some postures the laminae or spinal ligaments of osteoarthritic patients may grip the catheter as in a vice, making withdrawal very difficult. In this situation thin-walled catheters may become flattened and completely occluded, and patency may be restored only after flexion of the back (Kaufman and Reynolds, 1976). Forceful traction against the resistance may break the catheter. Methodical movement of the patient's back through extension, flexion or rotation of the spine with simultaneous gentle traction will usually find a posture that allows the catheter to slide out easily.

4. *Knotted catheters.* As mentioned in Chapter 7, this is an extremely rare phenomenon related to insertion of too great a length of catheter into the epidural space. We experienced one instance of this problem in over 30,000 epidural catheterizations. Most complications from catheters, such as foraminal escape, intravascular or intradural injection and

knots, are due to the mistake of inserting too much catheter into the epidural space. A length of 4 cm is quite sufficient and is short enough to keep out of serious trouble. If a knot should form, great gentleness, firmness and persistence are needed to ease out the knot without breaking the catheter.

Management of broken catheters

Traditionally, sequestered foreign bodies should be removed. If the material is inert, however, the risk of locating and removing it at open operation may outweigh the danger of leaving it behind in the body. Breaks at or just below the skin are easily dealt with by a small skin incision made under local anesthesia. The broken distal piece is grasped with a curved hemostat and drawn out by firm, gentle traction. Deep breaks within the spinal canal pose the more difficult question of whether to ignore the sequestered piece or remove it, possibly with the aid of radiography.

Opinions differ about the wisdom of using radiopaque catheters to aid localization. Personally, I have doubts and lean toward nonradiopaque catheters for the following reasons:

1. The visual density of currently available radiopaque catheters is so similar to bone that identification is difficult in a radiograph or with an image intensifier. For clear radiographic localization, the lumen of the catheter must be filled with contrast medium, such as Pantopaque or Hypaque.
2. Broken catheters in the lumbar region are very difficult to find at laminectomy, even with the help of X-rays.
3. A radiograph showing a broken piece of catheter is a permanent temptation for some enthusiast to subject the patient to a fruitless exploratory laminectomy, for the broken piece will almost certainly defy surgical search. This temptation is heightened if the patient complains of backache from any cause.
4. By the same token, in this age of prevalent litigation, a radiogram of a broken catheter might be regarded as a potential godsend by a lawyer looking for grounds to bring legal suit against the anesthesiologist.
5. A great deal of plastic material is deliberately buried in human tissues for prosthetic reasons every day with great success, and there is no evidence to support the assumption that a small segment of epidural catheter will cause any harm in the extradural space. Experiments with cats show that implanted epidural catheters become walled off by fibrous tissue after about three weeks, and a small piece of broken catheter will undergo the same kind of sequestration, remaining immured and innocuous within the epidural space. Very rarely, persistent symptoms may force an exploratory laminectomy and search for the foreign body. However, in the absence of symptoms, it is best to leave well enough alone.

Thus, a small piece of broken catheter in the lumbar region should probably be left where it is. A broken caudal catheter is somewhat different. Exploration of the caudal canal is technically easier than that of the lumbar spinal canal, and the prospects of finding a broken piece of catheter are greater if one enters through the sacrococcygeal membrane or a small trephination of the laminae of the sacrum (Chun and Karp, 1966).

In the event of a broken catheter, the patient should be informed and reassured, and the respective risks of masterly inactivity and enthusiastic exploration should be fully explained. The episode should be fully and carefully documented in the hospital record. If a radiopaque catheter has been used, then radiographs in two planes should become part of the permanent record.

NEUROLOGICAL COMPLICATIONS

Trauma

Damage to the spinal cord or nerve roots is one of the most feared complications of epidural anesthesia. Danger of direct trauma to the cord is exceedingly remote if epidural puncture is made below the tip of the conus medullaris. The adult spinal cord usually ends between the lower border of the first lumbar vertebra and the upper border of the second, but in infants the cord extends to L_3. Puncture below the second lumbar vertebra is therefore a prudent course for all but the highly skilled anesthesiologist.

Trauma to neural tissue by a needle or an epidural catheter is accompanied by pain. Any complaint of pain during induction or insertion of the catheter should be taken as an urgent signal to stop and wait until the patient can be questioned and the nature of the pain evaluated. Never persist in injecting solution or advancing a needle or catheter if the patient complains of pain or shows any signs of discomfort. The warning sign of pain is removed if the patient is asleep under general anesthesia, and for this reason it is wise to induce blockade with the patient fully conscious and responsive (Mostert, 1958). Very rarely, it may be necessary to induce epidural analgesia in an unconscious patient—an example of such a case is given on page 639—and then extreme care and gentleness should be used.

Bonica and his colleages (1957) reported one case of direct trauma to the cord in an analysis of 3,637 peridural blocks. Briefly, this case was as follows:

A resident anesthesiologist attempted a thoracic epidural puncture at the eighth thoracic interspace for anesthesia in a 76-year-old woman scheduled for cholecystectomy. Apparently the needle was placed correctly, but following a test dose of 3 ml of 2 per cent lidocaine, resistance to further injection was encountered. The needle was advanced deeper, using the loss-of-resistance test until the patient complained bitterly of severe lancinating pain in the right side of the trunk. The needle was withdrawn slightly and the pain stopped. No cerebrospinal fluid could be aspirated, but injection of saline did not meet any appreciable resistance. Concluding that the needle was now in the epidural space, 10 ml of 2 per cent lidocaine were injected. This was followed by all the signs of a massive subarachnoid injection, with apnea lasting 30 minutes and unconsciousness for one hour. The operation was cancelled, and on awakening there was lancinating pain in the left trunk, together with a sensory deficit from T_5–L_1 *on the right side and from* L_1–S_5 *on the left, with loss of the left patellar reflex. There were electromyographic signs of denervation, and the patient made a gradual recovery attended by complete alleviation of her gallbladder symptoms. The clinical outcome of this case was attributed to direct trauma to the right side of the thoracic cord.*

In trying to analyze the technical problems lying behind this accident, I would suspect that the patient was the victim of a sticky syringe during attempts at the loss-of-resistance test. The case emphasizes three practical points mentioned earlier.

1. Extreme caution must be exercised in the thoracic region. It is no place to blunder about, and the anesthesiologist should try another space if there is the slightest doubt about the accurate placement of his needle.

2. Complaints of lancinating pain are imperative calls to desist and to try elsewhere.

3. A sticky syringe is the major pons asinorum of the loss-of-resistance test, and for this reason an air-filled oscillating system is far safer than the theoretically ideal fluid-filled system, as explained in Chapter 6.

The following case history reported to me by the patient is another instance of possible mechanical trauma to the cord.

A healthy, vigorous man in his early forties received a single-injection epidural block for an upper abdominal operation. An injection of 20 ml of mepivacaine was made at the tenth thoracic interspace. During injection the patient experienced a lancinating pain in his left flank radiating down the left leg. Analgesia extended to the fourth thoracic segment. The operation was completely satisfactory, but postoperatively a bizarre type of sensory and motor loss remained, involving complete motor and sensory paralysis extending from T_{10}–L_5 on the left side only, with sympathetic paralysis from C_5–L_5 on both sides.

Sudomotor function gradually returned on the right but not on the left, and years later there was still a persistent sensory deficit from T_{10}–L_5 on the left. Motor paralysis slowly recovered, but weakness and wasting of the left vastus medialis remained. Thirteen years later there was still residual footdrop on the left side.

Comment

The precise nature and location of this lesion are highly speculative, but the complaint of sharp, radiating pain on induction suggests a traumatic origin, possibly to a spinal root, with tracking of injected solution into the subdural space and temporary pressure effects on neighboring roots and cord.

A third case of probable trauma to the cord again illustrates the common factor of a high site of puncture above the termination of the conus medullaris (Honkomp, 1966).

A 28-year-old woman was scheduled for right-sided nephropexy. Epidural analgesia was attempted at T_{11}–T_{12}, but the patient complained of severe pain in the back, and blood dripped from the needle. Bleeding did not stop after 10 ml of saline were flushed through the needle, so the block was abandoned, and the operation was performed under general anesthesia.

Postoperatively there was weakness, loss of sensation and areflexia of the left leg, and the abdominal reflexes were absent on the left side. Trophic ulcers developed over the left knee and ankle. A myelogram was not performed. Eighteen months later the neurological situation had not improved appreciably.

Comment

Evaluation of this case appears to have been somewhat incomplete. No radiographic or electromyographic investigations were reported. Nevertheless, direct trauma to the cord is suggested by the history of severe back pain during attempted epidural puncture, followed by localized sensory and motor loss on the opposite side to the site of operation.

These three cases emphasize a point that is self-evident but often forgotten—that is, inept attempts at epidural puncture at *any* level above the termination of the conus medullaris may lead to injury of the cord. This danger is avoided in adults by ensuring that the site of puncture is below the second lumbar vertebra, while in children the needle should be inserted even lower down because of the more caudal extension of the cord. Higher levels of puncture should be reserved strictly for experts with an irreproachable record of technical accuracy.

It cannot be repeated too often that great gentleness, precision and manual control are the basic essentials for technical success in epidural analgesia, and for avoiding trauma and complications. Textbook descriptions sometimes fail to emphasize this point and even go so far as to allow unconsciously violent phrases to creep into common parlance, such as "advance the needle until it *strikes* bone." Instructions of this sort are scarcely an encouragement to the precise gossamer touch that must be cultivated in any form of regional anesthesia. Some physicians do not possess the necessary psychomotor control to be let loose with a long, potentially dangerous needle, and if coordination is substandard it is wiser and kinder to guide the individual's skills to other fields.

Epidural Hematomas

Epidural hematomas may occur spontaneously in apparently normal patients and in the absence of anticoagulant therapy. Thirty-two cases of spontaneous epidural hematoma had been reported in the literature by 1960 (Lougheed and Hoffman, 1960), and by 1967 the total exceeded 50 cases (Bidzinski, 1966; Markham et al., 1967; Cooper, 1967). Spontaneous epidural hematomas are more likely to arise during anticoagulant therapy, and they may occur in the absence of any overt precipitating cause (Winer et al., 1959; Gold, 1963; Spurning, 1964; Jacobson et al., 1966; Binnert et al., 1971; Sreerama et al., 1973). Hematoma formation may also follow minimal trauma to epidural veins in the presence of clotting abnormalities (Bromage, 1954; Gingrich, 1968; Butler and Green, 1970; De Angelis, 1972; Cousins, 1972; Varkey and Brindle, 1974). The problem of choosing and managing epidural blockade in the face of heparinization is discussed more fully in Chapter 7. Increasing use of low-dose heparin prophylaxis against thromboembolism may make this decision more difficult in the future (Kakkar et al., 1975). A need exists for a reliable routine method for assay of plasma heparin (Yin et al., 1973; Denson and Bonnar, 1973; Cooke et al., 1976), so that safe criteria can be established for using both minimal-dose heparin and epidural analgesia when clinical indications exist for employing the two forms of therapy simultaneously. For example, obese patients undergoing major abdominal surgery are high-risk subjects both for deep vein thrombosis and for pulmonary complications arising from inadequate respiratory movements and retained tracheobronchial secretions. In this type of patient, continuous epidural blockade and low-dose heparin are both indicated; unfortunately, at present, routine methods of monitoring the coagulation system and factors that may lead to epidural hematoma formation are indirect and relatively imprecise (see Chapter 7, "Minidose Heparin Prophylaxis").

Spinal cord compression may develop rapidly from uncontrolled bleeding in the epidural space. During heparin administration, early myelographic examination should be done if the patient complains of pain in the back or legs or weakness of the legs, and urgent laminectomy should be performed if there are any clinical or radiological signs of spinal cord compression. Recovery is unlikely if laminectomy is delayed, and only two instances of spontaneous recovery have been recorded in over 100 cases that were not decompressed at an early stage (Harik et al., 1971).

Nerve palsy can also arise from hemorrhage outside the spinal canal. A case of right-sided femoral nerve palsy (L_2, L_3, L_4) has been described due to a spontaneous hematoma arising in the psoas muscle secondary to anticoagulant therapy unassociated with any surgery or anesthesia. The hematoma was evacuated, but no improvement had taken place six weeks later (Coupier et al., 1974).

The following case histories from the literature illustrate the sudden and often devastating course of spinal epidural hematoma associated with anticoagulant therapy:

CASE NO. 1 (FRUMIN AND SCHWARTZ, 1952)

Continuous epidural analgesia with a ureteric catheter was performed for femoral embolectomy and treatment of postoperative arterial spasm. An epidural hematoma developed after heparinization. Spinal cord compression resulted in prolonged loss of function in the lower part of the body.

CASE NO. 2 (BROMAGE, 1954)

Left femoral embolectomy was carried out in a 72-year-old man under continuous epidural block. The epidural catheter was left in place to prolong sympathetic blockade and promote vasodilatation. The patient was heparinized to avoid further clot formation in the femoral artery. Thirty-six hours after operation the patient died of massive hemorrhage into the left leg. At postmortem examination a large hematoma was also found in the epidural space, but this had not given rise to symptoms of cord compression in the last hours of life.

CASE NO. 3 (GINGRICH, 1968)

A 73-year-old patient presented with signs of left femoral artery occlusion three years after insertion of an aortoiliac Dacron prosthesis. Continuous epidural analgesia resulted in some improvement. Intravenous infusion of heparin was started 16 hours after the epidural catheter was inserted. The next day the patient complained of severe lumbar pain, and the epidural catheter was removed. Paralysis of the legs rapidly developed over the next six hours, with hypalgesia and paresis below T_{10}. Prompt surgical evacuation of an epidural hematoma was carried out. Partial recovery followed over the next few months.

CASE NO. 4 (BUTLER AND GREEN, 1970)

A left tibial embolectomy was performed in a 70-year-old man under continuous epidural analgesia. Intravenous heparinization with an initial dose of 10,000 units of heparin was started one hour after placement of the epidural catheter, and the catheter was removed after 13 hours. Twenty-four hours after operation the patient complained of severe back pain, but no neurological signs were evident for another hour, when the patient began to complain of numbness in the hands. Three hours after the initial complaint of back pain there was progressive numbness, dyspnea and sensory loss to the level of T_2. Myelography showed spinal compression at L_2 and C_3. Cervical and lumbar laminectomy showed a large liquid hematoma extending the whole length of the spine.

Postoperatively the sensory level dropped to T_8–T_9, but no further recovery occurred. The patient died three weeks later.

CASE NO. 5 (HELPERIN AND COHEN, 1971)

A 76-year-old man received a large dose of lidocaine (22 ml of 2 per cent lidocaine with 1/200,000 epinephrine and 0.2 per cent tetracaine) through a Cheng needle at L_3–L_4. A catheter was passed, and this caused transient paresthesia in the right leg, but no solution was injected up the catheter at any time. Seventy-five minutes later 5,000 units of heparin was given IV, and the epidural catheter was removed at the end of operation 70 minutes afterward. No blood was present in the catheter. A further 5,000 units of heparin were given at three hours and again at seven hours postoperatively. Twelve hours after operation the patient developed anesthesia of the saddle area and lower legs, with motor weakness of the right foot. A myelogram on the sixth day showed a spinal block at L_2–L_4. At laminectomy a large adherent hematoma was found on the right side of the spinal canal between L_2 and L_4. The patient regained very little function in his legs and died two years later.

CASE NO. 6 (De ANGELIS, 1972, QUOTING K. HELLMAN'S PERSONAL COMMUNICATION)

Exploratory laparotomy was performed under epidural anesthesia in an 80-year-old man. Two days later he suffered a myocardial infarction and was treated with anticoagulants. Paraplegia developed and death followed shortly afterward. A presumptive diagnosis of epidural hematoma was made. However, the paraplegia might also have been due to an embolus arising from the endocardial surface of the infarcted myocardium.

CASE NO. 7 (JANIS, 1971)

A 76-year-old man with chronic obstructive lung disease and hypertensive congestive failure underwent satisfactory open reduction of a fractured hip under continuous epidural analgesia. The epidural catheter was left in place to provide postoperative analgesia. Anticoagulant therapy was started three hours after operation with 100 mg heparin (i.e., 12,000 units), followed by 100 mg heparin every six hours for 24 hours. Protamine, 25 mg, was given 34 hours after heparin treatment was begun to reverse the anticoagulant effect, and the epidural catheter was removed two hours later. Fifteen hours after the catheter was removed, the patient was unable to move his legs, and there was sensory loss below T_{10}. In view of his poor condition, conservative therapy was tried, and epidural aspiration and lavage were carried out through 16-gauge needles at the first to fourth lumbar interspaces. Further epidural aspiration was carried out one hour later after myelography showed a block at L_1–L_2 and L_3–L_4. Steroid therapy was instituted, but no recovery took place.

CASE NO. 8 (VARKEY AND BRINDLE, 1974)

An active 70-year-old hypertensive farmer was given epidural analgesia through a Teflon catheter at L_3–L_4 for relief of pain following a left popliteal embolus. Pain relief was provided by administration of 5-ml doses of 1 per cent mepivacaine every three hours.

Intravenous heparin was started 20 minutes after induction of epidural analgesia and continued for the next 72 hours. Twenty-four hours after induction of epidural analgesia, the patient complained of urinary incontinence, and at 48 hours severe low back pain accompanied subsequent doses of epidural solution.

Above-the-knee amputation was performed at 72 hours, the same epidural catheter being used to provide operative epidural analgesia. Heparin was then *discontinued. The epidural catheter was left in place for a further 48 hours to provide postoperative pain relief and was then removed. Urinary incontinence again occurred, followed by fecal incontinence eight days later. Examination suggested a cauda equina lesion with sensory and motor reflex disturbance in the distribution of L_5–S_5. Myelography showed peridural compression at L_3–L_4. Laminectomy confirmed a well-defined epidural hematoma at the same level. The hematoma was evacuated, but this was not followed by any appreciable neurological improvement.*

Additional cases have been reported of spinal hemorrhage and compression following lumbar puncture for diagnostic reasons (De Angelis, 1972) or for subarachnoid block (Lerner et al., 1973). These reports confirm the need for great vigilance in patients who are given anticoagulant therapy and for urgency in making a prompt diagnosis and performing surgical decompression if back pain or any other signs of epidural hematoma should arise. Binnert et al. (1971) have reviewed 60 cases of spinal epidural hematoma from the literature, and they point out that ten of these patients who underwent laminectomy within 12 hours made satisfactory recoveries, whereas the remainder who were delayed beyond this point all suffered permanent paraplegia. A 12-hour delay is therefore maximum, and clearly it is desirable to relieve spinal compression at an even earlier stage.

Subdural Hematoma

Bleeding may also occur in the subdural space, and although hematoma at this site has not been documented as a complication of epidural anesthesia, the possibility should be borne in mind. Symptoms are very similar to those of epidural hematoma, and the need for prompt surgical exploration and decompression is equally urgent. The following case summary, unrelated to epidural blockade, illustrates the difficulty of making an accurate diagnosis, but at the same time it demonstrates the successful outcome of early decompression.

CASE NO. 9: ACUTE SPINAL SUBDURAL HEMATOMA (ZILKHA AND NICOLETTI, 1974)

A 26-year-old woman had an abscess of the occipital scalp drained. Two weeks later she fell on her back, but she had no immediate pain or weakness. Over the next week she gradually developed pain, weakness and numbness of the right leg, and she was unable to walk. She was found to have a fever of 104°F, weakness and diminished reflexes in both legs, and diminished sensation below L_3. There was tenderness over the second, third and fourth lumbar spines. Bleeding and clotting times were normal. Subsequent blood cultures grew Staphylococcus aureus. *The diagnosis appeared to be septicemia and lumbar epidural abscess secondary to scalp abscess. Antibiotic therapy was instituted, and lumbar laminectomy revealed a clear epidural space, but a purple, tense dura enclosed a subdural clot. Evacuation of the hematoma was followed by a complete neurological recovery. During the next few days the patient continued to have fever, and a fluctuant mass of the right thigh developed. This proved to be a deep abscess extending down to the periosteum of the right femur and containing 500 ml of staphylococcal pus.*

Comment

This case was not associated with epidural anesthesia, but the remarkably confusing clinical picture illustrates the great difficulty that is often experienced in pinpointing the precise origin of neurological sequelae to trauma, including possible trauma from epidural blockade. The case was investigated very thoroughly and efficiently, and its difficulty emphasizes one point of specific relevance that can be extended to complications following epidural blockade: it is futile to speculate about the etiology of neurological complications in the absence of sound investigation and proper documentation.

Although concurrent septicemia misled the diagnosis, in any event treatment was correct. Signs of compression from pus or blood in the spinal canal call for the same urgent approach—that is, immediate laminectomy and decompression.

Anterior Spinal Artery Syndrome

The vascular supply to the cord is tenuous and vulnerable to ischemic damage from atheroma or acute hypotension, particularly in "watershed" areas between the nutrient territory of the thoracic radicular artery and the radicularis magna of Adamkiewicz. The spinal arteries have very little resting tone, and they are poorly responsive to vasoactive agents in comparison with the rest of the circulation (Abraham et al., 1966; Mellander and Johansson, 1968). Thus, the spinal cord blood flow is largely determined by inflow pressure and outflow resistance. Dangerous impairment of cord capillary flow is most likely to occur if low arterial inflow pressure is associated with venous engorgement and a high outflow venous pressure from obstruction to major venous pathways, as may occur in compression of the inferior vena cava.

The anterior spinal artery syndrome is characterized by predominant motor weakness in the legs caused by ischemia of the anterior two thirds of the lower cord. The large motor cells lying deep in the anterior horn nuclei in the caudal parts of the cord are particularly liable to ischemic damage during low-flow states (Gilles and Nag, 1971). Any sensory loss is relatively minor and patchy, and due to associated ischemic necrosis of the posterior roots rather than to damage of sensory elements within the cord itself (Hughes and Brownell, 1966).

Epidural analgesia may come under suspicion as a contributing factor in the anterior spinal artery syndrome if epinephrine has been added to the injected solution and if arterial blood pressure has been low. At very low arterial pressure it is postulated that the local vasoconstrictor effect of the epinephrine might exceed the critical closing pressure of the anterior spinal artery, leading to collapse of the vessel and ischemia of its neural territory. At first sight this seems a likely explanation, especially in view of experimental work in dogs by Catterberg and Insausti (1964) showing slight paraplegia and spinal cord changes after epidural injections of epinephrine. However, in these animal experiments very large amounts of concentrated epinephrine were used in doses between 1.7 and 11.4 ml of 1 per cent epinephrine in dogs of 4.8 to 16 kg body weight. These experimental doses of epinephrine were about 100 to 600 times greater than those used in clinical practice, and it is doubtful if the results can be translated to the clinical situation in man. Moreover, radiographic studies by Margolis and his colleagues raise considerable doubts that epinephrine causes any appreciable degree of vasoconstriction in the larger vessels of the spinal cord (Abraham et al., 1966; Margolis, 1970). These investigators showed that the reactivity of the arterial tree of the cord is very weak in comparison with the much more powerful vasoconstrictive responses of vessels elsewhere. Experiments in monkeys performed by Wu and his colleagues (1954), in which very large amounts of intrathecal epinephrine in the range of 0.15 to 1.1 mg/kg were used, did not support the idea that these high doses of epinephrine cause paraplegia by spinal artery vasoconstriction; while some monkeys showed signs of temporary spinal analgesia lasting up to 60 minutes, all recovered completely without sequelae.

Unfortunately, a number of cases have been reported of an anterior spinal artery type of paraplegia following epidural analgesia, and the question arises, were these due to the epidural epinephrine or to effects arising from epidural blockade, or were they coincidental and due to other causes? In trying to arrive at an answer, one must remember the basic hemodynamic constraints of tissue flow within the cord and ask three preliminary questions:

1. Was the arterial supply to the cord compromised by surgical interruption of nutrient arteries (e.g., section, ligature or cautery of paravertebral vessels supplying the cord)?
2. Was flow jeopardized by excessive vascular hypotension?
3. Was flow jeopardized by venous congestion and outflow obstruction?

In addition, a postoperative anterior spinal artery syndrome must be viewed against the background incidence of spontaneous arterial insufficiency of the cord arising in a nonsurgical population. Accurate figures do not exist on this point, but today, degenerative arterial disease has supplanted syphilis as one of the commonest causes of spinal cord pathology. Published reports of spontaneous paraplegia due to "spinal stroke" are frequent enough to anticipate that spontaneous coincidental paraplegia will be associated with surgery from time to time in an elderly population (Lhermitte, 1907; Gruner and Lapresle, 1962; Garland et al., 1966; Henson and Parsons, 1967; Laguna and Cravioto, 1973; Silver and Buxton, 1974) and occasionally also in young patients as a result of acute viral infections and other causes entirely unrelated to surgery and anesthesia (Sinclair, 1954). These possible causes of cord ischemia will now be discussed more fully.

EPIDURAL EPINEPHRINE

There is very little convincing evidence that epidural epinephrine can lead to cord ischemia and paraplegia when given in modest concentrations of 1/300,000 to 1/200,000. Catterberg and Insausti (1964) collected reports of 11 cases of paraplegia in South America, all of which followed epidural blockade with epinephrine-containing solutions, and this report is often quoted in support of the thesis that epidural epinephrine is potentially harmful to the spinal cord. All but one of the patients were elderly and in the age range of 60 to 75 years, and the authors concluded that the vasoconstrictive action of epinephrine probably contributed to the paraplegia. Some of the case histories mention the strength of epinephrine used, and in one of them it was as concentrated as 1/80,000, but precise details of dosage, technique and operative course were not given, and it is impossible to form an opinion about the true cause of the tragedies on the data presented. At present, the weight of clinical and experimental evidence favors the judicious use of epinephrine as a routine epidural adjuvant. In dilutions of 1/200,000 to 1/300,000 epinephrine slows systemic absorption of local anesthetic and improves the quality and duration of blockade.

As has been pointed out before, the vasculature of the cord is less reactive to vasoconstrictor agents than vessels elsewhere in the body (Margolis, 1970), and there is little evidence to support the assumption that epinephrine in this degree of dilution can cause embarrassment to the arterial supply of the cord. Nevertheless, in spite of the absence of solid experimental data, suspicion remains that epidural epinephrine *may* contribute an element of vasoconstriction in prolonged low-flow states (Usubiaga, 1975). Therefore, in the present state of uncertain knowledge, it is probably prudent to avoid epidural epinephrine when epidural blockade is used to induce controlled hypotension in arteriosclerotic subjects.

SURGICAL AND RADIOLOGICAL CAUSES OF CORD DAMAGE

Surgical interruption of nutrient vessels to the spinal cord is a well-recognized cause of paraplegia after operations close to the aorta or the spinal column (Skillman et al., 1969; Pasternak et al., 1972). In cases in which the number of nutrient vessels to the cord is reduced by surgical intervention, it is of paramount importance to maintain a good head of arterial pressure so that perfusion of the surviving vessels may have a better chance of sustaining an adequate flow of blood within the cord. Usubiaga et al. (1970) described two cases of lower limb paralysis after this type of surgery. In both cases the operations were performed under epidural blockade, and the anesthesia was cleared of blame only by incontrovertible postmortem evidence showing infarction of the neural elements involved. A number of similar cases have been described in Usubiaga's monograph on Neurological Complications following Epidural Analgesia (1975), and the reader is referred to this work for further details.

Angiographic procedures of major blood vessels may deliver excessive amounts of toxic contrast material to the spinal cord, causing paraplegia. Margolis and his colleagues have pointed out the importance of the difference in reactivity of neural and extraneural vessels in this mechanism. Spinal cord blood vessels react very little to vasoconstrictor influences, either neural or humoral, so in the presence of vasopressor stimuli, injected contrast materials are forced in a neuripetal direction and into the substance of the cord, which is unable to protect itself against the raised inflow pressure caused by extraspinal vasoconstriction (Abraham et al., 1966; Margolis, 1970).

If epidural analgesia is chosen for major angiographic procedures, it should be in full knowledge that neurological sequelae may arise from the use of contrast media and that the anesthetic procedure is likely to be considered as a possible alternative cause for any complications that may occur. Clearly, if epidural analgesia is strongly indicated for some special reason, the anesthesiologist should not shirk the risk of this imputation. However, he should remember the basic problem of differential reactivity of neural and non-neural vasculature and ensure that the blood pressure is kept on the low side of normal, taking full advantage of the peripheral vasodilatation of the epidural blockade to encourage neurifugal rather than neuripetal flow of contrast material.

Vascular hypotension

It is generally considered that acute episodes of arterial hypotension are the cause of the anterior spinal artery syndrome, based on the simple application of the law of Laplace that collapse of a vessel occurs when the intraluminal pressure falls below the critical closing tension in the vessel wall.

Forrester (1959) described two cases of paraplegia following hypotension, one after epidural analgesia and the other after ganglionic blockade, both in patients with severe arteriosclerotic disease.

CASE NO. 10: HYPOTENSIVE SPINAL ISCHEMIA AFTER EPIDURAL ANESTHESIA (FORRESTER, 1959)

Right lumbar sympathectomy was performed in a man of 57 years for intermittent claudication of the right leg. Hypotensive conditions during surgery were provided by lumbar epidural blockade combined with nitrous oxide–oxygen anesthesia. Twenty-five ml of 1.5 per cent lidocaine (i.e., 375 mg lidocaine) with 1/160,000 epinephrine were injected at T_{12}–L_1. *A second bout of hypotension to a level of 70/40 mmHg occurred one hour after operation, but this was corrected with methamphetamine. Paraplegia was observed on the following day and was permanent.*

CASE NO. 11: HYPOTENSIVE SPINAL ISCHEMIA AFTER GANGLIONIC BLOCKADE (FORRESTER, 1959)

Laryngectomy was performed in a 56-year-old man suffering from hypertension (B.P. 240/160 mmHg) and left ventricular strain. Nitrous oxide–Trilene anesthesia was used, with pentolinium to produce hypotension. The blood pressure was maintained between 65/50 and 75/60 mmHg for 100 minutes. On the following day the patient was found to be paraplegic with a sensory level at T_{10}.

Hypotensive ischemia of the cord is most likely to occur in the presence of hypovolemia and severe arterial and venous vasoconstriction. However, the condition is less likely to arise if flow is preserved by vasodilatation and by maintaining a low outflow pressure on the venous side of the capillary bed. Scrutiny of case reports of postoperative paraplegia ascribed to the anterior spinal artery syndrome often reveal that a coincidental degree of venous obstruction existed during the operation and that this may have contributed to the outcome. One often quoted case of anterior spinal artery syndrome reported by Davies, Solomon and Levene (1958) illustrates the difficulty in ascribing any one factor to the genesis of the lesion.

CASE NO. 12

A 76-year-old man with congestive heart failure and elevated jugular venous pressure underwent a bowel resection for strangulated femoral hernia under epidural analgesia.

Analgesia was induced at the first lumbar interspace with 27 ml of 1.75 per cent lidocaine + 1/300,000 epinephrine (i.e., 472 mg lidocaine and 90 μg epinephrine). Blood pressure was maintained between 80 and 90 mmHg systolic, with a total dose of 100 mg ephedrine throughout an operation that lasted 45 minutes.

An anterior spinal artery type of neurological deficit followed, confirmed microscopically at postmortem examination nine months later.

Comment

The normal dose requirements of 2 per cent lidocaine for a 76-year-old patient are about 15.6 mg/segment. The actual dose of 472 mg would therefore be expected to produce a very extensive segmental block including the cervical segments, accompanied by total sympathetic blockade. Although the patient did receive a preoperative and intraoperative blood transfusion to a total of 820 ml, arterial pressure was maintained by a large dose of vasopressor rather than by augmentation of fluid volume to match the expanded circulatory bed. In addition, there was a pre-existing degree of venous congestion.

Was the neurological outcome due to:

1. Arterial hypotension?

2. The presence of 90 μg of epidural epinephrine?

3. The combination of arterial hypotension with generalized vasoconstriction and venous engorgement?

It is impossible to say, although arterial hypotension and venous engorgement remain the most likely causes.

The same authors quote a similar case reported to them of lower limb motor paresis in a 51-year-old man following total parotidectomy for carcinoma, in which epidural blockade was used to provide controlled hypotension and a dry surgical field. In this case 25 ml of 1.75 per cent lidocaine containing 1/80,000 epinephrine was injected at T_{12}–L_1. The systolic pressure was maintained at 80 mmHg for three hours. The patient had been treated for peripheral neuritis for some years before operation, and it is likely that the hypotension exacerbated a pre-existing neurological condition and precipitated the permanent paresis.

Venous congestion

Arterial insufficiency is not the only cause of spinal cord ischemia. Venous infarction may also be a major or a contributory factor in some neurological sequelae to surgical operations.

A persistently raised venous pressure impairs capillary flow, especially in the presence of low arterial pressure from hemorrhage or sympathetic paralysis. Under these circumstances compensatory vasoconstriction can no longer raise the pressure at the arterial end of the capillary bed, and if venous pressure remains high, capillary perfusion slows or may stop.

Thus, in low-pressure states it is imperative to be sure that obstruction of venous return does not cause venous congestion in the spinal cord. Obstruction of the inferior vena cava from any cause results in engorgement of the alternative vertebral or paravertebral venous pathways, and venous pressure rises in the cord. The following cases are examples quoted from the literature in which the evidence suggests that this mechanism was a substantial cause of the neurological outcome.

CASE NO. 13: PARAPLEGIA AFTER GENERAL ANESTHESIA (DITZLER AND McIVER, 1956)

A right upper lobectomy was performed on a hypertensive 67-year-old woman in the prone Overholt position. Cyclopropane and ether anesthesia were used. Respiration was difficult to control, and 75 minutes after induction a small dose of d-tubocurarine (4.5 mg) was given. This was rapidly followed by acute hypotension in spite of a total blood loss of less than 250 ml. The blood pressure was maintained between 70 and 90 mmHg systolic until the end of the operation, but the pressure rose to normal levels as soon as the patient was turned on her back. Postoperatively there was flaccid paralysis of the legs with patchy sensory loss from T_{12}–S_5. Myelography failed to show any obstruction to flow of contrast medium, thus ruling out the possibility of a metastatic tumor compressing the cord. A diagnosis of anterior spinal artery syndrome was made.

Comment

Here, arterial hypotension appears to have been associated with possible caval compression. The stormy anesthetic course suggests a postural fault with external abdominal compression that progressed to caval compression after relaxation of the abdominal musculature by curare.

CASE NO. 14: PARAPLEGIA FOLLOWING EPIDURAL ANALGESIA (URQUHART-HAY, 1969)

Retropubic prostatectomy was performed in a fit 62-year-old man under hypotensive epidural analgesia combined with light general anesthesia. The preoperative blood pressure was 170/90 mmHg. An injection of 25 ml of 1.5 per cent lidocaine with 1/200,000 epinephrine was made at L_3–L_4. Twenty minutes later the systolic pressure had not fallen below 100 mmHg, so 10 ml of the same analgesic mixture were injected in two increments of 5 ml, 15 minutes apart, with the object of lowering the blood pressure further. The systolic pressure then settled between 80 and 90 mmHg throughout the remainder of the operation. The patient was postured throughout the operation in a 10° head-down tilt, with the legs lowered 10° to extend the hips and raise the pubis.

On the next day the patient complained of severe pain in the knees and weakness of the legs, and the anesthesiologist observed neurological findings compatible with patchy involvement of L_2–L_4 spinal segments. The neurological deficit spread, and symmetrical motor weakness developed in all segments from L_1–S_1. Plantar reflexes were absent, but there was no obvious loss of cutaneous sensibility. X-ray of the spinal column showed hypertrophic lipping of vertebrae L_4, L_5, and S_1. The patient died 16 months later, and postmortem examination showed an infarction of the lower spinal cord involving bilateral necrosis of the dorsal nerve roots and the anterior horns and demyelination in the anterolateral columns in the lower lumbar cord. The anterior spinal artery appeared normal. The report concluded with the suggestion that the mechanism of infarction lay in the combination of hypotension and the vasoconstrictive action of the epidural epinephrine.

Comment

It is instructive to review this assertion in the light of a similar case reported by the same author five years later. It should be noted that the second case described below occurred in the absence *of epidural analgesia.*

CASE NO. 15: SPINAL THROMBOPHLEBITIS AFTER PROSTATECTOMY WITH HYPOTENSIVE ANESTHESIA (URQUHART-HAY AND TEAGUE, 1974)

Retropubic prostatectomy was performed in a male of 64 years with controlled congestive cardiac failure under nitrous oxide and relaxant anesthesia. Intravenous pentolinium tartrate was used to induce arterial hypotension. The systolic blood pressure was maintained at 65 mmHg during the operation and rose to 100 mmHg at the end.

Throughout the operation the patient was postured dorsally with a 10° head-down tilt and extension of the hips to make the pubis the highest point of the body, and the legs were lowered 10°.

The immediate postoperative course was uneventful, but after the sixth day neurological signs developed in the lumbar and sacral segments. At first there was bilateral motor involvement of L_2–L_4 with diminished sensation in L_5 and S_1, but by the thirteenth day there was hypalgesia in all segments below T_{11}. The legs were wasted and weak, with paresis more marked on the left. Lumbar puncture showed normal manometry and cerebrospinal fluid.

The patient died 91 days after operation. Postmortem examination showed no abnormality in the inferior vena cava or iliac veins, and the anterior and posterior spinal arteries were normal macroscopically and microscopically.

The lumbar and lower thoracic internal and external vertebral venous plexuses were prominent and tortuous and showed perivenous fibrosis and periphlebitis. The leptomeningeal veins in the lower thoracic and lumbar regions were also prominent and tortuous. The changes were considered to be consistent with spinal thrombophlebitis. In their discussion of the case the authors speculated that the hyperextended position of the spine might have caused an osteoarthritic process to impinge on the vertebral venous plexus with subsequent thrombosis and retrograde spread to involve the leptomeningeal veins.

An alternative mechanism to include both of these cases is proposed as a more frequent danger than generally appreciated (Bromage, 1974). Various abnormal postures may cause partial or complete obstruction of the inferior vena cava with consequent shunting of venous return through anastomotic vertebral and paravertebral pathways (Brigden et al., 1950). In routine anesthetic practice the following abnormal postures are most likely to cause this redistribution of venous return:

1. The lateral jackknife position lying on the right side; caval obstruction from lying on the left side has also been described (Malatinsky and Kadlic, 1974).
2. The prone position if the abdomen is compressed from inadequate bony support of the pelvis and thorax.
3. The dorsal position in pregnant women near term.
4. The exaggerated lordotic position.

Bull (1949) described the lordotic posture as a potent cause of proteinuria due to obstruction of venous outflow from the kidney, and Sharpey-Schafer's group (Brigden et al., 1950) confirmed the dramatic cardiovascular consequences that can result from this form of inferior vena caval obstruction. Radiography in the lordotic position shows that the principal site of caval obstruction is just below the diaphragm in the suprahepatic portion of the inferior vena cava (Ranniger and Switz, 1965; Doppman et al., 1966). In addition, a further site of obstruction lies more distally where the iliac veins are stretched over the rim of a backward-tilted pelvis.

In the face of severe caval obstruction, almost the entire venous return from the legs is forced to take the azygos path back to the heart. Although no harm will occur if arterial inflow pressure is adequate to maintain a normal head of perfusion pressure across the capillary bed of the spinal cord, nevertheless the margin of safety is narrowed by IVC compression in two ways. First, extradural pressures are 2 to 8 cmH_2O higher than normal in the presence of inferior vena caval obstruction (Galbert and Marx,

1974), and the resulting slight increase of venous pressure in the spinal cord will demand a comparably raised inflow pressure at the arterial end of the capillary bed to maintain normal tissue perfusion, and the cord will thereby become less tolerant of low levels of arterial hypotension. Second, distention of the vertebral venous plexus will be further increased by raised intrathoracic pressure from any cause, such as straining or raised airway pressure, and back-pressure on the cord will be transferred directly from the thorax through the azygos vein. This will further embarrass capillary perfusion in the cord, with the added possibility of vertebral venous thrombosis from stasis in the vertebral veins.

It seems likely that these conditions may have been operative both in Ditzler and McIver's case (Case No. 13) in which vascular collapse was relieved as soon as the patient was turned from the prone surgical position, and in Urquhart-Hay's two cases in which an exaggerated lordosis was combined with controlled arterial hypotension. In the last case (Case No. 15) the postmortem findings of tortuous engorged extradural veins are in accord with an episode of extradural venous stasis and infarction, brought about by an abnormal surgical posture in the presence of severe arterial hypotension.

The lession is surely clear. Unphysiological postures may compromise normal venous return to a serious degree and throw a heavy burden on the vertebral venous system, with the added risks of arterial or venous infarction to the cord. Provided serious hypotension is avoided and mean intrathoracic pressure is not raised, epidural analgesia should not influence the risks one way or the other.

It is inevitable that epidural analgesia will come under suspicion if the technique has been used in a case of spinal infarction. However, if blockade was carried out with care and asepsis, it is almost certain that the true cause will have lain elsewhere.

CASE NO. 16: POSSIBLE ISCHEMIC NEUROPATHY (BRAHAM AND SAIA, 1958)

A 66-year-old man was treated for bladder stones. Two epidural anesthetics were given one month apart. At the second operation epidural puncture was performed at L_2*–*L_3*, but no details of dosage, management or anesthetic course are given in the report.*

Motor power in the legs failed to return after operation. On examination, sensory and motor loss were not segmentally related. Motor paralysis involved the iliopsoas and quadriceps muscles but not the lower leg, while sensation was reduced in all segments below L_3*. The patient died of cardiopulmonary complications some weeks later. At postmortem examination a nodular growth of the spinal column was found at* T_{12} *from the remains of a chordoma that had been removed five years previously, and an extension the the size of a pea had invaded the subarachnoid space. No details of the microscopic or macroscopic appearance of the spinal cord or roots are given.*

The authors concluded that local hypersensitivity of nerve roots to the anesthetic agent or chemical changes or imptirities might have accounted for the permanent paralysis.

Comment

From the data available one cannot be sure about the cause of this man's neurological complication; however, the patchy distribution of the motor and sensory deficits is more suggestive of a vascular cause than a chemical or infective agency. The tumor at T_{12} *encroaching on the subarachnoid space above the termination of the conus medullaris could have set the scene for vascular insufficiency to arise from any minor disturbance of the local circulation in a cord already teetering on the brink of ischemia (Usubiaga, 1975). It seems likely that the same outcome could have resulted from a mild degree of hypotension associated with any type of general or regional anesthesia.*

Cord Compression by Vertebral Angiomas

Hemangiomas of the vertebrae and spinal cord are relatively common lesions. In a review of 3,829 vertebral columns, Junghanns (1932) demonstrated that hemangiomas occurred to some degree in about 10 per cent of the bodies examined. These vascular formations may enlarge under any circumstances that expose them to persistently increased intraluminal pressure, as in inferior vena caval obstruction and especially in pregnancy. The resulting enlargement may encroach upon the spinal canal, causing symptoms of cord compression (Newman, 1958; Nelson, 1964), or more rarely a "steal" phenomenon may occur as blood is drained away from a nutrient artery into the hemangiomatous malformation.

Vertebral angiomas may occur at any level, but they are most commonly found in the mid-thoracic region. As in any other compressive lesion of the spine, treatment of expanding angioma lies in urgent laminectomy. In the event of neurological complications, the anesthesiologist should be aware of the possibility of this entity, so that it can enter his list of differential diagnoses and appropriate treatment can be expedited.

The following case report (courtesy of Dr. A. Eisen, Montreal Neurological Institute) is typical of the long-standing but episodic nature of symptoms arising from this type of malformation. In this instance it was not compression but a "steal" phenomenon that caused localized cord ischemia.

Mrs. K.L., age 20, had a normal first pregnancy and spontaneously delivered a 7 lb 4 oz girl without regional or general anesthesia. She had a feeling of "stiffness all over" for ten days after delivery, but this wore off, and there were no residual effects.

During her second pregnancy at age 26, she had feelings of stiffness in the legs from the fourth month on. By the fifth month the legs became weak from the knees downward, and after the sixth month she began falling about. Labor was painless except for stabs of pain down the right leg from time to time, but progress was slow and forceps delivery of a large boy weighing 8 lb 5 oz was performed under general anesthesia. Right footdrop was apparent immediately after delivery, and she required a brace for six months. The right foot remained somewhat weaker than the other from then on, and her legs tired easily when walking, but otherwise she was symptom-free for the next 16 years. At the age of 41 her legs became weak again, and she became unsteady on her feet. She had some difficulty controlling her bladder, but rectal control was unimpaired. Sexual sensation was lost. There was some weakness of dorsiflexion of the right ankle and loss of pinprick sensation in the distribution of S_1*–*S_5 *on both sides, with patchy loss of* L_5 *on the right. The ankle jerks were absent. Myelography showed evidence of an arteriovenous malformation in the mid-thoracic region. Arterial angiography at the ninth left intercostal artery showed a long region of arteriovenous malformation extending from* T_1*–*T_9*. The artery of Adamkiewicz looped upward at* T_9 *with a large ascending branch feeding into the arteriovenous malformation. The descending branch going to the sacral part of the cord was a thin, fine line deprived of flow by the competing malformation above (see Figure 2–32). The arterial feeder to the arteriovenous malformation was subsequently clipped under epidural analgesia with the patient awake, and she made an excellent recovery with symptomatic improvement.*

It is easy to see how symptoms arising from this type of spinal cord pathology would almost certainly be attributed to an epidural anesthetic if one had been given during labor or at any other crucial time during the evolution of the sacral cord ischemia.

SPINAL CONTAMINANTS

Chemical Agents

The possibility of accidental dural puncture during epidural analgesia also implies that epidural anesthetic solution may find its way into the subarachnoid space. For this reason great care must be taken to ensure that anesthetic solutions are not only sterile but also free from chemical contaminants (Craig and Habib, 1977).

Winkelman (1952) pointed out that traces of cleaning detergents may cling to needles and syringes unless the subsequent rinsing routine is exceedingly thorough, and these traces may remain as a possible source of chemical contamination leading to myelitis if introduced into the subarachnoid space. Contamination of anesthetic solutions with metal ions released from metal containers by acid solutions has also been described (Lundqvist et al., 1948), but this is not likely to present a hazard in epidural blockade, in which local anesthetic solutions are usually drawn up directly from glass containers.

Methylene blue is useful for tracing tissue planes and tracks in difficult anatomical or surgical dissections, but it must be kept strictly away from any proximity to the spinal cord. Methylene blue is intensely neurotoxic, and a number of iatrogenic tragedies have arisen from its use in the subarachnoid space (Arief and Pyzik, 1960; Evans and Keegan, 1960). In the epidural space of cats, small quantities of 1 per cent methylene blue cause permanent paralysis with acute inflammation of leptomeninges and spinal roots (Poppers et al., 1970).

From time to time long-acting local anesthetic mixtures are proposed for prolonged pain relief but are later found to be extremely dangerous when injected near the spinal cord. Efocaine is an example of such a preparation that was introduced with enthusiastic reports (Iason and Shaftel, 1952; Ansbro et al., 1952); it was injected in numerous anatomical sites, including the caudal canal. Efocaine consisted essentially of procaine base dissolved in propylene glycol and polyethylene glycol, and the procaine was supposed to be deposited gradually in the tissues as a microprecipitate. However, the solvent vehicles of this mixture were later shown to be gravely neurotoxic, and several cases of intercostal thrombosis and cord damage arose from its use (Moore et al., 1954; Clarke, Morrison and Roberts, 1955). Efocaine is now remembered as a classic warning against the enthusiastic clinical use of potentially toxic materials.*

THERAPEUTIC NEUROLYTIC INJECTIONS

The deliberate use of neurolytic solutions in the epidural space for relief of widespread intractable malignant pain was discussed in Chapter 13.

---

*See page 620 concerning the possible neurolytic effects of polyethylene glycol in corticosteroid suspensions.

Again, the warning must be repeated that this is not a routine measure to be used lightly for all types of intractable pain. It is a desperate therapy for a desperate situation, and it must be approached with the same caution and deliberation as a destructive neurosurgical procedure. The dose of neurolytic solution required in the epidural space is many times larger and more destructive than would be chosen for discrete intrathecal injection, and the consequences of depositing such a large dose accidentally in the subarachnoid space would be catastrophic.

Infection

Epidural infection

Epidural infection is a rare event, usually arising endogenously from hematogenous metastatic spread secondary to infection elsewhere in the body (Dandy, 1926; Allen and Kahn, 1932; Rankin and Flothow, 1946; Heusner, 1948; Hulme and Dott, 1954; Baker et al., 1975). *Staphylococcus aureus* is the most common infecting organism (Hancock, 1973). The neurological outcome from thrombosis, spinal cord compression and subsequent paraplegia is grave, unless the complication is diagnosed promptly and followed by urgent surgical drainage and antibiotic therapy (Sarrell and Lafia, 1954). Very rarely, infection may be confined to the subdural space between the dura mater and the arachnoid (Fraser et al., 1973). The clinical course of subdural empyema is similar to that of epidural abscess.

When paraplegia due to epidural abscess does occur, the lesions of the cord are more extensive than can be accounted for by the mechanical effects of compression alone, and infective vasculitis is probably a major factor in the irreversible myelopathy. Baker and her associates (1975) reviewed 39 cases of spinal epidural abscess over a period of 27 years at the Massachusetts General Hospital. In 38 of these cases the epidural abscess was secondary to endogenous infection. Abscess was associated with epidural analgesia in only one case, and then there were no permanent sequelae. Females were involved twice as often as males. The salient features of the disease were classic and as follows:

Signs and Symptoms	***Incidence***
Severe back pain	100% (early symptom)
Local overlying tenderness	100%
Fever	100%
Leukocytosis	100%
Nuchal rigidity	50%

CSF: protein markedly elevated (average 464 mg/100 ml); leukocytosis (approximately 100 cells/mm^3)

Myelogram: always abnormal, with some degree of obstruction to the flow of contrast medium

The evolution of the acute disease was also classically rapid and inexorable, unless surgical decompression was performed at an early stage, and in this series the time course was roughly as follows:

Interval from onset of back pain to onset of root pain: 3 days

Interval from onset to lower limb weakness: 4½ days
Interval from weakness to paraplegia: 24 hours

Epidural infection may also arise from exogenous sources following contamination by spinal or caudal injection. Fortunately, the epidural space seems relatively resistant to exogenous infection compared to the very susceptible subarachnoid space; some grave liberties have been taken without incurring the infectious sequelae that might have been expected. Undoubtedly the widespread use of powerful antibiotics has prevented some accidents that might otherwise have occurred. For example:

A woman of 36 years had a vagotomy and pyloroplasty performed under segmental thoracic epidural analgesia and light thiopental–nitrous oxide–oxygen anesthesia, 12 ml of 2 per cent lidocaine with 1/200,000 epinephrine being injected at the sixth thoracic interspace. An epidural catheter was inserted and left in place for 2½ hours during the course of operation. The anesthesiologist failed to read the sterilization indicator on the needle container, and at the end of the operation it was discovered that the epidural needle used for insertion of the catheter had been clean but not sterilized. The patient was given prophylactic ampicillin and was watched closely for the next ten days. No back tenderness, fever or neurological signs developed, and the patient remained in good health at subsequent follow-up examinations.

Comment

This account should not be taken as an encouragement to slacken routine precautions. The anesthesiologist was negligent in failing to check the sterilization indicator on his equipment, and the fact that serious trouble was avoided was almost certainly due to the prompt and successful use of antibiotic therapy.

A number of less happy instances of epidural infection have been reported in the literature. Usubiaga (1975) collected reports of 13 cases in his monograph on complications, some of these being unpublished cases reported to him personally from a South American population. The following reported cases of six caudal infections and one epidural infection are collected from the early days of continuous peridural technique. The clinical course and outcome of some of these cases might have been very different if present-day antibiotic therapy had been available at the time.

CASE NO. 1 (MANALAN, 1942)

One case of caudal epidural infection arose among the first 46 reported cases of continuous caudal analgesia for obstetrics, in which an indwelling catheter was used. Obstetrical caudal analgesia was induced using a silk woven ureteral catheter. For analgesia 30 ml of 1 per cent procaine with epinephrine were used. Staphylococcal meningitis developed during the puerperium, but complete recovery followed a critical illness. Details of clinical course and treatment were not given.

CASE NO. 2 (EDWARDS AND HINGSON, 1943)

One infection occurred in 1,000 cases of continuous caudal analgesia for childbirth, in which a malleable needle was used. A caudal peridural abscess developed. Staphylococcus aureus *was the causative organism. The patient died 31 days after delivery in spite of sulfonamide therapy. No details of the case were reported.*

CASE NO. 3 (SIEVER AND MOUSEL, 1943)

One case of caudal epidural abscess arose in a series of 300 cases of continuous caudal analgesia for childbirth, in which a nylon catheter and 1.5 per cent procaine were used. The patient was seriously ill for three weeks and then recovered after treatment with large doses of sulfonamides. No details of the clinical course were reported.

CASE NO. 4 (PEACHER AND ROBERTSON, 1944)

Continuous caudal analgesia with a ureteric catheter was employed in a 26-year-old obstetrical patient during a long labor. A total of 960 mg of 1.5 per cent Metycaine was used. After delivery sacral pain radiating down both legs developed. One week after delivery hemolytic streptococci were cultured from the sacral canal, and pus was encountered at the fourth lumbar interspace. The patient recovered after treatment with sulfathiazole.

CASE NO. 5 (PEACHER AND ROBERTSON, 1944)

Continuous caudal analgesia with a ureteric catheter was performed in a 22-year-old obstetrical patient. During labor and delivery 335 mg of 1.5 per cent Metycaine were used. Nine days after delivery the patient complained of retention of urine, low back pain and a fever of 103°F. The patient appeared to improve under sulfadiazine therapy, but the condition progressed to diffuse arachnoiditis, confirmed by myelography and laminectomy.

CASE NO. 6 (BROWN, 1947)

A plastic caudal catheter was used for continuous analgesia in a 23-year-old obstetrical patient. Over a period of 5¾ hours 1500 mg of 1.5 per cent Metycaine were given. The next day there was a fever of 104°F, tenderness and hyperemia over the sacral area, and nuchal rigidity. Lumbar puncture yielded cloudy fluid at raised pressure, and polymorphonuclear leukocytes were present. A smear showed gram-positive organisms. After vigorous treatment with penicillin and sulfadiazine, the patient improved and the cerebrospinal fluid was clear six days later. There were no sequelae.

CASE NO. 7 (BÖDEN, 1954)

A 51-year-old man had two epidural anesthetics one month apart for urogenital surgery. The second epidural anesthetic was performed in the manner customary in Germany at that time, by filling the epidural space with a large volume of saline (80 ml in this case), followed by 10 ml of anesthetic solution, but the nature of the anesthetic solution is not stated in the report. On the day after the operation the patient complained of low lumbar and sacral pain. By 48 hours after operation there was a fever of 102°F, and the back pain had spread upward to the shoulders. Neurological signs became obvious on the fourth day, with stiffness of the back and bilateral hypoesthesia in the distribution of L_5*–*S_1*, as well as* S_2 *on the right. Lumbar epidural puncture revealed pus. Laminectomy between* L_2 *and* S_1 *showed the epidural space filled with creamy pus. The patient died on the operating table.*

Two more recent cases of epidural abscess must be added to this series. The second of these cases has several bizarre features that are only of interest from the point of view of unfortunate clinical management.

CASE NO. 8 (FERGUSON AND KIRSCH, 1974; ALSO REPORTED INDEPENDENTLY BY SAADY, 1976)

Epidural empyema extending from C_7 to T_{10} occurred in a 51-year-old man following insertion of a mid-thoracic epidural catheter for postoperative pain relief after vagotomy and pyloroplasty; the catheter was left in place for 48 hours. Symptoms began on the fourth postoperative day with cough, purulent sputum and right upper abdominal pain and meningeal irritation, and urinary retention occurred on the tenth day. Neurological consultation was not sought until the fourteenth day, when progressive leg weakness developed. Then, lumbar and cisternal myelography showed a complete extradural obstruction between C_7 and T_{10}. Decompressive laminectomy from C_7–T_{10} encountered epidural pus that grew a culture of Staphylococcus epidermidis. *Subsequently the patient made a partial neurological recovery.*

The following case history contains some bizarre features that illustrate the dangers of pelvic metastatic sepsis combined with local trauma and possibly direct infection of the epidural space.

CASE NO. 9: EPIDURAL ABSCESS FOLLOWING PELVIC PERITONITIS AND PROLONGED EPIDURAL CATHETERIZATION (MIKHAILOVICH ET AL., 1974)

Pelvic peritonitis and intestinal ileus occurred in a 23-year-old male five days after appendectomy for gangrenous appendicitis. Laparotomy and peritoneal drainage were performed under general anesthesia. The infecting organisms were not recorded. For reasons that are not stated in the report, it was decided to use prolonged epidural analgesia in the postoperative management. An epidural catheter was inserted at T_{10}–T_{11} and 10 ml of 2.5 per cent trimecaine were injected every four hours for a period of ten days. Pain was relieved, breathing improved and peristalsis returned.*

Epidural injections were stopped on the eleventh day, but by some mischance the catheter was forgotten and left in place until the nineteenth day, when signs of meningitis appeared. The epidural catheter was then removed. Antibiotic therapy was started, and two days later signs of epidural infection appeared in the lower thoracic spine. Three more days elapsed, and the patient became paraplegic. Finally, laminectomy was performed between the ninth thoracic and second lumbar arches. Thick pus was encountered. Antibiotic irrigation of the wound was continued for the next few days. The report states that the patient eventually recovered and that one year later no neurological sequelae remained.

In all these cases it seems likely that infection was carried in from outside, although in the last two cases metastatic infection from the peritoneal cavity or lung was probably a major contributory cause. The frequency of infection among the early series of continuous caudal anesthetics suggests that either sterilization of equipment or solutions were faulty, or there was some break in aseptic technique.

Epidural abscess is a potentially catastrophic event, and the triad of back pain made worse by movement, tenderness and fever should raise early suspicions. Treatment must be appropriate and urgent to avoid permanent neurological sequelae. While antibiotics may arrest an early infection, as some of the caudal cases show, there is no time to wait and see. The spinal canal must be opened and drained by laminectomy, for once neurological deficits

---

*Trimecaine, ω-diethylamino-2.4,6-trimethylacetanilide, is a local anesthetic very similar in properties to lidocaine and commonly used in eastern Europe (Löfgren, 1948; Goldberg, 1949).

have appeared, they are almost certainly signs of irreversible damage to the cord or spinal roots, and complete recovery is unlikely (Hulme and Dott, 1954).

Cases have also been reported that suggest subacute infection or some contaminating process that begins shortly after the epidural anesthetic and then either improves and leaves no sequelae or deteriorates to a picture of chronic adhesive arachnoiditis. It should be recalled that epidural abscesses usually occur spontaneously by endogenous metastatic spread and often from foci elsewhere in the body (Boongird et al., 1974). Pelvic peritonitis seems to be a potent cause. Hence, if epidural analgesia must be used in the face of peritoneal sepsis, it is wise to ensure that suitable antibiotic therapy is instituted.

The possibility of unrelated causes of epidural abscess should always be borne in mind, since a coincidental epidural anesthetic is almost certain to be wrongly blamed for the infection. The following case history is reproduced by kind permission of the authors (Male and Martin, 1973).

A 22-year-old woman was admitted for investigation of jaundice developing in the 39th week of her fourth pregnancy. Infectious hepatitis was diagnosed. Ten days after admission when the jaundice was fading, the patient was delivered of a healthy infant after a spontaneous labor lasting three hours. Epidural analgesia was not administered.

The postpartum course was uneventful until the sixth day, when the patient developed interscapular back pain and mild pyrexia. On the seventh day she developed paresthesias of the thighs and difficulty in walking. On the eighth day weakness and incoordination of the legs worsened and there was patchy loss of pinprick sensation in both legs. Bilateral ankle clonus was present. On the ninth day, three days after the onset of symptoms, she became paraplegic with a sensory level at T_6.

Several septic spots were present on the skin, and there was tenderness over the fourth, fifth and sixth thoracic spines. A diagnosis of epidural abscess was made. Contrast myelography showed a complete block at the level of the fourth thoracic vertebra. Emergency laminectomy in the upper thoracic region revealed a large epidural abscess and flattening of the dural tube. Staphylococcus aureus *sensitive to penicillin was isolated, and the patient was treated with penicillin systemically and by local irrigation. There was no improvement, and the patient remained a spastic paraplegic.*

Comment

In this case hematogenous spread of infection from the pyogenic skin lesions was the probable cause of the metastatic abscess. The evolution of the disease was more rapid than usual, and only 72 hours elapsed between the onset of symptoms and development of irreversible paraplegia, instead of the average period of $4\frac{1}{2}$ *to* $5\frac{1}{2}$ *days (Baker et al., 1975). No regional anesthesia was administered, but had an epidural block been given for relief of pain in labor, it would almost certainly have been wrongly imputed as the causative factor.*

SUBARACHNOID INFECTION

CASE NO. 1: ACUTE MENINGITIC REACTION WITH RECOVERY (ZÖHLEN, 1950)

A 27-year-old man received an epidural anesthetic for a urological procedure. An aberrant renal vessel had been resected under epidural analgesia one year previously without untoward effects.

Epidural puncture was carried out at the tenth thoracic interspace using a negative pressure method to identify the space, and an audible hiss was heard on entering the space. The needle was rotated through 180°, and no cerebrospinal fluid dripped back. The technique recommended by Buchholz was followed, and 20 ml of saline were injected, followed by 10 ml of viscous "Pantocaine plombe" injected very rapidly. The "plombe" consisted of 1.5 per cent Pantocaine in 6 per cent polyvinylpyrrolidone containing a bacteriostatic disinfectant.

Two hours later symptoms of meningitis appeared. Lumbar puncture was performed and the cerebrospinal fluid was cloudy, with white cells, but the protein was normal (28.8 mg/100 ml) and cultures were sterile.

The patient was treated with penicillin and recovered without sequelae.

Comment

The author suggested that the dura might have been traumatized when the epidural needle was rotated through 180° and that the PVP "plombe" might have been contaminated. As pointed out earlier in the chapter on Pharmacology, in my opinion the use of viscous "plombes" is undesirable. A mixture of 1.5 per cent tetracaine with 6 per cent polyvinylpyrrolidone is hyperosmolar and potentially dehydrating if it enters the subarachnoid space in appreciable quantities.

CASE NO. 2: ACUTE MENINGITIC REACTION WITH RECOVERY (JENICEK, 1955)

A 26-year-old man received a therapeutic epidural block for residual thrombophlebitis of the left leg following a healed fracture of the femur.

Seven ml of 0.8 per cent lidocaine were injected epidurally at the second lumbar interspace. The block appeared to be successful, and the leg became warm and pain-free.

Symptoms of meningitis, a chill and headache, developed four hours after the block. Nuchal rigidity appeared eight hours after the block, and the temperature rose to 101°F. Lumbar puncture produced cloudy cerebrospinal fluid with a high white cell count (9,600 polymorphonuclear cells/mm^3), but smears showed no organisms. Treatment with penicillin and streptomycin was started immediately. The cerebrospinal fluid cleared, and the patient steadily improved over the next few days. The solutions used for the block were cultured and reported sterile.

Comment

The author suggests that this was a case of aseptic meningitis due to chemical irritation from the solution used. However, lidocaine is not an irritating solution in the ordinary range of concentration used for clinical purposes, and a bacterial source of contamination seems more probable. The patient was fortunate to have had his condition diagnosed so promptly and to have received effective antibiotic therapy.

CASE NO. 3: ARACHNOIDITIS AND PARAPLEGIA (BRAHAM AND SAIA, 1958)

Cesarean section was performed in a 26-year-old asthmatic woman under epidural analgesia. The patient complained of headache and transient diplopia in the early postoperative period. Headache persisted for several weeks, and the patient noticed increasing difficulty in walking. Paresis of the legs developed, together with impaired sphincter control and loss of sensation in all segments below T_{11}. Myelography showed an obstruction at T_{11}. Laminectomy at T_{11}–L_1 revealed gross arachnoiditis extending cranially and caudally beyond the limits of the surgical exposure. The patient remained permanently crippled.

No details of the anesthetic technique and progress are given in the original report. However, the report mentions that the customary technique included the loss-of-resistance test followed by the injection of 25 to 30 ml of 2 per cent procaine.

Comment

In the absence of clinical details of the anesthetic management and postoperative course, it is impossible to do more than speculate on the nature of this case. Several mechanisms could be invoked to account for the extensive arachnoiditis, but the history of diplopia and persistent headache are suggestive of some form of subarachnoid contamination, either chemical or bacterial.

Adhesive Arachnoiditis of Uncertain Origin

Six cases of grave neurological complications have been reported from the region of Porto Alegre in the state of Rio Grande do Sul, Brazil (Kliemann, 1975). Four of the six cases were well documented and appeared to involve a form of acute chemical irritation leading to severe arachnoiditis and permanent neurological sequelae. Three of the patients were healthy young women receiving epidural analgesia for childbirth. The fourth was a 63-year-old male undergoing hernia repair. In all of these patients the analgesic agent was lidocaine hydrochloride in concentrations between 1.2 and 2 per cent with epinephrine 1/160,000 to 1/320,000. Details of the precise origin or analyses of the solutions are not available at the time of writing.

The cause of these tragedies remains undetermined. Samples of local anesthetic were submitted to biological testing by epidural injection in cats and rabbits at a laboratory in England. Preliminary histological results are reported as indicating severe inflammatory reaction in the spinal cord and meninges. On the basis of this evidence, it would appear that some form of chemical contamination may have been responsible for the disastrous outcome in these cases.

It is not generally appreciated that adhesive arachnoiditis may be found in association with numerous kinds of infection, including gynecological sepsis, as well as with spinal hemorrhage or trauma (Alpers and Mancall, 1971). In seeking an etiology for spinal arachnoiditis, a careful search should be made for associated infection elsewhere, whether acute or chronic, which may be present but not readily apparent and which may be amenable to treatment. There seem to be underlying geographical differences in etiology. For example, tuberculosis is a prevalent associated disease in India. In a lengthy review of 70 cases of adhesive arachnoiditis unrelated to spinal puncture, from the Bombay area, Wadia and Dastur (1969) found that 38 occurred in association with tuberculous infection. Thus, an epidural anesthetic preceding the onset of adhesive arachnoiditis should not immediately be presumed to be the cause. Such a facile conclusion may distract attention from more important associations and delay treatment of the true cause.

Summary

In comparison to the alarming incidence of infection from caudal catheters at the early period of their use, more recent practice has been remarkably fortunate in avoiding epidural infection. A number of factors have been responsible for this improvement. Catheter design is better, and the physical size is smaller. The continuous caudal approach has been largely replaced by the lumbar route, thus avoiding fecal contamination in obstetrical practice. Sterilization techniques are more standardized and reliable, and multidose vials of local anesthetics have been replaced by more hygienic single-dose ampules. Lastly, effective antibiotic therapy is readily available at the first suspicion of any trouble. Large series of lumbar peridural blocks have been performed without infectious complications. Lund (1966) reported over 12,000 cases, in which mostly multidose vials were used, without infection. More than 40,000 epidural and caudal blocks have been performed at the Royal Victoria Hospital, Montreal, since 1956, also without infection.

Attempts to culture microorganisms from indwelling epidural catheters in situ have been negative. Barretto (1962) examined 35 epidural catheters that had been in place for one to ten days. All aspirates from the catheters were sterile. Positive cultures were obtained from the tips of three catheters after they were removed. Two grew *Staphylococcus albus,* and the other aerobic gram-positive rods and *coli aerogens.* These were thought to be secondarily infected from the skin when the catheters were withdrawn. Strasser et al. (1974) examined 100 epidural catheters, some of which had been in place for 3½ days. None showed primary bacterial growth, but four were secondarily infected by skin organisms.

Freedom from infection demands scrupulous sterilization of equipment and anesthetic solutions. Aseptic techniques must be faultless, and sterile gloves must be donned carefully. Once the patient's skin has been prepared with an aseptic solution, sufficient time should be allowed for the antiseptic agent to perform its task. As far as possible, a no-touch technique should be cultivated, and the anesthesiologist should avoid unnecessary handling of parts of needles and catheters that will be inserted into the patient. Also, he should avoid touching the skin at the site of injection. Skin drapes should be used with discretion and good sense; often drapes defeat their own purpose by slipping out of place and contaminating a prepared area of skin, and in many instances it is better to avoid their use altogether (Chaplin and Renwick, 1958).

The introduction of micropore bacterial filters has added an extra line of defense against contamination in continuous epidural techniques (Desmond, 1972). While experience in large series has shown that their use is not essential to avoid infection nevertheless it is probably wise to include one of these little disposable filters between the syringe and the epidural catheter.

The remote possibility of unrelated or related epidural infection should always be borne in mind. Although epidural abscess is exceedingly rare, it is a very terrible development. The cardinal signs described earlier should be remembered, not only for the sake of the patient, so that prompt and appropriate action can be taken at an early stage while the process is still reversible, but also so that the anesthesiologist can ensure his own medicolegal well-being.

Etiologically the odds are that an epidural abscess will usually be due to endogenous metastatic spread rather than anesthetic causes. In Baker's series of 39 cases from the Massachusetts General Hospital, only one case associated with epidural analgesia arose over a period of 27 years (Baker et al., 1975). Nevertheless, the current medicolegal climate in North America is so emotionally biased and so predatory that court judgments are likely to be based on illogical post hoc, ergo propter hoc arguments rather than on the true probabilities of the case, and the anesthesiologist should have his facts well marshaled for his own protection.

ASSOCIATED PERIPHERAL NERVE LESIONS UNRELATED TO EPIDURAL ANALGESIA

Any postoperative neurological complications arising after regional anesthesia are likely to be attributed to the anesthetic. The nerve-blocking effects of subarachnoid and epidural anesthesia are so dramatic that it is perhaps natural to propose an etiology based on shallow assumptions of cause and effect. Other possible causes of neurological damage are frequently dismissed, either from ignorance, inadequate possession of the facts, inadequate examination of the patient, intellectual idleness or, occasionally, misinterpretation by a legal adversary. Examples have already been given of vascular lesions of the cord that would almost certainly have been attributed to an epidural anesthetic if one had been administered.

This section will consider peripheral nerve damage that may be wrongly attributed to the epidural anesthetic. The anesthesiologist should be fully aware of these possible lesions, not only for his own protection and defense in case of unjust accusation, but also, more importantly, so that he can perform his role as protector of the patient and be alert to potential and preventable causes that may require consultation and joint action with other members of the surgical team.

Summaries follow of some illustrative cases of peripheral nerve lesions in which suspicion originally fell upon associated epidural anesthesia, but in which physical examination and the subsequent clinical course left no doubt that other factors were the real cause. These cases will be followed by a brief review of published neurological sequelae of the lower limb in surgical and obstetrical practice unassociated with epidural analgesia, in order to emphasize the frequency with which associated but unrelated peripheral nerve damage is likely to arise in any large series of cases.

CASE NO. 1: POSTOPERATIVE FOOTDROP

Cholecystectomy was performed in a fit 32-year-old man under epidural analgesia and endotracheal nitrous oxide–oxygen anesthesia. Puncture was performed at the first lumbar interspace. An injection of 20 ml of 2 per cent mepivacaine with 1/200,000 epinephrine was made, and a catheter was inserted without eliciting any paresthesias. Analgesia spread to include all segments up to T_5 in 18 minutes, and 35 minutes after induction motor block was assessed as "partial" in both legs, that is, full movement at the ankle and partial flexion at the knee. At the end of operation it was noticed that the leg restraining strap had been placed below the knees instead of above them, and one of the metal buckles had been close to the head of the left fibula. A second dose of 20 ml of 2 per cent mepivacaine was given through the epidural catheter one hour after operation to relieve pain and facilitate postoperative breathing exercises. Again analgesia rose to T_5–T_6. This time there was no motor block in the right leg, but the left leg *became weak for the duration of the block, although some movement of the left toes and ankle persisted.*

Postoperatively there was left sided footdrop and hypoesthesia on the outer side of the left calf. The neurological lesion steadily improved, and 12 weeks later all signs and symptoms had disappeared.

Comment

Initially, the epidural block came under heavy suspicion. However, the distribution, subsequent course and recovery of the neurological deficit was typical of a compression lesion at the lateral popliteal nerve, probably caused by the buckle of the improperly placed restraining strap.

Although the epidural anesthetic was not to blame, the anesthesiologist was partly at fault for failing to check the proper placement of the restraining strap.

CASE NO. 2: POSTPARTUM SAPHENOUS NEURITIS

A 32-year-old secundagravida with a vertex presentation received epidural analgesia for labor. No other analgesic drugs were given. A catheter was inserted at the second lumbar interspace when the cervix was 4 cm dilated. A total cumulative dose of 65 mg of 0.5 per cent bupivacaine with 1/200,000 epinephrine gave satisfactory pain relief for labor, delivery and repair of episiotomy over a period of 4¾ hours. A male infant weighing 3,500 grams was delivered spontaneously, with an Apgar score of 9 at 1 minute. At delivery, analgesia extended from S_5–T_{10} on the right and to T_9 on the left. Motor block in the legs was assessed as "partial" on the right and "nil" on the left. After delivery, the patient complained of pain in the left leg in the distribution of the saphenous nerve. There was no loss of motor function or tendon reflexes and no sensory deficit. Symptoms gradually disappeared over the next two weeks.

Comment

Initially, epidural blockade was suspected as a cause of spinal nerve root irritation. However, the distribution of pain was not typical of root involvement, and no neurological signs accompanied the symptoms. The transient nature of the pain suggested a lesion of peripheral origin, probably due to compression by the inguinal ligament while the patient was in the lithotomy position.

CASE NO. 3: POSTOPERATIVE NUMBNESS OF THE THIGH (BIRKHAHN AND HEIFETZ, 1961)

Right ureteric stricture and hydronephrosis in a 44-year-old man were treated by partial cystectomy and reimplantation of the right ureter. The operation lasted 3 hours and 20 minutes. Epidural block was induced at the second lumbar interspace with 30 ml of 1.3 per cent lidocaine (400 mg) and 1/200,000 epinephrine. A catheter was inserted for 5 to 7 cm. Two top-up doses of plain 1.3 per cent lidocaine of 17 ml and 8 ml respectively were administered during the operation.

The patient complained of wound pain and pain in the back on the first day after operation. Back pain disappeared after 24 hours, but the patient then complained of a "queer sensation" in his right thigh. Examination showed hypalgesia and hypoesthesia on the anterolateral aspect of the right thigh in the distribution of the second lumbar dermatome, but not extending throughout the whole dermatome distribution. The neurological consultant commented that the numbness extended into L_3 territory. There was no motor loss or reflex disturbance. The area of sensory disturbance remained unchanged ten months later.

The authors considered meralgia paresthetica as a possibility but dismissed it in favor of damage to the root of L_2 by the epidural catheter. The neurological opinion also *favored trauma by the needle or catheter, and the possibility of operative trauma was not considered.*

Comment

This case is sometimes quoted as an instance of epidural trauma (Lund, 1966), but in my opinion this is not so. The area of numbness extended over the anterolateral aspect in part of the territory of L_2 *and* L_3*, on the side of the operation. The distribution of sensory loss combined with complete freedom from motor or reflex disturbance is not typical of root damage. However, it is completely typical of the cutaneous distribution found in meralgia paresthetica, arising from damage to the lateral femoral cutaneous nerve somewhere along its course between the lateral border of psoas and the inguinal ligament just medial to the anterior superior iliac spine. The course of this cutaneous nerve lies in close proximity to surgical manipulations and retractors used during the operation. As will be seen from the review to follow, surgical and obstetrical damage to nerves running across the pelvis and pelvic brim is a relatively common occurrence, and this mechanism appears to be the most likely etiology in this case.*

CASE NO. 4: POSTPARTUM BILATERAL FEMORAL NEUROPATHY FOLLOWING CONTINUOUS CAUDAL ANALGESIA (ADELMAN, GOLDBERG AND PUCKETT, 1973)

A 21-year-old primigravida received continuous caudal analgesia for the terminal stage of labor when the cervix was 8 cm dilated. An injection of 15 ml of 1.5 per cent lidocaine (225 mg) with 1/200,000 epinephrine was made, followed by administration of 10 ml (150 mg) lidocaine hourly. Analgesia extended to T_9–T_{10}*. The fetal head failed to descend in spite of Syntocinon administration, and after a prolonged labor cesarean section was carried out through a Pfannenstiel incision under general anesthesia. An 8 lb 4 oz infant was delivered (Apgar 8). No self-retaining retractors were used. Later, postoperative bleeding led to hemorrhagic shock, and the blood pressure fell to 60/40 mmHg. Twelve units of blood were transfused, and bleeding was arrested at a second operation under general anesthesia.*

On awakening from the second operation, the patient complained of inability to move her legs and dysesthesia over the front of the thighs. Sphincter control was normal.

Her motor and sensory deficit was bilateral and symmetrical. Sensation was diminished over the anteromedial surface of both thighs and the medial surface of the calves. Both quadriceps muscles were completely paralyzed, and patellar reflexes were absent. There was moderate weakness of hip flexion. There were no other neurological abnormalities. Lumbar puncture, myelography and spinal X-rays were all normal.

Initially, the bilateral symmetrical deficit suggested the possibility of a lesion of the spinal cord at the level of L_2–L_4*, from either some complication of the caudal anesthetic or possibly ischemia secondary to the period of hypotension and hemorrhagic shock. However, preservation of adductor movements of the thigh and partial iliopsoas activity (*L_2–L_3 *innervation) was against this.*

Recovery took place gradually and was complete in five months.

Comment

If this case had not been so thoroughly and competently investigated and followed up, it might well have been wrongly labeled as a complication of continuous caudal analgesia in accordance with the original suspicion.

In fact, the diagnosis was bilateral femoral neuropathy. The authors suggested that the cause was ischemia from a combination of factors, including pressure at the pelvic brim by the fetal head during prolonged labor, followed by significant hypotension.

Complete recovery in three to six months is typical of femoral neuropathy arising from compression ischemia during childbirth.

BRIEF LITERATURE REVIEW OF PERIPHERAL NERVE SEQUELAE UNASSOCIATED WITH EPIDURAL ANALGESIA

In the foregoing section all the cases of neurological sequelae were associated with epidural analgesia, but they were all attributable to other causes that exonerated the anesthetic technique. The cases presented in this section will illustrate typical neurological complications that arose spontaneously in the absence of epidural blockade or any other form of regional analgesia. At first sight this section may seem to be an irrelevant and anecdotal collection. However, these cases are included for the benefit of those who are interested in obtaining some conception of the frequency with which peripheral neurological sequelae occur in a "control" population. It may also be of value to physicians who find themselves the targets of legal suits for neurological sequelae arising from epidural analgesia. A summary review of this nature has little statistical value in a rigid sense, since it concerns haphazard retrospective information, but for this very reason the real frequency of coincidental peripheral nerve lesions unrelated to anesthesia is likely to be higher than the isolated reports lead one to suppose (Tillman, 1935; Rosenblum et al., 1966). Most of these reports are concerned with lesions attributable to trauma at childbirth, but a number also relate to routine surgical operations. These two causes will be dealt with separately.

The possibility of peripheral neurological sequelae to childbirth became apparent toward the middle of the nineteenth century. One of the earliest reports in English was described by Beatty in 1838 in his Second Report of the New Lying-In Hospital, Dublin.

Anne Kiernan, a 21-year-old primigravida, was delivered of a live infant on the 26th of November, 1836, after a seven-hour labor. On the second day she complained that her right leg felt numb and dead, and she could not move it. There was no pain or swelling, but sensation was diminished. Treatment consisted of turpentine frictions, but as there was no improvement, a line of blisters was applied along the course of the sciatic nerve. The report goes on to say that this restored power in the limb. In one month she was able to walk about the ward with a stick, but the leg dragged along with difficulty, "and the foot hung loose and vacillating, the toes pointing to the ground." In another month she had gained considerable power over the muscles, and sensation in the limb was almost entirely restored. "She continued to improve until the month of February, at which time she was walking about nearly well and preparing to leave the hospital, when puerperal fever made its appearance on the wards." The hospital was closed and cleared of all patients, but the woman, being very poor and more than two months having elapsed since her confinement, was allowed to remain. On the 5th of February, she was struck with alarming epigastric pain and dyspnea, and the next day she was transferred to another hospital where she died of pericarditis about a week later. Postmortem examination showed a considerable amount of seropurulent fluid in the pericardium.

This case illustrates most vividly a serious but reversible peripheral nerve lesion, probably of the lumbosacral trunk, with resultant footdrop, following an apparently easy and noninstrumental labor. It also conjures up the precarious nature of a hospital environment in those times, and the virulence of the infections that periodically raged through the wards.

Sixteen years later Fleetwood Churchill (1854) was able to collect another two cases from the European literature. One was a case of paraplegia of gradual onset, arising eight days after delivery and gradually spreading to involve the arms; it was probably an unrelated neurological process, possibly of infectious origin. The other was a second case of unilateral weakness and numbness of the leg with footdrop; this patient recovered in six months.

By 1892, the condition of postpartum palsy of the lower limb was well recognized, and Hünerman pointed out the special vulnerability of the lumbosacral trunk (L_4 and L_5) as it passes in front of the ala of the sacrum. Damage to the trunk leads to weakness of the muscles supplied by the external popliteal nerve and subsequent footdrop. In 1964 Murray was able to collect 201 cases of obstetrical palsy from the literature, and reports have continued to accumulate.

Obstetrical Peripheral Nerve Palsies

Injury to each of the nerves crossing the pelvic brim has been described from time to time. Many of these reports have been associated with maternofetal disproportion and difficult labor or instrumental delivery. However, about 25 per cent have followed easy, uncomplicated labors, and 15 per cent followed deliveries in which no instrumentation was used (Murray, 1964). In 1935 Tillman reported nine cases of peripheral nerve injury unassociated with regional anesthesia in 18,000 deliveries among a New York population—an incidence of 1:2,100 births. Twenty-seven years later Hill (1962) reported an incidence of 1:2,600 from a Californian population. Today's high rate of cesarean section in abnormal labor may have lowered the incidence somewhat, but the occurrence rate is still high enough to present a recurring problem of differential diagnosis and etiology in any large unit that makes extensive use of epidural analgesia.

LUMBOSACRAL TRUNK (L_4, L_5)

The lumbosacral trunk carrying fibers from L_4 and L_5 to join S_1 descends in front of the sacroiliac joint. Normally, it lies in the shelter of the sacral promontory and is protected against direct pressure from the fetal head, but in flat platypeloid pelves this protection is missing (Tillman, 1935), and the trunk is then exposed to trauma from forceps blades or pressure by the fetus. Injury often includes fibers from S_1, as well as the main lumbosacral trunk itself.

The resulting neurological syndrome is typical of denervation in the cutaneous and muscular territory of the lumbosacral trunk, that is, the territory of the lateral popliteal nerve, excluding its contribution from S_2, which usually escapes. Its features are:

1. Paralysis of the dorsiflexors of the ankle, with footdrop
2. Hypalgesia over the lateral aspect of the calf and foot (L_5 and S_1)
3. Slight weakness of quadriceps from loss of its L_4 component
4. Slight weakness of hip adductors from loss of L_4 and L_5 component to adductor magnus

Trauma to the lumbosacral trunk is one of the commonest peripheral nerve lesions of childbirth. Tillman (1935) described eight typical cases, and other series are described by Chalmers (1949) and Hill (1962). It is usually unilateral, and recovery takes from three to six months, but some residual footdrop may remain, with hypoesthesia over the lateral aspect of the calf.

FEMORAL NERVE (L_2, L_3 AND L_4)

This is not a common lesion in obstetrics, although it occurs relatively commonly after pelvic surgery. Damage to the femoral nerve results in quadriceps paralysis, loss of patellar reflex and hypalgesia over the front of the thigh and the medial aspect of the calf. King (1950) described a case that he attributed to kinking and ischemic pressure at Poupart's ligament from prolonged flexion in the lithotomy position.

Adelman et al. (1973) described an interesting case of bilateral femoral neuropathy after caudal analgesia for labor (see page 692). In this case damage was not due to the caudal anesthetic but was attributed to pressure from cephalopelvic disproportion, accompanied by hypotensive ischemia from hemorrhagic shock.

SCIATIC NERVE (L_4, L_5, S_1, S_2, S_3)

True sciatic nerve palsy of the entire nerve is a very rare complication of obstetrics. Paralysis of single roots within the sciatic distribution may arise relatively frequently from intervertebral disc protrusions pressing on sciatic roots during labor and delivery. O'Connell (1944) has described four cases, and others have been reported by Chalmers (1949) and Adler et al. (1956), but these are not true peripheral nerve injuries occurring in the intrapelvic course of the nerve.

OBTURATOR NERVE (L_2, L_3 AND L_4)

This is also very rare as an isolated injury. Hopf (1974) described one case in an obese patient weighing 106 kg.

LATERAL FEMORAL CUTANEOUS NERVE (L_2, L_3)

Complaints of transient numbness of the anterolateral part of one thigh in the distribution of the lateral femoral cutaneous nerve are encountered about as frequently as lesions of the lumbosacral trunk. Compression of the lateral femoral cutaneous nerve is usually considered to arise from prolonged posture in lithotomy stirrups leading to partial ischemia from kinking as the nerve passes under the lateral part of the inguinal ligament. External pressure over the inguinal ligament may cause the same condition, but this is more likely to arise from damage caused by retractors during surgical operations. Prolonged discomfort from damage to the lateral femoral cutaneous nerve (i.e., meralgia paresthetica) is very rare after delivery.

Lateral popliteal or common peroneal nerve (L_4, L_5, S_1, S_2)

The common peroneal nerve may be damaged by external pressure as it winds around the lateral surface of the head of the fibula. Pressure from improperly placed lithotomy poles or stirrups and from knee restraining straps is the usual cause of this injury, which results in footdrop accompanied by hypoesthesia over the lateral aspect of the lower leg. One such case arising after an abdominal operation has already been described on page 690.

Postoperative Peripheral Nerve Palsies

Recognition of peripheral nerve palsies secondary to surgical operations was slow to develop, and such reports did not become frequent until after 1950. The general subject of peripheral nerve injuries incident to anesthesia and operation has been well reviewed by Nicholson and Eversole (1957) and Britt and Gordon (1964). The review that follows will concern only those injuries that might be attributed to coincidental epidural analgesia, and it will be confined to palsies of the lower limb.

Surgical and radiological procedures close to the spine have already been discussed as possible causes of myelopathy and permanent paralysis that may be ascribed to coincidental epidural analgesia. Surgery in the abdomen and pelvis is also an occasional cause of less devastating and more reversible lesions to peripheral nerves as they course through the pelvis. The nerves most commonly damaged are those lying close to bony ridges or surfaces where retractors may press upon them, or where the nerve may be kinked as it passes under tight ligamentous structures. Local ischemia is the ultimate cause of the neuropathy, and in most cases it is reversible in three to six months. Predisposing conditions, such as diabetes or porphyria, may increase susceptibility of the nerves to damage and handicap their recovery, and these conditions should always be considered. Diabetes is more commonly involved in North America, while porphyria would be a more likely probability in a South African population (Dean, 1963). Goodman (1954) concluded that femoral neuropathy is the most common form of mononeuropathy in North American diabetics. Calverley and Mulder (1960) found that diabetes was present in 74 per cent of all femoral neuropathies that they studied.

Femoral nerve

The femoral nerve may be damaged at abdominal operation or during pelvic procedures, but the mechanism is different in the two approaches. In abdominal surgery injury from a retractor is usually the prime cause, and certain types of self-retaining retractors have a particularly bad record. In 1956 Adler et al. reported three cases, one of them bilateral, that had occurred following abdominal gynecological surgery under general anesthesia. All had typical weakness of the thigh and knee, absent patellar reflexes and sensory loss over the front of the thigh and inner calf. All recovered

TABLE 14–2 Features of Femoral Nerve Palsy

Site of Lesion	*Hip Flexors*	*Quadriceps*	*Patellar Reflex*	*Cutaneous Sensation (front of thigh and inner calf)*
At or below inguinal ligament	Normal	Paresis	Absent	Hypalgesia
Above inguinal ligament	Partially impaired (rarely complete)	Paresis	Absent	Hypalgesia

spontaneously in three to six months. Ruston and Polati (1958) also reported three cases which resulted from the use of the Mann self-retaining retractor; two of these patients were given spinal anesthesia, and initially the anesthetic came under suspicion as the cause of the paralysis. Winkelman (1958) reported six cases, all following general anesthesia, and Rosenblum et al. (1966) reported ten cases, six of which followed spinal anesthesia.

Femoral nerve palsy is less common following perineal surgery, but Hopper and Baker (1968) described three cases occurring after lengthy immobilization of the patient in the lithotomy position under general anesthesia. They concluded that the cause was ischemic due to prolonged pressure as the nerve became kinked around the inguinal ligament by acute flexion of the thigh. They also remarked that the lesion is time-dependent and more likely to occur in the hands of tardy surgeons than experienced ones—a trenchant observation that could be applied to many postoperative complications arising after prolonged surgery. Further, all three of their patients had abnormal glucose tolerances, and they point out that investigation of this type of case should include a search for possible underlying and predisposing causes of neuropathy, with a glucose tolerance test as a routine test for diabetes.

Differentiation between the site of femoral nerve lesions above or below the inguinal ligament hinges upon function in iliopsoas. Damage at the inguinal ligament is distal to the bifurcation of branches for iliopsoas and does not impair flexion at the hip. Damage higher up within the pelvis may interrupt the femoral nerve supply to iliacus and so interfere with hip flexion. However, some fibers to psoas usually arise separately from L_2 and L_3, and these often escape, so that even with intrapelvic lesions, flexion of the hip is seldom completely abolished. The main diagnostic features of femoral nerve damage are outlined in Table 14–2.

Lateral Femoral Cutaneous Nerve

The lateral femoral cutaneous nerve also runs a course that makes it vulnerable to trauma as it leaves the pelvis under the inguinal ligament. Direct pressure from surgical instruments or assistants' elbows, or kinking in the lithotomy position are possible causes of ischemic damage, and it is strange that this superficial nerve is not injured more often (Stenz, 1960). The symptoms of damage to this cutaneous nerve are so slight and so free of disability that most patients would ignore a temporary impairment of sensation over the outer part of the thigh. However, if the neuropathy is caused by severe ischemia, the cutaneous sensation may become unpleasant, in the form generally known as meralgia paresthetica, probably as a result of sprouting and regeneration of very fine C-fibers in the diameter range of 0.1 to 0.4 micron (Fowler and Ochoa, 1975). The case described by Birkhahn and Heifetz (1961), mentioned earlier on page 691, seems to be a typical example. The symptoms of that case were ascribed to a complication of epidural analgesia, but with what appears to be very little justification.

As with femoral neuropathy, a case of meralgia paresthetica should be investigated for possible disease underlying the neuropathy, with special emphasis on excluding diabetes as a cause of mononeuropathy in accordance with Hopper and Baker's (1968) recommendation. Prior to 1968 I encountered three cases of temporary impairment of the lateral femoral cutaneous nerve following epidural analgesia. All three patients had a return to normal sensation within a few weeks; unfortunately, however, at that time the possibility of mild diabetes was not considered, and glucose tolerance tests were not ordered.

DIFFERENTIAL DIAGNOSIS OF POSTEPIDURAL NEUROLOGICAL SEQUELAE

Sensory and motor disturbances may arise swiftly after surgery or childbirth, or premonitory signs may give gradual warning of their onset, as some of the foregoing reports have shown. The anesthesiologist should be alert to the interpretation and meaning of the various clinical pictures that may evolve, and he should have a clear scheme prepared in his mind so that he can quickly deploy any diagnostic or therapeutic resources that may be necessary.

Every effort should be made to unravel the incident in its entirety, so that appropriate treatment can be arranged. The questions to be answered in any case of neurological complications are: (a) what are the exact site, the nature and the cause of the deficit; (b) is the condition real or imagined; and (c) is there any associated cause that requires investigation or treatment? The formulation and organization of these inquiries are listed below in tabular form.

A. Possible site of nerve injury
   1. Cord
      a. Segmental distribution
      b. Axial distribution
   2. Subarachnoid space
   3. Subdural space
   4. Epidural space
   5. Nerve roots
   6. Nerve trunks
   7. Peripheral nerves
   8. Muscles
B. Possible nature of nerve injury
   1. Real or imagined
   2. Trauma

3. Ischemia
   a. Direct, avascular
   b. Indirect from pressure
4. Infection
5. Hemorrhage
6. Degeneration (e.g., prolapsed intervertebral disc, diabetic neuropathy, etc.)
7. Cysts or new growth

C. Possible cause of nerve injury
1. Anesthesia
   a. Needle trauma
   b. Toxic drugs
   c. Hypotension
2. Surgery
   a. Section or cautery of nutrient vessels to cord
   b. Faulty posture and caval obstruction
   c. Ischemic pressure from surgical retractors, or kinking of a nerve
   d. Accidental surgical section or suture of a nerve trunk or peripheral nerve
3. Radiological
   Toxic contrast media
4. Childbirth
   a. Spontaneous trauma
   b. Iatrogenic trauma (forceps)
5. Exacerbation of pre-existing disease

The first task is to establish the exact location and time of onset of the lesion. A thorough history and clinical examination are still the mainstay of investigation.

History

The history will help to determine the time of onset of the lesion by description of accompanying pain, paresthesia, or numbness and loss of power and the manner in which these symptoms appeared. The speed of onset is a particularly important indication of probable causes.

Sudden onset suggests trauma to the cord, roots or peripheral nerves or abrupt vascular occlusion to the cord by thrombosis, embolism or compression.

Rapid onset suggests developing expansion of some process compressing cord or roots, such as an epidural hematoma, abscess or new growth.

Slow onset suggests chronic inflammation or degenerative disease.

Physical Examination

The physical examination should include a thorough neurological examination, with particular emphasis on affected limbs, the back and spine,

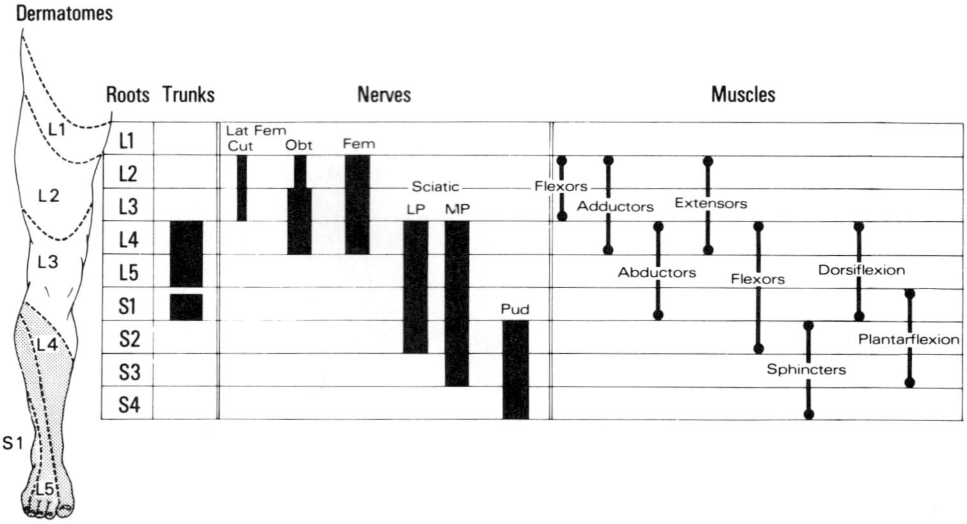

Figure 14–2. Cutaneous and muscular distribution of lumbar and sacral spinal segments, showing segmental disposition of lumbosacral trunk and peripheral nerves.

Lat Fem Cut = lateral femoral cutaneous
Obt = obturator
Fem = femoral
LP = lateral popliteal
MP = medial popliteal
Pud = pudendal

and the organ systems that may have etiological relevance. The resultant findings will usually define the site of the lesion within fairly close limits, especially when cutaneous and muscular deficits are considered together. Figure 14–2 outlines the cutaneous and muscular distribution of the lumbar and sacral spinal segments. Careful mapping of sensory and motor function will establish whether the lesion has the characteristics of a segmental or a peripheral nerve lesion and therefore whether the damage is likely to be at the level of the cord, spinal roots or somewhere along the path of a trunk or major nerve. Examination of the back will reveal any local tenderness that might raise suspicion of acute spinal infection.

Close spatial and temporal location of the lesion may require electromyographic evidence in some cases, and it is always wise to obtain EMG documentation as early as possible (Marinacci and Courville, 1958; Marinacci, 1962, 1968). Other ancillary tests that may be needed to identify the precise site and nature of the lesion include spinal X-rays, a coagulogram to exclude blood clotting abnormalities, lumbar or cisternal puncture, examination of the cerebrospinal fluid and myelography.

Investigation should also include other systems that may have causal significance. For example, metastatic lesions from the lung, breast or prostate commonly lodge in the spinal canal. An examination of the breast in the female and the prostate in the male should always be part of the routine physical examination. In peripheral nerve lesions a glucose tolerance test and examination of the urine or feces for porphyrins should be done to exclude diabetes or porphyria as an underlying cause of neuropathy. Dean's test for stercoporphyrins is a simple office screening procedure taking only a couple of minutes and a Wood's lamp to look for fluorescence (Dean, 1963).

Ancillary Investigations

Any one of the following ancillary tests may be crucial in clinching a diagnosis. Difficult and confusing cases may rarely require the whole gamut, but some specialized tests such as myelography and spinal angiography are notably invasive and carry with them a recognized and significant morbidity, and these should be reserved for cases in which they are clearly necessary. The following tests are listed in order of their invasiveness and in the order in which they would usually be applied.

X-RAY OF SPINE IN TWO PLANES

Spinal radiographs may reveal suspicious features compressing the cord or spinal roots, such as bony changes suggestive of new growths, tuberculosis or a vascular anomaly. Disc space abnormalities may suggest compression of roots by a ruptured annulus and an extruded disc.

COAGULOGRAM

Abnormalities of the clotting mechanism may suggest the possibility of an epidural hematoma in cases of early cord compression. This raises the nice question of whether to proceed with a diagnostic myelogram immediately and thus risk further bleeding, or whether to try to correct the bleeding tendency first. Time is vital in cases of cord compression from either blood or pus in the epidural space, and whatever course is taken, it should not be allowed to delay exploratory laminectomy if signs are progressive.

ELECTROMYOGRAPHY

Electromyography (EMG) may be of the greatest assistance in identifying neurological lesions both spatially and temporally. The technique requires considerable experience for accurate and intelligent interpretation, and it is only of real value when used in conjunction with a meticulous history and physical examination. An excellent and clear exposition of the subject will be found in the monograph *Electrodiagnosis of Neuromuscular Diseases* by Goodgold and Eberstein (1972). The medicolegal applications of EMG are discussed by Marinacci in a number of writings (Marinacci and Courville, 1958; Marinacci, 1962, 1968; Marinacci and Von Hagen, 1966). The basis for interpreting EMG changes in neurological lesions is summarized by Marinacci as follows. During early fetal development and before muscles and nerves have linked up, the isolated muscles lead an electrical life of their own, with disorderly incoordinate fibrillations recordable on the EMG. After innervation the muscles defer to neural instruction in an orderly coordinated manner. When a lower motor neuron is cut, the muscles supplied by it regress to their fetal state and the resultant electrical pattern is characteristic. This change does not happen immediately but takes time, and the elapsed time may be crucial in arriving at a medicolegal decision in compensation cases.

The electrical changes that occur in the denervated muscles seem to be dependent on the disappearance of some trophic substance within the distal stump of the cut nerve. Prolonged blockade of the nerve with local anesthetic for two weeks does not cause a fibrillation pattern to appear (Robert and Oester, 1970), as had been suggested by Sokoll et al. (1968), and it seems that physical rupture of the axon is the determining factor; patchy demyelination alone may slow conduction, but it does not cause a denervated pattern to appear.

The time between section of the nerve and the appearance of fibrillation depends on the store of trophic substance remaining in the distal stump, and this in turn depends on the length of the distal stump. Thus, the paraspinal muscles, with relatively short lower motor neurons, show denervation changes within eight to ten days of damage to their spinal root, whereas the appendicular nerves traveling in the anterior primary rami, and going to the distal parts of the limb, take about three weeks (see Figure 10–38). It must be emphasized that this interval of three weeks is an *average* estimate. In some patients changes may occur within two weeks, but in others it may take a month for electrical signs to appear in the lower leg (Goodgold and Eberstein, 1972). Thus, in attempting to pinpoint the exact date of onset of a lesion, the method does not have quite the degree of temporal precision that has been ascribed to it by some authors (Marinacci, 1968).

Electromyographic examination is conducted to discover:

1. Is the paralysis localized or general? That is, is the disordered EMG pattern confined only to the muscle groups allegedly paralyzed, or is the paralysis merely one manifestation of a generalized myopathy?

2. What muscle groups are involved?

3. Are the affected muscle groups distributed in a metameric fashion, or are they confined to the territory of a peripheral nerve? This question requires examination of the paraspinal muscles for an answer. If these are affected, the lesion is metameric and lies in the cord or roots; if not, then the lesion must lie extraspinally in the peripheral course of the lower motor neuron.

4. What is the precise time of onset of the lesion, and is it causally related to the anesthetic and operation? This question may require several repeated examinations for an exact answer.

For brevity, some of the various diagnostic possibilities are presented in diagrammatic form in Figure 14–3.

Interruption of a peripheral nerve is manifested only in the muscle groups supplied by that nerve, and a normal electromyographic pattern is found in other muscle groups, including the paraspinal muscles supplied by the posterior primary rami of the same metameric segments (see Fig. 14–3*B*). The reverse pattern may be seen in the early stages of metastatic tumors of the spine. In a series of 38 cases of malignant disease, LaBan and Grant (1971) found that the two primary rami are not equally involved initially, but there is a period of dissociation lasting for a week or a month, depending on the rate of tumor growth, when the posterior primary ramus is invaded while

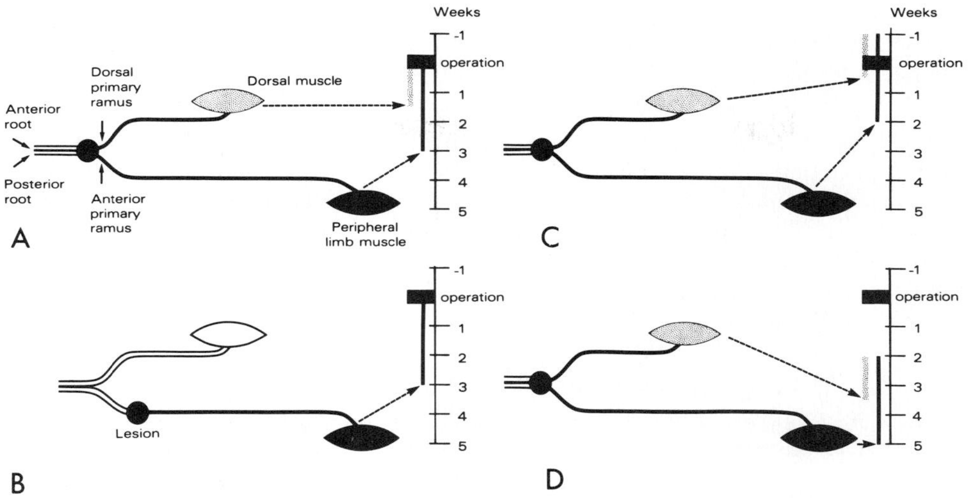

Figure 14-3. Electromyography in differential diagnosis of postoperative neurological complications. Diagram of spinal roots, dorsal and anterior primary rami, and peripheral nerves. Symbols:
● = Lesion
= Normal dorsal (paraspinal) muscle
= Denervated dorsal muscle
= Denervated peripheral limb muscle
= Normal nerve
= Damaged nerve distal to lesion
Vertical scale shows elapsed time in weeks from time of lesion to appearance of denervation EMG patterns in muscles.
A, Lesion of spinal roots at time of operation. Dorsal muscles show EMG changes $1^1/_2$ weeks later. Distal limb muscles show EMG changes three weeks later.
B, Lesion of peripheral nerve at time of operation. No change in dorsal muscle. Distal limb muscles show EMG changes three weeks later.
C, Associated but unrelated lesion of spinal roots one week before operation.
D, Lesion of spinal roots occurring two weeks after operation.

the anterior primary ramus remains unaffected. Later as the secondary growth enlarges, both rami become equally involved, and then a denervation pattern develops in the muscles supplied by both rami.

A lesion of the cord or spinal roots occurring at operation and due to anesthesia or surgery should result in a denervation pattern appearing in the segmental muscles of both the anterior and posterior primary rami in two to three weeks (see Fig. 14–3*A*). Thus, thorough testing of the paraspinal muscles, as well as the limb muscles, is crucial and should be carried out as soon as possible after the suspected injury and again at intervals of a week for the next three weeks. A denervation pattern in the muscles supplied by the anterior primary rami appearing earlier than two weeks after operation is strongly suggestive of a pre-existing pathology; this would indicate that the anesthesia was coincidental and not causally related (see Fig. 14–3*C*). On the other hand, a degeneration pattern that does not develop for a month or more suggests that the lesion arose after operation (see Fig. 14–3*D*). In this event it is possible that the lesion *may* have been related to some process initiated at the time of operation, for example, arachnoiditis, but equally well it may not have been, and other criteria must be sought to determine this point.

Marinacci and Courville (1958) applied these methods of analysis to

482 cases of spinal anesthesia, in which postoperative neurological complaints invited critical study. By their criteria, only 4 out of the 482 cases were found to have genuine anesthetic complications. In the remaining 478 patients, the neurological complaints were probably due to some concurrent and entirely unrelated condition. That is, in only 1 out of 120 cases (0.82 per cent) did the paralysis actually prove to be a genuine anesthetic complication; complications in the rest of the cases were considered to be counterfeits of postanesthetic complications.

Lumbar puncture

Diagnostic lumbar puncture should only be carried out if there are good grounds for suspecting a condition that requires it, such as localized compression above the lumbar region or infection in the subarachnoid space.

Suspected epidural infection should be treated more circumspectly, for such cases will not be helped by opening a track for infection to invade the subarachnoid space. In these cases diagnostic epidural or caudal puncture with a wide-bore needle is a more logical approach when pus is being sought in the extradural space. Any cerebrospinal fluid samples that are needed should be obtained by cisternal puncture, not by lumbar puncture.

Myelography

Contrast studies of the subarachnoid space may be extremely valuable in cases of suspected spinal compression. Myelography may reveal an unrelated lesion, such as a herniated intervertebral disc, that requires appropriate treatment, or it may show an epidural tumor or hematoma that requires urgent decompression. However, myelography is an invasive technique with a small but definite morbidity rate of its own, and it is therefore put low on the list of priorities in spite of its great potential value when there are genuine indications for its use.

Angiographic contrast studies

Very rarely, venous or arterial angiograms may be necessary to confirm the presence of a suspected angioma compressing the cord (Schobinger et al., 1961). Again, angiography of the cord carries a definite morbidity, both from the toxic effects of contrast media and from the risk of femoral artery thrombosis following femoral catheterization, and this type of study should be undertaken only by experts in the technique.

Surgical exploration

Surgical exploration as a diagnostic measure will obviously not be undertaken lightly, but there must be a lively awareness of the vital importance of early surgical decompression for expanding intraspinal lesions, whether they be from blood, pus or tumor. In the face of an epidural hematoma or epidural abscess, delay imposes an almost certain sentence of paraplegia, while prompt drainage is likely to be followed by complete recovery (Hulme and Dott, 1954).

Postmortem examination

A postmortem examination must be made if death should occur after a neurological complication. Sometimes, even when overt neurological symptoms have not arisen, examination of the spine may be instructive. The only epidural hematoma that I have encountered was asymptomatic and found when a special search was made after a heparinized patient had died of massive hemorrhage from another site (see Case 2 on page 669) (Bromage, 1954).

CONTRAINDICATIONS

Success in any field requires a balance of prudence and enough boldness to do what has to be done. In epidural analgesia, as in any other anesthetic technique, there are situations in which prudence demands that some other way be chosen.

Absolute Contraindications

Infection

Localized sepsis in the region of the proposed injection might be carried down to the epidural space and so produce a peridural cellulitis or abscess. Or, worse still, if the dura were accidentally punctured, meningitis might follow.

Chronic infection of the spine with pyogenic or acid-fast bacilli is an obvious reason to avoid a technique that might disturb and spread latent infection. This type of infection may easily be missed on rare occasions, and in cases of low back pain it is wise to obtain X-rays of the lumbar spine in two planes. I well remember seeing a fashionable London osteopath preparing to manipulate the lumbar spine of a 21-year-old girl for backache on the basis of a negative anteroposterior X-ray film. The osteopath was persuaded, somewhat reluctantly, to take a lateral film, and this picture revealed the typical fluffy pattern of tuberculous involvement of the first lumbar vertebra; the osteopath was dissuaded from carrying out manipulation, and the patient was referred to an orthopedic center for appropriate treatment. The possibility of chronic infection should be borne in mind, especially among populations in which tuberculosis is prevalent.

Nidation from systemic infection and distant foci is the commonest cause of spontaneous epidural abscess (Hulme and Dott, 1954). Metastatic infection from sources elsewhere may find a favorable nesting place in an area predisposed to infection by mild trauma or irritation from an epidural needle or indwelling catheter, and for this reason epidural analgesia is often considered to be contraindicated in the presence of systemic infection (Lund, 1966). Pelvic sepsis that may extend along the vertebral venous system and past the site of epidural puncture is another potential danger. However, provided the infection is well under control with appropriate antibiotic therapy, the risk of an epidural nidus would seem to be remote and acceptable if epidural analgesia is indicated.

Uncontrolled bleeding

Epidural analgesia is generally considered to be contraindicated in the presence of active bleeding. A disturbance of autonomic tone and compensatory vasoconstriction in the presence of an inadequate blood volume might precipitate complete cardiovascular collapse and cardiac arrest.

That is the orthodox view. However, my own experience in the past has included a number of cases in which epidural analgesia was deliberately induced in the presence of bleeding and in which compensatory vasoconstriction was provided when necessary by exogenous norepinephrine in very dilute solution (1 to 2 μg/ml), given intravenously as required. These patients all received blood as required, and all did well. *Provided blood volume can be maintained,* there seems to me to be no logical reason why controlled vasomotor tone should not be an acceptable part of the whole endeavor to control the patient's internal environment and to protect it from the effects of uncontrolled reflexes, including those of vasomotor origin.

Obviously, uncontrolled bleeding without adequate resources for blood replacement is an intrinsically lethal situation. Clearly, it would be imprudent to expand the vascular bed by vasodilatation and to hasten the end under circumstances in which adequate transfusion facilities are unavailable.

Clotting deficiencies

As pointed out earlier, severe disturbances of the clotting mechanism, whether by disease or anticoagulant therapy, carry an intrinsic risk of spontaneous hematomas, and these may arise within the spine or the calvarium. Marked increase of the partial thromboplastin time or rise of the blood heparin level above normal are prudent contraindications to regional anesthesia (see page 248 in Chapter 7).

Further study is needed of *minimum* dose regimens for heparin prophylaxis against postoperative thrombosis. Present evidence suggests the cautious use of epidural analgesia may be justified in the presence of subcoagulating doses of heparin, provided facilities are available to assess plasma heparin levels and provided the patient is closely watched for premonitory signs of epidural hematoma formation. The increasingly widespread use of heparin prophylaxis against deep vein thrombosis (Sharnoff and DeBlasio, 1970; Kakkar et al., 1975) will undoubtedly place a serious limitation on all types of regional analgesia for major elective surgery. It remains to be seen whether a safe compromise can be worked out between the two conflicting techniques of partial prophylactic heparinization and regional anesthesia involving the deep placement of needles and indwelling catheters.

Relative Contraindications

Existing neurological disease

This is sometimes listed as an absolute contraindication to epidural analgesia. As in subarachnoid anesthesia, it is probably wise to avoid the method in patients with obvious disease of the central nervous system, such as multiple sclerosis or spinal syphilis. Although it is difficult to see how an epidural block could have an adverse effect on these conditions, the anesthesiologist will avoid the possibility of becoming involved in a post hoc, ergo propter hoc litigation claim should a natural exacerbation of the disease develop after the operation.

If spinal disease were taken as an absolute contraindication under all circumstances, the prevalence of vascular degenerative disease would provide an almost universal and absurd reason for avoiding epidural analgesia in elderly patients. As we have seen in earlier chapters, the process of aging begins early and proceeds inexorably to death. Some individuals are physiologically older and closer to death than their chronological age would suggest. Neuraxial age is correspondingly advanced in these precociously geriatric patients, who are therefore prone to exhibit exaggerated spread of epidural blockade. However, there is no undue risk if dosage is adjusted to match advanced physiological age and reduced dosage requirements (Bromage, 1962).

Spinal deformities

Exceptionally severe spinal deformities may prevent a successful epidural puncture. Scoliosis need not present an insuperable technical difficulty, provided care and imagination are used to envisage the rotation of the vertebrae and the correct path for the needle.

Spina bifida, a congenital defect of the neural arch closure, may be a cause of technical difficulty and inadvertent dural puncture. The condition has an incidence of about 1 in 500 births (Matson, 1969). It is commonest at the level of L_5 or S_1, and may present as no more than a slight gap in the laminar arch of L_5. However, incomplete fusion of the laminae may extend further up the spinal column and along the whole length of the lumbar region. A fibrous pad tends to fill the gap between the unfused arches in spina bifida (Ingraham, 1944), and the dura mater may be anchored firmly to the overlying lipomatous tissue, so that the intervening epidural space is virtually obliterated. In the face of this abnormality, attempted epidural puncture at the level of the bifid spines is doomed to failure, as there is no posterior epidural space for the needle to encounter, and so an inadvertent subarachnoid tap is almost inevitable. In these cases epidural puncture must be attempted in some other region of the back, either above the level of the unfused spinal arches or below via the sacral hiatus.

Signs of underlying spina bifida may include one or more of the following stigmata:

1. Overlying tuft of hair.

2. Cutaneous angioma. A port-wine stain of the skin in the lumbosacral region is frequently associated with spina bifida occulta (Farmer, 1975).

3. Lipoma. A fatty swelling in the lumbosacral region should alert the anesthesiologist to the possibility of an underlying spina bifida occulta.

4. Dimple or furrow of skin overlying site of bifida.

Sensitivity to local anesthetic agents

Patients frequently present themselves with a history of sensitivity to local anesthetics, usually after some untoward experience in a dental chair. There are many possible causes for this kind of experience, but true sensitivity to the amide type of local anesthetics is seldom one of them (Aldrete and Johnson, 1970). It has been my practice to employ a screening intradermal test with lidocaine in these cases, normal saline being used as a control (see page 105). If the intradermal test is negative, I then proceed to use epidural analgesia, exercising great caution to induce blockade gradually, with small incremental doses, and having all necessary drugs prepared and drawn up in syringes in case of an allergic response. To date I have not seen an adverse reaction under these circumstances.

Certain cardiac conditions

Any cardiac condition with a low output may deteriorate and enter failure if venous return is reduced by vasodilatation. Constrictive pericarditis is the classic example in which venous return and cardiac output must be carefully maintained, and this condition would constitute a contraindication to epidural analgesia.

Partial heart block is sometimes considered a contraindication on the grounds that vascular uptake of local anesthetic may be sufficient to suppress surviving conduction tissue and precipitate complete heart block. This danger can be avoided by using low doses, preferably by segmental block, and by selecting an agent with high protein-binding characteristics, such as bupivacaine, that gives rise to very low plasma levels of free unbound drug.

SUMMARY

The list of complications collected over the years and the contraindications in this chapter may seem unduly formidable. However, they must be seen in historical perspective as a changing and attenuating hazard, lessened by improved techniques and drugs and by a better knowledge of how to apply these tools more safely. Also, they must be seen in perspective as part of a systematic choice of evils. No anesthetic is completely safe, and many fail to provide the unique set of conditions that epidural analgesia can produce. There is a range of options in selecting an anesthetic for any purpose, and each contains its own inherent dangers, in terms of both what it does and what it fails to do for the patient. In this light, the cost-effectiveness ratio of epidural analgesia ranks it among the most efficient anesthetic techniques.

The acute complications of today are less common and less florid than formerly. Improved understanding of dose requirements and the uptake and distribution of drugs from the epidural space has led to greater restraint in techniques and dosage. The practice of flooding the epidural space with volumes of 40 to 50 ml of potent solutions has given way to more cautious administration of anesthetics in a dosage properly related to age, and consequently the dramatic effects that follow accidental injection of bolus doses into the subarachnoid space or the vascular system are lessened.

Greater insight into the significance of related anatomy and physiology has opened the way for avoiding some mistakes of the past. One of the most important lessons has been the growing appreciation of the deleterious effects of obstruction of the inferior vena cava, especially in the presence of epidural analgesia. Cardiovascular depression, the possibility of venous congestion of the cord and uteroplacental insufficiency are all consequences that can now be avoided quite simply by proper use of posture or other maneuvers to relieve caval compression in any of the many situations that can cause it.

Increasingly thorough investigation of neurological complications that may occur in association with regional or general anesthesia has broadened the base of understanding for the natural history of such events and for the multiplicity of causes that may lead to them. Critical examination of published reports relating to neurological complications of epidural analgesia reveals the very slender evidence upon which a causal relationship has so often been assumed, without a thorough search for contributory factors or underlying disease. It can now be seen that many complications were wrongly ascribed to epidural analgesia on the basis of incomplete evidence and facile assumptions.

Statistical information can now be gathered in a more comprehensive and intelligible manner than was possible in the past, when so many of the coincidental variables were either unknown or unappreciated. With present methods of data collection, it should be possible to assemble the neurological complications arising in a non-epidural population of surgical and obstetrical patients and so assess the comparative frequency and significance of complications arising in an epidural population. Unfortunately, in a free society in which reporting is left to the individual physician, the practical fruition of such an ideal is almost doomed at the outset. The weakest link of any data collection system lies at the periphery, and if cases escape report because they are ignored, transferred to another hospital or simply concealed for fear of litigation, the statistical endeavor becomes an exercise in futility, and the results of the study will be dangerously misleading.

In 1971, a study of epidural complications was set up by the Association of Anaesthetists of Great Britain and Ireland in an attempt to look at the overall scene as objectively as possible; the outcome of this investigation should be of the greatest interest. Nevertheless, it seems likely that the free system of reporting upon which the study is based may restrict the results to a qualitative rather than a quantitative scale of values.

The future of epidural analgesia lies in guarding it from abuse in practice and in report. Training in its use must be thorough and craftsmanlike, Increasing use should be made of training simulator models, visual aids and cadavers, so that novices are not turned loose to gather a dismal harvest of dural punctures from their first endeavors. Initial clinical experience should be gained in a strict master-apprentice relationship, with tandem manual guidance as recommended by Lund (1966) and outlined in Chapter 15 on Teaching Techniques.

REFERENCES

Abraham, J., Margolis, G., O'Loughlin, J. C. and MacCarty, W. C.: Differential reactivity of neural and extraneural vasculature. I. Role in the pathogenesis of spinal cord damage from contrast media in experimental aortography. J. Neurosurg. *25*:257, 1966.

Adelman, J. U., Goldberg, G. S. and Puckett, J. D.: Postpartum bilateral femoral neuropathy. Obstet. Gynecol. *42*:845, 1973.

Adler, E., Jarus, A. and Magora, A.: Rare peripheral nerve complications in obstetrical and gynaecological conditions. Acta. Psych. Neurol. Scand. *31*:1, 1956.

Aldrete, J. A. and Johnson, D. A.: Evaluation of intracutaneous testing for investigation of allergy to local anesthetic agents. Anesth. Analg. *49*:173, 1970.

Allen, S. S. and Kahn, E. A.: Acute pyogenic infection of the spinal epidural space. J.A.M.A. *98*:875, 1932.

Alpers, B. J. and Mancall, E. J.: Clinical Neurology. 6th ed., Philadelphia, F. A. Davis Co., 1971, p. 418.

Ansbro, F. P., Iason, A. H., Shaftel, H. E., Halpern, A., Latteri, F. S. and Bodell, B.: The development of efocaine, a new approach to prolonged local anesthesia. Anesthesiology *13*:306, 1952.

Arieff, A. J. and Pyzik, S. W.: Quadriplegia after intrathecal injection of methylene blue. J.A.M.A. *173*:794, 1960.

Arner, O.: Complications following spinal anesthesia: Their significance and a technic to reduce their incidence. Acta Chir. Scand. Suppl. *167*:1, 1952.

Baker, A. S., Ojemann, R. G., Swartz, M. N. and Richardson, E. P.: Spinal epidural abscess. N. Engl. J. Med. *293*:463, 1975.

Barretto, R. S.: Bacteriological culture of indwelling epidural catheters. Anesthesiology *23*:643, 1962.

Beatty, T. E.: Second report of the new Lying-in-Hospital, Dublin. Dublin J. Med. Sci. *12*:273, 1838.

Bidzinski, J.: Spontaneous spinal epidural hematoma during pregnancy. Case report. J. Neurosurg. *24*:1017, 1966.

Binnert, D., Thierry, A., Michiels, R., Soichot, P. and Perrin, M.: Présentation d'un nouveau cas d'hématome extradural rachidien spontané observé au cours d'un accouchement. J. Med. Lyon *52*:1307, 1971.

Birkhahn, H. J. and Heifetz, M.: A complication following epidural anesthesia. Anesth. Analg. *40*:650, 1961.

Böden, O.: Letale Komplikation einer extraduralen Spinalanesthesie. Der Anaesthesist *3*:127, 1954.

Bonica, J. J., Backup, P. H., Anderson, C. E., Hadfield, D., Crepps, W. F. and Monk, B. F.: Peridural block: Analysis of 3,637 cases and a review. Anesthesiology *18*:723, 1957.

Boongird, P., Vimolchalao, M., Khantanaphar, S. and Bunyaratavej, S.: Acute spinal epidural abscess: A report of two cases, one with autopsy findings. J. Med. Assoc. Thailand *57*: 564, 1974.

Boys, J. E. and Norman, P. F.: Accidental subdural analgesia. Brit. J. Anaesth. *47*:1111, 1975.

Braham, J. and Saia, A.: Neurological complications of epidural anaesthesia. Brit. Med. J. *2*:657, 1958.

Brigden, W., Howarth, S. and Sharpey-Schafer, E. P.: Postural changes in the peripheral blood flow of normal subjects with observations on vaso-vagal fainting reactions as a result of tilting, the lordotic posture, pregnancy and spinal anaesthesia. Clin. Sci. *9*:79, 1950.

Britt, B. A. and Gordon, R. A.: Peripheral nerve injuries associated with anaesthesia. Canad. Anaesth. Soc. J. *11*:514, 1964.

Bromage, P. R.: Spinal Epidural Analgesia. Edinburgh, E. & S. Livingstone, Ltd., 1954, p. 102.

Bromage, P. R.: Exaggerated spread of epidural analgesia in arteriosclerotic patients. Dosage in relation to biological and chronological ageing. Brit. Med. J. *2*:1634, 1962.

Bromage, P. R.: Spinal thrombophlebitis after hypotensive anaesthesia. New Zealand Med. J. *80*:519, 1974.

Bromage, P. R. and Burfoot, M. F.: Quality of epidural blockade II: Influence of physico-chemical factors; hyaluronidase and potassium. Brit. J. Anaesth. *38*:857, 1966.
Brown, W. W. : Meningitis following continuous caudal anesthesia. Amer. J. Obstet. Gynecol. *53*:682, 1947.
Bull, G. M.: Postural proteinuria. Clin. Sci. 7:77, 1949.
Butler, A. E. and Green, C. D.: Haematoma following epidural anaesthesia. Canad. Anaesth. Soc. J. *17*:635, 1970.
Calverley, J. R. and Mulder, D. W.: Femoral neuropathy. Neurology *10*:963, 1960.
Catterberg, J. and Insausti, T.: Paraplejias consecutivas a anestesia peridural (estudio clinico y experimental). Rev. Assoc. Med. Argent *78*:1, 1964.
Chalmers, J. A.: Traumatic neuritis in the puerperium. J. Obstet. Gynecol. Brit. Emp. *56*:205, 1949.
Chaplin, R. A. and Renwick, W. A.: Lumbar epidural anaesthesia for vaginal delivery. Canad. Anaesth. Soc. J. *5*:414, 1958.
Chun, L. and Karp. M.: Unusual complications from placement of catheters in caudal canal in obstetrical anesthesia. Anesthesiology *27*:96, 1966.
Churchill, F.: On paralysis occurring during gestation and in childbed. Dublin. J. Quart. Med. *17*:259, 1854.
Clarke, E., Morrison, R. and Roberts, H.: Spinal cord damage by Efocaine. Lancet *1*:896, 1955.
Cooper, D. W.: Spontaneous spinal epidural hematoma. Case report. J. Neurosurg. *26*:343, 1967.
Coupier, L., Garbay, M. and Delègue, L.: Paralysie crurale par hématome spontané du psoas sous traitement anti-coagulant. Anesth. Analg. Réan. *31*:615, 1974.
Cousins, M. J.: Hematoma following epidural block. Anesthesiology *37*:263, 1972.
Craft, J. B., Epstein, B. S. and Coakley, C. S.: Prophylaxis of dural-puncture headache with epidural saline. Anesth. Analg. *52*:228, 1973.
Craig, D. B. and Habib, G. G.: Flaccid paraparesis following obstetrical epidural anesthesia: Possible role of benzyl alcohol. Anesth. Analg. *56*:219, 1977.
Crawford, J. S.: The prevention of headache consequent upon dural puncture. Brit. J. Anaesth. *44*:598, 1972.
Dandy, W. E.: Abscesses and inflammatory tumors in the spinal epidural space (so-called pachymeningitis externa). Arch. Surg. *13*:477, 1926.
Davies, A., Solomon, B. and Levene, A.: Paraplegia following epidural anaesthesia. Brit. Med. J. *2*:654, 1958.
Dean, G.: The Porphyrias: A Story of Inheritance and Environment. Philadelphia, J. B. Lippincott, 1963.
De Angelis, J.: Hazards of subdural and epidural anesthesia during anticoagulant therapy: A case report and review. Anesth. Analg. *51*:676, 1972.
Defalque, R. J.: Exaggerated spread of epidural block. Anesthesiology *28*:229, 1967.
Denson, K. W. E. and Bonnar, J.: The measurement of heparin. A method based on the potentiation of anti-factor Xa. Thrombos. Diathes. Haemorrh. (Stuttg.) *30*:471, 1973.
De Saram, M.: Accidental total spinal analgesia. Anaesthesia *11*:77, 1956.
Desmond, J.: The use of micropore filters in continuous epidural anaesthesia. Canad. Anaesth. Soc. J. *19*:97, 1972.
DiGiovanni, A. J. and Dunbar, B. S.: Epidural injections of autologous blood for postlumbar-puncture headache. Anesth Analg. *49*:268, 1970.
DiGiovanni, A. J., Galbert, M. W. and Wahle, W. M.: Epidural injections of autologous blood for postlumbar-puncture headache. II. Additional clinical experiences and laboratory investigation. Anesth. Analg. *51*:226, 1972.
Ditzler, J. W. and McIver, G.: Paraplegia following general anesthesia. Anesth. Analg. *35*:501, 1956.
Doppman, J., Rubinson, R. M., Rockoff, S. D., Vasko, J. S., Shapiro, R. and Morrow, A. G.: Mechanism of obstruction of the infradiaphragmatic portion of the inferior vena cava in the presence of increased intra-abdominal pressure. Invest. Radiol. *1*:37, 1966.
Duncalf, D. and Foldes, F. F.: The use of radio-iodinated serum albumin to confirm accidental intravascular insertion of epidural catheters. Anesthesiology *25*:564, 1964.
Edmonds-Seal, J.: An overdose of lignocaine: A case report on epidural analgesia for post-operative pain. Anesthesia *19*:222, 1964.
Edwards, W. B. and Hingson, R. A.: The present status of continuous caudal analgesia in obstetrics. Bull. N.Y. Acad. Med. *19*:507, 1943.
Evans, J. P. and Keegan, H. R.: Danger in the use of intrathecal methylene blue. J.A.M.A. *174*:856, 1960.
Farmer, T. W.: Pediatric Neurology. 2nd ed., Hagerstown, Md., Harper and Row, 1975, p. 428.
Ferguson, J. F. and Kirsch, W. M.: Epidural empyema following thoracic extradural block. J. Neurosurg. *41*:762, 1974.
Finch, C. A.: Methemoglobinemia and sulfhemoglobinemia. N. Engl. J. Med. *239*:470, 1948.
Forestner, J. E. and Raj, P. P.: Inadvertent epidural injection of thiopental: A case report. Anesth. Analg. *54*:406, 1975.

Forrester, A. C.: Mishaps in anaesthesia. Anaesthesia *14*:388, 1959.

Fowler, T. J. and Ochoa, J.: Unmyelinated fibres in normal and compressed peripheral nerves of the baboon: A quantitative electron microscopic study. Neuropathol. Appl. Neurobiol. *1*:247, 1975.

Fraser, R. A. R., Ratzan, K., Wolpert, S. M. and Weinstein, L.: Spinal subdural empyema. Arch. Neurol. *28*:235, 1973.

Frumin, M. J. and Schwartz, H.: Continuous segmental peridural anesthesia. Anesthesiology *13*:488, 1952.

Fujimori, M., Nishimura, K. and Goto, E.: Methemoglobinemia due to local anesthetics (a preliminary report). Far East J. Anesth. *4*:22, 1964.

Galbert, M. W. and Marx, G. F.: Extradural pressures in the parturient patient. Anesthesiology *40*:499, 1974.

Garland, H., Greenberg, J. and Harriman, D. G. F.: Infarction of the spinal cord. Brain *89*:645, 1966.

Gavin, R.: Continuous epidural analgesia. An unusual cause of dural perforation during catheterization of the epidural space. New Zealand J. Med. *64*:280, 1965.

Gilles, F. H. and Nag, D.: Vulnerability of human spinal cord in transient cardiac arrest. Neurology *21*:833, 1971.

Gillies, I. D. S. and Morgan, M.: Accidental total spinal analgesia with bupivacaine. Anaesthesia *28*:441, 1973.

Gingrich, T. F.: Spinal epidural hematoma following continuous epidural anesthesia. Anesthesiology *29*:162, 1968.

Gold, M. E.: Spontaneous spinal epidural hematoma. Radiology *80*:823, 1963.

Goldberg, L.: Studies on local anesthetics. Acta Physiol. Scand. *18*:1, 1949.

Goodgold, J. and Eberstein, A.: Electrodiagnosis of Neuromuscular Diseases. Baltimore, Williams & Wilkins Co. 1972, pp. 76, 164, 165, 169.

Goodman, J. I.: Femoral neuropathy in relation to diabetes mellitus: Report of 17 cases. Diabetes *3*:266, 1954.

Gordon Jones, R. G.: A complication of epidural technique. Anaesthesia *8*:242, 1953.

Gormley, J. B.: Treatment of postspinal headache. Anesthesiology *21*:565, 1960.

Grove, L. H.: Backache, headache and bladder dysfunction after delivery. Brit. J. Anaesth. *45*:1147, 1973.

Gruner, J. and Lapresle, J.: Etude anatomo-pathologique des médullopathies d'origine vasculaire. Rev. Neurol. *106*:592, 1962.

Hancock, D. O.: A study of 49 patients with acute spinal extradural abscess. Paraplegia *10*:285, 1973.

Harik, S. I., Raichle, M. E. and Reis, D. J.: Spontaneous remitting spinal epidural hematoma in a patient on anticoagulants. N. Engl. J. Med. *284*:1355, 1971.

Helperin, S. W. and Cohen, D. D.: Hematoma following epidural anesthesia: Report of a case. Anesthesiology *35*:641, 1971.

Henson, R. A. and Parsons, M.: Ischaemic lesions of the spinal cord: An illustrated review. Q. J. Med. *36*:205, 1967.

Heusner, A. P.: Nontuberculous spinal epidural infections. N. Engl. J. Med. *239*:845, 1948.

Hill, E. C.: Maternal obstetric paralysis. Amer. J. Obstet. Gynecol. *83*:1452, 1962.

Holmdahl, M. H., Sjögren, S., Ström, G. and Wright, B.: Clinical aspects of continuous epidural blockade for postoperative pain relief. Uppsala J. Med. Sci. *77*:47, 1972.

Honkomp, J.: Zur Begutachtung bleibender neurologischer Schaden nach Periduralanaesthesie. Der Anaesthesist *15*:246, 1966.

Hopf, H. C.: Obturatorius-Lähmung unter der Deburt. J. Neurol. *207*:165, 1974.

Hopper, C. L. and Baker, J. B.: Bilateral femoral neuropathy complicating vaginal hysterectomy. Obstet. Gynecol. *32*:543, 1968.

Hughes, J. T. and Brownell, B.: Spinal cord ischemia due to arteriosclerosis. Arch. Neurol. *15*:189, 1966.

Hulme, A. and Dott, N. M.: Spinal epidural abscess. Brit. Med. J. *1*:64, 1954.

Hünermann, S.: Oeber nervenlähmung im gebiete des nervus ischiadicus infolge von entbindungen. Arch. Gynäk. *42*:489, 1892.

Hylton, R. R., Eger, E. I. and Rovno, S. H.: Intravascular placement of epidural catheters. Anesth. Analg. *43*:379, 1964.

Iason, A. H. and Shaftel, H. E.: A new approach to the problem of postoperative pain. Amer. J. Surg. *83*:549, 1952.

Ingraham, F. C.: Spina Bifida and Cranium Bifidum. Cambridge, Mass., Harvard University Press, 1944, p. 44.

Jacobson, I., MacCabe, J. J., Harris, P. and Dott, N. M.: Spontaneous spinal epidural haemorrhage during anticoagulant therapy. Brit. Med. J. *1*:522, 1966.

Janis, K. M.: Epidural hematoma following postoperative epidural analgesia: A case report. Anesthesiology *51*:689, 1971.

Järvinen, P. A., Unnerus, C. E. and Vaananen, P.: Cystometric cystourethrographic studies during the puerperium. Ann. Chir. Gynaec. Fenn. *50*:237, 1961.
Jenicek, J. A.: Aseptic meningitis following lumbar epidural block: Case report. Anesthesiology *16*:464, 1955.
Junghanns, H.: Über die Häufigkeit gutartiger Geschwülste in den Wirbelkörpern (Angiome, Lipome, Osteome). Archiv. f. Klin. Chir. *169*:204, 1932.
Kakkar, V. V. et al.: Prevention of fatal postoperative pulmonary embolism by low doses of heparin: An International Multicentre Trial. Lancet *2*:45, 1975.
Kaplan, M. S. and Arrowood, J. G.: Prevention of headache following spinal anesthesia; use of epidural saline: A preliminary report. Anesthesiology *18*:103, 1952.
Kaufman, R. D. and Reynolds, R. C.: Occlusion of an epidural catheter secondary to osteoarthritis. Anesthesiology *44*:253, 1976.
King, A. B.: Neurologic conditions occurring as complications of pregnancy. Arch. Neurol. Psychiat. *63*:471, 610, 1950.
Kliemann, F. A. D.: Paraplegia and intercranial hypertension following epidural anesthesia. Report of four cases. Arquivos de Neuro-Psiquiatria *33*:217, 1975.
LaBan, M. M. and Grant, A. E.: Occult spinal metastases—early electromyographic manifestation. Arch. Phys. Med. Rehab. *52*:223, 1971.
Laguna, J. and Cravioto, H.: Spinal cord infarction secondary to occlusion of the anterior spinal artery. Arch. Neurol. *28*:134, 1973.
Lerner, S., Gutterman, P. and Jenkins, F.: Epidural hematoma and paraplegia after numerous lumbar punctures. Anesthesiology *39*:550, 1973.
Lhermitte, J.: Etude sur les paraplegies des vieillards. Thèse, Paris, 1907.
Löfgren, N.: Studies on Local Anaesthetics. Xylocaine, A New Synthetic Drug. Stockholm, Haeggströms, 1948.
Lougheed, W. M. and Hoffman, H. J.: Spontaneous spinal extradural hematoma. Neurology *10*:1059, 1960.
Lund, P. C.: Peridural Analgesia and Anesthesia. Springfield, Ill., Charles C Thomas, 1966, pp. 282, 163, 302, 326, 317.
Lundqvist, B., Löfgren, N., Persson, H. and Sjögren, B.: Metal ions as a cause of swelling after local anaesthesia in dental practice. Acta Chir. Scand. *97*:239, 1948.
Malatinsky, J. and Kadlic, T.: Inferior vena caval occlusion in the left lateral position. Brit. J. Anaesth. *46*:165, 1974.
Male, C. G. and Martin, R.: Puerperal spinal epidural abscess. Lancet *1*:608, 1973.
Manalan, S. A.: Caudal block anesthesia in obstetrics. J. Indiana Med. Assoc. *35*:564, 1942.
Mandlekar, V. M.: Accidental total spinal (intradural) block. A case with some unusual features. Anaesthesia *25*:393, 1970.
Mangelsdorff, A. F.: Treatment of methemoglobinemia. Arch. Ind. Health *14*:148, 1956.
Margolis, G.: Pathogenesis of contrast media injury: Insights provided by neurotoxicity studies. Invest. Radiol. *5*:392, 1970.
Marinacci, A. A.: The medicolegal application of electromyography in peripheral nerve injuries. Bull. Los Angeles Neurol. Soc. *27*:147, 1962.
Marinacci, A. A.: Applied Electromyography. Philadelphia, Lea & Febiger, 1968. pp. 163–180.
Marinacci, A. A. and Courville, C. B.: Electromyogram in evaluation of neurological complications of spinal anesthesia. J.A.M.A. *168*:1337, 1958.
Marinacci, A. A. and von Hagen, K. O.: Review article: Neurological complications occurring in hospitalized patients. Bull. Los Angeles Neurol. Soc. *31*:209, 1966.
Markham, J. W., Lynge, H. N. and Stahlman, G. E. B.: The syndrome of spontaneous spinal epidural hematoma. Report of three cases. J. Neurosurg. *26*:334, 1967.
Matson, D. D.: Neurosurgery of Infancy and Childhood. Springfield, Ill., Charles C Thomas, 1969, p. 6.
Mellander, S. and Johansson, B.: Control of resistance, exchange and capacitance functions in the peripheral circulation. Pharmacol. Rev. *20*:117, 1968.
Mikhailovich, V. A., Kotomina, G. L., Garmasher, I. A., et al.: Suppurative complication of prolonged peridural anaesthesia. Vestnik Khirurgii. *112(6)*:109, 1974.
Moir, D. D. and Davidson, S.: Postpartum complications of forceps delivery performed under epidural and pudendal nerve block. Brit. J. Anaesth. *44*:1197, 1972.
Moir, D. D. and Hesson, W. R.: Dural puncture by an epidural catheter. Anaesthesia *20*:373, 1965.
Moore, D. C.: Complications of regional anesthesia. *In* Bonica, J. J.: Clinical Anesthesia, Regional Anesthesia: Recent Advances and Current Status. Philadelphia, F. A. Davis Company, 1969, p. 234.
Moore, D. C., Bridenbaugh, L. D., Van Ackeren, E. G., Belda, F. B. and Cole, F. V.: Spread of radiopaque solutions in the epidural space of the human adult corpse. Anesthesiology *19*:377, 1958.
Moore, J. M. and Frew, I. D. O.: Peripheral vascular lesion in diabetes mellitus. Brit. Med. J. *2*:19, 1965.

Morrow, W. F. K.: Unexplained spread of epidural anaesthesia. Brit. J. Anaesth. *31*:359, 1959.
Mostert, J. W.: Coma contra-indicates spinal analgesia (Corr.). Anaesthesia *13*:242, 1958.
Mostert, J. W.: The risk of epidural block in old people. Brit. J. Anaesth. *32*:613, 1960.
Murray, R. R.: Maternal obstetrical paralysis. Amer. J. Obstet. Gynecol. *88*:399, 1964.
Nelson, D. A.: Spinal cord compression due to vertebral angiomas during pregnancy. Arch. Surg. *11*:408, 1964.
Newman, M. J. D.: Spinal angioma with symptoms in pregnancy. J. Neurol. Neurosurg. Psychiat. *21*:38, 1958.
Nicholson, M. J. and Eversole, U. H.: Nerve injuries incident to anesthesia and operation. Anesth. Analg. *36*(4):19, 1957.
O'Connell, J. E. A.: Maternal obstetrical paralysis. Surg. Gynecol. Obstet. *79*:374, 1944.
Ostheimer, G. W., Palahniuk, R. J. and Shnider, S. M.: Epidural blood patch for post-lumbar puncture headache. Anesthesiology *41*:307, 1974.
Pasternak, B. M., Boyd, D. P. and Ellis, F. H.: Spinal cord injury after procedures on the aorta. Surg. Gynecol Obstet. *135*:29, 1972.
Peacher, W. G. and Robertson, R. C. L.: Neurologic complications following the use of continuous caudal anesthesia. Arch. Neurol. Psychiat. *52*:531, 1944.
Philip, J. H. and Brown, W. U.: Total spinal anesthesia late in the course of obstetric bupivacaine epidural block. Anesthesiology *44*:340, 1976.
Poppers, P. J., Mastri, A. R., Lebeaux, M. and Covino, B. G.: The effect of methylene blue on neural tissue. Anesthesiology *33*:335, 1970.
Rankin, R. M. and Flothow, P. G.: Pyogenic infection in the spinal epidural space. West. J. Surg. Obstet. Gynecol. *54*:320, 1946.
Ranniger, K. and Switz, D. M.: Local obstruction of the inferior vena cava by massive ascites. Amer. J. Roentgenol. *93*:935, 1965.
Rice, G. G. and Dabbs, C. H.: The use of peridural and subarachnoid injections of saline solution in the treatment of severe postspinal headache. Anesthesiology *11*:17, 1950.
Robert, E. D. and Oester, Y. T.: Absence of supersensitivity to acetylcholine in innervated muscles subjected to a prolonged pharmacological nerve block. J. Pharmacol. Exp. Ther. *174*:133, 1970.
Rosenblum, J., Schwarz, G. A. and Bendler, E.: Femoral neuropathy—a neurological complication. J.A.M.A. *195*:409, 1966.
Ruston, F. G. and Polati, V. L.: Femoral nerve injury from abdominal retractors. Canad. Anaesth. Soc. J. *5*:428, 1958.
Ryan, D. W.: Accidental intravenous injection of bupivacaine: A complication of obstetrical epidural anaesthesia. Brit. J. Anaesth. *45*:907, 1973.
Saady, A.: Epidural abscess complicating thoracic epidural analgesia. Anesthesiology *44*:244, 1976.
Sarrell, W. G. and La Fia, D. J.: Acute lumbar epidural abscess; report of a case. N. Engl. J. Med. *250*:318, 1954.
Schobinger, R. A., Krueger, E. A. and Sobel, G. L.: Comparison of intraosseous vertebral venography and Pantopaque myelography in the diagnosis of surgical conditions of the lumbar spine and nerve roots. Radiology *77*:376, 1961.
Scott, D. B. and Kyles, J. R.: Lumbar epidural analgesia. Anaesthesia *16*:172, 1961.
Sharnoff, J. G. and DeBlasio, G.: Prevention of fatal postoperative thromboembolism by heparin prophylaxis. Lancet *2*:1006, 1970.
Sheffield, W. E., Kennedy, J. J. and Dornette, W. H. L.: Clinical experiences with mepivacaine hydrochloride. Anesth. Analg. *43*:192, 1964.
Siever, J. M. and Mousel, L. H.: Continuous caudal anesthesia in three hundred unselected obstetric cases. J.A.M.A. *122*:424, 1943.
Silver, J. R. and Buxton, P. H.: Spinal stroke. Brain *97*:539, 1974.
Sinclair, R. V.: Ascending spinal paralysis following hysterectomy under general anaesthesia. Anaesthesia *9*:286, 1954.
Skillman, J. J., Zervas, N. T., Weintraub, R. M. and Mayman, C. I.: Paraplegia after resection of aneurysms of the abdominal aorta. N. Engl. J. Med. *281*:422, 1969.
Sokoll, M. D., Sonesson, B. and Thesleff, S.: Denervation changes produced in an innervated skeletal muscle by long-continued treatment with a local anesthetic. Eur. J. Pharmacol. *4*:179, 1968.
Spurning, O. M.: Spinal epidural haematoma—two cases. Arch. Intern. Med. *114*:103, 1964.
Squire, A. W., Calvillo, O. and Bromage, P. R.: Painless intrathecal hypertonic saline. Canad. Anaesth. Soc. J. *21*:308, 1974.
Sreerama, V., Ivan, L. P., Dennery, J. M. and Richard, M. T.: Neurosurgical complications of anticoagulant therapy. Canad. Med. Assoc. J. *108*:305, 1973.
Stenz, K.: Kurze Mitteilungen über Meralgia paraesthetica nach gynäkologischer Lagerung. Z. Gynäk. *52*:2022, 1960.
Strasser, K., Hirsch, I. and Tomaschoff, E.: Bakteriologische Nachuntersuchungen von Epidural-Kathetern. Anaesthesist *23*:351, 1974.

Stringer, R. M.: Epidural anesthesia with Xylocaine. Anesth. Analg. *33*:195, 1954.
Sykes, M. K.: Delayed spinal analgesia. A complication of epidural analgesia. Anaesthesia *13*:78, 1958.
Taveras, J. M. and Wood, E. H.: Myelography: Technical Errors. *In* Robbins, L. L.: Golden's Diagnostic Roentgenology. Baltimore. Williams and Wilkins Co., 1972, Vol. I, pp. 836–840.
Tillman, A. J. B.: Traumatic neuritis in the puerperium. Amer. J. Obstet. Gynecol. *29*:660, 1935.
Urquhart-Hay, D.: Paraplegia following epidural analgesia. Anaesthesia. *24*:461, 1969.
Urquhart-Hay, D. and Teague, C. A.: Spinal thrombophlebitis after prostatectomy with hypotensive anaesthesia: Case report. New Zealand Med. J. *79*:654, 1974.
Usubiaga, J. E.: Neurological complications following epidural analgesia. Int. Anaesth. Clin. *13*(2):19, 50, 1975.
Usubiaga, J. E., Kolodny, J. and Usubiaga, L. E.: Neurological complications of prevertebral surgery under regional anesthesia. Surgery *68*:304, 1970.
Varkey, G. P. and Brindle, G. F.: Peridural anaesthesia and anti-coagulant therapy. Canad. Anaesth. Soc. J. *21*:106, 1974.
Wadia, N. H. and Dastur, D. K.: Spinal meningitides with radiculo-myelopathy. Part I. Clinical features. J. Neurol. Sci. *8*:239, 1969.
Winer, B. M., Horenstein, S. and Starr, A. M.: Spinal epidural hematoma during anticoagulant therapy. Circulation *19*:735, 1959.
Winkelman, N. W.: Neurologic symptoms following accidental intraspinal detergent injection. Neurology *2*:284, 1952.
Winkelman, N. W.: Femoral nerve complications after pelvic surgery. Amer. J. Obstet. Gynecol. *75*:1063, 1958.
Wu, J. J., Harnagel, D. L. A., Brizzee, K. R. and Smith, S. M.: Neurological effects following intrathecal administration of vasoconstrictor drugs in rhesus monkeys. Anesthesiology *15*:71, 1954.
Yin, E. T., Wessler, S. and Butler, J. V.: Plasma heparin: A unique, practical, submicrogram-sensitive assay. J. Lab. Clin. Med. *81*:298, 1973.
Youngman, H. R.: Toxic reactions in epidural anesthesia. Anesthesiology *17*:632, 1956.
Zilkha, A. and Nicoletti, J. M.: Acute spinal subdural hematoma. J. Neurosurg. *41*:627, 1974.
Zöhlen, E.: Periduralanästhesie mit Meningitis. Der. Chirurg. *21*:603, 1950.

chapter 15

Teaching Techniques

The aim of education or culture is merely the development of good taste in knowledge and good form in conduct. The cultured man or the ideal educated man is not necessarily one who is well-read or learned, but one who likes and dislikes the right things.

Lin Yutang
The Importance of Living (*1938*)

The manual skills of epidural puncture and epidural analgesia are not difficult to learn. As with all other skills, they must be well taught to protect the learner from acquiring bad habits, but at the same time patients must be protected from the tyro during his educative process. In the past, learning of this sort has been along traditional apprenticeship lines. The beginner prepared himself by appropriate introductory reading, and then apprentice and master approached the task together in the clinical setting, with live patients as the learning model.

Inevitably this method gave rise to a certain number of dural taps, and any resultant suffering on the part of the patient had to be accepted as a regrettable but inescapable part of a necessary teaching system committed to the future care of patients, as well as to the immediate present.

Today a number of protective learning devices can be placed between the beginner and the patient, and a fairly advanced degree of manual skill can be developed before the beginner even lays hands on a live model. As a consequence, the number of dural taps perpetrated by beginners during the learning phase can be reduced to a very small number.

Teaching aids may be classified as visual, audiovisual or tactile. Some techniques overlap and fall into more than one category, but broadly speaking this is a useful classification, and teaching aids should be used in this order, each step confirming, reinforcing and expanding knowledge and awareness gained from the preceding step.

VISUAL AIDS

Under this heading comes appropriate reading and study of the bony skeleton. A good tutor system should start at once to develop a sense of discrimination in the reader so that dogma is questioned and free thinking is encouraged on the one hand, while on the other certain immutable rules of behavior are laid down with an iron, uncompromising discipline. There are very few of the latter, but two absolute rules must be instilled at an early stage: gentleness and rigid manual control. Whatever else is argued or modified, there must be no compromise over these two absolutes. If the beginner is lacking in these qualities or is constitutionally incapable of comprehending their basic importance, he should be encouraged to seek some other métier at an early stage before he does unnecessary harm.

Early instruction in the essential differences between good and bad technique is important in preventing the beginner from indiscriminately accepting bad instruction at the next phase of audiovisual learning. There he will inevitably encounter a mixture in terms of quality. There are some excellent audiovisual productions that are sound in principle and design, but unfortunately there are others in which sloppy, undesirable technique has been committed to film and videotape.

Study of the skeleton should include the articulated skeleton as well as individual bones of the spinal column. Particular attention should be paid to the configuration of the lumbar and thoracic vertebrae. A large number of individual sacral bones should also be examined to provide concrete evidence of the widely varied capacity of the sacral canal and the contours of the sacral hiatus.

AUDIOVISUAL AIDS

Slide tape

Slide tape demonstrations are cheap to produce and easy to update. They are excellent for individual or small group instruction when a compact carousel screen projector, such as the Fairchild model, is used. Although slides throw a static picture, good script writing and design can impart a highly dynamic impression to a properly chosen sequence.

Videotape

Videotape has several advantages over film. It is cheaper to produce and easier to edit and update than film, and the sound track is easily modified. However, visual resolution is poorer than in film, and graphic material may have to be redrawn to suit the coarser resolution. The dynamic details of manual technique can be shown almost as clearly as on 16 mm film. Color videotape is now available in cassette form, and this medium is an economical and highly practical way to impart manual skills.

The reusable character of videotape lends it to individual tutorial methods in a wide variety of skills (Ravin, 1974). Athletic coaches have used this medium for many years, and ski schools commonly employ the method to point out individual errors of technique to beginners. A similar application of the medium to epidural puncture has a limited range of usefulness, as practical limitations of space and lighting usually confine the method to facsimile model teaching in a studio setting.

FILM

A number of films have been produced of variable quality, and some of these are listed at the end of the chapter. Film is an expensive but sophisticated medium for crystallizing an idea and for projecting a limited discrete message. The technique of film production has advanced enormously in latter years, but unhappily in some recently available films the trinity of Idea-Medium-Message sometimes becomes unbalanced in favor of the Medium, and the Idea and the Message are overshadowed by the technical beauty of production (Sayers, 1941).

While good films are a valuable adjunct to a well-conducted training program, in my view beginners should not be exposed to films and videotapes except in the presence of a highly critical and experienced tutor who is in a position to point out the hidden difficulties, dangers or technical faults that are sometimes obscured in a slick and polished production.

TACTILE METHODS

ANATOMICAL DISSECTION

The oldest and one of the best methods of acquiring a deep intuitive empathy for the tissues is still the laborious discipline of gross anatomy by personal dissection. Prosected wet specimens are also helpful in transferring the relevant three-dimensional relationships to the novice's inward eye.

FACSIMILE MODELS

Modern plastic materials have simplified the construction of three-dimensional training models that closely resemble the texture and feel of live human tissues. Component parts and the outer skin are replaceable when the original becomes worn by repeated use.

Figures 15–1 and 15–2 show this type of training model in use for lumbar epidural and caudal puncture, respectively. Students can practice their technique at leisure until confidence and dexterity have been gained and until they have become completely familiar with the orientation and characteristic sensation of the different layers of tissue. Then performance can be closely monitored by a tutor before the step is made toward contact with live patients under real clinical conditions. With this type of progressive learning process, the final transition to the clinical scene is pleasant and painless to learner and patient alike.

CLINICAL TUITION

The final step is a progression to the old apprenticeship situation in the clinical context. After absorbing the preliminary phases of visual, audio-visual and tactile experience, the pupil should have gained a high degree of

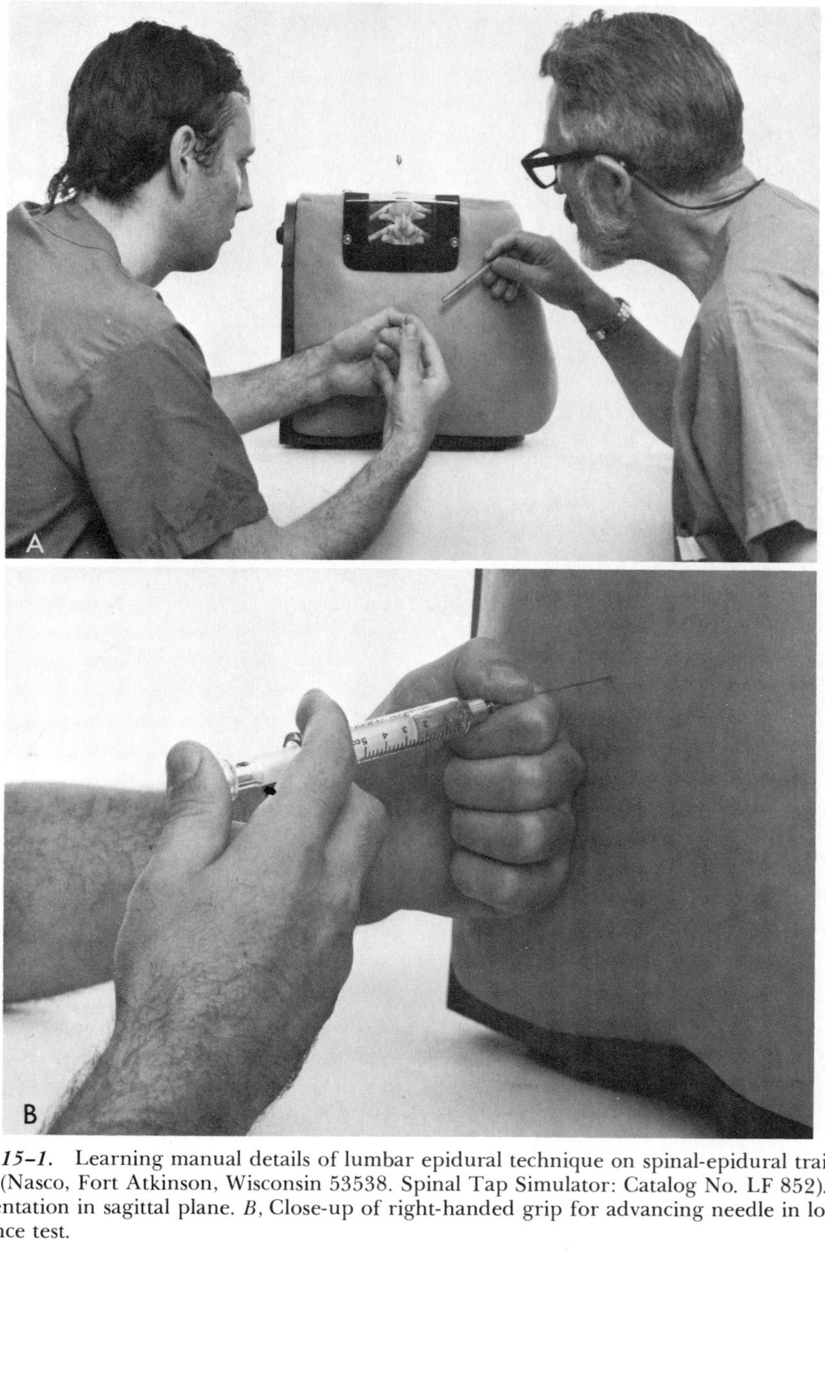

Figure 15–1. Learning manual details of lumbar epidural technique on spinal-epidural training model (Nasco, Fort Atkinson, Wisconsin 53538. Spinal Tap Simulator: Catalog No. LF 852). *A*, Orientation in sagittal plane. *B*, Close-up of right-handed grip for advancing needle in loss-of-resistance test.

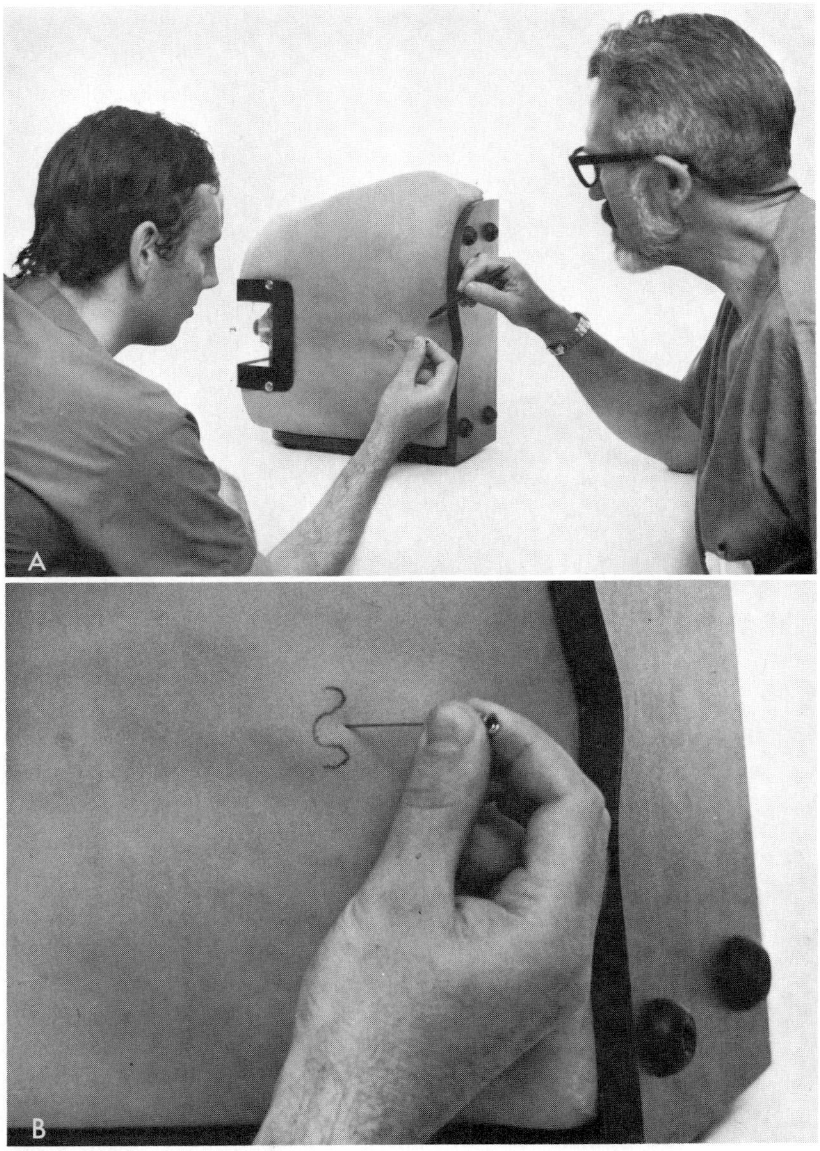

Figure 15–2. Learning manual technique of caudal puncture on spinal-epidural training model (Nasco, Fort Atkinson, Wisconsin 53538. Spinal Tap Simulator: Catalog No. LF 852). *A,* Orientation of needle. *B,* Close-up of puncture site in relation to underlying sacral hiatus (marked with erasable skin-pencil on plastic "skin").

coordination and needle control, and most of the uncertainty and anxiety should have been eliminated by the time the student approaches his first clinical epidural puncture. The attitude of mind in which this approach is made is important: confidence and responsibility are the keynotes. The student must be made to feel entirely confident on the basis of his preliminary grounding, but at the same time he must also be made to feel responsible in the knowledge that except under rare and unusual circumstances, dural punctures only occur through some technical shortcoming on the part of the operator.

LUMBAR EPIDURAL PUNCTURE

The first and most important phase of clinical tuition encompasses mastery of the loss-of-resistance test at levels below the termination of the conus medullaris. Only when the student has proved his ability by at least 50 consecutive and successful epidural anesthetics without a dural tap should any consideration be given to progressing to the hanging-drop technique in the thoracic region.

Pupil and tutor scrub and don sterile gloves and approach the first punctures together. The pupil makes all preliminary preparations, chooses the correct interspinous space and infiltrates the skin and deep tissues with local anesthetic. The pupil then inserts the epidural needle to a depth of 2 cm or so, and the tutor checks the orientation of the needle. From this point on, the task is divided in tandem. The tutor grips the needle and advances the point while the pupil exerts tremolo pressure movements on the plunger of the air-filled syringe until the epidural space is reached. The tutor then checks the loss of resistance and, if satisfied that the needle is correctly placed, he hands over control of the procedure to the pupil, keeping a strict supervisory eye open for care in details of advancing the catheter, removing the needle and performing an aspiration test through the catheter.

When the tutor is satisfied that the pupil has acquired a reliable sense of loss of resistance, the roles are reversed and the pupil advances the needle while the tutor performs tremolo movements on the plunger. Finally, the student is left to perform the whole operation single-handedly while the tutor, scrubbed and gloved, assumes a monitoring role, ready to initiate any corrections that may be necessary.

THORACIC EPIDURAL PUNCTURE

Not every trainee is suited to perform thoracic epidural puncture, and the risks of accidental cord damage from clumsy or uncontrolled movements of the needle are too great to put the technique in the hands of any but the most skilled and apt pupils. An elitist approach should be taken, and only those residents who have demonstrated consistent manual control and predictable success in a significantly large series of lumbar blocks should be encouraged to graduate to the thoracic region. A straight run of 50 uncomplicated lumbar blocks is a realistic criterion for this form of selection.

The nature of the technique demands that the pupil should have earned the tutor's complete confidence, for unlike the loss-of-resistance test, the hanging-drop technique cannot readily be done in tandem. The tutor must stand back while the pupil is left on his own to make the final crucial advance of the needle point through the ligamentum flavum into the epidural space.

The following sequence is recommended. For the first two or three occasions, the pupil should adopt a partially passive role, although he can perform the initial steps in conjunction with his tutor. The tutor allows the pupil to select a suitable paraspinous site and to infiltrate the skin and subcutaneous tissues with local anesthetic. Then the tutor performs the next step and infiltrates further, down to the lamina, using a 1½- or 2-inch 22-gauge needle, gently laying a barrage of local anesthetic at the periosteum. He allows the pupil to identify the surface of the lamina with the infiltrating needle, gradually walking the needle deeper in a cranial direction, until it is felt to glide forward on the upper surface of the lamina toward the ligamentum flavum. At this point the tutor takes over again, withdrawing the infiltrating needle and replacing it with the epidural needle and stylet. Needle and stylet are advanced until the lamina is reached, and the tutor allows the pupil to verify the bony landmark. At this point the tutor can correct any faults in needle control or posture of the pupil's hands. The stylet is now withdrawn and a hanging drop placed in the hub. The tutor completes the epidural puncture with the pupil watching closely to observe movements of the drop. When the tutor is satisfied that the pupil has gained reliable control of the needle at all times, the pupil may be allowed to proceed on his own, with the tutor verifying each step along the way. A resident's first thoracic puncture is always a moment of stress for both pupil and tutor, but in the right hands and with proper grounding, the risks become infinitesimal.

CRITIQUE OF VIDEOTAPE, FILM AND SLIDE TAPE DEMONSTRATIONS

Videotape

1. EPIDURAL ANALGESIA FOR OBSTETRICS

Author: P. R. Bromage

Produced by: McGill University Center for Development and Learning

Year of production: 1973

1-inch tape. Black and white: 53 minutes

Contents: A review of anatomy and pharmacology of epidural blockade related to obstetrical analgesia. The technique of induction and management of continuous epidural analgesia for labor and vaginal delivery is demonstrated, with emphasis on small-dose regimens.

Comments: This tape is too long; it attempts to cover both basic and applied elements in one sitting, when the material would be better divided into two parts. Importance of lateral position during labor is inadequately emphasized. Requires updating in color cassette format.

Films*

1. Technique of peridural anesthesia for thoracic surgery

Author: Oral B. Crawford (Springfield, Missouri)
Year of production: 1955
16 mm color: 25 minutes
Optical sound: English

Contents: Diagrammatic anatomical study of the epidural space, followed by demonstration of equipment, positioning and preparation of a patient for thoracic surgery under high thoracic epidural analgesia at the first thoracic interspace. The film demonstrates the possibility of excisional pulmonary surgery in the awake, spontaneously breathing patient, large volumes of a dilute analgesic solution being used—i.e., 30 ml of 0.8 per cent lidocaine and 0.07 per cent tetracaine.

Comments: Dr. Oral Crawford is a master of thoracic epidural analgesia, and this film is a classic in that it shows what many anesthesiologists have come to believe is impossible, that is, open chest surgery in the awake, nonintubated patient breathing spontaneously. Gentle surgery and proper management with positive-pressure oxygen by mask are the secrets. The technique only works in the hands of a team trained to use the method, and the technique is not recommended for ordinary use by teams unfamiliar with the method.

2. Cervical peridural anesthesia

Author: C. C. Wycoff (Los Angeles)
Year of production: 1957
16 mm color: 21 minutes
Optical sound: English

Contents: An anatomical study of the cervical and thoracic regions in cadaver material, followed by a demonstration of cervical epidural analgesia for thoracic surgery.

Comments: An old film but excellently produced. The anatomical demonstrations are clearly and convincingly done.

3. Epidural analgesia

Author: B. N. Dolan (Wellington Hospital, New Zealand)
Year of production: 1962
16 mm color: 22 minutes
Optical sound: English

Contents: Demonstration of anatomy of epidural analgesia in the cadaver. The Macintosh balloon and the Dogliotti loss-of-resistance methods

*The following films are available through the Astra Film Library, Astra Pharmaceuticals, Inc., Worcester, Massachusetts.

for identifying the epidural space are shown. Cases of suprapubic prostatectomy, hernia repair and cesarean section are demonstrated.

Comments: This film has some good explanatory diagrams; however, it should be viewed critically because the sound track is indistinct and sometimes difficult to follow without the written text, and a number of technical and factual errors are presented:

1. The statement is made that local anesthetics in the epidural space cannot spread to involve the intracranial contents. This is incorrect (as pointed out in Chapter 4).

2. Infiltration technique is poor: the infiltrating needle is advanced right up to the hub. This is an elementary fault that should be avoided in case the shaft should break off at the hub.

3. The epidural needle is rotated briskly after entering the epidural space. Rotational movements of this sort are unnecessary and potentially traumatic to veins and to dura, especially when a Huber point is used.

4. The precautionary aspiration test through the epidural catheter is omitted.

5. Cesarean section is shown without any degree of lateral tilt. However, it should be appreciated that this film was made in 1962, before the importance of uterine displacement was generally recognized. Also, the film fails to recommend the administration of 100 per cent oxygen to the mother as a routine precaution.

6. The film recommends that arterial hypotension during cesarean section be treated by vasopressor drugs. No mention is made of posture or volume expansion by prehydration. Again, this defect reflects current practice at the date of production (1962).

4. EPIDURAL ANALGESIA FOR CESAREAN SECTION

Authors: J. Bauman, J. M. Feeder and S. Steinberg
Year of production: 1961
16 mm color: 18 minutes
Optical sound: English

Contents: Management of epidural anaglesia for cesarean section based on experience with 400 cases. Sound emphasis is placed on safety and avoiding trouble. There is a thorough display of emergency equipment that should always be on hand before epidural analgesia is begun. A blood pressure cuff placed on the patient's arm emphasizes the need to monitor a normal arterial pressure until the baby is born. Left uterine displacement and raising the mother's legs are mentioned as aids in maintaining a normal maternal blood pressure.

Comments: Sound principles of alert anticipatory management are well portrayed in this film; however, the following criticisms must be pointed out:

1. The operator demonstrates a technically weak hold on the epidural needle, and there is too much mechanical compliance in the arrangement of the fingers. A grip of this sort is too unstable for most anesthesiologists to be able to exert the rigid micrometer control that is necessary to avoid dural puncture on all occasions.

2. The operator's hands are shown floating free during the injection of local anesthetic through the epidural needle, instead of being braced against the patient's back. Again, this presents an uncontrolled opportunity for inadvertent movement of the needle and possible accidental dural puncture.

3. Vasoxyl (methoxamine) is recommended as a prophylactic vasopressor. This recommendation reflects the date of production. Today prophylactic vasopressors are seldom necessary when maternal posture and prehydration are used properly. If a vasopressor were used, methoxamine would be the last choice, as its alpha-receptor action causes an inordinate reduction of placental blood flow (see Chapter 12).

5. Continuous caudal anaesthesia in obstetrics

Author: M. Pugh (Oxford)
Year of production: 1961
16 mm color: 26 minutes
Optical sound: English

Contents: Continuous caudal analgesia for labor and delivery using an indwelling catheter is explained by excellent animated diagrams and by clinical demonstration. A fixed induction dose of 20 ml of 1 per cent prilocaine with 1/200,000 epinephrine is recommended, followed by the same dose two hours later. There is a good display of emergency resuscitation equipment.

Comments: The photographic qualities of the film are excellent, with first-class animation. The following criticisms are offered:

1. The clinical demonstration shows a large-bore caudal needle being thrust into place without benefit of local anesthesia. This seems to be unnecessarily harsh treatment that could be softened by using a little local anesthetic in the skin without undue blurring of the anatomical landmarks.

2. The rather large amounts of epinephrine and prilocaine could lead to slowing of labor and methemoglobinemia if several successive doses were required, since each dose contains 100 μg of epinephrine and 200 mg of prilocaine.

3. The sound track states that patients are nursed on their backs in order to obtain symmetrical spread of analgesia and they are only turned on their sides if severe falls of blood pressure occur. This is bad practice, again reflecting the date of production of the film. Patients in labor should be nursed on their sides or in a tilted position, and they should not be allowed to be on their backs except for very brief periods (see Chapter 12).

6. Relief of postoperative pain: thoracic epidural blockade by continuous technique

Authors: M. Holmdahl, S. Sjögren and B. Wright (Uppsala)
Year of production: 1973
16 mm color: 18 minutes
Optical or magnetic sound: English

Contents: The Department of Anesthesia at Uppsala has accumulated a great deal of data on the physiological effects of lumbar and thoracic epidural blockade, as well as on the ability of epidural analgesia to modify respiratory performance after upper abdominal operations. The film uses animated sequences to summarize the salient features of this data, with special reference to thoracic epidural technique and dosage and to improved ventilatory performance after upper abdominal surgery using an infusion of 0.4 per cent lidocaine.

Comments: The photographic and artistic qualities of this film are outstanding (produced by Klinisk Film, Charlottenlund, Copenhagen). The animated sequences are clear and easy to follow, and the clinical scenes are well executed. The loss-of-resistance technique is demonstrated for thoracic puncture at the fifth thoracic interspace, but unfortunately the hanging-drop test is not shown. Nevertheless, the overall quality and content of this film are excellent. Copies of this film are available with either optical or magnetic sound track. The prospective viewer should check that his projection equipment is compatible with the type of sound track provided.

Slide Tape

1. Conduction Anesthesia, Spinal, Epidural, Caudal Blocks

Authors: J. F. Kaczmarek and J. S. Finch

Institution: University of Michigan Media Library, Towsley Center for Continuing Medical Education, University of Michigan, Ann Arbor, Michigan 48109

Year of production: 1975. Catalog No. 310

Duration: 100 slides, 25 minutes

Comments: An excellent programmed presentation of spinal, epidural and caudal anesthesia, with simple practical discussion of the physiology, technical aspects and clinical indications. This slide tape package includes seven pages of accompanying notes with a short list of selected reading. Two details of technique in the slide sequence must be criticized. First, sterility is less than stringent. The anesthesiologist is shown wearing rings and a wrist watch under his gloves while inducing subarachnoid and epidural blockade. Opinions may differ over this rather questionable standard of sterile technique as an example to be followed. Some will argue that they never perform a full surgical scrub before any type of regional anesthesia. Others will be more obsessively hygienic. My own view is that while a good social hand wash followed by careful sterile gloving is probably adequate for most types of block, a full ritual scrub should precede an elective subarachnoid block.

Second, manual control of the epidural needle for the loss-of-resistance test is less than ideal (slide No. 45 in the series). The slide depicts a grip that is not as viselike as it could be, and beginners who adopt this grip are likely to find that there is an appreciable degree of compliance or "give" in the system, leading to a higher incidence of dural punctures than necessary.

Aside from these two criticisms, the overall work is beautifully presented, and this module is a thoroughly worthwhile addition to the teaching resources of any anesthesiology department.

REFERENCES

Lin Yutang: The Importance of Living. William Heinemann Ltd., London, 1938, p. 325.

Ravin, M. B.: Teaching anesthesia motor skills by review of video taped performances. Anesth. Analg. *53*:698, 1974.

Sayers, D. L.: The Mind of the Maker. Chapter X: "Scalene Trinities." London, Methuen & Company, Ltd., 1941.

Index

NOTE: Page numbers in *italics* refer to illustrations. Page numbers followed by the letter *t* refer to tables.